BATES'
Guide to Physical Examination and History Taking

Chapter 2: Interviewing and the Health History revised and expanded by

Elizabeth H. Naumburg, MD
Associate Dean, Advising
Associate Professor of Family Medicine
University of Rochester School of Medicine and Dentistry
Rochester, New York

Chapter 12: The Pregnant Woman

Joyce Beebe Thompson, CNM, DrPH, FAAN, FACNM
Professor and Director, Retired
Graduate Program in Nurse Midwifery
School of Nursing
University of Pennsylvania
Philadelphia, Pennsylvania

Bernadine M. Lacey Professor of
Community Health Nursing
Bronson School of Nursing
Western Michigan University
Kalamazoo, Michigan

BATES' Guide to Physical Examination and History Taking

EIGHTH EDITION

Lynn S. Bickley, MD
Associate Professor of Internal Medicine and Neuropsychiatry
Texas Tech Health Sciences Center
Lubbock, Texas

Peter G. Szilagyi, MD, MPH
Professor of Pediatrics
Chief, Division of General Pediatrics
University of Rochester School of Medicine and Dentistry
Rochester, New York

LIPPINCOTT WILLIAMS & WILKINS
A **Wolters Kluwer** Company
Philadelphia • Baltimore • New York • London
Buenos Aires • Hong Kong • Sydney • Tokyo

Acquisitions Editor: Elizabeth Nieginski
Manager of Nursing Development: Jane Velker
Developmental Editor: Renee Gagliardi
Editorial Assistant: Jean Otsuki
Senior Production Editor: Sandra Cherrey Scheinin
Senior Production Manager: Helen Ewan
Art Director: Carolyn O'Brien
Designer: Melissa Olson
Illustration Coordinator: Brett MacNaughton
Interior Illustrator: Anne Rains
Manufacturing Manager: William Alberti
Indexer: Katherine Pitcoff
Compositor: Circle Graphics
Printer: Quebecor

Edition 8

9 8 7 6 5 4

Library of Congress Cataloging-in Publication Data

Bickley, Lynn S.
Bates' guide to physical examination and history taking.—8th ed. / Lynn S. Bickley. Peter G. Szilagyi.
p. ; cm.
Includes bibliographical references and index.
ISBN 0-7817-3511-4 (alk. paper)
1. Physical diagnosis. 2. Medical history taking. I. Title: Guide to physical examination and history taking. II. Szilagyi, Peter G. III. Title.
[DNLM: 1. Physical Examination—methods. 2. Medical History Taking—methods. WB 205 B583b 2003]
RC76 .B38 2003
616.07'54—dc21

2002141573

Care has been taken to confirm the accuracy of the information presented and to describe generally accepted practices. However, the authors, editors, and publisher are not responsible for errors or omissions or for any consequences from application of the information in this book and make no warranty, express or implied, with respect to the content of the publication.

The authors, editors, and publisher have exerted every effort to ensure that drug selection and dosage set forth in this text are in accordance with the current recommendations and practice at the time of publication. However, in view of ongoing research, changes in government regulations, and the constant flow of information relating to drug therapy and drug reactions, the reader is urged to check the package insert for each drug for any change in indications and dosage and for added warnings and precautions. This is particularly important when the recommended agent is a new or infrequently employed drug.

Some drugs and medical devices presented in this publication have Food and Drug Administration (FDA) clearance for limited use in restricted research settings. It is the responsibility of the health care provider to ascertain the FDA status of each drug or device planned for use in his or her clinical practice.

To Randolph Tecumseh Schiffer and Moira Ann Szilagyi,
whose cheer and forbearance helped bring forth this book.

Acknowledgments

For his extensive and thoughtful reshaping of *Chapter 17, Assessing Children: From Infancy Through Adolescence,* we acknowledge the important contribution of Peter Szilagyi, MD, MPH, our new pediatrics editor, to this eighth edition of *Bates' Guide to Physical Examination and History Taking.* We also extend our appreciation to Elizabeth H. Naumburg, MD, for her refinements of *Chapter 2, Interviewing and the Health History,* and to Joyce Beebe Thompson, CNM, author of *Chapter 12, The Pregnant Woman.* For their expertise and many helpful suggestions, we thank Christine Aronoff, MD, Dana Jeng, MD, Walter Lajara, MD, Fiona Prabhu, MD, Ron Rapini, MD, Randolph Schiffer, MD, and Jimmy Slaughterbeck, MD, from the Texas Tech School of Medicine, and Chloe Alexson, MD, Laurie Donahue, Jeffrey Kaczorowski, MD, Cheryl Kodjo, MD, Valerie Gilchrist, Brenda Lee, and Nancy Shafer-Clark, MD, from the University of Rochester School of Medicine and Dentistry. We also thank Libby Amos, Virginia Miller, Katherine Reavis, and Kathy Sridaromont, colleagues in the Texas Tech School of Nursing.

It has been rewarding and stimulating to work with a talented team at Lippincott Williams & Wilkins. Elizabeth Nieginski, Acquisitions Editor, has provided imagination and guidance, not only for the eighth edition, but for its new adjuncts, the Case Book, the Instructor's Resource CD-ROM, and the Connection Website for faculty and teachers. Jane Velker, Manager of Nursing Development, has brought patient, thoughtful, and meticulous care to additions and changes in both substance and format. Brett MacNaughton, Illustration Coordinator, has deftly handled the many challenges of coordinating both photographs and illustrations with layout and text. Sandra Scheinin, Senior Production Editor, deserves special mention for her patience and responsiveness. We remain grateful to these editors, as well as to the many other members of Lippincott Williams & Wilkins who have contributed so much to this edition.

For new color photography, often of complex composition, we are grateful for the skill of Steve Platten, medical photographer at Texas Tech Health Sciences Center, and Vince Sullivan, medical photographer at the University of Rochester. For the many small and large tasks that accompany manuscript preparation, we extend appreciation to Jacqulyn Staches and Britton Lui, and for invaluable computer expertise, to Tracy Tully.

Contents

List of Tables

Introduction

Bates' Guide to Physical Examination and History Taking is designed for students of health care who are learning to talk with patients, to perform their physical examinations, and to apply clinical reasoning to understand and assess their problems. The first chapter in the eighth edition provides an overview of the patient interview and physical examination and an example of how these essential components of patient assessment might appear in the written record. The second chapter guides students through the techniques of skilled and effective interviewing. Then follows a new chapter on the general survey of the patient and the vital signs that begin the physical examination. The subsequent chapters are devoted to the techniques of examination for the various body regions or systems. The regional examination chapters have the same sequence of topics. Each begins with a review of the anatomy and physiology relevant to its body system, followed by pertinent health history and information useful for health promotion and counseling, and a preview of examples of the written record for that system. Each regional examination chapter then continues with the techniques of examination and tables that help students recognize selected abnormalities. The chapter on assessing children summarizes history taking and examination for infants through adolescents. The final chapter concludes with insights about clinical reasoning and provides the written record of "Mrs. N," which demonstrates a sample assessment and plan.

We assume that our student readers have had basic courses in human anatomy and physiology. Our sections on these subjects are intended to help students apply their knowledge to interpreting symptoms, examining the human body, and understanding physical signs.

Throughout the book, we have emphasized common or important problems rather than the rare and esoteric. Occasionally, we have included a physical sign of a rare disorder when it occupies a solid niche in classic physical diagnosis, or when recognizing the disorder is especially important for the health or even the life of the patient.

Most students learn their examination skills first by practicing on one another. Most of the anatomy and physiology and many of the techniques of examination and abnormal findings are common to both adults and children. Dr. Szilagyi's chapter on the examination of infants and children describes variations that occur in younger age groups, together with signs or conditions that are unique to younger patients.

THE EIGHTH EDITION

The eighth edition brings several new departures to the *Guide to Physical Examination and History Taking.* In this edition, we introduce our new pediatrics editor, Peter Szilagyi MD, MPH, nationally known for his expertise in clinical pediatrics, particularly in the area of expanding immunization coverage for children. Dr. Szilagyi brings the insights of a distinguished career in general pediatrics to his lively, comprehensive, and readable text in *Chapter 17, Assessing Children: Infancy Through Adolescence.* We express grateful appreciation to Dr. Robert Hoekelman, retiring pediatrics editor, for his lucid and untiring efforts for the past two decades and seven editions of this book to unite developmental pediatrics with the techniques of physical examination and history taking for children.

In addition, readers of the eighth edition will find many new features in the text and tables. As with previous editions, the changes in the eighth edition spring from two sources: the queries of teachers and students, and the goal of making the book easier to read and more efficient to use. Readers will find several changes in the opening and closing chapters to improve overall organization and make the flow of information more logical.

- *Chapter 1, An Overview of Physical Examination and History Taking,* now provides an overview of "the road ahead," including the structure of the interview, the sequence of the physical examination, and a written example of the history and examination of a sample patient, "Mrs. N."

- *Chapter 2, Interviewing and the Health History,* focuses on the process and techniques of interviewing, with updated information on working with an interpreter, death and dying, and ethical aspects of patient care.

- *Chapter 18, Clinical Reasoning, Assessment, and Plan,* the closing chapter of the eighth edition, describes the steps of clinical reasoning and concludes with the written assessment and plan for the sample patient, "Mrs. N," introduced in Chapter 1.

It is also important for readers to recognize that in the eighth edition, health history information about symptoms (previously found in Chapter 2) is now incorporated into the regional examination chapter most relevant to those particular symptoms. *Each of the regional examination chapters now contains the following sections: Anatomy and Physiology, The Health History, Health Promotion and Counseling, Preview of the Written Record, Techniques of Examination,* and *Tables of Abnormalities.* For example, symptoms and tables pertaining to headache, earache, sinusitis, and difficulty swallowing are now in the Health History and Tables of Abnormalities sections of *Chapter 5, The Head and Neck;* symptoms and a Table of Abnormalities about diarrhea appear in *Chapter 9, The Abdomen.* Readers also will note that in the eighth edition the Mental Status Examination (previously found in Chapter 3) is now discussed in *Chapter 16, The Nervous System,* because the assessment of mental status plays such an important and integral role in neurologic evaluation.

Two chapters have been substantially rewritten to make important new information available to our readers. *Chapter 3, Beginning the Physical Examina-*

tion: General Survey and Vital Signs, begins with new material on the initial assessment of the patient, particularly nutritional status, use of the body mass index for measurements of height and weight, and current guidelines for determining excess weight and obesity. Chapter 3 contains a number of new tables to help clinicians with nutritional assessment, dietary recommendations, and recognition of low-weight conditions such as anorexia nervosa and bulimia. *Chapter 17, Assessing Children: Infancy Through Adolescence,* has been updated and rewritten by Dr. Szilagyi. He has added many new features to this important chapter, including a summary of normal child development (e.g., what an infant can do); tips on how to examine children; 67 new color photographs; and many new figures, tables, and boxes of clinical pearls to help you in your examination of children and adolescents. In addition, the sections on Health Promotion and Counseling throughout the book have been revised and expanded based on new information and guidelines, for example, for obesity, cholesterol screening, and childhood immunizations.

Color again demarcates chapter sections and tables more clearly and leads students more easily to examples of the written record: the history and examination of "Mrs. N" are color shaded in Chapter 1, as are her assessment and plan in Chapter 18. In this edition, color highlights special tips for challenging aspects of examination such as taking the blood pressure, assessing the jugular venous pressure, and keeping the patient comfortable during the examination of the pelvis. Color also highlights a new feature in each chapter, the preview of the written record for that chapter's regional examination. More than 200 new color photographs and drawings have been added to better illustrate key points in the accompanying text.

Readers will find several changes in techniques and standards of examination. National concern has directed attention to the prevention and early detection of pressure ulcers, now included in new text and in a Table of Abnormalities in *Chapter 4, The Skin.* New recommendations favoring "the strip method" for clinical and self-breast examinations are now incorporated in the Health Promotion and Counseling and Techniques of Examination sections of *Chapter 8, The Breasts and Axillae.*

Despite these changes, readers will recognize the basic core organization of the text. Students may study or review the Anatomy and Physiology sections according to their individual needs. They can study Techniques of Examination to learn how to do the relevant examination, then practice it under faculty guidance, and review it again afterward. Techniques for special situations are placed at the end of these sections so they do not interfere with the flow of the usual examination. Faculty may choose which of these Special Techniques to include in their expectations of students.

Students and faculty will also benefit from identifying common abnormal findings. Abnormalities appear in two places. The right-hand column of the book introduces students to abnormal findings that might be present. Distinguishing these findings from the normal, improves learners' observations. Further information on abnormalities is provided in the Tables of Abnormalities at the end of each of the regional examination chapters. These tables display or describe various abnormal conditions in a convenient format that allows students to compare and contrast related abnormalities in a single table.

SUGGESTIONS FOR USING THE BOOK

Although the health history and the physical examination are both essential for patient assessment and care, students often learn them separately, sometimes from different faculty members. Students learning interviewing are advised to return to *Chapter 2, Interviewing and the Health History,* as they gain experience talking with patients of different temperaments and ages. As they begin developing a smooth sequence of examination, students may wish to review the sequence of examination outlined in *Chapter 3, Beginning the Physical Examination: General Survey and Vital Signs.* Nevertheless, students must learn to integrate the patient's story and the patient's physical findings. We suggest that students study the relevant portions of the Health History as they learn successive parts of the examination. In a few areas, symptoms may lead to examination of more than one body system. For example, chest pain prompts evaluation of the thorax and lungs, as well as the cardiovascular system. The symptoms of the urinary tract are relevant to the chapters on the abdomen, the prostate, male genitalia, and female genitalia.

As students progress through the body systems and regions, they should make frequent reference to the Preview sections on the patient record and to the write-up of the sample patient, "Mrs. N," found in Chapter 1 and Chapter 18. This cross-checking will help them learn how to describe and organize information from the interview and physical examination into an understandable written format. Furthermore, studying *Chapter 18, Clinical Reasoning, Assessment, and Plan,* will help students to select and analyze the data they are learning to collect.

Skimming the Tables of Abnormalities makes students more familiar with what they should be looking for and why they are asking certain questions. They should not, however, try to memorize the details that are presented there. The best time to learn about abnormalities and diseases is when a patient, real or described, appears with a problem. Students should then use this book to try to analyze the concern or finding, and make use of other clinical texts or journals to pursue the patient's problems in as much depth as necessary. Students can refer to the *Bibliography* for additional relevant sources.

RELATED LEARNING MATERIAL

With the eighth edition, we introduce an accompanying Case Book to help students test their knowledge of symptoms and physical findings by applying principles of clinical reasoning and assessment to a series of common clinical vignettes. Also new for faculty and teachers are Lippincott's Connection Website and an Instructor's Resource CD-ROM.

In addition, *Bates' Pocket Guide to Physical Examination and History Taking* is an abbreviated version of this text, designed for portability, review, and convenience. This pocket guide does not stand alone; reference to the text and illustrations of *Bates' Guide to Physical Examination and History Taking* is required for a more comprehensive study and understanding of these subjects. *A Visual Guide to Physical Examination,* which is available in VHS, DVD, and streaming video formats, is a related product available from Lippincott Williams & Wilkins.

EQUIPMENT

Equipment necessary for a physical examination includes the following:

An ophthalmoscope and an otoscope. If the otoscope is to be used to examine children, it should allow for pneumatic otoscopy.
A flashlight or penlight
Tongue depressors
A ruler and flexible tape measure, preferably marked in centimeters
A thermometer
A watch with a second hand
A sphygmomanometer
A stethoscope with the following characteristics:

- Ear tips that fit snugly and painlessly. To get this fit, choose ear tips of the proper size, align the ear pieces with the angle of your ear canals, and adjust the spring of the connecting metal band to a comfortable tightness.
- Thick-walled tubing as short as feasible to maximize the transmission of sound: about 30 cm (12 inches) if possible and no longer than 38 cm (15 inches)
- A bell and a diaphragm with a good changeover mechanism

Gloves
Lubricant } For vaginal, rectal, and possibly oral examinations
Vaginal specula and equipment for cytological and perhaps bacteriological study
A reflex hammer
Tuning forks, ideally one of 128 Hz and one of 512 Hz
Safety pins or other disposable objects for testing two-point discrimination
Cotton for testing the sense of light touch
Two test tubes (optional) for testing temperature sensation
Paper and pen or pencil

BATES'

Guide to

Physical Examination

and History Taking

CHAPTER

An Overview of Physical Examination and History Taking

1

The techniques of physical examination and history taking that you are about to learn embody time-honored skills of healing and patient care. Your ability to gather a sensitive and nuanced history and to perform a thorough and accurate examination deepens your patient relationships, focuses your patient assessment, and sets the direction of your clinical thinking. The quality of your history and physical examination governs your next steps with the patient and guides your choices from the initially bewildering array of secondary testing and technology. Over the course of becoming an accomplished clinician, you will polish these important relational and clinical skills for a lifetime.

As you enter the realm of patient assessment, you begin integrating the essential elements of clinical care: empathic listening; the ability to interview patients of all ages, moods, and backgrounds; the techniques for examining the different body systems; and, finally, the process of clinical reasoning. Your experience with history taking and physical examination will grow and expand, and the steps of clinical reasoning will soon begin with the first moments of the patient encounter: identifying problem symptoms and abnormal findings; linking findings to an underlying process of pathophysiology or psychopathology; and establishing and testing a set of explanatory hypotheses. Working through these steps will reveal the multifaceted profile of the patient before you. Paradoxically, the very skills that allow you to assess all patients also shape the image of the unique human being entrusted to your care.

Clinical Assessment: The Road Ahead

This chapter provides a road map to clinical proficiency in three critical areas: the health history, the physical examination, and the written record, or "write-up." It describes the components of the health history and how to organize the patient's story; it gives an approach and overview to the physical examination and suggests a sequence for ensuring patient comfort; and, finally, it provides an example of the written record, showing documentation of findings from a sample patient history and physical examination. By studying the subsequent chapters of the book and perfecting the skills of examination and history taking described, you will cross into the world of patient assessment—gradually at first, but then with growing satisfaction and expertise.

After you work through this chapter to chart the tasks ahead, you will be directed by subsequent chapters in your journey to clinical competence. Chapter 2, Interviewing and the Health History, expands on the techniques and skills of good interviewing; Chapters 3 through 16 detail techniques for examining the different body systems. Once you master the elements of the adult history and examination, you will extend and adapt these techniques to children and adolescents. Children and adolescents evolve rapidly in both temperament and physiology; therefore, the special approaches to the interview and examination of children at different ages are consolidated in Chapter 17, Assessing Children: Infancy Through Adolescence. Finally, Chapter 18, Clinical Reasoning, Assessment, and Plan, explores the clinical reasoning process and how to document your evaluation, diagnoses, and plan. From this blend of mutual trust, respect, and clinical expertise emerges the timeless rewards of the clinical professions.

THE HEALTH HISTORY: STRUCTURE AND PURPOSES

As you read about successful interviewing, you will first learn the elements of the ***Comprehensive Health History.*** For adults, the comprehensive history includes *Identifying Data* and *Source of the History, Chief Complaint(s), Present Illness, Past History, Family History, Personal and Social History,* and *Review of Systems.* As you talk with the patient, you must learn to elicit and organize all of these elements of the patient's health. Bear in mind that during the interview this information will not spring forth in this order! However, you will quickly learn to identify where to fit in the different aspects of the patient's story.

As you gain experience assessing patients in different settings, you will find that new patients in the office or in the hospital merit a *comprehensive health history;* however, in many situations a more flexible *focused,* or *problem-oriented, interview* may be appropriate. Like a tailor fitting a special garment, you will adapt the scope of the health history to a number of factors: the patient's concerns and problems; your goals for assessment; the clinical setting (inpatient or outpatient; specialty or primary care); and the amount of time available. Knowing the content and relevance of all components of the comprehensive health history allows you to choose those elements that will be most helpful for addressing patient concerns in different contexts.

The components of the comprehensive health history structure the patient's story and the format of your written record, but the order shown here should not dictate the sequence of the interview. Usually the interview will be more fluid and will follow the patient's leads and cues, as described in Chapter 2. Each segment of the history has a specific purpose, which is summarized below.

These components of the comprehensive adult health history are more fully described in the next few pages. The *comprehensive pediatric history* appears in Chapter 17. These sample adult and pediatric health histories follow stan-

Components of the Health History

Identifying Data	■ *Identifying data*—such as age, gender, occupation, marital status ■ *Source of the history*—usually the patient, but can be family member, friend, letter of referral, or the medical record ■ If appropriate, establish *source of referral,* since a written report may be needed.
Reliability	Varies according to the patient's memory, trust, and mood
Chief Complaint(s)	The one or more symptoms or concerns causing the patient to seek care
Present Illness	■ Amplifies the *Chief Complaint,* describes how each symptom developed ■ Includes patient's thoughts and feelings about the illness ■ Pulls in relevant portions of the *Review of Systems* (see below) ■ May include *medications, allergies,* habits of *smoking* and *alcohol,* since these are frequently pertinent to the present illness
Past History	■ Lists childhood illnesses ■ Lists adult illnesses with dates for at least four categories: medical; surgical; obstetric/gynecologic; and psychiatric ■ Includes health maintenance practices such as: immunizations, screening tests, lifestyle issues, and home safety
Family History	■ Outlines or diagrams age and health, or age and cause of death, of siblings, parents, and grandparents ■ Documents presence or absence of specific illnesses in family, such as hypertension, coronary artery disease, etc.
Personal and Social History	Describes educational level, family of origin, current household, personal interests, and lifestyle
Review of Systems	Documents presence or absence of common symptoms related to each major body system

dard formats for written documentation, which will be useful for you to learn. As you review these histories, you will encounter a number of technical terms for symptoms. Definitions of terms, together with ways to ask about symptoms, can be found in each of the regional examination chapters.

As you acquire the techniques of the history taking and physical examination, remember the important differences between ***subjective information*** and ***objective information,*** as summarized in the table below. Knowing these differences helps you apply clinical reasoning and cluster patient information. These distinctions are equally important for organizing written and oral presentations concerning the patient.

Subjective Data	Objective Data
What the patient tells you	What you detect on the examination
The history, from Chief Complaint through Review of Systems	All physical examination findings
Example: Mrs. G is a 54-year-old hairdresser who reports pressure over her left chest "like an elephant sitting there," which goes into her left neck and arm.	*Example:* Mrs. G is an older white female, deconditioned, pleasant, and cooperative. BP 160/80, HR 96 and regular, respiratory rate 24, afebrile.

THE COMPREHENSIVE ADULT HEALTH HISTORY

Date and Time of History. The date is always important. You are strongly advised to routinely document the time you evaluate the patient, especially in urgent, emergent, or hospital settings.

Identifying Data. Includes age, gender, marital status, and occupation. The ***source of history*** or ***referral*** can be the patient, a family member or friend, an officer, a consultant, or the medical record. Patients requesting evaluations for schools, agencies, or insurance companies may have special priorities compared to patients seeking care on their own initiative. Designating the *source of referral* helps you to assess the type of information provided and any possible biases.

Reliability. Should be documented if relevant. For example, "The patient is vague when describing symptoms and unable to specify details." This judgment reflects the quality of the information provided by the patient and is usually made at the end of the interview.

Chief Complaint(s)

Make every attempt to quote the patient's own words. For example, "My stomach hurts and I feel awful." Sometimes patients have no overt complaints, in which case you should report their goals instead. For example, "I have come for my regular checkup"; or "I've been admitted for a thorough evaluation of my heart."

Present Illness

This section of the history is a complete, clear, and chronologic account of the problems prompting the patient to seek care. The narrative should include the onset of the problem, the setting in which it has developed, its manifestations, and any treatments. The principal symptoms should be well-characterized, with descriptions of (1) location, (2) quality, (3) quantity or severity, (4) timing, including onset, duration, and frequency, (5) the setting in which they occur, (6) factors that have aggravated or relieved the symptoms, and (7) associated manifestations. These ***seven attributes*** are invaluable for understanding all patient symptoms (see p. 27). It is also important to include "pertinent positives" and "pertinent negatives" from sections of the *Review of Systems* related to the *Chief Complaint(s)*. These designate the presence or absence of symptoms relevant to the *differential diagnosis,* which refers to the most likely diagnoses explaining the patient's condition. Other information is frequently relevant, such as risk factors for coronary artery disease in patients with chest pain, or current medications in patients with syncope. The *present illness* should reveal the patient's responses to his or her symptoms and what effect the illness has had on the patient's life. Always remember, *the data flows spontaneously from the patient, but the task of organization is yours.*

Medications should be noted, including name, dose, route, and frequency of use. Also list home remedies, nonprescription drugs, vitamins, mineral or herbal supplements, birth control pills, and medicines borrowed from family members or friends. It is a good idea to ask patients to bring in all of their medications so you can see exactly what they take. ***Allergies,*** including *specific reactions* to each medication, such as rash or nausea, must be recorded, as well as allergies to foods, insects, or environmental factors. Note ***tobacco*** use, including the type used. Cigarettes are often reported in pack-years (a person who has smoked 1½ packs a day for 12 years has an 18-pack-year history). If someone has quit, note for how long. ***Alcohol** and **drug** use* should always be queried (see pp. 43–44 for suggested questions). (Note that *tobacco, alcohol,* and *drugs* may also be included in the Personal and Social History; however, many clinicians find these habits pertinent to the Present Illness.)

Past History

Childhood illnesses, such as measles, rubella, mumps, whooping cough, chicken pox, rheumatic fever, scarlet fever, and polio are included in the Past History. Also included are any chronic childhood illnesses. You should provide information relative to ***Adult Illnesses*** in each of four areas: *Medical* (such as diabetes, hypertension, hepatitis, asthma, HIV disease, information about hospitalizations, number and gender of partners, at-risk sexual practices); *Surgical* (include dates, indications, and types of operations); *Obstetric/gynecologic* (relate obstetric history, menstrual history, birth control, and sexual function); and *Psychiatric* (include dates, diagnoses, hospitalizations, and treatments). You should also cover selected aspects of *Health Maintenance,* including *Immunizations,* such as tetanus, pertussis, diphtheria, polio, measles, rubella, mumps, influenza, hepatitis B, *Haemophilus influenza* type b, and pneumococcal vaccine (these can usually be obtained from prior medical records), and *Screening Tests,* such as tuberculin tests, Pap smears, mammograms, stools for occult blood, and cholesterol tests, together with the results and the dates they were last performed. If the patient does not know this information, written permission may be needed to obtain old medical records.

Family History

Under *Family History,* outline or diagram the age and health, or age and cause of death, of each immediate relative, including parents, grandparents, siblings, children, and grandchildren. Review each of the following conditions and record if they are present or absent in the family: hypertension, coronary artery disease, elevated cholesterol levels, stroke, diabetes, thyroid or renal disease, cancer (specify type), arthritis, tuberculosis, asthma or lung disease, headache, seizure disorder, mental illness, suicide, alcohol or drug addiction, and allergies, as well as symptoms reported by the patient.

Personal and Social History

The *Personal and Social History* captures the patient's personality and interests, sources of support, coping style, strengths, and fears. It should include: occupation and the last year of schooling; home situation and significant others; sources of stress, both recent and long-term; important life experiences, such as military service, job history, financial situation, and retirement; leisure activities; religious affiliation and spiritual beliefs; and activities of daily living (ADLs). Baseline level of function is particularly important in older or disabled patients (see p. 57 for the ADLs frequently assessed in older patients). The *Personal and Social History* also conveys lifestyle habits that promote health or create risk such as *exercise and diet,* including frequency of exercise, usual daily food intake, dietary supplements or restrictions, and use of coffee, tea, and other caffeine-containing beverages and *safety measures,* including use of seat belts, bicycle helmets, sunblock, smoke detectors, and other devices related to specific hazards. You may want to include any *alternative health care* practices.

You will come to thread personal and social questions throughout the interview to make the patient feel more at ease.

Review of Systems

Understanding and using *Review of Systems* questions is often challenging for beginning students. Think about asking series of questions going from "head to toe." It is helpful to prepare the patient for the questions to come by saying, "The next part of the history may feel like a million questions, but they are important and I want to be thorough." Most *Review of Systems* questions pertain to *symptoms,* but on occasion some clinicians also include diseases like pneumonia or tuberculosis. (If the patient remembers important illnesses as you ask questions within the *Review of Systems,* you should record or present such illnesses as part of the *Present Illness* or *Past History.*)

Start with a fairly general question as you address each of the different systems. This focuses the patient's attention and allows you to shift to more specific questions about systems that may be of concern. Examples of starting questions are: "How are your ears and hearing?" "How about your lungs and breathing?" "Any trouble with your heart?" "How is your digestion?"

"How about your bowels?" Note that you will vary the need for additional questions depending on the patient's age, complaints, general state of health, and your clinical judgment.

The *Review of Systems* questions may uncover problems that the patient has overlooked, particularly in areas unrelated to the *present illness*. Significant health events, such as a major prior illness or a parent's death, require full exploration. Remember that *major health events should be moved to the present illness or past history in your write-up*. Keep your technique flexible. Interviewing the patient yields a variety of information that you organize into formal written format only after the interview and examination are completed.

Some clinicians do the *Review of Systems* during the physical examination, asking about the ears, for example, as they examine them. If the patient has only a few symptoms, this combination can be efficient. However, if there are multiple symptoms, the flow of both the history and the examination can be disrupted and necessary note-taking becomes awkward. Listed below is a standard series of review-of-system questions. As you gain experience, the "yes or no" questions, placed at the end of the interview, will take no more than several minutes.

General. Usual weight, recent weight change, any clothes that fit more tightly or loosely than before. Weakness, fatigue, fever.

Skin. Rashes, lumps, sores, itching, dryness, color change, changes in hair or nails.

Head, Eyes, Ears, Nose, Throat (HEENT). ***Head:*** Headache, head injury, dizziness, lightheadedness. ***Eyes:*** Vision, glasses or contact lenses, last examination, pain, redness, excessive tearing, double vision, blurred vision, spots, specks, flashing lights, glaucoma, cataracts. ***Ears:*** Hearing, tinnitus, vertigo, earaches, infection, discharge. If hearing is decreased, use or nonuse of hearing aids. ***Nose and sinuses:*** Frequent colds, nasal stuffiness, discharge, or itching, hay fever, nosebleeds, sinus trouble. ***Throat (or mouth and pharynx):*** Condition of teeth, gums, bleeding gums, dentures, if any, and how they fit, last dental examination, sore tongue, dry mouth, frequent sore throats, hoarseness.

Neck. Lumps, "swollen glands," goiter, pain, or stiffness in the neck.

Breasts. Lumps, pain or discomfort, nipple discharge, self-examination practices.

Respiratory. Cough, sputum (color, quantity), hemoptysis, dyspnea, wheezing, pleurisy, last chest x-ray. You may wish to include asthma, bronchitis, emphysema, pneumonia, and tuberculosis.

Cardiovascular. Heart trouble, high blood pressure, rheumatic fever, heart murmurs, chest pain or discomfort, palpitations, dyspnea, orthopnea, paroxysmal nocturnal dyspnea, edema, past electrocardiographic or other heart test results.

Gastrointestinal. Trouble swallowing, heartburn, appetite, nausea, bowel movements, color and size of stools, change in bowel habits, rectal bleeding or black or tarry stools, hemorrhoids, constipation, diarrhea. Abdominal pain, food intolerance, excessive belching or passing of gas. Jaundice, liver or gallbladder trouble, hepatitis.

Urinary. Frequency of urination, polyuria, nocturia, urgency, burning or pain on urination, hematuria, urinary infections, kidney stones, incontinence; in males, reduced caliber or force of the urinary stream, hesitancy, dribbling.

Genital. ***Male:*** Hernias, discharge from or sores on the penis, testicular pain or masses, history of sexually transmitted diseases and their treatments. Sexual habits, interest, function, satisfaction, birth control methods, condom use, and problems. Exposure to HIV infection. ***Female:*** Age at menarche; regularity, frequency, and duration of periods; amount of bleeding, bleeding between periods or after intercourse, last menstrual period; dysmenorrhea, premenstrual tension; age at menopause, menopausal symptoms, postmenopausal bleeding. If the patient was born before 1971, exposure to diethylstilbestrol (DES) from maternal use during pregnancy. Vaginal discharge, itching, sores, lumps, sexually transmitted diseases and treatments. Number of pregnancies, number and type of deliveries, number of abortions (spontaneous and induced); complications of pregnancy; birth control methods. Sexual preference, interest, function, satisfaction, any problems, including dyspareunia. Exposure to HIV infection.

Peripheral Vascular. Intermittent claudication, leg cramps, varicose veins, past clots in the veins.

Musculoskeletal. Muscle or joint pains, stiffness, arthritis, gout, and backache. If present, describe location of affected joints or muscles, presence of any swelling, redness, pain, tenderness, stiffness, weakness, or limitation of motion or activity; include timing of symptoms (for example, morning or evening), duration, and any history of trauma.

Neurologic. Fainting, blackouts, seizures, weakness, paralysis, numbness or loss of sensation, tingling or "pins and needles," tremors or other involuntary movements.

Hematologic. Anemia, easy bruising or bleeding, past transfusions and/or transfusion reactions.

Endocrine. Thyroid trouble, heat or cold intolerance, excessive sweating, excessive thirst or hunger, polyuria, change in glove or shoe size.

Psychiatric. Nervousness, tension, mood, including depression, memory change, suicide attempts, if relevant.

THE PHYSICAL EXAMINATION: APPROACH AND OVERVIEW

In this section, we outline the ***comprehensive physical examination*** and provide an *overview* of all its components. You will conduct a comprehensive physical examination on most new patients or patients being admitted to the hospital. For more *problem-oriented*, or *focused, assessments*, the presenting complaints will dictate what segments of the examination you elect to perform. You will find a more extended discussion of the approach to the examination, its scope (comprehensive or focused), and a table summarizing the examination sequence in Chapter 3, Beginning the Physical Examination: General Survey and Vital Signs. Information about anatomy and physiology, interview questions, techniques of examination, and important abnormalities are detailed in Chapters 3 through 16 for each of the segments of the physical examination described below.

It is important to note that *the key to a thorough and accurate physical examination is developing a systematic sequence of examination.* At first, you may need notes to remember what to look for as you examine each region of the body; but with a few months of practice, you will acquire a routine sequence of your own. This sequence will become habit and often prompt you to return to an exam segment you may have inadvertently skipped, helping you to become thorough.

As you develop your own sequence of examination, *an important goal is to minimize the number of times you ask the patient to change position* from supine to sitting, or standing to lying supine. Some segments of the physical examination are best obtained while the patient is sitting, such as examinations of the head and neck and of the thorax and lungs, whereas others are best obtained supine, as are the cardiovascular and abdominal examinations. Some suggestions for patient positioning during the different segments of the examination are indicated in the right-hand column in *red.*

Most patients view the physical examination with at least some anxiety. They feel vulnerable, physically exposed, apprehensive about possible pain, and uneasy about what the clinician may find. At the same time, they appreciate the clinician's concern about their problems and respond to your attentiveness. With these considerations in mind, the skillful clinician is thorough without wasting time, systematic without being rigid, gentle yet not afraid to cause discomfort should this be required. In applying the techniques of inspection, palpation, auscultation, and percussion, the skillful clinician examines each region of the body, and at the same time senses the whole patient, notes the wince or worried glance, and shares information that calms, explains, and reassures.

For an overview of the physical examination, study the following example of the sequence of examination now. *Note that clinicians vary in where they place different segments of the examination, especially the examinations of the musculoskeletal system and the nervous system.* Some of these options are indicated below. With practice, you will develop your own sequence, keeping the need for thoroughness and patient comfort in mind. After you complete your study and practice the techniques described in the regional examination chapters, reread this overview to see how each segment of the examination fits into an integrated whole.

The Comprehensive Physical Examination

General Survey. Observe the patient's general state of health, height, build, and sexual development. Obtain the patient's weight. Note posture, motor activity, and gait; dress, grooming, and personal hygiene; and any odors of the body or breath. Watch the patient's facial expressions and note manner, affect, and reactions to persons and things in the environment. Listen to the patient's manner of speaking and note the state of awareness or level of consciousness.

The survey continues throughout the history and examination.

Vital Signs. Measure height and weight. Measure the blood pressure. Count the pulse and respiratory rate. If indicated, measure the body temperature.

The **patient is sitting** on the edge of the bed or examining table, unless this position is contraindicated. You should be standing in front of the patient, moving to either side as needed.

Skin. Observe the skin of the face and its characteristics. Identify any lesions, noting their location, distribution, arrangement, type, and color. Inspect and palpate the hair and nails. Study the patient's hands. Continue your assessment of the skin as you examine the other body regions.

Head, Eyes, Ears, Nose, Throat (HEENT). ***Head:*** Examine the hair, scalp, skull, and face. ***Eyes:*** Check visual acuity and screen the visual fields. Note the position and alignment of the eyes. Observe the eyelids and inspect the sclera and conjunctiva of each eye. With oblique lighting, inspect each cornea, iris, and lens. Compare the pupils, and test their reactions to light. Assess the extraocular movements. With an ophthalmoscope, inspect the ocular fundi. ***Ears:*** Inspect the auricles, canals, and drums. Check auditory acuity. If acuity is diminished, check lateralization (Weber test) and compare air and bone conduction (Rinne test). ***Nose and sinuses:*** Examine the external nose; using a light and a nasal speculum, inspect the nasal mucosa, septum, and turbinates. Palpate for tenderness of the frontal and maxillary sinuses. ***Throat (or mouth and pharynx):*** Inspect the lips, oral mucosa, gums, teeth, tongue, palate, tonsils, and pharynx. *(You may wish to assess the cranial nerves during this portion of the examination.)*

The room should be darkened for the ophthalmoscopic examination. This promotes pupillary dilation and visibility of the fundi.

Neck. Inspect and palpate the cervical lymph nodes. Note any masses or unusual pulsations in the neck. Feel for any deviation of the trachea. Observe sound and effort of the patient's breathing. Inspect and palpate the thyroid gland.

Move behind the sitting patient to feel the thyroid gland and to examine the back, posterior thorax, and the lungs.

Back. Inspect and palpate the spine and muscles of the back.

Posterior Thorax and Lungs. Inspect and palpate the spine and muscles of the *upper* back. Inspect, palpate, and percuss the chest. Identify the level of diaphragmatic dullness on each side. Listen to the breath sounds; identify any adventitious (or added) sounds, and, if indicated, listen to the transmitted voice sounds (see p. 229).

Breasts, Axillae, and Epitrochlear Nodes. In a woman, inspect the breasts with her arms relaxed, then elevated, and then with her hands pressed on her hips. In either sex, inspect the axillae and feel for the axillary nodes. Feel for the epitrochlear nodes.

The patient is **still sitting.** Move to the front again.

A Note on the Musculoskeletal System: By this time, you have made some preliminary observations of the musculoskeletal system. You have inspected the hands, surveyed the upper back, and at least in women, made a fair estimate of the shoulders' range of motion. Use these and subsequent observations to decide whether a full musculoskeletal examination is warranted. If indicated, *with the patient still sitting,* examine the hands, arms, shoulders, neck, and temporomandibular joints. Inspect and palpate the joints and check their range of motion. *(You may choose to examine upper extremity muscle bulk, tone, strength, and reflexes at this time, or you may decide to wait until later.)*

Palpate the breasts, while at the same time continuing your inspection.

The patient position is supine. Ask the patient to lie down. You should stand at the right side of the patient's bed.

Anterior Thorax and Lungs. Inspect, palpate, and percuss the chest. Listen to the breath sounds, any adventitious sounds, and, if indicated, transmitted voice sounds.

Cardiovascular System. Observe the jugular venous pulsations, and measure the jugular venous pressure in relation to the sternal angle. Inspect and palpate the carotid pulsations. Listen for carotid bruits.

Elevate the head of the bed to about 30° for the cardiovascular examination, adjusting as necessary to see the jugular venous pulsations.

Inspect and palpate the precordium. Note the location, diameter, amplitude, and duration of the apical impulse. Listen at the apex and the lower sternal border with the bell of a stethoscope. Listen at each auscultatory area with the diaphragm. Listen for the first and second heart sounds, and for physiologic splitting of the second heart sound. Listen for any abnormal heart sounds or murmurs.

Ask the patient to roll partly onto the left side while you listen at the apex. Then have the patient roll back to the supine position while you listen to the rest of the heart. The patient should sit, lean forward, and exhale while you listen for the murmur of aortic regurgitation.

Abdomen. Inspect, auscultate, and percuss the abdomen. Palpate lightly, then deeply. Assess the liver and spleen by percussion and then palpation. Try to feel the kidneys, and palpate the aorta and its pulsations. If you suspect kidney infection, percuss posteriorly over the costovertebral angles.

Lower the head of the bed to the flat position. **The patient should be supine.**

Lower Extremities. Examine the legs, assessing three systems while the patient is still supine. Each of these three systems can be further assessed when the patient stands.

The patient is **supine**.

Examination with the patient supine

- *Peripheral Vascular System.* Palpate the femoral pulses, and if indicated, the popliteal pulses. Palpate the inguinal lymph nodes. Inspect for lower extremity edema, discoloration, or ulcers. Palpate for pitting edema.

- *Musculoskeletal System.* Note any deformities or enlarged joints. If indicated, palpate the joints, check their range of motion, and perform any necessary maneuvers.

- *Nervous System.* Assess lower extremity muscle bulk, tone, and strength; also sensation and reflexes. Observe any abnormal movements.

Examination with the patient standing

The patient is **standing**. You should sit on a chair or stool.

- *Peripheral Vascular System.* Inspect for varicose veins.

- *Musculoskeletal System.* Examine the alignment of the spine and its range of motion, the alignment of the legs, and the feet.

- *Genitalia and Hernias in Men.* Examine the penis and scrotal contents and check for hernias.

- *Nervous System.* Observe the patient's gait and ability to walk heel-to-toe, walk on the toes, walk on the heels, hop in place, and do shallow knee bends. Do a Romberg test and check for pronator drift.

Nervous System. The complete examination of the nervous system can also be done at the end of the examination. It consists of the five segments described below: *mental status, cranial nerves* (including funduscopic examination), *motor system, sensory system,* and *reflexes.*

The patient is **sitting or supine.**

Mental Status. If indicated and not done during the interview, assess the patient's orientation, mood, thought process, thought content, abnormal perceptions, insight and judgment, memory and attention, information and vocabulary, calculating abilities, abstract thinking, and constructional ability.

Cranial Nerves. If not already examined, check sense of smell, strength of the temporal and masseter muscles, corneal reflexes, facial movements, gag reflex, and strength of the trapezia and sternomastoid muscles.

Motor System. Muscle bulk, tone, and strength of major muscle groups. *Cerebellar function:* rapid alternating movements (RAMs), point-to-point movements, such as finger-to-nose (F → N) and heel-to-shin (H → S); gait.

Sensory System. Pain, temperature, light touch, vibration, and discrimination. Compare right with left sides and distal with proximal areas on the limbs.

Reflexes. Including biceps, triceps, brachioradialis, patellar, Achilles deep tendon reflexes; also plantar reflexes or Babinski reflex (see pp. 591–592).

Additional Examinations. The *rectal* and *genital* examinations are often performed at the end of the physical examination. Patient positioning is as indicated.

Rectal Examination in Men. Inspect the sacrococcygeal and perianal areas. Palpate the anal canal, rectum, and prostate. If the patient cannot stand, examine the genitalia before doing the rectal examination.

The patient is **lying on his left side** for the rectal examination.

Genital and Rectal Examination in Women. Examine the external genitalia, vagina, and cervix. Obtain a Pap smear. Palpate the uterus and adnexa. Do a rectovaginal and rectal examination.

The patient is **supine in the lithotomy position**. You should be seated during examination with the speculum, then standing during bimanual examination of the uterus, adnexa, and rectum.

RECORDING YOUR FINDINGS

Now you are ready to review an actual written record documenting a patient's history and physical findings, illustrated below using the example of "Mrs. N." The history and physical examination form the database for your subsequent *assessment(s)* of the patient and your *plan(s)* with the patient for management and next steps. Your written record organizes the information from the history and physical examination and should clearly communicate the patient's clinical issues to all members of the health care team. You will find that following a standardized format is often the most efficient and helpful way to transfer this information.

Your written record should also facilitate clinical reasoning and communicate essential information to the many health professionals involved in your patient's care. Chapter 18, Clinical Reasoning, Assessment, and Plan, will provide more comprehensive information for formulating the *assessment* and *plan,* and additional guidelines for documentation.

If you are a beginner, organizing the *Present Illness* may be especially challenging, but do not get discouraged. Considerable knowledge is needed to cluster related symptoms and physical signs. If you are unfamiliar with hyperthyroidism, for example, it may not be apparent that muscular weakness, heat intolerance, excessive sweating, diarrhea, and weight loss, all represent a *Present Illness.* Until your knowledge and judgment grow, the patient's story and the seven key attributes of a symptom (see p. 27) are helpful and necessary guides to what to include in this portion of the record.

TIPS FOR A CLEAR AND ACCURATE WRITE-UP

You should write the record as soon as possible, before the data fade from your memory. At first, you will probably prefer to take notes when talking with the patient. As you gain experience, however, work toward recording the *Present Illness*, the *Past Medical History*, the *Family History*, the *Personal* and *Social History*, and the *Review of Systems* in final form during the interview. Leave spaces for filling in details later. During the *physical examination*, make note immediately of specific measurements, such as blood pressure and heart rate. On the other hand, recording multiple items interrupts the flow of the examination, and you will soon learn to remember your findings and record them after you have finished.

Several key features distinguish a clear and well-organized written record. Pay special attention to the *order* and the *degree of detail* as you review the record below and later when you construct your own write-ups. Remember that if handwritten, a good record is always legible!

Order of the Write-Up

The order should be consistent and obvious so that future readers, including yourself, can easily find specific points of information. Keep items of history in the history, for example, and do not let them stray into the physical examination. Offset your headings and make them clear by using indentations and spacing to accent your organization. Create emphasis by using asterisks and underlines for important points. Arrange the *present illness* in chronologic order, starting with the current episode and then filling in the relevant background information. If a patient with long-standing diabetes is hospitalized in a coma, for example, begin with the events leading up to the coma and then summarize the past history of the patient's diabetes.

Degree of Detail

The *degree of detail* is also a challenge. It should be pertinent to the subject or problem but not redundant. Review the record of Mrs. N, then turn to the checklist in Chapter 18 on pp. 796–798. Decide if you think the order and detail included meet the standards of a good medical record.

The Case of Mrs. N

8/30/02
Mrs. N is a pleasant, 54-year-old widowed saleswoman residing in Amarillo, Texas.
Referral. None
Source and Reliability. Self-referred; seems reliable.

Chief Complaint: "My head aches."

Present Illness

For about 3 months, Mrs. N has had increasing problems with frontal headaches. These are usually bifrontal, throbbing, and mild to moderately severe. She has missed work on several occasions due to associated nausea and vomiting. Headaches now average once a week, usually related to stress, and last 4 to 6 hours. They are relieved by sleep and putting a damp towel over the forehead. There is little relief from aspirin. No associated visual changes, motor-sensory deficits, or paresthesias.

"Sick headaches" with nausea and vomiting began at age 15, recurred throughout her mid-20s, then decreased to one every 2 or 3 months and almost disappeared.

The patient reports increased pressure at work from a new and demanding boss; she is also worried about her daughter (see *Personal and Social History*). Thinks her headaches may be like those in the past, but wants to be sure because her mother died of a stroke. She is concerned that they interfere with her work and make her irritable with her family. She eats three meals a day and drinks three cups of coffee per day; cola at night.

Medications. Aspirin, 1 to 2 tablets every 4 to 6 hours as needed. "Water pill" in the past for ankle swelling, none recently.

**Allergies.* Ampicillin causes rash.

Tobacco. About 1 pack of cigarettes per day since age 18 (36 pack-years).

Alcohol/drugs. Wine on rare occasions. No illicit drugs.

Past History

Childhood Illnesses. Measles, chickenpox. No scarlet fever or rheumatic fever.

Adult Illnesses. ***Medical:*** Pyelonephritis, 1982, with fever and right flank pain; treated with ampicillin; develop generalized rash with itching several days later. Reports kidney x-rays were normal; no recurrence of infection. ***Surgical:*** Tonsillectomy, age 6, appendectomy, age 13. Sutures for laceration, 1991, after stepping on glass. ***Ob/gyn:*** G3P3, with normal vaginal deliveries. 3 living children. Menarche age 12. Last menses 6 months ago. Little interest in sex, and not sexually active. No concerns about HIV infection. ***Psychiatric:*** None.

Health Maintenance. ***Immunizations:*** Oral polio vaccine, year uncertain; tetanus shots × 2, 1991, followed with booster 1 year later; flu vaccine, 2000, no reaction. ***Screening tests:*** Last Pap smear, 1998, normal. No mammograms to date.

Family History

A *note on recording the Family History*. There are two methods of recording the *Family History:* a diagram or a narrative. The diagram format is more helpful than the narrative for tracing genetic disorders. The negatives from the family history should follow either format.

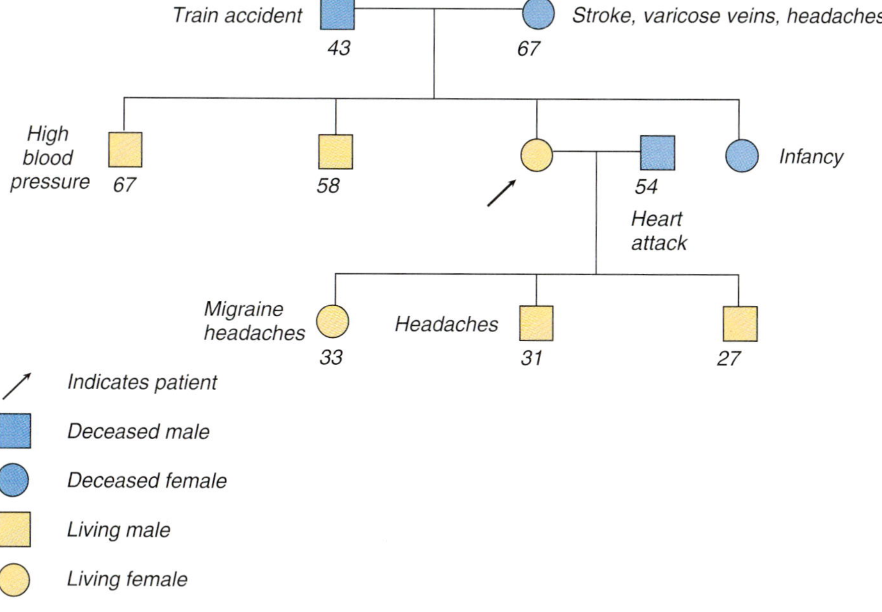

*Add an asterisk or underline important points.

or:

Father died at age 43 in train accident. Mother died at age 67 of stroke; had varicose veins, headaches
One brother, 61, with hypertension, otherwise well; one brother, 58, well except for mild arthritis; one sister, died in infancy of unknown cause
Husband died at age 54 of heart attack
Daughter, 33, with migraine headaches, otherwise well; son, 31, with headaches; son, 27, well

No family history of diabetes, tuberculosis, heart or kidney disease, cancer, anemia, epilepsy, or mental illness.

Personal and Social History

Born and raised in Lake City, finished high school, married at age 19. Worked as sales clerk for 2 years, then moved with husband to Amarillo, had 3 children. Returned to work 15 years ago because of financial pressures. Children all married. Four years ago Mr. N died suddenly of a heart attack, leaving little savings. Mrs. N has moved to small apartment to be near daughter, Dorothy. Dorothy's husband, Arthur, has an alcohol problem. Mrs. N's apartment now a haven for Dorothy and her 2 children, Kevin, 6 years, and Linda, 3 years. Mrs. N feels responsible for helping them; feels tense and nervous but denies depression. She has friends but rarely discusses family problems: "I'd rather keep them to myself. I don't like gossip." No church or other organizational support. She is typically up at 7:00 A.M., works 9:00 to 5:30, eats dinner alone.

Exercise and diet. Gets little exercise. Diet high in carbohydrates.
Safety measures. Uses seat belt regularly. Uses sunblock. Medications kept in an unlocked medicine cabinet. Cleaning solutions in unlocked cabinet below sink. Mr. N's shotgun and box of shells in unlocked closet upstairs.

Review of Systems

General. Has *gained* about 10 lb in the past 4 years.

Skin. No rashes or other changes.

Head, Eyes, Ears, Nose, Throat (HEENT). See *Present Illness*. No history of head injury. *Eyes:* Reading glasses for 5 years, last checked 1 year ago. No symptoms. *Ears:* Hearing good. No tinnitus, vertigo, infections. *Nose, sinuses:* Occasional mild cold. No hay fever, sinus trouble. **Throat (or *mouth and pharynx):*
Some bleeding of gums recently. Last dental visit 2 years ago. Occasional canker sore.

Neck. No lumps, goiter, pain. No swollen glands.

Breasts. No lumps, pain, discharge. Does self-breast exam sporadically.

Respiratory. No cough, wheezing, shortness of breath. Last chest x-ray, 1986, St. Mary's Hospital; unremarkable.

Cardiovascular. No known heart disease or high blood pressure; last blood pressure taken in 1998. No dyspnea, orthopnea, chest pain, palpitations. Has never had an electrocardiogram (ECG).

Gastrointestinal. Appetite good; no nausea, vomiting, indigestion. Bowel movement about once daily, though sometimes has hard stools for 2 to 3 days when especially tense; no diarrhea or bleeding. No pain, jaundice, gallbladder or liver problems.

Urinary. No frequency, dysuria, hematuria, or recent flank pain; nocturia × 1, large volume. Occasionally loses some urine when coughs hard.

Genital. No vaginal or pelvic infections. No dyspareunia.

Peripheral Vascular. Varicose veins appeared in both legs during first pregnancy. For 10 years, has had swollen ankles after prolonged standing; wears light elastic pantyhose; tried "water pill" 5 months ago, but it didn't help much; no history of phlebitis or leg pain.

Musculoskeletal. Mild, aching, low-back pain, often after a long day's work; no radiation down the legs; used to do back exercises but not now. No other joint pain.

Neurologic. No fainting, seizures, motor or sensory loss. Memory good.

Hematologic. Except for bleeding gums, no easy bleeding. No anemia.

Endocrine. No known thyroid trouble, temperature intolerance. Sweating average. No symptoms or history of diabetes.

Psychiatric. No history of depression or treatment for psychiatric disorders. See also *Present Illness* and *Personal and Social History.*

Physical Examination

Mrs. N is a short, moderately obese, middle-aged woman, who is animated and responds quickly to questions. She is somewhat tense, with moist, cold hands. Her hair is fixed neatly and her clothes are immaculate. Her color is good and she lies flat without discomfort.

Vital Signs. Ht (without shoes) 157 cm (5′2″). Wt (dressed) 65 kg (143 lb). BP 164/98 right arm, supine; 160/96 left arm, supine; 152/88 right arm, supine with wide cuff. Heart rate (HR) 88 and regular. Respiratory rate (RR) 18. Temperature (oral) 98.6°F.

Skin. Palms cold and moist, but color good. Scattered cherry angiomas over upper trunk. Nails without clubbing, cyanosis.

Head, Eyes, Ears, Nose, Throat (HEENT). *Head:* Hair of average texture. Scalp without lesions, normocephalic/atraumatic (NC/AT). *Eyes:* Vision 20/30 in each eye. Visual fields full by confrontation. Conjunctiva pink; sclera white. Pupils 4 mm constricting to 2 mm, round, regular, equally reactive to light. Extraocular movements intact. Disc margins sharp, without hemorrhages, exudates. No arteriolar narrowing or A-V nicking. *Ears:* Wax partially obscures right tympanic membrane (TM); left canal clear, TM with good cone of light. Acuity good to whispered voice. Weber midline. AC > BC. *Nose:* Mucosa pink, septum midline. No sinus tenderness. *Mouth:* Oral mucosa pink. Several interdental papillae red, slightly swollen. Dentition good. Tongue midline, with 3 × 4 mm shallow white ulcer on red base on undersurface near tip; tender but not indurated. Tonsils absent. Pharynx without exudates.

Neck. Neck supple. Trachea midline. Thyroid isthmus barely palpable, lobes not felt.

Lymph Nodes. Small (<1 cm), soft, nontender, and mobile tonsillar and posterior cervical nodes bilaterally. No axillary or epitrochlear nodes. Several small inguinal nodes bilaterally, soft and nontender.

Thorax and Lungs. Thorax symmetric with good excursion. Lungs resonant. Breath sounds vesicular with no added sounds. Diaphragms descend 4 cm bilaterally.

Cardiovascular. Jugular venous pressure 1 cm above the sternal angle, with head of examining table raised to 30°. Carotid upstrokes brisk, without bruits. Apical impulse discrete and tapping, barely palpable in the 5th left interspace,

8 cm lateral to the midsternal line. Good S_1, S_2; no S_3 or S_4. A II/VI medium-pitched midsystolic murmur at the 2nd right interspace; does not radiate to the neck. No diastolic murmurs.

Breasts. Pendulous, symmetric. No masses; nipples without discharge.

Abdomen. Obese. Well-healed scar, right lower quadrant. Bowel sounds active. No tenderness or masses. Liver span 7 cm in right midclavicular line; edge smooth, palpable 1 cm below right costal margin (RCM). Spleen and kidneys not felt. No costovertebral angle tenderness (CVAT).

Genitalia. External genitalia without lesions. Mild cystocele at introitus on straining. Vaginal mucosa pink. Cervix pink, parous, and without discharge. Uterus anterior, midline, smooth, not enlarged. Adnexa not palpated due to obesity and poor relaxation. No cervical or adnexal tenderness. Pap smear taken. Rectovaginal wall intact.

Rectal. Rectal vault without masses. Stool brown, negative for occult blood.

Extremities. Warm and without edema. Calves supple, nontender.

Peripheral Vascular. Trace edema at both ankles. Moderate varicosities of saphenous veins both lower extremities. No stasis pigmentation or ulcers. Pulses (2 + = brisk, or normal):

	Radial	Femoral	Popliteal	Dorsalis Pedis	Posterior Tibial
RT	2+	2+	2+	2+	2+
LT	2+	2+	2+	Absent	2+

Musculoskeletal. No joint deformities. Good range of motion in hands, wrists, elbows, shoulders, spine, hips, knees, ankles.

Neurologic. *Mental Status:* Tense but alert and cooperative. Thought coherent. Oriented to person, place, and time. *Cranial Nerves:* II–XII intact. *Motor:* Good muscle bulk and tone. Strength 5/5 throughout (see p. 574 for grading system). *Cerebellar:* Rapid alternating movements (RAMs), point-to-point movements intact. Gait stable, fluid. *Sensory:* Pinprick, light touch, position sense, vibration, and stereognosis intact. Romberg negative. *Reflexes:* Two methods of recording may be used, depending upon personal preference: a tabular form or a stick picture diagram, as shown below and at right. 2+ = brisk, or normal; see p. 587 for grading system.

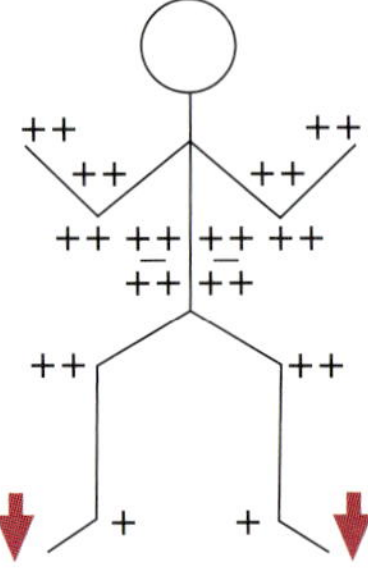

	Biceps	Triceps	Brachioradialis	Patellar	Achilles	Plantar
RT	2+	2+	2+	2+	1+	↓
LT	2+	2+	2+	2+/2+	1+	↓

Learning History Taking and Physical Examination

Now that you have surveyed the tasks ahead, the overviews of the health history and physical examination, and the patient record of Mrs. N, you are ready to turn to the chapters on history taking and physical examination. Chapter 18, Clinical Reasoning, Assessment, and Plan, provides more comprehensive information on how to formulate your *Assessment* and *Plan,* the final steps of patient assessment, and the remaining two sections of the written record. In Chapter 18 you will also find guidelines for documentation and the assessment and plan for Mrs. N. The rewards of mastering the skills of patient assessment lie just ahead!

CHAPTER

2

Interviewing and the Health History

The health history interview is a conversation with a purpose. As a clinician, you will draw on many of the interpersonal skills that you use every day, but with unique and important differences. Unlike social conversation, in which you express your own needs and interests with responsibility only for yourself, the primary goal of the clinician–patient interview is to improve the well-being of the patient. At its most basic level, the purpose of conversation with a patient is threefold: to establish a trusting and supportive relationship, to gather information, and to offer information. Communicating and relating therapeutically with patients are the most valued skills of clinical care. As a beginning clinician, you will focus your energies on gathering information. At the same time, by using techniques that promote trust and communication, you will allow the patient's story to unfold in its most full and detailed form. Establishing a supportive interaction enhances information-gathering and itself becomes part of the therapeutic process of patient care.

As a clinician facilitating the patient's story, you will come to generate a series of hypotheses about the nature of the patient's concerns. You will then test these various hypotheses by asking for more detailed information. You will also explore the patient's feelings and beliefs about his or her problem. Eventually, as your clinical experience grows, you will respond with your understanding of the patient's concerns. Even if you discover that little can be done for the patient's disease, discussing the patient's experience of being ill can be therapeutic. In the example that follows, a research protocol made the patient ineligible for treatment of her long-standing and severe arthritis.

> The patient had never talked about what the symptoms meant to her. She had never said "This means that I can't go to the bathroom by myself, put my clothes on, even get out of bed without calling for help."
>
> When we finished the physical examination, I said something like "Rheumatoid arthritis really has not been nice to you." She burst into tears, and so did her daughter, and I sat there, very close to losing it myself.
>
> She said "You know, no one has ever talked about it as a personal thing before. No one's ever talked to me as if this were a thing that mattered, a personal event."
>
> That was the significant thing about the encounter. I didn't really have much else to offer . . . But something really significant had happened between us, something that she valued and would carry away with her.[1]

---

[1]Hastings C: The lived experiences of the illness: Making contact with the patient. In Benner P, Wrubel J. The Primacy of Caring: Stress and Coping in Health and Illness. Menlo Park, CA, Addison-Wesley, 1989.

As you can see from this story, interviewing patients consists of much more than just asking a series of questions.

You will find that the interviewing process differs significantly from the format for the health history presented in Chapter 1. Both are fundamental to your work with patients, but each serves a different purpose. The health history format is a structured framework for organizing patient information in written or verbal form: it focuses the clinician's attention on specific pieces of information that must be obtained from the patient. The interviewing process that actually generates these pieces of information is more fluid. It requires knowledge of the information you need to obtain, the ability to elicit accurate and detailed information, and interpersonal skills that allow you to respond to the patient's feelings.

As you learned in Chapter 1, the kinds of questions you ask as you elicit the health history vary according to several factors. The scope and degree of detail depend on the patient's needs and concerns, the clinician's goals for the encounter, and the clinical setting (e.g., inpatient or outpatient, amount of time available, primary care or subspecialty). For new patients, regardless of the setting, you will do a *comprehensive health history,* described for adults in Chapter 1. For other patients who seek care for a specific complaint, such as a cough or painful urination, a more limited interview tailored to that specific problem may be indicated, sometimes known as a *problem-oriented history.* In a primary care setting, clinicians frequently choose to address issues of health promotion, such as tobacco cessation or reduction of high-risk sexual behaviors. A subspecialist may do an in-depth history to evaluate one problem that incorporates a wide range of areas of inquiry. Knowing the content and relevance of all the components of a comprehensive health history, reviewed for you below, enables you to select the kinds of information that will be most helpful for meeting both clinician and patient goals.

THE FORMAT OF THE COMPREHENSIVE HEALTH HISTORY

- Identifying Data
- Source and Reliability of History
- Chief Complaint
- History of Present Illness
  - Medications, Allergies, Tobacco, Alcohol and Drugs
- Past History
  - Childhood Illness
  - Adult Illness: Medical, Surgical, Ob/Gyn, Psychiatric, Health Maintenance
- Family History
- Personal and Social History
- Review of Systems

This chapter introduces you to the essential skills of interviewing for gathering the health history—skills that you will continually use and refine throughout your career. You will learn the guiding principles for how clinicians talk with patients and forge trusting relationships with them. You will read about preparing for the interview, the sequence of the interviewing process, important interviewing techniques, and strategies for addressing a variety of challenges that frequently arise in encounters with patients.

Getting Ready: The Approach to the Interview

Interviewing patients to obtain a health history requires planning. You are undoubtedly eager to begin your relationship with the patient, but you should first consider several points that are crucial to success.

Taking Time for Self-Reflection. As clinicians, we encounter a wide variety of people, each one of whom is unique. Establishing relationships with individuals from a broad spectrum of ages, social classes, races, ethnicities, and states of health or illness is an uncommon opportunity and privilege. Being consistently open and respectful toward individual differences is one of the clinician's challenges. Because we bring our own values, assumptions, and biases to every encounter, we must look inward to clarify how our own expectations and reactions may affect what we hear and how we behave. *Self-reflection is a continual part of professional development in clinical work. It brings a deepening personal awareness to our work with patients and is one of the most rewarding aspects of providing patient care.*

Reviewing the Chart. Before seeing the patient, review his or her medical record, or chart. The purpose of reviewing the chart is partly to gather information and partly to develop ideas about what to explore with the patient. Look closely at the identifying data (age, gender, address, health insurance), the problem list, the medication list, and other details, such as the documentation of allergies. The chart often provides valuable information about past diagnoses and treatments; however, you should not let the chart prevent you from developing new approaches or ideas. Remember that information in the chart comes from different observers, and that standardized forms reflect different institutional norms. Moreover, the chart often fails to capture the essence of the person you are about to meet. Data may be incomplete or even disagree with what you learn from the patient—understanding such discrepancies may prove helpful to the patient's care.

Setting Goals for the Interview. Before you begin talking with a patient, it is important to clarify your goals for the interview. As a student, your goal may be to obtain a complete health history so that you can submit a write-up to your teacher. As a clinician, your goals can range from completing forms needed by the health care facility or insurance companies to testing hypotheses generated by your review of the chart. A clinician must balance these provider-centered goals with patient-centered goals. There can be tension between the needs of the provider, the institution, and the patient and family. Part of the clinician's task is to consider these multiple agendas. By taking a few minutes to think through your goals ahead of time, you will find it easier to strike a healthy balance among the various purposes of the interview to come.

Reviewing Clinician Behavior and Appearance. Just as you observe the patient throughout the interview, the patient will be watching you. Consciously or not, you send messages through both your words and your behavior. Be sensitive to those messages and manage them as well as you can. Posture, gestures, eye contact, and tone of voice can all express interest, attention, acceptance, and understanding. The skilled interviewer seems calm and unhurried, even when time is limited. Reactions that betray disapproval, embarrassment, impatience, or boredom block communication, as do behaviors that condescend, stereotype, criticize, or belittle the patient. Although these types of negative feelings are unavoidable at times, you must take pains not to express them. Guard against them not only when talking to patients but also when discussing patients with your colleagues.

Your personal appearance can also affect your clinical relationships. Patients find cleanliness, neatness, conservative dress, and a name tag reassuring. Try to consider the patient's perspective. Remember that you want the patient to trust you.

Improving the Environment. Try to make the setting as private and comfortable as possible. Although you may have to talk with the patient under difficult circumstances, such as a two-bed room or the corridor of a busy emergency department, a proper environment improves communication. If there are privacy curtains, ask permission to pull them shut. Suggest moving to an empty room rather than having a conversation in a waiting area. *As the clinician, part of your job is to make adjustments to the location and seating that make the patient and you more comfortable.* Doing so is always worth the time.

Taking Notes. As a novice you will need to write down much of what you learn during the interview. Even though experienced clinicians seem to remember a great deal of the interview without taking notes, no one can remember all the details of a comprehensive history. Jot down short phrases, specific dates, or words rather than trying to put them into a final format. Do not, however, let note-taking or using written forms distract you from the patient. Maintain good eye contact, and whenever the patient is talking about sensitive or disturbing material, put down your pen. Most patients are accustomed to note-taking, but for those who find it uncomfortable, explore their concerns and explain your need to create an accurate record.

Learning About the Patient: The Process of Interviewing

Once you have devoted time and thought to preparing for the interview, you are fully ready to listen to the patient, elicit the patient's concerns, and learn about the patient's health. In general, an interview moves through several stages. *Throughout this sequence, you, as the clinician, must always be attuned to the patient's feelings, help the patient express them, respond to their content, and validate their significance.* A typical sequence follows.

THE SEQUENCE OF THE INTERVIEW

- Greeting the patient and establishing rapport
- Inviting the patient's story
- Establishing the agenda for the interview
- Expanding and clarifying the patient's story; generating and testing diagnostic hypotheses
- Creating a shared understanding of the problem(s)
- Negotiating a plan (includes further evaluation, treatment, and patient education)
- Planning for follow-up and closing the interview.

As a student, you will concentrate primarily on gathering the patient's story and creating a shared understanding of the problem. As you become a practicing clinician, negotiating a plan for further evaluation and treatment will become more important. Whether the interview is comprehensive or focused, you should move through this sequence while closely attending to the patient's feelings and affect.

Greeting the Patient and Establishing Rapport. The initial moments of your encounter with the patient lay the foundation for your ongoing relationship. How you greet the patient and other visitors in the room, provide for the patient's comfort, and arrange the physical setting all shape the patient's first impressions.

As you begin, *greet the patient* by name and introduce yourself, giving your own name. If possible, shake hands with the patient. If this is the first contact, explain your role, including your status as a student and how you will be involved in the patient's care. Repeat this part of the introduction on subsequent meetings until you are confident that the patient knows who you are. "Good morning, Mr. Peters. I'm Susan Jones, a 3rd-year medical student. You may remember me. I was here yesterday talking with you about your heart problems. I'm part of the medical team that's taking care of you."

Using a title to address the patient (e.g., Mr. O'Neil, Ms. Washington) is always best. Except with children or adolescents, avoid first names unless you have specific permission from the patient or family. Addressing an unfamiliar adult as "granny" or "dear" tends to depersonalize and demean. If you are unsure how to pronounce the patient's name, don't be afraid to ask. You can say "I'm afraid of mispronouncing your name. Could you say it for me?" Then repeat it to make sure that you heard it correctly.

When visitors are in the room, be sure to acknowledge and greet each one in turn, inquiring about each person's name and relationship to the patient. Whenever visitors are present, it is important for you to *maintain confidentiality.* Let the patient decide if visitors or family members should remain in the room, and ask for the patient's permission before conducting the interview in front of them. For example, "I'm comfortable with having your sister stay for the interview, Mrs. Jones, but I want to make sure that this is also what you want" or "Would you prefer if I spoke to you alone or with your sister present?"

It is important to *be attuned to the patient's comfort.* In the office or clinic, be sure there is a suitable place other than the patient's lap for coats and belongings. In the hospital, after greeting the patient, ask how the patient is feeling and if you are coming at a convenient time. Look for signs of discomfort, such as frequent changes of position or facial expressions that show pain or anxiety. Arranging the bed to make the patient more comfortable or allowing a few minutes for the patient to say goodbye to visitors or finish using the bedpan may be the shortest route to a good history.

Consider the best way to *arrange the room* and how far you should be from the patient. Remember that cultural background and individual taste influence preferences about interpersonal space. Choose a distance that facilitates conversation and good eye contact. You should probably be within several feet, close enough to be intimate but not intrusive. Pull up a chair and, if possible, try to sit at eye level with the patient. Move any physical barriers between you and the patient, such as desks or bedside tables, out of the way. In an outpatient setting, sitting on a rolling stool, for example, allows you to change distances in response to patient cues. Avoid arrangements that connote disrespect or inequality of power, such as interviewing a woman already positioned for a pelvic examination. Such arrangements are unacceptable. Lighting also makes a difference. If you sit between a patient and a bright light or window, although your view might be fine, the patient may have to squint uncomfortably to see you, making the interaction more like an interrogation than a supportive interview.

Give the patient your undivided attention. Try not to look down to take notes or read the chart, and spend enough time on small talk to put the patient at ease.

Inviting the Patient's Story. Now that you have established rapport, you are ready to pursue the patient's reason for seeking health care, or *chief complaint.* Begin with **open-ended questions** that allow full freedom of response. "What concerns bring you here today?" or "How can I help you?" Note that these questions encourage the patient to express any possible concerns and do not restrict the patient to a limited and minimally informative "yes" or "no" answer. Listen to the patient's answers without interrupting. After you have given the patient the opportunity to respond fully, inquire again or even several times, "Anything else?" You may need to lead the patient back several times to additional concerns or issues he or she may want to tell you about.

Some patients may want only a blood pressure check or routine examination, without having a specific complaint or problem. Others may say they just want a physical examination but feel uncomfortable bringing up an underlying concern. In all these situations, *it is still important to start with the patient's story.* Helpful open-ended questions are "Was there a specific health concern that prompted you to schedule this appointment?" and "What made you decide to come in for health care now?"

It is important to train yourself to *follow the patient's leads.* Good interviewing techniques include using verbal and nonverbal cues that prompt patients to recount their stories spontaneously. If you intervene too early and ask specific questions prematurely, you risk trampling on the very information you are seeking. Your role, however, is far from passive. You should listen actively and make use of *continuers,* especially at the outset. Examples include nodding your head and using phrases such as "uh huh," "go on," and "I see." Additional facilitative techniques (pp. 30–34) help keep you from missing any of the patient's concerns.

Establishing the Agenda for the Interview. The clinician often approaches the interview with specific goals in mind. The patient also has specific questions and concerns. It is important to identify all these issues at the beginning of the encounter. Doing so allows you to use the time available effectively and to make sure that you address all the patient's issues. As a student, you may have enough time to cover the breadth of both your concerns and the patient's in one visit. For a clinician, however, time management is almost always an issue. As a clinician, you may need to focus the interview by asking the patient which problem is most pressing. For example, "You have told me about several different problems that are important for us to discuss. I also wanted to review your blood pressure medication. We need to decide which problems to address today. Can you tell me which one you are most concerned about?" Then you can proceed with questions such as, "Tell me about that problem." Once you have agreed upon a manageable list, stating that the other problems are also important and will be addressed during a future visit gives the patient confidence in your ongoing collaboration.

Expanding and Clarifying the Health History (the Patient's Perspective). You can then guide the patient into elaborating areas of the health history that seem most significant. For the clinician, each symptom has attributes that must be clarified, including context, associations, and chronology, especially for complaints of pain. For all symptoms, it is critical to fully understand their essential characteristics. Always pursue the following elements.

THE SEVEN ATTRIBUTES OF A SYMPTOM

1. **Location.** Where is it? Does it radiate?
2. **Quality.** What is it like?
3. **Quantity or severity.** How bad is it? (For pain, ask for a rating on a scale of 1 to 10.)
4. **Timing.** When did (does) it start? How long did (does) it last? How often did (does) it come?
5. **Setting in which it occurs.** Include environmental factors, personal activities, emotional reactions, or other circumstances that may have contributed to the illness.
6. **Remitting or exacerbating factors.** Does anything make it better or worse?
7. **Associated manifestations.** Have you noticed anything else that accompanies it?

As you explore these attributes, be sure that you *use language that is understandable and appropriate* to the patient. Although you might ask a trained health professional about "dyspnea," the customary term to use for patients is "shortness of breath." It is easy to slip into using medical language with patients, but beware. Technical language confuses the patient and often blocks communication. Appropriate questions about symptoms are suggested in each of the chapters on the regional physical examinations. Whenever possible, however, *use the patient's words, making sure you clarify their meaning.*

To fill in specific details, learn to facilitate the patient's story by using different types of questions and the techniques of skilled interviewing described on pp. 30–39. Often you will need to use *directed questions* (see p. 31) that ask for specific information the patient has not already offered. *In general, an interview moves back and forth from an open-ended question to a directed question and then on to another open-ended question.*

Establishing the sequence and time course of the patient's symptoms is important. You can encourage a chronologic account by asking such questions as "What then?" or "What happened next?"

Generating and Testing Diagnostic Hypotheses (the Clinician's Perspective). As you listen to the patient's concerns, you will begin to *generate and test diagnostic hypotheses* about what disease process might be the cause. Identifying the various attributes of the patient's symptoms and pursuing specific details are fundamental to recognizing patterns of disease and differentiating one disease from another. As you learn more about diagnostic patterns, listening for and asking about these attributes will become more automatic. For additional data that will contribute to your analysis, use items from relevant sections of the *Review of Systems.* In these ways you build evidence for and against the various diagnostic possibilities. This kind of clinical thinking is illustrated by the tables on symptoms found in the regional examination chapters and further discussed in Chapter 18, Clinical Reasoning, Assessment, and Plan.

Creating a Shared Understanding of the Problem. Recent literature makes clear that delivering effective health care requires exploring the deeper meanings patients attach to their symptoms. While the "seven attributes of a symptom" add important details to the patient's history, the *disease/illness distinction model* helps you understand the full range of what every good interview needs to cover. This model acknowledges the dual but very different perspectives of the clinician and the patient. ***Disease*** is the explanation that the *clinician* brings to the symptoms. It is the way that the clinician organizes what he or she learns from the patient into a coherent picture that leads to a clinical diagnosis and treatment plan. ***Illness*** can be defined as how the *patient* experiences symptoms. Many factors may shape this experience, including prior personal or family health, the effect of symptoms on everyday life, individual outlook and style of coping, and expectations about medical care. *The health history interview needs to take into account both of these views of reality.*

Even a chief complaint as straightforward as sore throat can illustrate these divergent views. The patient may be most concerned about pain and difficulty swallowing, a cousin who was hospitalized with tonsillitis, or missing time from work. The clinician, however, may focus on specific points in the history that differentiate streptococcal pharyngitis from other etiologies or on a questionable history of allergy to penicillin. To understand the patient's expectations, the clinician needs to go beyond just the attributes of a symptom. Learning about the patient's perception of illness means asking patient-centered questions in the six domains listed below. Doing so is crucial to patient satisfaction, effective health care, and patient follow-through.

EXPLORING THE PATIENT'S PERSPECTIVE

- The patient's thoughts about the nature and the cause of the problem
- The patient's feelings, especially fears, about the problem
- The patient's expectations of the clinician and health care
- The effect of the problem on the patient's life
- Prior personal or family experiences that are similar
- Therapeutic responses the patient has already tried

The clinician should ask about the cause of the problem by saying, for example, "Why do you think you have this stomachache?" To uncover the patient's feelings, you might ask, "What concerns you most about the pain?" A patient may worry that the pain is a symptom of serious disease and want reassurance. Alternatively, the patient may be less concerned about the cause of the pain and just want relief. You need to find out what the patient expects from you, the clinician, or from health care in general . . . "I'm glad that the pain is almost gone. How specifically can I help you now?" Even if the stomach pain is almost gone, the patient may need a work excuse to take to an employer.

It may be helpful to ask the patient about previous experiences, what he or she has tried so far, and any related changes in daily activities.

> Clinician: "Has anything like this happened to you or your family before?"
>
> Patient: "I was worried that I might have appendicitis. My Uncle Charlie died from a ruptured appendix."

Explore what the patient has done so far to take care of the problem. Most patients will have tried over-the-counter medications, traditional remedies, or advice from friends or family. Ask how the illness has affected the patient's lifestyle and level of activity. This question is especially important for patients with chronic illness. "What can't you do now that you could do before?" "How has your backache (shortness of breath, etc.) affected your ability to work?" . . . "Your life at home?" . . . "Your social activities?" . . . "Your role as a parent?" . . . "Your role as a husband or wife?" . . . "The way you feel about yourself as a person?"

Negotiating a Plan. Learning about the disease and conceptualizing the illness give you and the patient the opportunity to create a complete picture of the problem. This multifaceted picture then forms the basis for planning further evaluation (physical examination, laboratory tests, consultations, etc.)

and negotiating a treatment plan. More specific techniques for negotiating a plan can be found in Chapter 18. Advanced skills, such as steps for motivating change and the therapeutic use of the clinician–patient relationship, are beyond the scope of this book.

Planning for Follow-Up and Closing. You may find that ending the interview is difficult. Patients often have many questions and, if you have done your job well, they are enjoying talking with you. Giving notice that the end of the interview is approaching allows time for the patient to ask any final questions. Make sure the patient understands the agreed-upon plans you have developed. For example, before gathering your papers or standing to leave the room, you can say "We need to stop now. Do you have any questions about what we've covered?" As you close, reviewing future evaluation, treatments, and follow-up is helpful. "So, you will take the medicine as we discussed, get the blood test before you leave today, and make a follow-up appointment for 4 weeks. Do you have any questions about this?" Address any related concerns or questions that the patient brings up.

The patient should have a chance to ask any final questions; however, the last few minutes are not the time to bring up new topics. If that happens (and the concern is not life-threatening), simply reassure the patient of your interest and make plans to address the problem at a future time. "That knee pain sounds concerning. Why don't you make an appointment for next week so we can discuss it?" Reaffirming that you will continue working to improve the patient's health is always appreciated.

Facilitating the Patient's Story: The Techniques of Skilled Interviewing

Skilled interviewing requires the use of specific learnable techniques. You need to practice these techniques and find ways to be observed or recorded so that you can receive feedback on your progress. Several of these fundamental skills are listed in the following box and described in more detail throughout this section.

THE TECHNIQUES OF SKILLED INTERVIEWING

- Active listening
- Adaptive questioning
- Nonverbal communication
- Facilitation
- Echoing
- Empathic responses
- Validation
- Reassurance
- Summarization
- Highlighting transitions

Active Listening. Underlying all these specific techniques is the practice of active listening. Active listening is the process of fully attending to what the patient is communicating, being aware of the patient's emotional state, and using verbal and nonverbal skills to encourage the speaker to continue and expand. Active listening takes practice. It is easy to drift into thinking about your next question or the differential diagnosis; however, you and the patient are best served by your concentration on listening.

Adaptive Questioning. There are several ways you can ask questions that add detail to the patient's story yet facilitate the flow of the interview. Learn to adapt your questioning to the patient's verbal and nonverbal cues.

ADAPTIVE QUESTIONING:
OPTIONS FOR CLARIFYING THE PATIENT'S STORY

- Directed questioning—from general to specific
- Questioning to elicit a graded response
- Asking a series of questions, one at a time
- Offering multiple choices for answers
- Clarifying what the patient means

Directed questioning is useful for drawing the patient's attention to specific areas of the history. It should follow several principles to be effective. *Directed questioning should proceed from the general to the specific.* A possible sequence, for example, might be "Tell me about your chest pain?" (Pause) "What else?" (Pause) "Where did you feel it?" (Pause) "Show me. Anywhere else?" (Pause) "Did it travel anywhere?" (Pause) "To which arm?" *Directed questions should not be leading questions* that call for a "yes" or "no" answer. If a patient says yes to "Did your stools look like tar?" you run the risk of turning your words into the patient's words. A better phrasing is "Please describe your stools."

If necessary, ask questions that require *a graded response* rather than a single answer. "What physical activity do you do that makes you short of breath?" is better than "How many steps can you climb before you get short of breath?" which is better than "Do you get short of breath climbing stairs?" Be sure to *ask one question at a time.* "Any tuberculosis, pleurisy, asthma, bronchitis, pneumonia?" may lead to a negative answer out of sheer confusion. Try "Do you have any of the following problems?" Be sure to pause and establish eye contact as you list each problem.

Sometimes patients seem quite unable to describe their symptoms without help. To minimize bias, *offer multiple-choice answers.* "Is your pain aching, sharp, pressing, burning, shooting, or what?" Almost any direct question can provide at least two possible answers. "Do you bring up any phlegm with your cough, or is it dry?"

At times patients use words that are ambiguous or have unclear associations. To understand their meaning, you need to *request clarification,* as in "Tell me exactly what you meant by 'the flu'" or "You said you were behaving just like your mother. What did you mean?"

Nonverbal Communication. Communication that does not involve speech occurs continuously and provides important clues to feelings and emotions. Becoming more sensitive to nonverbal messages allows you to both "read the patient" more effectively and to send messages of your own. Pay close attention to eye contact, facial expression, posture, head position and movement such as shaking or nodding, interpersonal distance, and placement of the arms or legs, such as crossed, neutral, or open. Matching your position to the patient's can be a sign of increasing rapport. Moving closer or engaging in physical contact (like placing your hand on the patient's arm) can convey empathy or help the patient gain control of feelings. Bringing nonverbal communication to the conscious level is the first step to using this crucial form of patient interaction. You also can mirror the patient's *paralanguage,* or qualities of speech such as pacing, tone, and volume, to increase rapport.

Facilitation. You use facilitation when, by posture, actions, or words, you encourage the patient to say more but do not specify the topic. Pausing with a nod of the head or remaining silent, yet attentive and relaxed, is a cue for the patient to continue. Leaning forward, making eye contact, and using continuers like "Mm-hmm," "Go on," or "I'm listening" all maintain the flow of the patient's story.

Echoing. Simple repetition of the patient's words encourages the patient to express both factual details and feelings, as in the following example:

> Patient: The pain got worse and began to spread. (Pause)
>
> Response: Spread? (Pause)
>
> Patient: Yes, it went to my shoulder and down my left arm to the fingers. It was so bad that I thought I was going to die. (Pause)
>
> Response: Going to die?
>
> Patient: Yes, it was just like the pain my father had when he had his heart attack, and I was afraid the same thing was happening to me.

This reflective technique has helped to reveal not only the location and severity of the pain but also its meaning to the patient. It did not bias the story or interrupt the patient's train of thought.

Empathic Responses. Conveying empathy is part of establishing and strengthening rapport with patients. As patients talk with you, they may express—with or without words—feelings they have not consciously acknowledged. These feelings are crucial to understanding their illnesses and to establishing a trusting relationship. *To empathize with your patient you must first identify his or her feelings.* When you sense important but unexpressed feelings from the patient's face, voice, words, or behavior, inquire about them rather than assume how the patient feels. You may simply ask "How did you feel about that?" Unless you let patients know that you are interested in feelings as well as in facts, you may miss important insights.

Once you have identified the feelings, respond with understanding and acceptance. Responses may be as simple as "I understand," "That sounds upsetting," or "You seem sad." Empathy may also be nonverbal—for example, offering a tissue to a crying patient or gently placing your hand on the patient's arm to show understanding. When you give an empathic response, be sure that you are responding correctly to what the patient is feeling. If your response acknowledges how upset a patient must have been at the death of a parent, when, in fact, the death relieved the patient of a long-standing financial and emotional burden, you have misunderstood the situation.

Validation. Another important way to make a patient feel accepted is to legitimize or validate his or her emotional experience. A patient who has been in a car accident but has no significant physical injury may still be experiencing distress. Stating something like "Being in that accident must have been very scary. Car accidents are always unsettling because they remind us of our vulnerability and mortality. That could explain why you still feel upset" reassures the patient. It helps the patient feel that such emotions are legitimate and understandable.

Reassurance. When you are talking with patients who are anxious or upset, it is tempting to reassure them. You may find yourself saying "Don't worry. Everything is going to be all right." While this may be appropriate in nonprofessional relationships, in your role as a clinician such comments are usually counterproductive. You may fall into reassuring the patient about the wrong thing. Moreover, premature reassurance may block further disclosures, especially if the patient feels that exposing anxiety is a weakness. Such admissions require encouragement, not a cover-up. *The first step to effective reassurance is identifying and accepting the patient's feelings without offering reassurance at that moment.* Doing so promotes a feeling of security. The actual reassurance comes much later after you have completed the interview, the physical examination, and perhaps some laboratory studies. At that point, you can interpret for the patient what you think is happening and deal openly with the real concerns.

Summarization. Giving a capsule summary of the patient's story in the course of the interview can serve several different functions. It indicates to the patient that you have been listening carefully. It can also identify what you know and what you don't know. "Now, let me make sure that I have the full story. You said you've had a cough for 3 days, it's especially bad at night, and you have started to bring up yellow phlegm. You have not had a fever or felt short of breath, but you do feel congested, with difficulty breathing through your nose." Following with an attentive pause or "Anything else?" lets the patient add other information and confirms that you have heard the story correctly. You can use summarization at different points in the interview to structure the visit, especially at times of transition (see below). This technique also allows you, the clinician, to organize your clinical reasoning and to convey your thinking to the patient, which makes the relationship more collaborative.

Highlighting Transitions. Patients have many reasons to feel worried and vulnerable. To put them more at ease, tell them when you are changing directions during the interview. This gives patients a greater sense of control. As you move from one part of the history to another and on to the physical examination, orient the patient with brief transitional phrases like "Now I'd like to ask some questions about your past health." Make clear what the patient should expect or do next . . . "Now I'd like to examine you. I'll step out for a few minutes. Please get completely undressed and put on this gown." Specifying that the gown should open in the back may earn the patient's gratitude and save you some time.

Adapting Interviewing Techniques to Specific Situations

Interviewing patients may precipitate several behaviors and situations that seem particularly vexing or perplexing. Your skill at handling these situations will evolve throughout your career. *Always remember the importance of listening to the patient and clarifying the patient's agenda.*

The Silent Patient. Novice interviewers may be uncomfortable with periods of silence and feel obligated to keep the conversation going. Silence has many meanings and many purposes. Patients frequently fall silent for short periods to collect thoughts, remember details, or decide whether they can trust you with certain information. The period of silence usually feels much longer to the clinician than it does to the patient. The clinician should appear attentive and give brief encouragement to continue when appropriate (see facilitative techniques on pp. 30–32). During periods of silence, watch the patient closely for nonverbal cues, such as difficulty controlling emotions. Alternatively, patients with depression or dementia may lose their usual spontaneity of expression, give short answers to questions, then quickly become silent afterwards. You may need to shift your inquiry to the symptoms of depression or begin an exploratory mental status examination (see Chapter 16, The Nervous System, pp. 560–565).

At times, silence may be the patient's response to how you are asking questions. Are you asking too many direct questions in rapid sequence? Have you offended the patient in any way, for example, by signs of disapproval or criticism? Have you failed to recognize an overwhelming symptom such as pain, nausea, or dyspnea? If so, you may need to ask the patient directly, "You seem very quiet. Have I done something to upset you?"

Finally, some patients are naturally laconic. Be accepting and try asking the patient for suggestions about other sources to help you gather more information. With the patient's permission, talking with family members or friends may be worthwhile.

The Talkative Patient. The garrulous, rambling patient may be just as difficult. Faced with limited time and the need to "get the whole story," you may grow impatient, even exasperated. Although this problem has no perfect solutions, several techniques are helpful. Give the patient free rein for the first 5 or 10 minutes and listen closely to the conversation. Perhaps the patient simply has lacked a good listener and is expressing pent-up concerns. Maybe the patient's style is to tell stories. Does the patient seem obsessively detailed or unduly anxious? Is there a flight of ideas or disorganized thought process that suggests a psychosis or confabulation?

Try to focus on what seems most important to the patient. Show your interest by asking questions in those areas. Interrupt if you must, but courteously. Remember that part of your task is to structure the interview. It is acceptable to be directive and set limits when necessary. A brief summary may help you change the subject yet validate any concerns. "Let me make sure that I understand. You've described many concerns. In particular, I heard about two different kinds of pain, one on your left side that goes into your groin and is fairly new, and one in your upper abdomen after you eat that you've had for months. Let's focus just on the side pain first. Can you tell me what it feels like?" Finally, do not show your impatience. If there is no more time, explain the need for a second meeting. Setting a time limit for the next appointment may be helpful. "I know we have much more to talk about. Can you come again next week? We'll have a full hour then."

The Anxious Patient. Anxiety is a frequent and normal reaction to sickness, treatment, and the health care system itself. For some patients, anxiety is a filter for all their perceptions and reactions; for others it may be part of their illness. Again, watch for nonverbal and verbal cues. Anxious patients may sit tensely, fidgeting with their fingers or clothes. They may sigh frequently, lick dry lips, sweat more than average, or actually tremble. Carotid pulsations may betray a rapid heart rate. Some anxious patients fall silent, unable to speak freely or confide. Others try to cover their feelings with words, busily avoiding their own basic problems. When you detect anxiety, reflect your impression back to the patient and encourage him or her to talk about any underlying concerns. Be careful not to transmit your own anxieties about completing the interview to the patient!

The Crying Patient. Crying signals strong emotions, ranging from sadness to anger or frustration. If the patient is on the verge of tears, pausing, gentle probing, or responding with empathy allows the patient to cry. Usually crying is therapeutic, as is your quiet acceptance of the patient's distress or pain. Offer a tissue and wait for the patient to recover. Make a facilitating or supportive remark like "I'm glad that you got that out." Most patients will soon compose themselves and resume their story. Aside from cases of acute grief or loss, it is unusual for crying to escalate and become uncontrollable.

Crying makes many people uncomfortable. If this is true for you, as a clinician, you will need to work through your feelings so that you can support patients at these significant times.

The Confusing Patient. Some patients are confusing because they have *multiple symptoms*. They seem to have every symptom that you ask about, or "a positive review of systems." Although they may have multiple medical illnesses, a somatization disorder is more likely. With these patients, focus on the meaning or function of the symptom and guide the interview into a psychosocial assessment. There is little profit to exploring each symptom in detail.

At other times you may be baffled, frustrated, and confused yourself. The history is vague and difficult to understand, ideas are poorly related to one another, and language is hard to follow. Even though you word your questions carefully, you cannot seem to get clear answers. The patient's manner of relating to you may also seem peculiar, distant, aloof, or inappropriate. Patients may describe symptoms in bizarre terms: "My fingernails feel too heavy" or "My stomach knots up like a snake." Using various facilitative techniques, try to learn more about the unusual qualities of the symptoms. Perhaps there is a mental status change such as psychosis or delirium, a mental illness such as schizophrenia, or a neurologic disorder (see Chapter 16, The Nervous System). Watch for delirium in acutely ill or intoxicated patients and for dementia in the elderly. Such patients give histories that are inconsistent and cannot provide a clear chronology about what has happened. Some may even confabulate to fill in the gaps in their memories.

When you suspect a psychiatric or neurologic disorder, do not spend too much time trying to get a detailed history. You will only tire and frustrate both the patient and yourself. Shift to the mental status examination, focusing on level of consciousness, orientation, and memory. You can work in the initial questions smoothly by asking "When was your last appointment at the clinic? Let's see . . . that was about how long ago?" "Your address now is . . . ? . . . and your phone number?" You can check these responses against the chart, assuming that the chart is accurate, or by getting permission to speak with family members or friends and then doing so.

The Angry or Disruptive Patient. Many patients have reasons to be angry: they are ill, they have suffered a loss, they lack their accustomed control over their own lives, and they feel relatively powerless in the health care system. They may direct this anger toward you. It is possible that hostility toward you is justified . . . were you late for your appointment, inconsiderate, insensitive, or angry yourself? If so, acknowledge the fact and try to make amends. More often, however, patients displace their anger onto the clinician as a reflection of their pain.

Accept angry feelings from patients and allow them to express such emotions without getting angry in return. Beware of joining such patients in their hostility toward another provider, the clinic, or the hospital, even when you are privately in sympathy. You can validate their feelings without agreeing with their reasons. "I understand that you felt very frustrated by the long wait and answering the same questions over and over. The complex nature of our health care system can seem very unsupportive when you're not feeling well." After the patient has calmed down, you can help find steps that will avert such situations in the future. Rational solutions to emotional problems are not always possible, however, and people need time to express and work through their angry feelings.

Some angry patients become hostile and disruptive. Few people can disrupt the clinic or emergency department more quickly than patients who are angry, belligerent, or uncontrolled. Before approaching such patients, alert the security staff—as a clinician, you have the right to feel and be safe. It is especially important to stay calm, appear accepting, and avoid being challenging in return. Keep your posture relaxed and nonthreatening and your hands loosely open. At first, do not try to make disruptive patients lower their voices or stop if they are cursing you or the staff. Listen carefully and try to understand what they are saying. Once you have established rapport, gently suggest moving to a different location that is not upsetting to other patients or families.

The Patient With a Language Barrier. Nothing will convince you more surely of the importance of the history than having to do without one. When your patient speaks a different language, make every possible effort to find an interpreter. A few broken words and gestures are no substitute for the full story. The ideal interpreter is a neutral objective person who is familiar with both languages and cultures. Beware of using family members or friends as interpreters—confidentiality may be violated, meanings may be distorted, and transmitted information may be incomplete. Untrained interpreters may try to speed up the interview by telescoping lengthy replies into a few words, losing much of what may be significant detail.

As you begin working with the interpreter, establish rapport and review what information would be most useful. Explain that you need the interpreter to translate everything, not to condense or summarize. *Make your questions clear, short, and simple.* You can also help the interpreter by outlining your goals for each segment of the history. After going over your plans with the interpreter, arrange the room so that you have easy eye contact and nonverbal communication with the patient. Then speak directly to the patient, asking "How long have you been sick?" rather than "How long has the patient been sick?" Having the interpreter close by keeps you from moving your head back and forth as though you were watching a tennis match!

When available, bilingual written questionnaires are invaluable, especially for the Review of Systems. First be sure patients can read in their language; otherwise, ask for help from the interpreter. Some clinical settings have speakerphone translators; use them if there are no better options.

GUIDELINES FOR WORKING WITH AN INTERPRETER

- Choose a professional interpreter in preference to a hospital worker, volunteer, or family member. Use the interpreter as a resource for cultural information.
- Orient the interpreter to the components you plan to cover in the interview; include reminders to translate everything the patient says.
- Arrange the room so that you and the patient have eye contact and can read each other's nonverbal cues.
- Seat the interpreter next to you and allow the interpreter and the patient to establish rapport.
- Address the patient directly. Reinforce your questions with nonverbal behaviors.
- Keep sentences short and simple. Focus on the most important concepts to communicate.
- Verify mutual understanding by asking the patient to repeat back what he or she has heard.
- Be patient. The interview will take more time and may provide less information.

The Patient With Reading Problems. Before giving written instructions, it is wise to assess the patient's ability to read. Literacy levels are highly variable, and marginal reading skills are more prevalent than commonly believed. People cannot read for many reasons, including language barriers, learning disorders, poor vision, or lack of education. Some people may try to hide their inability to read. Asking about educational level may be helpful but can be misleading. "I understand that this may be difficult to discuss, but do you have any trouble with reading?" Ask the patient to read whatever instructions you have written. Literacy skills may be the reason the patient has not followed through on taking medications or adhered to recommended treatments. Simply handing the patient written material upside-down to see if the patient turns it around may settle the question. Respond sensitively, and remember that illiteracy and lack of intelligence are not synonymous.

The Patient With Impaired Hearing. Communicating with the deaf presents many of the same challenges as communicating with patients who speak a different language. Even individuals with partial hearing may define themselves as Deaf, a distinct cultural group. Find out the patient's preferred method of communicating. Patients may use American Sign Language, which is a unique language with its own syntax, or various other communication forms combining signs and speech. Thus, communication is often truly cross-cultural. Ask when hearing loss occurred relative to the development of speech and other language skills and the kinds of schools that the patient has attended. These questions help you determine whether the patient identifies with the Deaf or the Hearing culture. If the patient prefers sign language, make every effort to find an interpreter and use the principles identified above. Although very time-consuming, handwritten questions and answers may be the only solution, though literacy skills may also be an issue.

When patients have partial hearing impairment or can read lips, face them directly, in good light. Speak at a normal volume and rate, and do not let your voice trail off at the ends of sentences. Avoid covering your mouth or looking down at papers while speaking. Remember that even the best lip readers comprehend only a percentage of what is said, so having patients repeat what you have said is important.

Hearing deficits vary. If the patient has a unilateral hearing loss, sit on the hearing side. If the patient has a hearing aid, find out if he or she is using it. Make sure it is working. Eliminate background noise such as television or hallway conversation as much as possible. Patients who wear glasses should use them so that they can pick up visual cues that will help them understand you better. Written questionnaires are also useful. When closing, supplement any oral instructions with written ones. A person who is *hard of hearing* may or may not be aware of the problem, a situation you will have to tactfully address.

The Patient With Impaired Vision. When meeting with a blind patient, shake hands to establish contact and explain who you are and why you are there. If the room is unfamiliar, orient the patient to the surroundings and report if anyone else is present. Remember to use words whenever you respond to such patients, because postures and gestures are unseen.

Encourage visually impaired patients to wear glasses, if available, to ease communication.

The Patient With Limited Intelligence. Patients of moderately limited intelligence can usually give adequate histories. In fact, you may even overlook their limitations and omit their dysfunction from disability evaluations or give them instructions they cannot understand. If you suspect such problems, pay special attention to the patient's schooling and ability to function independently. How far have such patients gone in school? If they didn't finish, why not? What kinds of courses are (were) they taking? How did they do? Have they had any testing done? Are they living alone? Do they get help with any activities, for example, transportation or shopping? The sexual history is equally important and often overlooked. Find out if the patient is sexually active and provide any information needed about pregnancy or sexually transmitted diseases. If you are unsure about the patient's level of intelligence, you can make a smooth transition to the mental status examination and assess simple calculations, vocabulary, memory, and abstract thinking (see Chapter 16).

For patients with severe mental retardation, you will have to obtain the history from the family or caregivers. Identify the person who accompanies them, but always show interest first in the patient. Establish rapport, make eye contact, and engage in simple conversation. As with children, avoid "talking down" or using affectations of speech or condescending behavior. The patient, family members, caretakers, or friends will notice and appreciate your respect.

The Poor Historian. Some patients are totally unable to give their own histories because of age, dementia, or other limitations. Others may be unable to relate certain parts of the history, such as events during a seizure. Under these circumstances, you must try to find a third person who can give you the story. Even when you have a reasonably comprehensive knowledge of the patient, other sources may offer surprising and important information. A spouse, for example, may report significant family strains, depressive symptoms, or drinking habits that the patient has denied.

For patients who are mentally competent, you must obtain their consent before you talk about their health with others. Assure patients that any information he or she has already told you is confidential, and clarify what can be shared. Even if patients can communicate only by facial expressions or gestures, you must maintain confidentiality and elicit their input. It is usually possible to divide the interview into two parts—one with the patient alone and the other with both the patient and the second person. Each part has its own value. Remember that data from others are also confidential.

The basic principles of interviewing apply to your conversations with relatives or friends. Find a private place to talk. Introduce yourself, state your purpose, inquire how they are feeling under the circumstances, and recognize and acknowledge their concerns. As you listen to their versions of the history, be alert to the quality of their relationship with the patient. It may color their credibility or give you helpful ideas for planning the patient's care. It is also important to establish how they know the patient. For example, when a child is brought in for health care, the accompanying adult may not be the primary or even frequent caregiver, just the most available ride. Always seek out the best-informed source. Occasionally, a relative or friend insists on being with the patient during your evaluation. Try to find out why and also the patient's wishes.

The Patient With Personal Problems. Patients may ask you for advice about personal problems outside the range of their health care. For example, should the patient quit a stressful job, move out of state, or have an abortion? Before responding, explore the different approaches the patient has considered and their pros and cons, whom else they have discussed the problem with, and what supports are available for different choices. Letting the patient talk through the problem with you is usually much more valuable and therapeutic than any answer you could give.

Special Aspects of Interviewing

Clinicians talk with patients about various subjects that are emotionally laden or sensitive. These discussions can be particularly difficult for inexperienced clinicians or during evaluations of patients clinicians do not know well. Even seasoned clinicians have some discomfort with certain topics: abuse of alcohol or drugs, sexual orientation or activities, death and dying, financial concerns, racial and ethnic experiences, family interactions, domestic violence, psychiatric illnesses, physical deformities, bowel function, and others. These areas are difficult to explore in part because of societal taboos. We all know, for example, that talking about bowel habits is not "polite table talk." In addition, many of these topics evoke strong cultural, societal, and personal values. Race, drug use, and homosexual practices are three obvious examples of issues that can raise biased attitudes and pose barriers during the interview. This section explores challenges to the clinician in these and other important and sometimes sensitive areas, including domestic violence, the dying patient, and mental illness.

Several basic principles can help guide your response to sensitive topics. *The single most important rule is to be nonjudgmental.* The clinician's role is to learn about the patient and help the patient achieve better health. Disapproval of behaviors or elements in the health history will only interfere with this goal. *Explain why you need to know certain information*—doing so makes patients less apprehensive. For example, say to patients "Because sexual practices put people at risk for certain diseases, I ask all of my patients the following questions." You should *use specific language.* Refer to genitalia with explicit words such as penis or vagina and avoid phrases like "private parts." *Choose words that the patient understands.* "By intercourse, I mean when a man inserts his penis into a woman's vagina." *Find opening questions for sensitive topics and learn the specific kinds of data needed for your assessments.*

Other strategies for becoming more comfortable with sensitive areas include general reading about these topics in medical and lay literature; talking to selected colleagues and teachers openly about your concerns; taking special courses that help you explore your own feelings and reactions; and ultimately, reflecting on your own life experience. Take advantage of all these resources. Whenever possible, listen to experienced clinicians, then practice similar discussions with your own patients. The range of topics that you can explore with comfort will widen progressively.

Cultural Competence. Developing the ability to interact and communicate effectively with patients from many backgrounds is a lifelong professional goal. The following examples illustrate how communication barriers, cultural differences, and unconscious biases can influence patient care.

> A 28-year-old taxi driver from Ghana who had recently moved to the United States complained to a friend about U.S. medical care. He had gone to the clinic because of fever and fatigue. He described being weighed, having his temperature taken, and having a cloth wrapped tightly, to the point of pain, around his arm. The clinician, a 36-year-old from Washington, DC, had asked the patient many questions, examined him, and wanted to take blood—which the patient had refused. The patient's final comment was " . . . and she didn't even give me chloroquine!"—his primary reason for seeking care. The man from Ghana was expecting few questions, no examination, and treatment for malaria, which is what fever usually means in Ghana.

In this example, cross-cultural miscommunication is understandable and unthreatening. Bias and miscommunication, however, occur in many clinical interactions and are usually subtler.

> A 16-year-old high school student came to the local teen health center because of painful menstrual cramps that were interfering with school. She was dressed in a tight top and short skirt and had multiple piercings, including in her eyebrow. The 30-year-old male clinician asked the following questions: "Are you passing all of your classes?" . . . "What kind of job do you want after high school?" . . . "What kind of birth control do you want?" The teenager felt pressured into accepting birth control pills, even though she had clearly stated that she had never had intercourse and planned to postpone it until she got married. She was an honor student, planning to go to college, but the clinician did not elicit these goals. The clinician glossed over her cramps by saying "Oh, you can just take some ibuprofen. Cramps usually get better as you get older." The patient will not take the birth control pills that were prescribed, nor will she seek health care soon again. She experienced the encounter as an interrogation, so failed to gain trust in her clinician. In addition, the questions implied incorrect assumptions about her health. She has received ineffective health care because of conflicting cultural values and clinician bias.

In both of these cases, the failure arises from the clinician's mistaken assumptions or biases. In the first case, the clinician did not consider the many variables that shape patient beliefs about health and expectations for medical care. In the second case, the clinician allowed stereotypes to dictate the agenda instead of listening to the patient and respecting her as an individual. Each of us has our own cultural background and our own biases. These do not simply fade away as we become clinicians.

As you provide care for an ever-expanding and diverse group of patients, it is increasingly important to understand how culture shapes not just the patient's beliefs, but your own. *Culture* is a system of shared ideas, rules, and meanings that influences how we view the world, experience it emotionally, and behave in relation to other people. It can be understood as the "lens" through which we perceive and make sense out of the world we inhabit. This definition of culture is broader than the term "ethnicity." The influence of culture is not limited to minority groups—it is relevant to everyone. While learning about specific cultural groups is important, without a framework, this may lead to its opposite, group stereotypes. For example, you may think that Asians have more rice in their diets than those from other cultural groups. For people of Asian descent in the United States, however, this may not be the case at all. Work on an appropriate and informed clinical approach to all patients by becoming aware of your own values and biases, developing communication skills that transcend cultural differences, and building therapeutic partnerships based on respect for each patient's life experience. This type of framework, described in the following section, will allow you to approach each patient as unique and distinct.

CLINICIAN GOALS FOR CULTURAL COMPETENCE

- **Self-awareness.** Learn about your own biases . . . we all have them.
- **Enhanced communication.** Work to eliminate assumptions about what is "normal." Learn directly from your patients—they are the experts on their culture and illness.
- **Collaborative partnerships.** Build your relationships with patients on respect and mutually acceptable plans.

Source: Cross-Cultural Education Committee, University of Rochester School of Medicine and Dentistry, Rochester, NY.

Self-awareness. Start by exploring your own cultural identity. How do you describe yourself in terms of ethnicity, class, region or country of origin, religion, and political affiliation? Don't forget the characteristics that we often take for granted—gender, life roles, sexual orientation, physical ability, and race—especially if you are from majority groups in these areas. What aspects of your family of origin do you identify with and how are you different from your family of origin? How do these identities influence your beliefs and behaviors?

Another more challenging aspect of learning about ourselves is the task of bringing our own values and biases to a conscious level. *Values* are the standards we use to measure our own and others' beliefs and behaviors. These may appear to be absolutes. *Biases* are the attitudes or feelings that we attach to perceived differences. Being attuned to difference is normal; in fact, in the distant past, detecting differences may have preserved life. Intuitively knowing members of one's own group is a survival skill that we have outgrown as a society but it is still actively at work. We often feel so guilty about our biases that it is hard to recognize and acknowledge them. Start with less threatening constructs, such as the way an individual relates to time, which can be a culturally determined phenomenon. Are you always on time—a positive value in the dominant Western culture? Or do you tend to run a little late? How do you feel about people whose habits are opposite to yours? Next time you attend a meeting or class, notice who is early, on time, or late. Is it predictable? Think about the role of physical appearance. Do you consider yourself thin, mid size, or heavy? How do you feel about your weight? What does prevailing U.S. culture teach us to value in physique? How do you feel about people who have different weights?

Enhanced Communication and Learning from the Patient. Given the complexity of culture, no one can possibly know the health beliefs and practices of every culture and subculture. Therefore, remember that your patients are the experts on their own unique cultural perspectives. Patients may not be able to identify or define their values or beliefs in the abstract but should be able to respond to specific questions. Find out about the patient's cultural background. Use some of the same questions discussed in "Expanding and Clarifying the Health History" (see p. 27). Maintain an open, respectful, and inquiring attitude. "What did you hope to get from this visit?" If you have established rapport and trust, patients will be willing to teach you. Be ready to acknowledge your ignorance or bias. "I know very little about Ghana. What would have happened at a clinic there if you had these concerns?" Or, with the second patient and with much more difficulty, "I mistakenly made assumptions about you that are not right. I apologize. Would you be willing to tell me more about yourself and your future goals?"

Learning about specific cultures is still valuable because it broadens what you, as a clinician, identify as areas you need to explore. Do some reading about the life experiences of individuals in ethnic or racial groups in your region. Go to movies that are made in different countries or explicitly present the perspective of different groups. Learn about the concerns of different consumer groups with visible health agendas. Seek out and establish collegial relationships with healers of different disciplines. Most importantly, be open to learning from your patients.

Collaborative Partnerships. Through continual work on self-awareness and seeing through the "lens" of others, the clinician lays the foundation for the collaborative relationship that best supports the patient's health. Communication based on trust, respect, and a willingness to reexamine assumptions helps allow patients to express concerns that may run counter to the dominant culture. These concerns may be associated with strong feelings such as anger or shame. You, the clinician, must be willing to listen to and to validate these feelings, and not let your own feelings prevent you from exploring painful areas. You must also be willing to reexamine your beliefs about what is the "right approach" to clinical care in a given situation. Make every effort to be flexible and creative in your plans, respectful of patients' knowledge about their own best interests, and consciously committed to clarifying the truly acute or life-threatening risks to the patient's health. Remember that if the patient stops listening, fails to follow your advice, or does not return, your health care has not been successful.

The Alcohol and Drug History. One difficult area for many clinicians is asking patients about their use of alcohol and drugs, either illegal or prescribed. Use of alcohol and drugs often directly contributes to symptoms and the need for care and treatment. Despite their high lifetime prevalence (in the United

States, more than 13% for alcohol and 4% for illegal drugs), substance abuse disorders are under diagnosed.

Do not let personal feelings interfere with your role as a clinician. It is your job to gather data, assess the impact on the patient's health, and plan a therapeutic response. Clinicians should routinely ask about current and past use of alcohol or drugs, patterns of use, and family history.

Questions about alcohol and other drugs follow naturally after questions about caffeine and cigarettes. "What do you like to drink?" or "Tell me about your use of alcohol" are good opening questions that avoid the easy yes or no response. Remember to ask what patients mean by alcohol, since for some patients the term does not include wine or beer. Asking about alcohol use may not be that helpful for detecting problem drinking, but you can make use of several well-validated short screening tools that do not take much time. Try two additional questions: "Have you ever had a drinking problem?" and "When was your last drink?" An affirmative answer to the first question, along with a drink within 24 hours, has been shown to suggest problem drinking. The most widely used screening questions are the CAGE questions about **C**utting down, **A**nnoyance if criticized, **G**uilty feelings, and **E**ye-openers.

THE CAGE QUESTIONNAIRE

- Have you ever felt the need to **Cut down** on drinking?
- Have you ever felt **Annoyed** by criticism of drinking?
- Have you ever felt **Guilty** about drinking?
- Have you ever taken a drink first thing in the morning **(Eye-opener)** to steady your nerves or get rid of a hangover?

Adapted from Mayfield D, McLeod G, Hall P: The CAGE questionnaire: Validation of a new alcoholism screening instrument. Am J Psychiatry 131:1121–1123, 1974.

Two or more affirmative answers to the CAGE Questionnaire suggest alcoholism. They indicate that you need to ask more questions about blackouts (loss of memory for events during drinking), seizures, accidents or injuries while drinking, job loss, marital conflict, or legal problems. Also ask specifically about drinking while driving or operating machinery.

Questions about drugs are similar. "How much marijuana do you use? Cocaine? Heroin? Amphetamines? (ask about each one by name). "How about prescription drugs such as sleeping pills?" "Diet pills?" "Pain-killers?" Another approach is to adapt the CAGE questions to screening for substance abuse by adding "or drugs" to each question. If the patient is using illegal substances, ask further questions such as "How do you feel when you take it?" . . . "Have you had any bad reactions?" "What happened?" . . . "Any drug-related accidents, injuries, or arrests?" "Job or family problems?" . . . "Have you ever tried to quit? Tell me about it."

Talking about drug use with adolescents can be even more challenging. It may be helpful to ask about substance use by friends or family members first.

"A lot of young people are using drugs these days. How about at your school? Any of your friends?" Once patients realize you are concerned and nonjudgmental, they may be more open about their own patterns of use. Remember that alcohol and drug use can start at young ages. These topics should be introduced, along with tobacco use, in front of the parent with children at ages 6 or 7.

The Sexual History. Asking questions about sexual function and practices can be life-saving. Sexual practices determine risks for pregnancy and sexually transmitted diseases (STDs), including AIDS—good interviewing helps prevent or reduce these risks. Sexual practices may be directly related to the patient's symptoms and integral to both diagnosis and treatment. Many patients have questions or concerns about sexuality that they would discuss more freely if you have asked about sexual health. Finally, sexual dysfunction may result from use of medication or from misinformation that, if recognized, may be readily addressed.

You can introduce questions about sexual function and practices at multiple points in a patient's history. If the Chief Complaint involves genitourinary symptoms, include the sexual history in the Present Illness. Chronic illness or serious symptoms such as pain or shortness of breath may also affect sexual function. For women, you can ask these questions as part of the Obstetric/Gynecologic section of the Past Medical History. You can include them during discussions about Health Maintenance, along with diet, exercise, and screening tests, or as part of the lifestyle issues or important relationships covered in the Personal and Social History. Or, in a comprehensive history, you can query about sexual practices during the Review of Systems.

An orienting sentence or two is often helpful. "Now I'd like to ask you some questions about your sexual health and practices." or "I routinely ask all patients about their sexual function." For more specific complaints, you might state "To figure out why you have this discharge and what we should do about it, I need to ask some questions about your sexual activity."

In general, ask about both specific sexual behaviors and satisfaction with sexual function. Specific questions are included in the chapters on Male Genitalia and Hernias (p. 370) and Female Genitalia (pp. 388–389). Be sure to ask such questions as:

- "When was the last time you had intimate physical contact with anyone?" "Did that contact include sexual intercourse?" Using the term "sexually active" can be ambiguous. Patients have been known to reply "No, I just lie there."
- "Do you have sex with men, women, or both?" The health implications of heterosexual, homosexual, or bisexual experiences are significant. Individuals may have sex with persons of the same gender, yet they may not consider themselves gay, lesbian, or bisexual.
- "How many sexual partners have you had in the last 6 months?" "In the last 5 years?" "In your lifetime?" Again, these questions give the patient an easy opportunity to acknowledge multiple partners.

- It is important to ask all patients "Do you have any concerns about HIV disease or AIDS?" because no explicit risk factors may be present. Ask also about routine use of condoms.

Note that these questions make no assumptions about marital status, sexual preference, or attitudes toward pregnancy or contraception. Listen to each of the patient's responses and ask additional questions as indicated. When patients are uncomfortable using sexual terminology, you may have to initiate more of the discussion.

Remember that sexual behavior, too, can start at a young age. Encourage parents to talk to their children about sexuality during their early years. It is frequently easier to discuss normal physiologic functions before children have been heavily socialized outside the home. For adolescents, because they often keep sexual behaviors from parents, be sensitive to the need for confidentiality (see p. 55, "Talking With Adolescents").

Domestic and Physical Violence. Because of the high prevalence of physical, sexual, and emotional abuse, many authorities recommend the routine screening of all female patients for domestic violence. Some men are also at risk. As with other sensitive topics, start this part of the interview with general "normalizing" questions: "Because abuse is common in many women's lives, I've begun to ask about it routinely." "Are there times in your relationships that you feel unsafe or afraid?" "Many women tell me that someone at home is hurting them in some way. Is this true for you?" "Within the last year, have you been hit, kicked, punched, or otherwise hurt by someone you know? If so, by whom?" As in other parts of the history, use a pattern that goes from general to specific, less difficult to more difficult.

Physical abuse—often not mentioned by either victim or perpetrator—should be considered in the following settings:

- If injuries are unexplained, seem inconsistent with the patient's story, are concealed by the patient, or cause embarrassment
- If the patient has delayed getting treatment for trauma
- If there is a past history of repeated injuries or "accidents"
- If the patient or a person close to the patient has a history of alcohol or drug abuse.

Also be suspicious if a partner tries to dominate the interview, will not leave the room, or seems unusually anxious or solicitous.

When you suspect abuse, it is important to spend part of the encounter alone with the patient. You can use the transition to the physical examination as an excuse to ask the other person to leave the room. If the patient is also resistant, you should not force the situation, potentially placing the victim in jeopardy. Be aware that certain diagnoses have a higher association with abuse, such as pregnancy and somatization disorder.

Child abuse is also common. Asking parents about their approach to discipline is a routine part of well-child care. You can also ask parents how they cope with a baby who will not stop crying or a child who misbehaves. "Most parents get very upset when their baby cries (or their child has been naughty). How do you feel when your baby cries?" "What do you do when your baby won't stop crying?" "Do you have any fears that you might hurt your child?" You should also inquire about how other caretakers or companions handle these situations.

The Mental Health History. Many cultures make ingrained distinctions between mental and physical illnesses causing marked differences in social acceptance and attitudes. Think how easily people talk about diabetes and taking insulin compared to discussing schizophrenia and using psychotropic medication. Use both open-ended and directed questions to elicit the individual and family history of mental illness. For example, you might begin by asking "Have you ever had any problem with emotional or mental illnesses?" Then move to more specific questions such as "Have you ever visited a counselor or psychotherapist?" . . . "Have you or has anyone in your family ever been hospitalized for an emotional or mental health problem?"

For patients with depression or thought disorders such as schizophrenia, a careful history is in order. Depression is common worldwide but still remains underdiagnosed and undertreated. For such patients, be open to their changes in mood or symptoms such as fatigue, unusual tearfulness, weight loss, insomnia, and vague somatic complaints. Two opening questions are "How have your mood or spirits been over the past month?" and "What about your level of interest or pleasure in each day's activities?" For serious depression, be sure to ask about thoughts of suicide . . . "Have you ever thought about hurting yourself or ending your life?" As with chest pain, you must evaluate severity—both are potentially lethal. For further approaches, turn to the mental status sections of Chapter 16, The Nervous System.

Many patients with schizophrenia or other psychotic disorders can function in the community and tell you about their diagnoses, symptoms, hospitalizations, and current medications. You should feel free to ask about symptoms and assess any impact on mood or daily activities.

Death and the Dying Patient. There is a growing and important focus in professional education and the literature on the need to address the issues of death and dying. Topics such as end-of-life decision-making, grief and bereavement, and advance directives are beyond the scope of this chapter. Basic concepts are appropriate even for beginning students, however, since you will care for patients near the end of their lives.

Many clinicians avoid the subject of death because of their own discomforts and anxieties. You will need to work through your own feelings with the help of reading and discussion. Kubler-Ross has described five stages in a person's response to loss or the anticipatory grief of impending death:

- Denial and isolation
- Anger
- Bargaining
- Depression or sadness
- Acceptance

These stages may occur sequentially or overlap in different combinations. At each stage, follow the same approach. Be alert to patients' feelings and to cues that they want to talk about them. Use facilitative techniques to help them to bring out their concerns. Make openings for them to ask questions: "I wonder if you have any concerns about the procedure?" . . . "Your illness?" . . . "What it will be like when you go home?" Explore these concerns and provide whatever information the patient requests. Be wary of inappropriate reassurance. If you can explore and accept patients' feelings, answer their questions, and demonstrate your commitment to staying with them throughout their illness, reassurance will grow where it really matters—within the patients themselves.

Dying patients rarely want to talk about their illnesses all the time, nor do they wish to confide in everyone they meet. Give them opportunities to talk and then listen receptively, but if they prefer to stay at a social level, you need not feel like a failure. Remember that illness—even a terminal one—is only one small part of the total person. A smile, a touch, an inquiry after a family member, a comment on the day's events, or even some gentle humor all recognize and affirm other areas of the patient's individuality and help sustain the living person. To communicate appropriately, you have to get to know the patient; that is part of the helping process.

Understanding the patient's wishes about treatment at the end of life is an important part of a clinician's role. Failing to establish this communication is widely viewed as a flaw in clinical care. Even if discussions of death and dying are difficult for you, you must learn to ask specific questions. The condition of the patient and the health care setting often determine what needs to be discussed. For patients who are acutely ill and in the hospital, discussing what the patient wants to have done in the event of a cardiac or respiratory arrest is usually mandatory. Asking about "*DNR status*" (Do Not Resuscitate) is often difficult when the clinician has no previous relationship with the patient and lacks knowledge of the patient's values or life experience. Patients may also be unrealistic about the effectiveness of resuscitation based on information in the media. Find out about the patient's frame of reference. "What experiences have you had with the death of a close friend or relative?" "What do you know about cardiopulmonary resuscitation (CPR)?" Educate patients about the likely success of CPR, especially if they are chronically ill or advanced in age. Assure them that relieving pain and taking care of their other spiritual and physical needs will be a priority.

In general, it is important to encourage any adult, but especially the elderly or chronically ill, to establish a *health proxy*, an individual who can act for the patient in life-threatening situations. This can be part of the interview aimed at a "values history" that identifies what is important to the patient and makes life worth living, and the point when living would no longer be worthwhile. Ask about how patients spend their time every day, what brings them joy, and what they look forward to. Make sure to clarify the meaning of statements like "You said that you don't want to be a burden to your family. What exactly do you mean by that?" In addition, explore the patient's religious or spiritual frame of reference so you and the patient can make the most appropriate decisions about health care.

Sexuality in the Clinician–Patient Relationship. Clinicians occasionally find themselves physically attracted to their patients. The emotional and physical intimacy of the clinician–patient relationship may lead to sexual feelings. If you become aware of such feelings, accept them as a normal human response and bring them to the conscious level so they will not affect your behavior. Denying these feelings makes it more likely for you to act inappropriately. *Any* sexual contact or romantic relationship with patients is *unethical;* keep your relationship with the patient within professional bounds and seek help if you need it.

Occasionally, clinicians meet patients who are frankly seductive or make sexual advances. Calmly but firmly make it clear that your relationship is professional, not personal. You may also wish to reflect on your image. Have you been overly warm with the patient? Expressed your affection physically? Sought his or her emotional support? Has your clothing or demeanor been unconsciously seductive? It is your responsibility to avoid these problems.

Ethical Considerations

You may wonder why an introductory chapter on interviewing contains a section on ethics. What is it about the process of talking with patients that calls for responses beyond our innate sense of morality? *Ethics* are a set of principles that have been created through reflection and discussion to guide our behavior. *Medical ethics*, which guide our professional behavior, are not static, but several principles have guided clinicians throughout the ages. Usually our ethical approach is instinctive, but even as students you will face situations that call for applications of ethical principles.

Some of the traditional and still fundamental maxims are as follows:

- ***Nonmaleficence*** or ***primum non nocere*** is commonly stated as "First, do no harm." In the context of an interview, giving information that is incorrect or not really related to the patient's problem can do harm. Avoiding relevant topics or creating barriers to open communication can also do harm. Your success in facilitating the patient's full expression of experiences, thoughts, and feelings determines the quality of your assessment.

- ***Beneficence*** is the dictum that the clinician needs to "do good" for the patient. As clinicians, our actions need to be motivated by what is in the patient's best interest.

- ***Autonomy*** reminds us that patients have the right to determine what is in their own best interest. This principle has become increasingly important over time and is consistent with collaborative rather than paternalistic patient relationships.

- ***Confidentiality*** can be one of the most challenging principles. As clinicians, we are obligated not to tell others what we learn from our patients. This privacy is fundamental to our professional relationships with patients. In the daily flurry of activity in a hospital, it must be carefully guarded.

Issues in health care that extend beyond our direct care of individual patients to complicated choices about the distribution of resources and the well-being of society continue to emerge. A broadly representative group that initially met in Tavistock Square in London in 1998 has continued to work on an evolving document of ethical principles to guide behavior in health care for both individuals and institutions. A current iteration of the Tavistock Principles is provided below.

THE TAVISTOCK PRINCIPLES

Rights: People have a right to health and health care.
Balance: Care of individual patients is central, but the health of populations is also our concern.
Comprehensiveness: In addition to treating illness, we have an obligation to ease suffering, minimize disability, prevent disease, and promote health.
Cooperation: Health care succeeds only if we cooperate with those we serve, each other, and those in other sectors.
Improvement: Improving health care is a serious and continuing responsibility.
Safety: Do no harm.
Openness: Being open, honest, and trustworthy is vital in health care.

As students you will learn about some of the ethical challenges that will confront you later as a practicing clinician. However, there are dilemmas unique to students that you will face from the time that you begin taking care of patients. The following vignettes capture some of the most common experiences. They raise a variety of ethical and practical issues that are overlapping.

Scenario #1

You are a 3rd-year medical student on your first clinical rotation in the hospital. It is late in the evening when you are finally assigned to the patient that you are responsible for "working up" and presenting the next day at preceptor rounds. You go to the patient's room and find the patient exhausted from the day's events and clearly ready to settle down for the night. You know that your intern and attending have already done their evaluations. Do you proceed with a history and physical examination that is likely to take 1 to 2 hours? Is this process only for your education? Do you ask permission before you start? What do you include?

Here you are confronted with the tension between *the need to learn by doing* and *doing no harm to patients*. There is a utilitarian ethical principle that reminds us that if clinicians-in-training do not learn, then there will be no future caregivers. Yet the dictums to do no harm and prioritize what is in the patient's best interests are clearly in conflict with that future need. As a student this dilemma will arise often.

Obtaining *informed consent* is the process for addressing this ethical dilemma. Making sure the patient realizes that you are in training and new at patient evaluation is always important. It is impressive how often patients willingly let students be involved in their care. It is an opportunity for patients to give back to their caregivers. Even when clinical activities appear to be purely for educational purposes, there may be a benefit to the patient. Multiple caregivers provide multiple perspectives. This scenario invokes the Tavistock Principles of *openness, balance, and safety*.

Scenario #2

You and your supervisor are on your way to draw an urgent blood sample from a patient. The patient was admitted with hypernatremia (a high sodium level) and needs to have his electrolytes monitored closely. It is already past the time for a repeat blood draw. Just then your supervisor is paged to an emergency and asks you to draw the sample on your own. You have seen several done but have only done one yourself and that was a few weeks ago.

In this situation you are being asked to be responsible for clinical care that exceeds your capability. This can happen in a number of situations, such as being asked to evaluate a clinical situation without proper backup or to complete DNR forms with a patient before you have been taught how. In the setting above, you may have the following thoughts: the patient will benefit by having a test that needs to be obtained; or, the risk to the patient from a venipuncture is more one of discomfort or pain rather than one that threatens his or her life, and you have already drawn blood once before. There is educational value to the learner in being pushed to the limits of his or her knowledge to solve problems and to gain confidence in functioning independently. But what is the right thing to do in this situation? In this scenario, think about the Tavistock Principles of *openness, cooperation, and safety*. You may need to find another person who is more qualified to do the procedure; or you may choose to attempt the venipuncture after alerting the patient to your inexperience and obtaining the patient's consent.

Scenario #3

You are assigned to a clinical team taking care of 25 patients who must be seen and have notes written on them before other commitments start at 7 A.M. There are four of you: the resident, an intern, a 4th-year medical student, and you, a mid-year clinical clerk. It is now 5:30 A.M. After the patients are divided among the three more senior members of the team, with time allowed for writing orders and notes, there are barely 5 minutes to assess each patient at the bedside. After seeing nine patients with the resident, you are asked to write three of the notes. You have questions about the care of several of the patients but realize that there is no time to ask. Feeling uncomfortable, you write the notes to the best of your ability.

This situation relates to the Tavistock Principles of *comprehensiveness, cooperation, openness, and improvement.* As these scenarios illustrate, clinical students are under pressure to go along with practices already in place. The context may be the way a team works on an in-patient service or the standard approach to patients in an emergency room or an outpatient clinic. You may find yourself choosing between cooperating as a member of a team and delivering care that is not consistent with your individual sense of quality. In addition, often you are working with clinicians who are evaluating your performance as a student. You may find yourself doing tasks that make you uncomfortable because of pressures to be a "team player."

As you can see, ethical dilemmas frequently occur in the life of clinical students. Because, as a student, you are often in a hierarchical situation where you have relatively less power, ethical conflicts that you have no control over may arise more often than when you are a practicing clinician. You can also see that often there are no clear or easy answers in such situations. What responses are available to you to address these and other quandaries?

You need to reflect on your beliefs and assess your level of comfort with a given situation. In some situations there may be alternative solutions. For example, in Scenario #1, the patient may really be willing to have the history and physical examination done at that hour, or perhaps you can renegotiate the time for the next morning. In Scenario #2, you might look for an alternative supervisor for the venipuncture. You will need to choose which situations warrant voicing your concerns, even at the risk of a bad evaluation. Seek out coaching on how to express your reservations in a way that ensures that they will be heard. As a clinical student, you will need settings for discussing these immediately relevant ethical issues with other students and with more senior trainees and faculty. Small groups that are structured to address these kinds of issues are particularly useful in providing validation and support. Avail yourself of these opportunities whenever possible.

Interviewing Patients of Different Ages

As patients move through different stages of life, you will need to make certain adaptations in your interviewing style. This section provides suggestions for talking with children, adolescents, and the elderly.

Talking With Children. Unlike adults, children usually are accompanied by a parent or caregiver. Even when adolescents are alone, they are often seeking health care at the request of their parents—indeed, the parent is usually sitting in the waiting room. When interviewing a child, you need to consider the needs and perspectives of both the child and the caregivers. In addition, the dictates of "well child care" may preset the clinician's agenda toward immunizations, anticipatory guidance, or developmental assessment.

Establishing Rapport. Begin the interview by greeting and establishing rapport with each person present. Refer to the infant or child by name rather than by "him," "her," or "the baby." Clarify the role or relationship of all the adults and children. "Now, are you Jimmy's grandmother?" "Please help me by telling me Jimmy's relationship to everyone here." Address the parents as "Mr. Smith" and "Ms. Smith" rather than by their first names or "Mom" or "Dad." When the family structure is not immediately clear, you may avoid embarrassment by asking directly about other members. "Who else lives in the home?" "Who is Jimmy's father?" "Do you live together?" Do not assume that just because parents are separated that only one parent is actively involved in the child's life.

To establish rapport, the key is to meet children on their own level. Use your personal experiences with children to guide how you interact in a health care setting. Maintaining eye contact at their level (for example, sit on the floor if needed), participating in playful engagement, and talking about what interests them are always good strategies. Ask children about their clothes, one of their toys, what book or TV show they like, or their adult companion in an enthusiastic but gentle style. Spending time at the beginning of the interview to calm down and connect with an anxious child or crying infant can put both the child and the caregiver at ease.

Working With Families. One of the biggest challenges when several people are present is deciding to whom to direct your questions. While eventually you need to get information from both the child and the parent(s), it is useful to start with the child if he or she can talk. Even at age 3 years, some children can tell you about the specific problem. Asking simple open-ended questions such as "Are you sick? . . . Tell me about it." followed by more specific questions often provides much of the History of the Present Illness. The parents can then verify the information, add details that give you the larger context, and identify other issues you need to address. You need to characterize symptom attributes the same way you do with adults. Sometimes children are embarrassed to begin, but once the parent has started the conversation, you can direct the questions back to the child.

- "Your mother tells me that you get a lot of stomachaches. Tell me about them."
- "Show me where you get the pain. What does it feel like?"
- "Is it sharp like a pinprick, or does it ache?"
- "Does it stay in the same spot, or does it move around?"
- "Anything else about feeling sick?"
- "What helps make it go away?"

- "What do you think causes it?"
- "How about missing school a lot?"

The presence of family members also provides a rich opportunity to observe how they interact with the child. As you talk with the parent, see how a young child relates to a new environment. It is normal for a toddler to open drawers, pull at paper, and wander around the room. An older child may be able to sit still or may get restless and start fidgeting. Watch how the parents set limits on the child or fail to set limits when appropriate.

MULTIPLE AGENDAS. Each individual in the room, including the clinician, may have a different idea about the nature of the problem and what needs to be done about it. It is your job to discover as many of these perspectives and agendas as possible. Family members who are not present (the absent parent or grandparent) may also have concerns. It is a good idea to ask about those concerns too. "If Suzie's father were here today, what questions or concerns would he have?" "Have you, Mrs. Jones, discussed this with your mother or anyone else?" "What does she think?" Mrs. Jones brings Suzie in for abdominal pain because she is worried that Suzie may have an ulcer. She is also worried about Suzie's eating habits. Suzie is not worried about the belly pain—it rarely interferes with what she wants to do. She is uneasy about the changes in her body, especially her belief that she is getting fat. Mr. Jones thinks that Suzie's schoolwork is not getting enough attention. You, as the clinician, need to balance these concerns with what you see as a healthy 12-year-old girl in early puberty with some mild functional abdominal pain. Your goals need to include helping the family to be realistic about the range of "normal" and uncovering the concerns of Mr. and Mrs. Jones and Suzie.

THE FAMILY AS A RESOURCE. Much of the information you obtain about a child comes from the family. In general, family members provide most of the care and are your natural allies in promoting the child's health. Being open to a wide range of parenting behaviors helps to make this alliance. Raising a child reflects cultural, socioeconomic, and family practices. It is important to respect the tremendous variation in these practices. A good strategy is to view the parents as experts in the care of their child and you as their consultant. This demonstrates respect for the parents' care and minimizes their likelihood of discounting or ignoring your advice. Most parents face many challenges raising children, so practitioners need to be supportive, not judgmental. Comments like "Why didn't you bring him in sooner?" or "What did you do that for!" do not improve your rapport with the parent. Statements acknowledging the hard work of parenting and praising successes are always appreciated.

HIDDEN AGENDAS. Finally, as with adults, the chief complaint may not relate to the real reason the parent has brought the child to see you. The complaint may be a "ticket to care" or bridge to concerns that may not seem legitimate. Try to create a trusting atmosphere that allows parents to be open about all their concerns. Ask facilitating questions like the following:

- "Do you have any other concerns about Randy that you would like to tell me about?"
- "What did you hope I would be able to do for you today?"
- "Was there anything else that you wanted to tell or ask me today?"

Talking With Adolescents. Adolescents, like most other people, usually respond positively to anyone who demonstrates a genuine interest in them. It is important to show interest early and then sustain the connection if communication is to be effective. Adolescents are more likely to open up when the interview is focused on them rather than on their problems. In contrast to most other interviews, *start with specific directed questions* to build trust and rapport and start the conversation. You may have to do more talking than usual. A good way to begin is to chat informally about friends, school, hobbies, and family. Using silence in an attempt to get adolescents to talk or asking about feelings directly is usually not a good idea. It is particularly important to use summarization and transitional statements (see pp. 33–34) and to explain what you are going to do during the physical examination. The physical examination can also be an opportunity to get the young person talking. Once you have established rapport, return to more open-ended questions. At that point, make sure to ask what concerns or questions the adolescent may have.

Remember also that adolescents' behavior is related to their developmental stage and not necessarily to chronologic age or physical maturation. Their age and appearance may fool you into assuming that they are functioning on a more future-oriented and realistic level. The reverse also can be true, especially in teens with delayed puberty or chronic illness.

Issues of *confidentiality* are important in adolescence. Explain to both parents and adolescents that the best health care allows adolescents some degree of independence and confidentiality. It helps if the clinician starts asking the parent to leave the room for part of the interview when the child is age 10 or 11 years. This prepares both caregivers and young people for future visits when the patient spends time alone with the clinician.

Before the parent leaves the room, get any relevant medical history from the parent, for example, certain elements of Past History, and clarify the parent's agenda for the visit. Also discuss the need for confidentiality. Explain that the purpose of confidentiality is to improve health care, not to keep secrets. Adolescents need to know that you will hold in confidence what they discuss with you. However, never make confidentiality unlimited. Always state explicitly that you may need to act on information that makes you concerned about safety . . . "I will not tell your parents what we talk about unless you give me permission or I am concerned about your safety—for example, if you were to talk to me about killing yourself and I thought there were a risk that you would actually try it."

Your goal is to help adolescents bring their concerns or questions to their parents. Encourage adolescents to discuss sensitive issues with their parents and offer to be present or help. While young people may believe that their parents would "kill them if they only knew," you may be able to promote more open dialogue. This entails a careful assessment of the parents' perspective and the young person's full and explicit consent.

Talking With Aging Patients. At the other end of the life cycle, aging patients also have special needs and concerns. Their hearing and vision may be impaired, their responses and explanations may be slow or lengthy, and they may have chronic illnesses with associated disabilities. Elderly people may not report their symptoms. Some may be afraid or embarrassed; others may be trying to avoid the medical expenses or the discomforts of diagnosis and treatment. They may think their symptoms are merely part of aging, or they may simply have forgotten about them. They may be inhibited by fears of losing their independence.

As you proceed with the interview, give elderly patients time to respond to your questions. Speak slowly and clearly but do not shout or raise your voice. A comfortable room, free of distractions and noise, is helpful. Ask about turning off the radio or television. Remember that visual cues may be important, so make sure that your face is well lit. If they wear glasses, make sure they put them on. Do not try to accomplish everything in one visit. Several visits may be less fatiguing and more productive.

From middle age on, people begin to measure their lives in terms of the years left rather than years lived. Older people often reminisce about the past and reflect upon previous experiences. Listening to this process of life review can give you important insights and help you support patients as they work through painful feelings or recapture joys or accomplishments.

Although some generalizations are useful, learn to recognize and avoid stereotypes that block your appreciation of each individual patient. Find out how patients see themselves and their situation, as well as each patient's unique priorities, goals, and patterns for handling problems. This knowledge will help you as you collaborate on treatment plans. For example, "Can you tell me how you feel about getting older?" "What kinds of things do you find most satisfying?" "What kinds of things worry you?" "What would you change if you could?"

Functional Assessment. Learning how the elderly, and those with chronic illness, function in terms of daily activities is essential and provides a baseline for future comparisons. There are two standard categories of assessment: physical activities of daily living (ADLs) and instrumental activities of daily living (IADLs).

Can the patients perform the ADLs independently, do they need some help, or are they entirely dependent? Instead of asking about each area separately, have the patient go through a typical day, in detail. Start with an open-ended

ACTIVITIES OF DAILY LIVING (ADLs)

Physical ADLs	*Instrumental ADLs*
Bathing	Using the telephone
Dressing	Shopping
Toileting	Preparing food
Transfers	Housekeeping
Continence	Laundry
Feeding	Transportation
Managing money	Taking medicine

request—"Tell me about your day yesterday"—and then guide the story to a greater level of detail. "You got up at 8? How is it getting out of bed?" "What did you do next?" Ask how things have changed, who is available for help, and what helpers actually do. Remember that increasing dependence on others is very difficult for most people to accept, but promoting safety is one of your important priorities.

CHAPTER

Beginning the Physical Examination: General Survey and Vital Signs

3

Once you understand the patient's concerns and have elicited a careful history, you are ready to begin the physical examination. At first you may feel unsure of how the patient will relate to you. With practice, your skills in physical examination will grow, and you will gain confidence. Through study and repetition the examination will flow more smoothly, and you will soon shift your attention from technique and how to handle instruments to what you hear, see, and feel. Touching the patient's body will seem more natural, and you will learn to minimize any discomfort to the patient. You will become more responsive to the patient's reactions and provide reassurance when needed. Before long, as you gain proficiency, what once took between 1 and 2 hours will take considerably less time.

This chapter addresses skills and techniques needed for initial assessment as you begin the physical examination. Under Anatomy and Physiology you will find information on how to measure height, weight, and Body Mass Index (BMI), and guidelines for nutritional assessment. There is clinical information on the relevant health history, health promotion and counseling, and a preview of how to record the patient's overall appearance. The section on Techniques of Examination describes the initial steps of the physical examination: preparing for the examination, conducting the general survey, and taking the vital signs.

ANATOMY AND PHYSIOLOGY

As you begin the physical examination, you will survey the patient's general appearance and measure the patient's height and weight. These data provide information about the patient's nutritional status and amount of body fat. Body fat consists primarily of adipose in the form of triglyceride and is stored in subcutaneous, intra-abdominal, and intramuscular fat depots. These stores are inaccessible and difficult to measure, so it will be important to compare your measurements of height and weight to standardized ranges of normal. In the past, tables of desirable weight-for-height have been based on life insurance data, which often did not adjust for the effects of smoking and selected weight-inducing medical conditions such as diabetes, and tended to overstate desirable weight. For those wishing to continue using such tables, see Table 3-1, p. 83.

More recently, however, many government and scientific health organizations have promoted use of the *Body Mass Index,* which incorporates estimated but more accurate measures of body fat than weight alone. BMI standards are derived from two surveys: the National Health Examination Survey, consisting of three survey cycles between 1960 and 1970, and the National Health and Nutrition Examination Survey, with three cycles from the 1970s to the 1990s.

More than half of U.S. adults are overweight (BMI >25), and nearly one fourth are obese (BMI >30), so assessing and educating patients about their BMI are vital for promoting health. Being overweight or obese are proven risk factors for diabetes, heart disease, stroke, hypertension, osteoarthritis, and some forms of cancer. Remember that these BMI criteria are not rigid cutpoints but guidelines for increasing risks for health and well-being. Note that persons over age 65 have a disproportionate risk of undernutrition when compared to younger adults.

Height and weight in childhood and adolescence reflect the many behavioral, cognitive, and physiologic changes of growth and development. Developmental milestones, markers for growth spurts, and sexual maturity ratings can be found in Chapter 17, Assessing Children: Infancy Through Adolescence. With aging, some of these changes reverse—height may decrease, posture may become more stooping from kyphosis of the thoracic spine, and extension of the knees and hips may diminish. The abdominal muscles may relax, changing the abdominal contour, and fat may accumulate at the hips and lower abdomen. Be alert to these changes and those described in the sections called "Changes With Aging" in the upcoming chapters.

Calculating the BMI. There are a number of ways to calculate the BMI. Choose the method most suited to your practice. The National Institute of Diabetes and Digestive and Kidney Diseases cautions that people who are very muscular may have a high BMI but still be healthy. Likewise, the BMI for elderly or other individuals with low muscle mass and reduced nutrition may appear inappropriately "normal." If you find the BMI difficult to use, you can use the nomogram on p. 62, which gives BMI values for weight in pounds or kilograms and height in feet or centimeters.

Methods to Calculate Body Mass Index (BMI)

Unit of Measure	Method of Calculation
Weight *in pounds,* height *in inches*	(1) Body Mass Index Chart (see table on p. 61) (2) Body Mass Index Nomogram (see table on p. 62) (3) $\dfrac{\left(\dfrac{\text{Weight (lbs)} \times 700^*}{\text{Height (inches)}}\right)}{\text{Height (inches)}}$
Weight *in kilograms,* height *in meters squared*	(4) $\dfrac{\text{Weight (kg)}}{\text{Height (m}^2\text{)}}$
Either	(5) "BMI Calculator" at website www.nhlbisupport.com/bmi

*Several organizations use 704.5, but the variation in BMI is negligible.

Conversion formulas: 2.2 lbs = 1 kg; 1.0 inch = 2.54 cm; 100 cm = 1 meter

Source: National Institute of Diabetes and Digestive and Kidney Diseases. www.niddk.nih.gov/health/nutrit/pubs/statobes.htm, Accessed 2/1/01.

Another option is to measure the patient's *waist circumference*. With the patient standing, measure the waist just above the hip bones. The patient may have excess body fat if the waist measures:

- ≥35 inches for women
- ≥40 inches for men

Interpreting and Acting on the BMI. If the BMI falls *above 25*, or the weight is greater than the upper limit of recommended weight for height, a nutrition assessment is in order. Engage the patient in a 24-hour dietary recall and compare the intake of food groups and number of servings per day with current recommendations. Or choose a screening tool and provide appropriate counseling or referral. You may wish to review the types of foods in different food groups, using the helpful diagram found in Table 3-5, "Food Guide Pyramid: A Guide to Daily Food Choices" (pp. 86–87). Remember that carbohydrates and protein furnish 4 calories per gram, and fat yields 9 calories per gram.

See also Table 3-1, Height and Weight Tables for Adults Age 25 and Over, p. 83.

See Table 3-2, Healthy Eating: Food Groups and Servings per Day, p. 84. For screening tools, see Table 3-3, Rapid Screen for Dietary Intake, p. 84, and Table 3-4, Nutrition Screening Checklist, p. 85.

If the BMI falls *below 17*, or the weight is less than the low end of the range of weight for height, be concerned about possible anorexia nervosa, bulimia, or other medical conditions. These conditions are summarized in Table 3-6, Eating Disorders and Excessively Low BMI, p. 88. (See also pp. 65–66 for health promotion and counseling for overweight or underweight patients.)

BODY MASS INDEX CHART

Height (inches)	19	20	21	22	23	24	25	26	27	28	29	30	31	32	33	34	35
	Body Weight (pounds)																
58	91	96	100	105	110	115	119	124	129	134	138	143	148	153	158	162	167
59	94	99	104	109	114	119	124	128	133	138	143	148	153	158	163	168	173
60	97	102	107	112	118	123	128	133	138	143	148	153	158	163	168	174	179
61	100	105	111	116	122	127	132	137	143	148	153	158	164	169	174	180	185
62	104	109	115	120	126	131	136	142	147	153	158	164	169	175	180	185	191
63	107	113	118	124	130	135	141	145	152	158	163	169	174	180	185	191	197
64	110	116	122	128	134	140	145	151	157	163	169	174	180	185	192	197	204
65	114	120	126	132	138	144	150	156	162	168	174	180	186	192	198	204	210
66	118	124	130	136	142	148	155	161	167	173	179	186	192	198	204	210	216
67	121	127	134	140	146	153	159	166	172	178	185	191	198	204	211	217	223
68	125	131	138	144	151	158	164	171	177	184	190	197	203	210	216	223	230
69	128	135	142	149	155	162	169	176	182	189	196	203	209	216	223	230	236
70	132	139	146	153	160	167	174	181	188	189	196	203	209	216	223	230	236
71	136	143	150	157	165	172	179	186	193	200	208	215	222	229	236	243	250
72	140	147	154	162	169	177	184	191	199	206	213	221	228	235	242	250	258
73	144	151	159	166	174	182	189	197	204	212	219	227	235	242	250	257	265
74	148	155	163	171	179	186	194	202	210	218	225	233	241	249	256	264	272
75	152	160	168	176	184	192	200	208	216	224	232	240	248	256	264	272	279
76	156	164	172	180	189	197	205	213	221	230	238	246	254	263	271	279	287

Source: Clinical Guidelines on the Identification, Evaluation, and Treatment of Overweight and Obesity in Adults, National Institutes of Health and National Heart, Lung, and Blood Institute. June 1998.

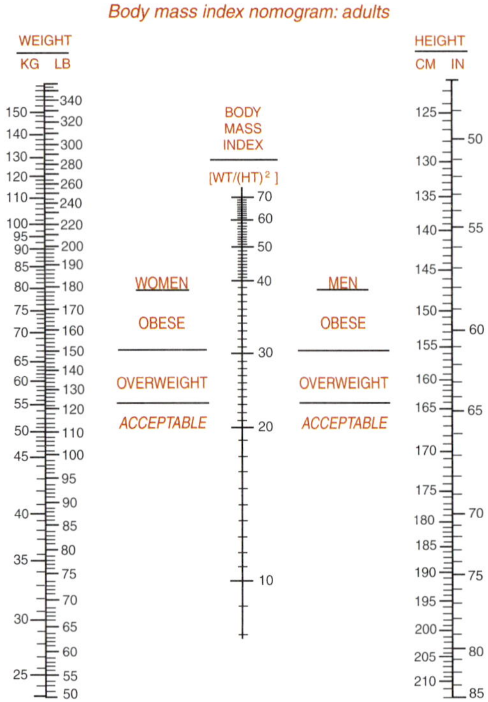

Source: Katz DL: Nutrition in Clinical Practice. Philadelphia, Lippincott Williams & Wilkins, 2001:340.

THE HEALTH HISTORY

Common or Concerning Symptoms

- Changes in weight
- Weakness and fatigue
- Fever, chills, night sweats

Changes in Weight. Changes in weight result from changes in body tissues or body fluid. *Weight gain* occurs when caloric intake exceeds caloric expenditure over a period of time and typically appears as increased body fat. Weight gain may also reflect abnormal accumulation of body fluids. When the retention of fluid is relatively mild, it may not be visible, but several pounds of fluid usually appear as *edema*.

Rapid changes in weight (over a few days) suggest changes in body fluids, not tissues.

Good opening questions include "How often do you check your weight?" "How is it compared to a year ago?" For changes, ask "Why do you think it has changed?" "What would you like to weigh?" If weight gain or loss appears to be a problem, ask about the amount of change, its timing, the setting in which it occurred, and any associated symptoms.

In the overweight patient, for example, when did the weight gain begin? Was the patient heavy as an infant or a child? Using milestones appropriate to the patient's age, inquire about weight at the following times: birth, kindergarten, high school or college graduation, discharge from military service, marriage, after each pregnancy, menopause, and retirement. What were the patient's life circumstances during the periods of weight gain? Has the patient tried to lose weight? How? With what results?

Weight loss is an important symptom that has many causes. Mechanisms include one or more of the following: decreased intake of food for reasons such as anorexia, dysphagia, vomiting, and insufficient supplies of food; defective absorption of nutrients through the gastrointestinal tract; increased metabolic requirements; and loss of nutrients through the urine, feces, or injured skin. A person may also lose weight when a fluid-retaining state improves or responds to treatment.

Causes of weight loss include: gastrointestinal diseases, endocrine disorders (diabetes mellitus, hyperthyroidism, adrenal insufficiency), chronic infections; malignancy; chronic cardiac, pulmonary, or renal failure; depression; and anorexia nervosa or bulimia (see Table 3-6, Eating Disorders and Excessively Low BMI, p. 88).

Try to determine if the drop in weight is proportional to any change in food intake, or whether it has remained normal or even increased.

Weight loss with relatively high food intake suggests diabetes mellitus, hyperthyroidism, or malabsorption. Consider also binge eating (bulimia) with clandestine vomiting.

Symptoms associated with weight loss often suggest a cause, as does a good psychosocial history. Who cooks and shops for the patient? Where does the patient eat? With whom? Are there any problems with obtaining, storing, preparing, or chewing food? Does the patient avoid or restrict certain foods for medical, religious, or other reasons?

Poverty, old age, social isolation, physical disability, emotional or mental impairment, lack of teeth, ill-fitting dentures, alcoholism, and drug abuse increase the likelihood of malnutrition.

Throughout the history, be alert for signs of malnutrition. Symptoms may be subtle and nonspecific, such as weakness, easy fatigability, cold intolerance, flaky dermatitis, and ankle swelling. Securing a good history of eating patterns and quantities is mandatory. It is important to ask general questions about intake at different times throughout the day, such as "Tell me what you typically eat for lunch." "What do you eat for a snack?" "When?"

See Table 3-4, Nutrition Screening Checklist, p. 85.

Fatigue and Weakness. Like weight loss, *fatigue* is a relatively nonspecific symptom with many causes. It refers to a sense of weariness or loss of energy that patients describe in various ways. "I don't feel like getting up in the morning" . . . "I don't have any energy" . . . "I just feel blah". . . . "I'm all done in" . . . "I can hardly get through the day" . . . "By the time I get to the office I feel as if I've done a day's work." Because fatigue is a normal response to hard work, sustained stress, or grief, try to elicit the life cir-

Fatigue is a common symptom of depression and anxiety states, but also consider infections (such as hepatitis, infectious mononucleosis, and tuberculosis); endocrine disorders (hypothyroidism, adrenal insufficiency, diabetes mellitus,

cumstances in which it occurs. When fatigue is unrelated to such situations, further investigation is needed.

panhypopituitarism); heart failure; chronic disease of the lungs, kidneys, or liver; electrolyte imbalance; moderate to severe anemia; malignancies; nutritional deficits; medications.

Use open-ended questions to explore the attributes of the patient's fatigue, and encourage the patient to fully describe what he or she is experiencing. Important clues about etiology are often found in a good psychosocial history, exploration of sleep patterns, and a thorough review of systems.

Infants and children cannot describe fatigue verbally, so inquire about any changes in behavior, such as withdrawal from normal activities, irritability, loss of interest in their surroundings, and excessive sleeping.

Weakness is different from fatigue. It denotes a demonstrable loss of muscle power and will be discussed later with other neurologic symptoms (see pp. 550–551).

Weakness, especially if localized in a neuroanatomic pattern, suggests possible neuropathy or myopathy.

Fever and Chills. *Fever* refers to an abnormal elevation in body temperature (see p. 81 for definitions of normal). Ask about fever if patients have an acute or chronic illness. Find out whether the patient has used a thermometer to measure the temperature. (Errors in technique can lead to unreliable information.) Has the patient felt feverish or unusually hot, noted excessive sweating, or felt chilly and cold? Try to distinguish between subjective *chilliness* and a *shaking chill,* with shivering throughout the body and chattering of teeth.

Recurrent shaking chills suggest more extreme swings in temperature and systemic bacteremia.

Feeling cold, goosebumps, and shivering accompany a rising temperature, while feeling hot and sweating accompany a falling temperature. Normally the body temperature rises during the day and falls during the night. When fever exaggerates this swing, *night sweats* occur. Malaise, headache, and pain in the muscles and joints often accompany fever.

Feelings of heat and sweating also accompany menopause. Night sweats occur in tuberculosis and malignancy.

Fever has many causes. Focus your questions on the timing of the illness and its associated symptoms. Become familiar with patterns of infectious diseases that may affect your patient. Inquire about travel, contact with sick persons, or other unusual exposures. Be sure to inquire about medications, since they may cause fever. In contrast, recent ingestion of aspirin, acetaminophen, corticosteroids, and nonsteroidal anti-inflammatory drugs may mask it and affect the temperature recorded at the time of the physical examination.

HEALTH PROMOTION AND COUNSELING

Important Topics for Health Promotion and Counseling

- Optimal weight and nutrition
- Exercise
- Blood pressure and diet

Optimal Weight and Nutrition. Less than half of U.S. adults maintain a healthy weight (BMI ≥19 but ≤25). Obesity has increased in every segment of the population, regardless of age, gender, income, ethnicity, or socioeconomic group. More than half of people with non-insulin-dependent diabetes and roughly 20% of those with hypertension or elevated cholesterol are overweight or obese. Increasing obesity in children has been linked to rising rates of childhood diabetes. Once excess weight or unhealthy nutritional patterns are detected, take advantage of the excellent materials available to promote weight loss and good nutrition. Even reducing weight by 5% to 10% can improve blood pressure, lipid levels, and glucose tolerance and reduce the risk of developing diabetes or hypertension.

Once you have assessed food intake and nutritional status and the patient's motivation to change eating behaviors, you are ready to begin health counseling. First, explain the components of a healthy diet and encourage patients to select appropriately sized servings from each of the five major food groups: grains such as bread, cereal, rice, and pasta; fruits; vegetables; dairy products; and meat and beans. Be prepared to help adolescents and adults over age 50 identify foods rich in calcium. Advise pregnant women to increase intake of iron and folic acid, and older adults to increase intake of vitamin D.

See Table 3-2, Healthy Eating: Food Groups and Servings per Day, p. 84, and Table 3-5. Food Guide Pyramid, pp. 86–87.

See Table 3-7, Nutrition Counseling: Sources of Nutrients, p. 89.

Exercise. Fitness is a key component of both weight control and weight loss. Currently, 30 minutes of moderate activity, defined as walking 2 miles in 30 minutes on most days of the week or its equivalent, is recommended. Patients can increase exercise by such simple measures as parking further away from their place of work or using stairs instead of elevators. A safe goal for weight loss is ½ to 2 pounds per week.

Blood Pressure and Diet. With respect to blood pressure, there is reliable evidence that regular and frequent exercise, decreased sodium intake and increased potassium intake, and maintaining a healthy weight will reduce risk of developing hypertension as well as lower blood pressure in adults who are already hypertensive. Explain to patients that most of the sodium in our diet comes from salt (sodium chloride). Inform your patients that the recommended daily allowance (RDA) of sodium is

See Table 3-8, Patients With Hypertension: Recommended Changes in Diet, p. 89.

<2400 mg, or 1 teaspoon, per day. Patients need to read food labels closely, especially the Nutrition Facts panel. Low sodium foods are those with sodium listed at less than 5% of the RDA of <2400 mg. For nutritional interventions to reduce risk of cardiac disease, turn to p. 89.

Preview: Recording the Physical Examination— The General Survey and Vital Signs

Your write-up of the physical examination begins with a general description of the patient's appearance, based on the General Survey. Note that initially you may use sentences to describe your findings; later you will use phrases. The style below contains phrases appropriate for most write-ups. Unfamiliar terms are explained in the next section, "Techniques of Examination." Choose vivid and graphic adjectives, as if you are painting a picture in words. Avoid cliches such as "well-developed" or "well-nourished" or "in no acute distress," since they could apply to any patient and do not convey the special features of the patient before you.

Record the vital signs taken at the time of your examination. They are preferable to those taken earlier in the day by other providers. (Common abbreviations for blood pressure, heart rate, and respiratory rate are self-explanatory.)

> "Mrs. Scott is a young, healthy-appearing woman, well-groomed, fit, and in good spirits. Height is 5′4″, weight 135 lbs, BP 120/80, HR 72 and regular, RR 16, temperature 37.5°C."
>
> **OR:**
>
> "Mr. Jones is an elderly male who looks pale and chronically ill. He is alert, with good eye contact but unable to speak more than two or three words at a time due to shortness of breath. He has intercostal muscle retraction when breathing and sits upright in bed. He is thin, with diffuse muscle wasting. Height is 6′2″, weight 175 lbs, BP 160/95, HR 108 and irregular, RR 32 and labored, temperature 101.2°F."

TECHNIQUES OF EXAMINATION

Beginning the Examination: Setting the Stage

Preparing for the Physical Examination

- Reflect on your approach to the patient
- Decide on the scope of the examination
- Choose the examination sequence
- Adjust the lighting and the environment
- Make the patient comfortable

Before you begin the physical examination, take time to prepare for the tasks ahead. Think through your approach to the patient, your professional demeanor, and how to make the patient feel comfortable and relaxed. Review the measures that promote the patient's physical comfort and make any adjustments needed in the lighting and the surrounding environment. *Make sure that you wash your hands in the presence of the patient before beginning the examination. This is a subtle yet much appreciated gesture of concern for the patient's welfare.*

Approaching the Patient. When first examining patients, feelings of insecurity are inevitable, but these will soon diminish with experience. Be straightforward. Let the patient know you are a student and try to appear calm, organized, and competent, even when you feel differently. If you forget to do part of the examination, this is not uncommon, especially at first! Simply examine those areas out of sequence, but smoothly. It is not unusual to go back to the bedside and ask to check one or two items that you might have overlooked.

As a beginner, you will need to spend more time than experienced clinicians on selected portions of the examination, such as the ophthalmoscopic examination or cardiac auscultation. To avoid alarming the patient, warn the patient ahead of time by saying, for example, "I would like to spend extra time listening to your heart and the heart sounds, but this doesn't mean I hear anything wrong."

Over time, you will begin sharing your findings with the patient. Clinicians have different approaches as to how and when this occurs. As a beginner, you should avoid interpreting your findings. You are not the patient's primary caretaker, and your views may be conflicting or in error. As you grow in experience and responsibility, sharing findings will become more appropriate. If the patient has specific concerns, you may even provide reassurance as you finish examining the relevant area. Be selective, however—if you find an unexpected abnormality, you may wish you had kept a judicious silence. At times, you may discover abnormalities such as an ominous mass or a deep oozing ulcer. Always avoid showing distaste, alarm, or other negative reactions.

Scope of the Examination: How Complete Should It Be? There is no simple answer to this common question. Chapter 1 provided some guidelines to help you choose whether to do a *comprehensive* or *focused examination*. As a general principle, a new patient warrants a complete examination, regardless of chief complaint or setting. You may choose to abbreviate the examination for patients making routine office visits or seeking urgent care. A more limited examination may also be appropriate for patients with symptoms restricted to a specific body system or with patients you know well.

A *comprehensive examination* does more than assess the body systems. The physical examination is a source of fundamental and personalized knowledge about the patient and strengthens the clinician–patient relationship. Most people seeking health care have specific worries or symptoms. The physical examination helps to identify or rule out related physical causes. It gives information for answering patient questions and serves as a baseline for future comparisons. The physical examination also provides important opportunities for health promotion through education and counseling, and increases the credibility and conviction of the clinician's reassurance and advice. Furthermore, students must repeatedly perform such examinations to gain proficiency, and clinicians need ongoing practice to maintain their skills. How to best divide the usually limited time allotted to a patient visit between listening, discussion, or counseling on the one hand, and the physical examination on the other, takes both judgment and experience.

For the *focused examination*, select the methods relevant to assessing the problem as precisely and carefully as possible. The patient's symptoms, age, and health history help determine the scope of your examination, as does your knowledge of disease patterns. Out of all the patients with sore throat, for example, you will need to decide who may have infectious mononucleosis and warrants careful palpation of the liver and spleen and who, in contrast, has a common cold and does not need this examination. The clinical thinking that underlies and guides such decisions is discussed in Chapter 18.

What about the need for a *periodic physical examination* for screening and prevention? The utility of the comprehensive physical examination for the purposes of screening and prevention of illness, in contrast to evaluation of symptoms, has been scrutinized in a number of studies. Studies have validated a number of physical examination techniques: blood pressure measurement, assessment of central venous pressure from the jugular venous pulse, listening to the heart for evidence of valvular disease, the clinical breast examination, detection of hepatic and splenic enlargement, and the pelvic examination with Papanicolaou smears. Recommendations for examination and screening have been further expanded by various consensus panels and expert advisory groups. Bear in mind, however, that when used for screening (rather than assessment of complaints), not all components of the examination have been validated as ways to reduce future morbidity and mortality.

Choosing the Examination Sequence, Examining Position, and Handedness. Remember that the sequence of the comprehensive or focused examination should maximize the patient's comfort, avoid unnecessary changes in position, and enhance the clinician's efficiency. In general, move from "head to toe." An important goal for you as a student is to develop your own sequence of examination with these principles in mind. For example, avoid examining the patient's feet or genital areas before checking the face or mouth.

Turn back to Chapter 1, pp. 10–13, to review a suggested examination sequence, and look over the outline of such a sequence below.

THE PHYSICAL EXAMINATION: SUMMARY OF SUGGESTED SEQUENCE

- General survey
- Vital signs
- Skin: upper torso, anterior and posterior
- Head and neck, including thyroid and lymph nodes
- *Optional:* nervous system (mental status, cranial nerves, upper extremity motor strength, bulk, tone; cerebellar function)
- Thorax and lungs
- Breasts
- Musculoskeletal as indicated: upper extremities
- Cardiovascular, including JVP, carotid upstrokes and bruits, PMI, etc.
- Cardiovascular, for S_3 and murmur of mitral stenosis
- Cardiovascular, for murmur of aortic insufficiency
- *Optional:* thorax and lungs — anterior
- Breasts and axillae
- Abdomen
- Peripheral vascular; *Optional:* skin-lower torso and extremities
- Nervous system: lower extremity motor strength, bulk, tone: sensation; reflexes; Babinskis
- Musculoskeletal, as indicated
- *Optional:* skin, anterior and posterior
- *Optional:* nervous system, including gait
- *Optional:* musculoskeletal, comprehensive
- *Women:* pelvic and rectal examination
- *Men:* prostate and rectal examination

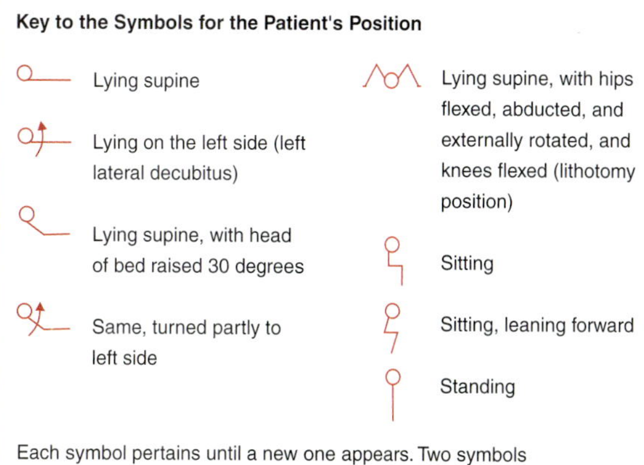

Key to the Symbols for the Patient's Position
Lying supine
Lying on the left side (left lateral decubitus)
Lying supine, with head of bed raised 30 degrees
Same, turned partly to left side
Lying supine, with hips flexed, abducted, and externally rotated, and knees flexed (lithotomy position)
Sitting
Sitting, leaning forward
Standing
Each symbol pertains until a new one appears. Two symbols separated by a slash indicate either or both positions.

This book recommends examining the patient from the patient's right side, moving to the opposite side or foot of the bed or examining table as necessary. This is the standard position for the physical examination and has several advantages compared to the left side: It is more reliable to estimate jugular venous pressure from the right, the palpating hand rests more comfortably on the apical impulse, the right kidney is more frequently palpable than the left, and examining tables are frequently positioned to accommodate a right-handed approach.

Left-handed students are encouraged to adopt right-sided positioning, even though at first it may seem awkward. It still may be easier to use the left hand for percussing or for holding instruments such as the otoscope or reflex hammer.

Often you will need to examine *the supine patient.* This may dictate changes in your sequence of examination. Some patients, for example, are unable to sit up in bed or stand. You can examine the head, neck, and anterior chest with the patient lying supine. Then roll the patient onto each side to listen to the lungs, examine the back, and inspect the skin. Roll the patient back and finish the rest of the examination with the patient again in the supine position.

Adjusting Lighting and the Environment. Surprisingly, a number of environmental factors affect the calibre and reliability of your physical findings. To achieve superior techniques of examination, it is important to "set the stage" so that both you and the patient are comfortable. As the examiner, you will find that awkward positions impair the quality of your observations. Take the time to adjust the bed to a convenient height (but be sure to lower it when finished!), and ask the patient to move toward you if this makes it easier to examine a region of the body more carefully.

Good lighting and a quiet environment make important contributions to what you see and hear but may be hard to arrange. Do the best you can. If a television interferes with listening to heart sounds, politely ask the nearby patient to lower the volume. Most people cooperate readily. Be courteous and remember to thank them as you leave.

Tangential lighting is optimal for inspecting a number of structures such as the jugular venous pulse, the thyroid gland, and the apical impulse of the heart. It casts light across body surfaces that throws contours, elevations, and depressions, whether moving or stationary, into sharper relief.

When light is perpendicular to the surface or diffuse, as shown on the next page, shadows are reduced and subtle undulations across the surface are lost. Experiment with focused, tangential lighting across the tendons on the back of your hand; try to see the pulsations of the radial artery at your wrist.

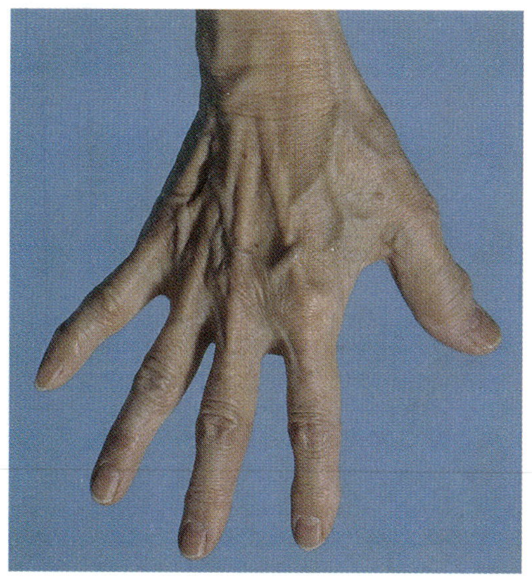

TANGENTIAL LIGHTING

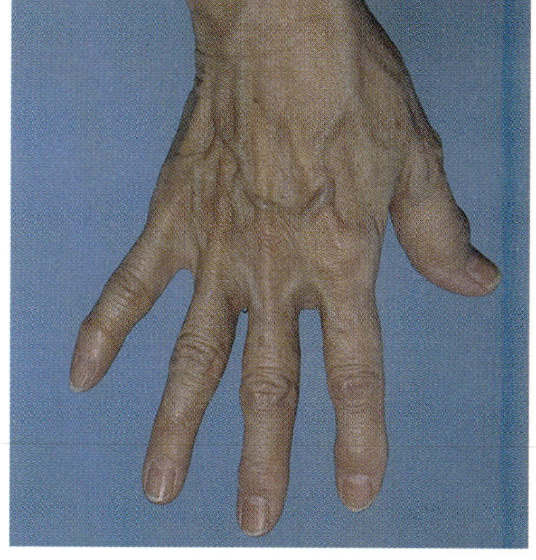

PERPENDICULAR LIGHTING

Promoting the Patient's Comfort. Your access to the patient's body is a unique and time-honored privilege of your role as a clinician. Showing concern for privacy and patient modesty must be ingrained in your professional behavior. These attributes help the patient feel respected and at ease. Be sure to close nearby doors and draw the curtains in the hospital or examining room before the examination begins.

You will acquire the art of *draping the patient* with the gown or draw sheet as you learn each segment of the examination in the chapters ahead. *Your goal is to visualize one area of the body at a time.* This preserves the patient's modesty but also helps you to focus on the area being examined. With the patient sitting, for example, untie the gown in back to better listen to the lungs. For the breast examination, uncover the right breast but keep the left chest draped. Redrape the right chest, then uncover the left chest and proceed to examine the left breast and heart. For the abdominal examination, only the abdomen should be exposed. Adjust the gown to cover the chest and place the sheet or drape at the inguinal area.

To help the patient prepare for segments that might be awkward, it is considerate to briefly describe your plans before starting the examination. As you proceed with the examination, keep the patient informed, especially when you anticipate embarrassment or discomfort, as when checking for the femoral pulse. Also try to gauge how much the patient wants to know. Is the patient curious about the lung findings or your method for assessing the liver or spleen?

Make sure your instructions to the patient at each step in the examination are courteous and clear. For example, "I would like to examine your heart now, so please lie down."

As in the interview, be sensitive to the patient's feelings and physical comfort. Watching the patient's facial expressions and even asking "Is it okay?"

as you move through the examination often reveals unexpressed worries or sources of pain. To ease discomfort, it may help to adjust the slant of the patient's bed or examining table. Rearranging the pillows or adding blankets for warmth shows your attentiveness to the patient's well-being.

When you have completed the examination, tell the patient your general impressions and what to expect next. For hospitalized patients, make sure the patient is comfortable and rearrange the immediate environment to the patient's satisfaction. Be sure to lower the bed to avoid risk of falls, reapply any restraints you may have removed, and raise the bedrails if needed. As you leave, wash your hands, clean your equipment, and dispose of any waste materials.

THE GENERAL SURVEY

The *General Survey* of the patient's build, height, and weight begins with the opening moments of the patient encounter, but you will find that your observations of the patient's appearance crystallize as you start the physical examination. The best clinicians continually sharpen their powers of observation and description, like naturalists identifying birds from silhouettes backlit against the sky. It is important to heighten the acuity of your clinical perceptions of the patient's mood, build, and behavior. These details enrich and deepen your emerging clinical impression. A skilled observer can depict distinguishing features of the patient's general appearance so well in words that a colleague could spot the patient in a crowd of strangers.

Many factors contribute to the patient's body habitus—socioeconomic status, nutrition, genetic makeup, degree of fitness, mood state, early illnesses, gender, geographic location, and age cohort. Recall that many of the characteristics you scrutinize during the *General Survey* are affected by the patient's nutritional status: height and weight, blood pressure, posture, mood and alertness, facial coloration, dentition and condition of the tongue and gingiva, color of the nail beds, and muscle bulk, to name a few. Be sure to make the assessment of height, weight, BMI, and risk of obesity a routine part of your clinical practice.

You should now recapture the observations you have been making since the first moments of your interaction and sharpen them throughout your assessment. Does the patient hear you when greeted in the waiting room or examination room? Rise with ease? Walk easily or stiffly? If hospitalized when you first meet, what is the patient doing—sitting up and enjoying television? . . . or lying in bed? . . . What occupies the bedside table—a magazine? . . . a flock of "get well" cards? . . . a Bible or a rosary? . . . an emesis basin? . . . or nothing at all? Each of these observations should raise one or more tentative hypotheses about the patient for you to consider during future assessments.

Apparent State of Health. Try to make a general judgment based on observations made throughout the encounter. Support it with the significant details.

Acutely or chronically ill, frail, feeble, robust, vigorous

Level of Consciousness. Is the patient awake, alert, and responsive to you and others in the environment?

If not, promptly assess the level of consciousness (see p. 558).

Signs of Distress. For example, does the patient show evidence of these problems?

- Cardiac or respiratory distress

Clutching the chest, pallor, diaphoresis; labored breathing, wheezing, cough

- Pain

Wincing, sweating, protectiveness of painful area

- Anxiety or depression

Anxious face, fidgety movements, cold moist palms; inexpressive or flat affect, poor eye contact, psychomotor slowing

Height and Build. If possible, measure the patient's height in stocking feet. Is the patient unusually short or tall? Is the build slender and lanky, muscular, or stocky? Is the body symmetric? Note the general body proportions and look for any deformities.

Very short stature is seen in Turner's syndrome, childhood renal failure, achondroplastic and hypopituitary dwarfism. Long limbs in proportion to the trunk is seen in hypogonadism and Marfan's syndrome

Weight. Is the patient emaciated, slender, plump, obese, or somewhere in between? If the patient is obese, is the fat distributed evenly or concentrated over the trunk, the upper torso, or around the hips?

Generalized fat in simple obesity; truncal fat with relatively thin limbs in Cushing's syndrome and syndrome X

Whenever possible, weigh the patient with shoes off. Weight provides one index of caloric intake, and changes over time yield other valuable diagnostic data. Remember that changes in weight can occur with changes in body fluid status, as well as in fat or muscle mass.

Causes of weight loss include malignancy, diabetes mellitus, hyperthyroidism, chronic infection, depression, diuresis, and successful dieting

Skin Color and Obvious Lesions. See Chapter 4, The Skin, for details.

Pallor, cyanosis, jaundice, rashes, bruises

Dress, Grooming, and Personal Hygiene. How is the patient dressed? Is clothing appropriate to the temperature and weather? Is it clean, properly buttoned, and zipped? How does it compare with clothing worn by people of comparable age and social group?

Excess clothing may reflect the cold intolerance of hypothyroidism, hide skin rash or needle marks, or signal personal lifestyle preferences.

Glance at the patient's shoes. Have holes been cut in them? Are the laces tied? Or is the patient wearing slippers?

Cut-out holes or slippers may indicate gout, bunions, or other painful foot conditions. Untied laces or slippers also suggest edema.

Is the patient wearing any unusual jewelry? Where? Is there any body piercing?

Copper bracelets are sometimes worn for arthritis. Body piercing may appear on any part of the body.

Note the patient's hair, fingernails, and use of cosmetics. They may be clues to the patient's personality, mood, or lifestyle. Nail polish and hair coloring that have "grown out" may signify decreased interest in personal appearance.

"Grown-out" hair and nail polish can help you estimate the length of an illness if the patient cannot give a history. Fingernails chewed to the quick may reflect stress.

Do personal hygiene and grooming seem appropriate to the patient's age, lifestyle, occupation, and socioeconomic group? These are norms that vary widely, of course.

Unkempt appearance may be seen in depression and dementia, but this appearance must be compared with the patient's probable norm.

Facial Expression. Observe the facial expression at rest, during conversation about specific topics, during the physical examination, and in interaction with others. Watch for eye contact. Is it natural? Sustained and unblinking? Averted quickly? Absent?

The stare of hyperthyroidism; the immobile face of parkinsonism; the flat or sad affect of depression. Decreased eye contact may be cultural, or may suggest anxiety, fear, or sadness.

Odors of the Body and Breath. Odors can be important diagnostic clues, such as the fruity odor of diabetes or the scent of alcohol. (For the scent of alcohol, the CAGE questions, p. 44, will help you determine possible misuse.)

Breath odors of alcohol, acetone (diabetes), pulmonary infections, uremia, or liver failure

Never assume that alcohol on a patient's breath explains changes in mental status or neurologic findings.

Alcoholics may have other serious and potentially correctable problems such as hypoglycemia, subdural hematoma, or post-ictal state

Posture, Gait and Motor Activity. What is the patient's preferred posture?

Preference for sitting up in left-sided heart failure, and for leaning forward with arms braced in chronic obstructive pulmonary disease

Is the patient restless or quiet? How often does the patient change position? How fast are the movements?

Fast, frequent movements of hyperthyroidism; slowed activity of hypothyroidism

Is there any apparent involuntary motor activity? Are some body parts immobile? Which ones?

Tremors or other involuntary movements; paralyses. See Table 16-8, Involuntary Movements, (pp. 608–609).

Does the patient walk smoothly, with comfort, self-confidence, and balance, or is there a limp or discomfort, fear of falling, loss of balance, or any movement disorder?

See Table 16-13, Abnormalities of Gait and Posture (pp. 618–619).

THE VITAL SIGNS

Now you are ready to measure the *Vital Signs*—the blood pressure, heart rate, respiratory rate, and temperature. You may find that the vital signs are already taken and recorded in the chart; if abnormal, you may wish to repeat them yourself. (You can also make these important measurements later as you start the cardiovascular and thorax and lung examinations, but often they provide important initial information that influences the direction of your evaluation.)

Check either the blood pressure or the pulse first. If the blood pressure is high, measure it again later in the examination. Count the radial pulse with your fingers, or the apical pulse with your stethoscope at the cardiac apex. Continue either of these techniques and count the respiratory rate without alerting the patient. (Breathing patterns may change if patient becomes aware that someone is watching.) The temperature is taken with glass thermometers, tympanic thermometers, or digital electronic probes. Further details on techniques for ensuring accuracy of the vital signs are provided in the following pages.

See Table 3-9, Abnormalities of the Arterial Pulse and Pressure Waves (p. 90). See Table 3-12 Abnormalities in Rate and Rhythm of Breathing (p. 93).

Blood Pressure

Choice of Blood Pressure Cuff (Sphygmomanometer). As many as 50 million Americans have elevated blood pressure. To measure blood pressure accurately, you must carefully choose a cuff of appropriate size. The guidelines below will help you advise patients wishing to purchase blood pressure cuffs as well.

Cuffs that are too short or too narrow may give falsely high readings. Using a regular-size cuff on an obese arm may lead to a false diagnosis of hypertension.

SELECTING THE CORRECT BLOOD PRESSURE CUFF

- Width of the inflatable bladder of the cuff should be about 40% of upper arm circumference (about 12–14 cm in the average adult)
- Length of inflatable bladder should be about 80% of upper arm circumference (almost long enough to encircle the arm)
- If anaeroid, recalibrate periodically before use

The blood pressure cuff may be either the aneroid or the mercury type. Because an aneroid instrument often becomes inaccurate with repeated use, it should be recalibrated regularly.

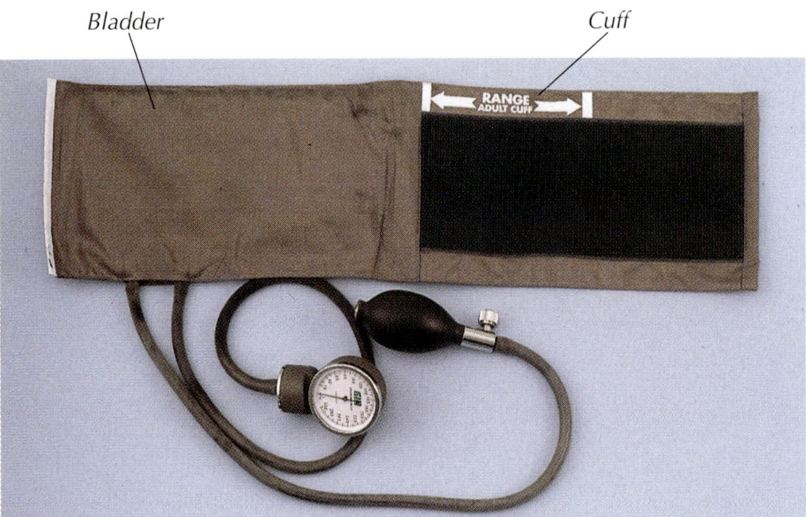

Technique. Before assessing the blood pressure, you should take several steps to make sure your measurement will be accurate. Once these steps are taken, you are ready to measure the blood pressure. Proper technique is important and reduces the inherent variability arising from the patient or examiner, the equipment, and the procedure itself.

GETTING READY TO MEASURE BLOOD PRESSURE

- Ideally, ask the patient to avoid smoking or drinking caffeinated beverages for 30 minutes before the blood pressure is taken and to rest for at least 5 minutes.
- Check to make sure the examining room is quiet and comfortably warm.
- Make sure the arm selected is *free of clothing.* There should be no arteriovenous fistulas for dialysis, scarring from prior brachial artery cutdowns, or signs of lymphedema (seen after axillary node dissection or radiation therapy).
- Palpate the brachial artery to confirm that it has a viable pulse.
- Position the arm so that the brachial artery, at the antecubital crease, is *at heart level*—roughly level with the 4th interspace at its junction with the sternum.
- If the patient is seated, rest the arm on a table a little above the patient's waist; if standing, try to support the patient's arm at the midchest level.

If the brachial artery is much below heart level, blood pressure appears falsely high. The patient's own effort to support the arm may raise the blood pressure.

Now you are ready to measure the blood pressure. Center the inflatable bladder over the brachial artery. The lower border of the cuff should be about 2.5 cm above the antecubital crease. Secure the cuff snugly. Position the patient's arm so that it is slightly flexed at the elbow.

A loose cuff or a bladder that balloons outside the cuff leads to falsely high readings.

To determine how high to raise the cuff pressure, first estimate the systolic pressure by palpation. As you feel the radial artery with the fingers of one hand, rapidly inflate the cuff until the radial pulse disappears. Read this pressure on the manometer and add 30 mm Hg to it. Use of this sum as the target for subsequent inflations prevents discomfort from unnecessarily high cuff pressures. It also avoids the occasional error caused by an auscultatory gap—a silent interval that may be present between the systolic and the diastolic pressures.

An unrecognized auscultatory gap may lead to serious underestimation of systolic pressure (e.g., 150/98 in the example below) or overestimation of diastolic pressure.

Deflate the cuff promptly and completely and wait 15 to 30 seconds.

Now place the bell of a stethoscope lightly over the brachial artery, taking care to make an air seal with its full rim. Because the sounds to be heard (*Korotkoff sounds*) are relatively low in pitch, they are heard better with the bell.

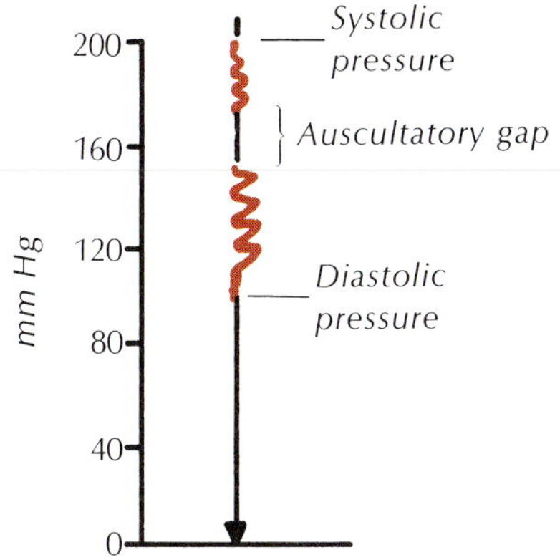

If you find an auscultatory gap, record your findings completely (e.g., 200/98 with an auscultatory gap from 170–150).

Inflate the cuff rapidly again to the level just determined, and then deflate it slowly at a rate of about 2 to 3 mm Hg per second. Note the level at which you hear the sounds of at least two consecutive beats. This is the systolic pressure.

Continue to lower the pressure slowly until the sounds become muffled and then disappear. To confirm the disappearance of sounds, listen as the pressure falls another 10 to 20 mm Hg. Then deflate the cuff rapidly to zero. The disappearance point, which is usually only a few mm Hg below the muffling point, enables the best estimate of true diastolic pressure in adults.

In some people, the muffling point and the disappearance point are farther apart. Occasionally, as in aortic regurgitation, the sounds never disappear. If there is more than 10 mm Hg difference, record both figures (e.g., 154/80/68).

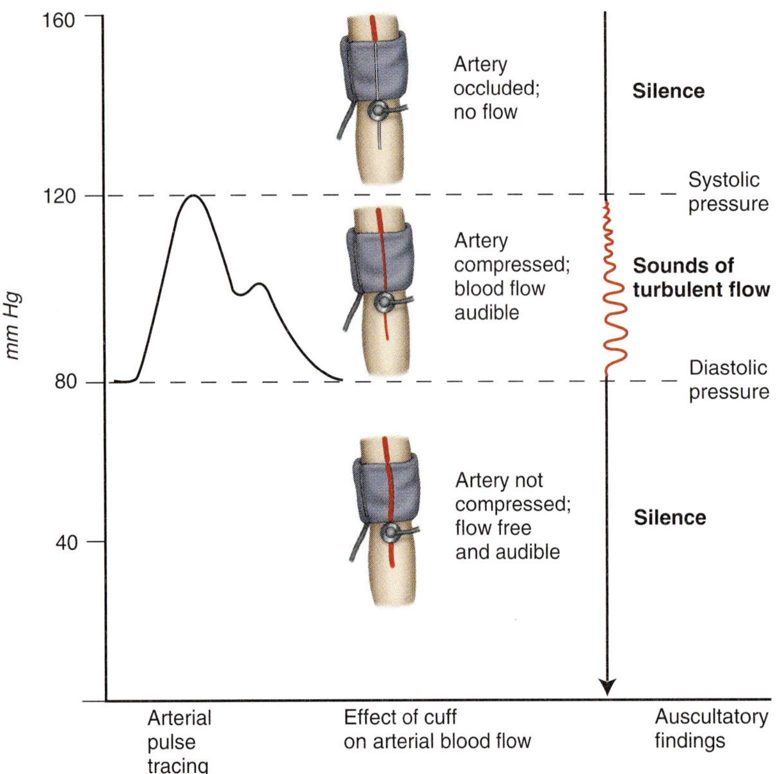

Read both the systolic and the diastolic levels to the nearest 2 mm Hg. Wait 2 or more minutes and repeat. Average your readings. If the first two readings differ by more than 5 mm Hg, take additional readings.

When using a mercury sphygmomanometer, keep the manometer vertical (unless you are using a tilted floor model) and make all readings at eye level with the meniscus. When using an aneroid instrument, hold the dial so that it faces you directly. Avoid slow or repetitive inflations of the cuff, because the resulting venous congestion can cause false readings.

By making the sounds less audible, venous congestion may produce artificially low systolic and high diastolic pressures.

Blood pressure should be taken in both arms at least once. Normally, there may be a difference in pressure of 5 mm Hg and sometimes up to 10 mm Hg. Subsequent readings should be made on the arm with the higher pressure.

Pressure difference of more than 10–15 mm Hg suggests arterial compression or obstruction on the side with the lower pressure.

In patients taking antihypertensive medications or patients with a history of fainting, postural dizziness, or possible depletion of blood volume, take the blood pressure in three positions—supine, sitting, and standing (unless contraindicated). Normally, as the patient rises from the horizontal to a standing position, systolic pressure drops slightly or remains unchanged while diastolic pressure rises slightly. Another measurement after 1 to 5 minutes of standing may identify orthostatic hypotension missed by earlier readings. This repetition is especially useful in the elderly.

A fall in systolic pressure of 20 mm Hg or more, especially when accompanied by symptoms, indicates orthostatic (postural) hypotension. Causes include drugs, loss of blood, prolonged bed rest, and diseases of the autonomic nervous system.

Definitions of Normal and Abnormal Levels. In 1997, the Joint National Committee on Detection, Evaluation, and Treatment of High Blood Pressure recommended that hypertension should be diagnosed only when a higher than normal level has been found on at least two or more visits after initial screening. Either the diastolic blood pressure (DBP) or the systolic blood pressure (SBP) may be considered high. For adults (aged 18 or over), the Committee has categorized six levels of DBP and SBP:

*Blood Pressure Classification (Adults)**

Category	Systolic (mm Hg)	Diastolic (mm Hg)
Hypertension		
Stage 3 (severe)	≥180	≥110
Stage 2 (moderate)	160–179	100–109
Stage 1 (mild)	140–159	90–99
High Normal	130–139	85–89
Normal	<130	<85
Optimal	<120	<80

*When the systolic and diastolic levels indicate different categories, use the higher category. For example, 170/92 mm Hg is moderate hypertension and 170/120 mm Hg is severe hypertension.

In *isolated systolic hypertension,* systolic pressure is 140 mm Hg or more and diastolic pressure is less than 90 mm Hg.

Assessment of hypertension also includes its effects on target organs—the eyes, the heart, the brain, and the kidneys. Look for evidence of hypertensive retinopathy, left ventricular hypertrophy, and neurologic deficits suggesting a stroke. (Renal assessment requires urinalysis and blood tests.)

Relatively low levels of blood pressure should always be interpreted in the light of past readings and the patient's present clinical state.

A pressure of 110/70 would usually be normal, but could also indicate significant hypotension if past pressures have been high.

Special Problems

The Apprehensive Patient. Anxiety is a frequent cause of high blood pressure, especially during an initial visit. Try to relax the patient. Repeat your measurements later in the encounter. Some patients will say their blood pressure is only elevated in the office ("white coat hypertension") and may need to have their blood pressure measured several times at home or in a community setting.

The Obese or Very Thin Arm. For the obese arm, it is important to use a wide cuff (15 cm). If the arm circumference exceeds 41 cm, use a thigh cuff (18 cm wide). For the very thin arm, a pediatric cuff may be indicated.

Leg Pulses and Pressures. To rule out coarctation of the aorta, two observations should be made at least once with every hypertensive patient:

- Compare the volume and timing of the radial and femoral pulses.
- Compare blood pressures in the arm and leg.

To determine blood pressure in the leg, use a wide, long thigh cuff that has a bladder size of 18 × 42 cm, and apply it to the midthigh. Center the bladder over the posterior surface, wrap it securely, and listen over the popliteal artery. If possible, the patient should be prone. Alternatively, ask the supine patient to flex one leg slightly, with the heel resting on the bed. When cuffs of the proper size are used for both the leg and the arm, blood pressures

A femoral pulse that is smaller and later than the radial pulse suggests coarctation of the aorta or occlusive aortic disease. Blood pressure is lower in the legs than in the arms in these conditions.

should be equal in the two areas. (The usual arm cuff, improperly used on the leg, gives a falsely high reading.) A systolic pressure lower in the legs than in the arms is abnormal.

Weak or Inaudible Korotkoff Sounds. Consider technical problems such as erroneous placement of your stethoscope, failure to make full skin contact with the bell, and venous engorgement of the patient's arm from repeated inflations of the cuff. Consider also the possibility of shock.

When you cannot hear Korotkoff sounds at all, you may be able to estimate the systolic pressure by palpation. Alternative methods such as Doppler techniques or direct arterial pressure tracings may be necessary.

To intensify Korotkoff sounds, one of the following methods may be helpful:

- Raise the patient's arm before and while you inflate the cuff. Then lower the arm and determine the blood pressure.
- Inflate the cuff. Ask the patient to make a fist several times, and then determine the blood pressure.

Arrhythmias. Irregular rhythms produce variations in pressure and therefore unreliable measurements. Ignore the effects of an occasional premature contraction. With frequent premature contractions or atrial fibrillation, determine the average of several observations and note that your measurements are approximate.

Heart Rate and Rhythm

By examining arterial pulses, you can count the rate of the heart and determine its rhythm, assess the amplitude and contour of the pulse wave, and sometimes detect obstructions to blood flow.

Heart Rate. The radial pulse is commonly used to assess the heart rate. With the pads of your index and middle fingers, compress the radial artery until a maximal pulsation is detected. If the rhythm is regular and the rate seems normal, count the rate for 15 seconds and multiply by 4. If the rate is unusually fast or slow, however, count it for 60 seconds.

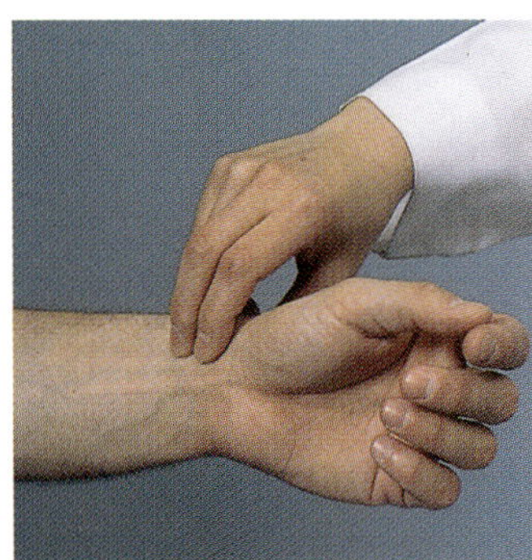

When the rhythm is irregular, the rate should be evaluated by cardiac auscultation, because beats that occur earlier than others may not be detected peripherally and the heart rate can thus be seriously underestimated.

Irregular rhythms include atrial fibrillation and atrial or ventricular premature contractions.

Rhythm. To begin your assessment of rhythm, feel the radial pulse. If there are any irregularities, check the rhythm again by listening with your stethoscope at the cardiac apex. Is the rhythm regular or irregular? If irregular, try to identify a pattern: (1) Do early beats appear in a basically regular rhythm? (2) Does the irregularity vary consistently with respiration? (3) Is the rhythm totally irregular?

Palpation of an irregularly irregular rhythm reliably indicates atrial fibrillation. For all other irregular patterns, an ECG is needed to identify the arrhythmia.

See Table 3-10, Selected Heart Rates and Rhythms (p. 91) and Table 3-11, Selected Irregular Rhythms (p. 92).

Respiratory Rate and Rhythm

Observe the *rate, rhythm, depth,* and *effort of breathing.* Count the number of respirations in 1 minute either by visual inspection or by subtly listening over the patient's trachea with your stethoscope during your examination of the head and neck or chest. Normally, adults take 14 to 20 breaths a minute in a quiet regular pattern. An occasional sigh is normal. Check to see if expiration is prolonged.

See Table 3-12, Abnormalities in Rate and Rhythm of Breathing (p. 93).

Prolonged expiration suggests narrowing in the bronchioles.

Temperature

Although you may choose to omit measuring the temperature in ambulatory patients, it should be checked whenever you suspect an abnormality. The average *oral temperature,* usually quoted at 37°C (98.6°F), fluctuates considerably. In the early morning hours it may fall as low as 35.8°C (96.4°F), and in the late afternoon or evening it may rise as high as 37.3°C (99.1°F). *Rectal temperatures* are *higher* than oral temperatures by an average of 0.4 to 0.5°C (0.7 to 0.9°F), but this difference is also quite variable. (In contrast, *axillary temperatures* are *lower* than oral temperatures by approximately 1 degree, but take 5 to 10 minutes to register and are generally considered less accurate than other measurements.)

Fever or pyrexia refers to an elevated body temperature. *Hyperpyrexia* refers to extreme elevation in temperature, above 41.1°C (106°F), while *hypothermia* refers to an abnormally low temperature, below 35°C (95°F) rectally.

Most patients prefer oral to rectal temperatures. However, taking oral temperatures is not recommended when patients are unconscious, restless, or unable to close their mouths. Temperature readings may be inaccurate and thermometers may be broken by unexpected movements of the patient's jaws.

Rapid respiratory rates tend to increase the discrepancy between oral and rectal temperatures. In this situation, rectal temperatures are more reliable.

For *oral temperatures,* you may choose either a glass or electronic thermometer. When using a glass thermometer, shake the thermometer down to 35°C (96°F) or below, insert it under the tongue, instruct the patient to close both lips, and wait 3 to 5 minutes. Then read the thermometer, reinsert it for a minute, and read it again. If the temperature is still rising, repeat this procedure until the reading remains stable. Note that hot or cold liquids, and even smoking, can alter the temperature reading. In these situations it is best to delay measuring the temperature for 10 to 15 minutes.

Causes of *fever* include infection, trauma (such as surgery or crush injuries), malignancy, blood disorders (such as acute hemolytic anemia), drug reactions, and immune disorders (such as collagen vascular disease).

If using an electronic thermometer, carefully place the disposable cover over the probe and insert the thermometer under the tongue. Ask the patient to close both lips, and then watch closely for the digital readout. An accurate temperature recording usually takes about 10 seconds.

For a *rectal temperature*, ask the patient to lie on one side with the hip flexed. Select a rectal thermometer with a stubby tip, lubricate it, and insert it about 3 cm to 4 cm (1½ inches) into the anal canal, in a direction pointing to the umbilicus. Remove it after 3 minutes, then read. Alternatively, use an electronic thermometer after lubricating the probe cover. Wait about 10 seconds for the digital temperature recording to appear.

Taking the *tympanic membrane temperature* is an increasingly common practice and is quick, safe, and reliable if performed properly. Make sure the external auditory canal is free of cerumen. Position the probe in the canal so that the infrared beam is aimed at the tympanic membrane (otherwise the measurement will be invalid). Wait 2 to 3 seconds until the digital temperature reading appears. This method measures core body temperature, which is higher than the normal oral temperature by approximately 0.8°C (1.4°F).

The chief cause of *hypothermia* is exposure to cold. Other predisposing causes include reduced movement as in paralysis, interference with vasoconstriction as from sepsis or excess alcohol, starvation, hypothyroidism, and hypoglycemia. Elderly people are especially susceptible to hypothermia and also less likely to develop fever.

TABLE 3-1 ■ Height and Weight Tables for Adults Age 25 and Over

Height (without shoes)	Weight in Pounds (without clothing)		
	Small Frame	*Medium Frame*	*Large Frame*
Men			
5′1″	105–113	111–122	119–134
5′2″	108–116	114–126	122–137
5′3″	111–119	117–129	125–141
5′4″	114–122	120–132	128–145
5′5″	117–126	123–136	131–149
5′6″	121–130	127–140	135–154
5′7″	125–134	131–145	140–159
5′8″	129–138	135–149	144–163
5′9″	133–143	139–153	148–167
5′10″	137–147	143–158	152–172
5′11″	141–151	147–163	157–177
6′0″	145–155	151–168	161–182
6′1″	149–160	155–173	168–187
6′2″	153–164	160–178	171–192
6′3″	157–168	165–183	175–197
Women			
4′9″	90–97	94–106	102–118
4′10″	92–100	97–109	106–121
4′11″	95–103	100–112	108–124
5′0″	98–106	103–116	111–127
5′1″	101–109	106–118	114–130
5′2″	104–112	109–122	117–134
5′3″	107–115	112–126	121–138
5′4″	110–119	116–131	125–142
5′5″	114–123	120–136	129–146
5′6″	118–127	124–139	133–150
5′7″	122–131	128–143	137–154
5′8″	126–136	132–147	141–159
5′9″	130–140	136–151	145–164
5′10″	134–144	140–155	149–169

From Clinician's Handbook of Preventive Services. Washington, DC: U.S. Department of Health and Human Services, 1994:142–143.

These data are derived from an insured population. Note that assessment of the size of the body frame is subjective and must be estimated visually. Weights at the lower end of the range of normal may be advisable for patients with cardiovascular disease and diabetes.

TABLE 3-2 ■ Healthy Eating: Food Groups and Servings per Day

Food Group	Women, Some Older Adults, Children Ages 2–6 yrs (about 1,600 cal)*	Active Women, Most Men, Older Children, Teen Girls (about 2,200 cal)*	Active Men, Teen Boys (about 2,800 cal)*
Bread, rice, cereal, pasta (grains) group, especially whole grain	6	9	11
Vegetable group	3	4	5
Fruit group	2	3	4
Milk, yogurt, and cheese (dairy) group—preferably fat free or low fat	2–3**	2–3**	2–3**
Dry beans, eggs, nuts, fish, and meat and poultry group—preferably lean or low fat	2, for a total of 5 oz	2, for a total of 6 oz	3, for a total of 7 oz

Source: Adapted from U.S. Department of Agriculture, Center for Nutrition Policy and Promotion. The Food Guide Pyramid, Home and Garden Bulletin Number 252, 1996.
*These are the calorie levels if low-fat, lean foods are chosen from the 5 major food groups and foods from the fats, oil, and sweets group are used sparingly.
**Older children and teenagers (ages 9–18 yrs) and adults over the age of 50 need 3 servings daily. During pregnancy and lactation, the recommended number of dairy group servings is the same as for nonpregnant women.

TABLE 3-3 ■ Rapid Screen for Dietary Intake

	Portions Consumed by Patient	Recommended
Grains, cereals, bread group	_____	6–11
Fruit group	_____	2–4
Vegetable group	_____	3–5
Meat/meat substitute group	_____	2–3
Dairy group	_____	2–3
Sugars, fats, snack foods	_____	—
Soft drinks	_____	—
Alcoholic beverages	_____	<2

Instructions. Ask the patient for a 24-hour dietary recall (perhaps two of these) before completing the form.

Source: Nestle M. Nutrition. In: Woolf SH, Jonas S, Lawrence RS, eds. *Health Promotion and Disease Prevention in Clinical Practice.* Baltimore: Williams & Wilkins, 1996.

TABLE 3-4 ■ Nutrition Screening Checklist

I have an illness or condition that made me change the kind and/or amount of food I eat.	Yes (2 pts) _____
I eat fewer than 2 meals per day.	Yes (3 pts) _____
I eat few fruits or vegetables, or milk products.	Yes (2 pts) _____
I have 3 or more drinks of beer, liquor, or wine almost every day.	Yes (2 pts) _____
I have tooth or mouth problems that make it hard for me to eat.	Yes (2 pts) _____
I don't always have enough money to buy the food I need.	Yes (4 pts) _____
I eat alone most of the time.	Yes (1 pt) _____
I take 3 or more different prescribed or over-the-counter drugs each day.	Yes (1 pt) _____
Without wanting to, I have lost or gained 10 pounds in the last 6 months.	Yes (2 pts) _____
I am not always physically able to shop, cook and/or feed myself.	Yes (2 pts) _____
	TOTAL _____

Instructions. Check "yes" for each condition that applies, then total the nutritional score. For total scores between 3–5 points (moderate risk) or ≥6 points (high risk), further evaluation is needed (especially for the elderly).

Source: The Nutrition Screening Initiative, American Academy of Family Physicians. *aafp.org/nsi/e-check1.html.* Accessed 7/22/01.

TABLE 3-5 ■ Food Guide Pyramid: A Guide to Daily Food Choices

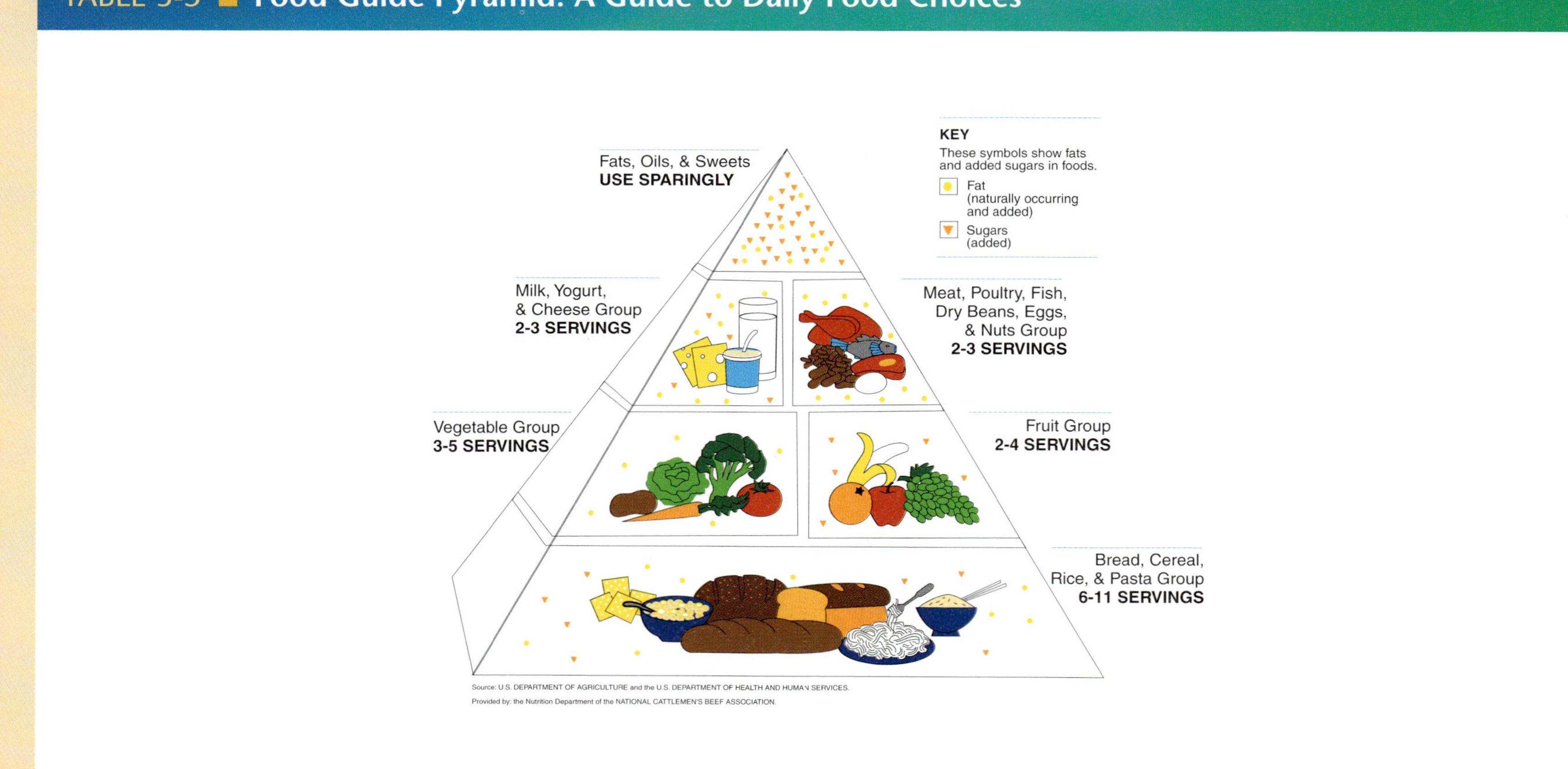

TABLE 3-5 ■ Food Guide Pyramid: A Guide to Daily Food Choices

How Many Servings Do You Need?

The *Food Guide Pyramid* shows a range of daily servings for each food group. The number of servings that is right for you depends on how many calories you need. Calories are a way to measure food energy. The energy your body needs depends on your age, sex, and size. It also depends on how active you are.

In general, daily intake should be:

- 1,600 calories for most women and older adults
- 2,200 calories for children, teen girls, active women, and most men
- 2,800 calories for teen boys and active men.

Those with lower calorie needs should select the lower number of servings from each food group. Their diet should include 2 servings of protein for a total of 5 ounces. Those with average calorie needs should select the middle number of servings from each food group. They should include 2 servings of protein for a total of 6 ounces. Those with higher calorie needs should select the higher number of servings from each food group. Their diet should include 3 servings of protein for a total of 7 ounces. Also, pregnant or breast-feeding women, teens, and young adults up to age 24 should consume 3 servings of dairy foods daily.

The amount of food that counts as one serving is listed below. If you eat a larger portion, it is more than one serving. For example a slice of bread is one serving. A hamburger bun is two servings.

For mixed foods, estimate the food group servings of the main ingredients. For example, a large piece of sausage pizza would count in the bread group (crust), the milk group (cheese), the meat group (sausage), and the vegetable group (tomato sauce). Likewise, a helping of beef stew would count in the meat group and the vegetable group.

What Counts as a Serving?

Bread, Cereal, Rice, & Pasta	*Vegetable*	*Fruit*	*Milk, Yogurt, & Cheese*	*Meat, Poultry, Fish, Dry Beans, Eggs, & Nuts*	*Fats, Oils, & Sweets*
1 slice bread 1 tortilla ½ c cooked rice, pasta or cereal 1 oz ready-to-eat cereal ½ hamburger roll, bagel or English muffin 3–4 plain crackers (sm) 1 pancake (4″) ½ croissant (lg) ½ doughnut or danish (med) 1/16 cake (average) 2 cookies (med) 1/12 pie (2-crust, 8″)	½ c chopped raw or cooked vegetables 1 c raw, leafy vegetables ¾ c vegetable juice ½ c scalloped potatoes ½ c potato salad 10 French fries	1 piece fruit or melon wedge ¾ c fruit juice ½ c chopped, cooked or canned fruit ¼ c dried fruit	1 c milk or yogurt 1½ oz natural cheese 2 oz process cheese 1½ c ice cream or ice milk 1 c frozen yogurt	2 ½ to 3 oz cooked lean beef, pork, lamb, veal, poultry or fish ½ c cooked beans or 1 egg or 2 T peanut butter or ⅓ c nuts count as 1 oz of meat *Lean Beef Choices* Eye of round Top round Round tip Top sirloin Bottom round Top loin Tenderloin	Use sparingly

Adapted from U.S. Department of Agriculture, Human Nutrition Service. The Food Guide Pyramid, Home and Garden Bulletin Number 252, 1996.

TABLE 3-6 ■ Eating Disorders and Excessively Low BMI

In the United States an estimated 5 to 10 million women and one million men suffer from eating disorders. These severe disturbances of eating behavior are often difficult to detect, especially in teens wearing baggy clothes, or in individuals who binge then induce vomiting or evacuation. Be familiar with the two principal eating disorders, *anorexia nervosa* and *bulimia nervosa*. Both conditions are characterized by distorted perceptions of body image and weight. Early detection is important, since prognosis improves when treatment occurs in the early stages of these disorders.

Clinical Features

Anorexia Nervosa

- Refusal to maintain minimally normal body weight (or BMI above 17.5 kg/m^2)
- Afraid of appearing fat
- Frequently starving but in denial; lacking insight
- Often brought in by family members
- May present as failure to make expected weight gains in childhood or adolescence, amenorrhea in women, loss of libido or potency in men
- Associated with depressive symptoms such as depressed mood, irritability, social withdrawal, insomnia, decreased libido
- Additional features supporting diagnosis: self-induced vomiting or purging, excessive exercise, use of appetite suppressants and/or diuretics
- Biological complications
  - *Neuroendocrine changes:* amenorrhea, increased corticotropin-releasing factor, cortisol, growth hormone, serotonin; decreased diurnal cortisol fluctuation, luteinizing hormone, follicle-stimulating hormone, thyroid-stimulating hormone
  - *Cardiovascular disorders:* bradycardia, hypotension, arrhythmias, cardiomyopathy
  - *Metabolic disorders:* hypokalemia, hypochloremic metabolic alkalosis, increased BUN, edema
  - *Other:* dry skin, dental caries, delayed gastric emptying, constipation, anemia, osteoporosis

Bulimia Nervosa

- Repeated binge eating followed by self-induced vomiting, misuse of laxatives, diuretics or other medications, fasting; or excessive exercise
- Overeating at least twice a week during 3-month period; large amounts of food consumed in short period (~2 hrs)
- Preoccupation with eating; craving and compulsion to eat; lack of control over eating; alternating with periods of starvation
- Dread of fatness but may be obese
- Subtypes of
  - *Purging:* bulimic episodes accompanied by self-induced vomiting or use of laxatives, diuretics, or enemas
  - *Nonpurging:* bulimic episodes accompanied by compensatory behavior such as fasting, exercise but without purging
- Biological complications

  See changes listed for anorexia nervosa, especially weakness, fatigue, mild cognitive disorder; also erosion of dental enamel, parotitis, pancreatic inflammation with elevated amylase, mild neuropathies, seizures, hypokalemia, hypochloremic metabolic acidosis, hypomagnesemia

Sources: World Health Organization: The ICD-10 Classification of Mental and Behavioral Disorders: Diagnostic Criteria for Research. At World Health Organization, Geneva, 1993. American Psychiatric Association: DSM-IV-TR: Diagnostic and Statistical Manual of Mental Disorders, 4th ed. American Psychiatric Association, Washington, DC, 1994. Halmi, KA: Eating Disorders: In: Kaplan, HI, Sadock BJ, eds. Comprehensive Textbook of Psychiatry, 7th ed. Philadelphia, Lippincott Williams & Wilkins; 2000:1663–1676.

TABLE 3-7 ■ Nutrition Counseling: Sources of Nutrients

Nutrient	Food Source
Calcium	Dairy foods such as yogurt, milk, and natural cheeses Breakfast cereal, fruit juice with calcium supplements Dark green leafy vegetables such as collards, turnip greens
Iron	Shellfish Lean meat, dark turkey meat Cereals with iron supplements Spinach, peas, lentils Enriched and whole-grain bread
Folate	Cooked dried beans and peas Oranges, orange juice Dark-green leafy vegetables
Vitamin D	Milk (fortified) Eggs, butter, margarine Cereals (fortified)

Source: Adapted from Dietary Guidelines Committee, 2000 Report. "Nutrition and Your Health: Dietary Guidelines for Americans," Washington, DC, Agricultural Research Service, U.S. Department of Agriculture.

TABLE 3-8 ■ Patients With Hypertension: Recommended Changes in Diet

Dietary Change	Food Source
Increase foods high in potassium	Baked white or sweet potatoes, cooked greens such as spinach Bananas, plantains, many dried fruits, orange juice
Decrease foods high in sodium	Canned foods (soups, tuna fish) Pretzels, potato chips, pickles, olives Many processed foods (frozen dinners, ketchup, mustard) Batter-fried foods Table salt, including for cooking

Source: Adapted from Dietary Guidelines Committee, 2000 Report. "Nutrition and Your Health: Dietary Guidelines for Americans," Washington, DC, Agricultural Research Service, U.S. Department of Agriculture.

TABLE 3-9 ■ Abnormalities of the Arterial Pulse and Pressure Waves

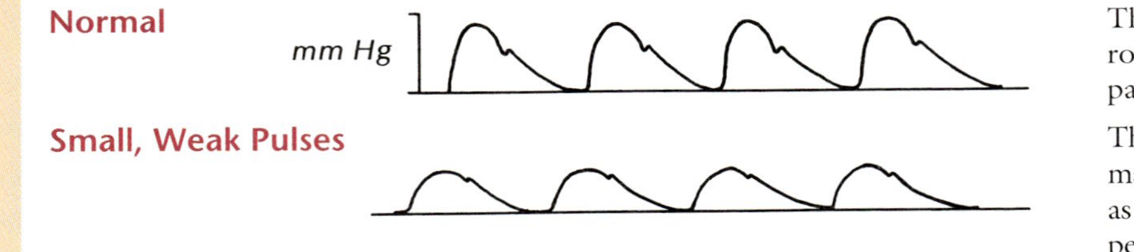

Normal

The pulse pressure is about 30–40 mm Hg. The pulse contour is smooth and rounded. (The notch on the descending slope of the pulse wave is not palpable.)

Small, Weak Pulses

The pulse pressure is diminished, and the pulse feels weak and small. The upstroke may feel slowed, the peak prolonged. Causes include (1) decreased stroke volume, as in heart failure, hypovolemia, and severe aortic stenosis, and (2) increased peripheral resistance, as in exposure to cold and severe congestive heart failure.

Large, Bounding Pulses

The pulse pressure is increased and the pulse feels strong and bounding. The rise and fall may feel rapid, the peak brief. Causes include (1) an increased stroke volume, a decreased peripheral resistance, or both, as in fever, anemia, hyperthyroidism, aortic regurgitation, arteriovenous fistulas, and patent ductus arteriosus, (2) an increased stroke volume due to slow heart rates, as in bradycardia and complete heart block, and (3) decreased compliance (increased stiffness) of the aortic walls, as in aging or atherosclerosis.

Bisferiens Pulse

A bisferiens pulse is an increased arterial pulse with a double systolic peak. Causes include pure aortic regurgitation, combined aortic stenosis and regurgitation, and, though less commonly palpable, hypertrophic cardiomyopathy.

Pulsus Alternans

The pulse alternates in amplitude from beat to beat even though the rhythm is basically regular (and must be for you to make this judgment). When the difference between stronger and weaker beats is slight, it can be detected only by sphygmomanometry. Pulsus alternans indicates left ventricular failure and is usually accompanied by a left-sided S_3.

Bigeminal Pulse

Premature contractions

This is a disorder of rhythm that may masquerade as pulsus alternans. A bigeminal pulse is caused by a normal beat alternating with a premature contraction. The stroke volume of the premature beat is diminished in relation to that of the normal beats, and the pulse varies in amplitude accordingly.

Paradoxical Pulse

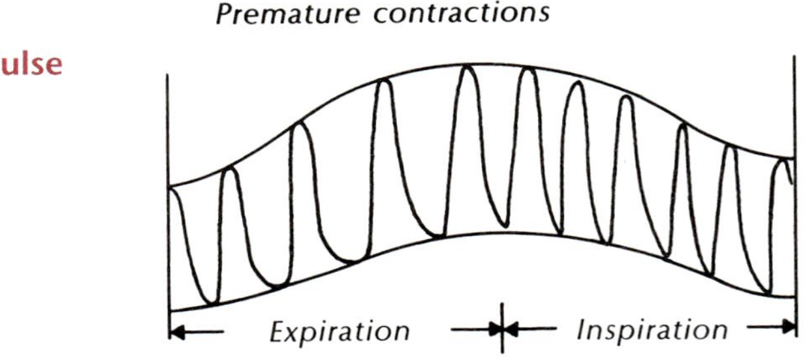

A paradoxical pulse may be detected by a palpable decrease in the pulse's amplitude on quiet inspiration. If the sign is less pronounced, a blood-pressure cuff is needed. Systolic pressure decreases by more than 10 mm Hg during inspiration. A paradoxical pulse is found in pericardial tamponade, constrictive pericarditis (though less commonly), and obstructive lung disease.

TABLE 3-10 ■ Selected Heart Rates and Rhythms

Cardiac rhythms may be classified as regular or irregular. When rhythms are irregular or rates are fast or slow, an ECG is required to identify the origin of the beats (sinus node, AV node, atrium, or ventricle) and the pattern of conduction. Note that with AV (atrioventricular) block, arrhythmias may have a fast, normal, or slow ventricular rate.

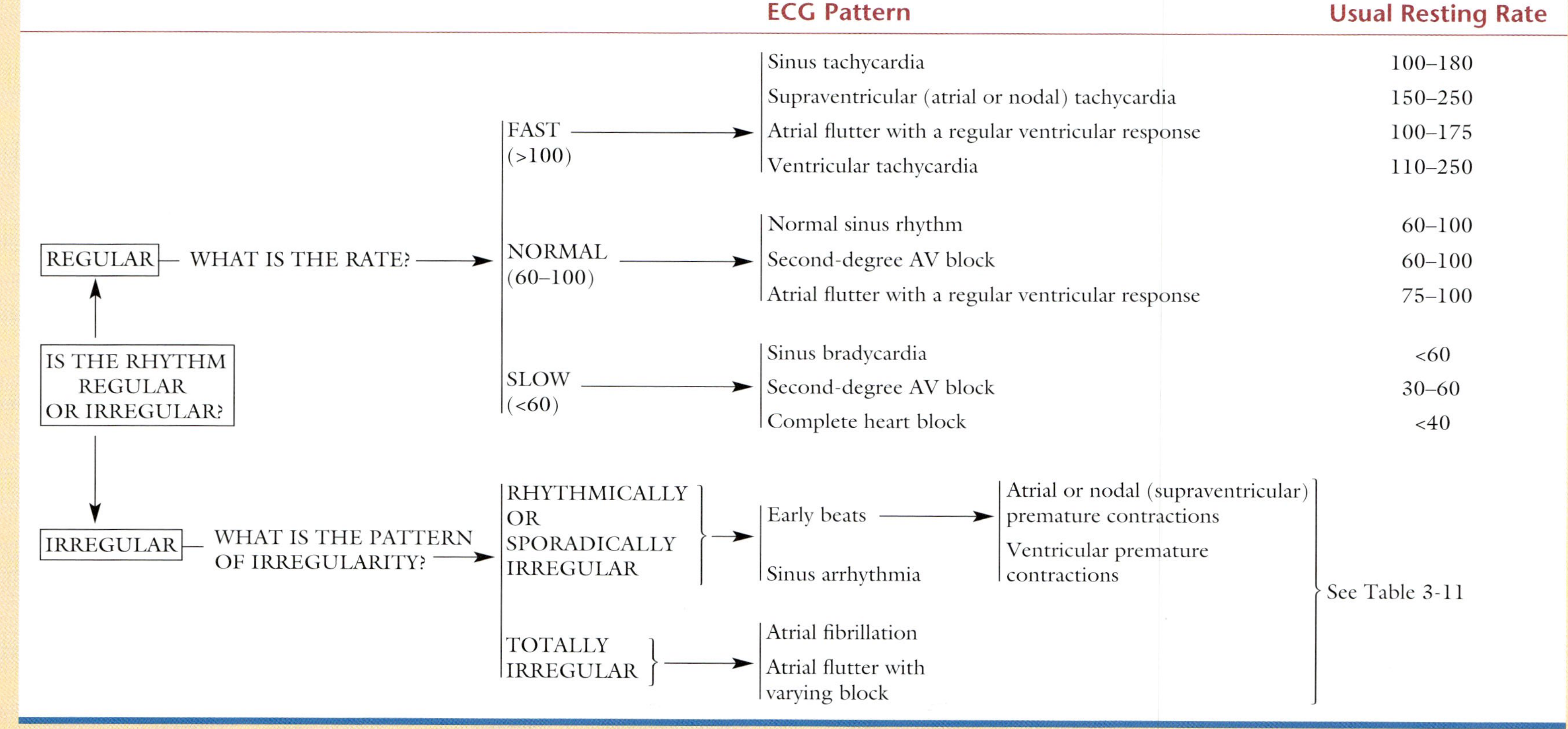

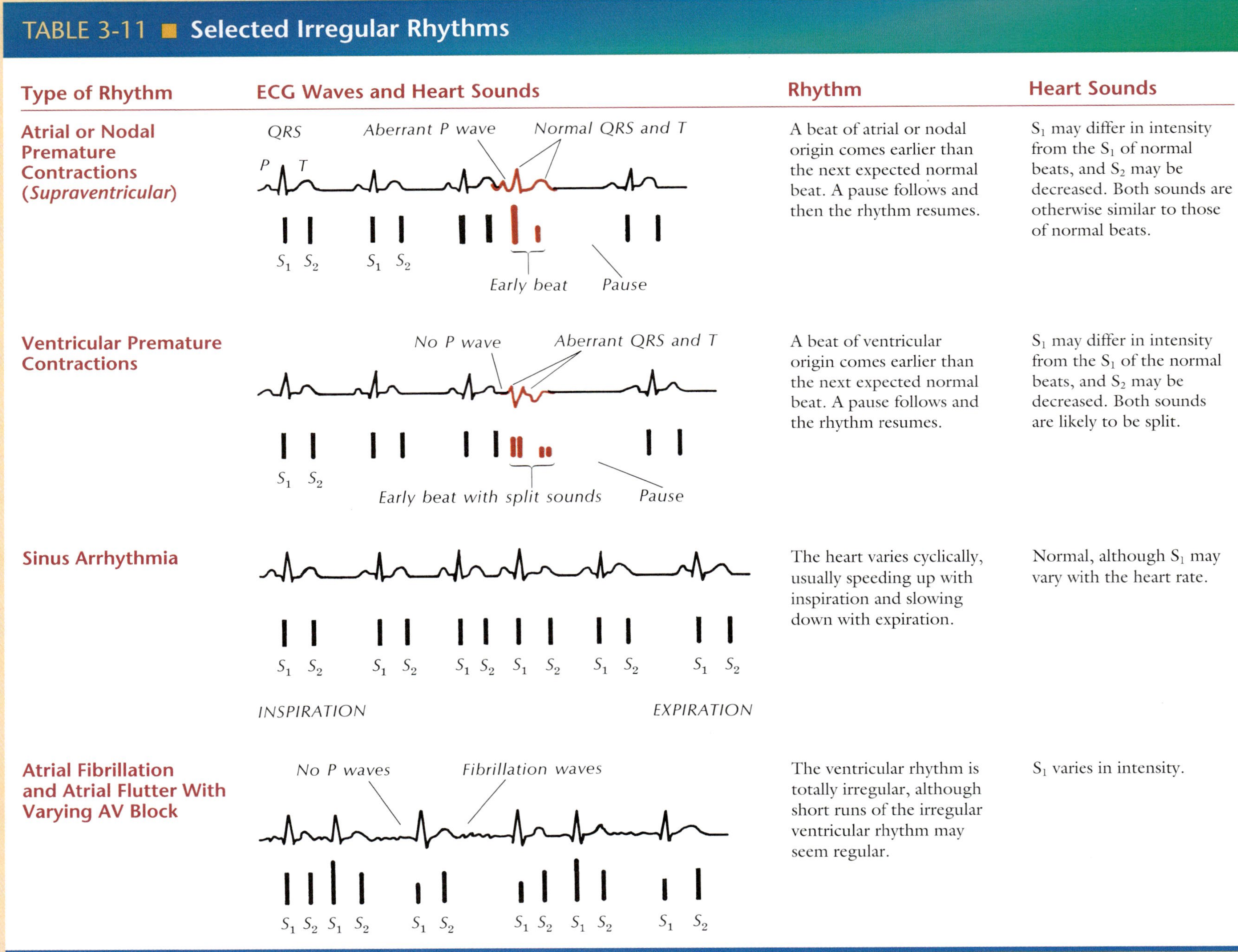

TABLE 3-11 ■ Selected Irregular Rhythms

Type of Rhythm	ECG Waves and Heart Sounds	Rhythm	Heart Sounds
Atrial or Nodal Premature Contractions (*Supraventricular*)	*QRS, P, T, Aberrant P wave, Normal QRS and T; S_1 S_2, S_1 S_2; Early beat, Pause*	A beat of atrial or nodal origin comes earlier than the next expected normal beat. A pause follows and then the rhythm resumes.	S_1 may differ in intensity from the S_1 of normal beats, and S_2 may be decreased. Both sounds are otherwise similar to those of normal beats.
Ventricular Premature Contractions	*No P wave, Aberrant QRS and T; S_1 S_2; Early beat with split sounds, Pause*	A beat of ventricular origin comes earlier than the next expected normal beat. A pause follows and the rhythm resumes.	S_1 may differ in intensity from the S_1 of the normal beats, and S_2 may be decreased. Both sounds are likely to be split.
Sinus Arrhythmia	*S_1 S_2, S_1 S_2, S_1 S_2, S_1 S_2, S_1 S_2, S_1 S_2; INSPIRATION, EXPIRATION*	The heart varies cyclically, usually speeding up with inspiration and slowing down with expiration.	Normal, although S_1 may vary with the heart rate.
Atrial Fibrillation and Atrial Flutter With Varying AV Block	*No P waves, Fibrillation waves; S_1 S_2 S_1 S_2, S_1 S_2, S_1 S_2 S_1 S_2, S_1 S_2*	The ventricular rhythm is totally irregular, although short runs of the irregular ventricular rhythm may seem regular.	S_1 varies in intensity.

TABLE 3-12 ■ Abnormalities in Rate and Rhythm of Breathing

When observing respiratory patterns, think in terms of *rate, depth,* and *regularity* of the patient's breathing. Describe what you see in these terms. Traditional terms, such as tachypnea, are given below so that you will understand them, but simple descriptions are recommended for use.

Normal

The respiratory rate is about 14–20 per min in normal adults and up to 44 per min in infants.

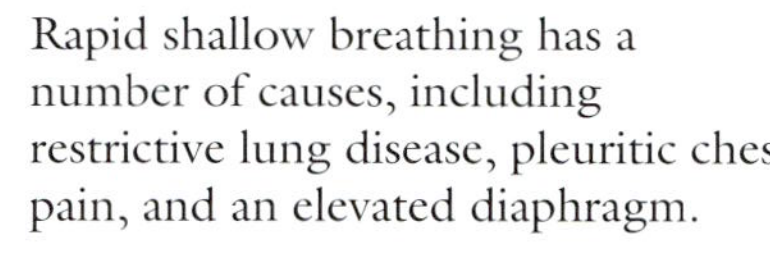

Rapid Shallow Breathing (*Tachypnea*)

Rapid shallow breathing has a number of causes, including restrictive lung disease, pleuritic chest pain, and an elevated diaphragm.

Rapid Deep Breathing (*Hyperpnea, Hyperventilation*)

Rapid deep breathing has several causes, including exercise, anxiety, and metabolic acidosis. In the comatose patient, consider infarction, hypoxia, or hypoglycemia affecting the midbrain or pons. *Kussmaul breathing* is deep breathing due to metabolic acidosis. It may be fast, normal in rate, or slow.

Slow Breathing (*Bradypnea*)

Slow breathing may be secondary to such causes as diabetic coma, drug-induced respiratory depression, and increased intracranial pressure.

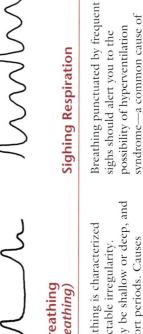

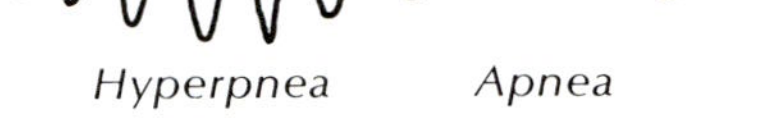

Cheyne–Stokes Breathing

Periods of deep breathing alternate with periods of apnea (no breathing). Children and aging people normally may show this pattern in sleep. Other causes include heart failure, uremia, drug-induced respiratory depression, and brain damage (typically on both sides of the cerebral hemispheres or diencephalon).

Ataxic Breathing (*Biot's Breathing*)

Ataxic breathing is characterized by unpredictable irregularity. Breaths may be shallow or deep, and stop for short periods. Causes include respiratory depression and brain damage, typically at the medullary level.

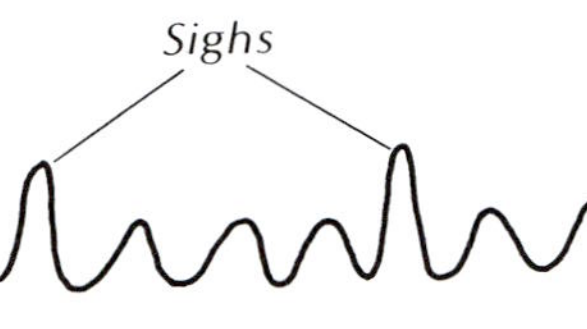

Sighing Respiration

Breathing punctuated by frequent sighs should alert you to the possibility of hyperventilation syndrome—a common cause of dyspnea and dizziness. Occasional sighs are normal.

Obstructive Breathing

In obstructive lung disease, expiration is prolonged because narrowed airways increase the resistance to air flow. Causes include asthma, chronic bronchitis, and COPD.

CHAPTER

4

The Skin

ANATOMY AND PHYSIOLOGY

The major function of the skin is to keep the body in homeostasis despite the daily assaults of the environment. It provides boundaries for body fluids while protecting underlying tissues from microorganisms, harmful substances, and radiation. It modulates body temperature and synthesizes vitamin D.

The skin is the heaviest single organ of the body, accounting for approximately 16% of body weight and covering an area of roughly 1.2 to 2.3 meters squared. It contains three layers: the epidermis, the dermis, and the subcutaneous tissues.

The most superficial layer, the *epidermis,* is thin, devoid of blood vessels, and itself divided into two layers: an outer horny layer of dead keratinized cells and an inner cellular layer where both melanin and keratin are formed.

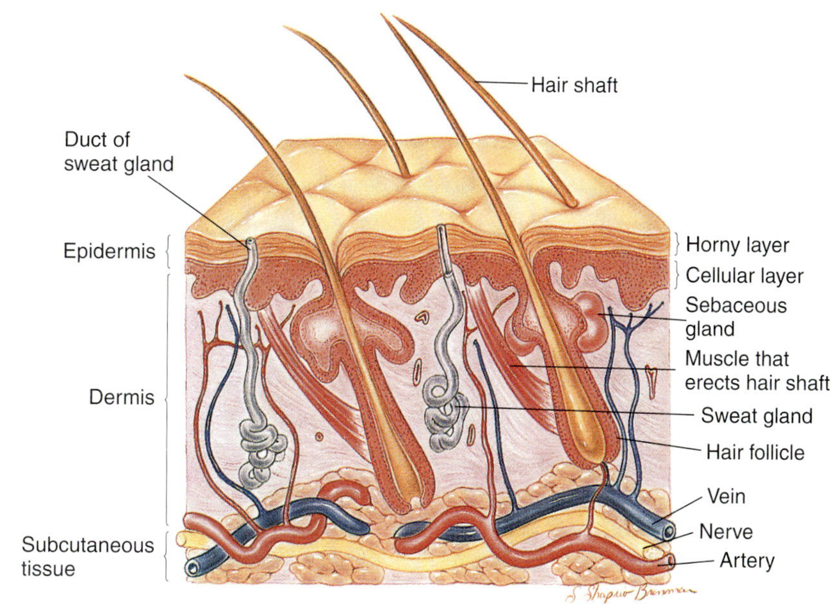

The epidermis depends on the underlying *dermis* for its nutrition. The dermis is well supplied with blood. It contains connective tissue, sebaceous glands, sweat glands, and hair follicles. It merges below with *subcutaneous tissue,* or *adipose,* also known as fat.

Hair, nails, and *sebaceous* and *sweat glands* are considered appendages of the skin. Adults have two types of hair: *vellus hair,* which is short, fine, inconspicuous, and relatively unpigmented; and *terminal hair,* which is coarser, thicker, more conspicuous, and usually pigmented. Scalp hair and eyebrows are examples of terminal hair.

Nails protect the distal ends of the fingers and toes. The firm, rectangular, and usually curving *nail plate* gets its pink color from the vascular *nail bed* to which the plate is firmly attached. Note the whitish moon (*lunula*) and the free edge of the nail plate. Roughly a fourth of the nail plate (the *nail root*) is covered by the *proximal nail fold*. The *cuticle* extends from this fold and, functioning as a seal, protects the space between the fold and the plate from external moisture. *Lateral nail folds* cover the sides of the nail plate. Note that the angle between the proximal nail fold and the nail plate is normally less than 180°.

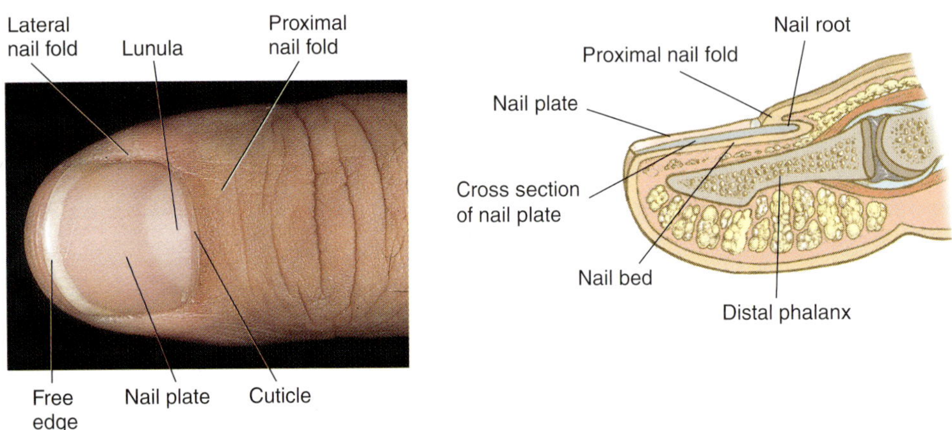

Fingernails grow at about 0.1 mm daily; toenails grow more slowly.

Sebaceous glands produce a fatty substance that is secreted onto the skin surface through the hair follicles. These glands are present on all skin surfaces except the palms and soles. *Sweat glands* are of two types: eccrine and apocrine. The *eccrine glands* are widely distributed, open directly onto the skin surface, and by their sweat production help to control body temperature. In contrast, the *apocrine glands* are found chiefly in the axillary and genital regions, usually open into hair follicles, and are stimulated by emotional stress. Bacterial decomposition of apocrine sweat is responsible for adult body odor.

The color of normal skin depends primarily on four pigments: melanin, carotene, oxyhemoglobin, and deoxyhemoglobin. The amount of *melanin*, the brownish pigment of the skin, is genetically determined and is increased by sunlight. *Carotene* is a golden yellow pigment that exists in subcutaneous fat and in heavily keratinized areas such as the palms and soles.

Hemoglobin, which circulates in the red cells and carries most of the oxygen of the blood, exists in two forms. *Oxyhemoglobin,* a bright red pigment, predominates in the arteries and capillaries. An increase in blood flow through the arteries to the capillaries of the skin causes a reddening of the skin, while the opposite change usually produces pallor. The skin of light-colored persons is normally redder on the palms, soles, face, neck, and upper chest.

As blood passes through the capillary bed, some of the oxyhemoglobin loses its oxygen to the tissues and changes to *deoxyhemoglobin*—a darker and somewhat bluer pigment. An increased concentration of deoxyhemoglobin in cutaneous blood vessels gives the skin a bluish cast known as *cyanosis.*

Cyanosis is of two kinds, depending on the oxygen level in the arterial blood. If this level is low, cyanosis is *central.* If it is normal, cyanosis is *peripheral.* Peripheral cyanosis occurs when cutaneous blood flow decreases and slows, and tissues extract more oxygen than usual from the blood. Peripheral cyanosis may be a normal response to anxiety or a cold environment.

Skin color is affected not only by pigments but also by the scattering of light as it is reflected back through the turbid superficial layers of the skin or vessel walls. This scattering makes the color look more blue and less red. The bluish color of a subcutaneous vein is a result of this effect; it is much bluer than the venous blood obtained on venipuncture.

Changes With Aging

As people age their skin wrinkles, becomes lax, and loses turgor. The vascularity of the dermis decreases and the skin of light-skinned persons tends to look paler and more opaque. *Comedones* (blackheads) often appear on the cheeks or around the eyes. Where skin has been exposed to the sun it looks weatherbeaten: thickened, yellowed, and deeply furrowed. Skin on the backs of the hands and forearms appears thin, fragile, loose, and transparent, and may show whitish, depigmented patches known as pseudoscars. Well-demarcated, vividly purple macules or patches, termed actinic purpura, may also appear in the same areas, fading after several weeks. These purpuric spots come from blood that has leaked through poorly supported capillaries and has spread within the dermis. Dry skin (asteatosis)—a common problem—is flaky, rough, and often itchy. It is frequently shiny, especially on the legs, where a network of shallow fissures often creates a mosaic of small polygons.

Some common benign lesions often accompany aging: cherry angiomas (p. 106), which often appear early in adulthood, seborrheic keratoses (p. 107), and, in sun-exposed areas, actinic lentigines or "liver spots" and actinic keratoses (p. 107). Elderly people may also develop two common skin cancers: basal cell carcinoma and squamous cell carcinoma (p. 107).

Nails lose some of their luster with age and may yellow and thicken, especially on the toes.

Hair on the scalp loses its pigment, producing the well-known graying. As early as 20, a man's hairline may start to recede at the temples; hair loss at the vertex follows. Many women show a less severe loss of hair in a similar pattern. Hair loss in this distribution is genetically determined.

In both sexes, the number of scalp hairs decreases in a generalized pattern, and the diameter of each hair diminishes.

Less familiar, but probably more important clinically, is the normal hair loss elsewhere on the body: the trunk, pubic areas, axillae, and limbs.

These changes will be discussed in later chapters. Coarse facial hairs appear on the chin and upper lip of many women by about the age of 55, but do not increase further thereafter.

Many of the observations described here pertain to lighter-skinned persons and do not necessarily apply to others. For example, Native American men have relatively little facial and body hair compared to lighter-skinned men, and should be evaluated according to their own norms.

THE HEALTH HISTORY

Common or Concerning Symptoms

- Hair loss
- Rash
- Moles

Start your inquiry about the skin with a few open-ended questions: "Have you noticed any changes in your skin?". . . your hair? . . . your nails?. . . "Have you had any rashes? . . . sores? . . . lumps? . . . itching?" "Have you noticed any moles that have changed in appearance?" "Where?" "When?"

Causes of generalized itching without obvious reason include dry skin, aging, pregnancy, uremia, jaundice, lymphomas and leukemia, drug reaction, and lice.

It is usually best to defer further questions about the skin until the physical examination, when you can see what the patient is talking about.

HEALTH PROMOTION AND COUNSELING

Important Topics for Health Promotion and Counseling

- Risk factors for melanoma
- Avoidance of excessive sun exposure

Clinicians play an important role in counseling patients about protective measures for skin care and the hazards of excessive sun exposure. Basal cell and squamous cell carcinomas are the most common cancers in the United States and are found most frequently in sun-exposed areas, particularly the head, neck, and hands. Malignant melanoma, although rare, is the most rapidly increasing U.S. malignancy, now occurring in 1 in 74 Americans. Although melanoma often arises in non–sun-exposed areas, it is associated with intermittent and intense sun exposure and blistering sunburns in childhood. Other risk factors include family history of melanoma, light skin, presence of atypical moles (dysplastic nevi) or ≥50 common moles, and immunosuppression.

Protective measures are three-fold: avoiding unnecessary sun exposure, using sunscreen, and inspecting the skin. Caution patients to minimize direct sun exposure, especially at midday when ultraviolet B rays (UV-B), the most common cause of skin cancer, are most intense. Sunscreens fall into two categories—thick pastelike ointments that block all solar rays, and light-absorbing sunscreens rated by "sun protective factor" (SPF). The SPF is a ratio of the number of minutes for treated versus untreated skin to redden with exposure to UV-B. An SPF of at least 15 is recommended and protects against 93% of UV-B. (There is no scale for UV-A, which causes photoaging, or UV-C, the most carcinogenic ray but blocked in the atmosphere by ozone.) Water-resistant sunscreens that remain on the skin for prolonged periods are preferable.

Detection of skin cancer rests on visual inspection, preferably of the total body surface. Current detection rates are higher for clinicians than patients, but the benefits of self-examination are not well studied. Recommendations about screening intervals are variable. The American Cancer Society recommends monthly self-examination, clinician screening at 3-year intervals for persons aged 20 to 39, and annual clinical examination for persons over age 40. Clinicians and patients should know the "ABCDEs" for melanoma: **A** for *a*symmetry, **B** for irregular *b*orders, **C** for *c*olor variation or change (especially blue or black), **D** for *d*iameter larger than 6 mm, and **E** for *e*levation. Look in sun-exposed areas for ulcerated nodules with translucent or pearly surfaces (seen in basal cell carcinoma) and roughened patches of skin with accompanying erythema (common in squamous cell carcinoma). Patients with suspicious lesions should be referred to a dermatologist for further evaluation and biopsy.

Preview: Recording the Physical Examination—The Skin

Note that initially you may use sentences to describe your findings; later you will use phrases. The style below contains phrases appropriate for most write-ups. Unfamiliar terms are explained in the next section, "Techniques of Examination."

"Color good. Skin warm and moist. Nails without clubbing or cyanosis. No suspicious nevi. No rash, petechiae, or ecchymoses."

OR

"Marked facial pallor, with circumoral cyanosis. Palms cold and moist. Cyanosis in nailbeds of fingers and toes. One raised blue-black nevus, 1 × 2 cm, with irregular border on right forearm. No rash."

Suggests central cyanosis and possible melanoma

OR

"Facial plethora. Skin icteric. Spider angioma over anterior torso. Single pearly papule with depressed center and telangiectasias, 1 × 1 cm, on posterior neck above collarline. No suspicious nevi. Nails with clubbing but no cyanosis."

Suggests possible liver disease and basal cell carcinoma

TECHNIQUES OF EXAMINATION

Observe the skin and related structures during the General Survey and throughout the rest of your examination. The entire skin surface should be inspected in good light, preferably natural light or artificial light that resembles it. Correlate your findings with observations of the mucous membranes. Diseases may manifest themselves in both areas, and both are necessary for assessing skin color. Techniques of examining these membranes are described in later chapters.

Artificial light often distorts colors and masks jaundice.

To make your observations more astute, acquaint yourself now with some of the skin lesions and colors that you may encounter.

See Table 4-1, Basic Types of Skin Lesions (pp. 103–104), and Table 4-2, Skin Colors (p. 105).

Skin

Inspect and palpate the skin. Note these characteristics:

Color. Patients may notice a change in their skin color before the clinician does. Ask about it. Look for increased pigmentation (brownness), loss of pigmentation, redness, pallor, cyanosis, and yellowing of the skin.

The red color of oxyhemoglobin and the pallor due to a lack of it are best assessed where the horny layer of the epidermis is thinnest and causes the least scatter: the fingernails, the lips, and the mucous membranes, particularly those of the mouth and the palpebral conjunctiva. In dark-skinned persons, inspecting the palms and soles may also be useful.

Pallor due to decreased redness is seen in anemia and in decreased blood flow, as in fainting or arterial insufficiency.

Central cyanosis is best identified in the lips, oral mucosa, and tongue. The lips, however, may turn blue in the cold, and melanin in the lips may simulate cyanosis in darker-skinned people.

Causes of central cyanosis include advanced lung disease, congenital heart disease, and abnormal hemoglobins.

Cyanosis of the nails, hands, and feet may be central or peripheral in origin. Peripheral cyanosis may be caused by anxiety or a cold examining room.

Cyanosis in congestive heart failure is usually peripheral, reflecting decreased blood flow, but in pulmonary edema it may also be central. Venous obstruction may cause peripheral cyanosis.

Look for the yellow color of jaundice in the sclera. Jaundice may also appear in the palpebral conjunctiva, lips, hard palate, undersurface of the tongue, tympanic membrane, and skin. To see jaundice more easily in the lips, blanch out the red color by pressure with a glass slide.

Jaundice suggests liver disease or excessive hemolysis of red blood cells.

For the yellow color that accompanies high levels of carotene, look at the palms, soles, and face.

Carotenemia

Moisture. Examples are dryness, sweating, and oiliness.

Dryness in hypothyroidism; oiliness in acne

Temperature. Use the backs of your fingers to make this assessment. In addition to identifying generalized warmth or coolness of the skin, note the temperature of any red areas.

Generalized warmth in fever, hyperthyroidism; coolness in hypothyroidism. Local warmth of inflammation or cellulitis

Texture. Examples are roughness and smoothness.

Roughness in hypothyroidism

Mobility and Turgor. Lift a fold of skin and note the ease with which it lifts up (mobility) and the speed with which it returns into place (turgor).

Decreased mobility in edema, scleroderma; decreased turgor in dehydration

Lesions. Observe any lesions of the skin, noting their characteristics:

- Their *anatomic location and distribution* over the body. Are they generalized or localized? Do they, for example, involve the exposed surfaces, the intertriginous (skin fold) areas, or areas exposed to specific allergens or irritants such as wrist bands, rings, or industrial chemicals?

Many skin diseases have typical distributions. Acne affects the face, upper chest, and back; psoriasis, the knees and elbows (among other areas); and *Candida* infections, the intertriginous areas.

- Their *arrangement.* For example, are they linear, clustered, annular (in a ring), arciform (in an arc), or dermatomal (covering a skin band that corresponds to a sensory nerve root; see pp. 546–547)?

Vesicles in a unilateral dermatomal pattern are typical of herpes zoster.

- The *type(s) of skin lesions* (e.g., macules, papules, vesicles, nevi). If possible, find representative and recent lesions that have not been traumatized by scratching or otherwise altered. Inspect them carefully and feel them.
- Their *color.*

See Table 4-1, Basic Types of Skin Lesions (pp. 103–104); Table 4-3, Vascular and Purpuric Lesions of the Skin (p. 106); Table 4-4, Skin Tumors (p. 107); and Table 4-5, Benign and Malignant Nevi (p. 108).

EVALUATING THE BEDBOUND PATIENT

People who are confined to bed, especially when they are emaciated, elderly, or neurologically impaired, are particularly susceptible to skin damage and ulceration. *Pressure sores* result when sustained compression obliterates arteriolar and capillary blood flow to the skin. Sores may also result from the shearing forces created by bodily movements. When a person slides down in bed from a partially sitting position, for example, or is dragged rather than lifted up from a supine position, the movements may distort the soft tissues of the buttocks and close off the arteries and arterioles within. Friction and moisture further increase the risk.

See Table 4-6, Pressure Ulcers (p. 109).

Assess every susceptible patient by carefully inspecting the skin that overlies the sacrum, buttocks, greater trochanters, knees, and heels. Roll the patient onto one side to see the sacrum and buttocks.

Local redness of the skin warns of impending necrosis, although some deep pressure sores develop without antecedent redness. Ulcers may be seen.

Nails

Inspect and palpate the fingernails and toenails. Note their color and shape, and any lesions. Longitudinal bands of pigment may be seen in the nails of normal people who have darker skin.

See Table 4-7, Findings In or Near the Nails (pp. 110–111).

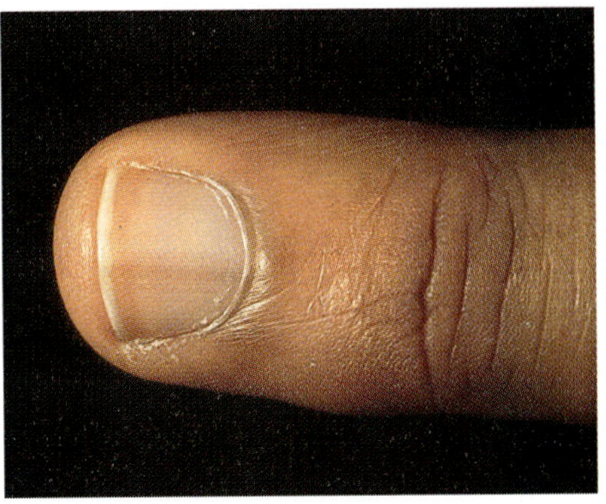

Hair

Inspect and palpate the hair. Note its quantity, distribution, and texture.

Alopecia refers to hair loss—diffuse, patchy, or total.

Sparse hair in hypothyroidism; fine silky hair in hyperthyroidism

Skin Lesions in Context

After familiarizing yourself with the basic types of lesions, review their appearances in Table 4-8 and in a well-illustrated textbook of dermatology. Whenever you see a skin lesion, look it up in such a text. The type of lesions, their location, and their distribution, together with other information from the history and the examination, should equip you well for this search and, in time, for arriving at specific dermatologic diagnoses.

See Table 4-8, Skin Lesions in Context (pp. 112–113).

TABLE 4-1 ■ Basic Types of Skin Lesions

Primary Lesions *(May Arise From Previously Normal Skin)*

Circumscribed, Flat, Nonpalpable Changes in Skin Color

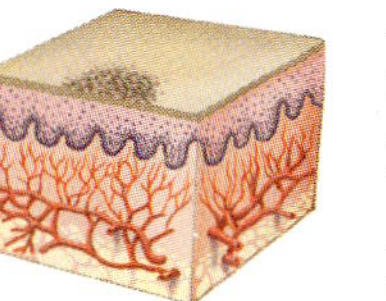

Macule—Small flat spot, up to 1.0 cm

Examples: freckle, petechia

Patch—Flat spot, 1.0 cm or larger

Palpable Elevated Solid Masses

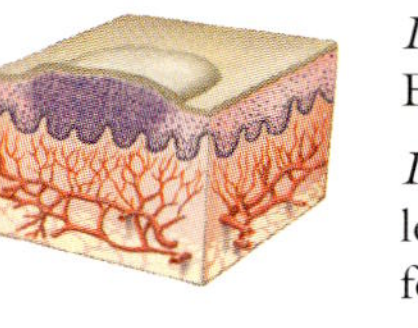

Papule—Up to 1.0 cm. Example: an elevated nevus

Plaque—Elevated superficial lesion 1.0 cm or larger, often formed by coalescence of papules

Nodule—Marble-like lesion larger than 0.5 cm, often deeper and firmer than a papule

Wheal—A somewhat irregular, relatively transient, superficial area of localized skin edema. Examples: mosquito bite, hive

Circumscribed Superficial Elevations of the Skin Formed by Free Fluid in a Cavity Within the Skin Layers

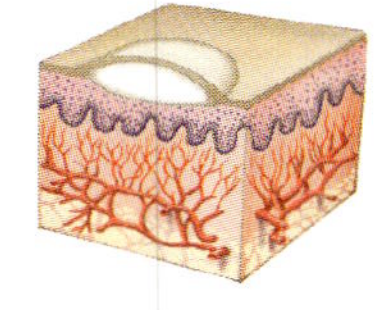

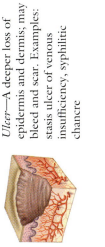

Vesicle—Up to 1.0 cm; filled with serous fluid. Example: herpes simplex

Bulla—1.0 cm or larger; filled with serous fluid. Example: 2nd-degree burn

Pustule—Filled with pus. Examples: acne, impetigo

Secondary Lesions *(Result From Changes in Primary Lesions)*

Loss of Skin Surface

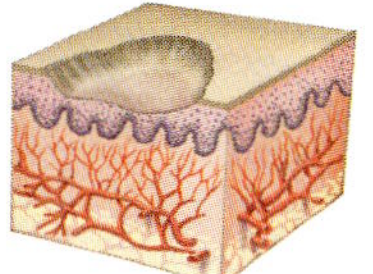

Erosion—Loss of the superficial epidermis; surface is moist but does not bleed. Example: moist area after the rupture of a vesicle, as in chickenpox

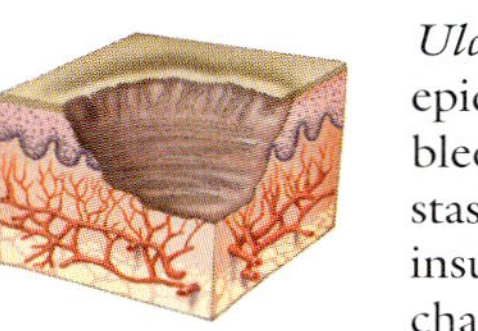

Ulcer—A deeper loss of epidermis and dermis; may bleed and scar. Examples: stasis ulcer of venous insufficiency, syphilitic chancre

Fissure—A linear crack in the skin. Example: athlete's foot

Material on the Skin Surface

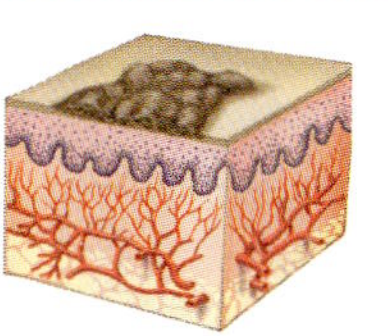

Crust—The dried residue of serum, pus, or blood. Example: impetigo

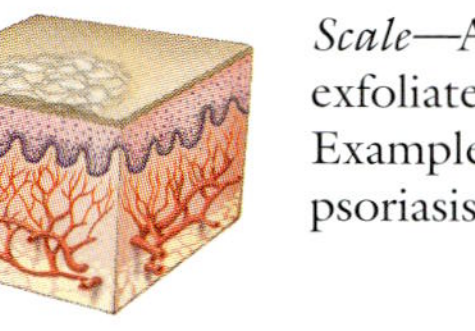

Scale—A thin flake of exfoliated epidermis. Examples: dandruff, dry skin, psoriasis

(table continues next page)

TABLE 4-1 ■ Basic Types of Skin Lesions *(Continued)*

Miscellaneous Lesions

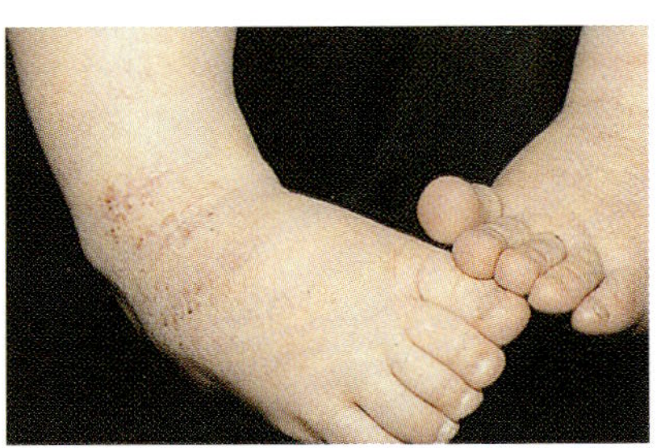

Lichenification—Thickening and roughening of the skin with increased visibility of the normal skin furrows. Example: atopic dermatitis

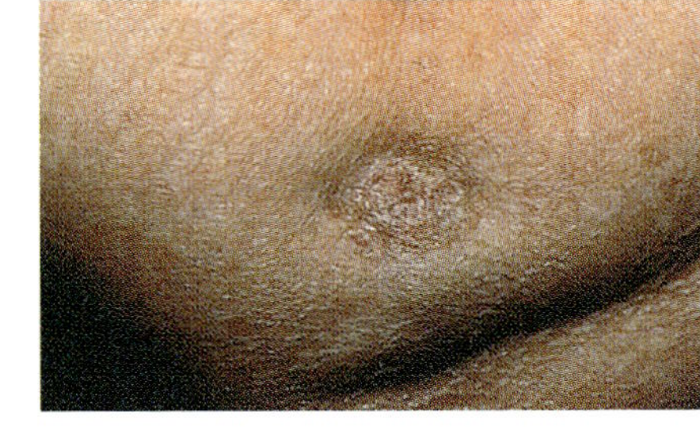

Atrophy—Thinning of the skin with loss of the normal skin furrows; the skin looks shinier and more translucent than normal. Example: arterial insufficiency

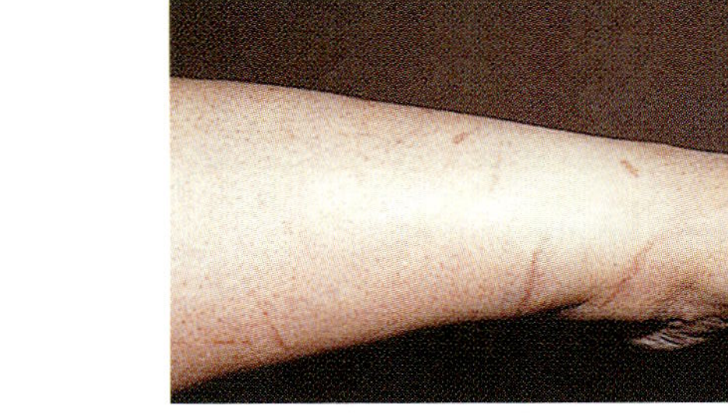

Excoriation—An abrasion or scratch mark. It may be linear, as illustrated, or rounded, as in a scratched insect bite.

Scar—Replacement of destroyed tissue by fibrous tissue. May be thick and pink (hypertrophic) or thin and white (atrophic), but does not extend beyond the injured area

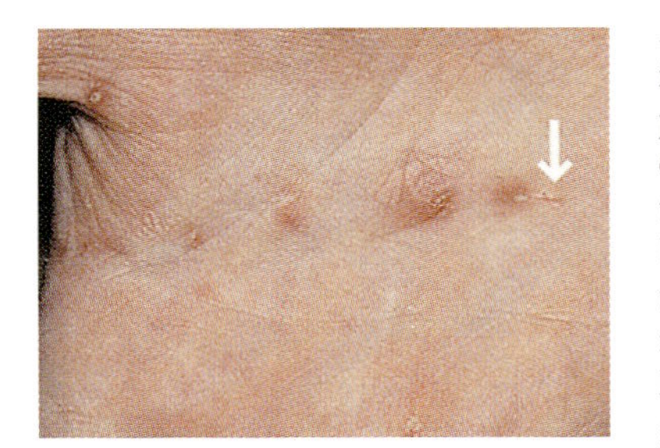

Burrow of Scabies—A person with scabies has intense itching. Skin lesions include small papules, pustules, lichenified areas, and excoriations. With a magnifying lens, look for the *burrow* of the mite that causes it. A burrow is a minute, slightly raised tunnel in the epidermis and is commonly found on the finger webs and on the sides of the fingers. It looks like a short (5–15 mm), linear or curved, gray line and may end in a tiny vesicle.

Additional Lesions:

- *Comedo*—The common blackhead that marks the plugged opening of a sebaceous gland, frequently seen with acne
- *Nevus*—The common mole; appears flat to slightly elevated, round and evenly pigmented; however, some nevi look quite different, as in the pigmented nevi of melanoma.
- *Telangiectasias*—Dilated small vessels (can be venules, arterioles, including spider angiomas, or capillaries) that look either red or bluish. May appear by themselves or as parts of other lesions, as in a basal cell carcinoma or radiodermatitis (skin injury from ionizing radiation).

(Sources of photos: *Lichenification, Excoriation, Scar, Burrow of Scabies*—Goodheart HP: A Photoguide of Common Skin Disorders: Diagnosis and Management. Philadelphia, Lippincott Williams & Wilkins, 1999; *Atrophy*—Fitzpatrick JE, Aeling JL: Dermatology Secrets in Color, 2nd ed. Philadelphia, Lippincott Williams & Wilkins, 2000)

TABLE 4-2 ■ Skin Colors

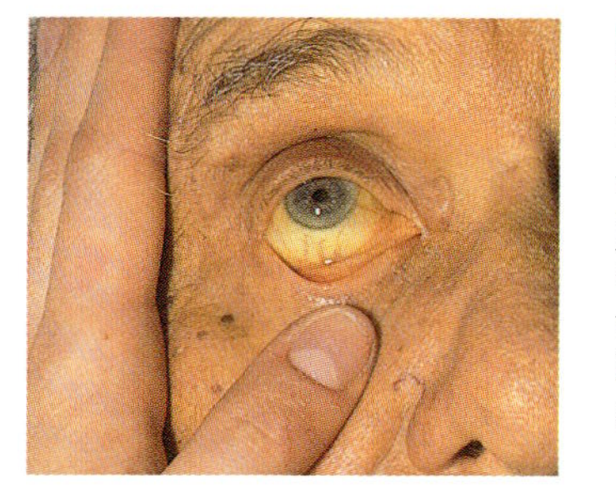

Jaundice

Jaundice makes the skin diffusely yellow. Note this patient's skin color, contrasted with the examiner's hand. The color of jaundice is seen most easily and reliably in the sclera, as shown here. It may also be visible in mucous membranes. Causes include liver disease and hemolysis of red blood cells.

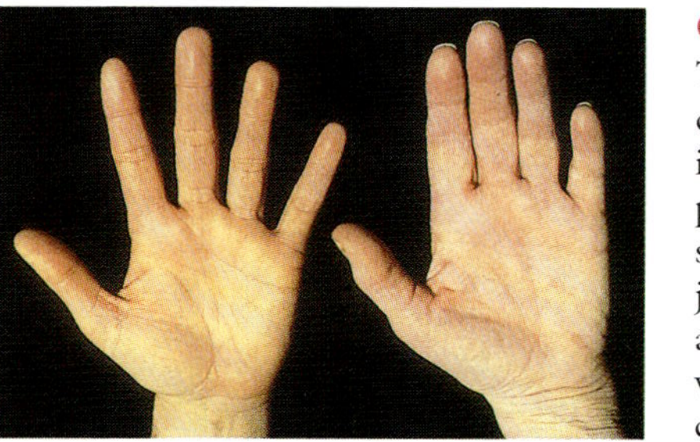

Carotenemia

The yellowish palm of carotenemia, shown on the left, is compared with a normally pink palm—a useful technique for a sometimes subtle finding. Unlike jaundice, carotenemia does not affect the sclera, which remains white. The cause is a diet high in carrots and other yellow vegetables or fruits. Carotenemia is not harmful, but indicates the need for assessing dietary intake.

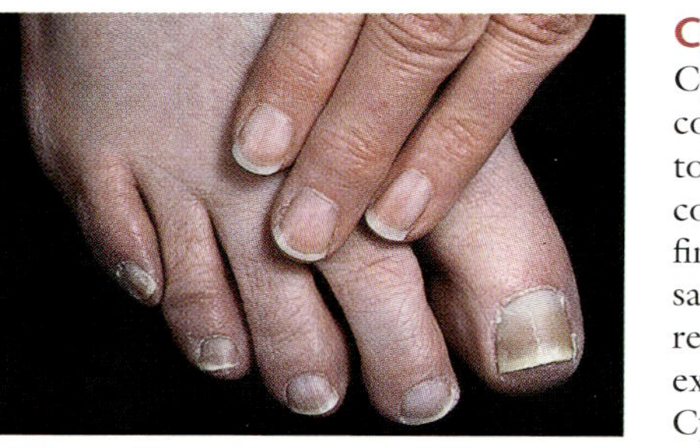

Cyanosis

Cyanosis is the somewhat bluish color that is visible in these toenails and toes. Compare this color with the normally pink fingernails and fingers of the same patient. Impaired venous return in the leg caused this example of peripheral cyanosis. Cyanosis, especially when slight, may be hard to distinguish from normal skin color.

Changes in Melanin

A widespread increase in melanin may be caused by Addison's disease (hypofunction of the adrenal cortex) or some pituitary tumors. More common are local areas of increased or decreased pigment:

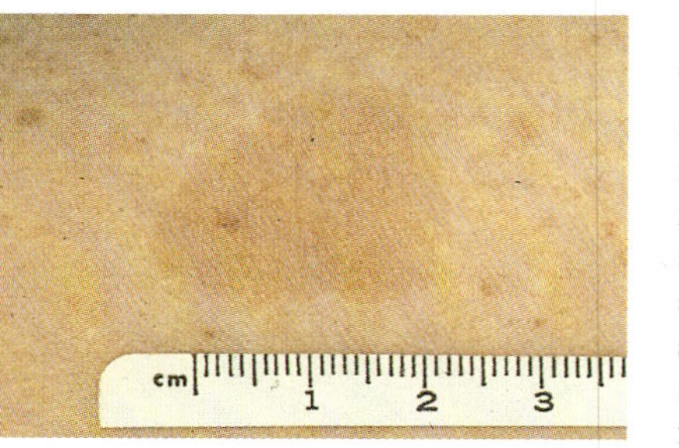

Café-Au-Lait Spot

The common café-au-lait spot is a slightly but uniformly pigmented macule or patch with a somewhat irregular border. Most of these spots are 0.5 cm to 1.5 cm in diameter and are of no consequence. Six or more such spots, each with a diameter of >1.5 cm, however, suggest neurofibromatosis (p. 113). (The small, darker macules are unrelated.)

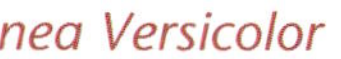

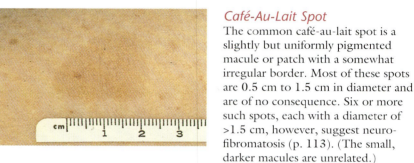

Tinea Versicolor

More common than vitiligo is this superficial fungus infection of the skin. It causes hypopigmented, slightly scaly macules on the trunk, neck, and upper arms. They are easier to see in darker skin and may become more obvious after tanning. In lighter skin, the macules may look reddish or tan instead of pale. The macules may be much more numerous than in this example.

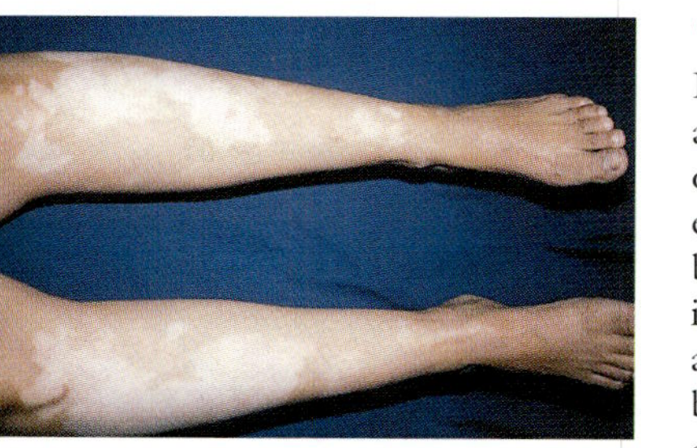

Vitiligo

In vitiligo, depigmented macules appear on the face, hands, feet, and other regions and may coalesce into extensive areas that lack melanin. The brown pigment on this woman's legs is her normal skin color; the pale areas are due to vitiligo. The condition may be hereditary. These changes may be distressing to the patient.

TABLE 4-3 ■ Vascular and Purpuric Lesions of the Skin

	Vascular			Purpuric	
	Spider Angioma	*Spider Vein*	*Cherry Angioma*	*Petechia/Purpura*	*Ecchymosis*
Color	Fiery red	Bluish	Bright or ruby red; may become brownish with age	Deep red or reddish purple, fading away over time	Purple or purplish blue, fading to green, yellow, and brown with time
Size	From very small to 2 cm	Variable, from very small to several inches	1–3 mm	Petechia, 1–3 mm; purpura, larger	Variable, larger than petechiae
Shape	Central body, sometimes raised, surrounded by erythema and radiating legs	Variable. May resemble a spider or be linear, irregular, cascading	Round, flat or sometimes raised, may be surrounded by a pale halo	Rounded, sometimes irregular; flat	Rounded, oval, or irregular; may have a central subcutaneous flat nodule (a hematoma)
Pulsatility	Often demonstrable in the body of the spider, when pressure with a glass slide is applied	Absent	Absent	Absent	Absent
Effect of Pressure	Pressure on the body causes blanching of the spider.	Pressure over the center does not cause blanching, but diffuse pressure blanches the veins.	May show partial blanching, especially if pressure is applied with the edge of a pinpoint	None	None
Distribution	Face, neck, arms, and upper trunk; almost never below the waist	Most often on the legs, near veins; also on the anterior chest	Trunk; also extremities	Variable	Variable
Significance	Liver disease, pregnancy, vitamin B deficiency; also occurs normally in some people	Often accompanies increased pressure in the superficial veins, as in varicose veins	None; increase in size and numbers with aging	Blood outside the vessels; may suggest a bleeding disorder or, if petechiae, emboli to skin	Blood outside the vessels; often secondary to bruising or trauma; also seen in bleeding disorders

(Sources of photos: *Spider Angioma*—Marks R: Skin Disease in Old Age. Philadelphia, JB Lippincott, 1987; *Petechia/Purpura*—Kelley WN: Textbook of Internal Medicine. Philadelphia, JB Lippincott, 1989)

TABLE 4-4 ■ Skin Tumors

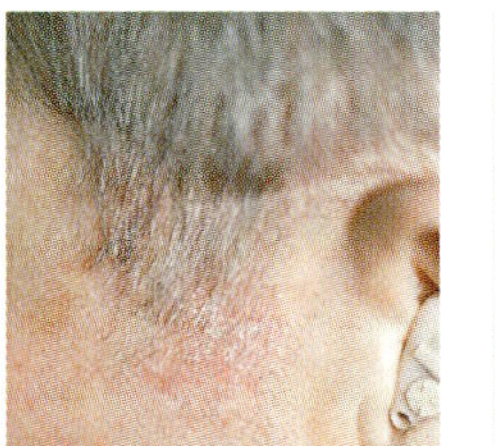

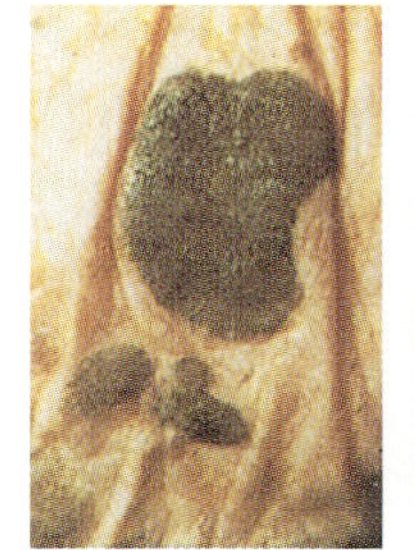

Actinic Keratosis

Actinic keratoses are superficial, flattened papules covered by a dry scale. Often multiple, they may be round or irregular, and are pink, tan, or grayish. They appear on sun-exposed skin of older, fair-skinned persons. Though themselves benign, these lesions may give rise to squamous cell carcinoma (suggested by rapid growth, induration, redness at the base, and ulceration). Keratoses on face and hand, typical locations, are shown.

Seborrheic Keratosis

Seborrheic keratoses are common, benign, yellowish to brown, raised lesions that feel slightly greasy and velvety or warty. Typically multiple and symmetrically distributed on the trunk of older people, they may also appear on the face and elsewhere. In black people, often younger women, they may appear as small, deeply pigmented papules on the cheeks and temples (dermatosis papulosa nigra).

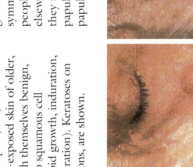

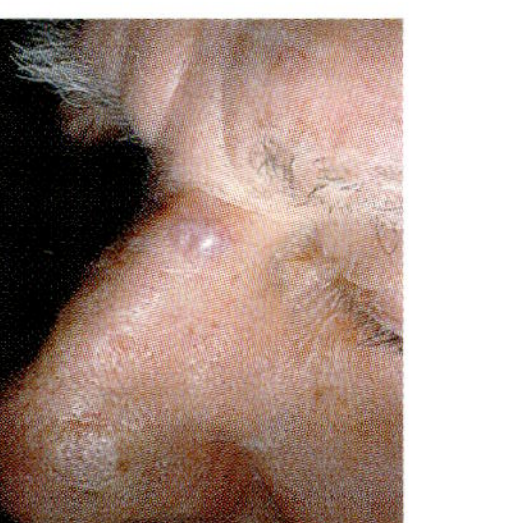

Basal Cell Carcinoma

A basal cell carcinoma, though malignant, grows slowly and seldom metastasizes. It is most common in fair-skinned adults over age 40, and usually appears on the face. An initial translucent nodule spreads, leaving a depressed center and a firm, elevated border. Telangiectatic vessels are often visible.

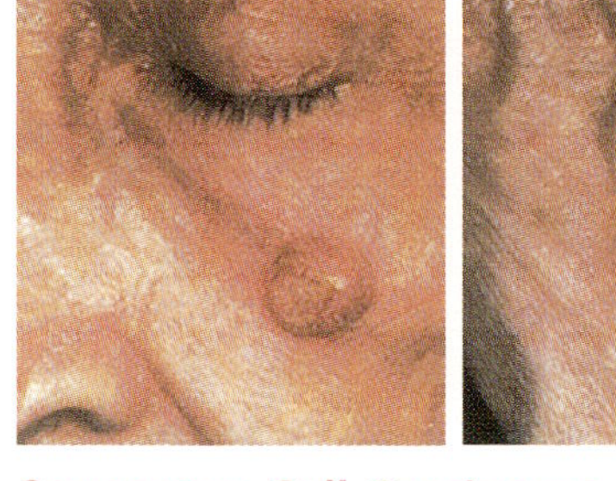

Squamous Cell Carcinoma

Squamous cell carcinoma usually appears on sun-exposed skin of fair-skinned adults over 60. It may develop in an actinic keratosis. It usually grows more quickly than a basal cell carcinoma, is firmer, and looks redder. The face and the back of the hand are often affected, as shown here.

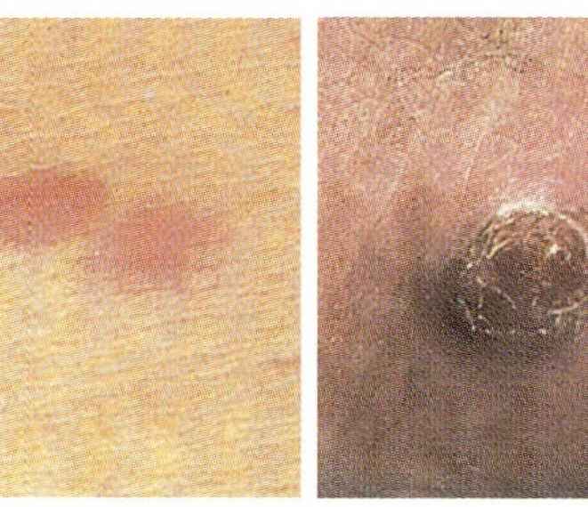

Kaposi's Sarcoma in AIDS

When Kaposi's sarcoma, a malignant tumor, accompanies AIDS, it may appear in many forms: macules, papules, plaques, or nodules almost anywhere on the body. Lesions are often multiple and may involve internal structures. On the left are ovoid, pinkish red plaques that typically lengthen along the skin lines. They may become pigmented. On the right is a purplish red nodule on the foot.

(Sources of photos: *Basal Cell Carcinoma:* Rapini R. *Squamous Cell Carcinoma, Actinic Keratosis,* and *Seborrheic Keratosis*—Sauer GC: Manual of Skin Diseases, 5th ed. Philadelphia, JB Lippincott, 1985; *Kaposi's Sarcoma in AIDS*—DeVita VT Jr, Hellman S, Rosenberg SA [eds]: AIDS: Etiology, Diagnosis, Treatment, and Prevention. Philadelphia, JB Lippincott, 1985)

TABLE 4-5 ■ Benign and Malignant Nevi

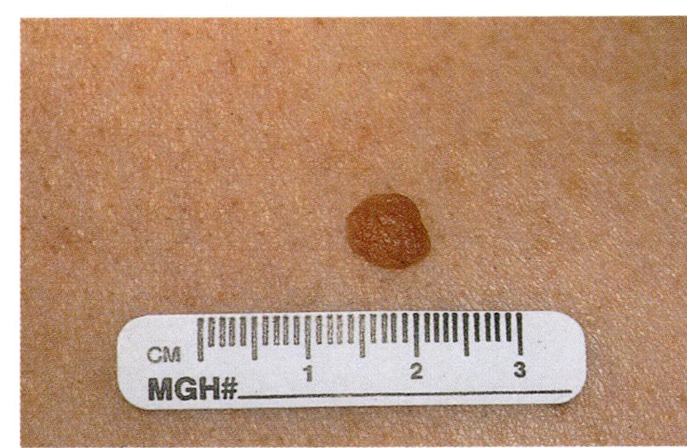

Benign Nevus

The *benign nevus,* or common mole, usually appears in the first few decades. Several nevi may arise at the same time, but their appearance usually remains unchanged. Note the following typical features and contrast them with those of atypical nevi and melanoma:

- Round or oval shape
- Sharply defined borders
- Uniform color, especially tan or brown
- Diameter < 6 mm
- Flat or raised surface

Changes in these features raise the the spectre of *atypical (dysplastic) nevi,* or melanoma. Atypical nevi are varied in color but often dark and larger than 6 mm, with irregular borders that fade into the surrounding skin. Look for atypical nevi primarily on the trunk. They may number more than 50 to 100.

Malignant Melanoma

Learn the "**ABCDEs**" of melanoma from these reference standard photographs from the American Cancer Society:

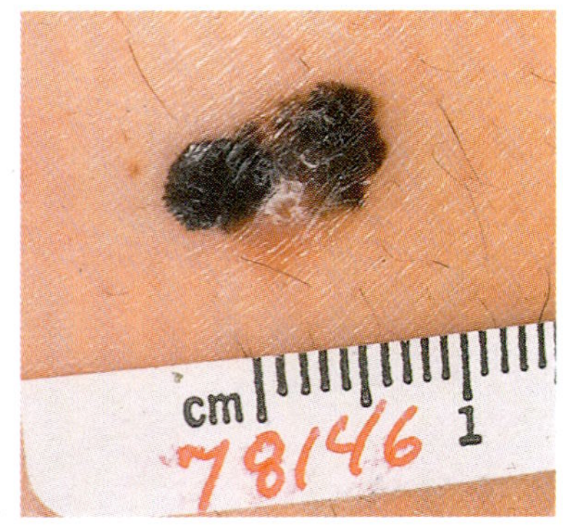

A

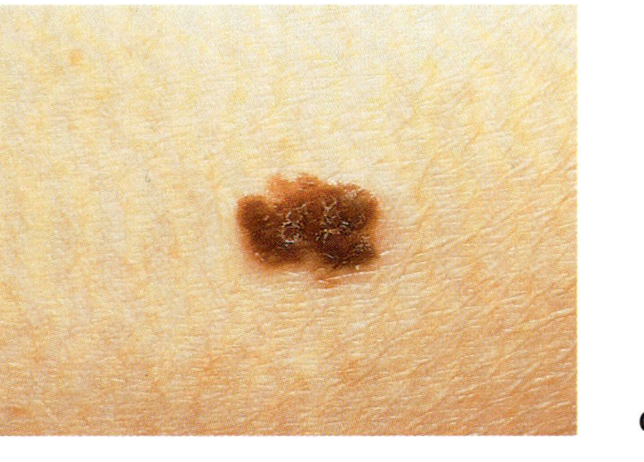
B

C

- *Asymmetry* (Fig. A)
- Irregular ***Borders***, especially notching (Fig. B)
- Variation in ***Color***, especially mixtures of black, blue, and red (Figs. B, C)
- ***Diameter*** >6 mm (Fig. C)
- ***Elevation***, though also may be flat (Fig. C).

Review *melanoma risk factors* such as intense year-round sun exposure, blistering sunburns in childhood, fair skin that freckles or burns easily (especially if blond or red hair), family history of melanoma, and nevi that are changing or atypical, especially if >50. Changing nevi may have new swelling or redness beyond the border, scaling, oozing, or bleeding, or sensations such as itching, burning, or pain.

On darker skin, look for melanomas under the nails, on the hands, or on the soles of the feet.

(Courtesy of American Cancer Society; American Academy of Dermatology)

TABLE 4-6 ■ Pressure Ulcers

Pressure ulcers, also termed *decubitus* ulcers, usually develop over body prominences subject to unrelieved pressure, resulting in ischemic damage to underlying tissue. Prevention is as important as identification and treatment: inspect the skin thoroughly for *early warning signs* of erythema that blanches with pressure, especially in patients with risk factors. Pressure ulcers form most commonly over the sacrum, ischial tuberosities, greater trochanters, and heels. A commonly applied staging system, based on depth of destroyed tissue, is illustrated below. However, *note:* in Stage I the skin is still intact and is not yet an ulcer; ulcers with necrosis or eschar must be débrided before they can be staged; and ulcers do not necessarily progress sequentially through the four stages. Inspect ulcers for signs of infection, including drainage, odor, cellulitis, or necrosis. Fever, chills, and pain suggest possible underlying osteomyelitis. Assessment should address the patient's overall physical and mental health, including: *comorbid conditions* such as vascular disease, diabetes, immune deficiencies, collagen vascular disease, malignancy, psychosis, or depression; nutritional status; pain and level of analgesia; risk of recurrence; psychosocial factors such as learning ability, social supports, and lifestyle; and any evidence of polypharmacy, overmedication, or abuse of alcohol, tobacco, or illicit drugs.

Risk Factors for Pressure Ulcers

- Decreased mobility, especially if accompanied by increased pressure or movement causing friction or shear stress
- Decreased sensation, from brain or spinal cord lesions or peripheral nerve disease
- Decreased blood flow from hypotension or microvascular disease such as diabetes or atherosclerosis
- Fecal or urinary incontinence
- Presence of fracture
- Poor nutritional status or low albumin

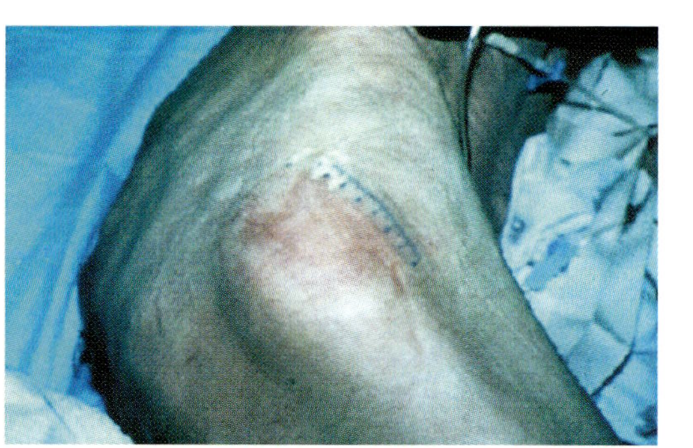

Stage I

Pressure-related alteration of intact skin, with changes in temperature (warmth or coolness), consistency (firm or boggy), sensation (pain or itching), or color (red, blue, or purple on darker skin; red on lighter skin)

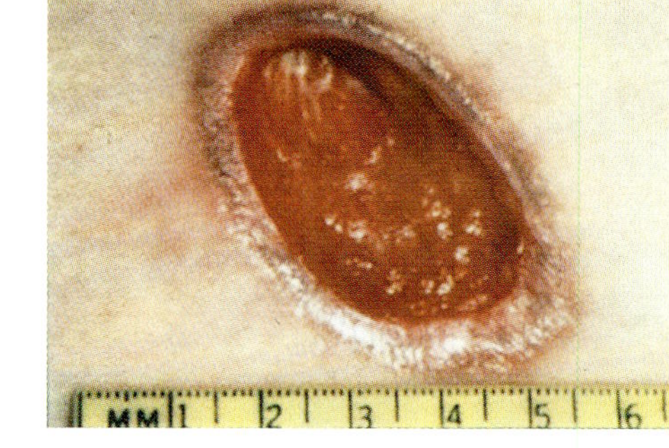

Stage III

Full-thickness skin loss, with damage to or necrosis of subcutaneous tissue that may extend to, but not through, underlying muscle

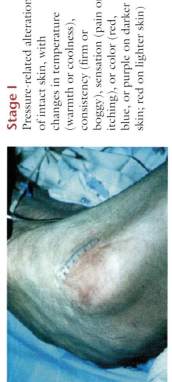

Stage II

Partial-thickness skin loss or ulceration involving the epidermis, dermis, or both

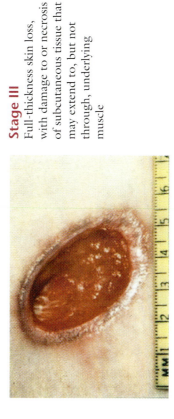

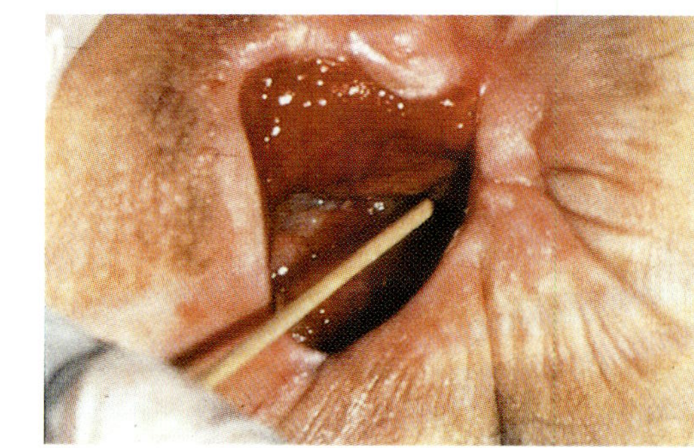
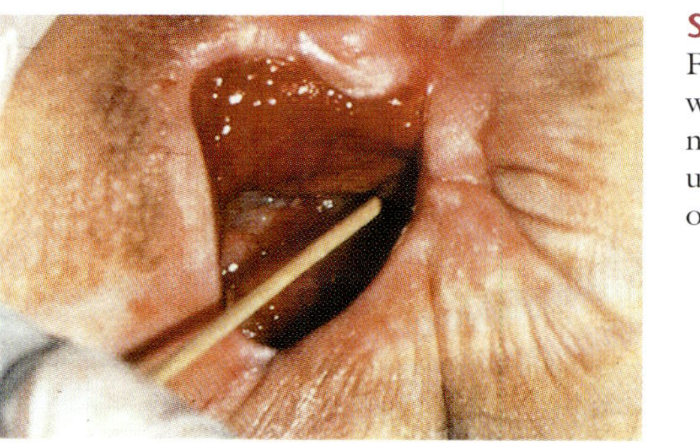
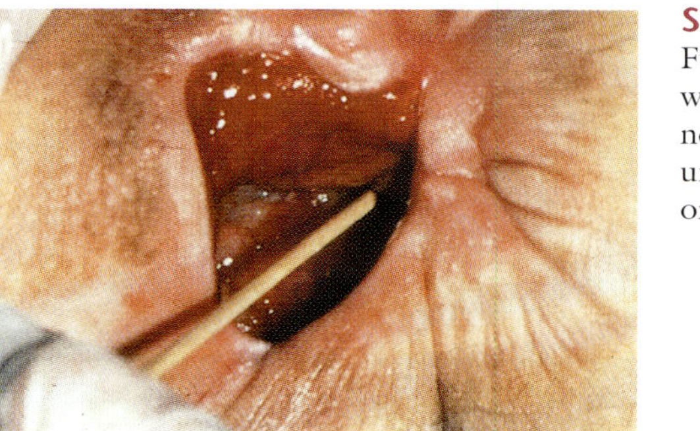

Stage IV

Full-thickness skin loss, with destruction, tissue necrosis, or damage to underlying muscle, bone, or supporting structures

(Source of photos: National Pressure Ulcer Advisory Panel. Reston, VA)

TABLE 4-7 ■ Findings in or Near the Nails

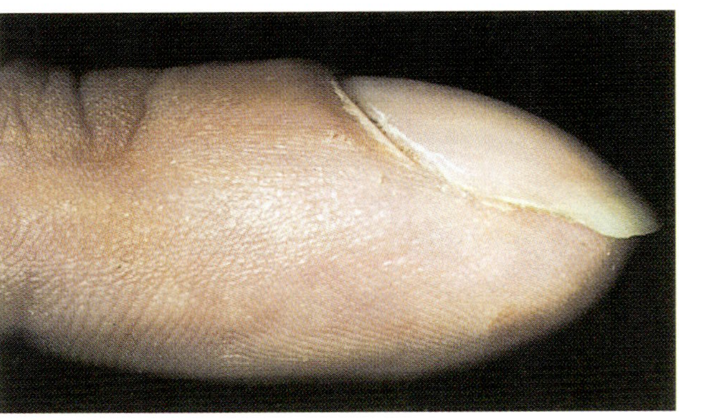

Clubbing of the Fingers

In clubbing, the distal phalanx of each finger is rounded and bulbous. The nail plate is more convex, and the angle between the plate and the proximal nail fold increases to 180° or more. The proximal nail fold, when palpated, feels spongy or floating. Causes are many, including chronic hypoxia from heart disease or lung cancer and hepatic cirrhosis.

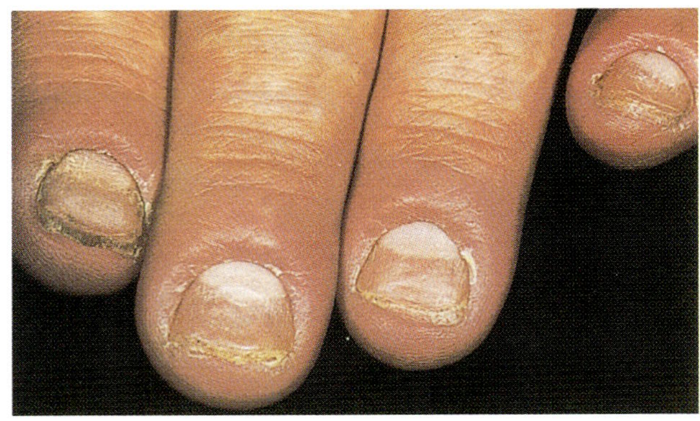

Paronychia

A paronychia is an inflammation of the proximal and lateral nail folds. It may be acute or, as illustrated, chronic. The folds are red, swollen, and often tender. The cuticle may not be visible. People who frequently immerse their nails in water are especially susceptible. Multiple nails are often affected.

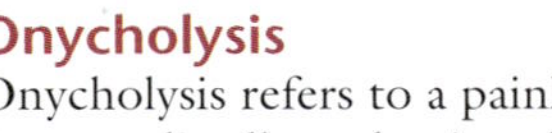

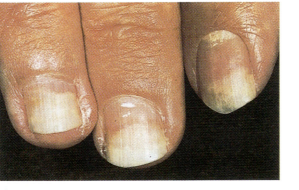

Onycholysis

Onycholysis refers to a painless separation of the nail plate from the nail bed. It starts distally, enlarging the free edge of the nail to a varying degree. Several or all nails are usually affected. Causes are many.

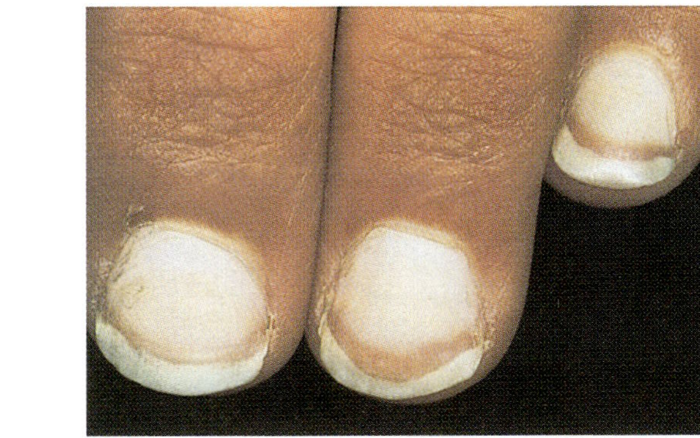

Terry's Nails

Terry's nails are mostly whitish with a distal band of reddish brown. The lunulae of the nails may not be visible. These nails may be seen with aging and in people with chronic diseases such as cirrhosis of the liver, congestive heart failure, and non-insulin-dependent diabetes.

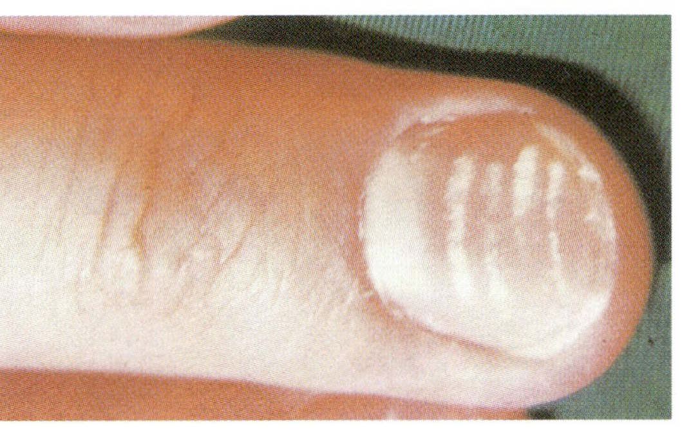

White Spots *(Leukonychia)*

Trauma to the nails is commonly followed by white spots that grow slowly out with the nail. Spots in the pattern illustrated are typical of overly vigorous and repeated manicuring. The curves in this example resemble the curve of the cuticle and proximal nail fold.

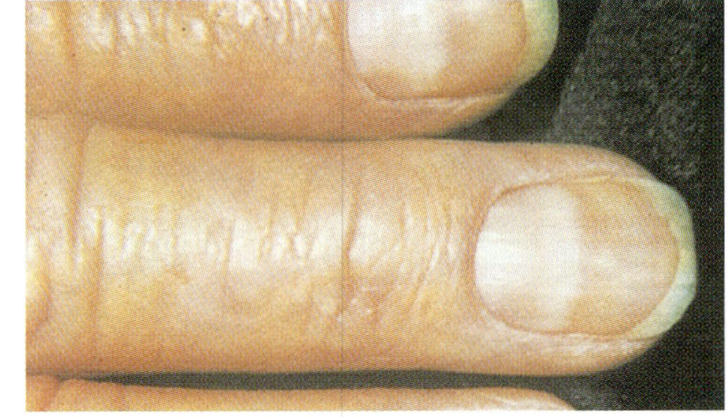

Transverse White Lines *(Mees' Lines)*

These are transverse lines, not spots, and their curves are similar to those of the lunula, not the cuticle. These uncommon lines may follow an acute or severe illness. They emerge from under the proximal nail folds and grow out with the nails.

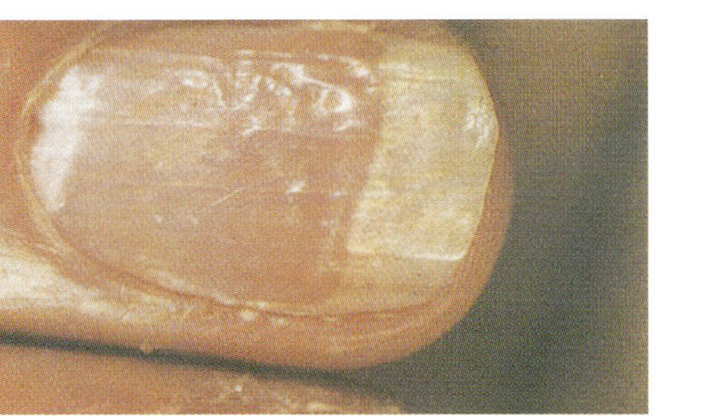

Psoriasis

Small pits in the nails may be early signs of psoriasis but are not specific for it. Additional findings, not shown here, include onycholysis and a circumscribed yellowish tan discoloration known as an "oil spot" lesion. Marked thickening of the nails may develop.

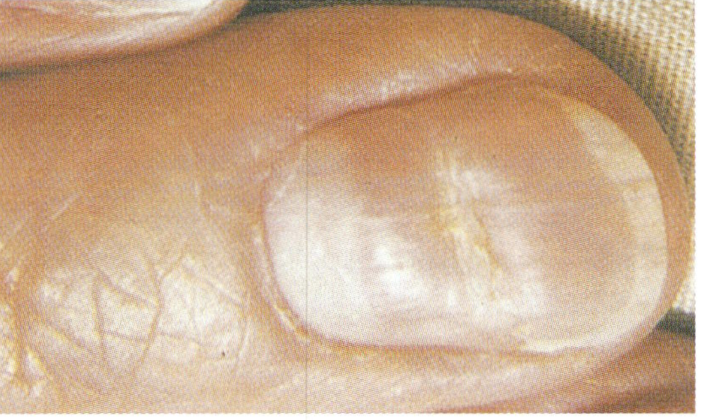

Beau's Lines

Beau's lines are transverse depressions in the nails associated with acute severe illness. The lines emerge from under the proximal nail folds weeks later and grow gradually out with the nails. As with Mees' lines, clinicians may be able to estimate the timing of a causal illness.

(Sources of photos: *Clubbing of the Fingers, Paronychia, Onycholyis, Terry's Nails*—Habif TP: Clinical Dermatology: A Color Guide to Diagnosis and Therapy, 2nd ed. St. Louis, CV Mosby, 1990; *White Spots, Transverse White Lines, Psoriasis, Beau's Lines*—Sams WM Jr, Lynch PJ: Principles and Practice of Dermatology. New York, Churchill Livingstone, 1990)

TABLE 4-8 ■ Skin Lesions in Context

This table shows a variety of primary and secondary skin lesions. Try to identify them, including those indicated by letters, before reading the accompanying text.

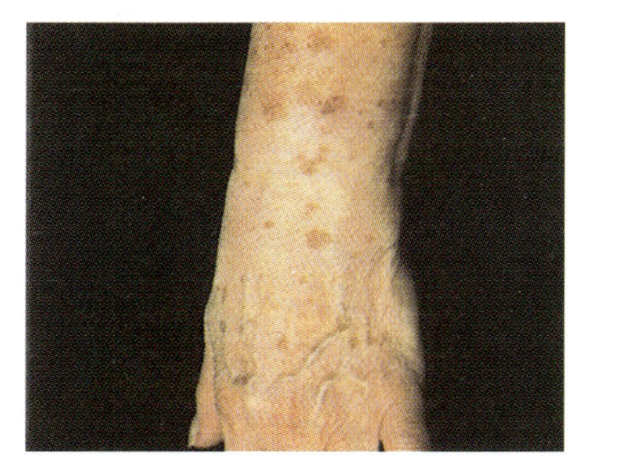

Macules on the dorsum of the hand, wrist, and forearm (actinic lentigines)

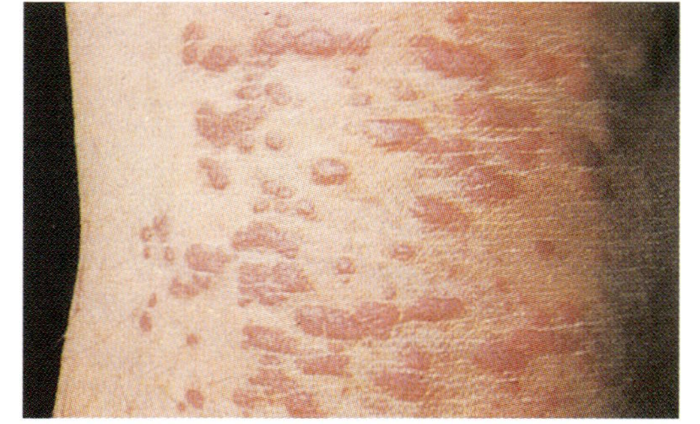

Papules on the knee (in lichen planus)

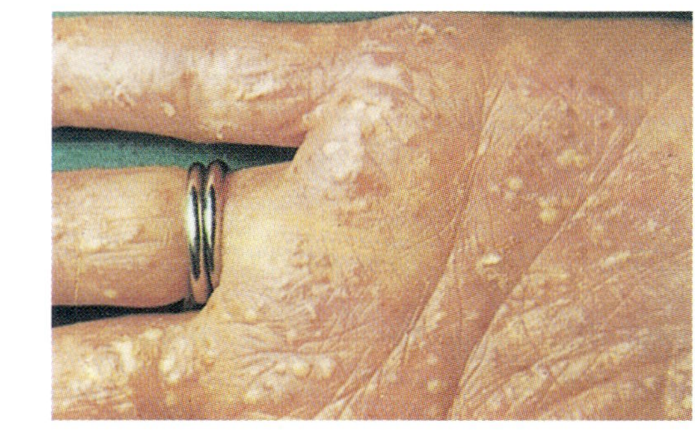

Pustules on the palm (in pustular psoriasis)

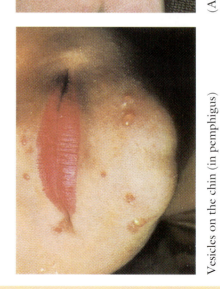

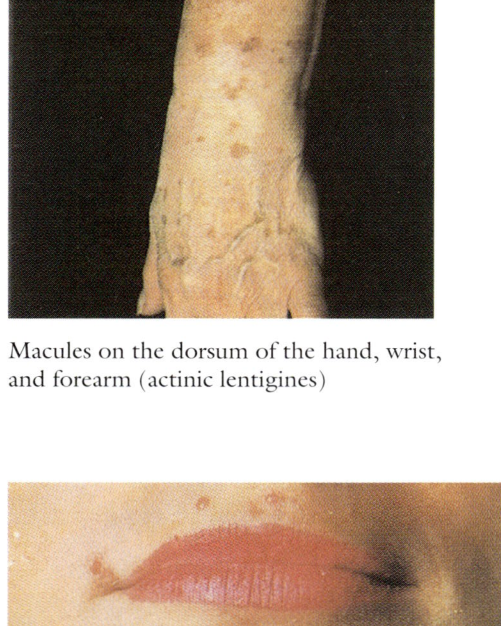

Vesicles on the chin (in pemphigus)

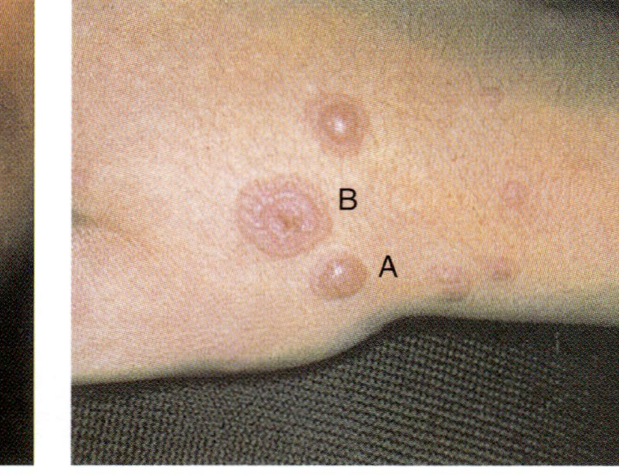

(A) Bulla,
(B) Target (or iris) lesion (in erythema multiforme)

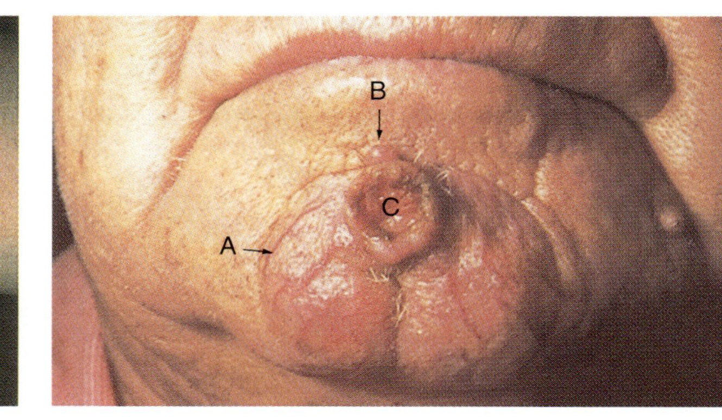

(A) Telangiectasia, (B) nodule, (C) ulcer (in squamous cell carcinoma)

Wheals (urticaria) in a drug eruption in an infant

(A) Patch, (B) nodules—a combination typical of neurofibromatosis. This patch is a café-au-lait spot.

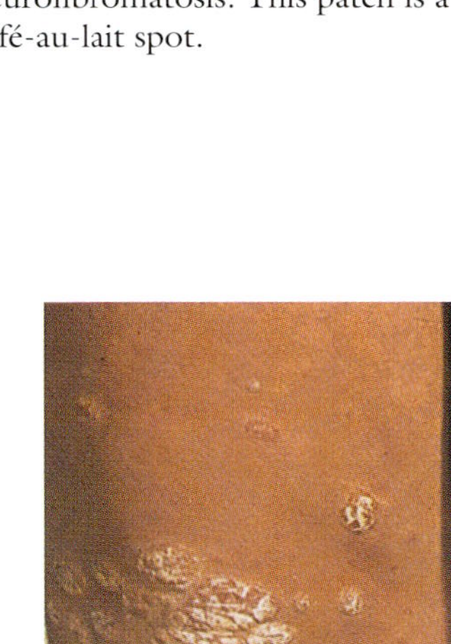

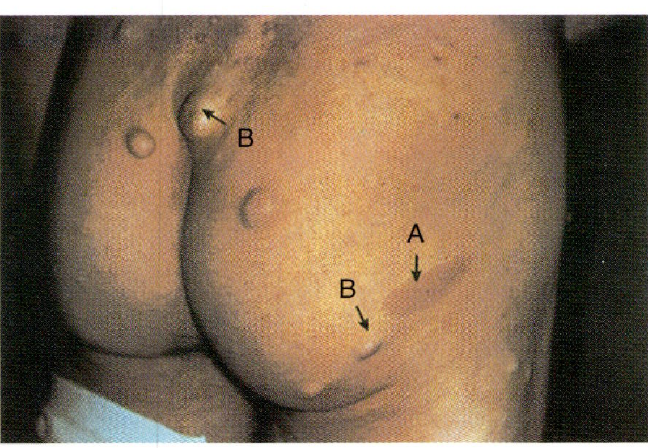

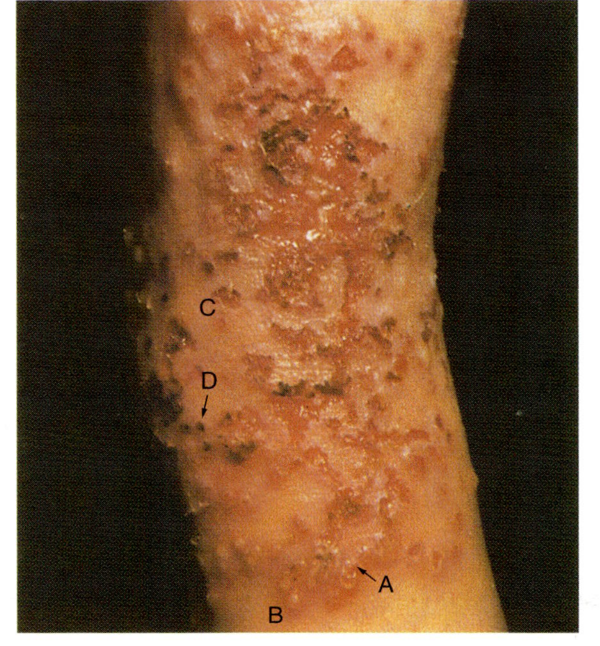

(A) Vesicle, (B) pustule, (C) erosions, (D) crust, on the back of a knee (in infected atopic dermatitis)

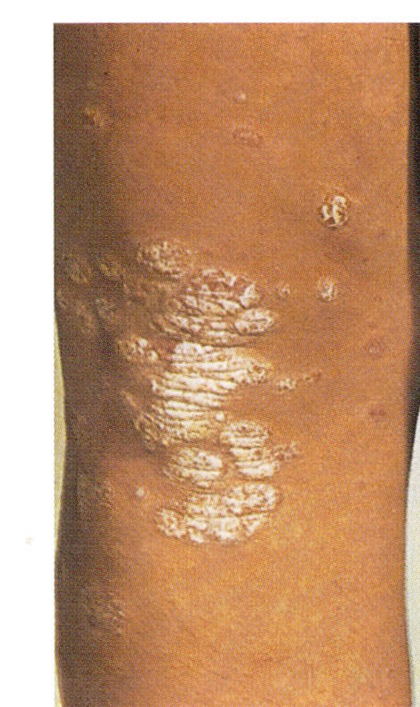

Plaques with scales on the front of a knee (in psoriasis)

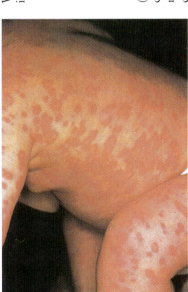

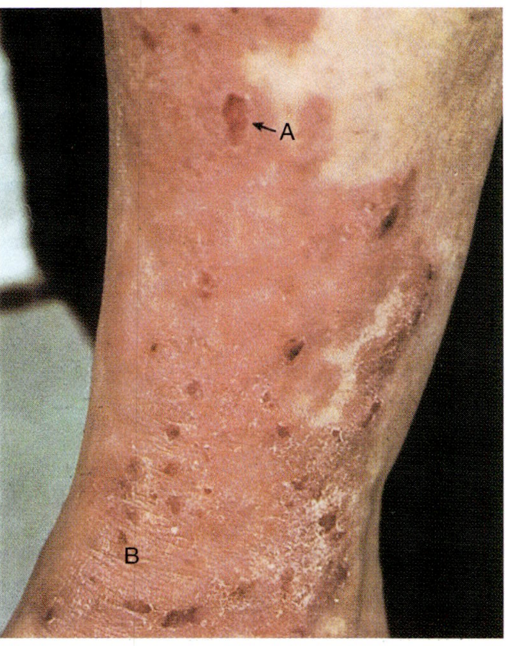

(A) Excoriation, (B) lichenification on the leg (in atopic dermatitis)

(Source of all photos except for *Macules:* Sauer GC: Manual of Skin Diseases, 5th ed. Philadelphia, JB Lippincott, 1985)

CHAPTER

5

The Head and Neck

ANATOMY AND PHYSIOLOGY

The Head

Regions of the head take their names from the underlying bones of the skull (e.g., frontal area). Knowing this anatomy helps to locate and describe physical findings.

Two paired salivary glands lie near the mandible: the *parotid gland*, superficial to and behind the mandible (both visible and palpable when enlarged), and the *submandibular gland*, located deep to the mandible. Feel for the latter as you bow and press your tongue against your lower incisors. Its lobular surface can often be felt against the tightened muscle. The openings of the parotid and submandibular ducts are visible within the oral cavity (see p. 130).

The *superficial temporal artery* passes upward just in front of the ear, where it is readily palpable. In many normal people, especially thin and elderly ones, the tortuous course of one of its branches can be traced across the forehead.

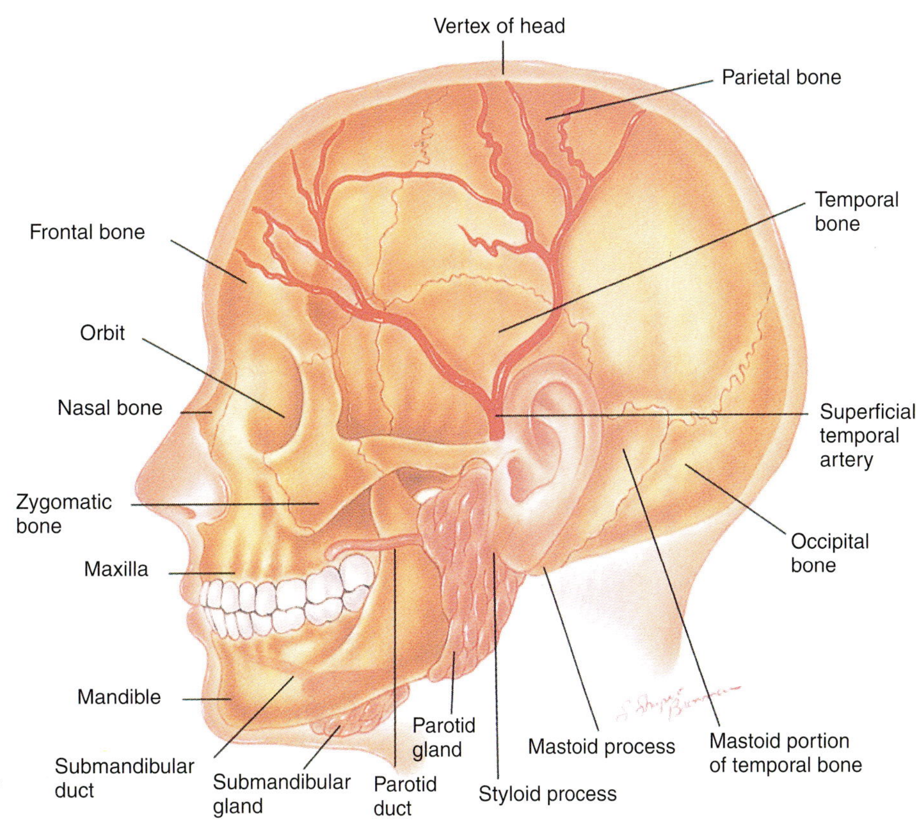

The Eye

Gross Anatomy. Identify the structures illustrated. Note that the upper eyelid covers a portion of the iris but does not normally overlap the pupil.

The opening between the eyelids is called the *palpebral fissure*. The white *sclera* may look somewhat buff-colored at its extreme periphery. Do not mistake this color for jaundice, which is a deeper yellow.

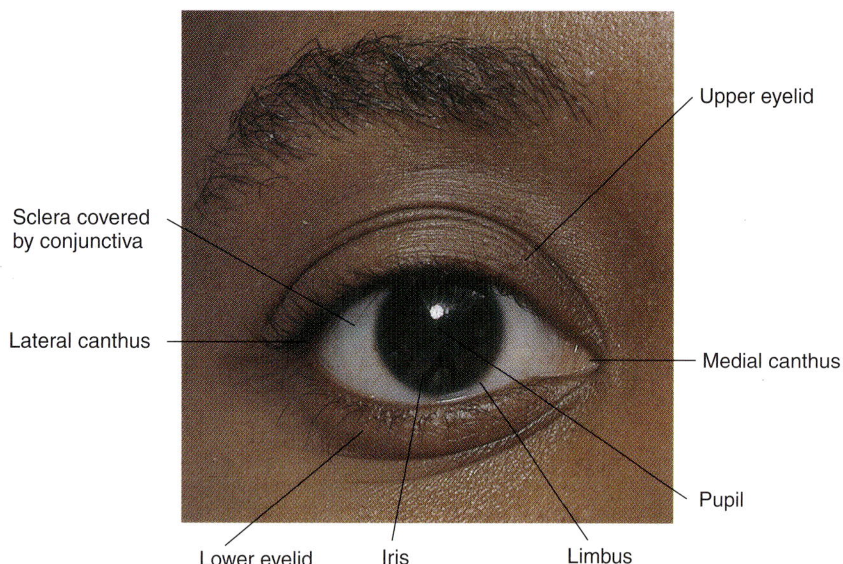

The *conjunctiva* is a clear mucous membrane with two easily visible components. The *bulbar conjunctiva* covers most of the anterior eyeball, adhering loosely to the underlying tissue. It meets the cornea at the *limbus*. The *palpebral conjunctiva* lines the eyelids. The two parts of the conjunctiva merge in a folded recess that permits the eyeball to move.

Within the *eyelids* lie firm strips of connective tissue called *tarsal plates*. Each plate contains a parallel row of *meibomian glands*, which open on the lid margin. The *levator palpebrae muscle*, which raises the upper eyelid, is innervated by the oculomotor nerve (Cranial Nerve III). Smooth muscle, innervated by the sympathetic nervous system, contributes to raising this lid.

A film of *tear fluid* protects the conjunctiva and cornea from drying, inhibits microbial growth, and gives a smooth optical surface to the cornea. This fluid comes from three sources: meibomian glands, conjunctival glands, and the lacrimal gland. The *lacrimal gland* lies mostly within the bony orbit, above and lateral to the eyeball. The tear fluid spreads across the eye and drains medially through two tiny holes called *lacrimal puncta*. The tears then pass into the *lacrimal sac* and on into the nose through the *nasolacrimal duct*. (You can easily find a punctum atop the small elevation of the lower lid medially. You cannot detect the lacrimal sac, which rests in a small depression inside the bony orbit.)

The eyeball is a spherical structure that focuses light on the neurosensory elements within the retina. The muscles of the *iris* control pupillary size. Muscles of the *ciliary body* control the thickness of the lens, allowing the eye to focus on near or distant objects.

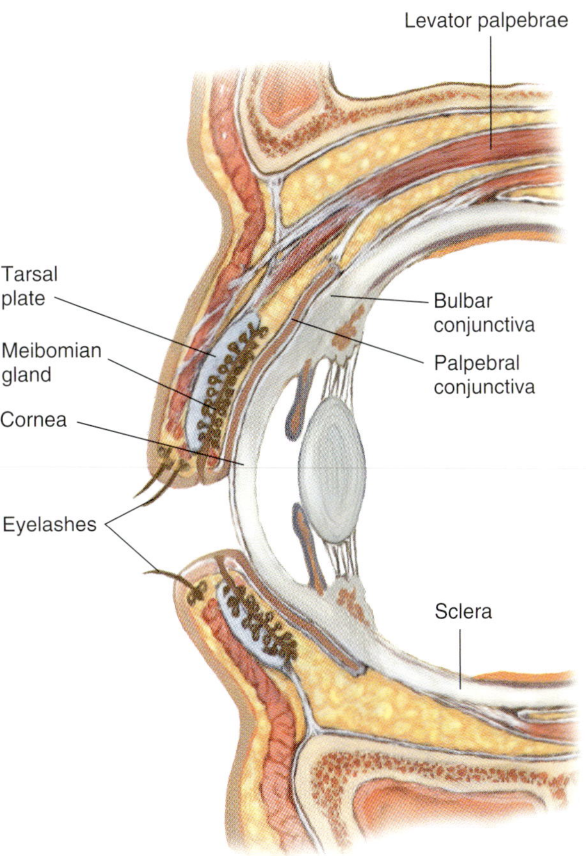

SAGITTAL SECTION OF ANTERIOR EYE WITH LIDS CLOSED

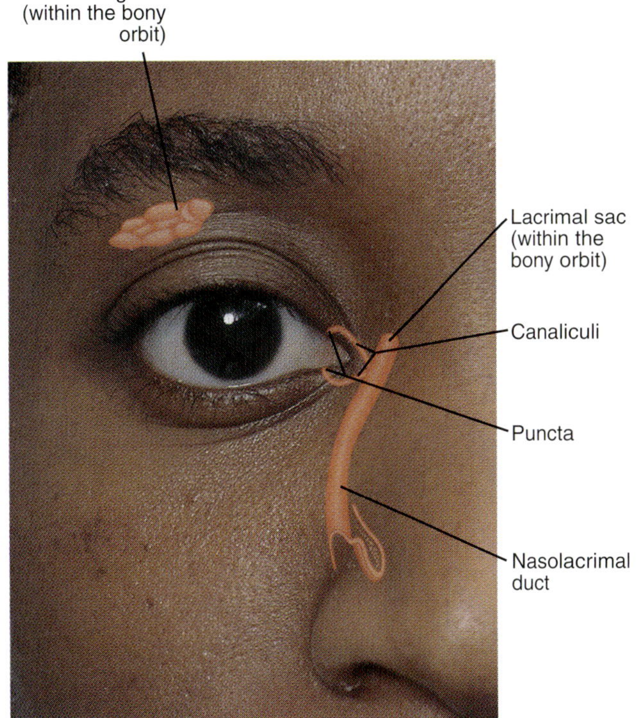

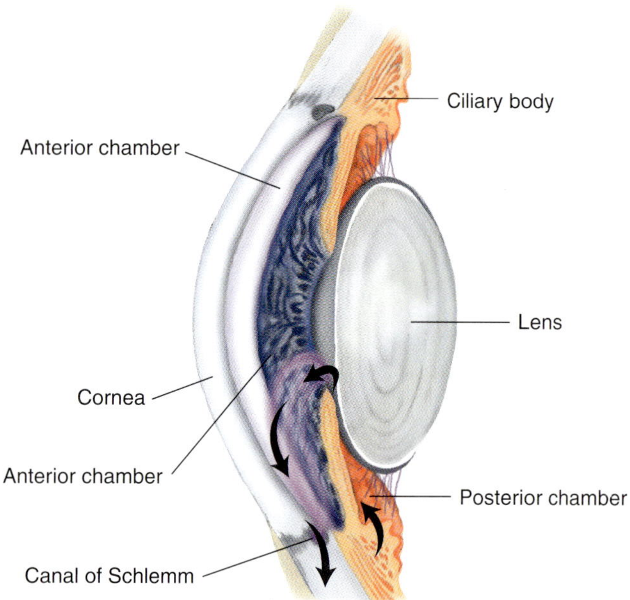

CIRCULATION OF AQUEOUS HUMOR

A clear liquid called *aqueous humor* fills the anterior and posterior chambers of the eye. Aqueous humor is produced by the ciliary body, circulates from the posterior chamber through the pupil into the anterior chamber, and drains out through the canal of Schlemm. This circulatory system helps to control the pressure inside the eye.

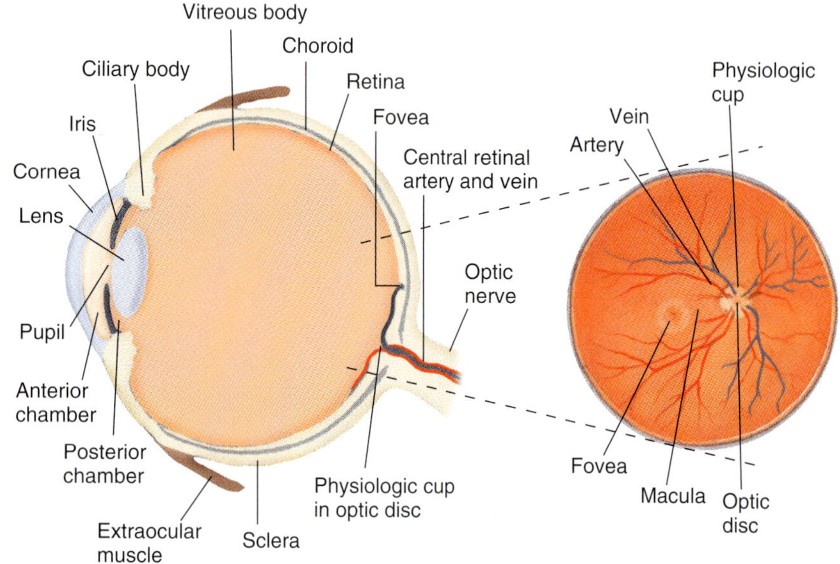

CROSS SECTION OF THE RIGHT EYE FROM ABOVE SHOWING A PORTION OF THE FUNDUS COMMONLY SEEN WITH THE OPHTHALMOSCOPE

The posterior part of the eye that is seen through an ophthalmoscope is often called the *fundus* of the eye. Structures here include the retina, choroid, fovea, macula, optic disc, and retinal vessels. The optic nerve with its retinal vessels enters the eyeball posteriorly. You can find it with an ophthalmoscope at the *optic disc*. Lateral and slightly inferior to the disc, there is a small depression in the retinal surface that marks the point of central vision. Around it is a darkened circular area called the *fovea*. The roughly circular *macula* (named for a microscopic yellow spot) surrounds the fovea but has no discernible margins. It does not quite reach the optic disc. You do not usually see the normal *vitreous body,* a transparent mass of gelatinous material that fills the eyeball behind the lens. It helps to maintain the shape of the eye.

Visual Fields. A *visual field* is the entire area seen by an eye when it looks at a central point. Fields are conventionally diagrammed on circles from the patient's point of view. The center of the circle represents the focus of gaze. The circumference is 90° from the line of gaze. Each visual field, shown by the white areas below, is divided into quadrants. Note that the fields extend farthest on the temporal sides. Visual fields are normally limited by the brows above, by the cheeks below, and by the nose medially. A lack of retinal receptors at the optic disc produces an oval blind spot in the normal field of each eye, 15° temporal to the line of gaze.

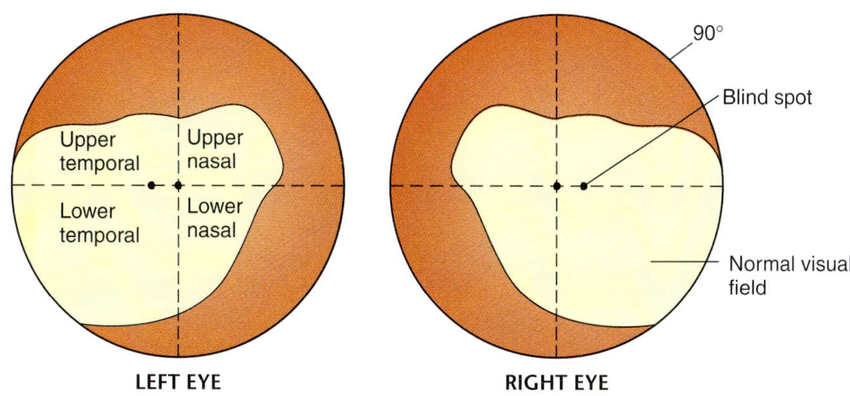

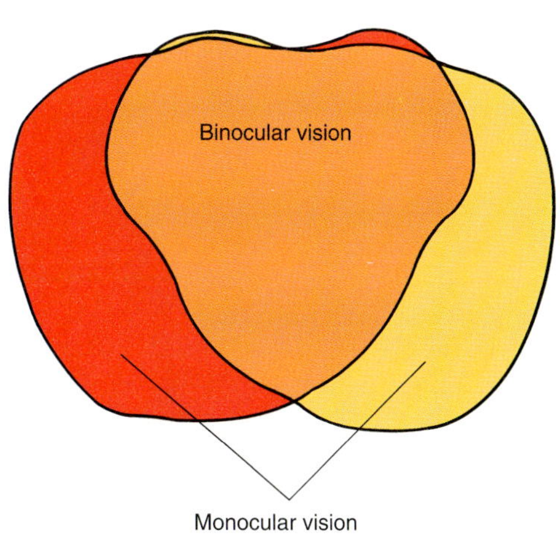

When a person is using both eyes, the two visual fields overlap in an area of binocular vision. Laterally, vision is monocular.

Visual Pathways. For an image to be seen, light reflected from it must pass through the pupil and be focused on sensory neurons in the retina. The image projected there is upside down and reversed right to left. An

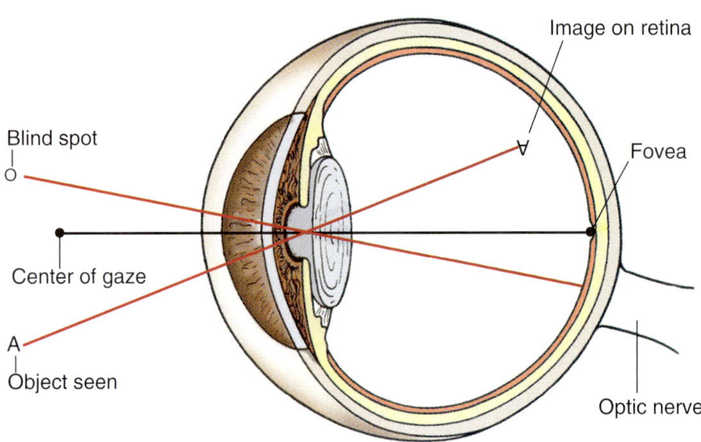

image from the upper nasal visual field thus strikes the lower temporal quadrant of the retina.

Nerve impulses, stimulated by light, are conducted through the retina, optic nerve, and optic tract on each side, and then on through a curving tract called the *optic radiation*. This ends in the visual cortex, a part of the occipital lobe.

Pupillary Reactions. Pupillary size changes in response to light and to the effort of focusing on a near object.

The Light Reaction. A light beam shining onto one retina causes pupillary constriction in both that eye (the *direct reaction* to light) and the opposite eye (the *consensual reaction*). The initial sensory pathways are similar to those described for vision: retina, optic nerve, and optic tract. The pathways diverge in the midbrain, however, and impulses are transmitted through the oculomotor nerve to the constrictor muscles of the iris of each eye.

The Near Reaction. When a person shifts gaze from a far object to a near one, the pupils constrict. This response, like the light reaction, is mediated by the oculomotor nerve. Coincident with this pupillary reaction (but not part of it) are (1) *convergence of the eyes,* an extraocular movement, and (2) *accommodation,* an increased convexity of the lenses caused by contraction of the ciliary muscles. This change in shape of the lenses brings near objects into focus but is not visible to the examiner.

Autonomic Nerve Supply to the Eyes. Fibers traveling in the oculomotor nerve and producing pupillary constriction are part of the parasympathetic nervous system. The iris is also supplied by sympathetic fibers. When these are stimulated, the pupil dilates and the upper eyelid rises a little, as if from fear. The sympathetic pathway starts in the hypothalamus and passes down through the brainstem and cervical cord into the neck. From there, it follows the carotid artery or its branches into the

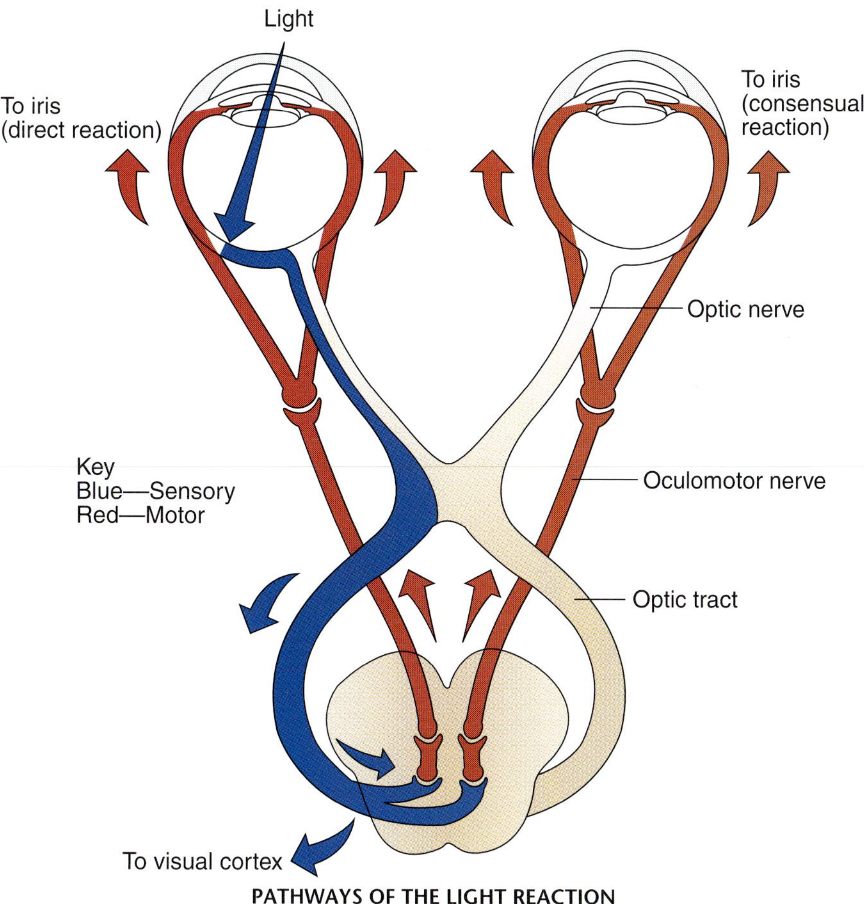

PATHWAYS OF THE LIGHT REACTION

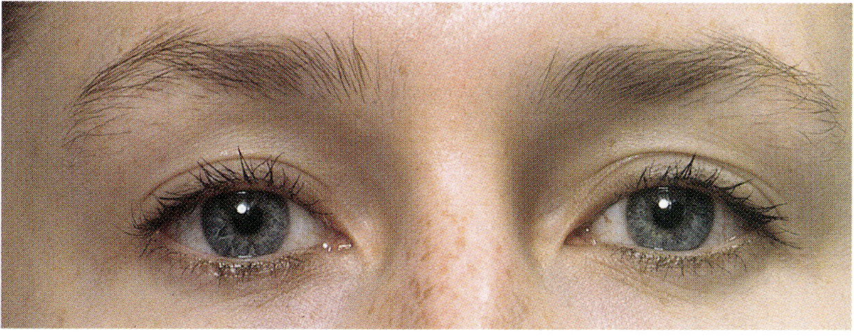

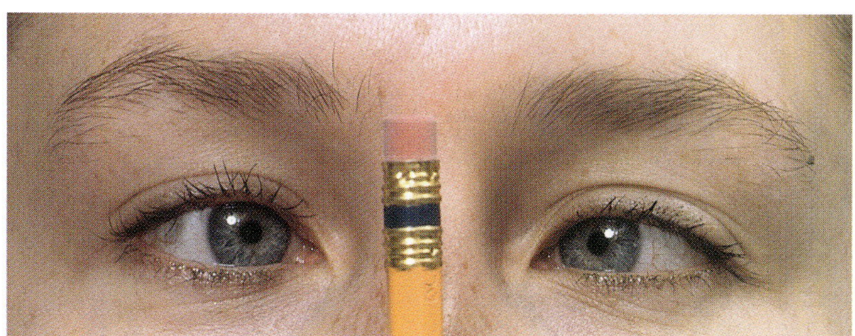

THE NEAR REACTION

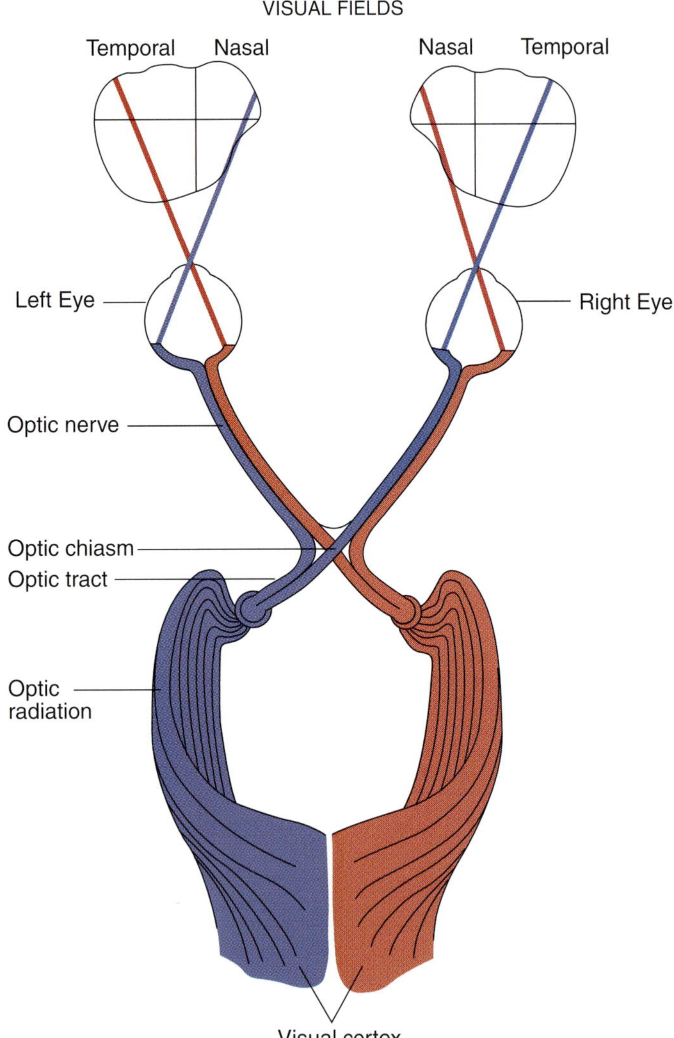

VISUAL PATHWAYS FROM THE RETINA TO THE VISUAL CORTEX

orbit. A lesion anywhere along this pathway may impair sympathetic effects on the pupil.

Extraocular Movements. The movement of each eye is controlled by the coordinated action of six muscles, the four rectus and two oblique muscles. You can test the function of each muscle and the nerve that supplies it by asking the patient to move the eye in the direction controlled by that muscle. There are six such *cardinal directions,* indicated by the lines on the figure on p. 123. When a person looks down and to the right, for example, the right inferior rectus (Cranial Nerve III) is principally responsible for moving the right eye, while the left superior oblique (Cranial Nerve IV) is principally responsible for moving the left. If one of these muscles is paralyzed, the eye will deviate from its normal position in that direction of gaze and the eyes will no longer appear conjugate, or parallel.

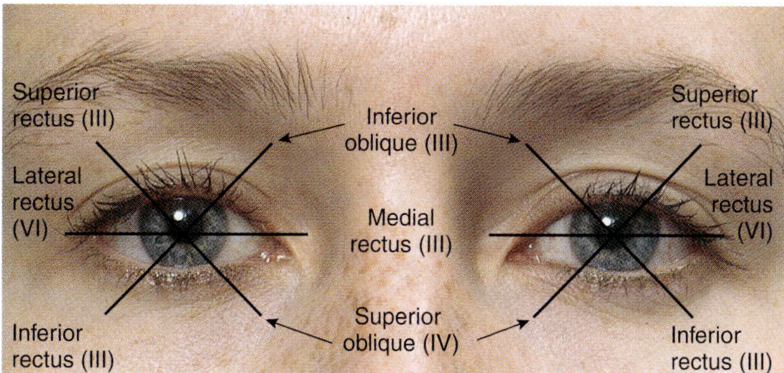

CARDINAL DIRECTIONS OF GAZE

The Ear

Anatomy. The ear has three compartments: the external ear, the middle ear, and the inner ear.

The *external ear* comprises the auricle and ear canal. The *auricle* consists chiefly of cartilage covered by skin and has a firm, elastic consistency.

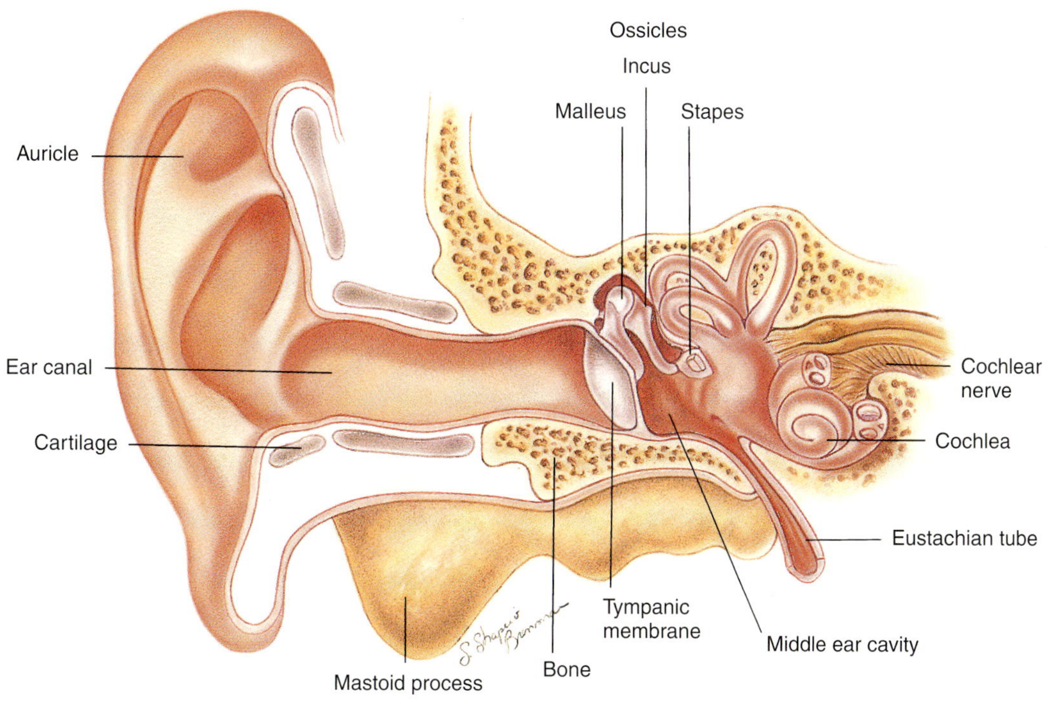

The *ear canal* opens behind the tragus and curves inward about 24 mm. Its outer portion is surrounded by cartilage. The skin in this outer portion is hairy and contains glands that produce cerumen (wax). The inner portion of the canal is surrounded by bone and lined by thin, hairless skin. Pressure on this latter area causes pain—a point to remember when you examine the ear.

The bone behind and below the ear canal is the mastoid part of the temporal bone. The lowest portion of this bone, the mastoid process, is palpable behind the lobule.

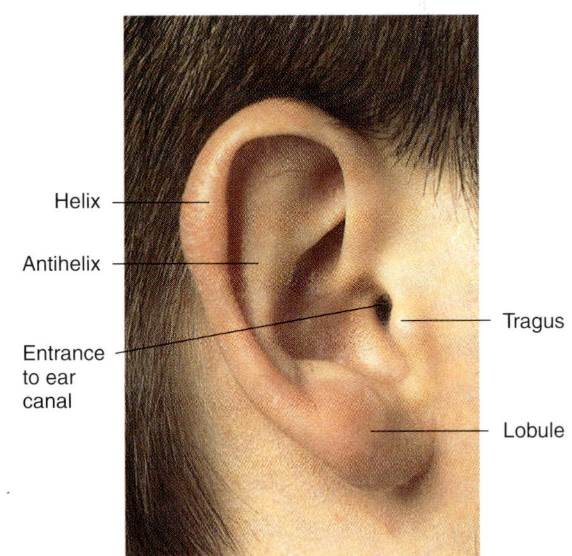

At the end of the ear canal lies the *tympanic membrane* (eardrum), marking the lateral limits of the middle ear. The *middle ear* is an air-filled cavity that transmits sound by way of three tiny bones, the ossicles. It is connected by the eustachian tube to the nasopharynx.

The eardrum is an oblique membrane held inward at its center by one of the ossicles, the *malleus.* Find the *handle* and the *short process* of the malleus—the two chief landmarks. From the *umbo,* where the eardrum meets the tip of the malleus, a light reflection called the *cone of light* fans downward and anteriorly. Above the short process lies a small portion of the eardrum called the *pars flaccida.* The remainder of the drum is the *pars tensa.* Anterior and posterior malleolar folds, which extend obliquely upward from the short process, separate the pars flaccida from the pars tensa but are usually invisible unless the eardrum is retracted. A second ossicle, the incus, can sometimes be seen through the drum.

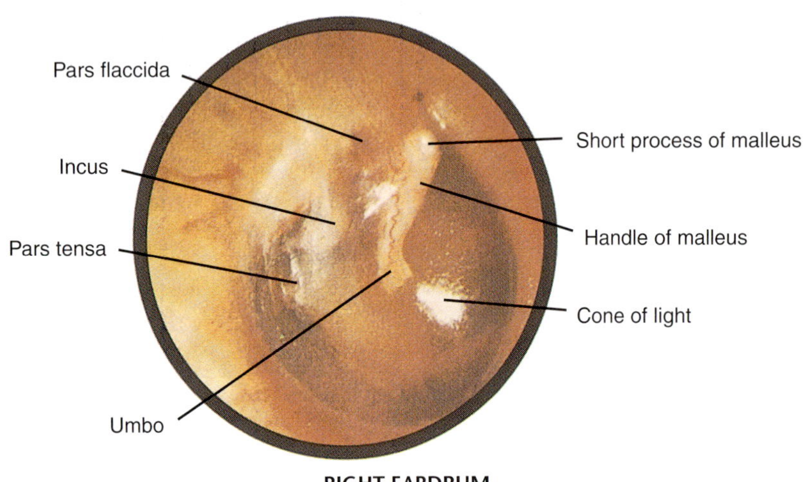

RIGHT EARDRUM

Much of the middle ear and all of the inner ear are inaccessible to direct examination. Some inferences concerning their condition can be made, however, by testing auditory function.

Pathways of Hearing. Vibrations of sound pass through the air of the external ear and are transmitted through the eardrum and ossicles of the middle ear to the cochlea, a part of the inner ear. The cochlea senses and codes the vibrations, and nerve impulses are sent to the brain through the cochlear nerve. The first part of this pathway—from the external ear through the middle ear—is known as the *conductive* phase, and a disorder here causes conductive hearing loss. The second part of the pathway, involving the cochlea and the cochlear nerve, is called the *sensorineural* phase; a disorder here causes sensorineural hearing loss.

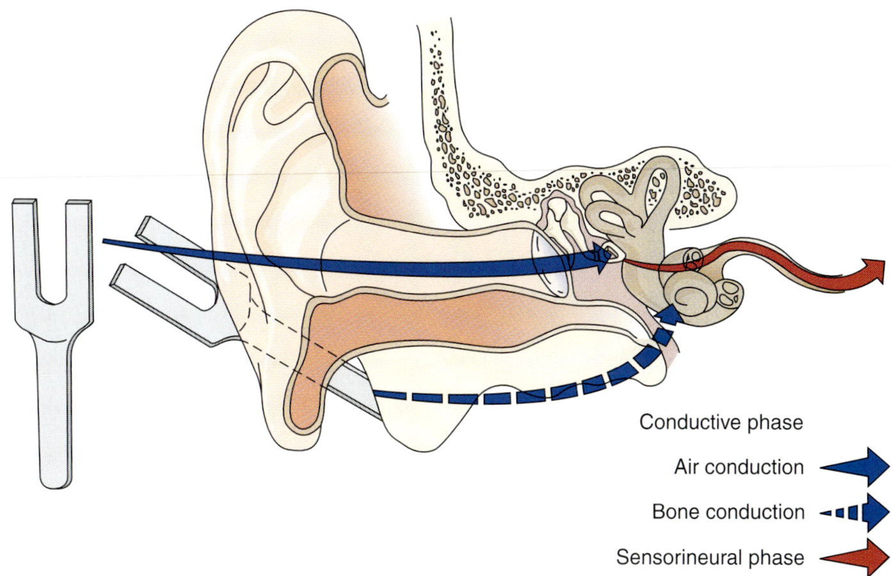

Air conduction describes the normal first phase in the hearing pathway. An alternate pathway, known as *bone conduction,* bypasses the external and the middle ear and is used for testing purposes. A vibrating tuning fork, placed on the head, sets the bone of the skull into vibration and stimulates the cochlea directly. In a normal person, air conduction is more sensitive.

Equilibrium. The labyrinth within the inner ear senses the position and movements of the head and helps to maintain balance.

The Nose and Paranasal Sinuses

Review the terms used to describe the external anatomy of the nose.

Approximately the upper third of the nose is supported by bone, the lower two thirds by cartilage. Air enters the nasal cavity by way of the *anterior naris* on either side, then passes into a widened area known as the *vestibule* and on through the narrow nasal passage to the nasopharynx. The medial wall of each nasal cavity is formed by the *nasal septum* which, like the external nose, is supported by both bone and cartilage. It is covered by a mucous membrane well supplied with blood. The vestibule, unlike the rest of the nasal cavity, is lined with hair-bearing skin, not mucosa.

Laterally, the anatomy is more complex. Curving bony structures, the *turbinates,* covered by a highly vascular mucous membrane, protrude into the nasal cavity. Below each turbinate is a groove, or meatus, each named according to the turbinate above it. Into the inferior meatus drains the nasolacrimal duct; into the middle meatus drain most of the paranasal sinuses. Their openings are not usually visible.

The additional surface area provided by the turbinates and the mucosa covering them aids the nasal cavities in their principal functions: cleansing, humidification, and temperature control of inspired air.

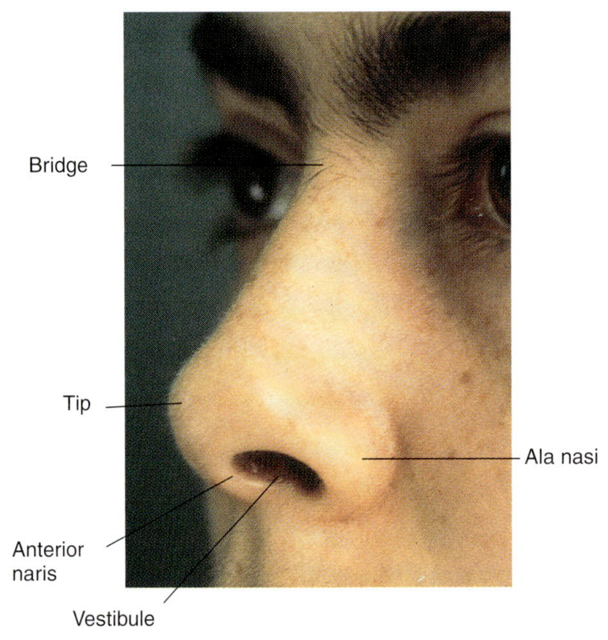

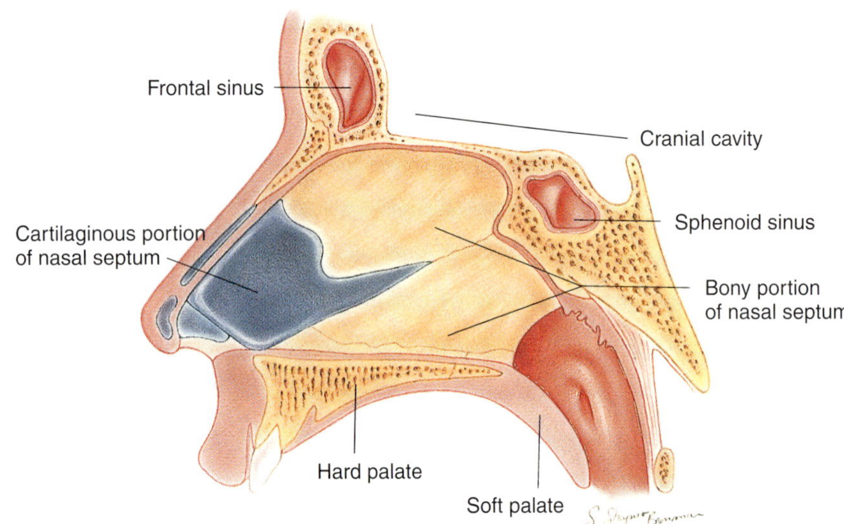

MEDIAL WALL—LEFT NASAL CAVITY (MUCOSA REMOVED)

Inspection of the nasal cavity through the anterior naris is usually limited to the vestibule, the anterior portion of the septum, and the lower and middle turbinates. Examination with a nasopharyngeal mirror is required for detection of posterior abnormalities. This technique is beyond the scope of this book.

The *paranasal sinuses* are air-filled cavities within the bones of the skull. Like the nasal cavities into which they drain, they are lined with mucous membrane. Their locations are diagrammed below. Only the frontal and maxillary sinuses are readily accessible to clinical examination.

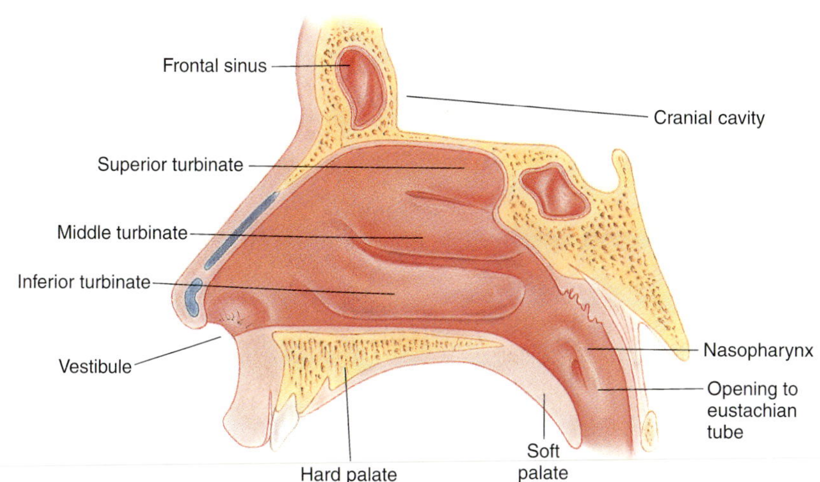

LATERAL WALL—RIGHT NASAL CAVITY

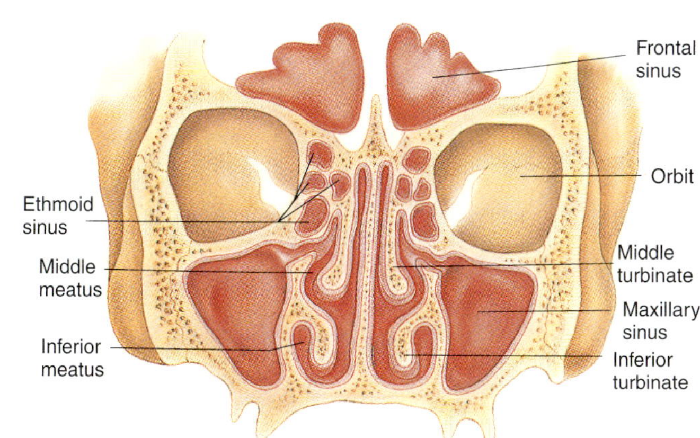

CROSS SECTION OF NASAL CAVITY—ANTERIOR VIEW

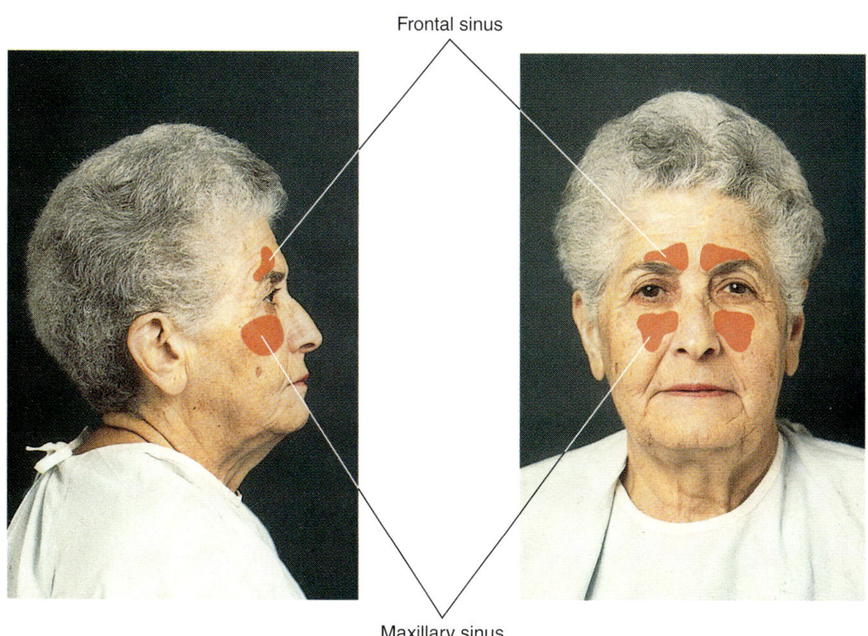

The Mouth and Pharynx

The *lips* are muscular folds that surround the entrance to the mouth. When opened, the gums (gingiva) and teeth are visible. Note the scalloped shape of the *gingival margins* and the pointed *interdental papillae.*

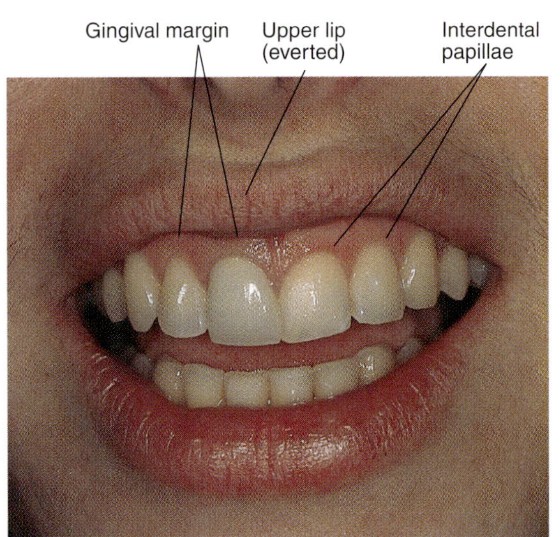

The *gingiva* is firmly attached to the teeth and to the maxilla or mandible in which they are seated. In lighter-skinned people, the gingiva is pale or coral pink and lightly stippled. In darker-skinned people, it maybe diffusely or partly brown as shown below. A midline mucosal fold, called a *labial frenulum,* connects each lip with the gingiva. A shallow *gingival sulcus* between the gum's thin margin and each tooth is not readily visible (but is probed and measured by dentists). Adjacent to the gingiva is the *alveolar mucosa,* which merges with the *labial mucosa* of the lip.

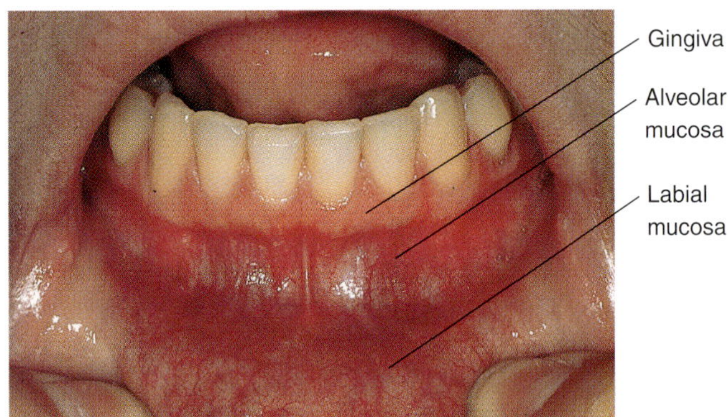

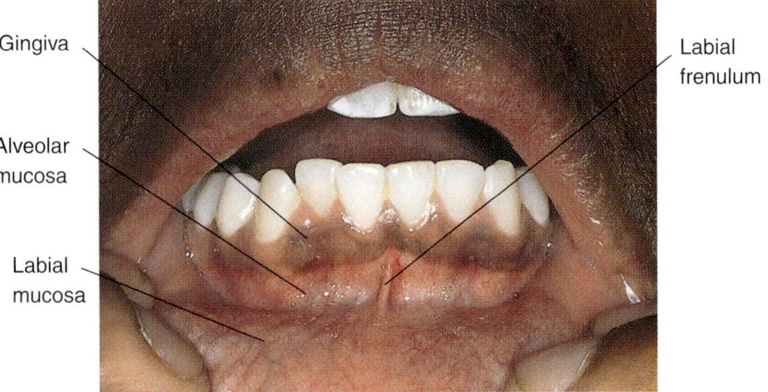

Each *tooth*, composed mostly of dentin, lies rooted in a bony socket with only its enamel-covered crown exposed. Small blood vessels and nerves enter the tooth through its apex and pass into the pulp canal and pulp chamber.

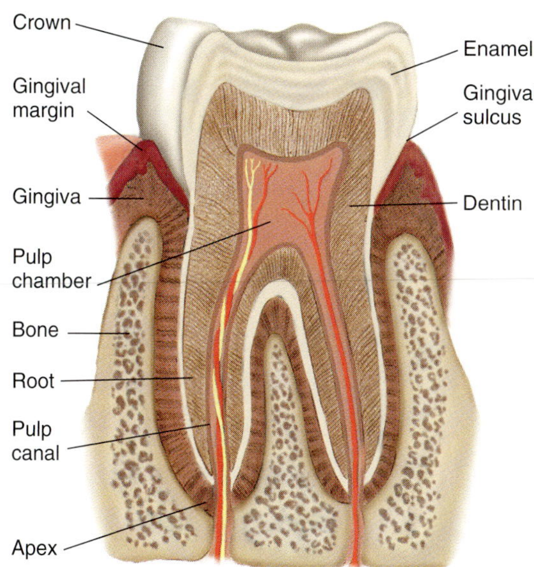

The 32 adult teeth (16 in each jaw) are identified below.

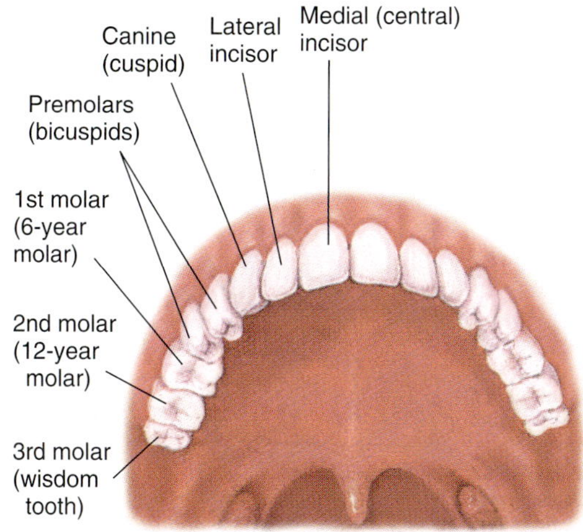

The dorsum of the *tongue* is covered with papillae, giving it a rough surface. Some of these papillae look like red dots, which contrast with the thin white coat that often covers the tongue. The undersurface of the tongue has no papillae. Note the midline *lingual frenulum* that connects the tongue to the floor of the mouth. At the base of the tongue the *ducts of the submandibu-*

lar gland (Wharton's ducts) pass forward and medially. They open on papillae that lie on each side of the lingual frenulum.

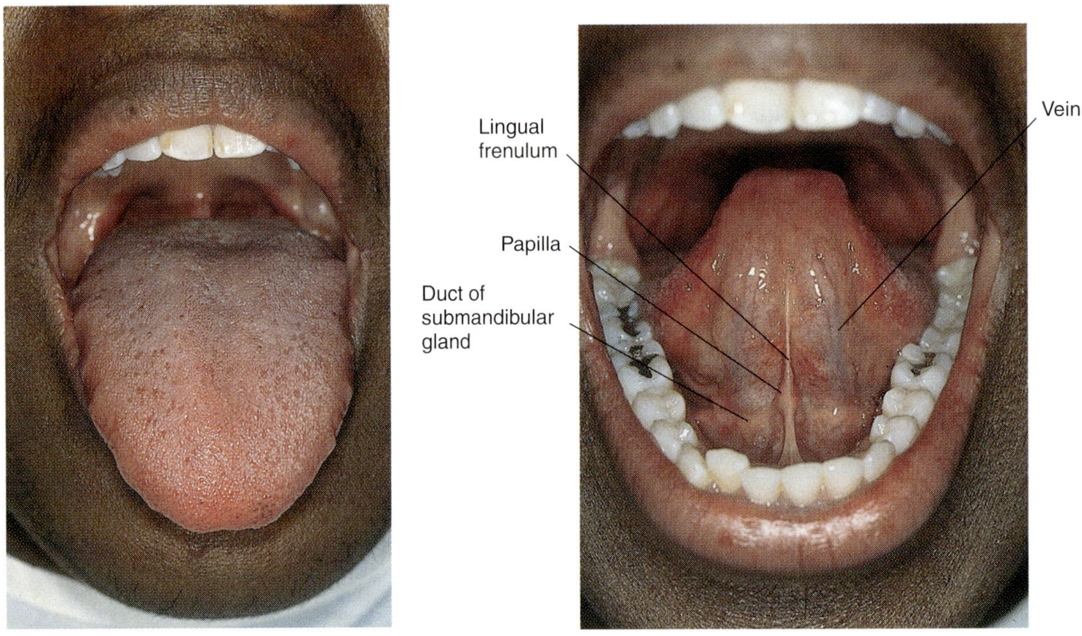

Each *parotid duct* (Stensen's duct) empties into the mouth near the upper 2nd molar, where its location is frequently marked by a small papilla. The *buccal mucosa* lines the cheeks.

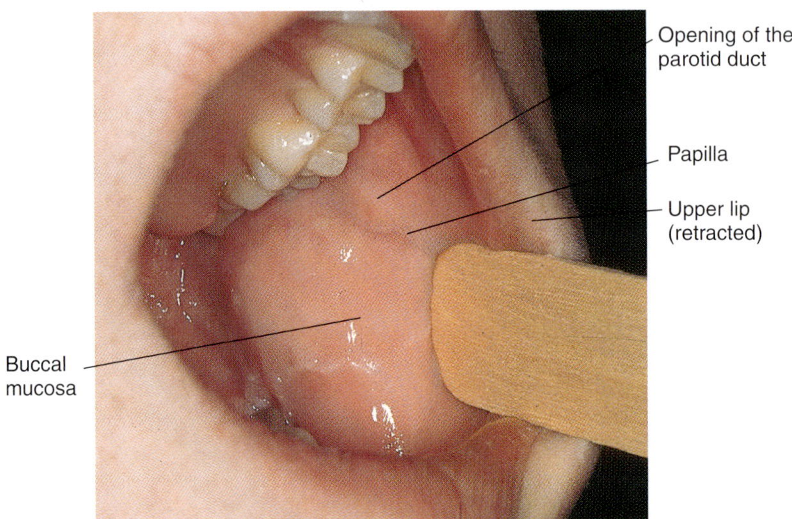

Above and behind the tongue rises an arch formed by the *anterior* and *posterior pillars, soft palate,* and *uvula*. In the following example, the right *tonsil* can be seen in its fossa (cavity) between the anterior and posterior pillars. In adults, tonsils are often small or absent, as exemplified on the left side here. A meshwork of small blood vessels may web the soft palate. Between the soft palate and tongue the *pharynx* is visible.

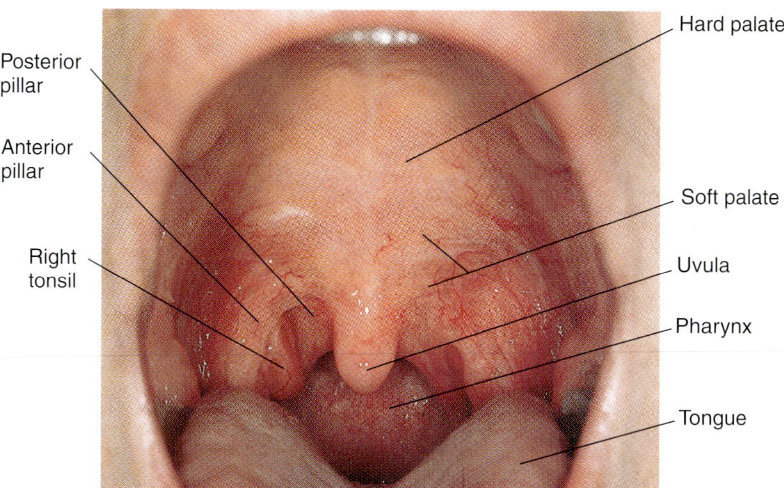

The Neck

For descriptive purposes, each side of the neck is divided into two triangles by the sternomastoid (sternocleidomastoid) muscle. The *anterior triangle* is bounded above by the mandible, laterally by the sternomastoid, and medially by the midline of the neck. The *posterior triangle* extends from the ster-

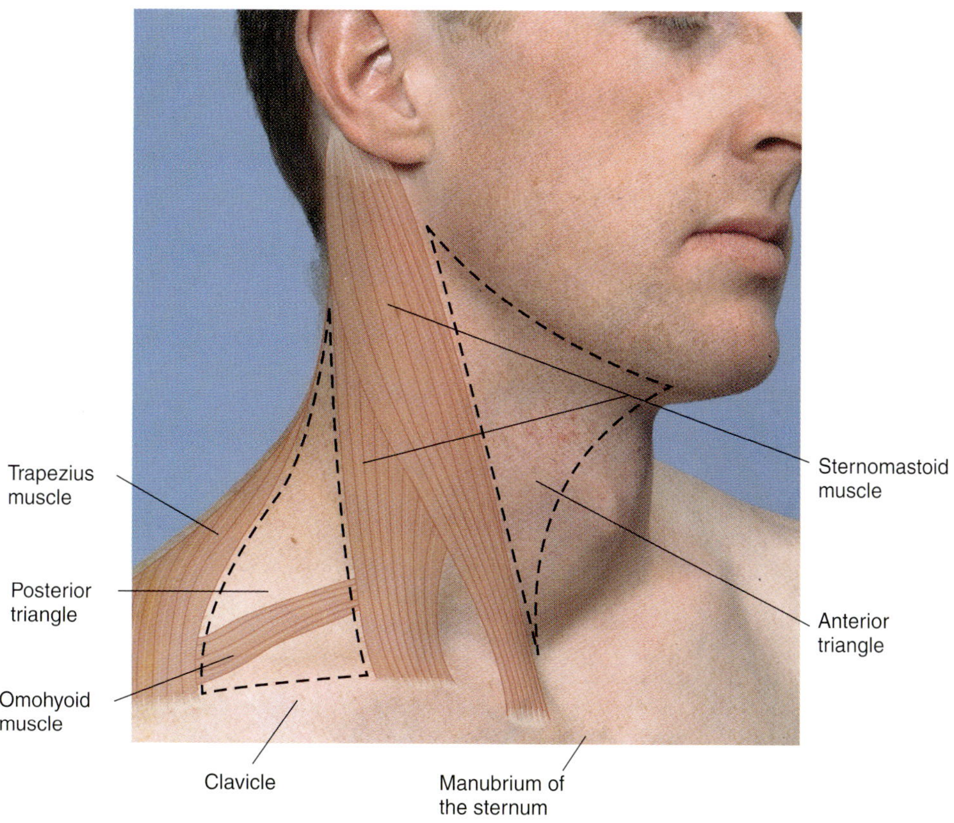

nomastoid to the trapezius and is bounded below by the clavicle. A portion of the omohyoid muscle crosses the lower portion of the posterior triangle and can be mistaken by the uninitiated for a lymph node or mass.

Deep to the sternomastoids run the great vessels of the neck: the *carotid artery* and *internal jugular vein*. The *external jugular vein* passes diagonally over the surface of the sternomastoid.

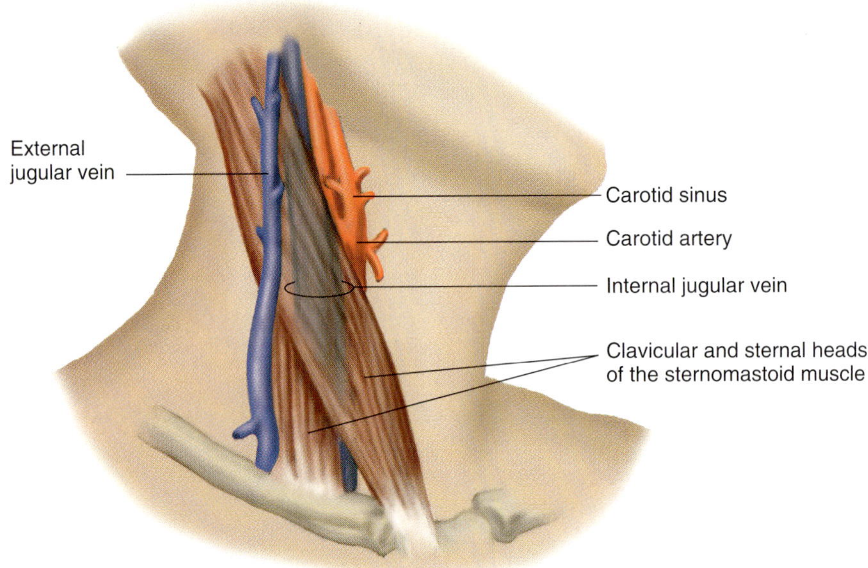

Now identify the following midline structures: (1) the mobile *hyoid bone* just below the mandible, (2) the *thyroid cartilage,* readily identified by the notch on its superior edge, (3) the *cricoid cartilage,* (4) the *tracheal rings,* and (5) the *thyroid gland.* The isthmus of the thyroid gland lies across the trachea

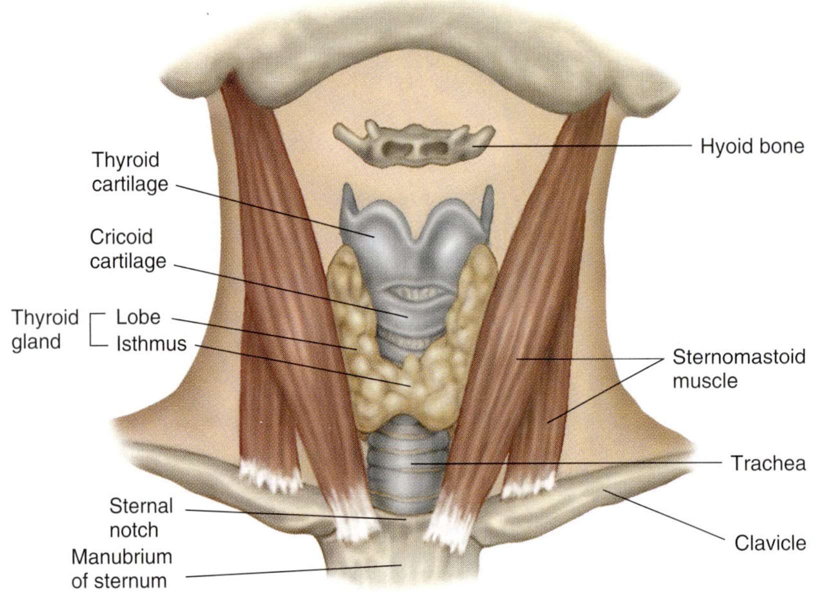

below the cricoid. The lateral lobes of this gland curve posteriorly around the sides of the trachea and the esophagus. Except in the midline, the thyroid gland is covered by thin straplike muscles, among which only the sternomastoids are visible.

Women have larger and more easily palpable glands than men.

The *lymph nodes* of the head and neck have been classified in a variety of ways. One classification is shown here, together with the directions of lymphatic drainage. The deep cervical chain is largely obscured by the overlying sternomastoid muscle, but at its two extremes the tonsillar node and supraclavicular nodes may be palpable. The submandibular nodes lie superficial to the submandibular gland, from which they should be differentiated. Nodes are normally round or ovoid, smooth, and smaller than the gland. The gland is larger and has a lobulated, slightly irregular surface (see p. 115).

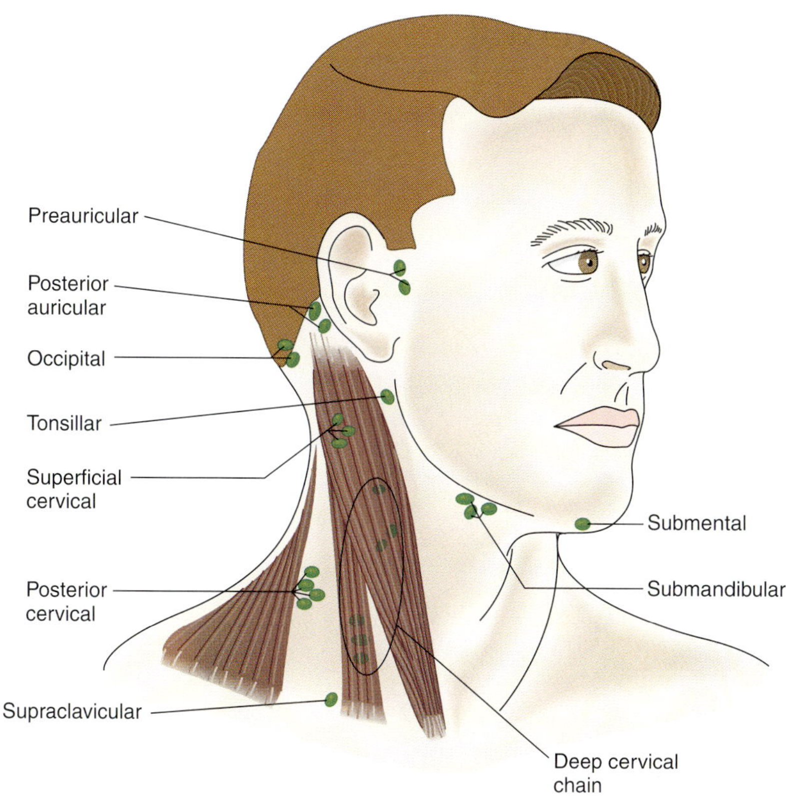

Note that the tonsillar, submandibular, and submental nodes drain portions of the mouth and throat as well as the face.

Knowledge of the lymphatic system is important to a sound clinical habit: whenever a malignant or inflammatory lesion is observed, look for involvement of the regional lymph nodes that drain it; whenever a node is enlarged or tender, look for a source such as infection in the area that it drains.

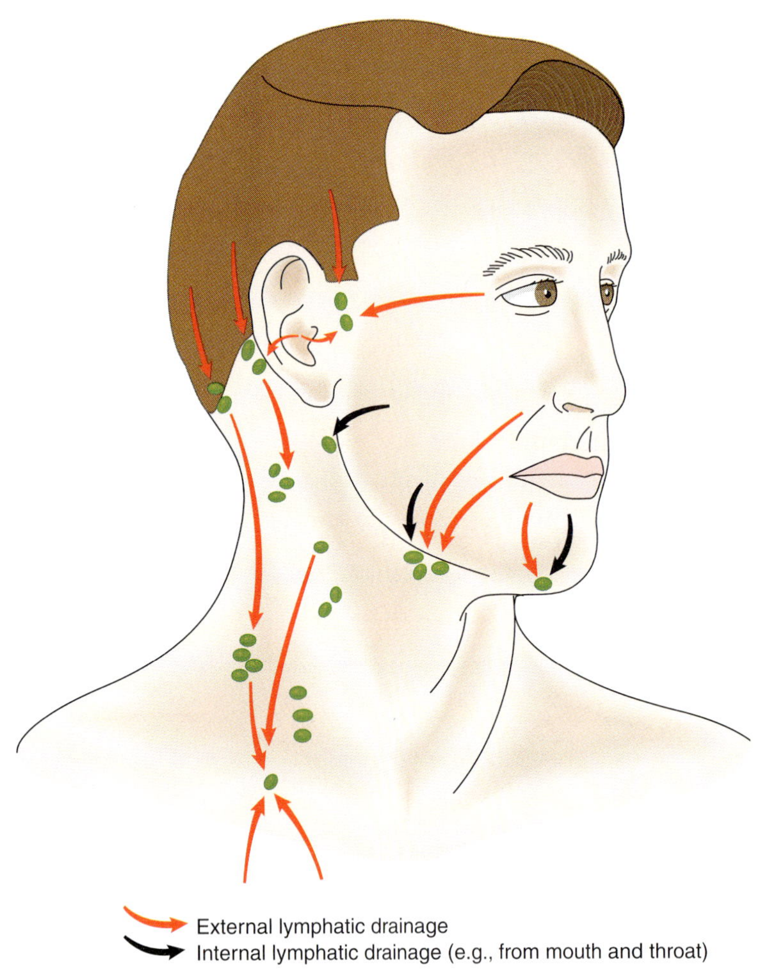

Changes With Aging

Tonsils, which are also composed of lymphoid tissue, become gradually smaller after the age of 5 years. In adulthood, they become inconspicuous or invisible. The frequency of palpable cervical nodes gradually diminishes with age, and according to one study falls below 50% sometime between the ages of 50 and 60. In contrast to the lymph nodes, the submandibular glands become easier to feel in older people.

The eyes, ears, and mouth bear the brunt of old age. Visual acuity remains fairly constant between the ages of 20 and 50 and then diminishes, gradually until about age 70 and then more rapidly. Nevertheless, most elderly people retain good to adequate vision—20/20 to 20/70 as measured by standard charts. Near vision, however, begins to blur noticeably for virtually everyone. From childhood on, the lens gradually loses its elasticity and the eye grows progressively less able to focus on nearby objects. This loss of accommodative power, called *presbyopia,* usually becomes noticeable in one's 40s.

Aging also affects the tissues in and around the eyes. In some elderly people the fat that surrounds and cushions the eye within the bony orbit atrophies, allowing the eyeball to recede somewhat in the orbit. The skin of the eyelids becomes wrinkled, occasionally hanging in loose folds. Fat may push the fascia of the eyelids forward, creating soft bulges, especially in the lower lids and the inner third of the upper ones (p. 175). Combinations of a weakened levator palpebrae, relaxation of the skin, and increased weight of the upper eyelid may cause a senile ptosis (drooping). More important, the lower lid may fall outward away from the eyeball or turn inward onto it, resulting in ectropion and entropion, respectively (p. 177). Because their eyes produce fewer lacrimal secretions, aging patients may complain of dryness of the eyes.

Corneal arcus (*arcus senilis*) is common in elderly persons and in them has no clinical significance (p. 180). The corneas lose some of their luster. The pupils become smaller—a characteristic that makes it more difficult to examine the fundi of elderly people. The pupils may also become slightly irregular but should continue to respond to light and near effort. Except for possible impairment in upward gaze, extraocular movements should remain intact.

Lenses thicken and yellow with age, impairing the passage of light to the retinas, and elderly people need more light to read and do fine work. When the lens of an elderly person is examined with a flashlight it frequently looks gray, as if it were opaque, when in fact it permits good visual acuity and looks clear on ophthalmoscopic examination. Do not depend on your flashlight alone, therefore, to make a diagnosis of cataract—a true opacity of the lens (p. 180). Cataracts do become relatively common, however, affecting 1 out of 10 people in their 60s and 1 out of 3 in their 80s. Because the lens continues to grow over the years, it may push the iris forward, narrowing the angle between iris and cornea and increasing the risk of *narrow-angle glaucoma* (p. 148).

Ophthalmoscopic examination reveals fundi that have lost their youthful shine and light reflections. The arteries look narrowed, paler, straighter, and less brilliant (p. 190). *Drusen* (colloid bodies) may be seen (p. 187). On a more anterior plane you may be able to see some vitreous floaters—degenerative changes that may cause annoying specks or webs in the field of vision. You may also find evidence of other, more serious, conditions that occur more often in elderly people than in younger ones: macular degeneration, glaucoma, retinal hemorrhages, or possibly retinal detachment.

Acuity of hearing, like that of vision, usually diminishes with age. Early losses, which start in young adulthood, involve primarily the high-pitched sounds beyond the range of human speech and have relatively little functional significance. Gradually, however, loss extends to sounds in the middle and lower ranges. When a person fails to catch the upper tones of words while hearing the lower ones, words sound distorted and are difficult to understand, especially in noisy environments. Hearing loss associated with aging, known as *presbycusis,* becomes increasingly evident, usually after the age of 50.

Diminished salivary secretions and a decreased sense of taste have been attributed to aging, but medications or various diseases probably account for most of these changes. Teeth may wear down or become abraded over time, or they may be lost to dental caries or other conditions (pp. 203–205). Periodontal disease is the chief cause of tooth loss in most adults (p. 203). If a person has no teeth, the lower portion of the face looks small and sunken, with accentuated "purse-string" wrinkles radiating out from the mouth. Overclosure of the mouth may lead to maceration of the skin at the corners—*angular cheilitis* (p. 198). The bony ridges of the jaws that once surrounded the tooth sockets are gradually resorbed, especially in the lower jaw.

THE HEALTH HISTORY

Common or Concerning Symptoms

- Headache
- Change in vision: hyperopia, presbyopia, myopia, scotomas
- Double vision, or diplopia
- Hearing loss, earache; tinnitus
- Vertigo
- Nosebleed, or epistaxis
- Sore throat; hoarseness
- Swollen glands
- Goiter

The Head

Headache is an extremely common symptom that always requires careful evaluation, since a small fraction of headaches arise from life-threatening conditions. It is important to elicit a full description of the headache and all seven attributes of the patient's pain (see p. 27). Is the headache one-sided or bilateral? Steady or throbbing? Continuous or comes and goes? After your usual open-ended approach, ask the patient to *point to the area of pain or discomfort.*

See Table 5-1, Headaches, pp. 170–173. Tension and migraine headaches are the most common kinds of recurring headaches.

Tension headaches often arise in the temporal areas; cluster headaches may be retro-orbital.

The most important attributes of headache are the *chronologic pattern* and *severity.* Is the problem new and acute? Chronic and recurring, with little change in pattern? Chronic and recurring but with recent change in pattern or progressively severe? Does the pain recur at the same time every day?

Changing or progressively severe headaches increase the likelihood of tumor, abscess, or other mass lesion. Extremely severe headaches suggest subarachnoid hemorrhage or meningitis.

Ask about associated symptoms. Inquire specifically about associated nausea and vomiting and neurologic symptoms such as change in vision or motor-sensory deficits.

Visual aura or scintillating scotomas with migraine. Nausea and vomiting common with migraine but also occur with brain tumors and subarachnoid hemorrhage.

Ask whether coughing, sneezing, or changing the position of the head have any effect (better, worse, or no effect) on the headache.

Such maneuvers may increase pain from brain tumor and acute sinusitis.

Ask about family history.

Family history may be positive in patients with migraine.

The Eyes

Start your inquiry about eye and vision problems with open-ended questions such as "How is your vision?" and "Have you had any trouble with your eyes?" If the patient reports a change in vision, pursue the related details:

Refractive errors most commonly explain gradual blurring. High blood sugar levels may cause blurring.

- Is the onset sudden or gradual?

Sudden visual loss suggests retinal detachment, vitreous hemorrhage, or occlusion of the central retinal artery.

- Is the problem worse during close work or at distances?

Difficulty with close work suggests *hyperopia* (farsightedness) or *presbyopia* (aging vision); with distances, *myopia* (near-sightedness).

- Is there blurring of the entire field of vision or only parts of it? If the visual field defect is partial, is it central, peripheral, or only on one side?

Slow central loss in nuclear cataract (p. 180), macular degeneration (p. 155); peripheral loss in advanced open-angle glaucoma (p. 148); one-sided loss in hemianopsia and quadrantic defects (p. 145).

- Are there specks in the vision or areas where the patient cannot see (*scotomas*)? If so, do they move around in the visual field with shifts in gaze or are they fixed?

Moving specks or strands suggest vitreous floaters; fixed defects (scotomas) suggest lesions in the retinas or visual pathways.

- Has the patient seen lights flashing across the field of vision? This symptom may be accompanied by vitreous floaters.

Flashing lights or new vitreous floaters suggest detachment of vitreous from retina. Prompt eye consultation is indicated.

- Does the patient wear glasses?

Ask about *pain* in or around the eyes, *redness,* and *excessive tearing or watering.*

See Table 5-7, Red Eyes, p. 179.

Check for presence of *diplopia,* or double vision. If present, find out whether the images are side by side (horizontal diplopia) or on top of each other (vertical diplopia). Does diplopia persist with one eye closed? Which eye is affected?

One kind of horizontal diplopia is physiologic. Hold one finger upright about 6 inches in front of your face, a second at arm's length. When you focus on either finger, the image of the other is double. A patient who notices this phenomenon can be reassured.

Diplopia in adults may arise from a lesion in the brainstem or cerebellum, or from weakness or paralysis of one or more extraocular muscles as in horizontal diplopia from palsy of CN III or VI, or vertical diplopia from palsy of CN III or IV. Diplopia in one eye, with the other closed, suggests a problem in the cornea or lens.

The Ears

Opening questions for the ears are "How is your hearing?" and "Have you had any trouble with your ears?" If the patient has noticed a *hearing loss,* does it involve one or both ears? Did it start suddenly or gradually? What are the associated symptoms, if any?

See Table 5-19, Patterns of Hearing Loss, pp. 196–197.

Try to distinguish between two basic types of hearing impairment: *conductive loss,* which results from problems in the external or middle ear, and *sensorineural loss,* from problems in the inner ear, the cochlear nerve, or its central connections in the brain. Two questions may be helpful . . . Does the patient have special difficulty understanding people as they talk? . . . What difference does a noisy environment make?

Persons with sensorineural loss have particular trouble understanding speech, often complaining that others mumble; noisy environments make hearing worse. In conductive loss, noisy environments may help.

Infants may fail to respond to the parent's voice or to sounds in the environment (see p. 677). Toddlers may exhibit a delay in developing speech. Such findings deserve thorough investigation.

Symptoms associated with hearing loss, such as earache or vertigo, help you to assess likely causes. In addition, inquire specifically about medications that might affect hearing and ask about sustained exposure to loud noise.

Medications that affect hearing include aminoglycosides, aspirin, NSAIDs, quinine, furosemide, and others.

Complaints of *earache,* or *pain in the ear,* are especially common in office visits. Ask about associated fever, sore throat, cough, and concurrent upper respiratory infection.

Pain suggests a problem in the external ear, such as *otitis externa,* or, if associated with symptoms of respiratory infection, in the inner ear, as in *otitis media.* It may also be referred from other structures in the mouth, throat, or neck.

Ask about *discharge from the ear*, especially if associated with earache or trauma.

Unusually soft wax, debris from inflammation or rash in the ear canal, or discharge through a perforated eardrum secondary to acute or chronic otitis media

Tinnitus is a perceived sound that has no external stimulus—commonly, a musical ringing or a rushing or roaring noise. It can involve one or both ears. Tinnitus may accompany hearing loss and often remains unexplained. Occasionally, popping sounds originate in the temporomandibular joint, or vascular noises from the neck may be audible.

Tinnitus is a common symptom, increasing in frequency with age. When associated with hearing loss and vertigo it suggests Ménière's disease.

Vertigo refers to the perception that the patient or the environment is rotating or spinning. These sensations point primarily to a problem in the labyrinths of the inner ear, peripheral lesions of CN VIII or lesions in its central pathways, or nuclei in the brain.

See Table 5-2, Vertigo, p. 174.

Vertigo is a challenging symptom for you as clinician, since patients differ widely in what they mean by the word "dizzy." "Are there times when you feel dizzy?" is an appropriate first question, but patients often find it difficult to be more specific. Ask "Do you feel unsteady, as if you are going to fall or black out? . . . Or do you feel the room is spinning (true vertigo)?" Get the story without biasing it. You may need to offer the patient several choices of wording. Ask if the patient feels pulled to the ground or off to one side. And if the dizziness is related to a change in body position. Pursue any associated feelings of clamminess or flushing, nausea, or vomiting. Check if any medications may be contributing.

Feeling unsteady, light-headed, or "dizzy in the legs" sometimes suggests a cardiovascular etiology. A feeling of being pulled suggests true vertigo from an inner ear problem or a central or peripheral lesion of CN VIII.

The Nose and Sinuses

Rhinorrhea refers to drainage from the nose and is often associated with *nasal congestion*, a sense of stuffiness or obstruction. These symptoms are frequently accompanied by *sneezing*, watery eyes, and throat discomfort, and also by *itching* in the eyes, nose, and throat.

Causes include viral infections, allergic rhinitis ("hay fever"), and vasomotor rhinitis. Itching favors an allergic cause.

Assess the chronology of the illness. Does it last for a week or so, especially when common colds and related syndromes are prevalent, or does it occur seasonally when pollens are in the air? Is it associated with specific contacts or environments? What remedies has the patient used? For how long? And how well do they work?

Relation to seasons or environmental contacts suggests allergy.

Excessive use of decongestants can worsen the symptoms.

Inquire about drugs that might cause stuffiness.

Oral contraceptives, reserpine, guanethidine, and alcohol

Are there symptoms in addition to rhinorrhea or congestion, such as pain and tenderness in the face or over the sinuses, local headache, or fever?

These together suggest sinusitis.

Is the patient's nasal congestion limited to one side? If so, you may be dealing with a different problem that requires careful physical examination.

Consider a deviated nasal septum, foreign body, or tumor.

Epistaxis means bleeding from the nose. The blood usually originates from the nose itself, but may come from a paranasal sinus or the nasopharynx. The history is usually quite graphic! However, in patients who are lying down, or whose bleeding originates in posterior structures, blood may pass into the throat instead of out the nostrils. You must identify the source of the bleeding carefully—is it from the nose or has it been coughed up or vomited? Assess the site of bleeding, its severity, and associated symptoms. Is it a recurrent problem? Has there been easy bruising or bleeding elsewhere in the body?

Local causes of epistaxis include trauma (especially nose picking), inflammation, drying and crusting of the nasal mucosa, tumors, and foreign bodies.

Bleeding disorders may contribute to epistaxis.

The Mouth, Throat, and Neck

Sore throat is a frequent complaint, usually developing in the setting of acute upper respiratory symptoms.

Fever, pharyngeal exudates, and anterior lymphadenopathy, especially in the absence of cough, suggest streptococcal pharyngitis, or *strep throat* (p. 200)

A *sore tongue* may be caused by local lesions as well as by systemic illness.

Aphthous ulcers (p. 207); sore smooth tongue of nutritional deficiency (p. 206).

Bleeding from the gums is a common symptom, especially when brushing teeth. Ask about local lesions and any tendency to bleed or bruise elsewhere.

Bleeding gums are most often caused by gingivitis (p. 203).

Hoarseness refers to an altered quality of the voice, often described as husky, rough, or harsh. The pitch may be lower than before. Hoarseness usually arises from disease of the larynx, but may also develop as extralaryngeal lesions press on the laryngeal nerves. Check for overuse of the voice, allergy, smoking or other inhaled irritants, and any associated symptoms. Is the problem acute or chronic? If hoarseness lasts more than 2 weeks, visual examination of the larynx by indirect or direct laryngoscopy is advisable.

Overuse of the voice (as in cheering) and acute infections are the most likely causes.

Causes of chronic hoarseness include smoking, allergy, voice abuse, hypothyroidism, chronic infections such as tuberculosis, and tumors.

Asking "Have you noticed any swollen glands or lumps in your neck?" is advisable, since patients are more familiar with the lay terms than with "*lymph nodes.*"

Enlarged tender lymph nodes commonly accompany pharyngitis.

Assess thyroid function and ask about any evidence of an enlarged thyroid gland or *goiter*. To evaluate thyroid function, ask about *temperature intolerance* and *sweating*. Opening questions include "Do you prefer hot or cold weather?" "Do you dress more warmly or less warmly than other people?" "What about blankets . . . do you use more or fewer than others at home?" "Do you perspire more or less than others?" "Any new palpitations or change in weight?" Note that as people grow older, they sweat less, have less tolerance for cold, and tend to prefer warmer environments.

With goiter, thyroid function may be increased, decreased, or normal.

Intolerance to cold, preference for warm clothing and many blankets, and decreased sweating suggest hypothyroidism; the opposite symptoms, palpitations and involuntary weight loss suggest hyperthyroidism (p. 208).

HEALTH PROMOTION AND COUNSELING

Important Topics for Health Promotion and Counseling

- Changes in vision: cataracts, macular degeneration, glaucoma
- Hearing loss
- Oral health

Vision and hearing, critical senses for experiencing the world around us, are two areas of special importance for health promotion and counseling. Oral health, often overlooked, also merits clinical attention.

Disorders of vision shift with age. Healthy young adults generally have refractive errors. Up to 25% of adults over 65 have refractive errors; however, cataracts, macular degeneration, and glaucoma become more prevalent. These disorders reduce awareness of the social and physical environment and contribute to falls and injuries. To improve detection of visual defects, test visual acuity with a Snellen chart or handheld card (p. 675). Examine the lens and fundi for clouding of the lens (*cataracts*); mottling of the *macula,* variations in the retinal pigmentation, subretinal hemorrhage or exudate (*macular degeneration*); and change in size and color of the optic cup (*glaucoma*). After diagnosis, review effective treatments—corrective lenses, cataract surgery, photocoagulation for choroidal neovascularization in macular degeneration, and topical medications for glaucoma.

Surveillance for glaucoma is especially important. Glaucoma is the leading cause of blindness in African Americans and the second leading cause of blindness overall. There is gradual loss of vision with damage to the optic nerve, loss of visual fields beginning usually at the periphery, and pallor and increasing size of the optic cup (enlarging to more than half the diameter of the optic disc). Elevated intraocular pressure (IOP) is seen in up to 80% of cases and is linked to damage of the optic nerve. Risk factors include age over 65, African American origin, diabetes mellitus, myopia, family history of glaucoma, and ocular hypertension (IOP $\geq$ 21 mm Hg). Screening tests include tonometry to measure IOP, ophthalmoscopy or slit-lamp examination of the optic nerve head, and perimetry to map the visual fields. In the hands of general clinicians, however, all three tests lack accuracy, so attention to risk factors and referral to eye specialists remain important tools for clinical care.

Hearing loss can also trouble the later years. More than a third of adults over age 65 have detectable hearing deficits, contributing to emotional isolation and social withdrawal. These losses may go undetected—unlike vision prerequisites for driving and vision, there is no mandate for widespread testing and many seniors avoid use of hearing aids. Questionnaires and hand-held audioscopes work well for periodic screening. Less sensitive are the clinical "whisper test," rubbing fingers, or use of the tuning fork. Groups at risk are those with a history of congenital or familial hearing loss, syphilis, rubella, meningitis, or exposure to hazardous noise levels at work or on the battlefield.

Clinicians should play an active role in promoting oral health: up to half of all children ages 5 to 17 have from one to eight cavities, and the average US adult has 10 to 17 teeth that are decayed, missing, or filled. In adults, the prevalence of gingivitis and periodontal disease is 50% and 80% respectively. In the U.S., more than half of all adults over age 65 have no teeth at all!* Effective screening begins with careful examination of the mouth. Inspect the oral cavity for decayed or loose teeth, inflammation of the gingiva, and signs of periodontal disease (bleeding, pus, recession of the gums, and bad breath). Inspect the mucous membranes, the palate, the oral floor, and the surfaces of the tongue for ulcers and leukoplakia, warning signs for oral cancer and HIV disease.

To improve oral health, counsel patients to adopt daily hygiene measures. Use of fluoride-containing toothpastes reduces tooth decay, and brushing and flossing retard periodontal disease by removing bacterial plaques. Urge patients to seek dental care at least annually to receive the benefits of more specialized preventive care such as scaling, planing of roots, and topical fluorides.

Diet, tobacco and alcohol use, changes in salivary flow from medication, and proper use of dentures should also be addressed.** As with children, adults should avoid excessive intake of foods high in refined sugars, such as sucrose, which enhance attachment and colonization of cariogenic bacteria. Use of all tobacco products and excessive alcohol, the principal risk factors for oral cancers, should be avoided.

Saliva cleanses and lubricates the mouth. Many medications reduce salivary flow, increasing risk of tooth decay, mucositis, and gum disease from xerostomia, especially for the elderly. For those wearing dentures, be sure to counsel removal and cleaning each night to reduce bacterial plaque and risk of malodor. Regular massage of the gums relieves soreness and pressure from dentures on the underlying soft tissue.

*U.S. Preventive Services Task Force: Guide to Clinical Preventive Services (2nd ed), pp. 711–721. Baltimore, Williams & Wilkins, 1996.

**Greene JC, Greene AR: Chapter 15: Oral Health. In Woolf SH, Jonas S, Lawrence RS (eds): Health Promotion and Disease Prevention in Clinical Practice, pp. 315–334. Baltimore, Williams & Wilkins, 1996.

Preview: Recording the Physical Examination—The Head, Eyes, Ears, Nose, and Throat (HEENT)

Note that initially you may use sentences to describe your findings; later you will use phrases. The style below contains phrases appropriate for most write-ups. Unfamiliar terms are explained in the next section, Techniques of Examination.

HEENT: Head—The skull is normocephalic/atraumatic (NC/AT). Hair with average texture. *Eyes*—Visual acuity 20/20 bilaterally. Sclera white, conjunctiva pink. Pupils are 4 mm constricting to 2 mm, equally round and reactive to light and accommodations. Disc margins sharp; no hemorrhages or exudates, no arteriolar narrowing. *Ears*—Acuity good to whispered voice. Tympanic membranes (TMs) with good cone of light. Weber midline. AC > BC. *Nose*—Nasal mucosa pink, septum midline; no sinus tenderness. *Throat (or Mouth)*—Oral mucosa pink, dentition good, pharynx without exudates.

Neck—Trachea midline. Neck supple; thyroid isthmus palpable, lobes not felt.

Lymph Nodes—No cervical, axillary, epitrochlear, inguinal adenopathy.

OR

Head—The skull is normocephalic/atraumatic. Frontal balding. *Eyes*—Visual acuity 20/100 bilaterally. Sclera white; conjunctiva infected. Pupils constrict 3 mm to 2 mm, equally round and reactive to light and accommodation. Disc margins sharp; no hemorrhages or exudates. Arteriolar-to-venous ratio (AV ratio) 2:4; no A-V nicking. *Ears*—Acuity diminished to whispered voice; intact to spoken voice. TMs clear. *Nose*—Mucosa swollen with erythema and clear drainage. Septum midline. Tender over maxillary sinuses. *Throat*—Oral mucosa pink, dental caries in lower molars, pharynx erythematous, no exudates.

Neck—Trachea midline. Neck supple; thyroid isthmus midline, lobes palpable but not enlarged.

Lymph Nodes—Submandibular and anterior cervical lymph nodes tender, 1 × 1 cm, rubbery and mobile; no posterior cervical, epitrochlear, axillary, or inguinal lymphadenopathy.

Suggests myopia and mild arteriolar narrowing. Also upper respiratory infection.

TECHNIQUES OF EXAMINATION

The Head

Because abnormalities covered by the hair are easily missed, ask if the patient has noticed anything wrong with the scalp or hair. If you note a hairpiece or wig, ask the patient to remove it.

Examine:

The Hair. Note its quantity, distribution, texture, and pattern of loss, if any. You may see loose flakes of dandruff.

Fine hair in hyperthyroidism; coarse hair in hypothyroidism. Tiny white ovoid granules that adhere to hairs may be nits, or eggs of lice.

The Scalp. Part the hair in several places and look for scaliness, lumps, nevi, or other lesions.

Redness and scaling in seborrheic dermatitis, psoriasis; pilar cysts (wens)

The Skull. Observe the general size and contour of the skull. Note any deformities, depressions, lumps, or tenderness. Familiarize yourself with the irregularities in a normal skull, such as those near the suture lines between the parietal and occipital bones.

Enlarged skull in hydrocephalus, Paget's disease of bone. Tenderness after trauma

The Face. Note the patient's facial expression and contours. Observe for asymmetry, involuntary movements, edema, and masses.

See Table 5-3, Selected Facies (p. 175).

The Skin. Observe the skin, noting its color, pigmentation, texture, thickness, hair distribution, and any lesions.

Acne in many adolescents. Hirsutism (excessive facial hair) in some women

The Eyes

Important Areas of Examination

- Visual acuity
- Visual fields
- Conjunctiva and sclera
- Cornea, lens, and pupils
- Extraocular movements
- Fundi, including
  - Optic disc and cup
  - Retina
  - Retinal vessels

Visual Acuity. To test the acuity of central vision use a Snellen eye chart, if possible, and light it well. Position the patient 20 feet from the chart. Patients who use glasses other than for reading should put them on. Ask

Vision of 20/200 means that at 20 feet the patient can read print that a person with normal vision

the patient to cover one eye with a card (to prevent peeking through the fingers) and to read the smallest line of print possible. Coaxing to attempt the next line may improve performance. A patient who cannot read the largest letter should be positioned closer to the chart; note the intervening distance. Determine the smallest line of print from which the patient can identify more than half the letters. Record the visual acuity designated at the side of this line, along with use of glasses, if any. Visual acuity is expressed as two numbers (e.g., 20/30): the first indicates the distance of patient from chart, and the second, the distance at which a normal eye can read the line of letters.

could read at 200 feet. The larger the second number, the worse the vision. "20/40 corrected" means the patient could read the 40 line with glasses (a correction).

Myopia is impaired far vision.

Testing near vision with a special handheld card helps to identify the need for reading glasses or bifocals in patients over age 45. You can also use this card to test visual acuity at the bedside. Held 14 inches from the patient's eyes, the card simulates a Snellen chart. You may, however, let patients choose their own distance.

Presbyopia is the impaired near vision, found in middle-aged and older people. A presbyopic person often sees better when the card is farther away.

If you have no charts, screen visual acuity with any available print. If patients cannot read even the largest letters, test their ability to count your upraised fingers and distinguish light (such as your flashlight) from dark.

In the United States, a person is usually considered legally blind when vision in the better eye, corrected by glasses, is 20/200 or less. Legal blindness also results from a constricted field of vision: 20° or less in the better eye.

Visual Fields by Confrontation

Screening. Screening starts in the temporal fields because most defects involve these areas. Imagine the patient's visual fields projected onto a

Field defects that are all or partly temporal include *homonymous hemianopsia,*

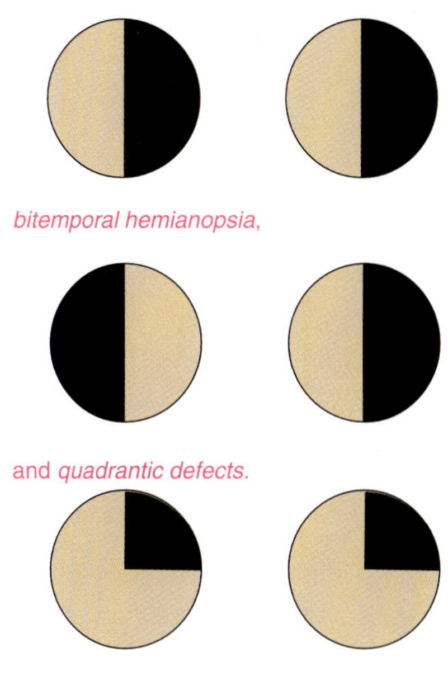

bitemporal hemianopsia,

and *quadrantic defects.*

Review these patterns in Table 5-4, Visual Field Defects, p. 176.

glass bowl that encircles the front of the patient's head. Ask the patient to look with both eyes into your eyes. While you return the patient's gaze, place your hands about 2 feet apart, lateral to the patient's ears. Instruct the patient to point to your fingers as soon as they are seen. Then slowly move the wiggling fingers of both your hands along the imaginary bowl and toward the line of gaze until the patient identifies them. Repeat this pattern in the upper and lower temporal quadrants.

Normally, a person sees both sets of fingers at the same time. If so, fields are usually normal.

Further Testing. If you find a defect, try to establish its boundaries. Test one eye at a time. If you suspect a temporal defect in the left visual field, for example, ask the patient to cover the right eye and, with the left one, to look into your eye directly opposite. Then slowly move your wiggling fingers from the defective area toward the better vision, noting where the patient first responds. Repeat this at several levels to define the border.

When the patient's left eye repeatedly does not see your fingers until they have crossed the line of gaze, a left temporal hemianopsia is present. It is diagrammed from the patient's viewpoint.

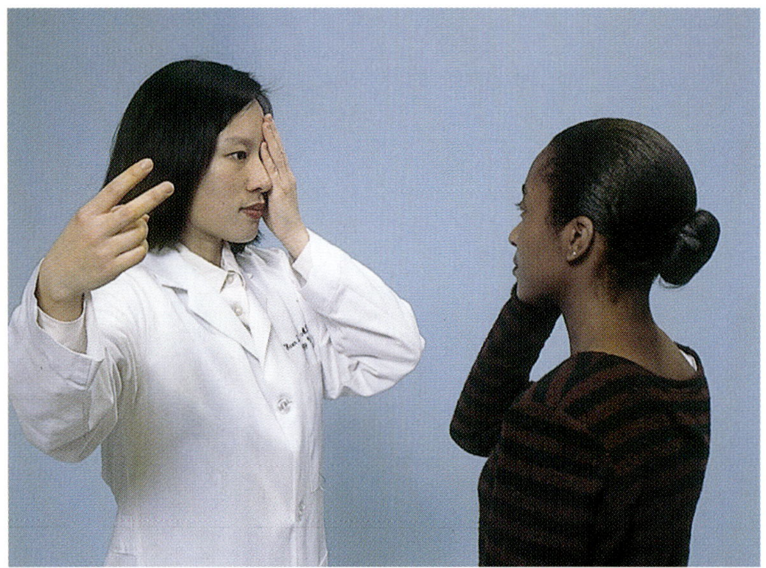

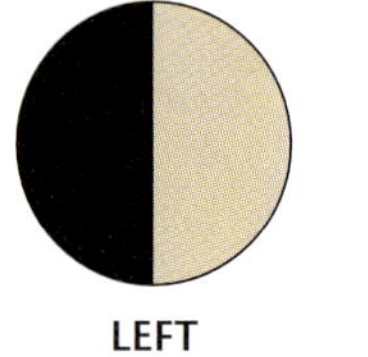

LEFT

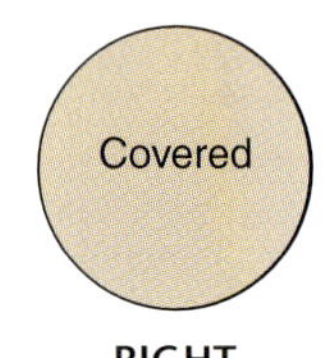

RIGHT

A temporal defect in the visual field of one eye suggests a nasal defect in the other eye. To test this hypothesis, examine the other eye in a similar way, again moving from the anticipated defect toward the better vision.

A left homonymous hemianopsia may thus be established.

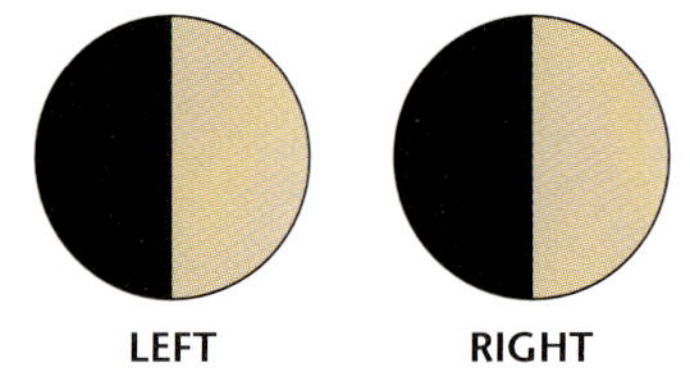

Small visual field defects and enlarged blind spots require a finer stimulus. Using a small red object such as a red-headed matchstick or the red eraser on a pencil, test one eye at a time. As the patient looks into your eye directly opposite, move the object about in the visual field. The normal blind spot can be found 15° temporal to the line of gaze. (Find your own blind spots for practice.)

An enlarged blind spot occurs in conditions affecting the optic nerve, e.g., glaucoma, optic neuritis, and papilledema.

Position and Alignment of the Eyes. Stand in front of the patient and survey the eyes for position and alignment with each other. If one or both eyes seem to protrude, assess them from above (see p. 167).

Inward or outward deviation of the eyes; abnormal protrusion in Graves' disease or ocular tumors

Eyebrows. Inspect the eyebrows, noting their quantity and distribution and any scaliness of the underlying skin.

Scaliness in seborrheic dermatitis; lateral sparseness in hypothyroidism

Eyelids. Note the position of the lids in relation to the eyeballs. Inspect for the following:

- Width of the palpebral fissures
- Edema of the lids
- Color of the lids (e.g., redness)
- Lesions
- Condition and direction of the eyelashes
- Adequacy with which the eyelids close. Look for this especially when the eyes are unusually prominent, when there is facial paralysis, or when the patient is unconscious.

See Table 5-5, Variations and Abnormalities of the Eyelids (p. 177). *Blepharitis* is an inflammation of the eyelids along the lid margins, often with crusting or scales.

Failure of the eyelids to close exposes the corneas to serious damage.

Lacrimal Apparatus. Briefly inspect the regions of the lacrimal gland and lacrimal sac for swelling.

See Table 5-6, Lumps and Swellings In and Around the Eyes (p. 178).

Look for excessive tearing or dryness of the eyes. Assessment of dryness may require special testing by an ophthalmologist. To test for nasolacrimal duct obstruction, see pp. 167–168.

Excessive tearing may be due to increased production or impaired drainage of tears. In the first group, causes include conjunctival inflammation and corneal irritation; in the second, ectropion (p. 177) and nasolacrimal duct obstruction.

Conjunctiva and Sclera. Ask the patient to look up as you depress both lower lids with your thumbs, exposing the sclera and conjunctiva. Inspect the sclera and palpebral conjunctiva for color, and note the vascular pattern against the white scleral background. Look for any nodules or swelling.

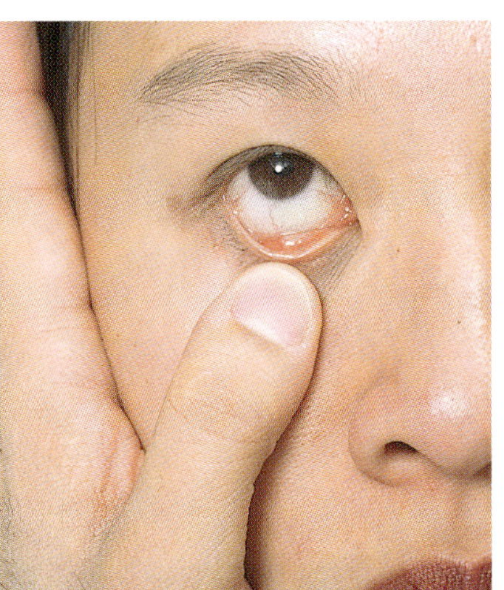

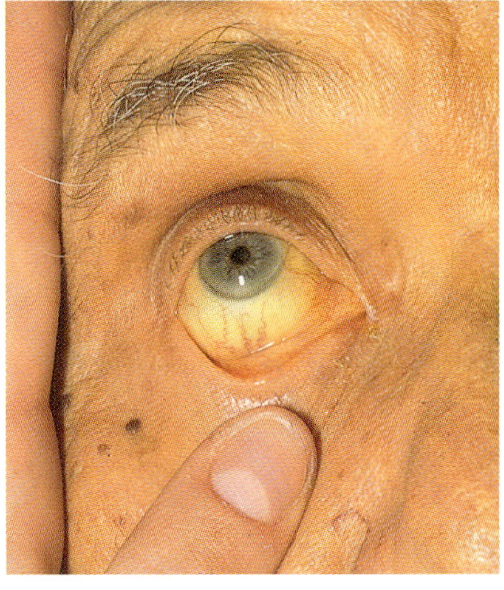

A yellow sclera indicates jaundice.

If you need a fuller view of the eye, rest your thumb and finger on the bones of the cheek and brow, respectively, and spread the lids.

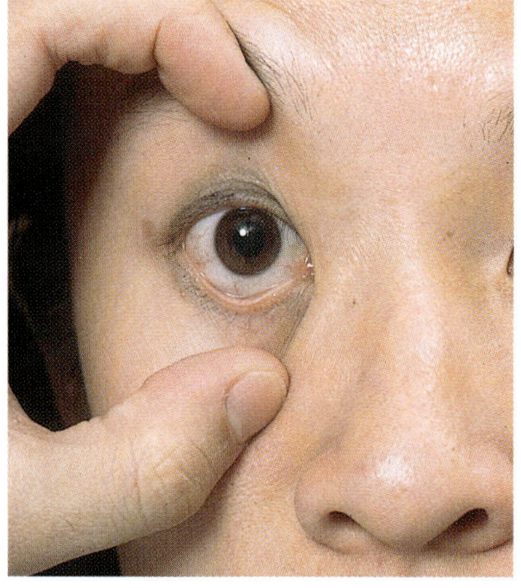

Ask the patient to look to each side and down. This technique gives you a good view of the sclera and bulbar conjunctiva, but not of the palpebral conjunctiva of the upper lid. For this purpose, you need to evert the lid (see p. 168).

The local redness below is due to nodular episcleritis:

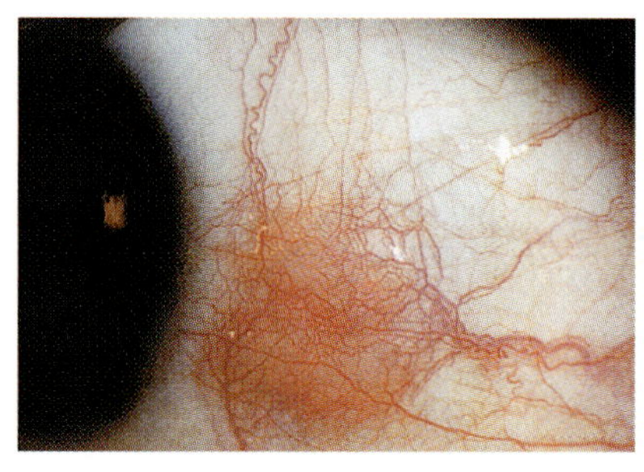

For comparisons, see Table 5-7, Red Eyes (p. 179).

Cornea and Lens. With oblique lighting, inspect the cornea of each eye for opacities and note any opacities in the lens that may be visible through the pupil.

See Table 5-8, Opacities of the Cornea and Lens (p. 180).

Iris. At the same time, inspect each iris. The markings should be clearly defined. With your light shining directly from the temporal side, look for a crescentic shadow on the medial side of the iris. Since the iris is normally fairly flat and forms a relatively open angle with the cornea, this lighting casts no shadow.

Occasionally the iris bows abnormally far forward, forming a very narrow angle with the cornea. The light then casts a crescentic shadow.

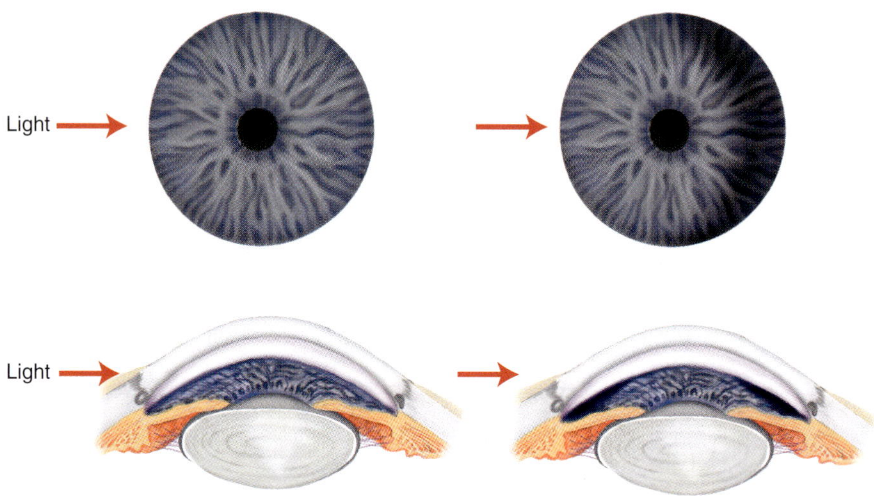

In open-angle glaucoma—the common form of glaucoma—the normal spatial relation between iris and cornea is preserved and the iris is fully lit.

This narrow angle increases the risk of acute *narrow-angle glaucoma*—a sudden increase in intraocular pressure when drainage of the aqueous humor is blocked.

Pupils. Inspect the *size, shape,* and *symmetry* of the pupils. If the pupils are large (>5 mm), small (<3 mm), or unequal, measure them. A card with black circles of varying sizes facilitates measurement.

Miosis refers to constriction of the pupils, *mydriasis* to dilation.

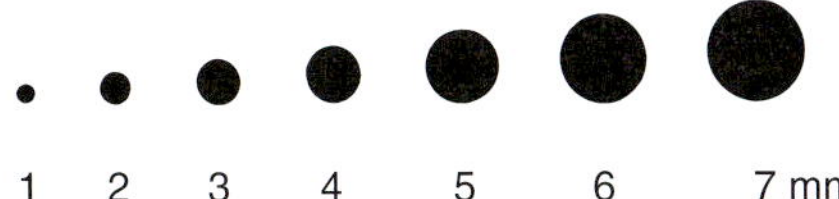

Pupillary inequality of less than 0.5 mm (*anisocoria*) is visible in about 20% of normal people. If pupillary reactions are normal, anisocoria is considered benign.

Compare benign anisocoria with Horner's syndrome, oculomotor nerve paralysis, and tonic pupil. See Table 5-9, Pupillary Abnormalities (p. 181).

Test the *pupillary reactions to light*. Ask the patient to look into the distance, and shine a bright light obliquely into each pupil in turn. (Both the distant gaze and the oblique lighting help to prevent a near reaction.) Look for:

- The direct reaction (pupillary constriction in the same eye)
- The consensual reaction (pupillary constriction in the opposite eye)

Always darken the room and use a bright light before deciding that a light reaction is absent.

If the reaction to light is impaired or questionable, test the *near reaction* in normal room light. Testing one eye at a time makes it easier to concentrate on pupillary responses, without the distraction of extraocular movement. Hold your finger or pencil about 10 cm from the patient's eye. Ask the patient to look alternately at it and into the distance directly behind it. Watch for pupillary constriction with near effort.

Testing the near reaction is helpful in diagnosing Argyll Robertson and tonic (Adie's) pupils (see p. 181).

Extraocular Muscles. From about 2 feet directly in front of the patient, shine a light onto the patient's eyes and ask the patient to look at it. *Inspect the reflections in the corneas.* They should be visible slightly nasal to the center of the pupils.

Asymmetry of the corneal reflections indicates a deviation from normal ocular alignment. A temporal light reflection on one cornea, for example, indicates a nasal deviation of that eye. See Table 5-10, Deviations of the Eyes (p. 182).

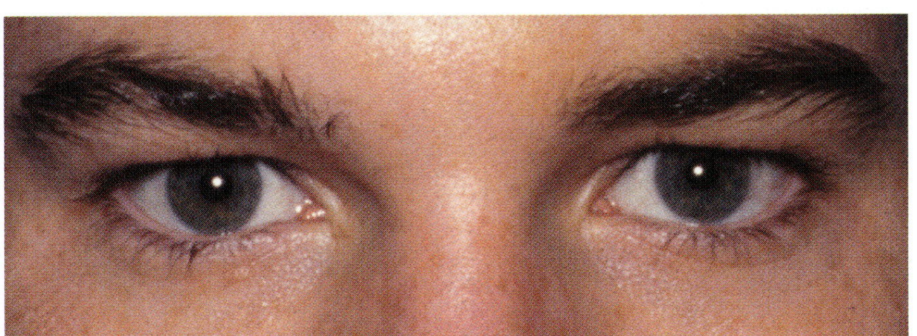

A *cover–uncover test* may reveal a slight or latent muscle imbalance not otherwise seen (see p. 182).

Now *assess the extraocular movements*, looking for:

- The normal *conjugate movements* of the eyes in each direction, or any *deviation* from normal

See Table 5-10, Deviations of the Eyes (p. 182).

- *Nystagmus,* a fine rhythmic oscillation of the eyes. A few beats of nystagmus on extreme lateral gaze are within normal limits. If you see it, bring your finger in to within the field of binocular vision and look again.

Sustained nystagmus within the binocular field of gaze is seen in a variety of neurologic conditions. See Table 16-9, Nystagmus (pp. 610–611).

- A *lid lag* as the eyes move from above downward.

Lid lag of hyperthyroidism

To make these observations, *ask the patient to follow your finger or pencil* as you sweep through the six cardinal directions of gaze. Making a wide H in the air, lead the patient's gaze (1) to the patient's extreme right, (2) to the right and upward, and (3) down on the right; then (4) without pausing in the middle, to the extreme left, (5) to the left and upward, and (6) down on the left. Pause during upward and lateral gaze to detect nystagmus. Move your finger or pencil at a comfortable distance from the patient. Because middle-aged or older people may have difficulty focusing on near objects, make this distance greater for them than for young people. Some patients move their heads to follow your finger. If necessary, hold the head in the proper midline position.

In paralysis of the CN VI, illustrated below, the eyes are conjugate in right lateral gaze but not in left lateral gaze (left infranuclear ophthalmoplegia)

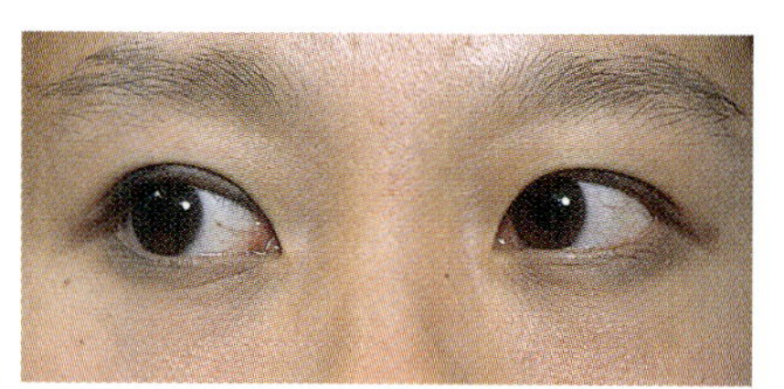

1

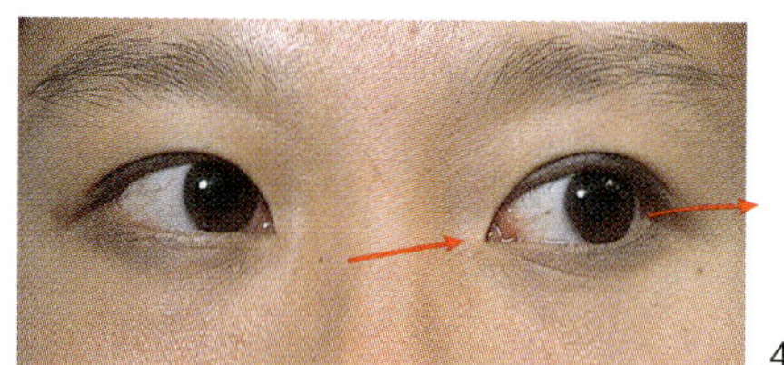

4

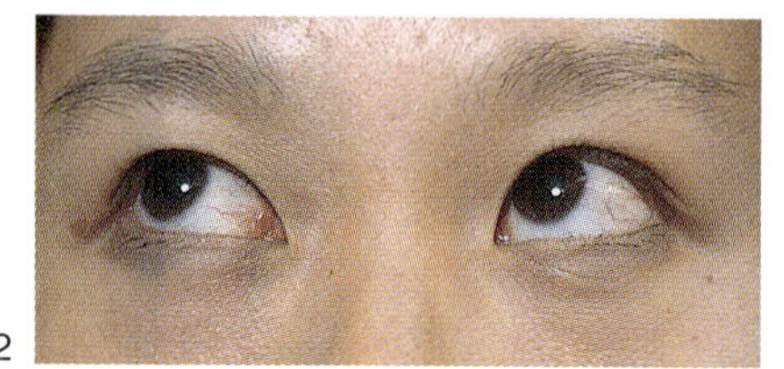

2

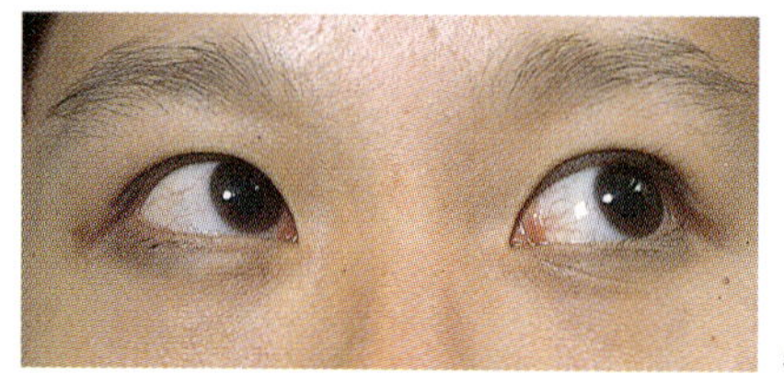

5

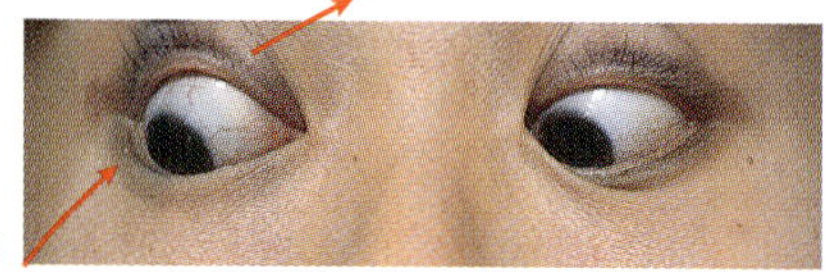

3

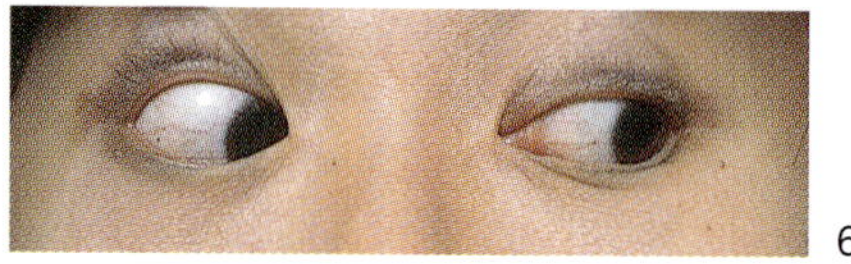

6

LOOKING RIGHT

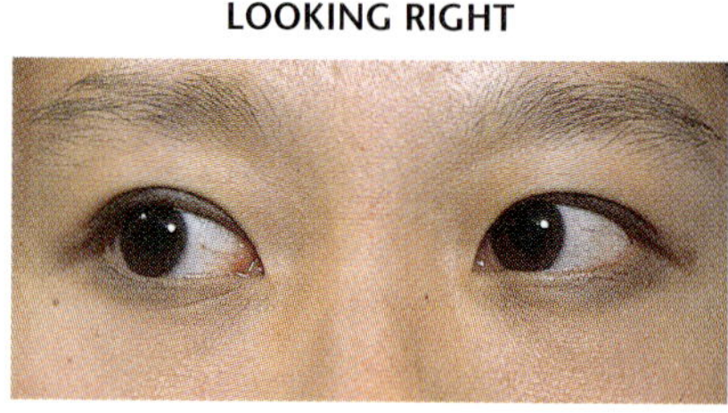

LOOKING LEFT

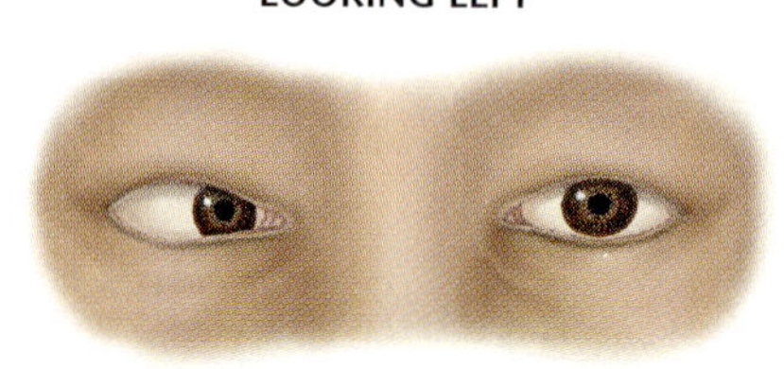

If you suspect a lid lag or hyperthyroidism, ask the patient to follow your finger again as you move it slowly from up to down in the midline. The lid should overlap the iris slightly throughout this movement.

In the lid lag of hyperthyroidism, a rim of sclera is seen between the upper lid and iris; the lid seems to lag behind the eyeball.

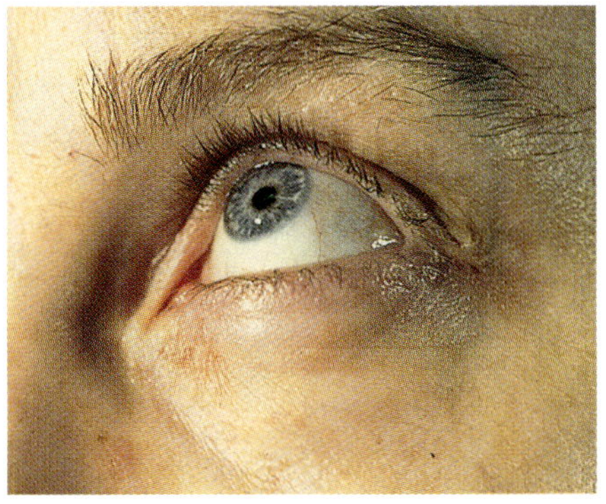

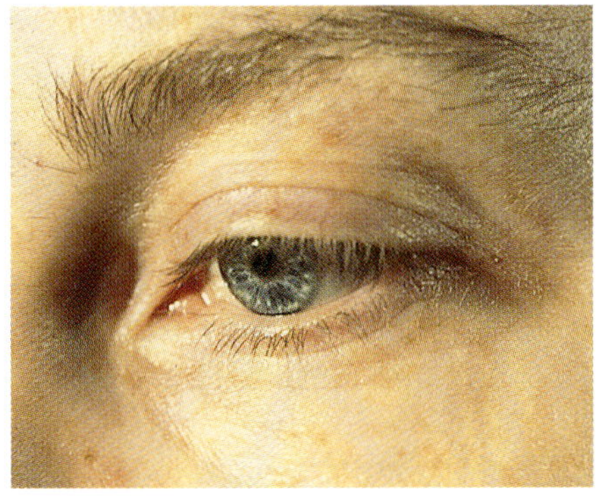

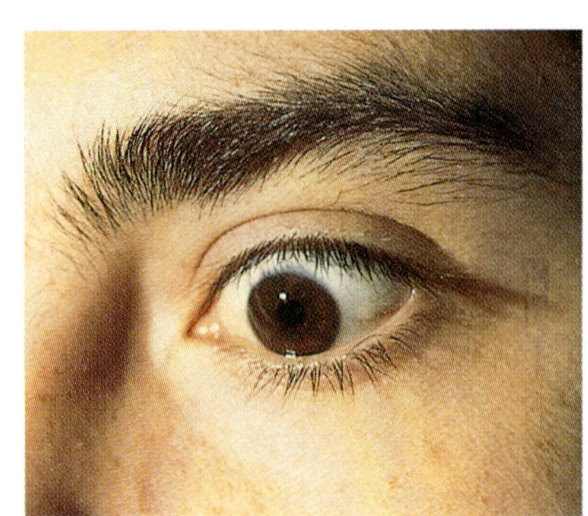

Finally, test for *convergence*. Ask the patient to follow your finger or pencil as you move it in toward the bridge of the nose. The converging eyes normally follow the object to within 5 cm to 8 cm of the nose.

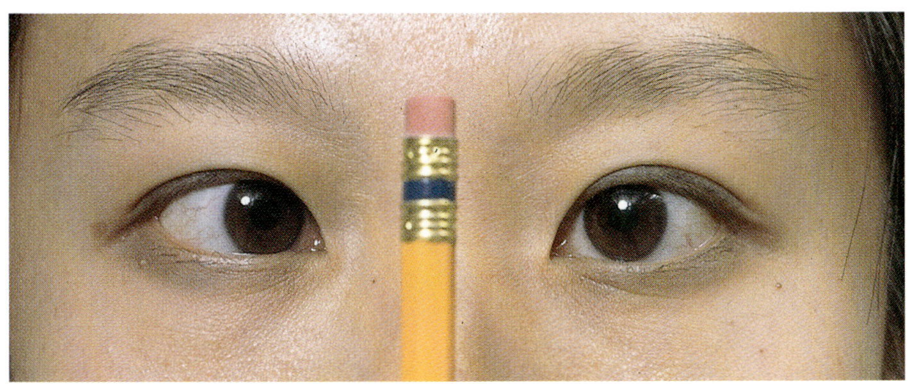

CONVERGENCE

Poor convergence in hyperthyroidism

Ophthalmoscopic Examination. In general health care, you should usually examine your patients' eyes without dilating their pupils. Your view is therefore limited to the posterior structures of the retinal surface. To see more peripheral structures, to evaluate the macula well, or to investigate unexplained visual loss, ophthalmologists dilate the pupils with mydriatic drops unless this is contraindicated.

Contraindications for mydriatic drops include (1) head injury and coma, in which continuing observations of pupillary reactions are essential, and (2) any suspicion of narrow-angle glaucoma.

At first, using the ophthalmoscope may seem awkward, and it may be difficult to visualize the fundus. With patience and practice of proper technique, the fundus will come into view, and you will be able to assess important structures such as the optic disc and the retinal vessels. Remove your glasses unless you have marked nearsightedness or severe astigmatism. (However, if the patient's refractive errors make it difficult to focus on the fundi, it may be easier to keep your glasses on.)

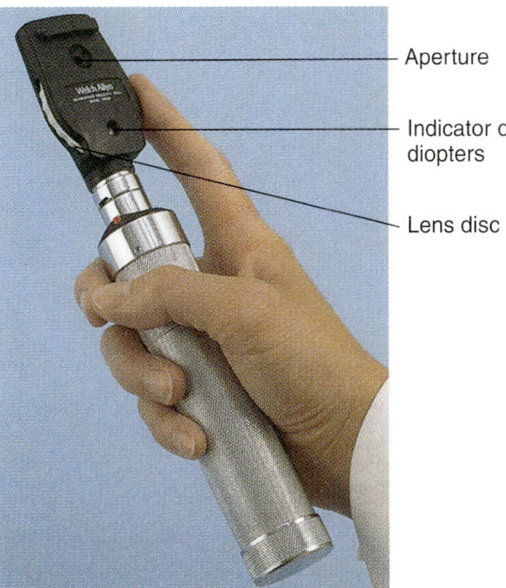

Review the components of the ophthalmoscope pictured on the previous page. Then follow the steps for using the ophthalmoscope, and your examination skills will improve over time.

STEPS FOR USING THE OPHTHALMOSCOPE

- Darken the room. Switch on the ophthalmoscope light and turn the lens disc until you see the large round beam of white light.* Shine the light on the back of your hand to check the type of light, its desired brightness, and the electrical charge of the ophthalmoscope.
- Turn the lens disc to the 0 diopter (a diopter is a unit that measures the power of a lens to converge or diverge light). At this diopter the lens neither converges nor diverges light. Keep your finger on the edge of the lens disc so you can turn the disc to focus the lens when you examine the fundus.
- Remember, hold the ophthalmoscope *in your right hand* to examine *the patient's right eye;* hold it *in your left hand* to examine *the patient's left eye.* This keeps you from bumping the patient's nose and gives you more mobility and closer range for visualizing the fundus. At first, you may have difficulty using the nondominant eye, but this will abate with practice.
- Hold the ophthalmoscope firmly braced against the medial aspect of your bony orbit, with the handle tilted laterally at about a 20° slant from the vertical. Check to make sure you can see clearly through the aperture. Instruct the patient to look slightly up and over your shoulder at a point directly ahead on the wall.
- Place yourself about 15 inches away from the patient and at an angle 15° lateral to the patient's line of vision. Shine the light beam on the pupil and look for the orange glow in the pupil—the *red reflex.* Note any opacities interrupting the red reflex.
- Now, place the thumb of your other hand across the patient's eyebrow (this technique helps keep you steady but is not essential). Keeping the light beam focused on the red reflex, move in with the ophthalmoscope on the 15° angle toward the pupil until you are very close to it, almost touching the patient's eyelashes.

Try to keep both eyes open and relaxed, as if gazing into the distance, to help minimize any fluctuating blurriness as your eyes attempt to accommodate.

You may need to lower the brightness of the light beam to make the examination more comfortable for the patient, avoid *hippus* (spasm of the pupil), and improve your observations.

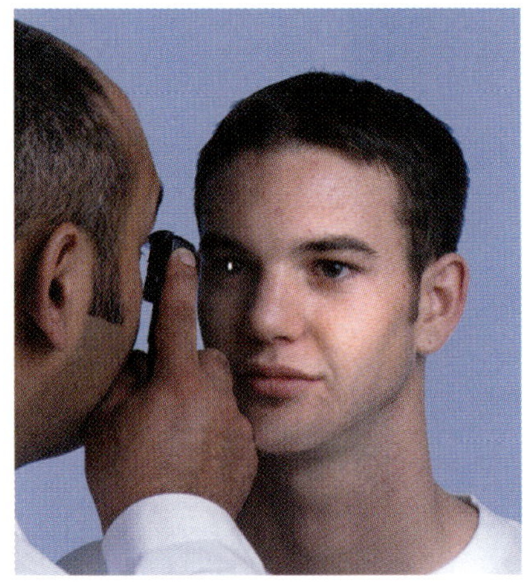

Absence of a *red reflex* suggests an opacity of the lens (cataract) or possibly of the vitreous. Less commonly, a detached retina or, in children, a retinoblastoma may obscure this reflex. Do not be fooled by an artificial eye, which, of course, has no red reflex.

* Some clinicians like to use the large round beam for large pupils, the small round beam for small pupils. The other beams are rarely helpful. The slitlike beam is sometimes used to assess elevations or concavities in the retina, the green (or red-free) beam to detect small red lesions, and the grid to make measurements. Ignore the last three lights and practice with the large round white beam.

Now you are ready to inspect the *optic disc* and the *retina*. You should be seeing the optic disc—a yellowish orange to creamy pink oval or round structure that may fill your field of gaze or even exceed it. Of interest, the ophthalmoscope magnifies the normal retina about 15 times and the normal iris about 4 times. The optic disc actually measures about 1.5 mm.

When the lens has been removed surgically, its magnifying effect is lost. Retinal structures then look much smaller than usual, and you can see a much larger expanse of fundus.

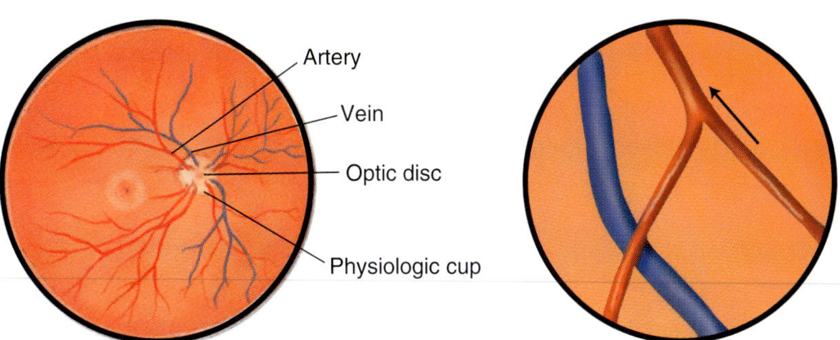

Follow the steps below for this important segment of the physical examination:

STEPS FOR EXAMINING THE OPTIC DISC AND THE RETINA

- First, *locate the optic disc.* Look for the round yellowish orange structure described above. If you do not see it at first, follow a blood vessel centrally until you do. You can tell which direction is central by noting the angles at which vessels branch—the vessel size becomes progressively larger at each junction as you approach the disc.

- Now, *bring the optic disc into sharp focus* by adjusting the lens of your ophthalmoscope. If both you and the patient have no refractive errors, the retina should be in focus at 0 diopters. (A diopter is a unit that measures the power of a lens to converge or diverge light.) If structures are blurred, rotate the lens disc until you find the sharpest focus.

In a refractive error, light rays from a distance do not focus on the retina. In myopia, they focus anterior to it; in hyperopia, posterior to it. Retinal structures in a myopic eye look larger than normal.

  For example, if the patient is myopic (nearsighted), rotate the lens disc counterclockwise to the minus diopters; in a hyperopic (farsighted) patient, move the disc clockwise to the plus diopters. You can correct your own refractive error in the same way.

- *Inspect the optic disc.* Note the following features:

  – *The sharpness or clarity of the disc outline.* The nasal portion of the disc margin may be somewhat blurred, a normal finding.

  – *The color of the disc,* normally yellowish orange to creamy pink. White or pigmented crescents may ring the disc, a normal finding.

  – *The size of the central physiologic cup,* if present. It is usually yellowish white. The horizontal diameter is usually less than half the horizontal diameter of the disc.

See Table 5-11, Normal Variations of the Optic Disc (p. 183), and Table 5-12, Abnormalities of the Optic Disc (p. 184).

An enlarged cup suggests chronic open-angle glaucoma.

– *The presence of venous pulsations.* In a normal person, pulsations in the retinal veins as they emerge from the central portion of the disc may or may not be present.

Loss of venous pulsations in pathologic conditions like head trauma, meningitis, or mass lesions may be an early sign of elevated intracranial pressure.

– *The comparative symmetry of the eyes* and findings in the fundi

- *Inspect the retina,* including arteries and veins as they extend to the periphery, arteriovenous crossings, the fovea, and the macula. Distinguish arteries from veins based on the features listed below.

	Arteries	Veins
Color	Light red	Dark red
Size	Smaller (2/3 to 4/5 the diameter of veins)	Larger
Light Reflex (*reflection*)	Bright	Inconspicuous or absent

- *Follow the vessels peripherally in each of four directions,* noting their relative sizes and the character of the arteriovenous crossings. Identify any lesions of the surrounding *retina* and note their size, shape, color, and distribution. As you search the retina, move your head and instrument as a unit, using the patient's pupil as an imaginary fulcrum. At first, you may repeatedly lose your view of the retina because your light falls out of the pupil. You will improve with practice.

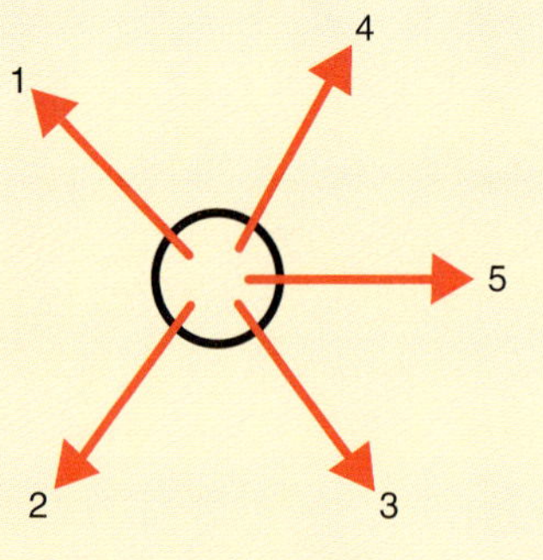

Sequence of inspection from disc to macula
LEFT EYE

See Table 5-13, Retinal Arteries and Arteriovenous Crossings: Normal and Hypertensive (p. 185).

See Table 5-14, Red Spots and Streaks in the Fundi (p. 186).

See Table 5-15, Light-Colored Spots in the Fundi (pp. 187–188).

See Table 5-16, Ocular Fundi (pp. 189–191).

- Finally, by directing your light beam laterally or by asking the patient to look directly into the light, inspect the *fovea* and surrounding *macula.* Except in older people, the tiny bright reflection at the center of the fovea helps to orient you. Shimmering light reflections in the macular area are common in young people.

- Lesions of the retina can be measured in terms of "disc diameters" from the optic disc. For example, among the cotton-wool patches illustrated on the next page, note the irregular patches between 11 and 12 o'clock, 1 to 2 disc diameters from the disc. It measures about one-half by one-half disc diameters.

Macular degeneration is an important cause of poor central vision in the elderly. Types include *dry atrophic* (more common but less severe) and *wet exudative,* or neovascular. Undigested cellular debris, called *drusen,* may be hard and sharply defined, or soft and confluent with altered pigmentation, as seen on the following page.

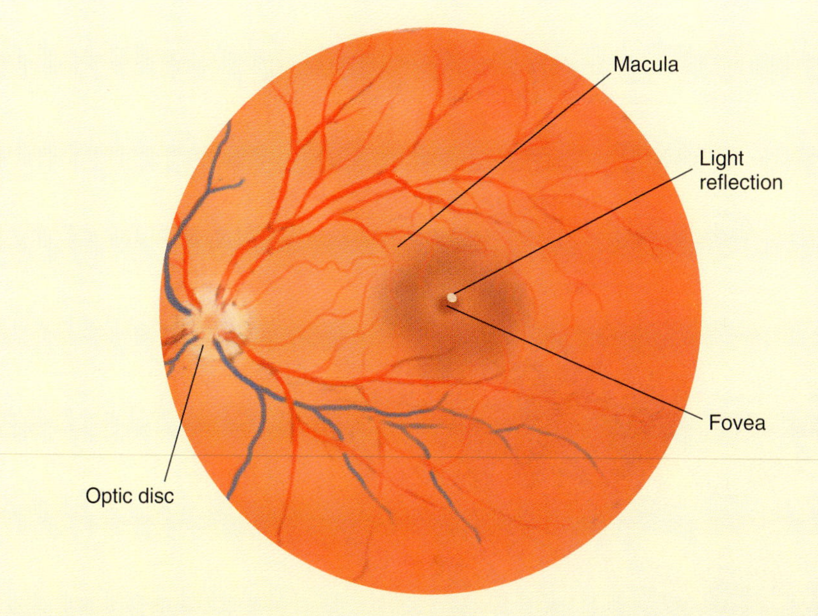

LEFT EYE

Tasman W, Jaeger E (eds): The Wills Eye Hospital Atlas of Clinical Ophthalmology, 2nd ed. Philadelphia, Lippincott Williams & Wilkins, 2001.

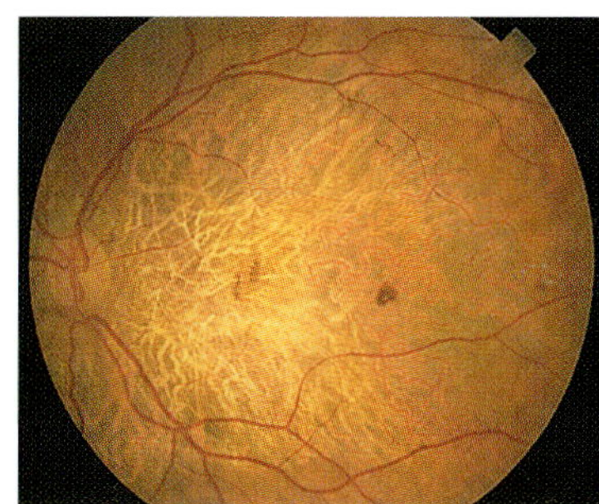

MACULAR DEGENERATION OF AGING

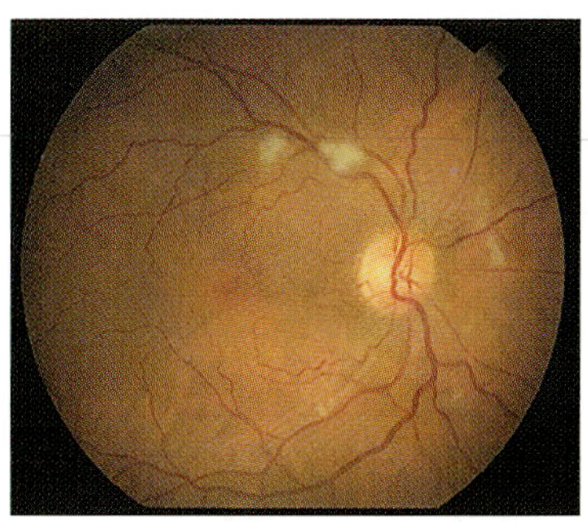

COTTON WOOL PATCHES

- The elevated optic disc of papilledema can be measured by noting the differences in diopters of the two lenses used to focus clearly on the disc and on the uninvolved retina. Note that at the retina, 3 diopters of elevation +1 mm.

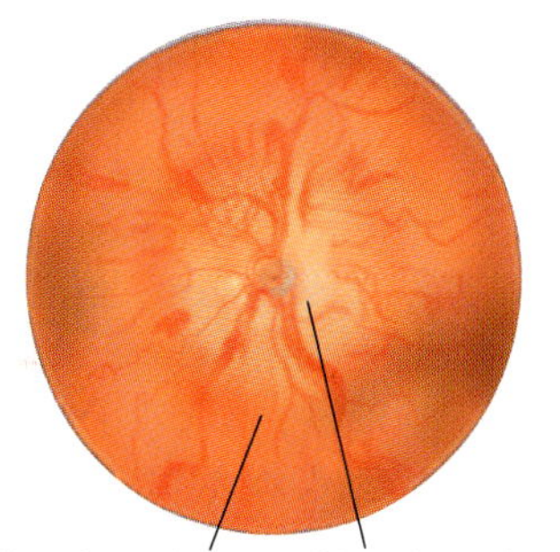

PAPILLEDEMA

Photos above from Tasman W, Jaeger E (eds): The Wills Eye Hospital Atlas of Clinical Ophthalmology, 2nd ed. Philadelphia, Lippincott Williams & Wilkins, 2001.

Papilledema signals increased intracranial pressure from such serious conditions as trauma, mass lesions, subarachnoid hemorrhage, or meningitis.

- *Inspect the anterior structures.* Look for opacities in the *vitreous* or *lens* by rotating the lens disc progressively to diopters of around +10 or +12. This technique allows you to focus on the more anterior structures in the eye.

Vitreous floaters may be seen as dark specks or strands between the fundus and the lens. Cataracts are densities in the lens (see p. 180).

The Ears

The Auricle. Inspect each auricle and surrounding tissues for deformities, lumps, or skin lesions.

See Table 5-17, Lumps On or Near the Ear (pp. 192–193).

If ear pain, discharge, or inflammation is present, move the auricle up and down, press the tragus, and press firmly just behind the ear.

Movement of the auricle and tragus (the "tug test") is painful in acute *otitis externa* (inflammation of the ear canal), but not in *otitis media* (inflammation of the middle ear). Tenderness behind the ear may be present in otitis media.

Ear Canal and Drum. To see the ear canal and drum, use an otoscope with the largest ear speculum that the canal will accommodate. Position the patient's head so that you can see comfortably through the instrument. To straighten the ear canal, grasp the auricle firmly but gently and pull it upward, backward, and slightly away from the head.

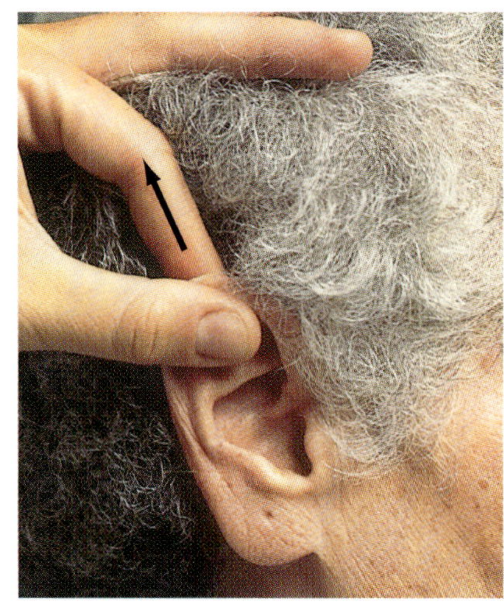

Holding the otoscope handle between your thumb and fingers, brace your hand against the patient's face. Your hand and instrument thus follow unexpected movements by the patient. (If you are uncomfortable switching hands for the left ear, as shown below, you may reach over that ear to pull it up and back with your left hand and rest your otoscope-holding right hand on the head behind the ear.)

Insert the speculum gently into the ear canal, directing it somewhat down and forward and through the hairs, if any.

Nontender nodular swellings covered by normal skin deep in the ear canals suggest *exostoses.* These are nonmalignant overgrowths, which may obscure the drum.

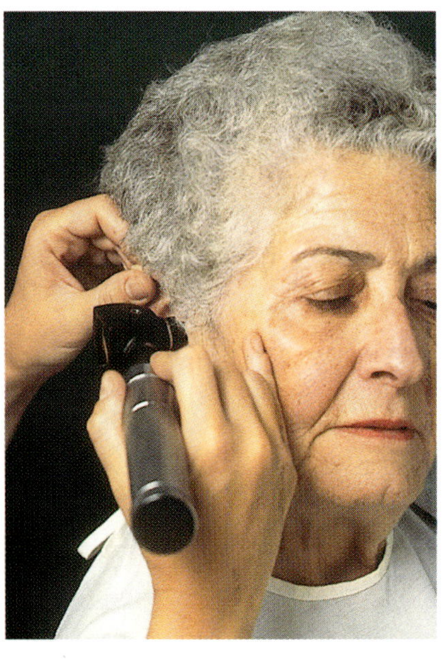

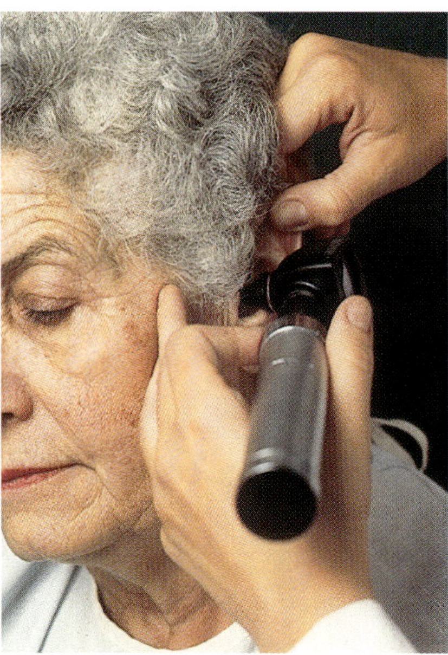

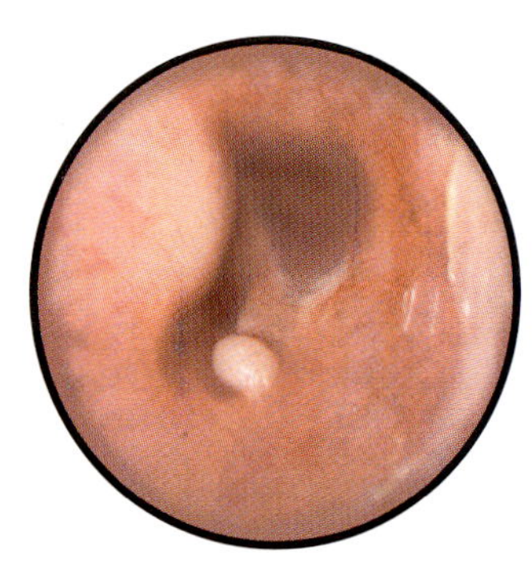

Inspect the ear canal, noting any discharge, foreign bodies, redness of the skin, or swelling. Cerumen, which varies in color and consistency from yellow and flaky to brown and sticky or even to dark and hard, may wholly or partly obscure your view.

In acute *otitis externa*, shown below, the canal is often swollen, narrowed, moist, pale, and tender. It may be reddened.

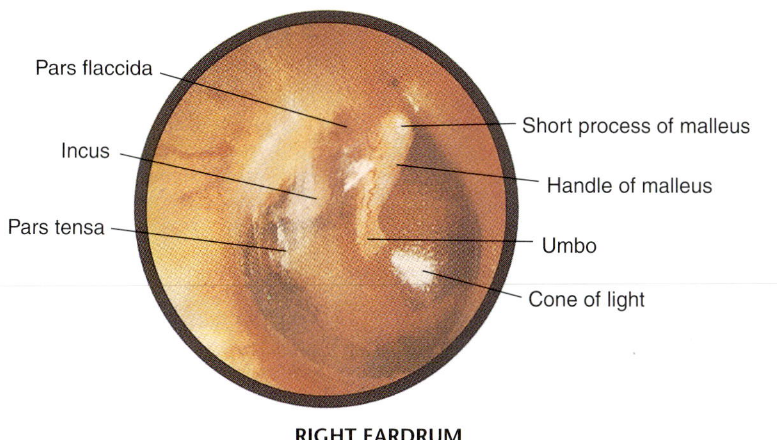

RIGHT EARDRUM

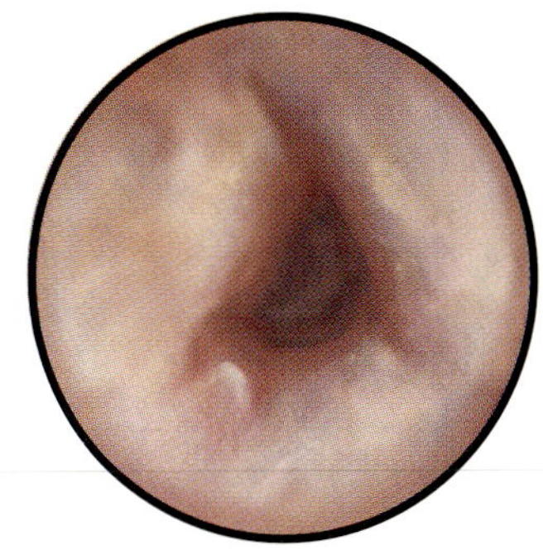

In *chronic otitis externa*, the skin of the canal is often thickened, red, and itchy.

Inspect the eardrum, noting its color and contour. The cone of light—usually easy to see—helps to orient you.

Red bulging drum of acute purulent otitis media, amber drum of a serous effusion

Identify the *handle of the malleus,* noting its position, and inspect the *short process of the malleus.*

An unusually prominent short process and a prominent handle that looks more horizontal suggest a retracted drum.

Gently move the speculum so that you can see as much of the drum as possible, including the pars flaccida superiorly and the margins of the pars tensa. Look for any perforations. The anterior and inferior margins of the drum may be obscured by the curving wall of the ear canal.

See Table 5-18, Abnormalities of the Eardrum (pp. 194–195).

Mobility of the eardrum can be evaluated with a pneumatic otoscope.

A serous effusion, a thickened drum, or purulent otitis media may decrease mobility.

Auditory Acuity. To estimate hearing, test one ear at a time. Ask the patient to occlude one ear with a finger or, better still, occlude it yourself. When auditory acuity on the two sides is different, move your finger rapidly, but gently, in the occluded canal. The noise so produced will help to prevent the occluded ear from doing the work of the ear you wish to test. Then, standing 1 or 2 feet away, exhale fully (so as to minimize the intensity of your voice) and whisper softly toward the unoccluded ear. Choose numbers or other words with two equally accented syllables, such as "nine-four," or "baseball." If necessary, increase the intensity of your voice to a medium whisper, a loud whisper, and then a soft, medium, and loud voice. To make sure the patient does not read your lips, cover your mouth or obstruct the patient's vision.

Air and Bone Conduction. If hearing is diminished, *try to distinguish between conductive and sensorineural hearing loss.* You need a quiet room and a tuning fork, preferably of 512 Hz or possibly 1024 Hz. These frequencies fall within the range of human speech (300 Hz to 3000 Hz)—functionally the most important range. Forks with lower pitches may lead to overestimating bone conduction and can also be felt as vibration.

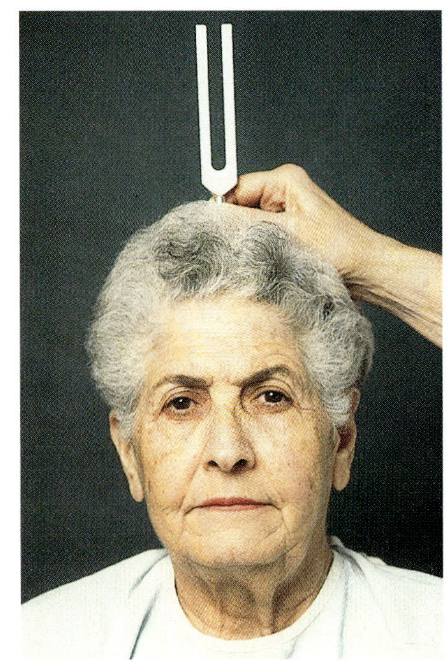

Set the fork into light vibration by briskly stroking it between thumb and index finger or by tapping it on your knuckles.

- *Test for lateralization* (Weber test). Place the base of the lightly vibrating tuning fork firmly on top of the patient's head or on the midforehead.

  Ask where the patient hears it: on one or both sides. Normally the sound is heard in the midline or equally in both ears. If nothing is heard, try again, pressing the fork more firmly on the head.

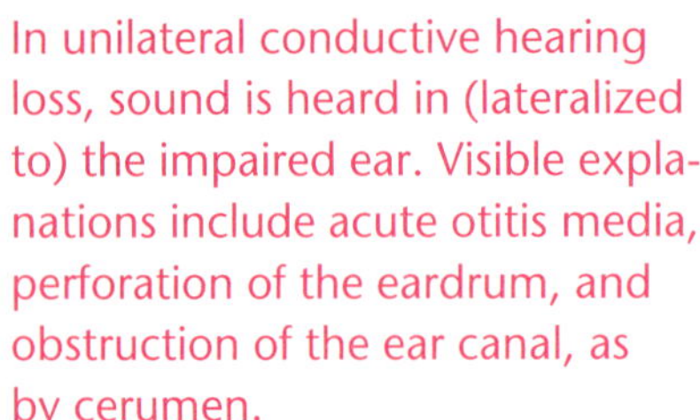

In unilateral conductive hearing loss, sound is heard in (lateralized to) the impaired ear. Visible explanations include acute otitis media, perforation of the eardrum, and obstruction of the ear canal, as by cerumen.

In unilateral sensorineural hearing loss, sound is heard in the good ear.

- *Compare air conduction (AC) and bone conduction (BC)* (Rinne test). Place the base of a lightly vibrating tuning fork on the mastoid bone, behind the ear and level with the canal. When the patient can no longer hear the sound, quickly place the fork close to the ear canal and ascertain whether the sound can be heard again. Here the "U" of the fork should face forward, thus maximizing its sound for the patient. Normally the sound is heard longer through air than through bone (AC > BC).

In conductive hearing loss, sound is heard through bone as long as or longer than it is through air (BC = AC or BC > AC). In sensorineural hearing loss, sound is heard longer through air (AC > BC). See Table 5-19, Patterns of Hearing Loss (pp. 196–197).

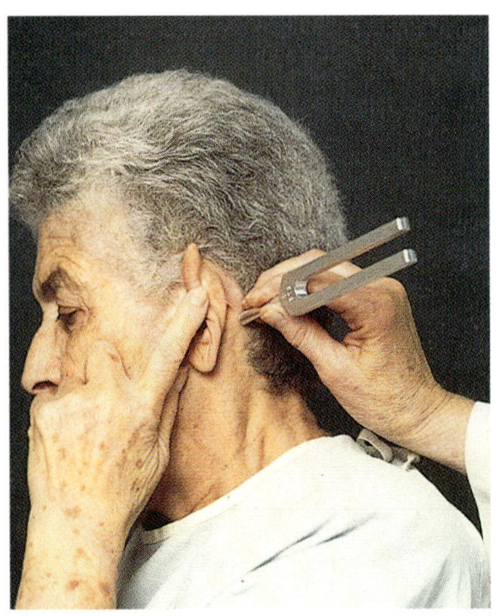

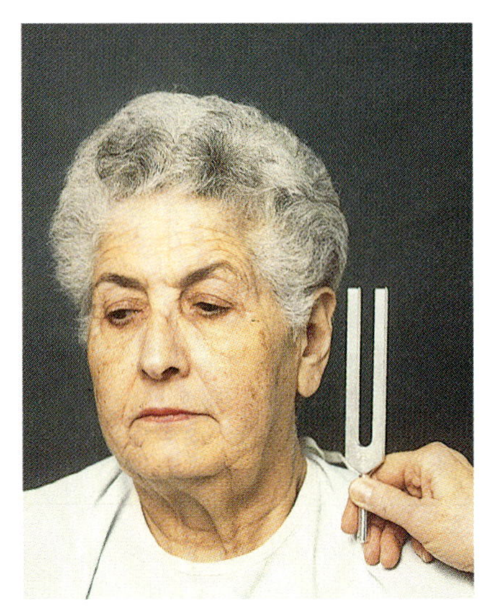

The Nose and Paranasal Sinuses

Inspect the anterior and inferior surfaces of the nose. Gentle pressure on the tip of the nose with your thumb usually widens the nostrils and, with the aid of a penlight or otoscope light, you can get a partial view of each nasal vestibule. If the tip is tender, be particularly gentle and manipulate the nose as little as possible.

Tenderness of the nasal tip or alae suggests local infection such as a furuncle.

Note any asymmetry or deformity of the nose.

Deviation of the lower septum is common and may be easily visible, as illustrated below. Deviation seldom obstructs air flow.

Test for nasal obstruction, if indicated, by pressing on each ala nasi in turn and asking the patient to breathe in.

Inspect the inside of the nose with an otoscope and the largest ear speculum available.‡ Tilt the patient's head back a bit and insert the speculum gently into the vestibule of each nostril, avoiding contact with the sensitive nasal septum. Hold the otoscope handle to one side to avoid the patient's chin and improve your mobility. By directing the speculum posteriorly, then upward in small steps, try to see the inferior and middle turbinates, the nasal septum, and the narrow nasal passage between them. Some asymmetry of the two sides is normal.

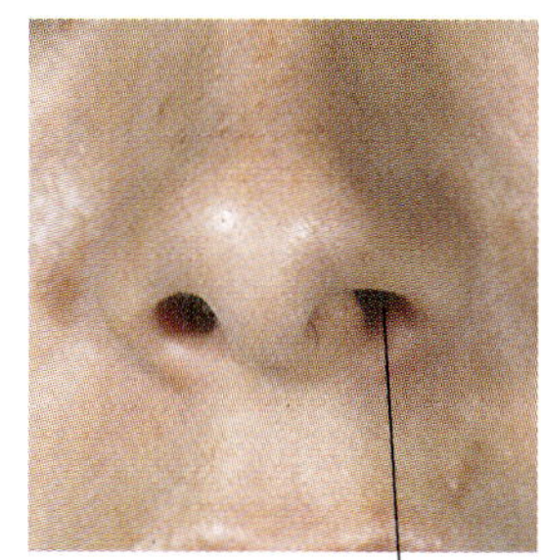

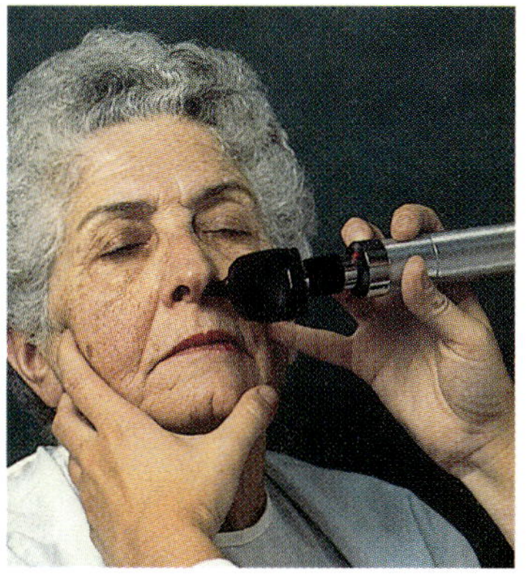

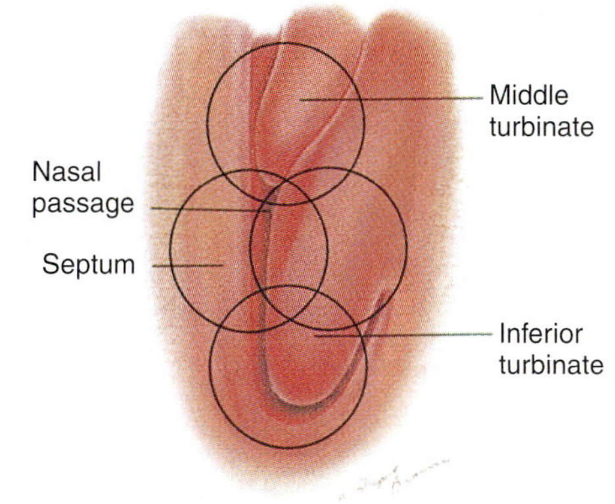

Observe:

- The *nasal mucosa* that covers the septum and turbinates. Note its color and any swelling, bleeding, or exudate. If exudate is present, note its character: clear, mucopurulent, or purulent. The nasal mucosa is normally somewhat redder than the oral mucosa.

In viral rhinitis the mucosa is reddened and swollen; in allergic rhinitis it may be pale, bluish, or red.

‡A nasal illuminator, equipped with a short wide nasal speculum but lacking an otoscope's magnification, may also be used, but structures look much smaller. Otolaryngologists use special equipment not widely available to others.

- The *nasal septum*. Note any deviation, inflammation, or perforation of the septum. The lower anterior portion of the septum (where the patient's finger can reach) is a common source of *epistaxis* (nosebleed).

Fresh blood or crusting may be seen. Causes of septal perforation include trauma, surgery, and the intranasal use of cocaine or amphetamines.

- Any *abnormalities* such as ulcers or polyps.

Polyps are pale, semitranslucent masses that usually come from the middle meatus. Ulcers may result from nasal use of cocaine.

Make it a habit to place all nasal and ear specula outside your instrument case after use. Then discard them or clean and disinfect them appropriately. (Check the policies of your institution.)

Palpate for sinus tenderness. Press up on the *frontal sinuses* from under the bony brows, avoiding pressure on the eyes. Then press up on the *maxillary sinuses.*

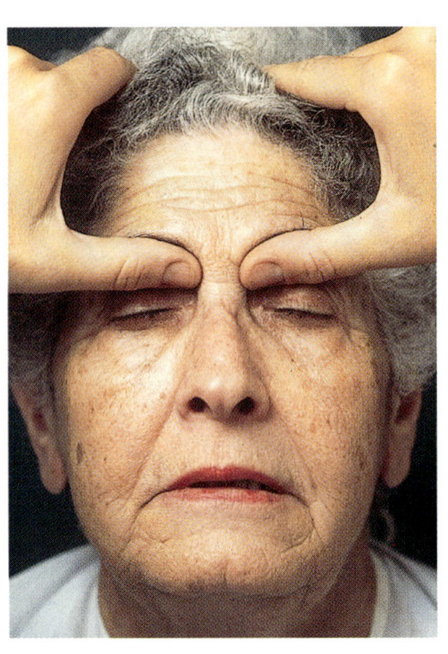

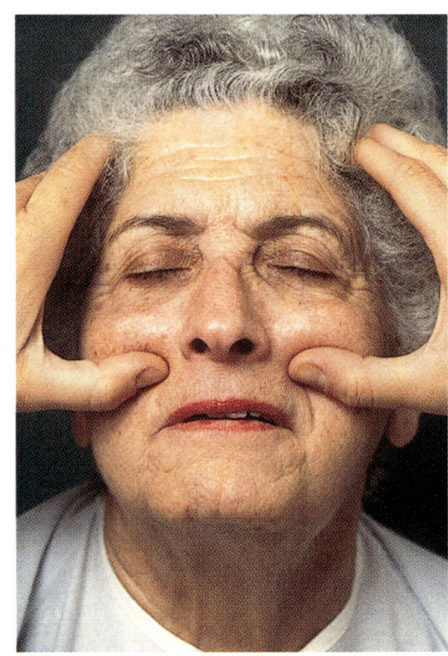

Local tenderness, together with symptoms such as pain, fever, and nasal discharge, suggests acute sinusitis involving the frontal or maxillary sinuses. Transillumination may be diagnostically useful. For this technique, see p. 169.

The Mouth and Pharynx

If the patient wears dentures, offer a paper towel and ask the patient to remove them so that you can see the mucosa underneath. If you detect any suspicious ulcers or nodules, put on a glove and palpate any lesions, noting especially any thickening or infiltration of the tissues that might suggest malignancy.

Bright red edematous mucosa underneath a denture suggests denture sore mouth. There may be ulcers or papillary granulation tissue.

Inspect the following:

The Lips. Observe their color and moisture, and note any lumps, ulcers, cracking, or scaliness.

Cyanosis, pallor. See Table 5-20, Abnormalities of the Lips (pp. 198–199).

The Oral Mucosa. Look into the patient's mouth and, with a good light and the help of a tongue blade, inspect the oral mucosa for color, ulcers, white patches, and nodules. The wavy white line on this buccal mucosa developed where the upper and lower teeth meet. Irritation from sucking or chewing may cause or intensify it.

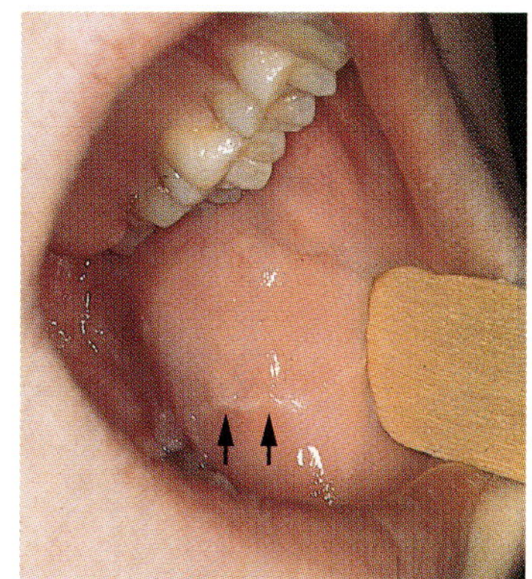

An aphthous ulcer on the labial mucosa is shown by the patient.

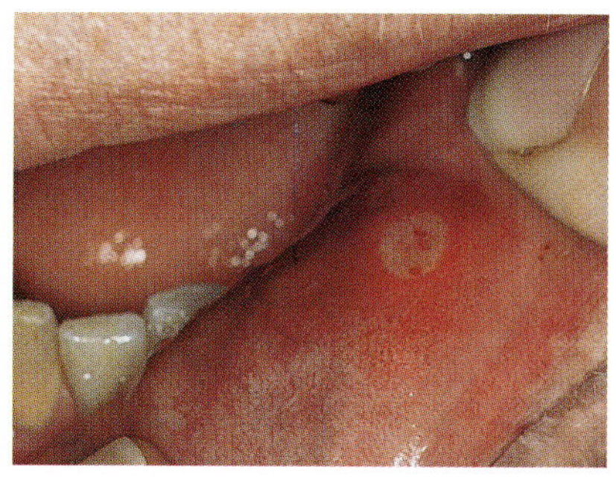

See p. 207 and Table 5-21, Findings in the Pharynx, Palate, and Oral Mucosa (pp. 200–202).

The Gums and Teeth. Note the color of the gums, normally pink. Patchy brownness may be present, especially but not exclusively in black people.

Redness of gingivitis, black line of lead poisoning

Inspect the gum margins and the interdental papillae for swelling or ulceration.

Swollen interdental papillae in gingivitis. See Table 5-22, Findings in the Gums and Teeth (pp. 203–205).

Inspect the teeth. Are any of them missing, discolored, misshapen, or abnormally positioned? You can check for looseness with your gloved thumb and index finger.

The Roof of the Mouth. Inspect the color and architecture of the hard palate.

Torus palatinus, a midline lump (see p. 201)

The Tongue and the Floor of the Mouth. Ask the patient to put out his or her tongue. Inspect it for symmetry—a test of the hypoglossal nerve (Cranial Nerve XII).

Note the color and texture of the dorsum of the tongue.

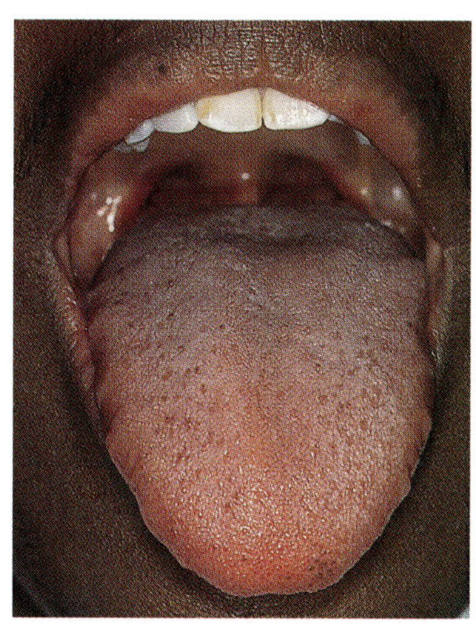

Asymmetric protrusion suggests a lesion of Cranial Nerve XII, as shown below.

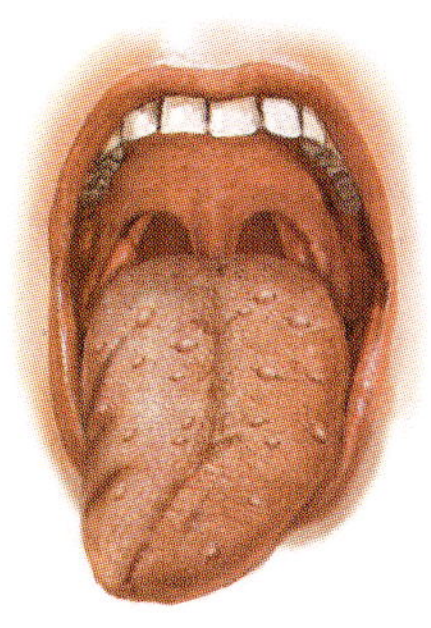

Inspect the sides and undersurface of the tongue and the floor of the mouth. These are the areas where cancer most often develops. Note any white or reddened areas, nodules, or ulcerations. Because cancer of the tongue is

Cancer of the tongue is the second most common cancer of the mouth, second only to cancer of

more common in men over age 50, especially in those who use tobacco and drink alcohol, palpation is indicated for these patients. Explain what you plan to do and put on gloves. Ask the patient to protrude his tongue. With your right hand, grasp the tip of the tongue with a square of gauze and gently pull it to the patient's left. Inspect the side of the tongue, and then palpate it with your gloved left hand, feeling for any induration (hardness). Reverse the procedure for the other side.

the lip. Any persistent nodule or ulcer, red or white, must be suspect. Induration of the lesion further increases the possibility of malignancy. Cancer occurs most often on the side of the tongue, next most often at its base.

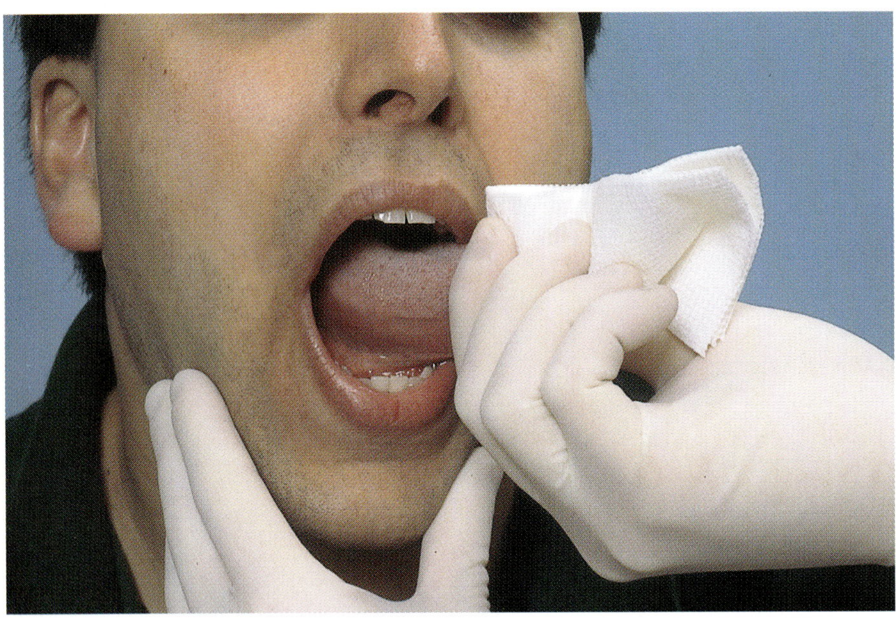

A carcinoma on the left side of a tongue:

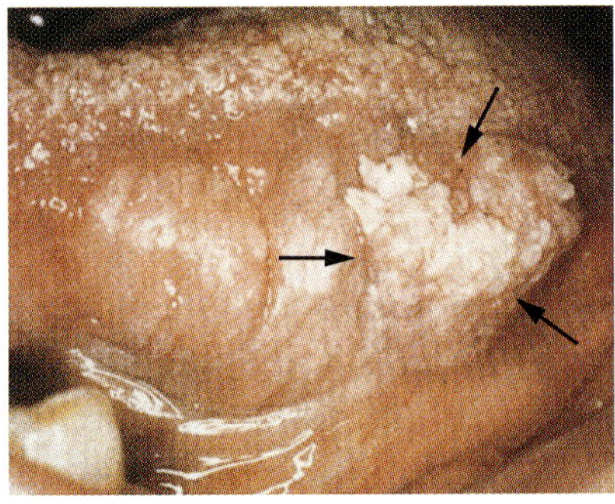

(Photo reprinted by permission of the New England Journal of Medicine, 328: 186, 1993—arrows added)

See Table 5-23, Findings In or Under the Tongue (pp. 206–207).

The Pharynx. Now, with the patient's mouth open but the tongue not protruded, ask the patient to say "ah" or yawn. This action may let you see the pharynx well. If not, press a tongue blade firmly down upon the midpoint of the arched tongue—far enough back to get good visualization of the pharynx but not so far that you cause gagging. Simultaneously, ask for an "ah" or a yawn. Note the rise of the soft palate—a test of Cranial Nerve X (the vagal nerve).

In Cranial Nerve X paralysis, the soft palate fails to rise and the uvula deviates to the opposite side.

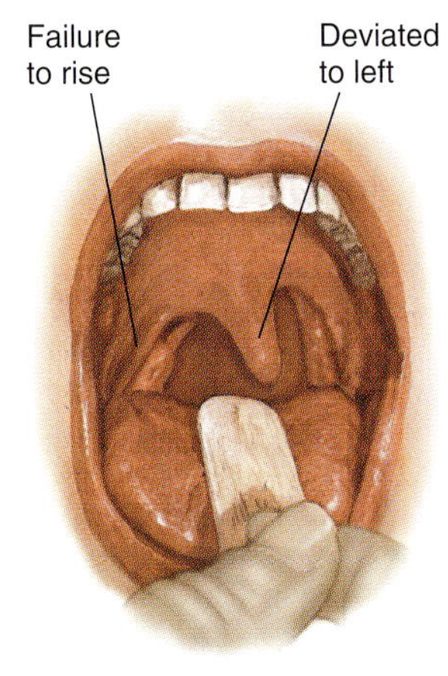

Inspect the soft palate, anterior and posterior pillars, uvula, tonsils, and pharynx. Note their color and symmetry and look for exudate, swelling, ulceration, or tonsillar enlargement. If possible, palpate any suspicious area for induration or tenderness. Tonsils have crypts, or deep infoldings of squamous epithelium. Whitish spots of normal exfoliating epithelium may sometimes be seen in these crypts.

See Table 5-21, Findings in the Pharynx, Palate, and Oral Mucosa (pp. 200–202).

Discard your tongue blade after use.

The Neck

Inspect the neck, noting its symmetry and any masses or scars. Look for enlargement of the parotid or submandibular glands, and note any visible lymph nodes.

A scar of past thyroid surgery may be the clue to unsuspected thyroid disease.

Lymph Nodes. *Palpate the lymph nodes.* Using the pads of your index and middle fingers, move the skin over the underlying tissues in each area. The patient should be relaxed, with neck flexed slightly forward and, if needed, slightly toward the side being examined. You can usually examine both sides at once. For the submental node, however, it is helpful to feel with one hand while bracing the top of the head with the other.

Feel in sequence for the following nodes:

1. Preauricular—in front of the ear
2. Posterior auricular—superficial to the mastoid process
3. Occipital—at the base of the skull posteriorly
4. Tonsillar—at the angle of the mandible
5. Submandibular—midway between the angle and the tip of the mandible. These nodes are usually smaller and smoother than the lobulated submandibular gland against which they lie.
6. Submental—in the midline a few centimeters behind the tip of the mandible
7. Superficial cervical—superficial to the sternomastoid
8. Posterior cervical—along the anterior edge of the trapezius
9. Deep cervical chain—deep to the sternomastoid and often inaccessible to examination. Hook your thumb and fingers around either side of the sternomastoid muscle to find them.
10. Supraclavicular—deep in the angle formed by the clavicle and the sternomastoid

A "tonsillar node" that pulsates is really the carotid artery. A small, hard, tender "tonsillar node" high and deep between the mandible and the sternomastoid is probably a styloid process.

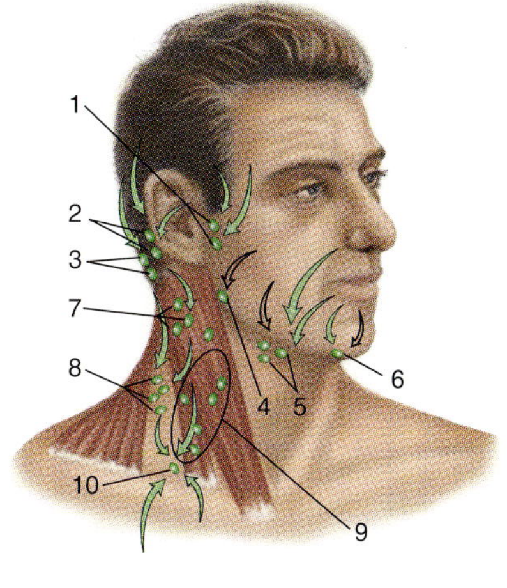

Enlargement of a supraclavicular node, especially on the left, suggests possible metastasis from a thoracic or an abdominal malignancy.

Note their size, shape, delimitation (discrete or matted together), mobility, consistency, and any tenderness. Small, mobile, discrete, nontender nodes, sometimes termed "shotty," are frequently found in normal persons.

Tender nodes suggest inflammation; hard or fixed nodes suggest malignancy.

Using the pads of the 2nd and 3rd fingers, palpate the preauricular nodes with a gentle rotary motion. Then examine the posterior auricular and occipital lymph nodes.

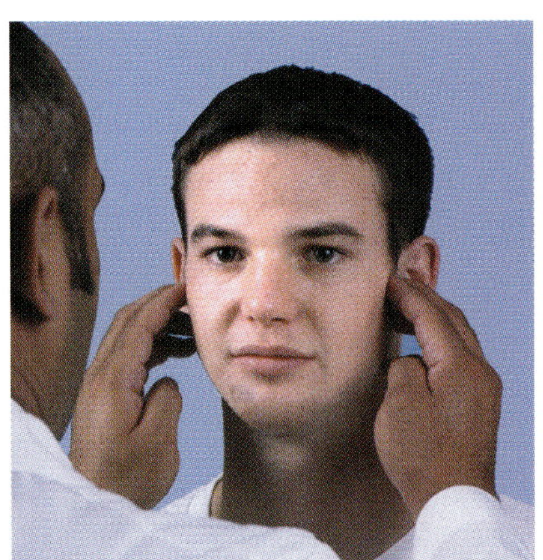

Palpate the anterior cervical chain, located anterior and superficial to the sternomastoid. Then palpate the posterior cervical chain along the trapezius (anterior edge) and along the sternomastoid (posterior edge). Flex the patient's neck slightly forward toward the side being examined. Examine the supraclavicular nodes in the angle between the clavicle and the sternomastoid.

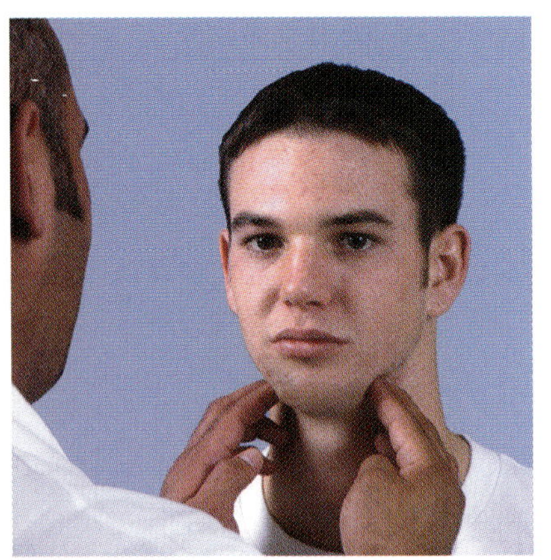

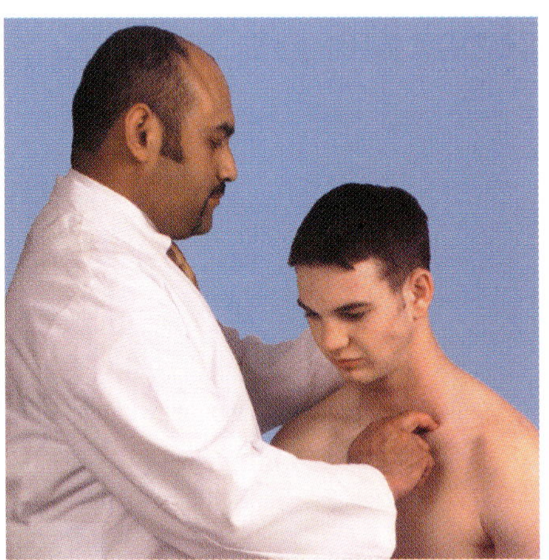

Enlarged or tender nodes, if unexplained, call for (1) reexamination of the regions they drain, and (2) careful assessment of lymph nodes elsewhere so that you can distinguish between regional and generalized lymphadenopathy.

Occasionally you may mistake a band of muscle or an artery for a lymph node. You should be able to roll a node in two directions: up and down, and side to side. Neither a muscle nor an artery will pass this test.

Diffuse lymphadenopathy raises the suspicion of infection from human immunodeficiency virus (HIV) or acquired immunodeficiency syndrome (AIDS).

The Trachea and the Thyroid Gland. To orient yourself to the neck, identify the thyroid and cricoid cartilages and the trachea below them.

- *Inspect the trachea* for any deviation from its usual midline position. Then *feel for any deviation.* Place your finger along one side of the trachea and note the space between it and the sternomastoid. Compare it with the other side. The spaces should be symmetric.

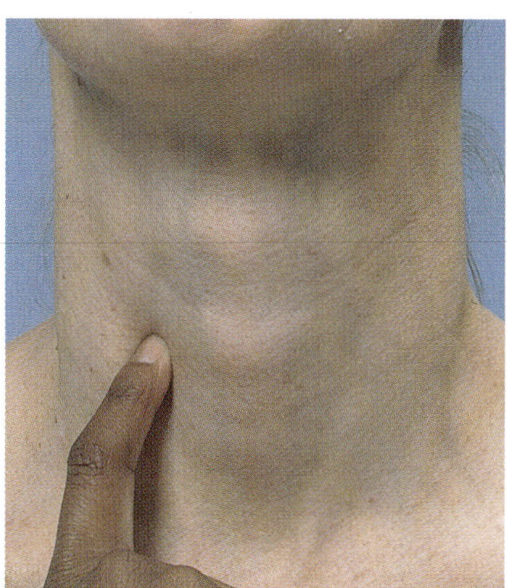

Masses in the neck may push the trachea to one side. Tracheal deviation may also signify important problems in the thorax, such as a mediastinal mass, atelectasis, or a large pneumothorax (see p. 243).

- *Inspect the neck for the thyroid gland.* Tip the patient's head back a bit. Using tangential lighting directed downward from the tip of the patient's chin, inspect the region *below the cricoid cartilage* for the gland. The lower, shadowed border of each thyroid gland shown here is outlined by arrows.

The lower border of this large thyroid gland is outlined by tangential lighting. *Goiter* is a general term for an enlarged thyroid gland.

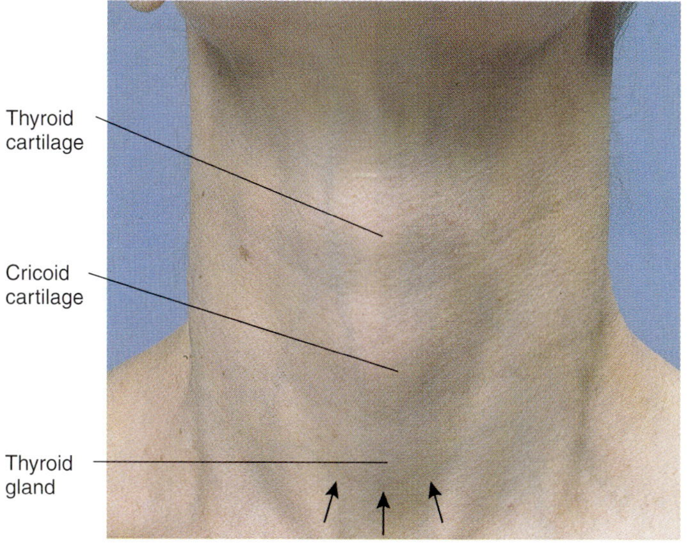

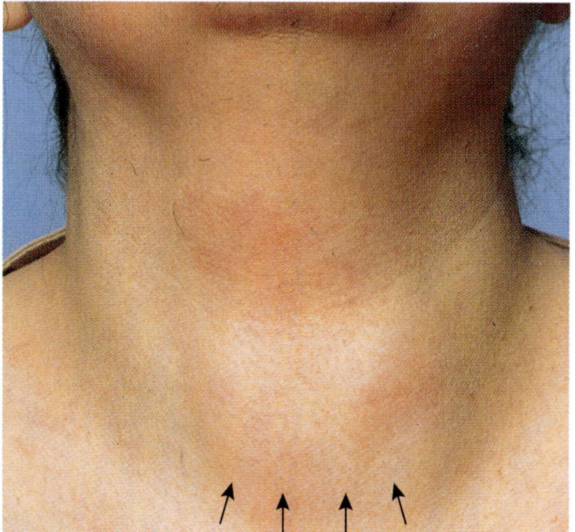

AT REST

Ask the patient to sip some water and to extend the neck again and swallow. Watch for upward movement of the thyroid gland, noting its contour and symmetry. The thyroid cartilage, the cricoid cartilage, and the thyroid gland all rise with swallowing and then fall to their resting positions.

With swallowing, the lower border of this large gland rises and looks less symmetrical.

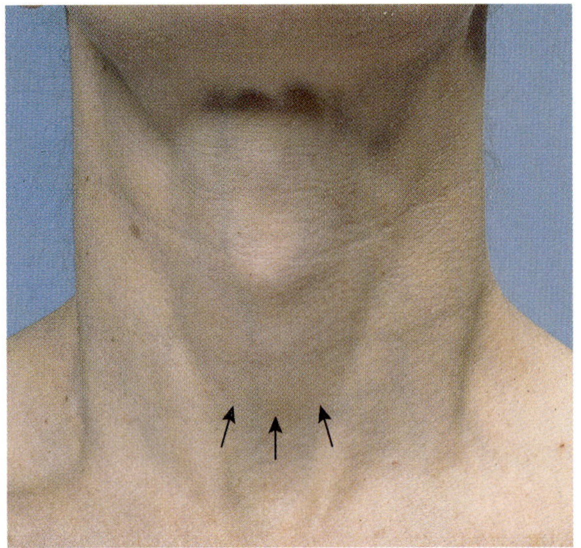

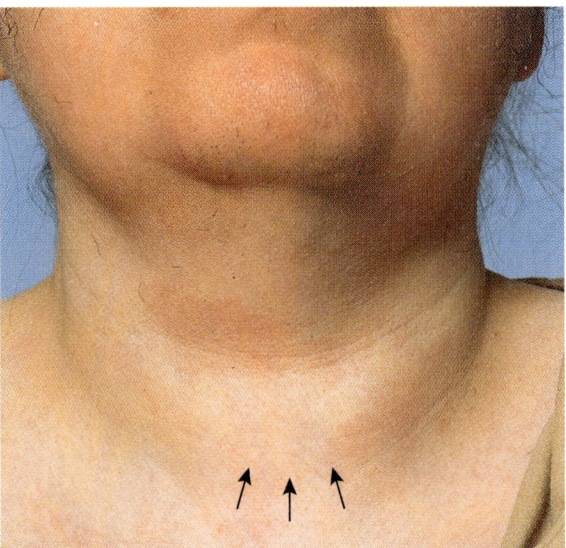

SWALLOWING

Until you become familiar with this examination, check your visual observations with your fingers from in front of the patient. This will orient you to the next step.

You are now ready to *palpate the thyroid gland*. This may seem difficult at first. Use the cues from visual inspection. Find your landmarks, adopt good technique, and follow the steps on the next page, which outline the posterior approach (technique for the anterior approach is similar). With experience you will become more adept. The thyroid gland is usually easier to feel in a long slender neck than in a short stocky one. In shorter necks, added extension of the neck may help. In some persons, however, the thyroid gland is partially or wholly substernal and not amenable to physical examination.

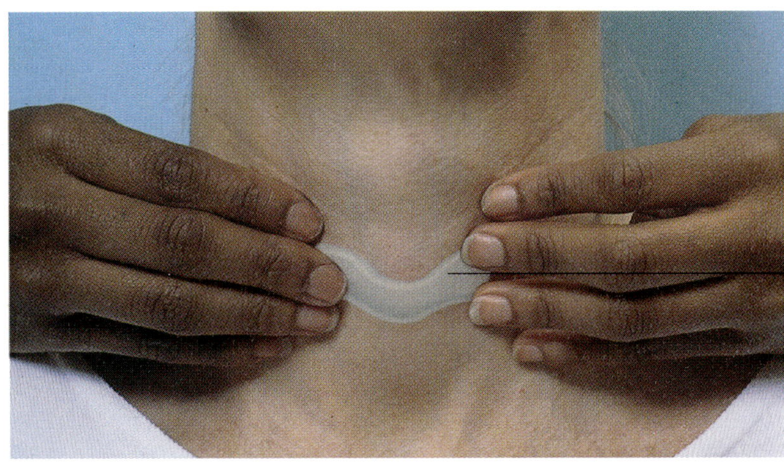

STEPS FOR PALPATING THE THYROID GLAND

- Ask the patient to flex the neck slightly forward to relax the sternomastoid muscles.
- Place the fingers of both hands on the patient's neck so that your index fingers are just below the cricoid cartilage.
- Ask the patient to sip and swallow water as before. Feel for the thyroid isthmus rising up under your finger pads. It is often but not always palpable.
- Displace the trachea to the right with the fingers of the left hand; with the right-hand fingers, palpate laterally for the right lobe of the thyroid in the space between the displaced trachea and the relaxed sternomastoid. Find the lateral margin. In similar fashion, examine the left lobe.

  The lobes are somewhat harder to feel than the isthmus, so practice is needed. The anterior surface of a lateral lobe is approximately the size of the distal phalanx of the thumb and feels somewhat rubbery.

Although physical characteristics of the thyroid gland, such as size, shape, and consistency, are diagnostically important, they tell you little if anything about thyroid function. Assessment of thyroid function depends upon symptoms, signs elsewhere in the body, and laboratory tests. See Table 5-24, Thyroid Enlargement and Function (p. 208).

- Note the *size, shape,* and *consistency* of the gland and identify any *nodules* or *tenderness.*

Soft in Graves' disease; firm in Hashimoto's thyroiditis, malignancy. Benign and malignant nodules, tenderness in thyroiditis

If the thyroid gland is enlarged, listen over the lateral lobes with a stethoscope to detect a bruit, a sound similar to a cardiac murmur but of noncardiac origin.

A localized systolic or continuous bruit may be heard in hyperthyroidism.

The Carotid Arteries and Jugular Veins. You will probably defer a detailed examination of these vessels until the patient lies down for the cardiovascular examination. Jugular venous distention, however, may be visible in the sitting position and should not be overlooked. You should also be alert to unusually prominent arterial pulsations. See Chapter 7 for further discussion.

Special Techniques

For Assessing Prominent Eyes. Inspect unusually prominent eyes from above. Standing behind the seated patient, draw the upper lids gently upward, and then compare the positions of the eyes and note the relationship of the corneas to the lower lids. Further assessment can be made with an exophthalmometer, an instrument that measures the prominence of the eyes from the side. The upper limits of normal for eye prominence are increased in African Americans.

Exophthalmos is an abnormal protrusion of the eye (see p. 177).

For Nasolacrimal Duct Obstruction. This test helps to identify the cause of excessive tearing. Ask the patient to look up. Press on the lower lid close to the medial canthus, just *inside* the rim of the bony orbit. You are thus compressing the lacrimal sac.

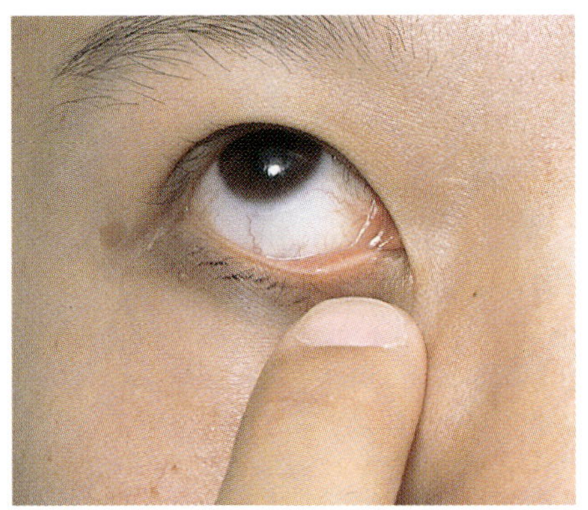

Look for fluid regurgitated out of the puncta into the eye. Avoid this test if the area is inflamed and tender.

Regurgitation of mucopurulent fluid from the puncta suggests an obstructed nasolacrimal duct.

For Inspection of the Upper Palpebral Conjunctiva. Adequate examination of the eye in search of a foreign body requires eversion of the upper eyelid. Follow these steps:

- Instruct the patient to look down. Get the patient to relax the eyes—by reassurance and by gentle, assured, and deliberate movements. Raise the upper eyelid slightly so that the eyelashes protrude, and then grasp the upper eyelashes and pull them gently down and forward.

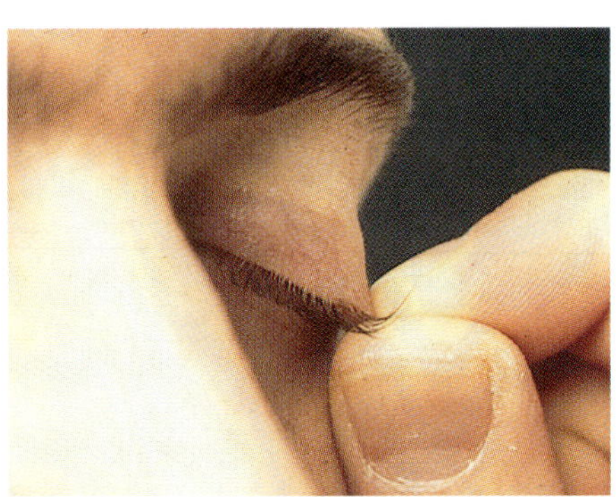

- Place a small stick such as an applicator or a tongue blade at least 1 cm above the lid margin (and therefore at the upper border of the tarsal plate). Push down on the stick as you raise the edge of the lid, thus everting the eyelid or turning it "inside out." Do not press on the eyeball itself.

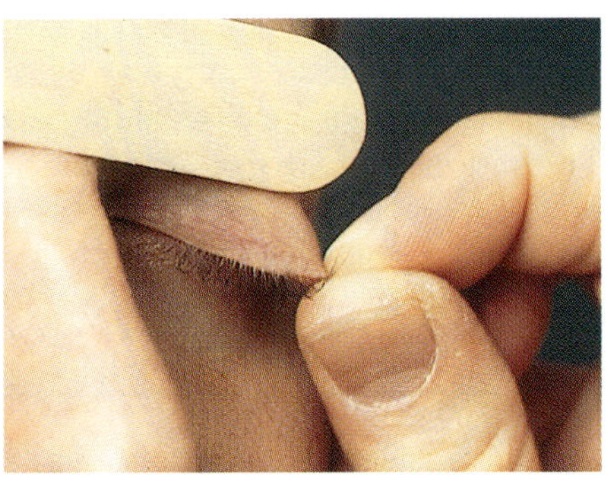

- Secure the upper lashes against the eyebrow with your thumb and inspect the palpebral conjunctiva. After your inspection, grasp the upper eyelashes and pull them gently forward. Ask the patient to look up. The eyelid will return to its normal position.

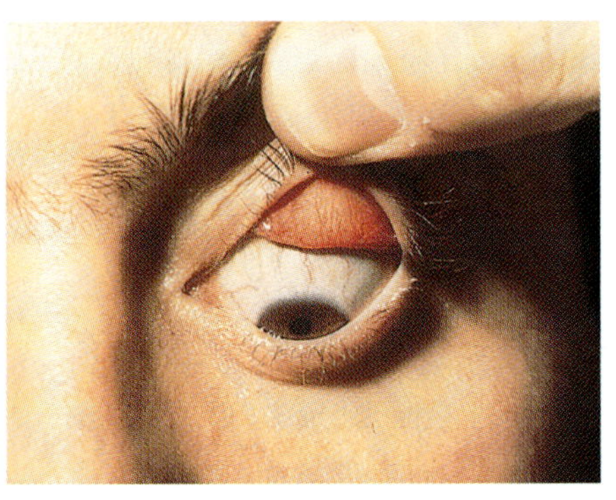

This view allows you to see the upper palpebral conjunctiva and look for a foreign body that might be lodged there.

Swinging Flashlight Test. This test helps you to decide whether reduced vision is due to ocular disease or to optic nerve disease. For an adequate test, vision must not be entirely lost. In dim room light, note the size of the pupils. After asking the patient to gaze into the distance, swing the beam of a penlight back and forth from one pupil to the other, each time concentrating on the pupillary size and reaction in the eye that is lit. Normally, each illuminated eye looks or promptly becomes constricted. The opposite eye also constricts consensually.

When the optic nerve is damaged, as in the left eye below, the sensory (afferent) stimulus sent to the midbrain is reduced. The pupil, responding less vigorously, dilates from its prior constricted state. This response is an *afferent pupillary defect* (Marcus Gunn pupil). The opposite eye responds consensually.

When ocular disease, such as a cataract, impairs vision, the pupils respond normally.

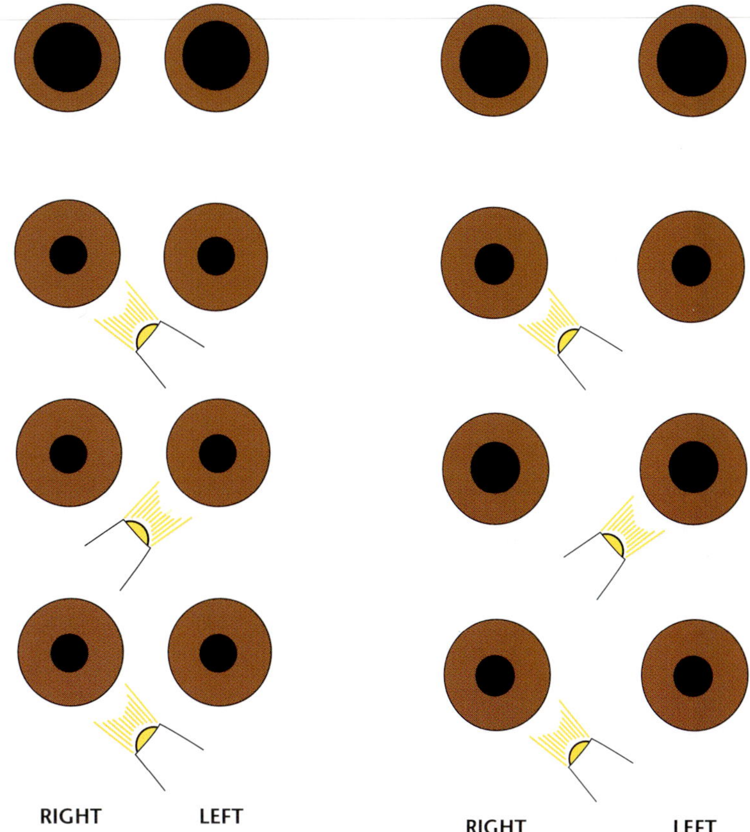

Transillumination of the Sinuses. When sinus tenderness or other symptoms suggest sinusitis, this test can at times be helpful but is not highly sensitive or specific for diagnosis. The room should be thoroughly darkened. Using a strong, narrow light source, place the light snugly deep under each brow, close to the nose. Shield the light with your hand. Look for a dim red glow as light is transmitted through the air-filled frontal sinus to the forehead.

Absence of glow on one or both sides suggests a thickened mucosa or secretions in the frontal sinus, but it may also result from developmental absence of one or both sinuses.

Ask the patient to tilt his or her head back with mouth opened wide. (An upper denture should first be removed.) Shine the light downward from just below the inner aspect of each eye. Look through the open mouth at the hard palate. A reddish glow indicates a normal air-filled maxillary sinus.

Absence of glow suggests thickened mucosa or secretions in the maxillary sinus. See p. 681 for an alternative method of transilluminating the maxillary sinuses.

TABLE 5-1 ■ Headaches

Problem	Process	Location	Quality and Severity	Timing	
				Onset	*Duration*
Tension Headaches	Unclear	Usually bilateral; may be generalized or localized to the back of the head and upper neck or to the frontotemporal area	Mild and aching or a nonpainful tightness and pressure	Gradual	Variable: hours or days, but often weeks or months
Migraine Headaches *("Classic migraine" in contrast to "common migraine" is distinguished by visual or neurologic symptoms during the half hour before the headache.)*	Dilatation of arteries outside or inside the skull, possibly of biochemical origin; often familial	Typically frontal or temporal, one or both sides, but also may be occipital or generalized. "Classic migraine" is typically unilateral.	Throbbing or aching, variable in severity	Fairly rapid, reaching a peak in 1–2 hours	Several hours to 1–2 days
Toxic Vascular Headaches *due to fever, toxic substances, or drug withdrawal*	Dilatation of arteries, mainly inside the skull	Generalized	Aching, of variable severity	Variable	Depends on cause
Cluster Headaches	Unclear	One-sided; high in the nose, and behind and over the eye	Steady, severe	Abrupt, often 2–3 hours after falling asleep	Roughly 1–2 hours
Headaches With Eye Disorders					
Errors of Refraction (farsightedness and astigmatism, but not nearsightedness)	Probably the sustained contraction of the extraocular muscles, and possibly of the frontal, temporal, and occipital muscles	Around and over the eyes, may radiate to the occipital area	Steady, aching, dull	Gradual	Variable
Acute Glaucoma	Sudden increase in intraocular pressure (see p. 148)	In and around one eye	Steady, aching, often severe	Often rapid	Variable, may depend on treatment

Blanks appear in these tables when the categories are not applicable or are not usually helpful in assessing the problem.

Course	Associated Symptoms	Factors That Aggravate or Provoke	Factors That Relieve	Convenient Categories of Thought
Often recurrent or persistent over long periods	Symptoms of anxiety, tension, and depression may be present.	Sustained muscular tension, as in driving or typing; emotional	Possible massage, relaxation	
Often begins between childhood and early adulthood. Typically recurrent at intervals of weeks, months, or years, usually decreasing with pregnancy and advancing age	Often nausea and vomiting. A minority of patients have preceding visual disturbances (local flashes of light, blind spots) or neurologic symptoms (local weakness, sensory disturbances, and other symptoms).	May be provoked by alcohol, certain foods, or tension. More common premenstrually. Aggravated by noise and bright light	Quiet, dark room; sleep; sometimes transient relief from pressure on the involved artery, if early in the course	The two most common kinds of headache
Depends on cause	Depends on cause	Fever, carbon monoxide, hypoxia, withdrawal of caffeine, other causes	Depends on cause	Vascular headaches
Typically clustered in time, with several each day or week and then relief for weeks or months	Unilateral stuffy, runny nose, and reddening and tearing of the eye	During a cluster, may be provoked by alcohol		
Variable	Eye fatigue, "sandy" sensations in the eyes, redness of the conjunctiva	Prolonged use of the eyes, particularly for close work	Rest of the eyes	
Variable, may depend on treatment	Diminished vision, sometimes nausea and vomiting	Sometimes provoked by drops that dilate the pupils		Face pains

(table continues next page)

TABLE 5-1 ■ Headaches *(Continued)*

Problem	Process	Location	Quality and Severity	Timing: *Onset*	Timing: *Duration*
Headaches With Acute Paranasal Sinusitis	Mucosal inflammation of the paranasal sinuses and their openings	Usually above the eye (frontal sinus) or in the cheekbone area (maxillary sinus), one or both sides	Aching or throbbing, variable in severity	Variable	Often several hours at a time, recurring over days or longer
Trigeminal Neuralgia	Mechanism variable, often unknown	Cheek, jaws, lips, or gums (second and third divisions of the trigeminal nerve)	Sharp, short, brief, lightninglike jabs; very severe	Abrupt	Each jab is transient, but jabs recur in clusters at intervals of seconds or minutes
Giant Cell Arteritis	Chronic inflammation of the cranial arteries, cause unknown, often associated with polymyalgia rheumatica	Localized near the involved artery (most often the temporal, also the occipital); may become generalized	Aching, throbbing, or burning, often severe	Gradual or rapid	Variable
Chronic Subdural Hematoma	Bleeding into the subdural space after trauma, followed by slow accumulation of fluid that compresses the brain	Variable	Steady, aching	Gradual onset weeks to months after the injury	Often depends on surgical intervention
Post-concussion Syndrome	Mechanism unclear	May be localized to the injured area, but not necessarily	Variable	Within a few hours of the injury	Weeks, months, or even years
Meningitis	Infection of the meninges that surround the brain	Generalized	Steady or throbbing, very severe	Fairly rapid	Variable, usually days
Subarachnoid Hemorrhage	Bleeding, most often from a ruptured intra-cranial aneurysm	Generalized	Very severe, "the worst of my life"	Usually abrupt. Prodromal symptoms may occur	Variable, usually days
Brain Tumor	Displacement of or traction on pain-sensitive arteries and veins or pressure on nerves, all within the skull	Varies with the location of the tumor	Aching, steady, variable in intensity	Variable	Often brief

Course	Associated Symptoms	Factors That Aggravate or Provoke	Factors That Relieve	Convenient Categories of Thought
Often recurrent in a repetitive daily pattern: starting in the morning (frontal) or in the afternoon (maxillary)	Local tenderness, nasal congestion, discharge, and fever	May be aggravated by coughing, sneezing, or jarring the head	Nasal decongestants	Face pains
Pain may be troublesome for months, then disappears for months, but often recurs. It is uncommon at night.	Exhaustion from recurrent pain	Typically triggered by touching certain areas of the lower face or mouth, or by chewing, talking, or brushing teeth		
Recurrent or persistent over weeks to months	Tenderness of the adjacent scalp; fever, malaise, fatigue, and anorexia; muscular aches and stiffness; visual loss or blindness			Consider these three in older adults.
Progressively severe but may be obscured by clouded consciousness	Alterations in consciousness, changes in personality, and hemiparesis (weakness on one side of the body). The injury is often forgotten.			Headaches following head trauma
Tends to diminish over time	Poor concentration, giddiness or vertigo, irritability, restlessness, tenseness, and fatigue	Mental and physical exertion, straining, stooping, emotional excitement, alcohol	Rest	
A persistent headache in an acute illness	Fever, stiff neck			Acute illnesses with very severe headaches
A persistent headache in an acute illness	Nausea, vomiting, possibly loss of consciousness, neck pain			
Often intermittent, but progressive	Neurologic and mental symptoms and nausea and vomiting may develop.	May be aggravated by coughing, sneezing, or sudden movements of the head		An underlying concern of patient and clinician alike

TABLE 5-2 ■ Vertigo

Problem	Timing: Onset	Timing: Duration	Timing: Course	Hearing	Tinnitus	Other Associated Symptoms
Benign Positional Vertigo	Sudden, on rolling over onto the affected side or tilting the head up	Brief, a few seconds to minutes	Persists a few weeks, may recur	Not affected	Absent	Sometimes nausea and vomiting
Vestibular Neuronitis *(acute labyrinthitis)*	Sudden	Hours to days, up to 2 weeks	May recur over 12–18 months	Not affected	Absent	Nausea, vomiting
Ménière's Disease	Sudden	Several hours to a day or more	Recurrent	Sensorineural hearing loss that improves and recurs, eventually progresses; one or both sides*	Present, fluctuating*	Nausea, vomiting, pressure or fullness in the affected ear
Drug Toxicity *(as from amino-glycosides or alcohol intoxication)*	Insidious or acute	May or may not be reversible Partial adaptation occurs		May be impaired, both sides	May be present	Nausea, vomiting
Tumor, Pressing on the 8th Nerve	Insidious**	Variable	Variable	Impaired, one side	Present	Those of pressure on Cranial Nerves V, VI, and VII

Additional disorders of the brainstem or cerebellum may also cause vertigo. These include ischemia secondary to atherosclerosis, tumors, and multiple sclerosis. Additional neurologic symptoms and signs are usually present.

*Hearing impairment, tinnitus, and rotary vertigo do not always develop concurrently. Time is often required to make this diagnosis.
**Persistent unsteadiness is more common, but vertigo may occur.

TABLE 5-3 ■ Selected Facies

Acromegaly

The increased growth hormone of acromegaly produces enlargement of both bone and soft tissues. The head is elongated, with bony prominence of the forehead, nose, and lower jaw. Soft tissues of the nose, lips, and ears also enlarge. The facial features appear generally coarsened.

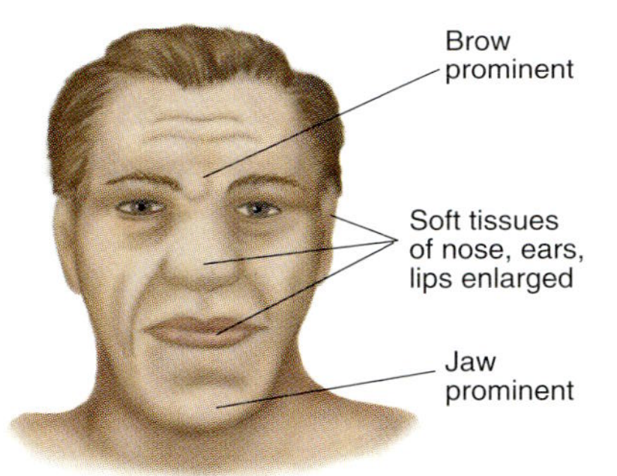

Myxedema

The patient with severe hypothyroidism (*myxedema*) has a dull, puffy facies. The edema, often particularly pronounced around the eyes, does not pit with pressure. The hair and eyebrows are dry, coarse, and thinned. The skin is dry.

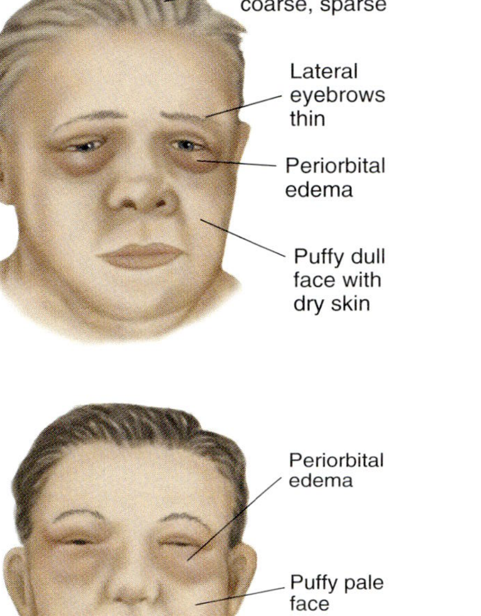

Nephrotic Syndrome

The face is edematous and often pale. Swelling usually appears first around the eyes and in the morning. The eyes may become slitlike when edema is severe.

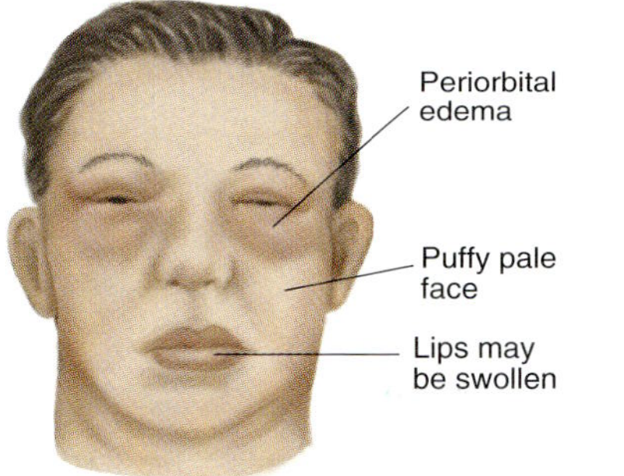

Cushing's Syndrome

The increased adrenal hormone production of Cushing's syndrome produces a round or "moon" face with red cheeks. Excessive hair growth may be present in the mustache and sideburn areas and on the chin.

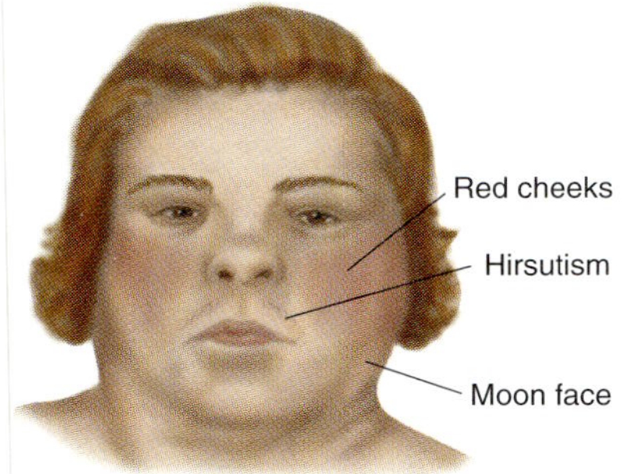

Parotid Gland Enlargement

Chronic bilateral asymptomatic parotid gland enlargement may be associated with obesity, diabetes, cirrhosis, and other conditions. Note the swellings anterior to the ear lobes and above the angles of the jaw. Gradual unilateral enlargement suggests neoplasm. Acute enlargement is seen in mumps.

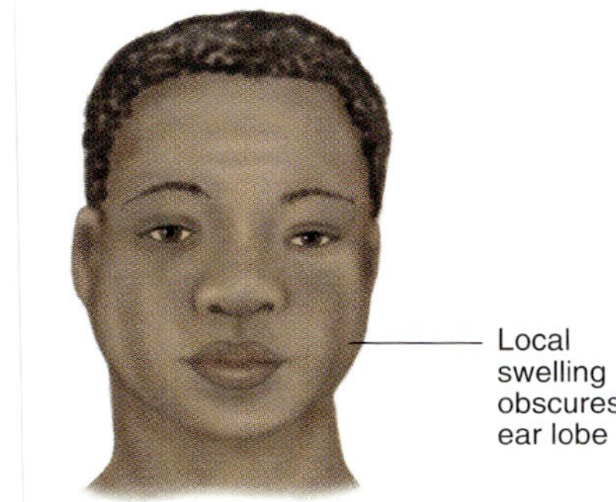

Parkinson's Disease

Decreased facial mobility blunts expression. A masklike face may result, with decreased blinking and a characteristic stare. Since the neck and upper trunk tend to flex forward, the patient seems to peer upward toward the observer. Facial skin becomes oily, and drooling may occur.

Stare

Decreasd mobility

TABLE 5-4 ■ Visual Field Defects

Visual Pathway Lesions

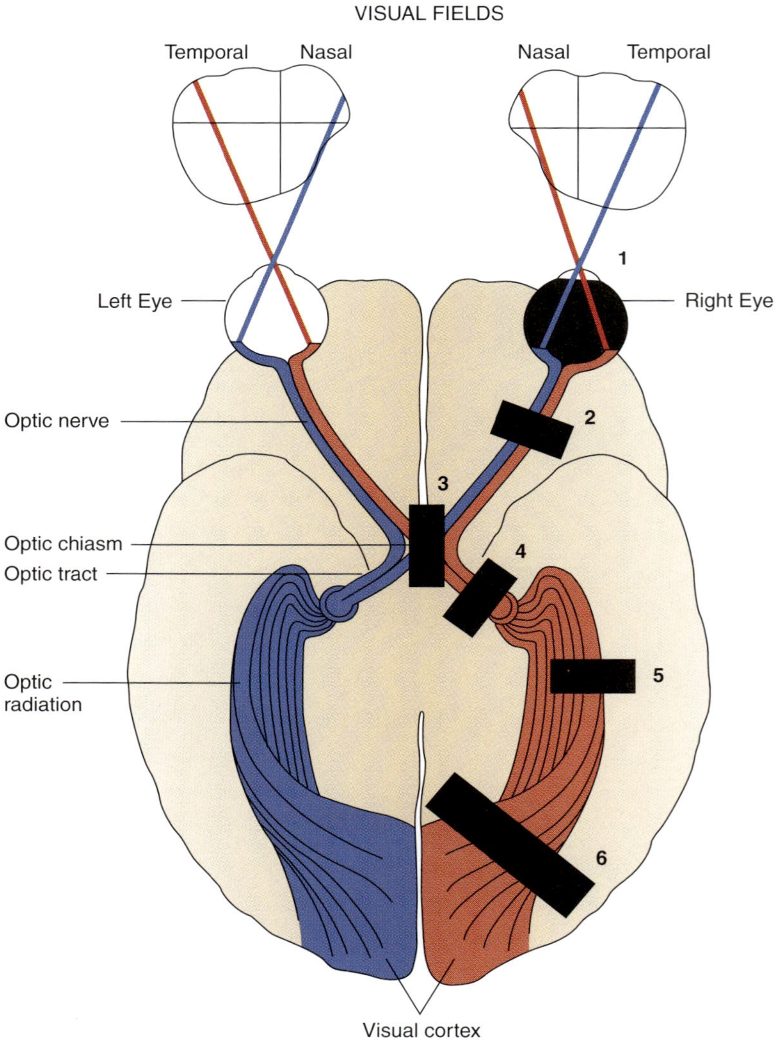

VISUAL FIELDS
Temporal
Nasal
Nasal
Temporal
Left Eye
Right Eye
Optic nerve
Optic chiasm
Optic tract
Optic radiation
Visual cortex
1
2
3
4
5
6

Visual Field Defects

1 Horizontal Defect

Occlusion of a branch of the central retinal artery may cause a horizontal (altitudinal) defect. Shown is the lower field defect associated with occlusion of the superior branch of this artery.

2 Blind Right Eye (right optic nerve)

A lesion of the optic nerve, and of course of the eye itself, produces unilateral blindness.

3 Bitemporal Hemianopsia (optic chiasm)

A lesion at the optic chiasm may involve only the fibers that are crossing over to the opposite side. Since these fibers originate in the nasal half of each retina, visual loss involves the temporal half of each field.

4 Left Homonymous Hemianopsia (right optic tract)

A lesion of the optic tract interrupts fibers originating on the same side of both eyes. Visual loss in the eyes is therefore similar (homonymous) and involves half of each field (hemianopsia).

5 Homonymous Left Superior Quadrantic Defect (right optic radiation, partial)

A partial lesion of the optic radiation may involve only a portion of the nerve fibers, producing, for example, a homonymous quadrantic defect.

6 Left Homonymous Hemianopsia (right optic radiation)

A complete interruption of fibers in the optic radiation produces a visual defect similar to that produced by a lesion of the optic tract.

Diagrammed From Patient's Viewpoint

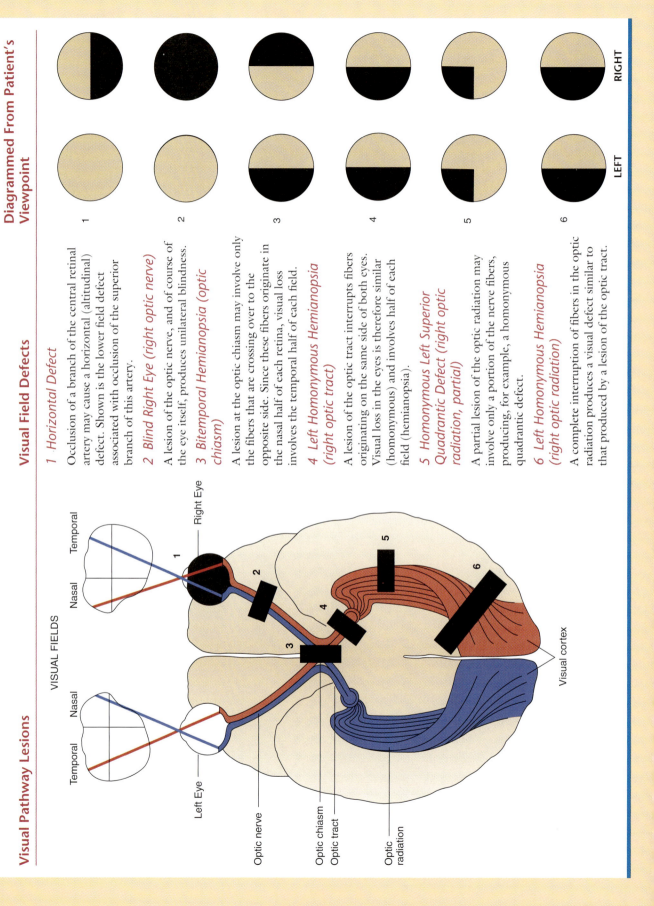

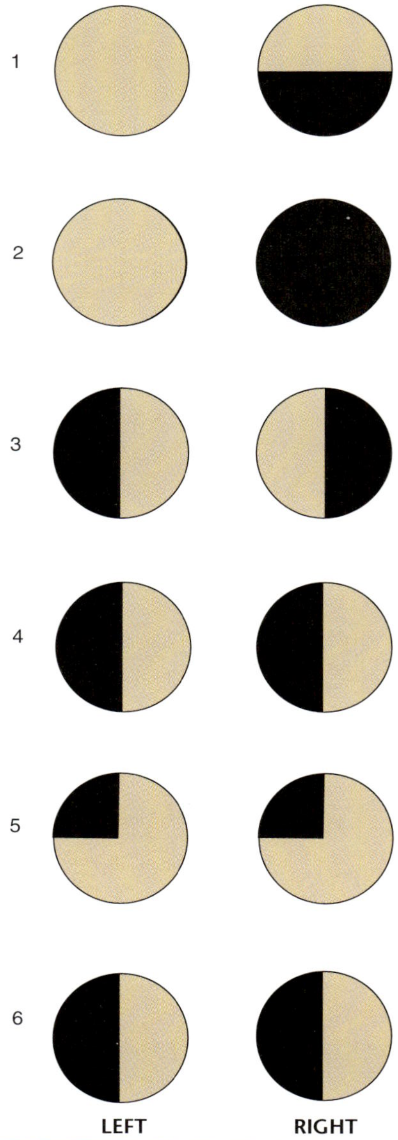

1
2
3
4
5
6
LEFT
RIGHT

TABLE 5-5 ■ Variations and Abnormalities of the Eyelids

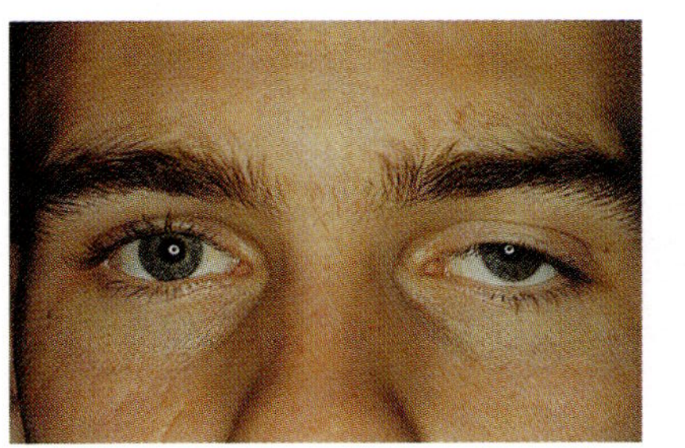

Ptosis

Ptosis is a drooping of the upper lid. Causes include myasthenia gravis, damage to the oculomotor nerve, and damage to the sympathetic nerve supply (*Horner's syndrome*). A weakened muscle, relaxed tissues, and the weight of herniated fat may cause senile ptosis. Ptosis may also be congenital.

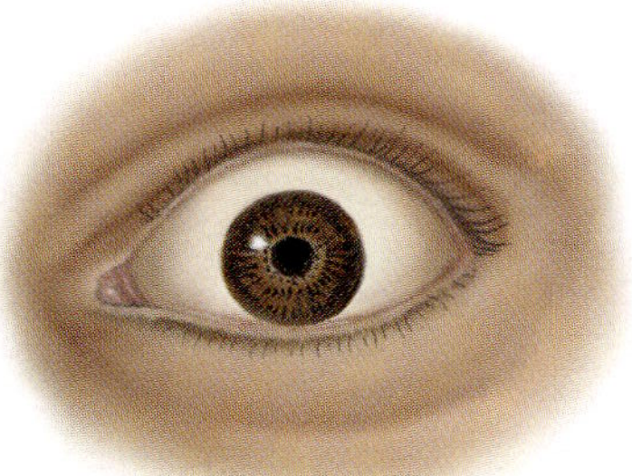

Retracted Lid

A wide-eyed stare suggests retracted eyelids—in this case, the upper lid. Note the rim of sclera between the upper lid and the iris. Retracted lids and a lid lag (p. 150) are often due to hyperthyroidism but may be seen in normal people. The eye does not protrude forward unless exophthalmos coexists.

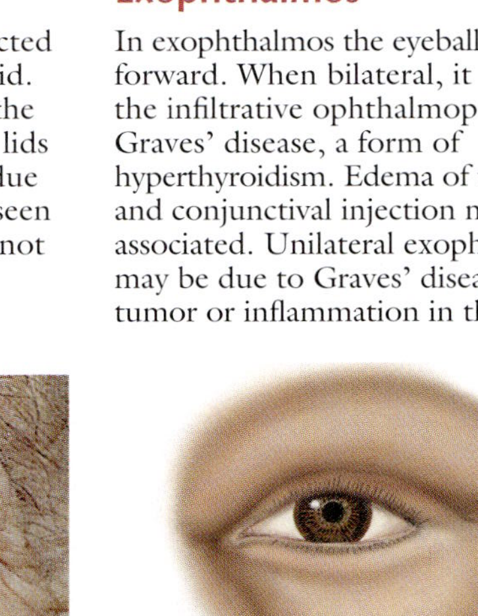

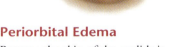

Exophthalmos

In exophthalmos the eyeball protrudes forward. When bilateral, it suggests the infiltrative ophthalmopathy of Graves' disease, a form of hyperthyroidism. Edema of the eyelids and conjunctival injection may be associated. Unilateral exophthalmos may be due to Graves' disease or to a tumor or inflammation in the orbit.

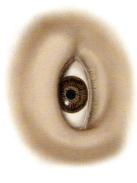

Epicanthus

An epicanthus (epicanthal fold) is a vertical fold of skin that lies over the medial canthus. It is normal among many Asian peoples. These folds are also seen in Down's syndrome and in a few other congenital conditions. They may falsely suggest a convergent strabismus (see p. 182).

Ectropion

In ectropion the margin of the lower lid is turned outward, exposing the palpebral conjunctiva. When the punctum of the lower lid turns outward, the eye no longer drains satisfactorily and tearing occurs. Ectropion is more common in the elderly.

Entropion

Entropion, more common in the elderly, is an inward turning of the lid margin. The lower lashes, which are often invisible when turned inward, irritate the conjunctiva and lower cornea. Asking the patient to squeeze the lids together and then open them may reveal an entropion that is not obvious.

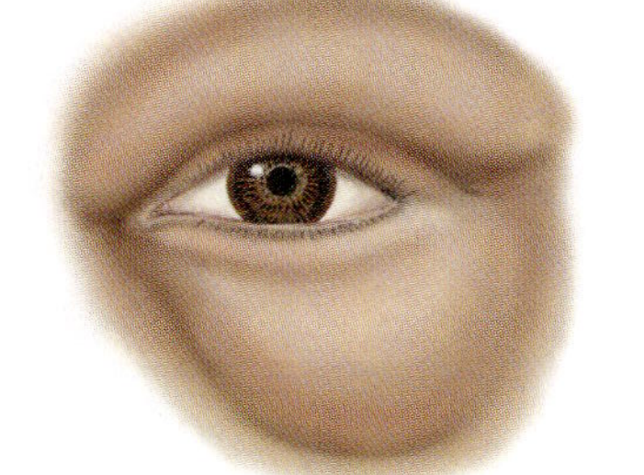

Periorbital Edema

Because the skin of the eyelids is loosely attached to underlying tissues, edema tends to accumulate there easily. Causes include allergies, local inflammation, cellulitis, myxedema, and fluid-retaining states such as the nephrotic syndrome.

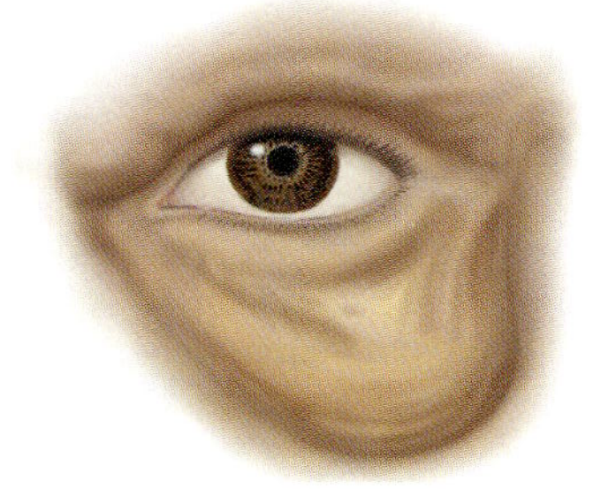

Herniated Fat

Puffy eyelids may be caused by fat. It pushes weakened fascia in the eyelids forward, producing bulges that involve the lower lids, the inner third of the upper ones, or both. These bulges appear more often in elderly people but may affect younger ones.

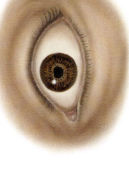

(Source of photos: *Ptosis, Ectropion, Entropion*—Tasman W, Jaeger E (eds): The Wills Eye Hospital Atlas of Clinical Ophthalmology, 2nd ed. Philadelphia, Lippincott Williams & Wilkins, 2001.)

TABLE 5-6 ■ Lumps and Swellings In and Around the Eyes

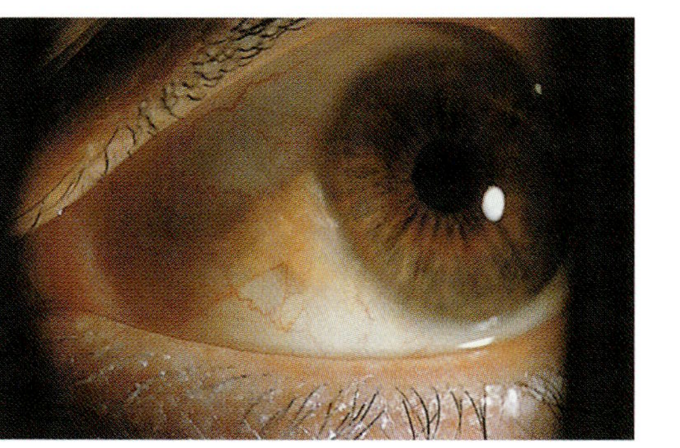

Pinguecula

A yellowish, somewhat triangular nodule in the bulbar conjunctiva on either side of the iris, a pinguecula is harmless. Pingueculae appear frequently with aging, first on the nasal and then on the temporal side.

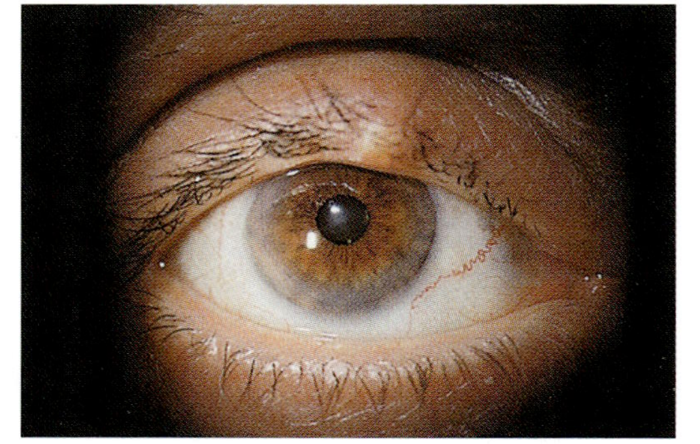

Sty (Acute Hordeolum)

A painful, tender, red infection in a gland at the margin of the eyelid, a sty looks like a pimple or boil pointing on the lid margin.

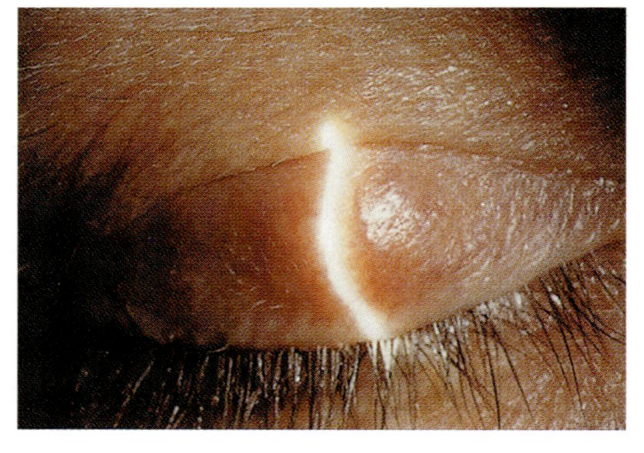

Chalazion

A chalazion is a subacute nontender nodule involving a meibomian gland. A beady nodule in an otherwise normal lid, it is usually painless. Occasionally a chalazion becomes acutely inflamed but, unlike a sty, usually points inside the lid rather than on the lid margin.

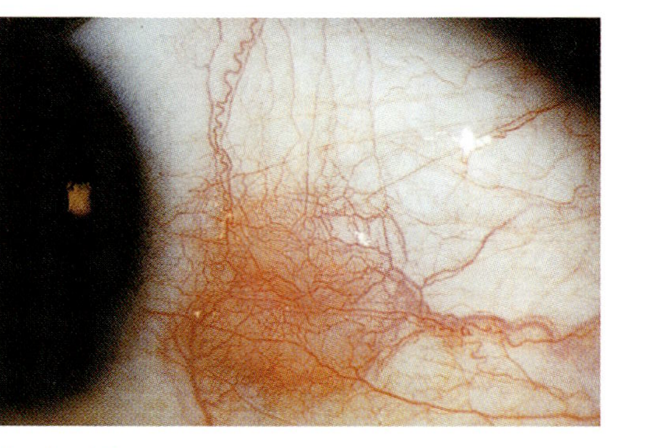

Episcleritis

Episcleritis is a localized ocular redness from inflammation of the episcleral vessels. In natural light, vessels appear salmon pink and are movable over the scleral surface. Usually benign and self-limited, episcleritis may be nodular, as shown here, or may show only redness and dilated vessels.

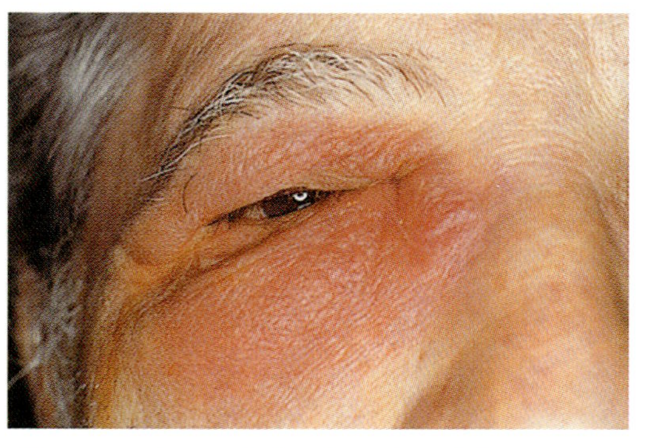

Inflammation of the Lacrimal Sac (Dacryocystitis)

A swelling between the lower eyelid and nose suggests inflammation of the lacrimal sac. An *acute* inflammation (illustrated) is painful, red, and tender. *Chronic* inflammation is associated with obstruction of the nasolacrimal duct. Tearing is prominent, and pressure on the sac produces regurgitation of material through the puncta of the eyelids.

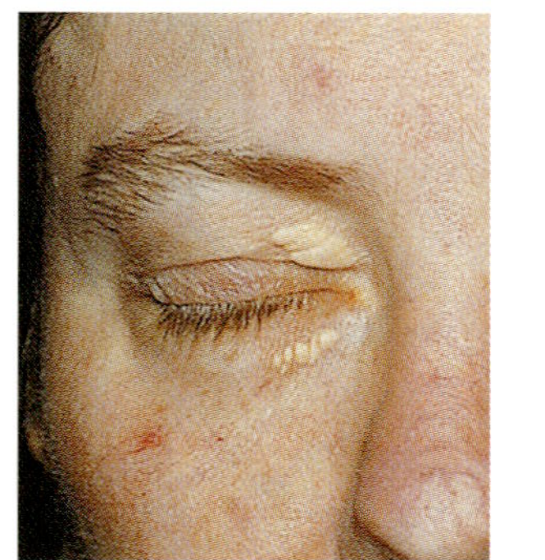

Xanthelasma

Slightly raised, yellowish, well-circumscribed plaques in the skin, xanthelasmas appear along the nasal portions of one or both eyelids. They may accompany lipid disorders (e.g., hypercholesterolemia), but may also occur independently.

(Source of photos: Tasman W, Jaeger E (eds): The Wills Eye Hospital Atlas of Clinical Ophthalmology, 2nd ed. Philadelphia, Lippincott Williams & Wilkins, 2001.)

TABLE 5-7 ■ Red Eyes

	Conjunctivitis	Corneal Injury or Infection	Acute Iritis	Glaucoma	Subconjunctival Hemorrhage
Pattern of Redness	Conjunctival injection: diffuse dilatation of conjunctival vessels with redness that tends to be maximal peripherally	Ciliary infection: dilation of deeper vessels that are visible as radiating vessels or a reddish violet flush around the limbus. Ciliary infection is an important sign of these three conditions but may not be apparent. The eye may be diffusely red instead. Other clues of these more serious disorders are pain, decreased vision, unequal pupils, and a less than perfectly clear cornea.			Leakage of blood outside of the vessels, producing a homogeneous, sharply demarcated, red area that fades over days to yellow and then disappears
Pain	Mild discomfort rather than pain	Moderate to severe, superficial	Moderate, aching, deep	Severe, aching, deep	Absent
Vision	Not affected except for temporary mild blurring due to discharge	Usually decreased	Decreased	Decreased	Not affected
Ocular Discharge	Watery, mucoid, or mucopurulent	Watery or purulent	Absent	Absent	Absent
Pupil	Not affected	Not affected unless iritis develops	May be small and, with time, irregular	Dilated, fixed	Not affected
Cornea	Clear	Changes depending on cause	Clear or slightly clouded	Steamy, cloudy	Clear
Significance	Bacterial, viral, and other infections; allergy; irritation	Abrasions, and other injuries; viral and bacterial infections	Associated with many ocular and systemic disorders	Acute increase in intraocular pressure—an emergency	Often none. May result from trauma, bleeding disorders, or a sudden increase in venous pressure, as from cough

TABLE 5-8 ■ Opacities of the Cornea and Lens

Corneal Arcus

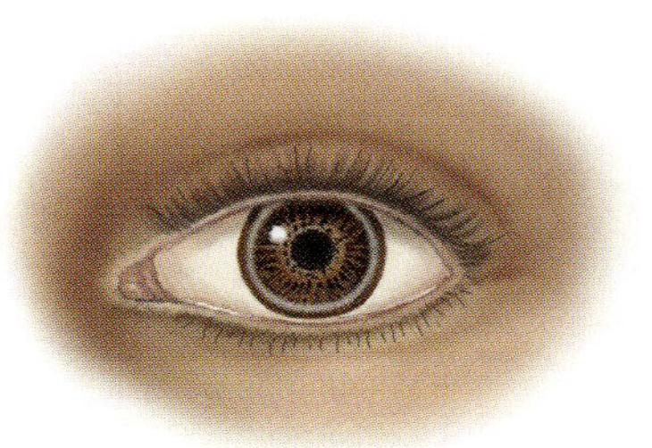

A corneal arcus is a thin grayish white arc or circle not quite at the edge of the cornea. It accompanies normal aging but may also be seen in younger people, especially African Americans. In young people, a corneal arcus suggests the possibility of hyperlipoproteinemia but does not prove it. Some surveys have revealed no relationship.

Corneal Scar

A corneal scar is a superficial grayish white opacity in the cornea, secondary to an old injury or to inflammation. Size and shape are variable. It should not be confused with the opaque lens of a cataract, visible on a deeper plane and only through the pupil.

Pterygium

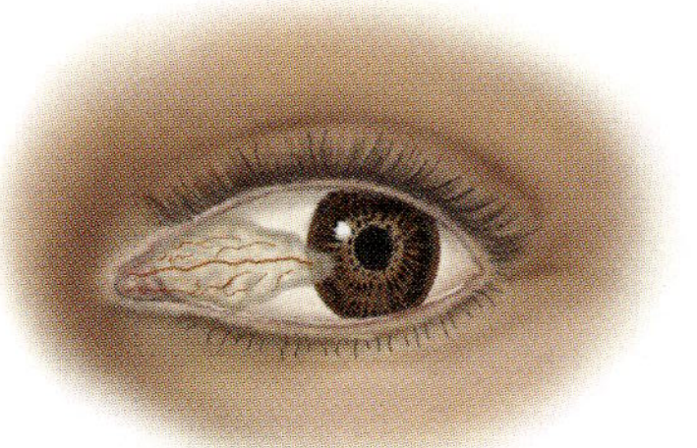

A pterygium is a triangular thickening of the bulbar conjunctiva that grows slowly across the outer surface of the cornea, usually from the nasal side. Reddening may occur intermittently. A pterygium may interfere with vision as it encroaches upon the pupil.

Cataracts

Cross Section of Lens

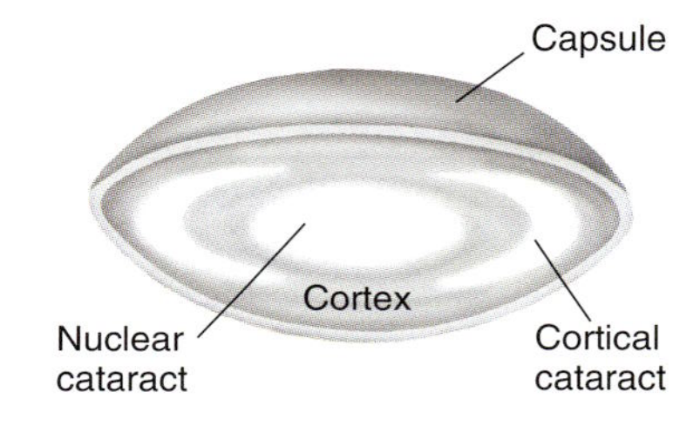

A cataract is an opacity of the lens and is seen through the pupil. Cataracts are classified in many ways, including cause and location. Old age is the most common cause. Two kinds of age-related cataract are illustrated below. In each example, the pupil has been widely dilated.

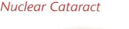

Nuclear Cataract

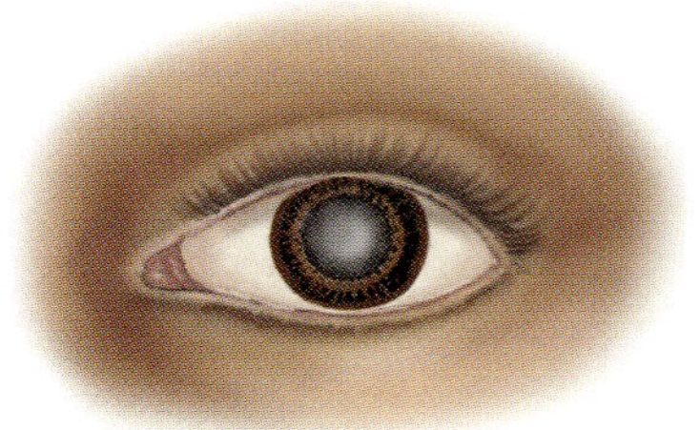

A nuclear cataract looks gray when seen by a flashlight. If the pupil is widely dilated, the gray opacity is surrounded by a black rim. Through an ophthalmoscope, the cataract looks black against the red reflex.

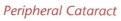

Peripheral Cataract

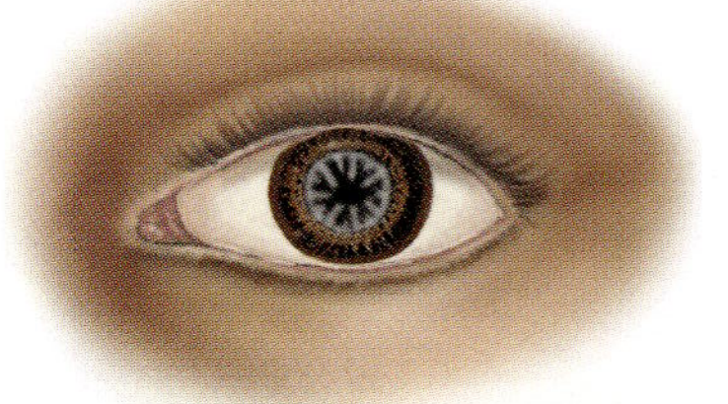

A peripheral cataract produces spokelike shadows that point inward—gray against black as seen with a flashlight, or black against red with an ophthalmoscope. A dilated pupil, as shown here, facilitates this observation.

TABLE 5-9 ■ Pupillary Abnormalities

Unequal Pupils (*Anisocoria*)

When anisocoria is greater in bright light than in dim light, the larger pupil cannot constrict properly. Causes include blunt trauma to the eye, open-angle glaucoma (p. 148), and impaired parasympathetic nerve supply to the iris, as in tonic pupil and oculomotor nerve paralysis. When anisocoria is greater in dim light, the smaller pupil cannot dilate properly, as in Horner's syndrome, which is caused by an interruption of the sympathetic nerve supply.

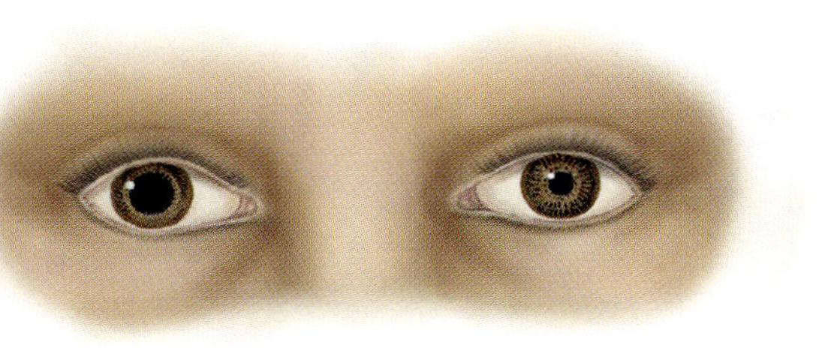

Tonic Pupil (*Adie's Pupil*)

A tonic pupil is large, regular, and usually unilateral. Its reaction to light is severely reduced and slowed, or even absent. The near reaction, though very slow, is present. Slow accommodation causes blurred vision. Deep tendon reflexes are often decreased.

Oculomotor Nerve (CN III) Paralysis

The dilated pupil (about 6–7 mm) is fixed to light and near effort. Ptosis of the upper eyelid and lateral deviation of the eye, as shown here, are often but not always present. (An even more dilated [8–9 mm] and fixed pupil may be due to local application of atropine-like agents.)

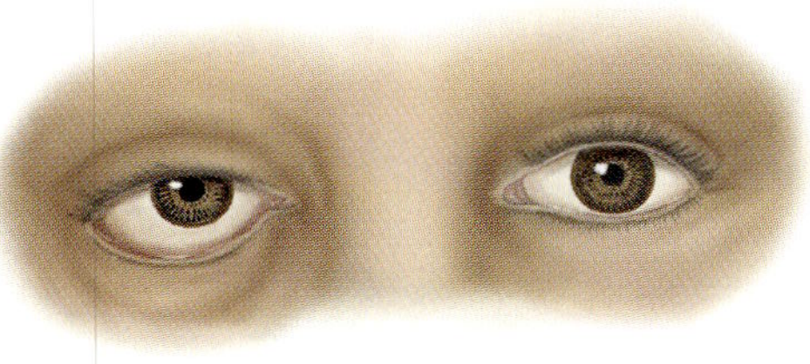

Horner's Syndrome

The affected pupil, though small, reacts briskly to light and near effort. Ptosis of the eyelid is present, perhaps with loss of sweating on the forehead of the same side. In congenital Horner's syndrome, the involved iris is lighter in color than its fellow (*heterochromia*).

Equal Pupils and One Blind Eye

Unilateral blindness does not cause anisocoria as long as the sympathetic and parasympathetic innervation to both irises is normal. A light directed into the seeing eye produces a direct reaction in that eye and a consensual reaction in the blind eye. A light directed into the blind eye, however, causes no response in either eye.

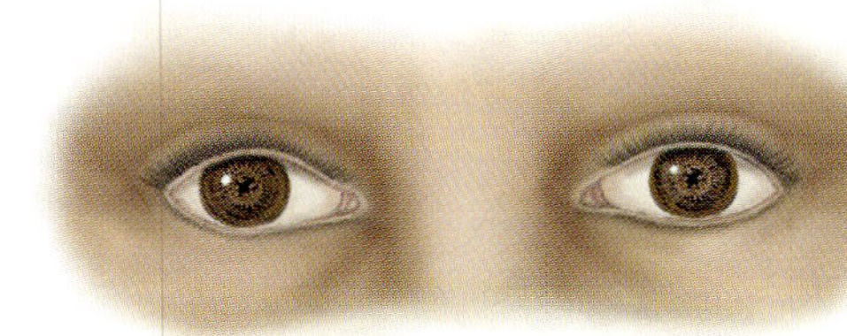

Small Irregular Pupils

Small, irregular pupils that do not react to light but do react to near effort indicate *Argyll Robertson pupils.* They are usually but not always caused by central nervous system syphilis.

See also Table 16-15, Pupils in Comatose Patients, p. 621.

TABLE 5-10 ■ Deviations of the Eyes

Deviation of the eyes from their normally conjugate position is termed *strabismus* or *squint.* Strabismus may be classified into two groups: (1) *nonparalytic,* in which the deviation is constant in all directions of gaze, and (2) *paralytic,* in which the deviation varies depending on the direction of gaze.

Nonparalytic Strabismus

Nonparalytic strabismus is caused by an imbalance in ocular muscle tone. It has many causes, may be hereditary, and usually appears early in childhood. Deviations are further classified according to direction:

Convergent Strabismus (Esotropia)

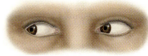

Divergent Strabismus (Exotropia)

COVER–UNCOVER TEST

A cover–uncover test may be helpful. Here is what you would see in the right monocular esotropia illustrated above.

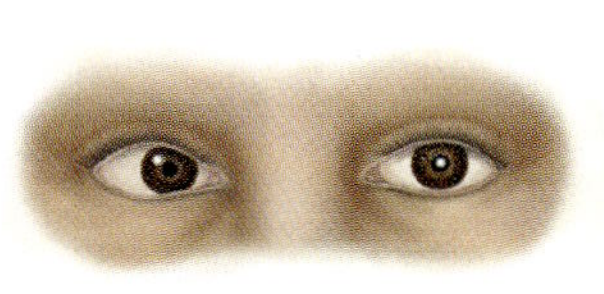

Corneal reflections are asymmetric.

COVER

The right eye moves outward to fix on the light. (The left eye is not seen but moves inward to the same degree.)

UNCOVER

The left eye moves outward to fix on the light. The right eye deviates inward again.

Paralytic Strabismus

Paralytic strabismus is usually caused by weakness or paralysis of one or more extraocular muscles. Determine the direction of gaze that maximizes the deviation. For example:

A Left Cranial Nerve VI Paralysis

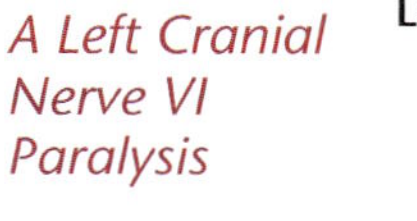

LOOKING TO THE RIGHT

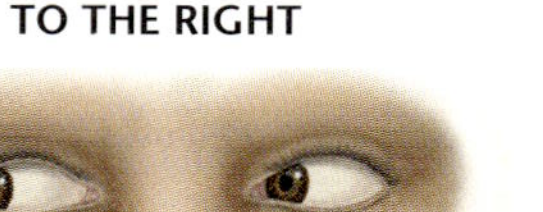

Eyes are conjugate.

LOOKING STRAIGHT AHEAD

Esotropia appears.

LOOKING TO THE LEFT

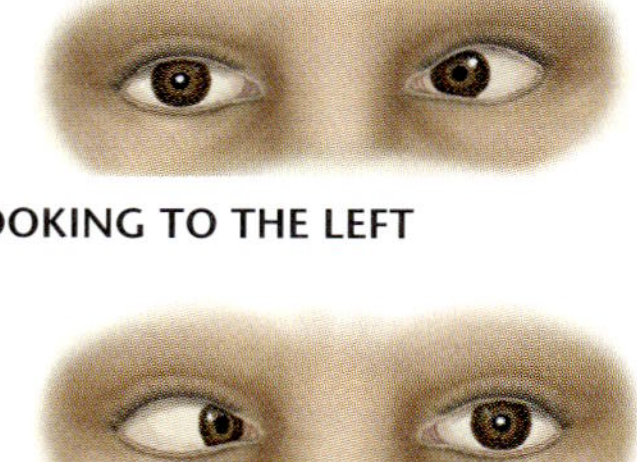

Esotropia is maximum.

A Left Cranial Nerve IV Paralysis

LOOKING DOWN AND TO THE RIGHT

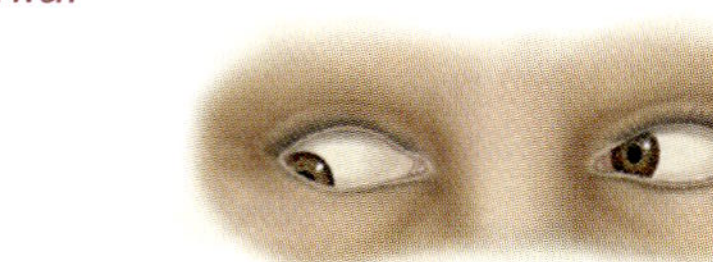

The left eye cannot look down when turned inward. Deviation is maximum in this direction.

A Left Cranial Nerve III Paralysis

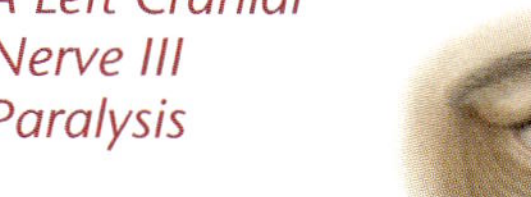

LOOKING STRAIGHT AHEAD

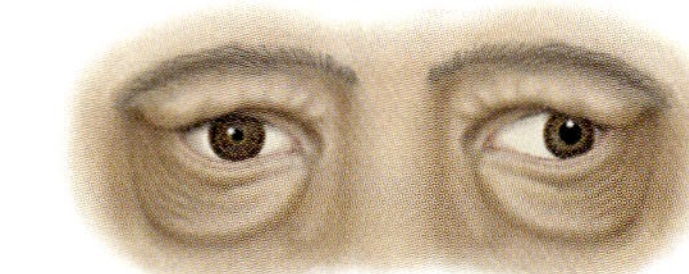

The eye is pulled outward by action of the 6th nerve. Upward, downward, and inward movements are impaired or lost. Ptosis and pupillary dilation may be associated.

TABLE 5-11 ■ Normal Variations of the Optic Disc

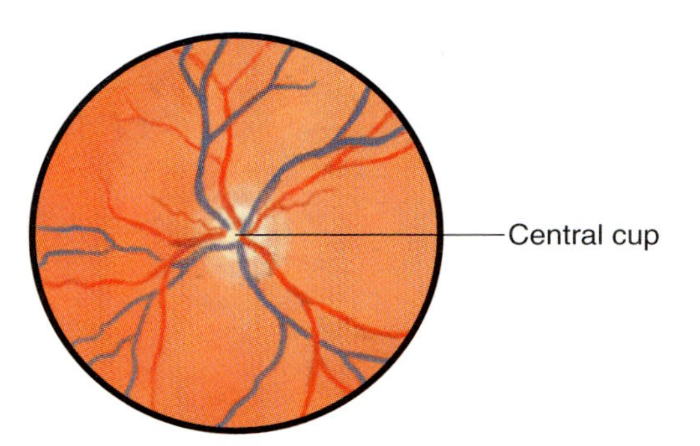

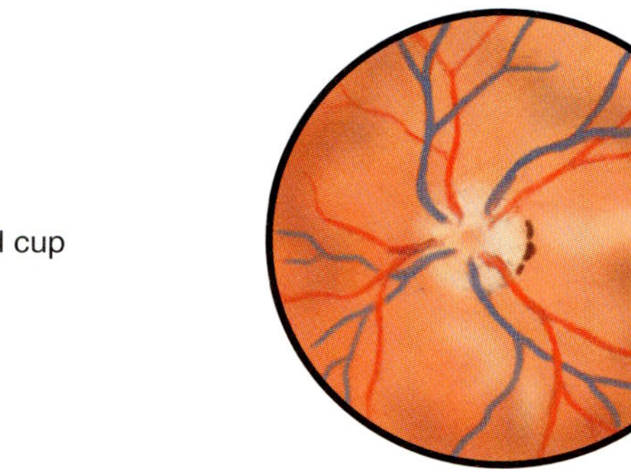

Physiologic Cupping

The physiologic cup is a small whitish depression in the optic disc from which the retinal vessels appear to emerge. Although sometimes absent, the cup is usually visible either centrally or toward the temporal side of the disc. Grayish spots are often seen at its base.

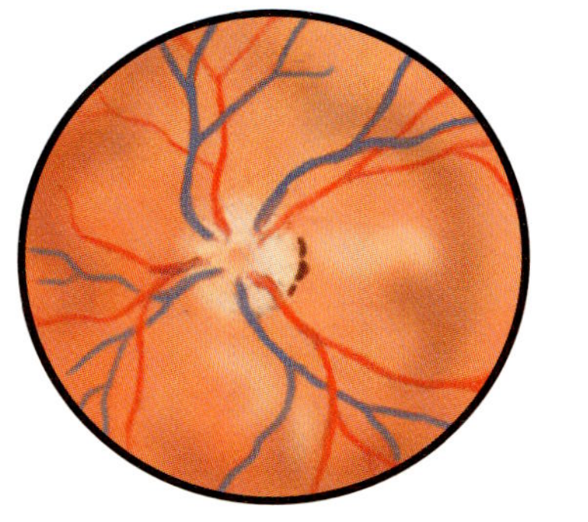

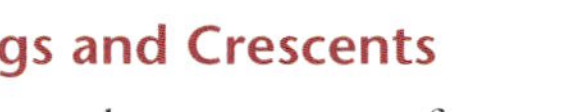

Rings and Crescents

Rings and crescents are often seen around the optic disc. These are developmental variations in which you can glimpse either white sclera, black retinal pigment, or both, especially along the temporal border of the disc. Rings and crescents are not part of the disc itself and should not be included in your estimates of disc diameters.

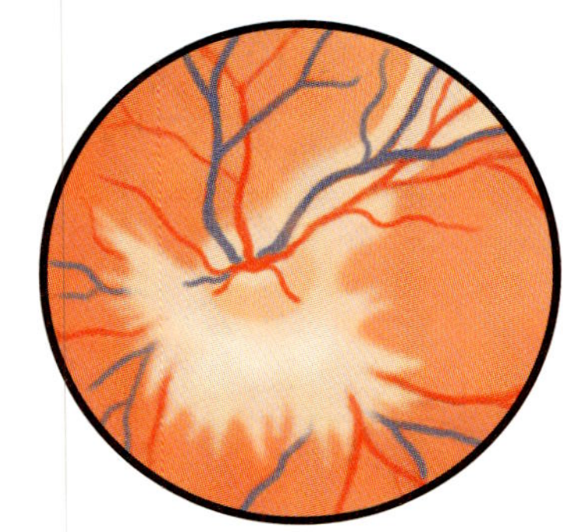

Medullated Nerve Fibers

Medullated nerve fibers are a much less common but dramatic finding. Appearing as irregular white patches with feathered margins, they obscure the disc edge and retinal vessels. They have no pathologic significance.

TABLE 5-12 ■ Abnormalities of the Optic Disc

	Normal	Optic Atrophy	Papilledema	Glaucomatous Cupping
Process	Tiny disc vessels give normal color to the disc.	Death of optic nerve fibers leads to loss of the tiny disc vessels.	Venous stasis leads to engorgement and swelling.	Increased pressure within the eye leads to increased cupping (backward depression of the disc) and atrophy.
Appearance	Color yellowish orange to creamy pink	Color white	Color pink, hyperemic	The base of the enlarged cup is pale.
	Disc vessels tiny	Disc vessels absent	Disc vessels more visible, more numerous, curve over the borders of the disc	
	Disc margins sharp (except perhaps nasally)		Disc swollen with margins blurred	
	The physiologic cup is located centrally or somewhat temporally. It may be conspicuous or absent. Its diameter from side to side is usually less than half that of the disc.		The physiologic cup is not visible.	The physiologic cup is enlarged, occupying more than half of the disc's diameter, at times extending to the edge of the disc. Retinal vessels sink in and under it, and may be displaced nasally.

(Source of photos: Tasman W, Jaeger E (eds): The Wills Eye Hospital Atlas of Clinical Ophthalmology, 2nd ed. Philadelphia, Lippincott Williams & Wilkins, 2001.)

TABLE 5-13 ■ Retinal Arteries and Arteriovenous Crossings: Normal and Hypertensive

Normal Retinal Artery and Arteriovenous (A-V) Crossing

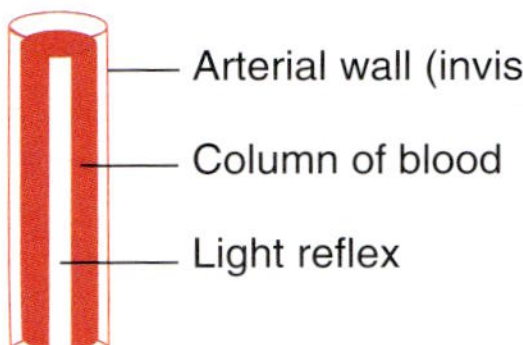

The normal arterial wall is transparent. Only the column of blood within it can usually be seen. The normal light reflex is narrow—about one fourth the diameter of the blood column.

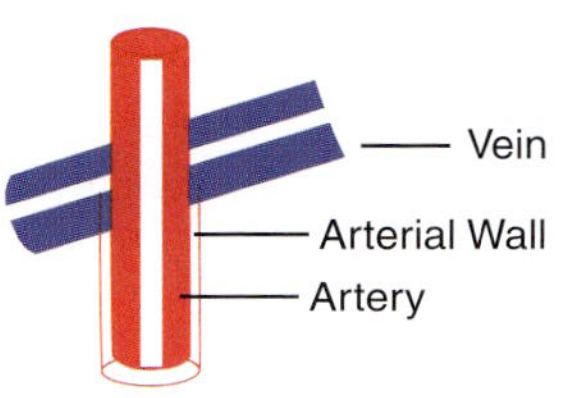

Because the arterial wall is transparent, a vein crossing beneath the artery can be seen right up to the column of blood on either side.

Retinal Arteries in Hypertension

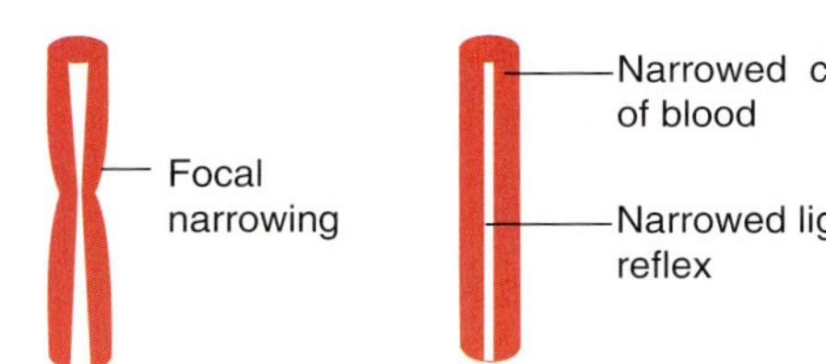

In hypertension, the arteries may show areas of focal or generalized narrowing. The light reflex is also narrowed. Over many months or years, the arterial wall thickens and becomes less transparent.

Sometimes the arteries, especially those close to the disc, become full and somewhat tortuous and develop an increased light reflex with a bright coppery luster. Such a vessel is called a copper wire artery.

Occasionally a portion of a narrowed artery develops such an opaque wall that no blood is visible within it. It is then called a silver wire artery. This change typically occurs in the smaller branches.

Arteriovenous Crossing

When the arterial walls lose their transparency, changes appear in the arteriovenous crossings. Decreased transparency of the retina probably also contributes to the first two changes shown below.

TAPERING

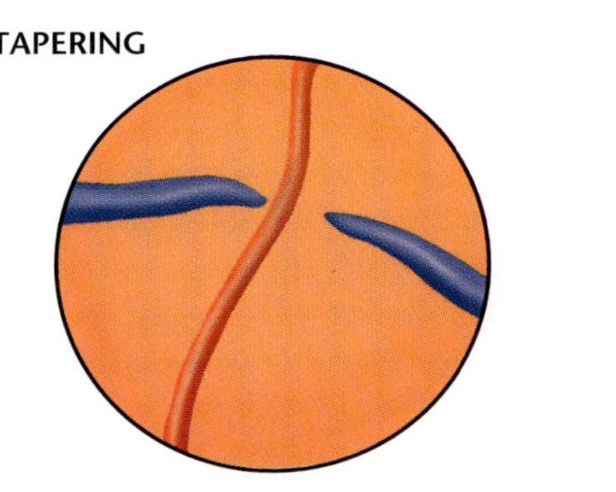

The vein appears to taper down on either side of the artery.

CONCEALMENT OR A–V NICKING

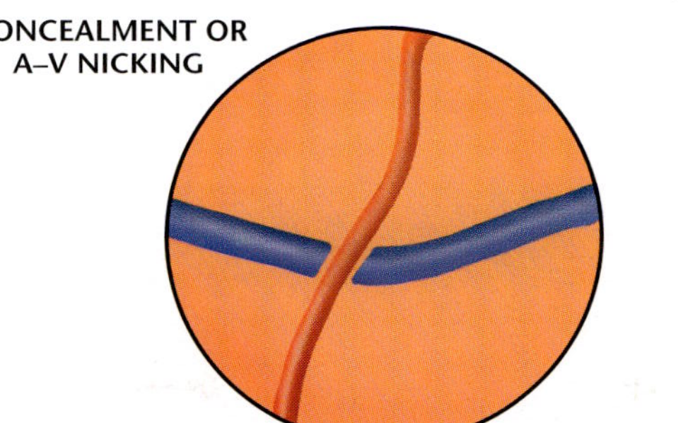

The vein appears to stop abruptly on either side of the artery.

BANKING

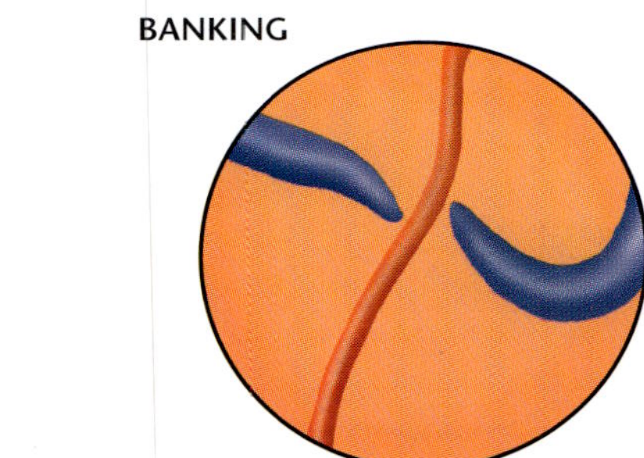

The vein is twisted on the distal side of the artery and forms a dark, wide knuckle.

TABLE 5-14 ■ Red Spots and Streaks in the Fundi

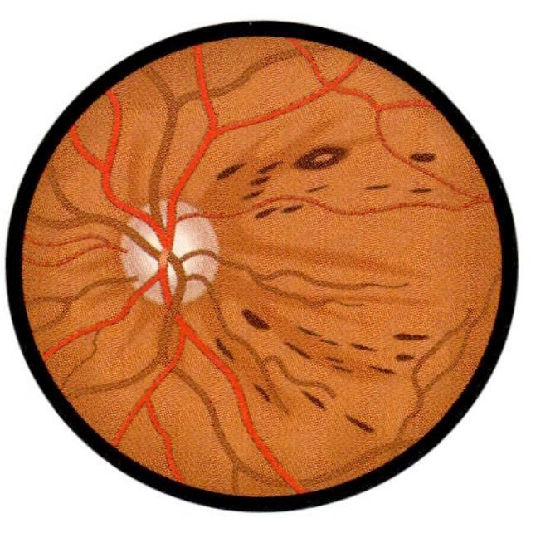

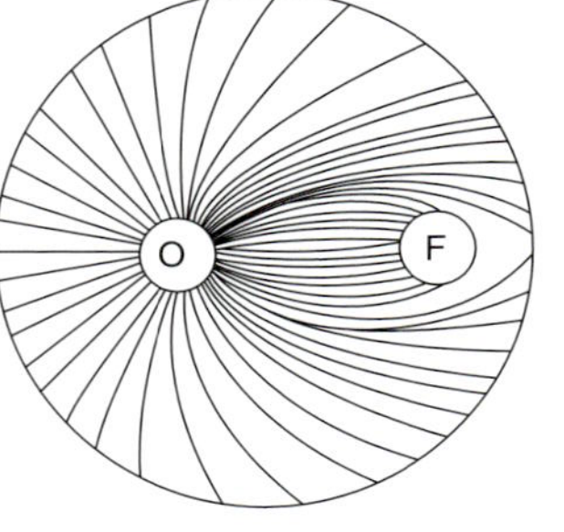

Superficial Retinal Hemorrhages

Superficial retinal hemorrhages are small, linear, flame-shaped, red streaks in the fundi. They are shaped by the superficial bundles of nerve fibers that radiate from the optic disc in the pattern illustrated (O = optic disc; F = fovea). Sometimes the hemorrhages occur in clusters and then simulate a larger hemorrhage, but the linear streaking at the edges shows their true nature. Superficial hemorrhages are seen in severe hypertension, papilledema, and occlusion of the retinal vein, among other conditions.

An occasional superficial hemorrhage has a white center consisting of fibrin. White-centered retinal hemorrhages have many causes.

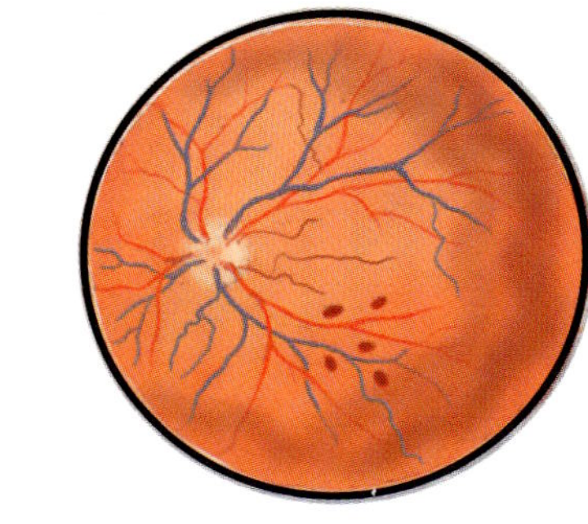

Deep Retinal Hemorrhages

Deep retinal hemorrhages are small, rounded, slightly irregular red spots that are sometimes called dot or blot hemorrhages. They occur in a deeper layer of the retina than flame-shaped hemorrhages. Diabetes mellitus is a common cause.

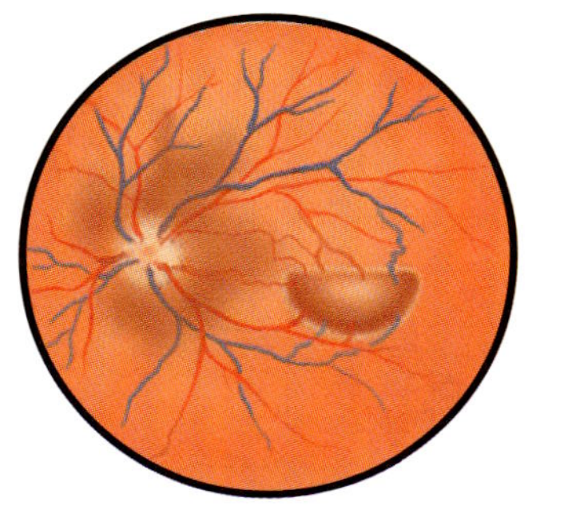

Preretinal Hemorrhage

A preretinal (subhyaloid) hemorrhage develops when blood escapes into the potential space between retina and vitreous. This hemorrhage is typically larger than retinal hemorrhages. Because it is anterior to the retina, it obscures any underlying retinal vessels. In an erect patient, red cells settle, creating a horizontal line of demarcation between plasma above and cells below. Causes include a sudden increase in intracranial pressure.

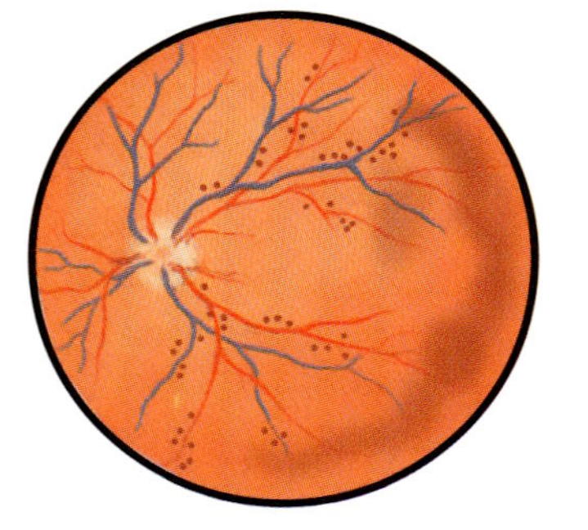

Microaneurysms

Microaneurysms are tiny, round, red spots seen commonly but not exclusively in and around the macular area. They are minute dilatations of very small retinal vessels, but the vascular connections are too small to be seen ophthalmoscopically. Microaneurysms are characteristic of diabetic retinopathy but not specific to it.

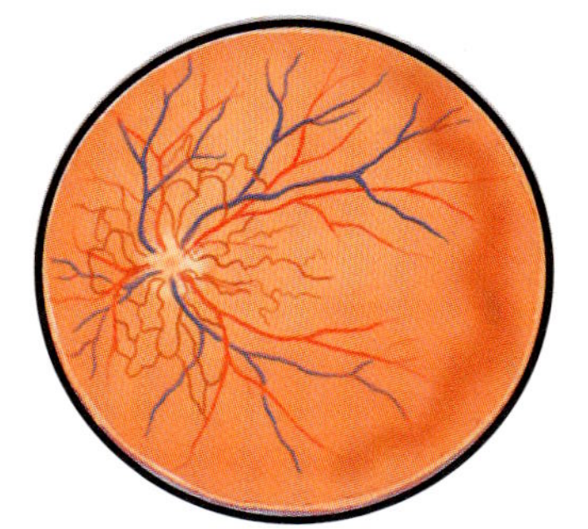

Neovascularization

Neovascularization refers to the formation of new blood vessels. They are more numerous, more tortuous, and narrower than other blood vessels in the area and form disorderly looking red arcades. A common cause is the late, proliferative stage of diabetic retinopathy. The vessels may grow into the vitreous, where retinal detachment or hemorrhage may cause loss of vision.

TABLE 5-15 ■ Light-Colored Spots in the Fundi

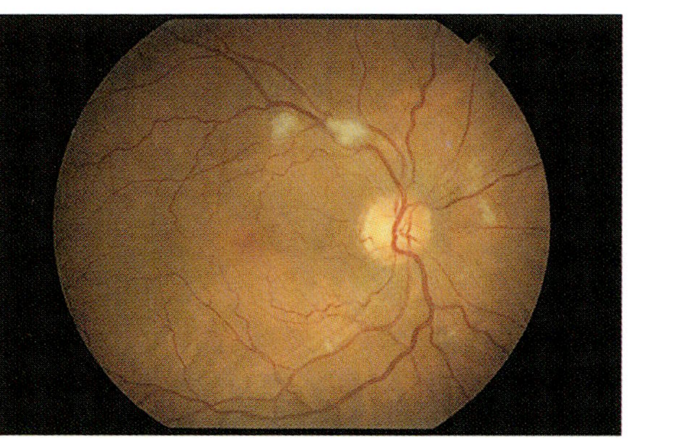

Cotton-Wool Patches (*Soft Exudates*)

Cotton-wool patches are white or grayish, ovoid lesions with irregular (thus "soft") borders. They are moderate in size but usually smaller than the disc. They result from infarcted nerve fibers and are seen with hypertension and many other conditions.

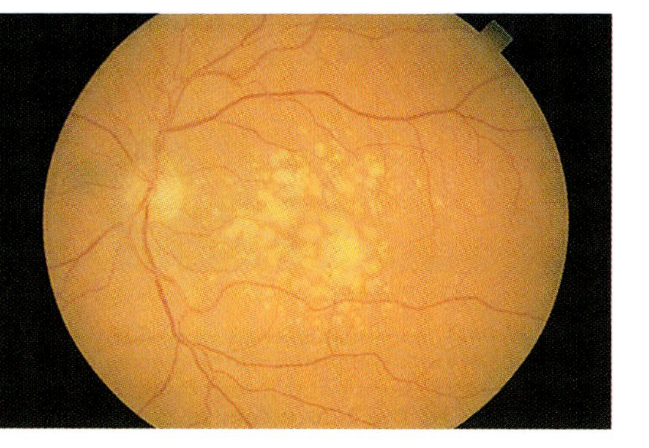

Drusen

Drusen are yellowish round spots that vary from tiny to small. The edges may hard, as here, or soft. They are haphazardly distributed but may concentrate at the posterior pole. Drusen appear with normal aging but may also accompany various conditions, including age-related macular degeneration.

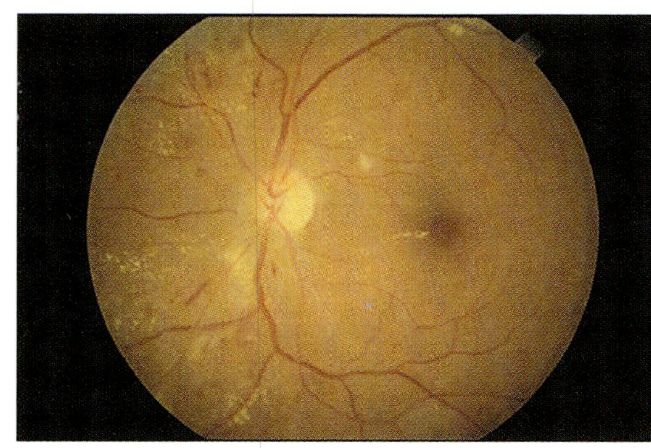

Hard Exudates

Hard exudates are creamy or yellowish, often bright lesions with well-defined (thus "hard") borders. They are small and round (as shown in the lower group of exudates) but may coalesce into larger irregular spots (as shown in the upper group). They often occur in clusters or in circular, linear, or star-shaped patterns. Causes include diabetes and hypertension.

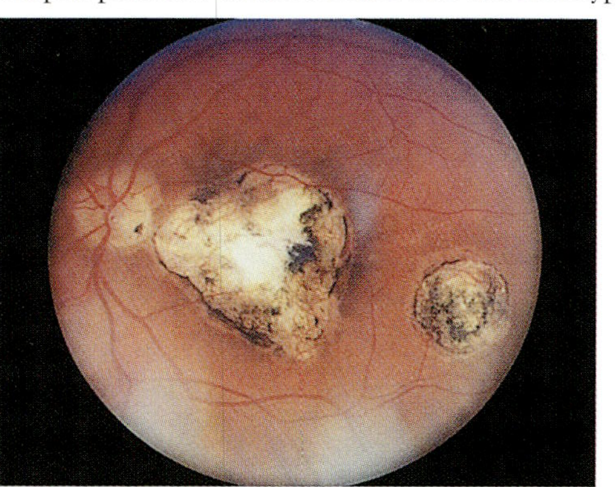

Healed Chorioretinitis

Here inflammation has destroyed the superficial tissues to reveal a well-defined, irregular patch of white sclera marked with dark pigment. Size varies from small to very large. Toxoplasmosis is illustrated. Multiple, small, somewhat similar-looking areas may be due to laser treatments. Here there is also a temporal scar near the macula.

(*table continues next page*)

TABLE 5-15 ■ Light-Colored Spots in the Fundi *(Continued)*

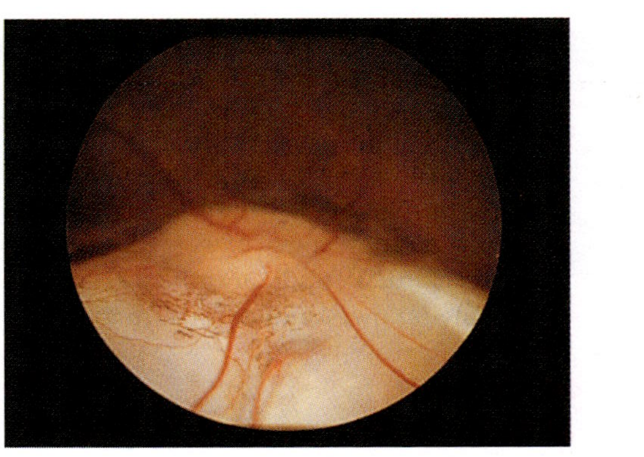

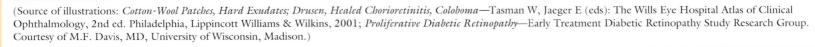

Coloboma

A coloboma of the choroid and retina is a developmental abnormality. A well demarcated, moderate-sized to large, white oval of sclera is visible below the disc, often extending well beyond the limits of your examination. Its borders may be pigmented.

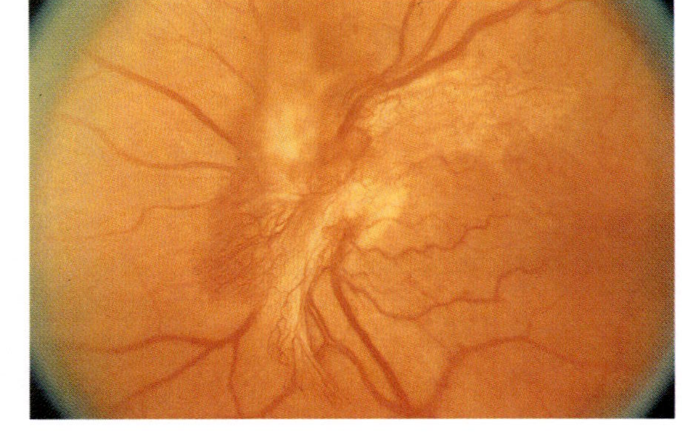

Proliferative Diabetic Retinopathy

Bands or strands of white fibrous tissue develop in the late proliferative stage of diabetic retinopathy. They lie anterior to the retinal vessels and therefore obscure them. Neovascularization (p. 186) is typically associated.

(Source of illustrations: *Cotton-Wool Patches, Hard Exudates; Drusen, Healed Chorioretinitis, Coloboma*—Tasman W, Jaeger E (eds): The Wills Eye Hospital Atlas of Clinical Ophthalmology, 2nd ed. Philadelphia, Lippincott Williams & Wilkins, 2001; *Proliferative Diabetic Retinopathy*—Early Treatment Diabetic Retinopathy Study Research Group. Courtesy of M.F. Davis, MD, University of Wisconsin, Madison.)

TABLE 5-16 ■ Ocular Fundi

Out of a piece of paper, cut a circle about the size of an optic disc shown below. The circle simulates an ophthalmoscope's light beam. Lay it on each illustration, and inspect each fundus systematically.

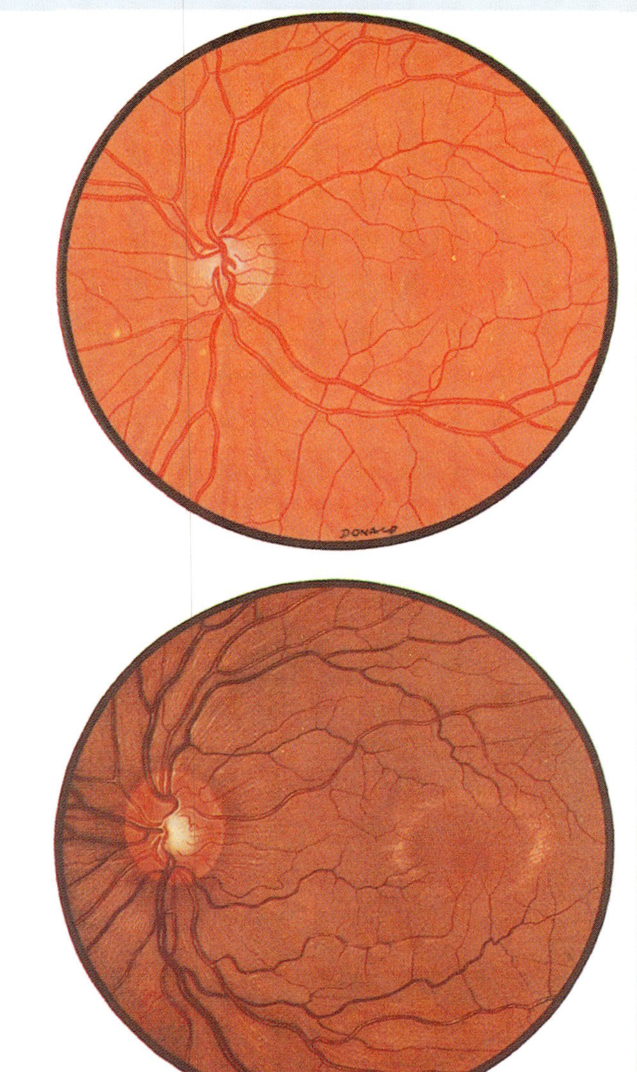

Normal Fundus of a Fair-Skinned Person

Find and inspect the optic disc. Follow the major vessels in four directions, noting their relative sizes and the nature of the arteriovenous crossings—both normal here. Inspect the macular area. The slightly darker fovea is just discernible; no light reflex is visible in this subject. Look for any lesions in the retina. Note the striped, or tessellated, character of the fundus, especially in the lower field. This comes from normal choroidal vessels that are unobscured by pigment.

Normal Fundus of a Dark-Skinned Person

Again, inspect the disc, the vessels, the macula, and the retinal background. The ring around the fovea is a normal light reflection. Compare the color of the fundus to that in the illustration above. It has a grayish brownish, almost purplish cast, which comes from pigment in the retina and the choroid. This pigment characteristically obscures the choroidal vessels, and no tessellation is visible. In contrast to either of these two figures, the fundus of a light-skinned person with brunette coloring is redder.

(table continues next page)

TABLE 5-16 ■ Ocular Fundi *(Continued)*

Normal Fundus of an Older Person

Inspect the fundus as before. What differences do you observe? Two characteristics of the aging fundus can be seen in this example. The blood vessels are straighter and narrower than those in younger people, and the choroidal vessels can be seen easily. In this person the optic disc is less pink, and pigment may be seen temporal to the disc and in the macular area.

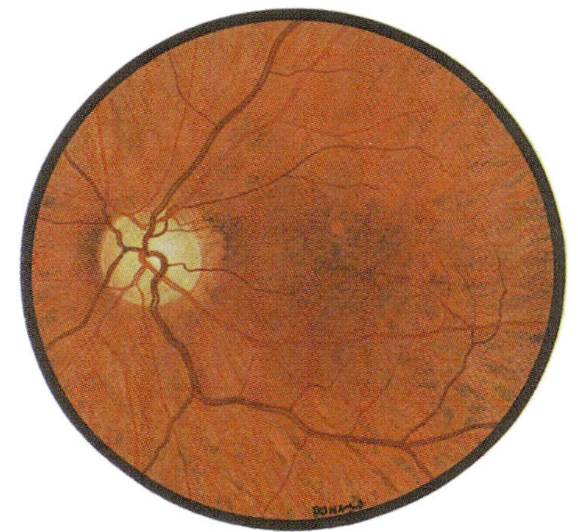

Hypertensive Retinopathy

Inspect the fundus. The nasal border of the optic disc is blurred. The light reflexes from the arteries just above and below the disc are increased. Note venous tapering—at the A–V crossing, about 1 disc diameter above the disc. Note tapering and banking at 4:30 o'clock, 2 disc diameters from the disc, also punctate hard exudates and a few deep hemorrhages.

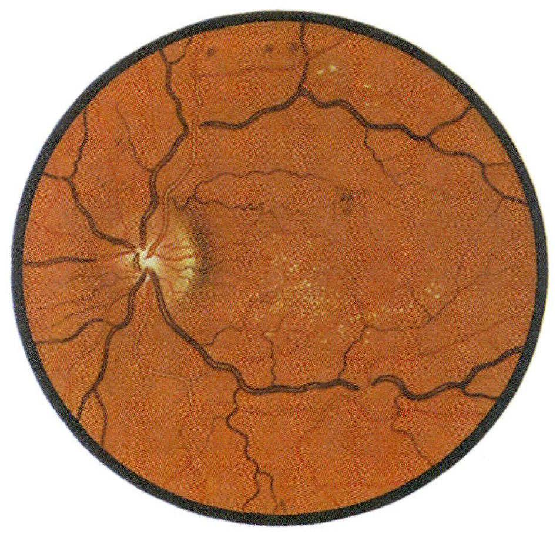

Hypertensive Retinopathy With Macular Star

Punctate exudates are readily visible: some are scattered; others radiate from the fovea to form a macular star. Note the two small, soft exudates about 1 disc diameter from the disc. Find the flame-shaped hemorrhages sweeping toward 4 o'clock and 5 o'clock; a few more may be seen toward 2 o'clock. These fundi show changes typical of accelerated (malignant) hypertension and are often accompanied by a papilledema (p. 184).

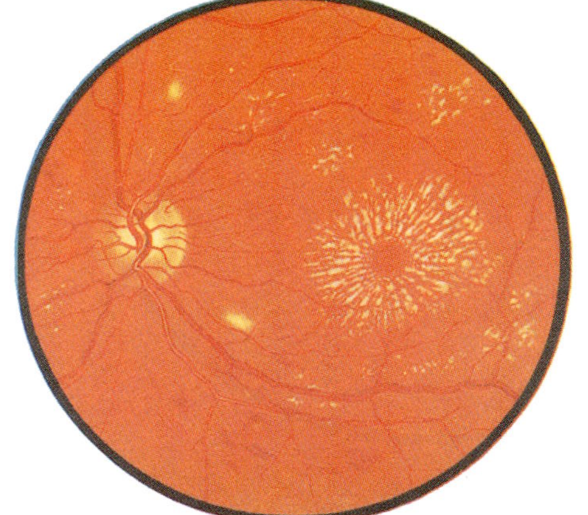

(Source of illustrations: *Normal Fundus of a Fair-Skinned Person, Normal Fundus of a Dark-Skinned Person, Normal Fundus of an Older Person, Hypertensive Retinopathy, Hypertensive Retinopathy With Macular Star*—Michaelson IC: Textbook of the Fundus of the Eye [3rd ed.], Edinburgh, Churchill Livingstone, 1980.)

Diabetic Retinopathy

Study carefully the fundi in the series of photographs below. They represent a national standard used by ophthalmologists to assess diabetic retinopathy.

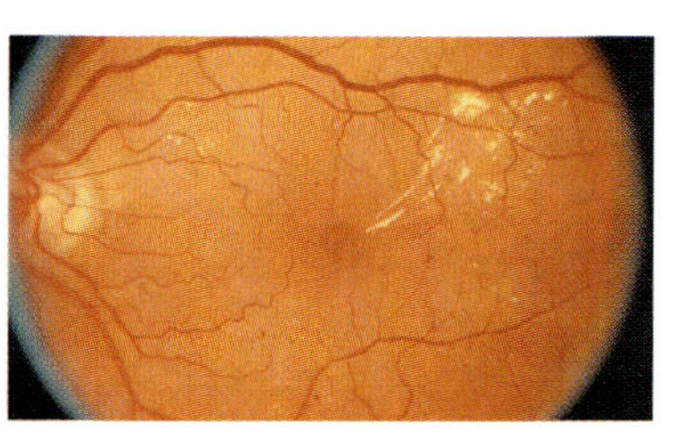

Nonproliferative Retinopathy, Moderately Severe

Note tiny red dots or microaneurysms. Note also the ring of hard exudates (white spots) located supero-temporally. Retinal thickening or edema in the area of the hard exudates can impair visual acuity if it extends into the center of the macula (detection requires specialized stereoscopic examination).

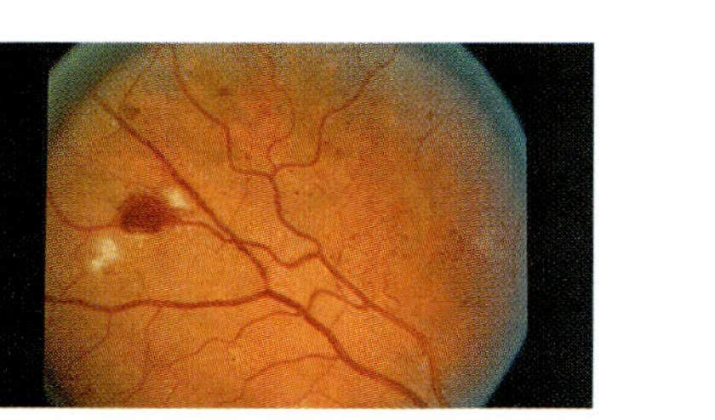

Nonproliferative Retinopathy, Severe

In the superior temporal quadrant, note the large retinal hemorrhage between two cotton-wool patches, beading of the retinal vein just above them, and tiny tortuous retinal vessels above the superior temporal artery.

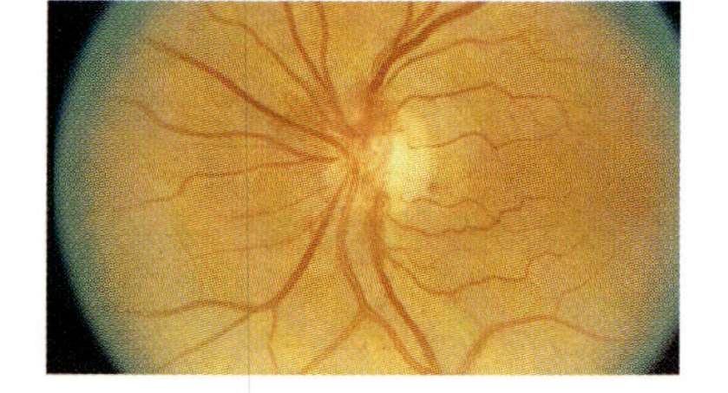

Proliferative Retinopathy, With Neovascularization

Note new preretinal vessels arising on the disc and extending across the disc margins. Visual acuity is still normal, but the risk of visual loss is high (photocoagulation reduces this risk by >50%).

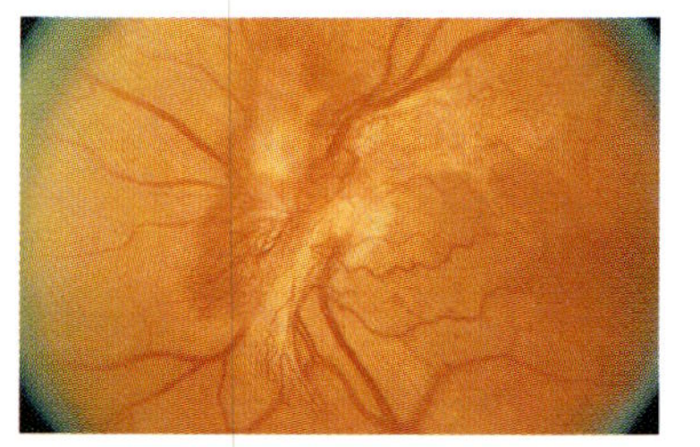

Proliferative Retinopathy, Advanced

This is the same eye, but 2 years later and without treatment. Neovascularization has increased, now with fibrous proliferations, distortion of the macula, and reduced visual acuity.

(Source of photos: *Nonproliferative Retinopathy, Moderately Severe; Proliferative Retinopathy, With Neovascularization; Nonproliferative Retinopathy, Severe; Proliferative Retinopathy, Advanced*—Early Treatment Diabetic Retinopathy Study Research Group. Courtesy of MF Davis, MD, University of Wisconsin, Madison.)

TABLE 5-17 ■ Lumps On or Near the Ear

Chondrodermatitis Helicis

This chronic inflammatory lesion starts as a painful, tender papule that is usually on the helix but may be on the antihelix. Typically the lesion is single, but in this case two are visible. The lower papule is an early lesion; the upper lesion illustrates the later stage of ulceration and crusting. Reddening may occur. Older men are usually affected. To distinguish chondrodermatitis from carcinoma, a biopsy is needed.

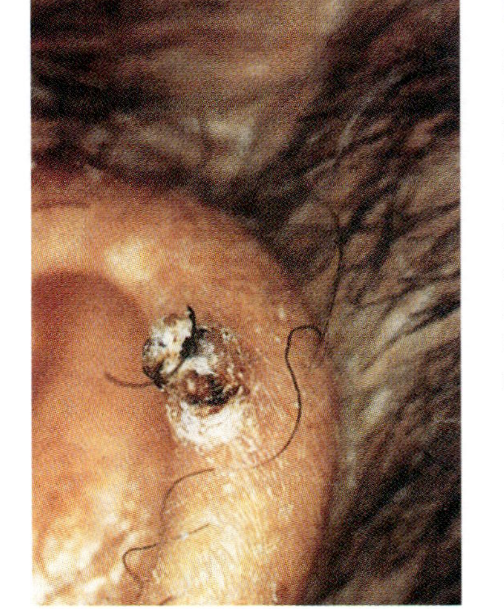

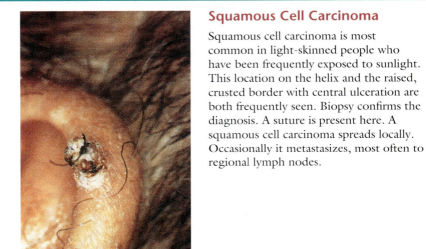

Squamous Cell Carcinoma

Squamous cell carcinoma is most common in light-skinned people who have been frequently exposed to sunlight. This location on the helix and the raised, crusted border with central ulceration are both frequently seen. Biopsy confirms the diagnosis. A suture is present here. A squamous cell carcinoma spreads locally. Occasionally it metastasizes, most often to regional lymph nodes.

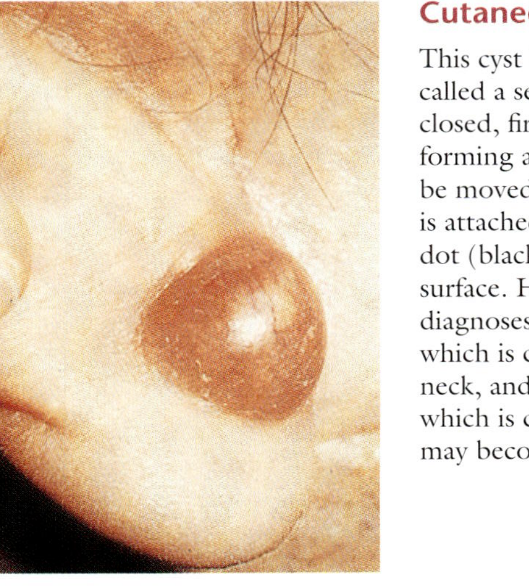

Cutaneous Cyst

This cyst behind the ear used to be called a sebaceous cyst. It is a benign, closed, firm sac that lies in the dermis, forming a dome-shaped lump. It can be moved over underlying tissues but is attached to the epidermis. A dark dot (blackhead) may be visible on its surface. Histologically, one of two diagnoses is likely: (1) *epidermoid* cyst, which is common on the face and neck, and (2) *pilar (trichilemmal)* cyst, which is common in the scalp. Each may become inflamed.

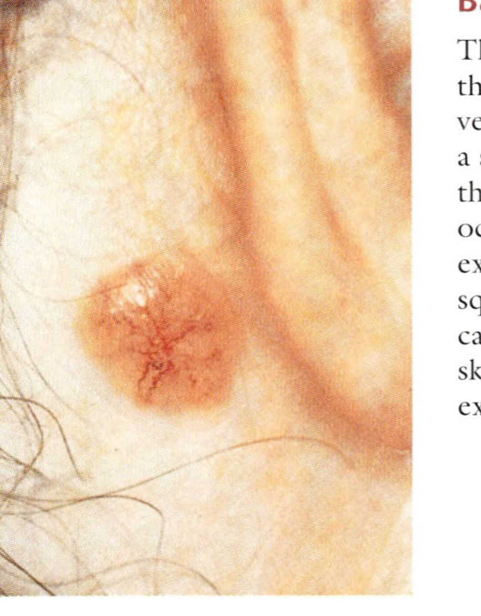

Basal Cell Carcinoma

The raised nodule behind this ear shows the lustrous surface and telangiectatic vessels that suggest basal cell carcinoma, a slow-growing and common malignancy that rarely metastasizes. Ulceration may occur, and in the absence of treatment extends in width and depth. Like squamous cell carcinoma, basal cell carcinoma occurs more frequently in fair-skinned people who have been much exposed to sunlight.

(Sources of photos: *Chondrodermatitis Helicis, Cutaneous Cyst*—Young EM Jr, Newcomer VD, Kligman AM: Geriatric Dermatology: Color Atlas and Practitioner's Guide. Philadelphia, Lea & Febiger, 1993; *Squamous Cell Carcinoma, Basal Cell Carcinoma*—Reprinted, by permission of the N Engl J Med, 326:169–170, 1992.)

Tophi

A tophus is a deposit of uric acid crystals characteristic of chronic tophaceous gout. Tophi appear as hard nodules in the helix or antihelix and may discharge their chalky white crystals through the skin. Tophi may also appear near the joints, as in the hands (p. 530), feet, and other areas. Tophi usually develop only after years of sustained high blood levels of uric acid. With better control of hyperuricemia by drugs, tophi are becoming less common.

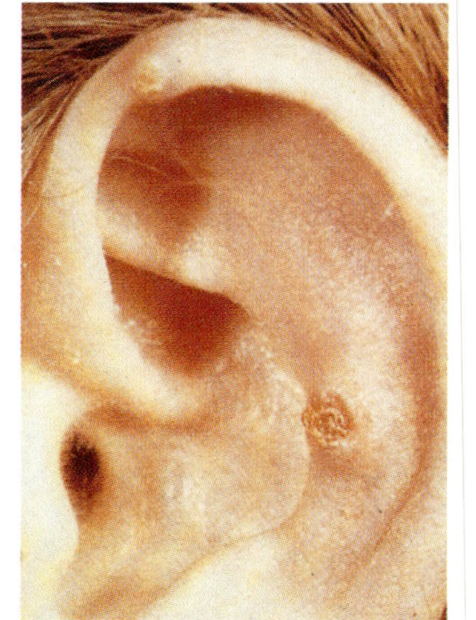
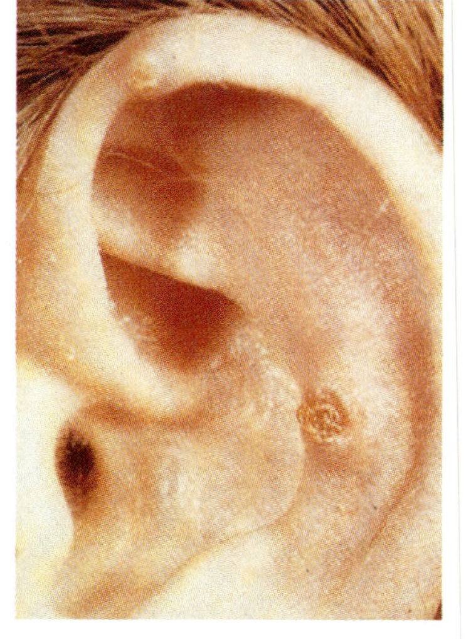

Rheumatoid Nodules

In a patient with chronic arthritis, one or more small lumps on the helix or antihelix may be rheumatoid nodules of rheumatoid arthritis, as shown here. Do not mistake such lumps for tophi. Look for additional nodules elsewhere, e.g., on the hands, along the surface of the ulna distal to the elbow (pp. 528, 529), on the knees, and on the heels. Ulceration may result from repeated small injuries. Rheumatoid nodules may antedate the arthritis.

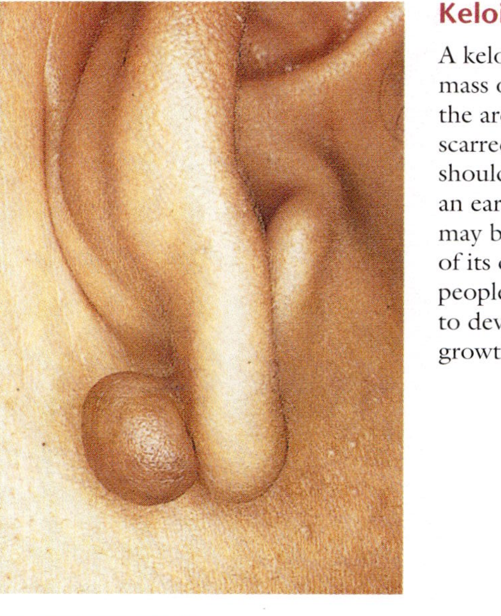

Keloid

A keloid is a firm, nodular, hypertrophic mass of scar tissue that extends beyond the area of injury. It may develop in any scarred area, but is most common on the shoulders and upper chest. A keloid on an earlobe that was pierced for earrings may be especially troublesome because of its cosmetic effects. Darker-skinned people are more likely than lighter ones to develop keloids. Recurrence of the growth may follow treatment.

Lepromatous Leprosy

The ear is one of the sites for lepromatous leprosy, a form of Hansen's disease, which results from infection by *Mycobacterium leprae.* The multiple papules and nodules on this auricle are due to this chronic infection. Similar lesions would probably be visible on the face and elsewhere in the body. Now seldom seen in the United States, leprosy is still a worldwide problem. Other forms of the disease have different manifestations.

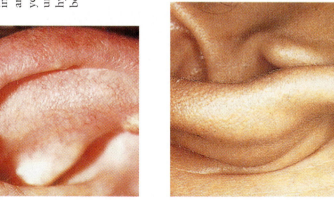

(Sources of photos: *Tophi, Lepromatous Leprosy*—From Atlas of Clinical Dermatology, 2nd ed, by Anthony du Vivier. London, UK, Gower Medical Publishing, 1993; *Rheumatoid Nodules*—Champion RH, Burton JL, Ebling FJG (eds): Rook/Wilkinson/Ebling Textbook of Dermatology, 5th ed. Oxford, Blackwell Scientific Publications Limited, 1992; *Keloid*—Sams WM Jr, Lynch PJ (eds): Principles and Practice of Dermatology. Edinburgh, Churchill Livingstone, 1990.)

TABLE 5-18 ■ Abnormalities of the Eardrum

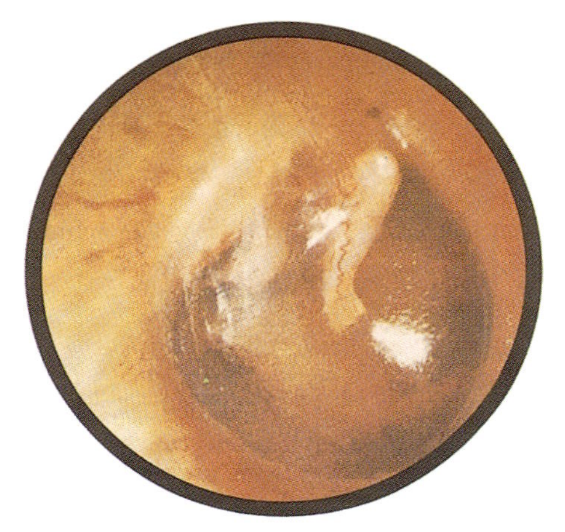

Normal Eardrum

This normal right eardrum (tympanic membrane) is pinkish gray. The handle of the malleus lies in a somewhat oblique position behind the upper part of the drum. The short process of the malleus pushes the membrane laterally, creating a small white elevation. Above the short process lies a small portion of the eardrum called the pars flaccida. The remainder of the drum is the pars tensa. Anterior and posterior malleolar folds, which extend obliquely upward from the short process, separate the pars flaccida from the pars tensa, but they are often invisible unless the eardrum is retracted. From the umbo the bright cone of light fans anteriorly and downward. Other light reflections seen in this photo are artifactual. Posterior to the malleus, part of the incus is visible behind the drum. The small blood vessels that course along the handle of the malleus are within the range of normal and do not indicate inflammation. The ear canal, which surrounds the eardrum, looks flatter than it really is because of distortion inherent in the photographic technique.

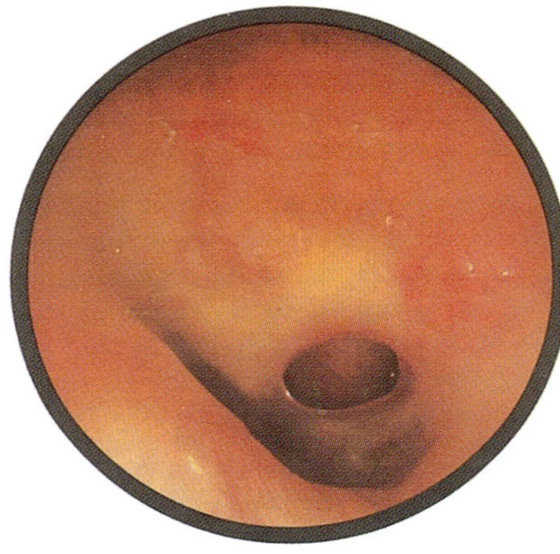

Perforation of the Drum

Perforations are holes in the eardrum that usually result from purulent infections of the middle ear. They are classified as *central* perforations, which do not extend to the margin of the drum, and *marginal* perforations, which do involve the margin.

The more common central perforation is illustrated here. In this case a reddened ring of granulation tissue surrounds the perforation, indicating a chronic infectious process. The eardrum itself is scarred and no landmarks are discernible. Discharge from the infected middle ear may drain out through such a perforation, but none is visible here.

A perforation of the eardrum often closes in the healing process, as illustrated in the next photo. The membrane covering the hole may be exceedingly thin and transparent.

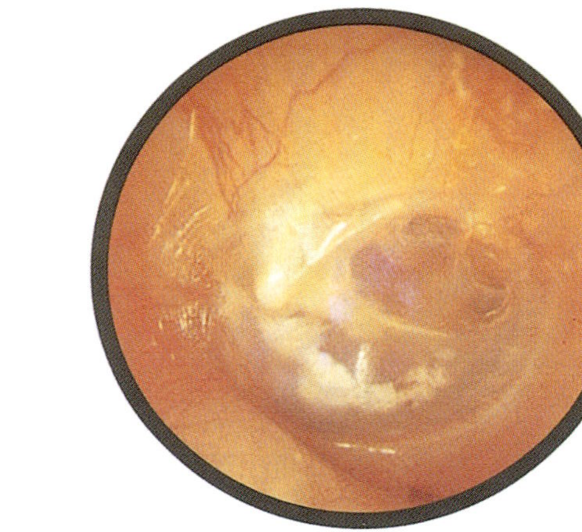

Tympanosclerosis

In the inferior portion of this left eardrum there is a large, chalky white patch with irregular margins. It is typical of tympanosclerosis: a deposition of hyaline material within the layers of the tympanic membrane that sometimes follows a severe episode of otitis media. It does not usually impair hearing, and is seldom clinically significant.

Other abnormalities in this eardrum include a *healed perforation* (the large oval area in the upper posterior drum) and signs of a *retracted drum.* A retracted drum is pulled medially, away from the examiner's eye, and the malleolar folds are tightened into sharp outlines. The short process often protrudes sharply, and the handle of the malleus, pulled inward at the umbo, looks foreshortened and more horizontal.

(Sources of photos: *Normal Eardrum*—Hawke M, Keene M, Alberti PW: Clinical Otoscopy: A Text and Colour Atlas. Edinburgh, Churchill Livingstone, 1984; *Perforation of the Drum, Tympanosclerosis*—Courtesy of Michael Hawke, MD, Toronto, Canada.)

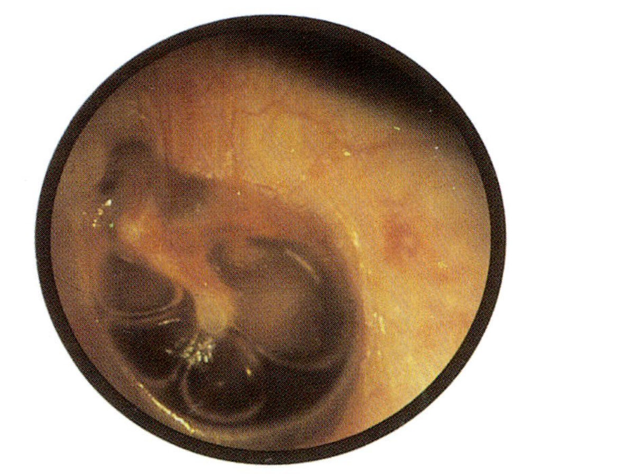

Serous Effusion

Serous effusions are usually caused by viral upper respiratory infections (*otitis media with serous effusion*) or by sudden changes in atmospheric pressure as from flying or diving (*otitic barotrauma*). The eustachian tube cannot equalize the air pressure in the middle ear with that of the outside air. Air is partly or completely absorbed from the middle ear into the bloodstream, and serous fluid accumulates there instead. Symptoms include fullness and popping sensations in the ear, mild conduction hearing loss, and perhaps some pain.

Amber fluid behind the eardrum is characteristic, as in this left drum of a patient with otitic barotrauma. A fluid level, a line between air above and amber fluid below, can be seen on either side of the short process. Air bubbles (not always present) can be seen here within the amber fluid.

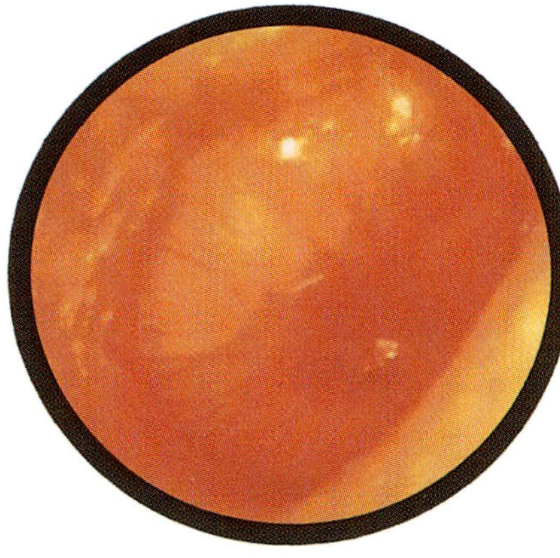

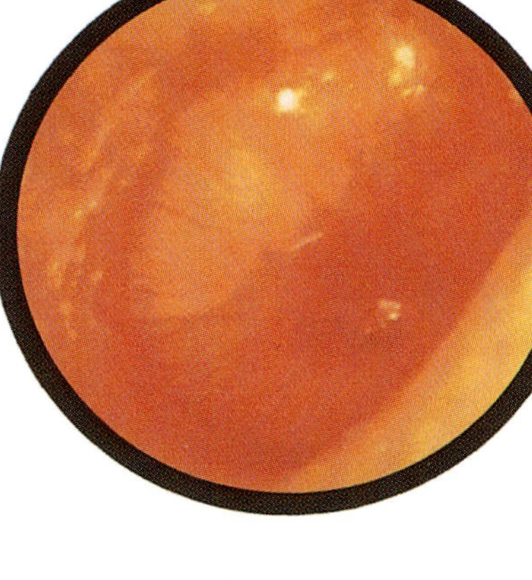

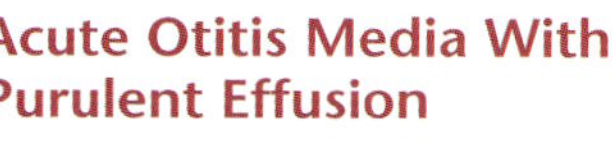

Acute Otitis Media With Purulent Effusion

Acute otitis media with purulent effusion is caused by bacterial infection. Symptoms include earache, fever, and hearing loss. The eardrum reddens, loses its landmarks, and bulges laterally, toward the examiner's eye.

In this right ear the drum is bulging and most landmarks are obscured. Redness is most obvious near the umbo, but dilated vessels can be seen in all segments of the drum. A diffuse redness of the entire drum often develops. Spontaneous rupture (perforation) of the drum may follow, with discharge of purulent material into the ear canal.

Moving the auricle and pressing on the tragus do not cause pain in otitis media as they usually do in acute otitis externa. Hearing loss is of the conductive type. Acute purulent otitis media is much more common in children than in adults.

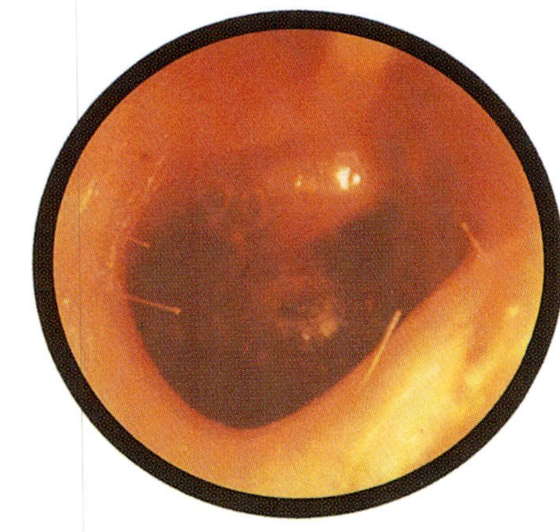

Bullous Myringitis

Bullous myringitis is a viral infection characterized by painful hemorrhagic vesicles that appear on the tympanic membrane, the ear canal, or both. Symptoms include earache, blood-tinged discharge from the ear, and hearing loss of the conductive type.

In this right ear, at least two large vesicles (bullae) are discernible on the drum. The drum is reddened, and its landmarks are obscured. Several different viruses may cause this condition.

(Sources of photos: *Serous Effusion*—Hawke M, Keene M, Alberti PW: Clinical Otoscopy: A Text and Colour Atlas. Edinburgh, Churchill Livingstone, 1984; *Acute Otitis Media, Bullous Myringitis*—The Wellcome Trust, National Medical Slide Bank, London, UK.)

TABLE 5-19 ■ Patterns of Hearing Loss

Hearing loss is of two major types. In *conductive hearing loss,* a disorder of the external or middle ear impairs the conduction of sound to the inner ear. In *sensorineural hearing loss,* a disorder of the inner ear, the cochlear nerve, or its central connections impairs the transmission of nerve impulses to the brain. A *mixed hearing loss* has both deficits.

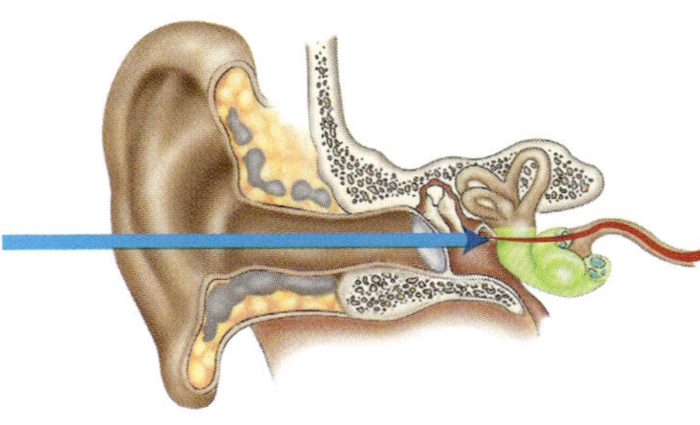

	Conductive Loss	Sensorineural Loss
Distortion of Sounds That Impairs the Understanding of Words	Relatively minor	Often present as the upper tones of words are disproportionately lost
Effect of a Noisy Environment	Hearing may seem to improve.	Hearing typically worsens.
Patient's Own Voice	Tends to be soft: the patient's voice is conducted through bone to a normal inner ear and cochlear nerve.	May be loud: the patient has trouble hearing his or her own voice.
Usual Age of Onset	Most often in childhood and young adulthood, up to age 40	Most often in the middle or later years.
Ear Canal and Drum	An abnormality is usually visible, except in otosclerosis.	The problem is not visible.

Weber Test *(in unilateral hearing loss)*

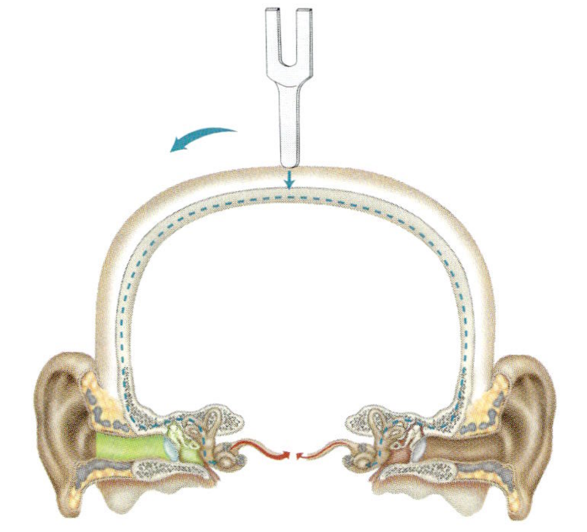

The sound lateralizes to the impaired ear. Because this ear is not distracted by room noise, it can detect the tuning fork's vibrations better than normal. (Test yourself while plugging one ear with your finger.) This lateralization disappears in an absolutely quiet room.

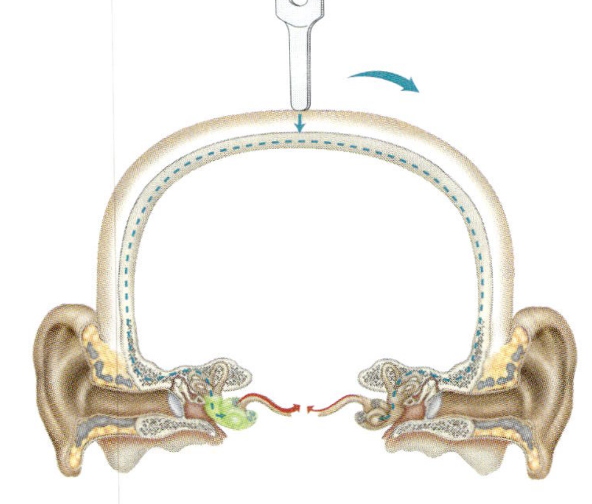

The sound lateralizes to the good ear. The impaired inner ear or cochlear nerve is less able to transmit impulses no matter how the sound reaches the cochlea. The sound is therefore heard in the better ear.

Rinne Test

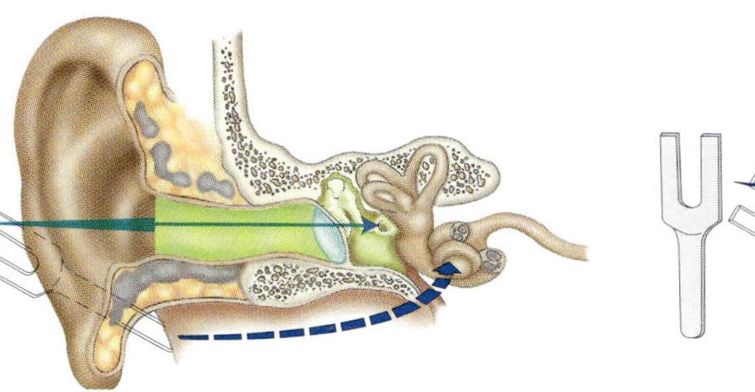

Bone conduction lasts longer than or is equal to air conduction (BC > AC or BC = AC). While air conduction through the external or middle ear is impaired, vibrations through bone bypass the problem to reach the cochlea.

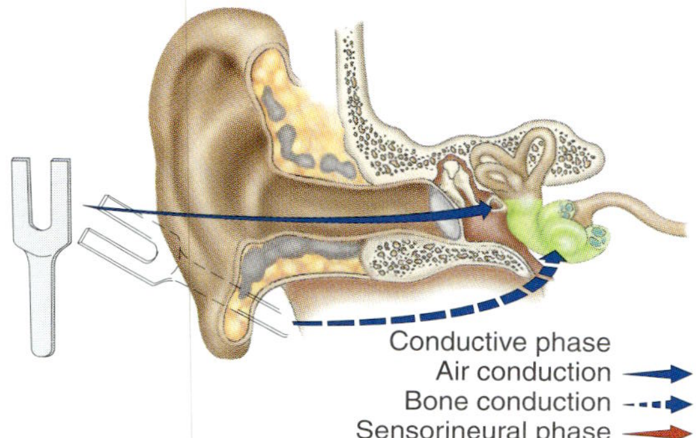

Air conduction lasts longer than bone conduction (AC > BC). The inner ear or cochlear nerve is less able to transmit impulses regardless of how the vibrations reach the cochlea. The normal pattern prevails.

Causes Include:

Obstruction of the ear canal, otitis media, a perforated or relatively immobilized eardrum, and otosclerosis (a fixation of the ossicles by bony overgrowth)

Sustained exposure to loud noise, drugs, infections of the inner ear, trauma, tumors, congenital and hereditary disorders, and aging (presbycusis)

Further evaluation is done by audiometry and other specialized procedures.

TABLE 5-20 ■ Abnormalities of the Lips

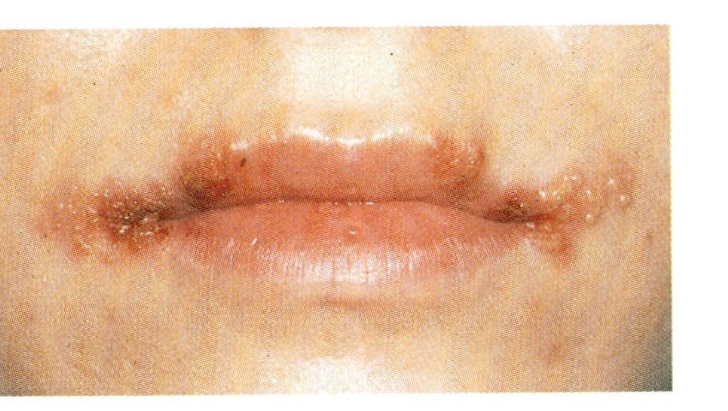

Herpes Simplex *(Cold Sore, Fever Blister)*

The herpes simplex virus (HSV) produces recurrent and painful vesicular eruptions of the lips and surrounding skin. A small cluster of vesicles first develops. As these break, yellow-brown crusts form, and healing ensues within 10 to 14 days. Both of these stages are visible here.

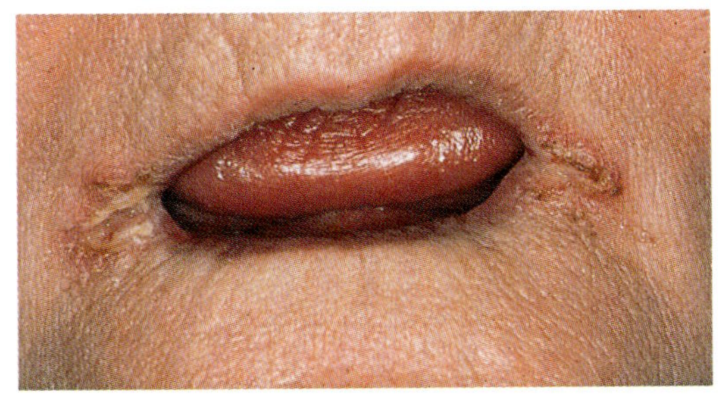

Angular Cheilitis

Angular cheilitis starts with softening of the skin at the angles of the mouth, followed by fissuring. It may be due to nutritional deficiency or, more commonly, to overclosure of the mouth, as in persons with no teeth or with ill-fitting dentures. Saliva wets and macerates the infolded skin, often leading to secondary infection with *Candida,* as in this example.

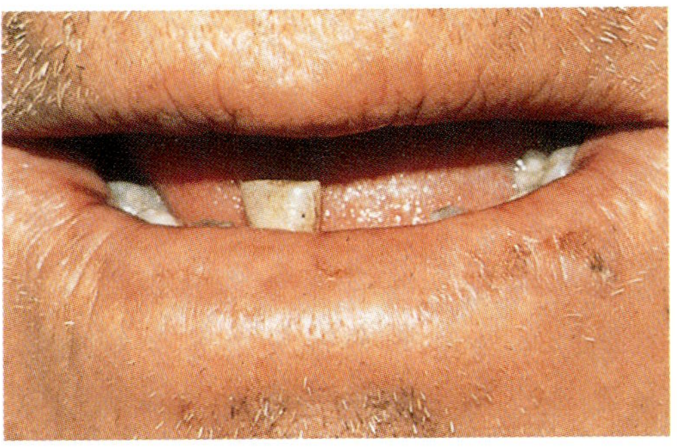

Actinic Cheilitis

Actinic cheilitis results from excessive exposure to sunlight and affects primarily the lower lip. Fair-skinned men who work outdoors are most often affected. The lip loses its normal redness and may become scaly, somewhat thickened, and slightly everted. Because solar damage also predisposes to carcinoma of the lip, be alert to this possibility.

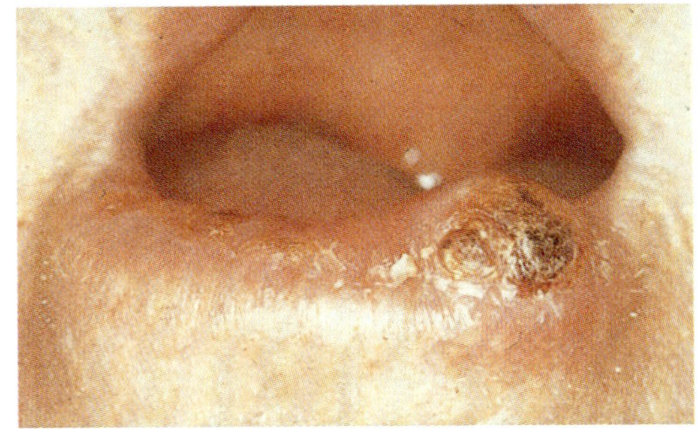

Carcinoma of the Lip

Like actinic cheilitis, carcinoma usually affects the lower lip. It may appear as a scaly plaque, as an ulcer with or without a crust, or as a nodular lesion, illustrated here. Fair skin and prolonged exposure to the sun are common risk factors.

(Sources of photos: *Herpes Simplex, Angular Cheilitis*—From Neville B et al: Color Atlas of Clinical Oral Pathology. Philadelphia, Lea & Febiger, 1991. Used with permission; *Actinic Cheilitis*—From Langlais RP, Miller CS: Color Atlas of Common Oral Diseases. Philadelphia, Lea & Febiger, 1992. Used with permission; *Carcinoma of the Lip*—Tyldesley WR: A Colour Atlas of Orofacial Diseases, 2nd ed. London, Wolfe Medical Publications, 1991.)

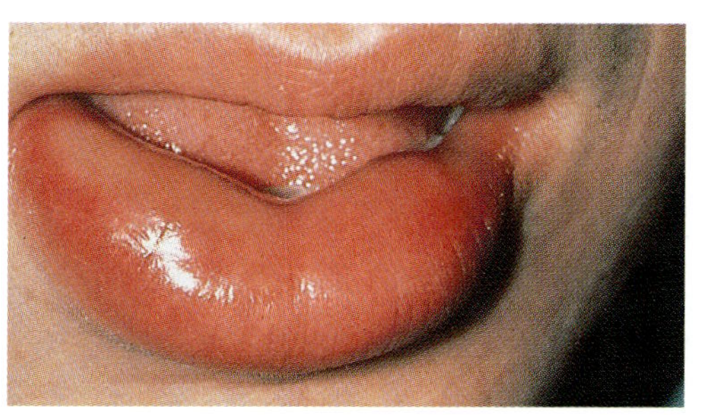

Angioedema

Angioedema is a diffuse, nonpitting, tense swelling of the dermis and subcutaneous tissue. It develops rapidly, and typically disappears over subsequent hours or days. Although usually allergic in nature and sometimes associated with hives, angioedema does not itch.

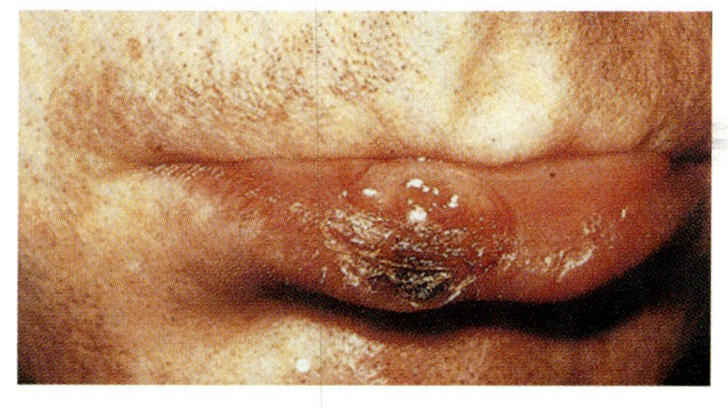

Chancre of Syphilis

This lesion of primary syphilis may appear on the lip rather than on the genitalia. It is a firm, buttonlike lesion that ulcerates and may become crusted. A chancre may resemble a carcinoma or a crusted cold sore. Because it is infectious, use gloves to feel any suspicious lesion.

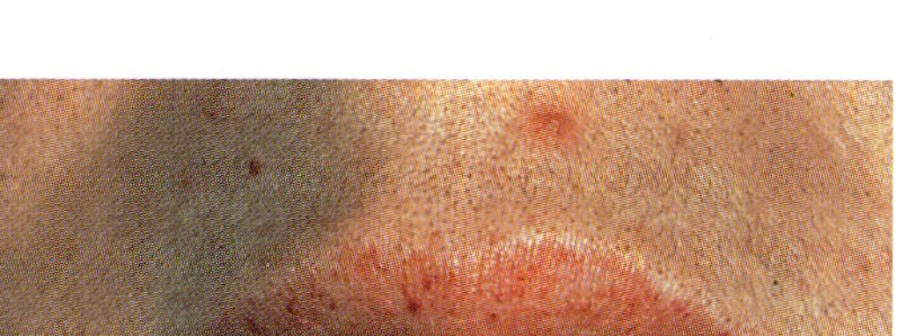

Hereditary Hemorrhagic Telangiectasia

Multiple small red spots on the lips strongly suggest hereditary hemorrhagic telangiectasia. Spots may also be visible on the face and hands and in the mouth. The spots are dilated capillaries and may bleed when traumatized. Affected people often have nosebleeds and gastrointestinal bleeding.

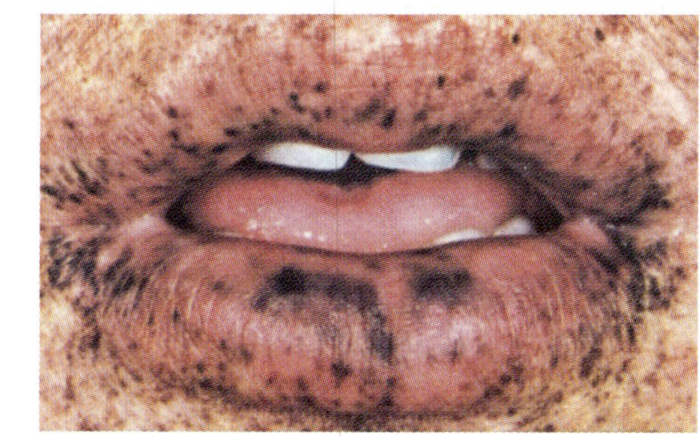

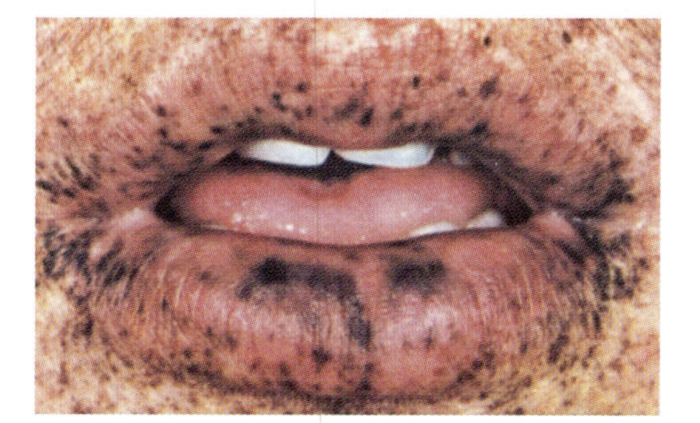

Peutz-Jeghers Syndrome

When pigmented spots on the lips are more prominent than freckling of the surrounding skin, suspect this syndrome. Pigment in the buccal mucosa helps to confirm the diagnosis. Pigmented spots may also be found on the face and hands. Multiple intestinal polyps are often associated.

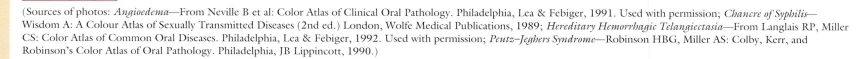

(Sources of photos: *Angioedema*—From Neville B et al: Color Atlas of Clinical Oral Pathology. Philadelphia, Lea & Febiger, 1991. Used with permission; *Chancre of Syphilis*—Wisdom A: A Colour Atlas of Sexually Transmitted Diseases (2nd ed.) London, Wolfe Medical Publications, 1989; *Hereditary Hemorrhagic Telangiectasia*—From Langlais RP, Miller CS: Color Atlas of Common Oral Diseases. Philadelphia, Lea & Febiger, 1992. Used with permission; *Peutz-Jeghers Syndrome*—Robinson HBG, Miller AS: Colby, Kerr, and Robinson's Color Atlas of Oral Pathology. Philadelphia, JB Lippincott, 1990.)

TABLE 5-21 ■ Findings in the Pharynx, Palate, and Oral Mucosa

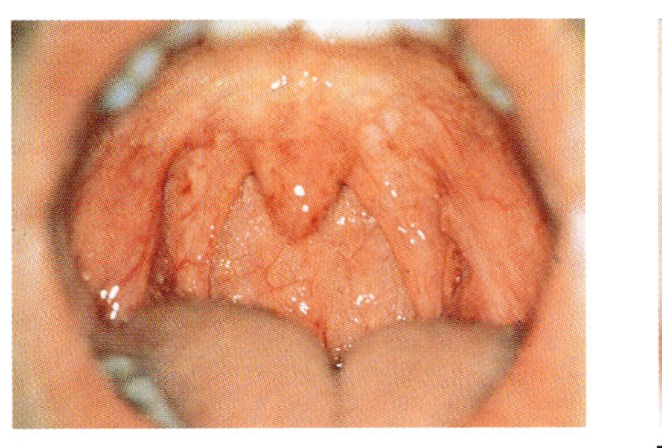

A

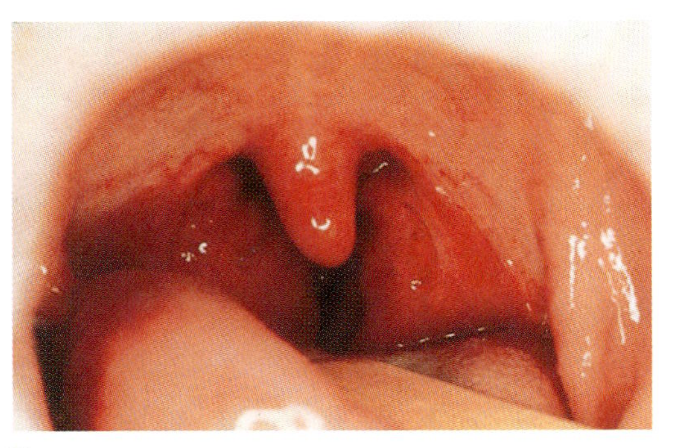

B

Pharyngitis

These two photos show reddened throats without exudate. In ***A***, redness and vascularity of the pillars and uvula are mild to moderate. In ***B***, redness is diffuse and intense. Each patient would probably complain of a sore throat, or at least a scratchy one. Possible causes include several kinds of viruses and bacteria. If the patient has no fever, exudate, or enlargement of cervical lymph nodes, the chances of infection by either of two common and important causes—*group A streptococci* and *Epstein-Barr virus* (infectious mononucleosis)—are very small.

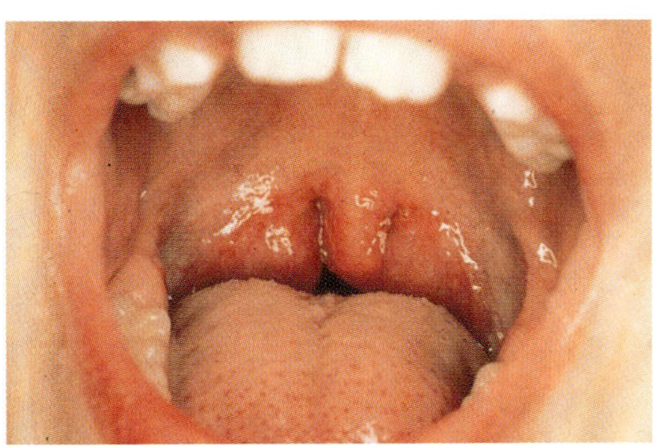

Large Normal Tonsils

Normal tonsils may be large without being infected, especially in children. They may protrude medially beyond the pillars and even to the midline. Here they touch the sides of the uvula and obscure the pharynx. Their color is within normal limits. The white marks are light reflections, not exudate.

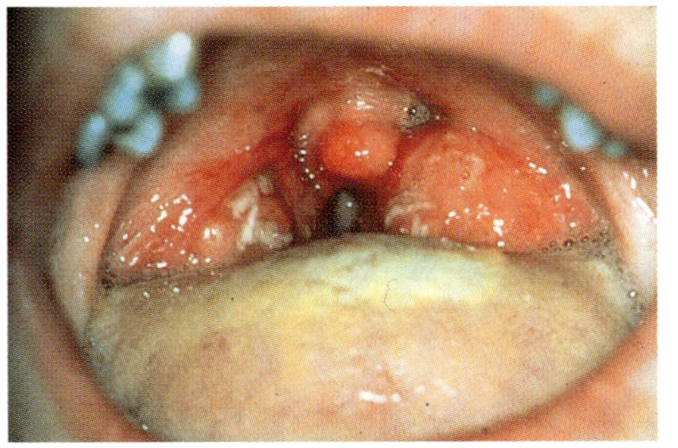

Exudative Tonsillitis

This red throat has a white exudate on the tonsils. This, together with fever and enlarged cervical nodes, increases the probability of *group A streptococcal infection*, or infectious mononucleosis. Some anterior cervical lymph nodes are usually enlarged in the former, posterior nodes in the latter.

(Sources of photos: *Pharyngitis [A and B], Large Normal Tonsils, Exudative Tonsillitis*—The Wellcome Trust, National Medical Slide Bank, London, UK.)

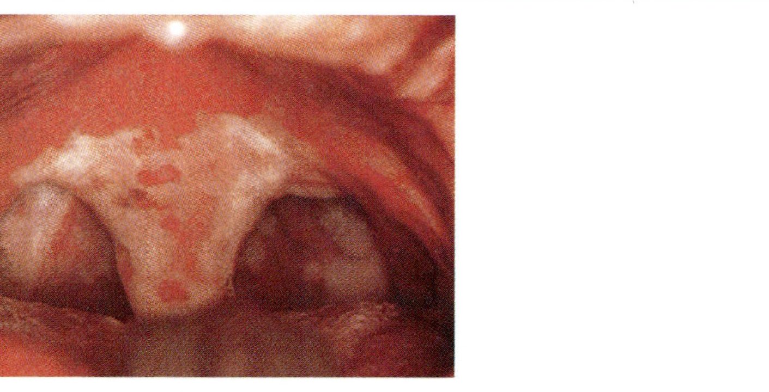

Diphtheria

Diphtheria (an acute infection caused by *Corynebacterium diphtheriae*) is now rare but still important. Prompt diagnosis may lead to life-saving treatment. The throat is dull red, and a gray exudate (pseudomembrane) is present on the uvula, pharynx, and tongue. The airway may become obstructed.

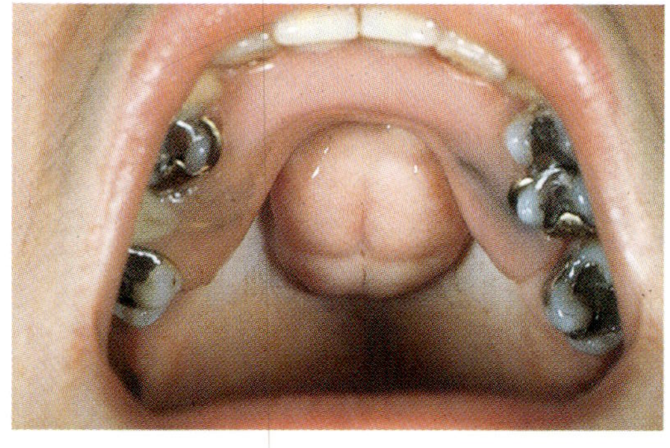

Torus Palatinus

A torus palatinus is a midline bony growth in the hard palate that is fairly common in adults. Its size and lobulation vary. Although alarming at first glance, it is harmless. In this example, an upper denture has been fitted around the torus.

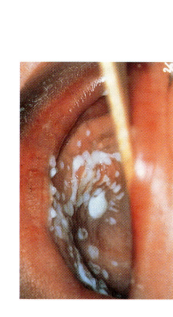

Thrush on the Palate (Candidiasis)

Thrush is a yeast infection due to *Candida*. Shown here on the palate, it may appear elsewhere in the mouth (see p. 206). Thick, white plaques are somewhat adherent to the underlying mucosa. Predisposing factors include (1) prolonged treatment with antibiotics or corticosteroids, and (2) AIDS.

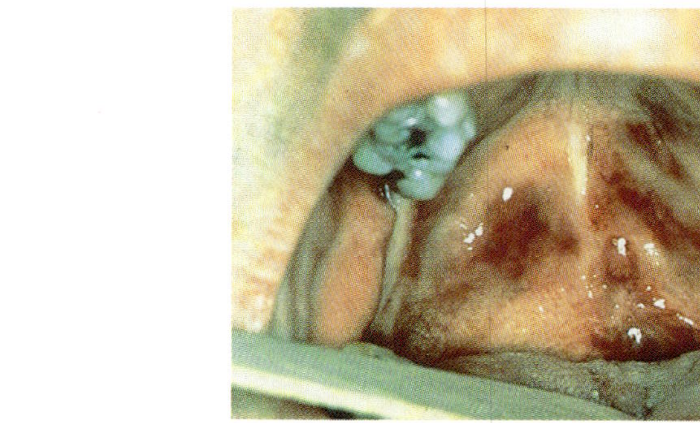

Kaposi's Sarcoma in AIDS

The deep purple color of these lesions, although not necessarily present, strongly suggests Kaposi's sarcoma. The lesions may be raised or flat. Among people with AIDS, the palate, as illustrated here, is a common site for this tumor.

(Sources of photos: *Diphtheria*—Reproduced with permission from Harnisch JP et al: Diphtheria among alcoholic urban adults. Ann Intern Med 1989; 111:77; *Thrush on the Palate*—The Wellcome Trust, National Medical Slide Bank, London, UK; *Kaposi's Sarcoma in AIDS*—Ioachim HL: Textbook and Atlas of Disease Associated With Acquired Immune Deficiency Syndrome. London, UK, Gower Medical Publishing, 1989.)

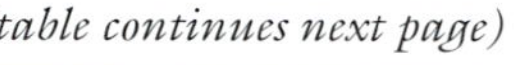

(table continues next page)

TABLE 5-21 ■ Findings in the Pharynx, Palate, and Oral Mucosa *(Continued)*

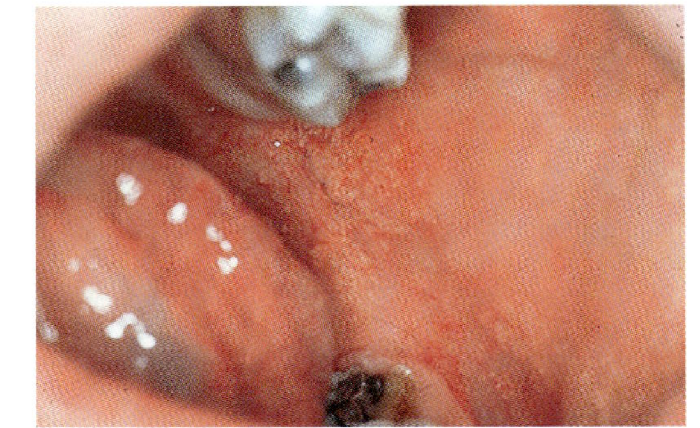

Koplik's Spots

Koplik's spots are an early sign of measles (rubeola). Search for small white specks that resemble grains of salt on a red background. They usually appear on the buccal mucosa near the first and second molars. In this photo, look also in the upper third of the mucosa. The rash of measles appears within a day.

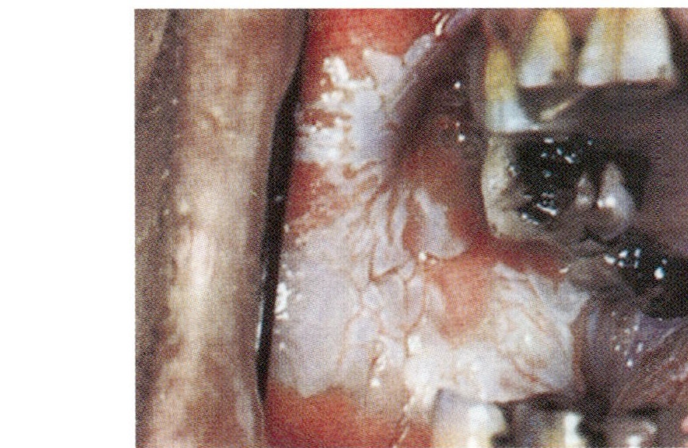

Fordyce Spots *(Fordyce Granules)*

Fordyce spots are normal sebaceous glands that appear as small yellowish spots in the buccal mucosa or on the lips. A worried person who has suddenly noticed them may be reassured. Here they are seen best anterior to the tongue and lower jaw. These spots are usually not so numerous.

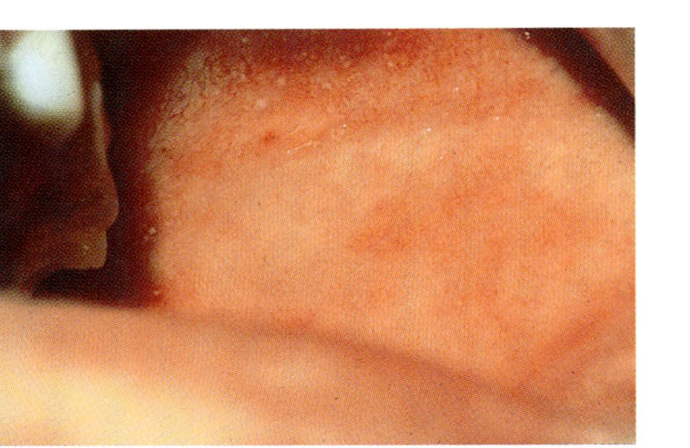

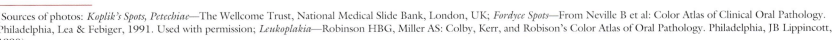

Petechiae

Petechiae are small red spots that result when blood escapes from capillaries into the tissues. Petechiae in the buccal mucosa, as shown, are often caused by accidentally biting the cheek. Oral petechiae may be due to infection or decreased platelets, as well as to trauma.

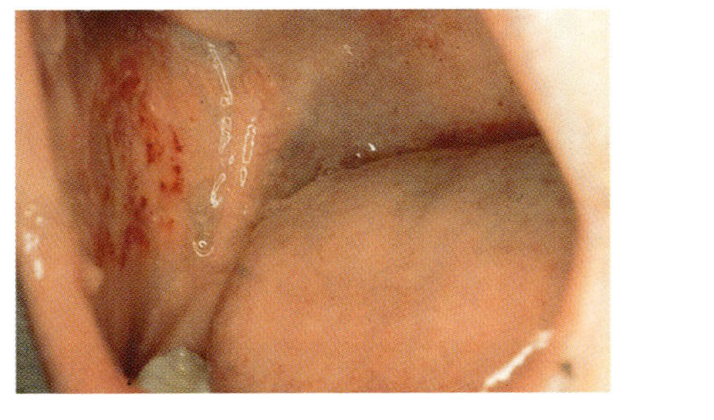

Leukoplakia

A thickened white patch (*leukoplakia*) may occur anywhere in the oral mucosa. The extensive example shown on this buccal mucosa resulted from frequent chewing of tobacco, a local irritant. This kind of irritation may lead to cancer.

(Sources of photos: *Koplik's Spots, Petechiae*—The Wellcome Trust, National Medical Slide Bank, London, UK; *Fordyce Spots*—From Neville B et al: Color Atlas of Clinical Oral Pathology. Philadelphia, Lea & Febiger, 1991. Used with permission; *Leukoplakia*—Robinson HBG, Miller AS: Colby, Kerr, and Robison's Color Atlas of Oral Pathology. Philadelphia, JB Lippincott, 1990)

TABLE 5-22 ■ Findings in the Gums and Teeth

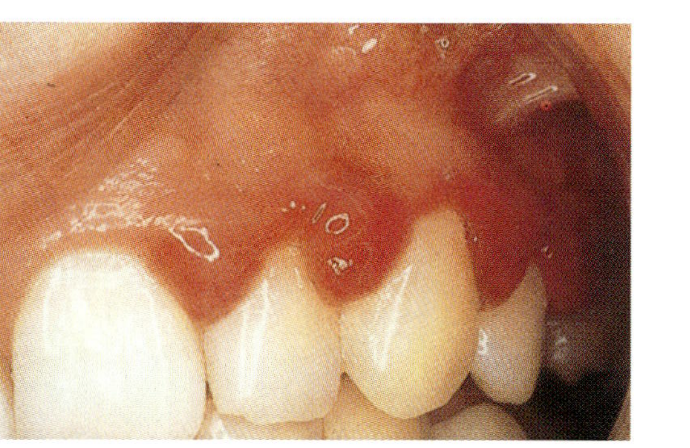

Marginal Gingivitis

Marginal gingivitis is common among teenagers and young adults. The gingival margins are reddened and swollen, and the interdental papillae are blunted, swollen, and red. Brushing the teeth often makes the gums bleed. *Plaque*—the soft white film of salivary salts, protein, and bacteria that covers the teeth and leads to gingivitis—is not readily visible.

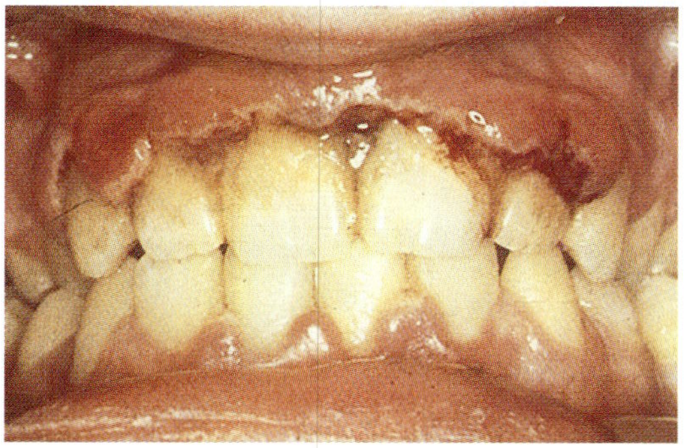

Acute Necrotizing Ulcerative Gingivitis

This uncommon form of gingivitis occurs suddenly in adolescents and young adults and is accompanied by fever, malaise, and enlarged lymph nodes. Ulcers develop in the interdental papillae. Then the destructive (necrotizing) process spreads along the gum margins, where a grayish pseudomembrane develops. The red, painful gums bleed easily; the breath is foul.

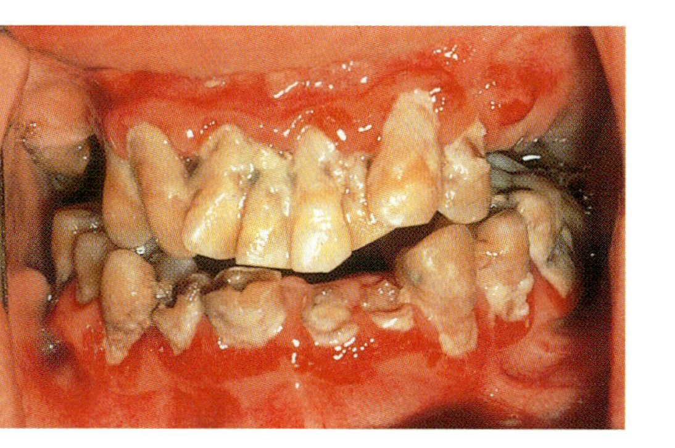

Chronic Gingivitis and Periodontitis

Chronic, untreated gingivitis may progress to periodontitis—inflammation of the deeper tissues, that normally hold the teeth in place. Attachments between gums and teeth are gradually destroyed, the gum margins recede, and the teeth eventually loosen. *Calculus* (calcified plaque), seen here as hard, cream-colored deposits on the teeth, contributes to the inflammation.

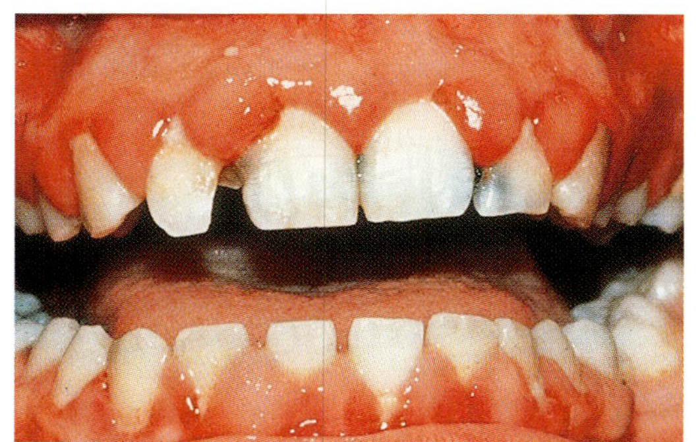

Gingival Hyperplasia

Gums enlarged by hyperplasia are swollen into heaped-up masses that may even cover the teeth. The redness of inflammation may coexist, as in this example. Causes include Dilantin therapy (as in this case), puberty, pregnancy, and leukemia.

(Sources of photos: *Marginal Gingivitis, Acute Necrotizing Ulcerative Gingivitis*—Tyldesley WR: A Colour Atlas of Orofacial Diseases, 2nd ed. London, Wolfe Medical Publications, 1991; *Chronic Gingivitis and Periodontitis* (Courtesy of Dr. Tom McDavid), *Gingival Hyperplasia* (Courtesy of Dr. James Cottone)—From Langlais RP, Miller CS: Color Atlas of Common Oral Diseases. Philadelphia, Lea & Febiger, 1992. Used with permission.)

(table continues next page)

TABLE 5-22 ■ Findings in the Gums and Teeth *(Continued)*

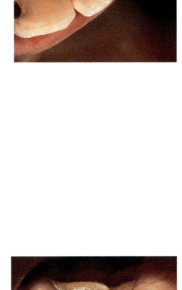

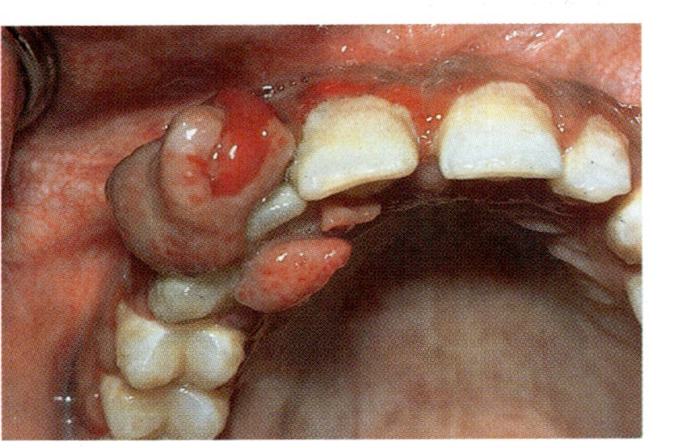

Pregnancy Tumor (Epulis, Pyogenic Granuloma)

Gingival enlargement may be localized, forming a tumorlike mass that usually originates in an interdental papilla. It is red and soft and usually bleeds easily. The estimated incidence of this lesion in pregnancy is about 1%. Note the accompanying gingivitis in this example.

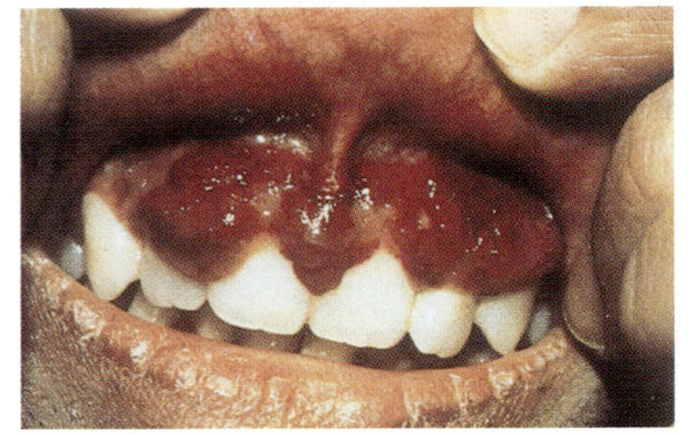

Kaposi's Sarcoma in AIDS

In people with AIDS, Kaposi's sarcoma may appear in the gums, as in other structures. The shape of the lesions in this advanced example might suggest hyperplasia, but the color suggests Kaposi's sarcoma. Be alert for less obvious lesions.

Lead Line

Now rare, a bluish-black line on the gums may signal chronic lead poisoning. The line is about 1 mm from the gum margin, follows its contours, and is absent where there are no teeth. In this example, as is common, periodontitis coexists.

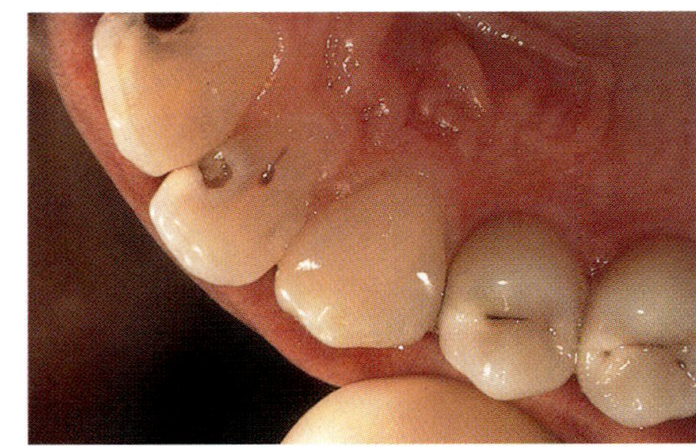

Dental Caries

Dental caries is first visible as a chalky white area in the enamel surface of a tooth. This area may then turn brown or black, become soft, and cavitate. Special dental techniques, including x-rays, are necessary for early detection.

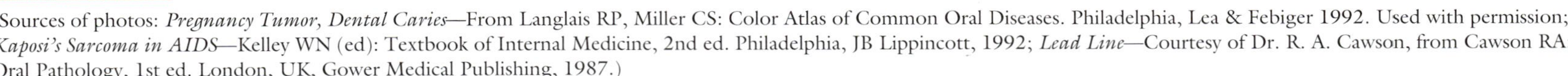

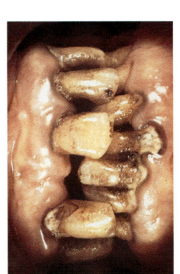

(Sources of photos: *Pregnancy Tumor, Dental Caries*—From Langlais RP, Miller CS: Color Atlas of Common Oral Diseases. Philadelphia, Lea & Febiger 1992. Used with permission; *Kaposi's Sarcoma in AIDS*—Kelley WN (ed): Textbook of Internal Medicine, 2nd ed. Philadelphia, JB Lippincott, 1992; *Lead Line*—Courtesy of Dr. R. A. Cawson, from Cawson RA: Oral Pathology, 1st ed. London, UK, Gower Medical Publishing, 1987.)

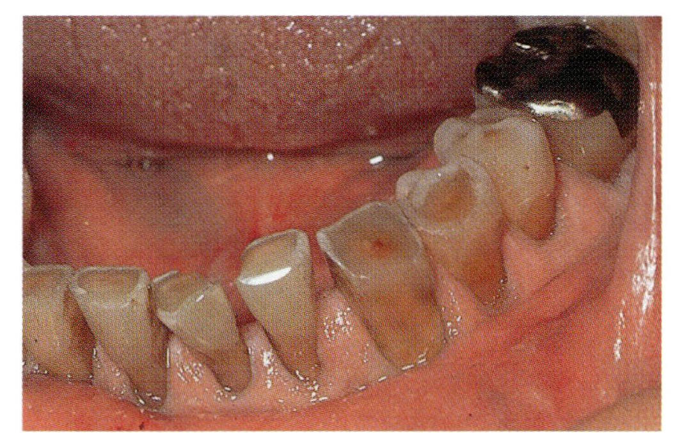

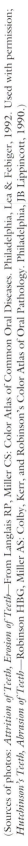

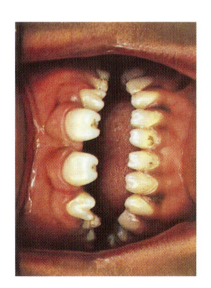

Attrition of Teeth; Recession of Gums

In many elderly people, the chewing surfaces of the teeth have been worn down by repetitive use so that the yellow-brown dentin becomes exposed—a process called *attrition*. Note also the *recession of the gums,* which has exposed the roots of the teeth, giving a "long in the tooth" appearance.

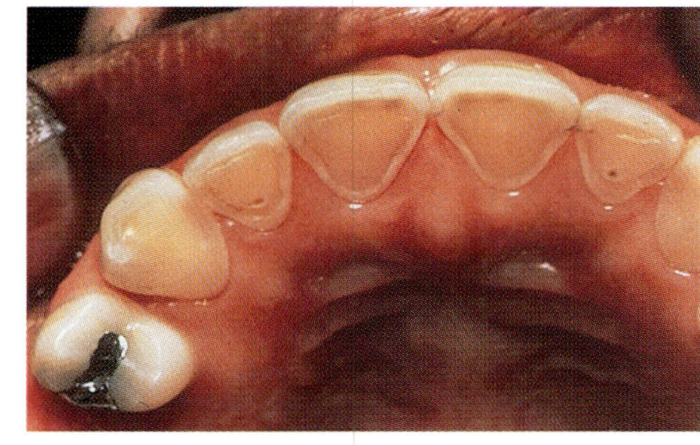

Erosion of Teeth

Teeth may be eroded by chemical action. Note here the erosion of the enamel from the lingual surfaces of the upper incisors, exposing the yellow-brown dentin. This results from recurrent regurgitation of stomach contents, as in bulimia.

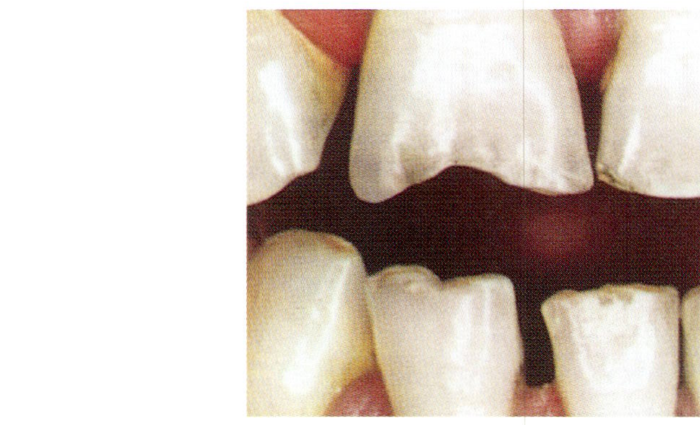

Hutchinson's Teeth

Hutchinson's teeth are smaller and more widely spaced than normal and are notched on their biting surfaces. The sides of the teeth taper toward the biting edges. The upper central incisors of the permanent (not the deciduous) teeth are most often affected. These teeth are a sign of congenital syphilis.

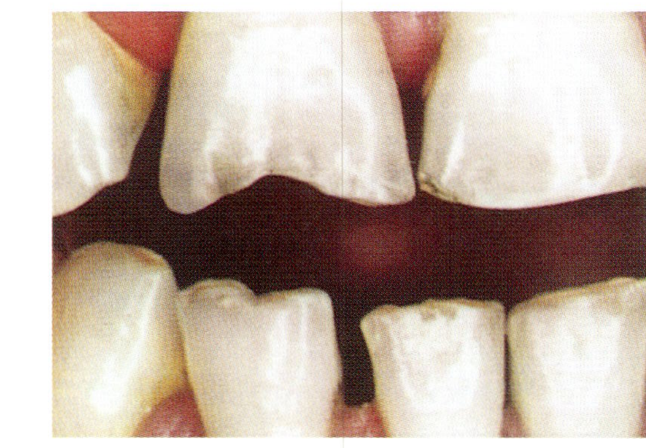

Abrasion of Teeth With Notching

The biting surface of the teeth may become abraded or notched by recurrent trauma, such as holding nails or opening bobby pins between the teeth. Unlike Hutchinson's teeth, the sides of these teeth show normal contours; size and spacing of the teeth are unaffected.

(Sources of photos: *Attrition of Teeth, Erosion of Teeth*—From Langlais RP, Miller CS: Color Atlas of Common Oral Diseases. Philadelphia, Lea & Febiger, 1992. Used with permission; *Hutchinson's Teeth, Abrasion of Teeth*—Robinson HBG, Miller AS: Colby, Kerr, and Robinson's Color Atlas of Oral Pathology. Philadelphia, JB Lippincott, 1990.)

TABLE 5-23 ■ Findings In or Under the Tongue

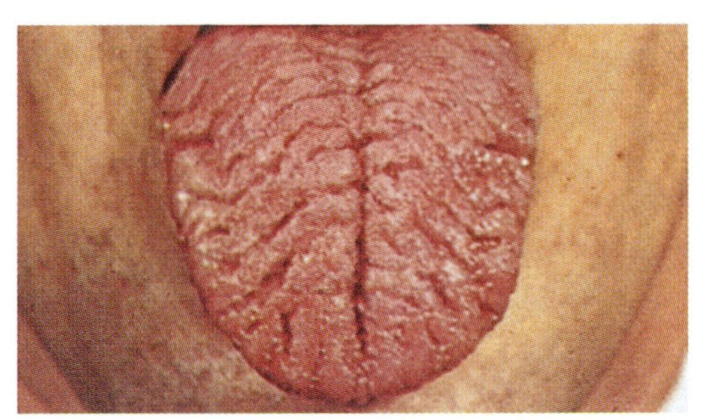

Fissured Tongue

Fissures may appear in the tongue with increasing age. Their appearance has led to the alternate term, *scrotal tongue*. Although food debris may accumulate in the crevices and become irritating, a fissured tongue usually has little significance.

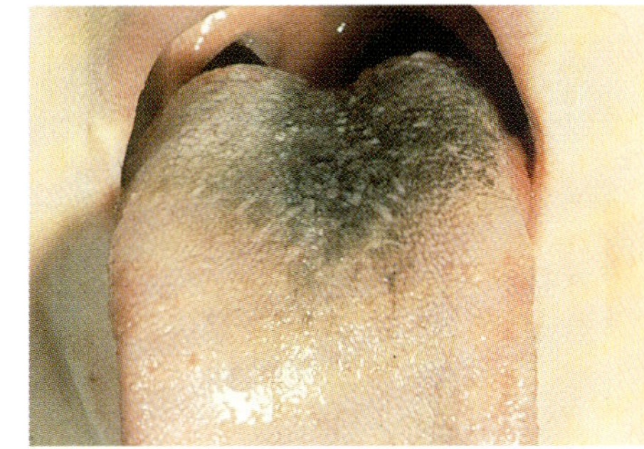

Hairy Tongue

The "hair" of hairy tongue consists of elongated papillae on the dorsum of the tongue, and is yellowish to brown or black. Hairy tongue may follow antibiotic therapy but may also occur spontaneously, without known cause. It is harmless.

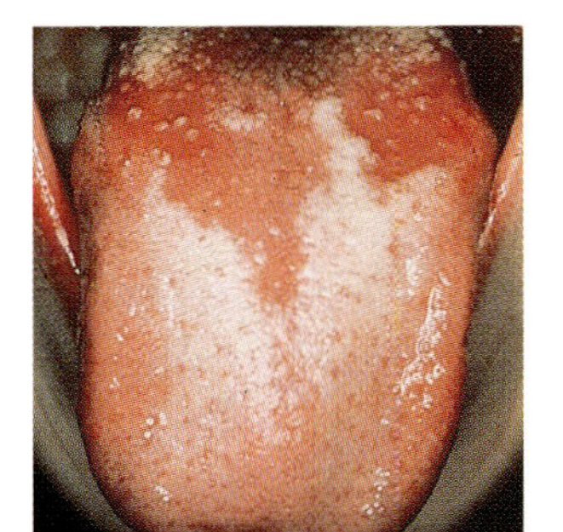

Geographic Tongue

The dorsum of a geographic tongue shows scattered smooth red areas that are denuded of papillae. Together with the normal rough and coated areas, they give a maplike pattern that changes over time. Of unknown cause, the condition is benign.

Smooth Tongue *(Atrophic Glossitis)*

A smooth and often sore tongue that has lost its papillae suggests a deficiency in riboflavin, niacin, folic acid, vitamin B_{12}, pyridoxine, or iron. Specific diagnosis is often difficult. Anticancer drugs may also be responsible.

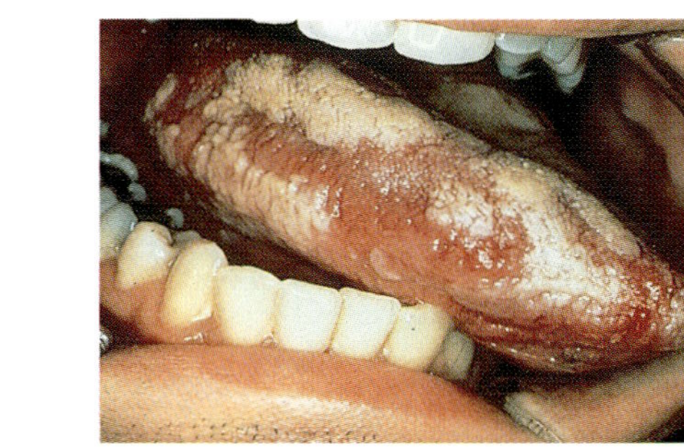

Hairy Leukoplakia

Whitish raised areas that have a feathery or corrugated pattern suggest hairy leukoplakia. Unlike candidiasis, these areas cannot be scraped off. The sides of the tongue are most often affected. This lesion is seen in HIV infection and AIDS.

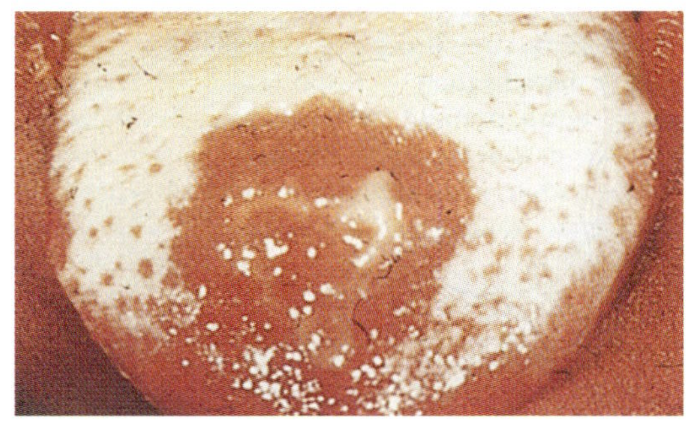

Candidiasis

The thick white coat on this tongue is due to *Candida* infection. A raw red surface is left where the coat was scraped off. This infection may also cause redness of the tongue without the white coat. AIDS, among other factors, predisposes to this condition.

(Sources of photos: *Fissured Tongue, Candidiasis*—Robinson HBG, Miller AS: Colby, Kerr, and Robinson's Color Atlas of Oral Pathology. Philadelphia, JB Lippincott, 1990; *Smooth Tongue*—Courtesy of Dr. R. A. Cawson, from Cawson RA: Oral Pathology, 1st ed. London, UK, Gower Medical Publishing, 1987; *Geographic Tongue*—The Wellcome Trust, National Medical Slide Bank, London, UK; *Hairy Leukoplakia*—Ioachim HL: Textbook and Atlas of Disease Associated With Acquired Immune Deficiency Syndrome. London, UK, Gower Medical Publishing, 1989.)

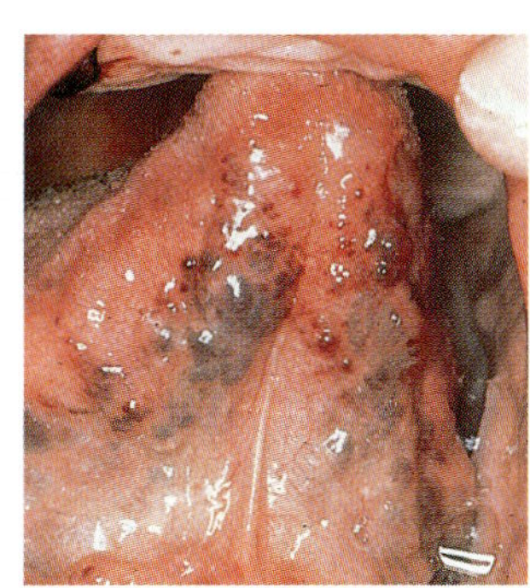

Varicose Veins

Small purplish or blue-black round swellings may appear under the tongue with age. They are dilatations of the lingual veins and have no clinical significance. Reassure a worried patient. These varicosities are also called *caviar lesions.*

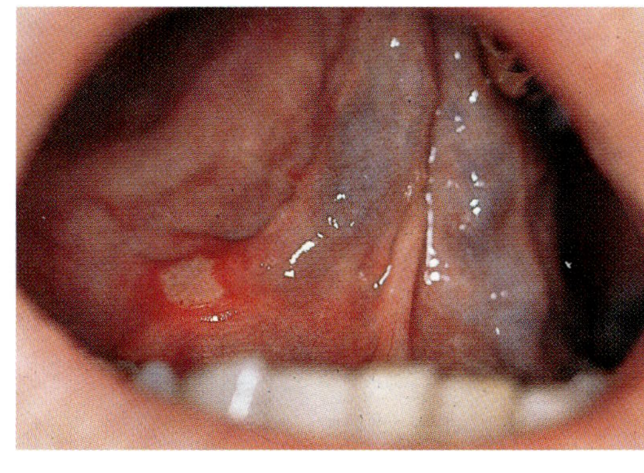

Aphthous Ulcer *(Canker Sore)*

A painful, small, round or oval ulcer that is white or yellowish gray and surrounded by a halo of reddened mucosa typifies the common aphthous ulcer. These ulcers may be single or multiple. They heal in 7 to 10 days, but may recur.

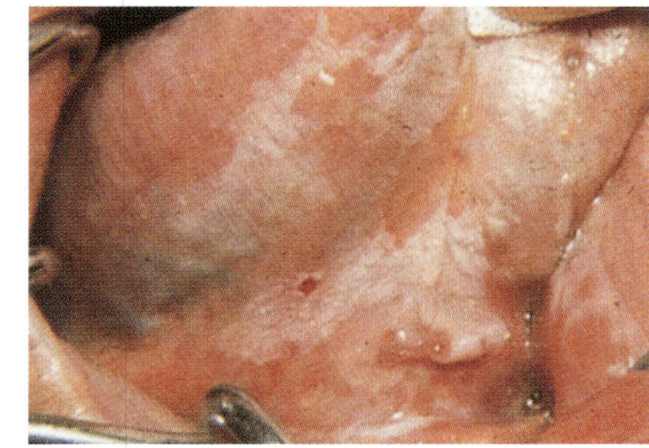

Leukoplakia

A persisting painless white patch in the oral mucosa is often called leukoplakia until biopsy reveals its nature. Here, the undersurface of the tongue looks as if it had been painted white. Smaller patches are more common. Leukoplakia of any size raises the possibility of malignant change.

Mucous Patch of Syphilis

This painless lesion occurs in the secondary stage of syphilis and is highly infectious. It is slightly raised, oval, and covered by a grayish membrane. Mucous patches may be multiple and occur elsewhere in the mouth.

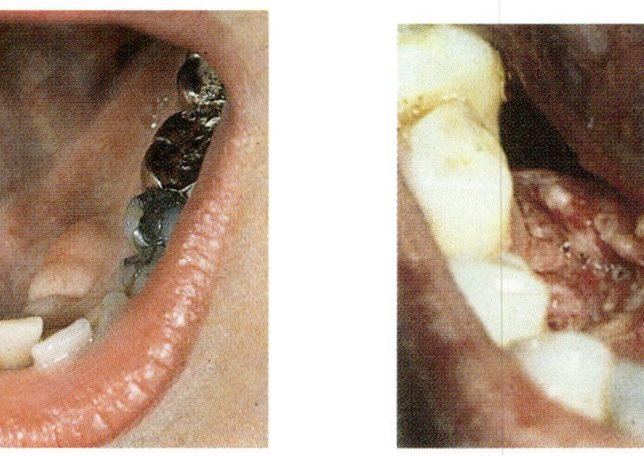

Tori Mandibulares

Tori mandibulares are rounded bony protuberances that grow from the inner surfaces of the mandible. They are typically bilateral and asymptomatic. The overlying mucosa is normal in color. Like a torus palatinus (p. 201), these tori are harmless.

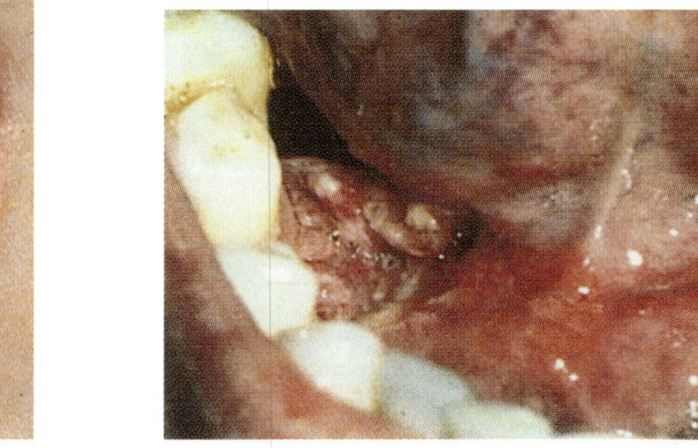

Carcinoma, Floor of the Mouth

This ulcerated lesion is in a common location for carcinoma, which also occurs on the side of the tongue. Medial to the carcinoma, note the reddened area of mucosa, called *erythroplakia*. Like leukoplakia, erythroplakia warns of possible malignancy.

(Sources of photos: *Mucous Patch, Leukoplakia, Carcinoma*—Robinson HBG, Miller AS: Colby, Kerr, and Robinson's Color Atlas of Oral Pathology. Philadelphia, JB Lippincott, 1990; *Varicose Veins*—From Neville B et al: Color Atlas of Clinical Oral Pathology. Philadelphia, Lea & Febiger, 1991. Used with permission.)

TABLE 5-24 ■ Thyroid Enlargement and Function

Evaluation of the thyroid gland includes a description of the gland and a functional assessment.

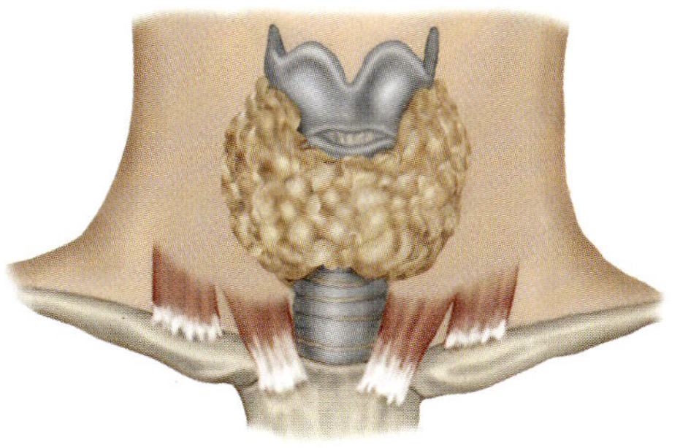

Diffuse Enlargement

A diffusely enlarged gland includes the isthmus and the lateral lobes, but there are no discretely palpable nodules. Causes include Graves' disease, Hashimoto's thyroiditis, and endemic goiter (related to iodine deficiency, now uncommon in the United States). Sporadic goiter refers to an enlarged gland with no apparent cause.

Multinodular Goiter

This term refers to an enlarged thyroid gland that contains two or more identifiable nodules. Multiple nodules suggest a metabolic rather than a neoplastic process, but irradiation during childhood, a positive family history, enlarged cervical nodes, or continuing enlargement of one of the nodules raises the suspicion of malignancy.

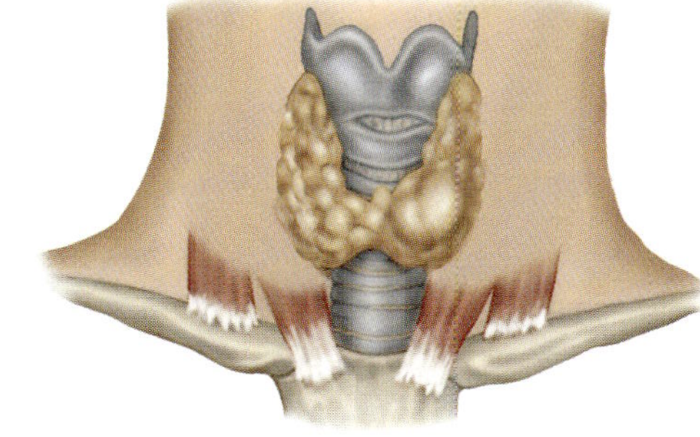

Single Nodule

A clinically single nodule may be a cyst, a benign tumor, or one nodule within a multinodular gland, but it also raises the question of a malignancy. Prior irradiation, hardness, rapid growth, fixation to surrounding tissues, enlarged cervical nodes, and occurrence in males increase the probability of malignancy.

Symptoms of Thyroid Dysfunction		Signs of Thyroid Dysfunction	
Hyperthyroidism	*Hypothyroidism*	*Hyperthyroidism*	*Hypothyroidism*
Nervousness	Fatigue, lethargy	Tachycardia or atrial fibrillation	Bradycardia and, in late stages, hypothermia
Weight loss despite an increased appetite	Modest weight gain with anorexia	Increased systolic and decreased diastolic blood pressures	Decreased systolic and increased diastolic blood pressures
Excessive sweating and heat intolerance	Dry, coarse skin and cold intolerance	Hyperdynamic cardiac pulsations with an accentuated S_1	Intensity of heart sounds sometimes decreased
Palpitations	Swelling of face, hands, and legs	Warm, smooth, moist skin	Dry, coarse, cool skin, sometimes yellowish from carotene, with nonpitting edema and loss of hair
Frequent bowel movements	Constipation	Tremor and proximal muscle weakness	Impaired memory, mixed hearing loss, somnolence, peripheral neuropathy, carpal tunnel syndrome
Muscular weakness of the proximal type and tremor	Weakness, muscle cramps, arthralgias, paresthesias, impaired memory and hearing	With Graves' disease, eye signs such as stare, lid lag, and exophthalmos	Periorbital puffiness

CHAPTER

6

The Thorax and Lungs

ANATOMY AND PHYSIOLOGY

Study the *anatomy of the chest wall*, identifying the structures illustrated. Note that an interspace between two ribs is numbered by the rib above it.

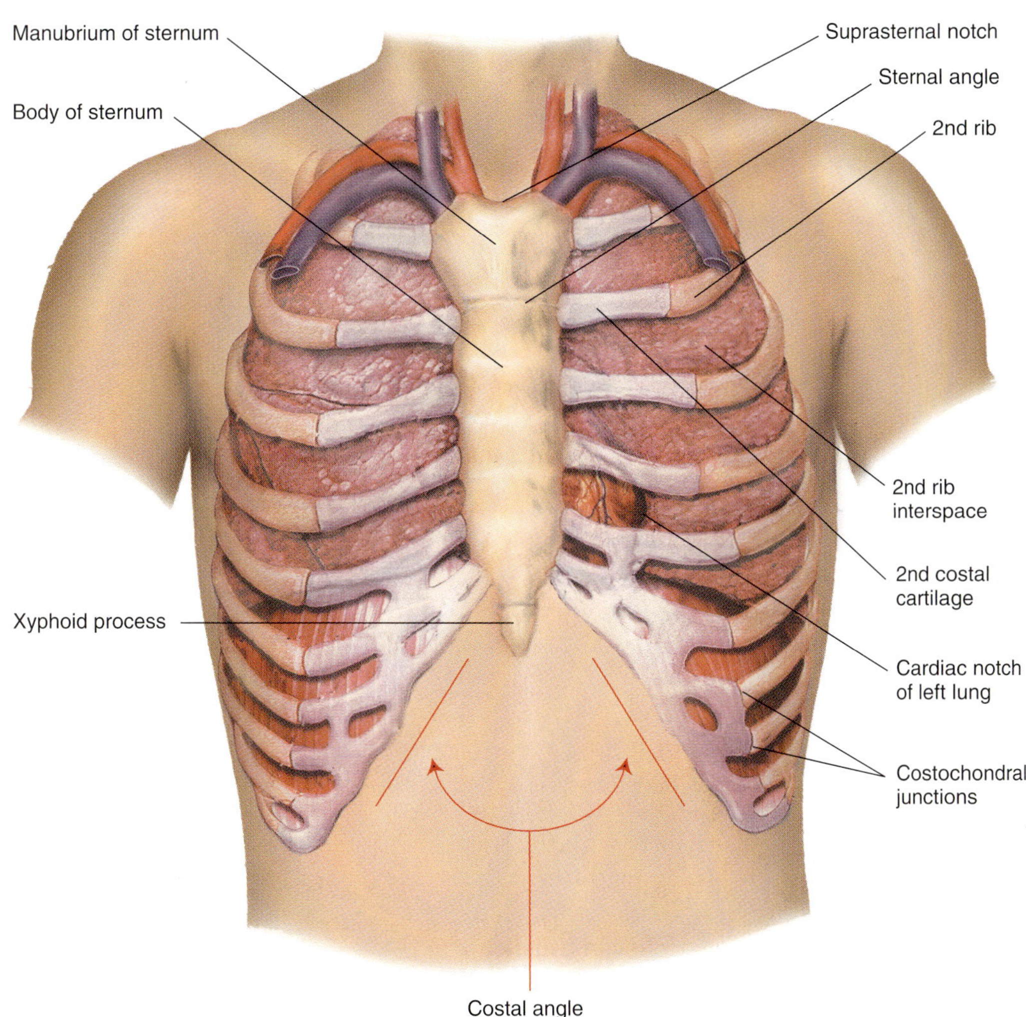

Locating Findings on the Chest. Describe abnormalities of the chest in two dimensions: *along the vertical axis* and *around the circumference of the chest.*

To make *vertical* locations, you must be able to count the ribs and interspaces. The *sternal angle,* also termed the angle of Louis, is the best guide: place your finger in the hollow curve of the suprasternal notch, then move your finger down about 5 cm to the horizontal bony ridge joining the manubrium to the body of the sternum. Then move your finger laterally and find the adjacent 2nd rib and costal cartilage. From here, using two fingers, you can "walk down the interspaces," one space at a time, on an oblique line illustrated by the red numbers below. Do not try to count interspaces along the lower edge of the sternum; the ribs there are too close together. In a woman, to find the interspaces either displace the breast laterally or palpate a little more medially than illustrated. Avoid pressing too hard on tender breast tissue.

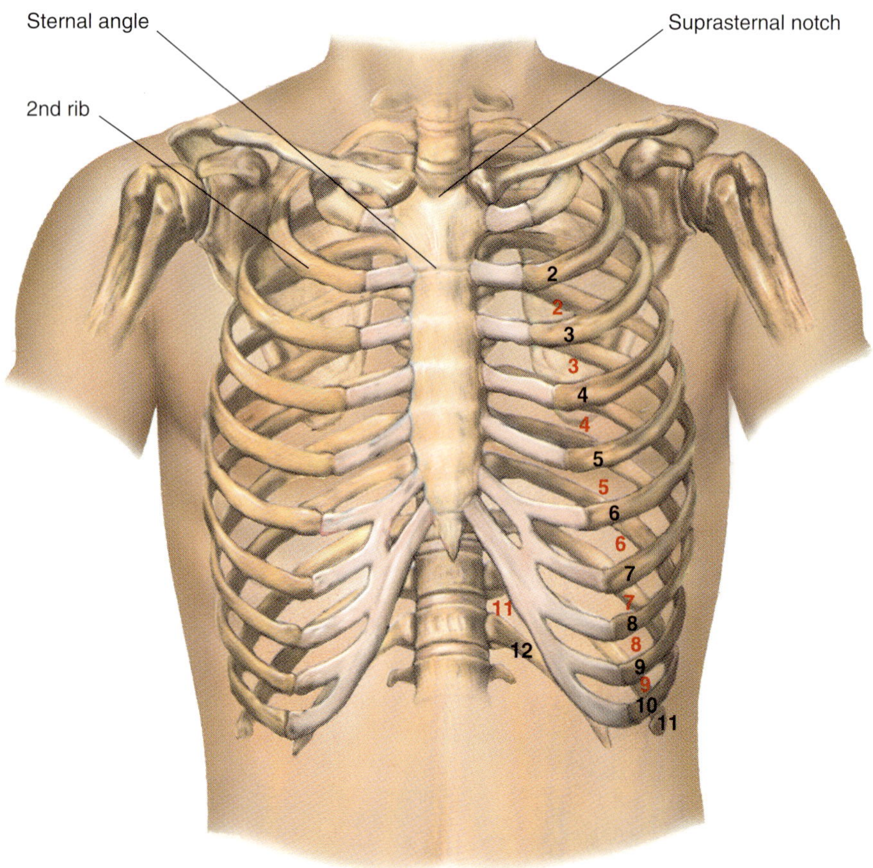

Note that the costal cartilages of the first seven ribs articulate with the sternum; the cartilages of the 8th, 9th, and 10th ribs articulate with the costal cartilages just above them. The 11th and 12th ribs, the "floating ribs," have no anterior attachments. The cartilaginous tip of the 11th rib can usually be felt laterally, and the 12th rib may be felt posteriorly. On palpation, costal cartilages and ribs feel identical.

Posteriorly, the 12th rib is another possible starting point for counting ribs and interspaces: it helps locate findings on the lower posterior chest and provides an option when the anterior approach is unsatisfactory. With the fingers of one hand, press in and up against the lower border of the 12th rib, then "walk up" the interspaces numbered in red below, or follow a more oblique line up and around to the front of the chest.

The inferior tip of the scapula is another useful bony marker—it usually lies at the level of the 7th rib or interspace.

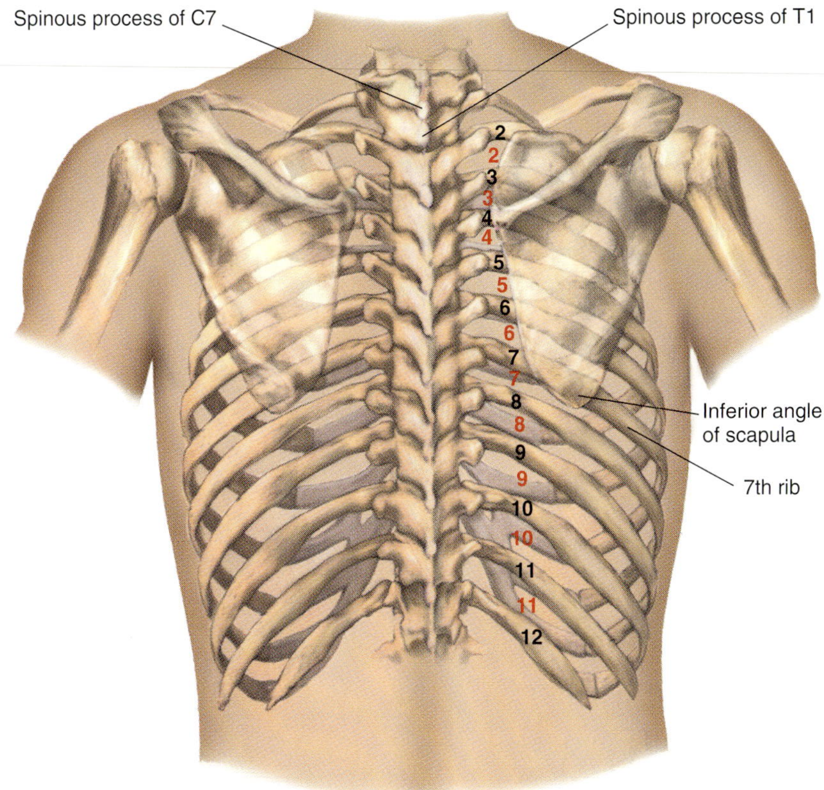

The spinous processes of the vertebrae are also useful anatomic landmarks. When the neck is flexed forward, the most protruding process is usually the vertebra of C7. If two processes are equally prominent, they are C7 and T1. You can often palpate and count the processes below them, especially when the spine is flexed.

To locate findings around the circumference of the chest, use a series of vertical lines, shown in the next three illustrations. The *midsternal and vertebral lines* are precise; the others are estimated. The *midclavicular line* drops vertically from the midpoint of the clavicle. To find it, you must identify both ends of the clavicle accurately (see p. 469). The *anterior and posterior axillary lines* drop vertically from the anterior and posterior axillary folds, the muscle masses that border the axilla. The *midaxillary line* drops from the apex of the axilla.

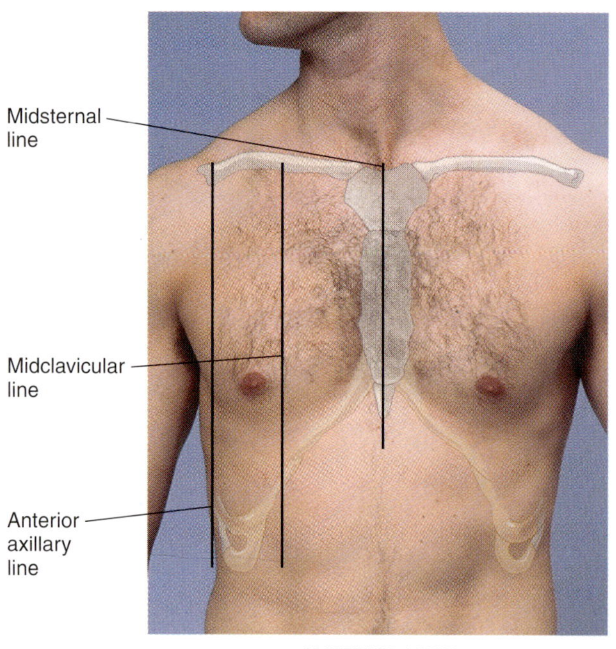

ANTERIOR VIEW

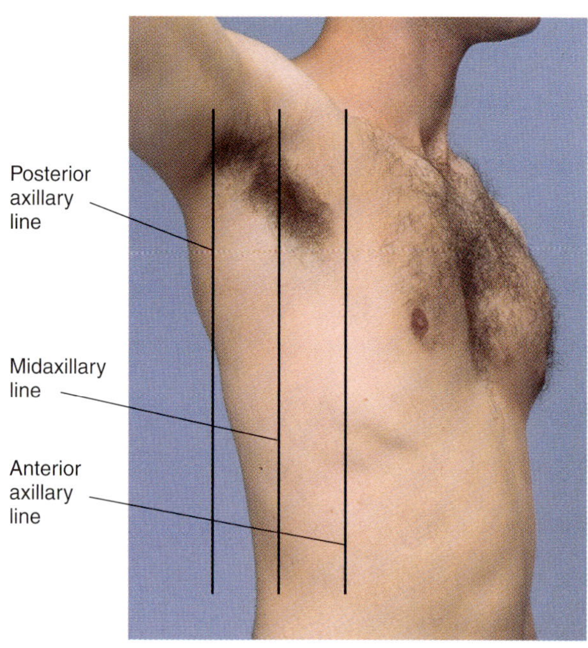

RIGHT ANTERIOR OBLIQUE VIEW

Posteriorly, the *vertebral line* overlies the spinous processes of the vertebrae. The scapular line drops from the inferior angle of the scapula.

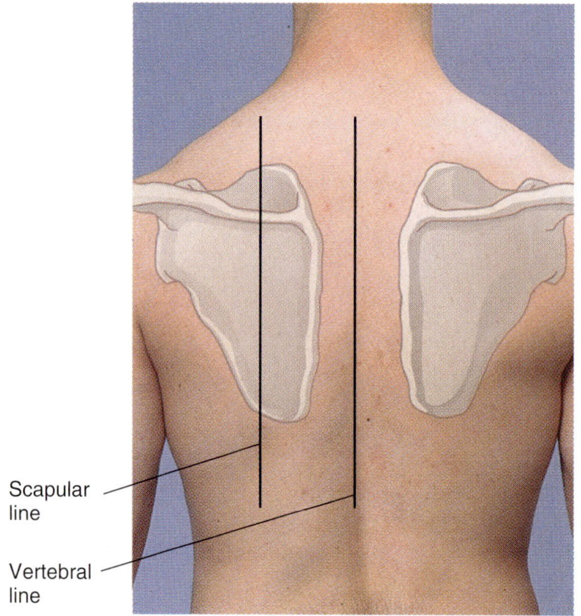

POSTERIOR VIEW

Lungs, Fissures, and Lobes. The lungs and their fissures and lobes can be mentally pictured on the chest wall. Anteriorly, the apex of each lung rises about 2 cm to 4 cm above the inner third of the clavicle. The lower border of the lung crosses the 6th rib at the midclavicular line and the 8th rib at the midaxillary line. (Because ribs slant, a fairly horizontal line can drop a rib or more as it passes across the chest.) Posteriorly, the lower border of the lung lies at about the level of the T10 spinous process. On inspiration, it descends farther.

Each lung is divided roughly in half by an *oblique (major) fissure*. This fissure may be approximated by a string that runs from the T3 spinous process obliquely down and around the chest to the 6th rib at the midclavicular line. The right lung is further divided by the *horizontal (minor) fissure*. Anteriorly, this fissure runs close to the 4th rib and meets the oblique fissure in the midaxillary line near the 5th rib.

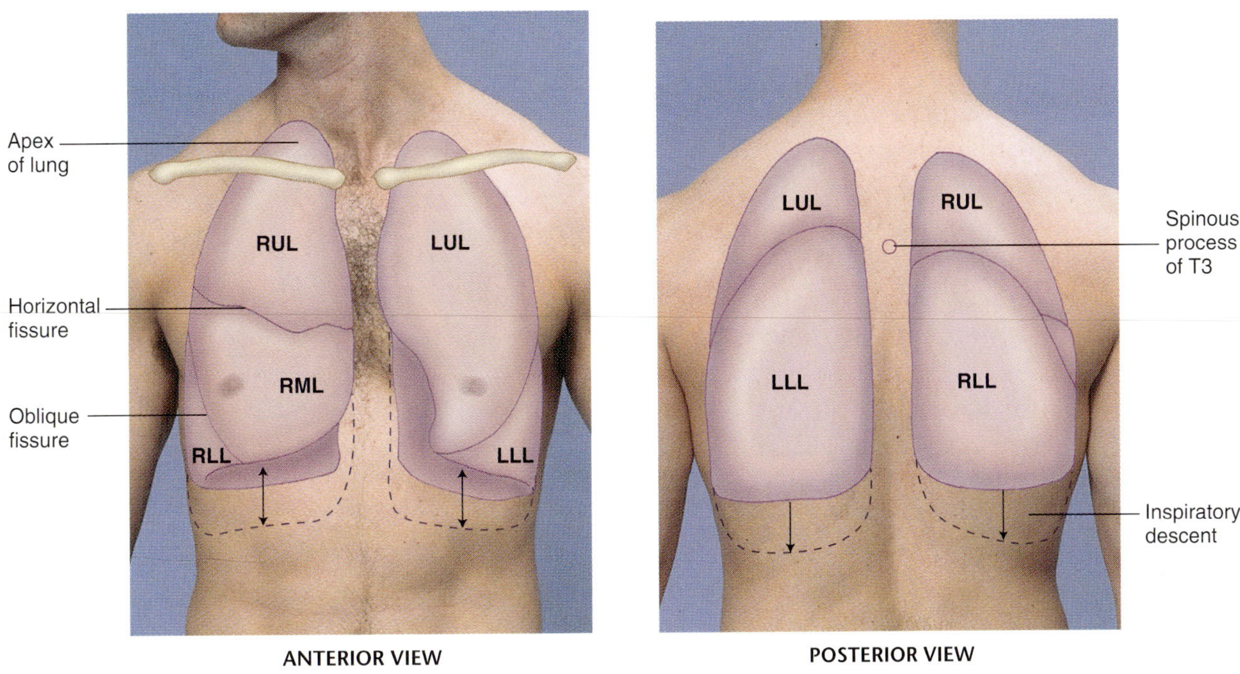

ANTERIOR VIEW

POSTERIOR VIEW

The right lung is thus divided into *upper, middle, and lower lobes.* The left lung has only two lobes, upper and lower.

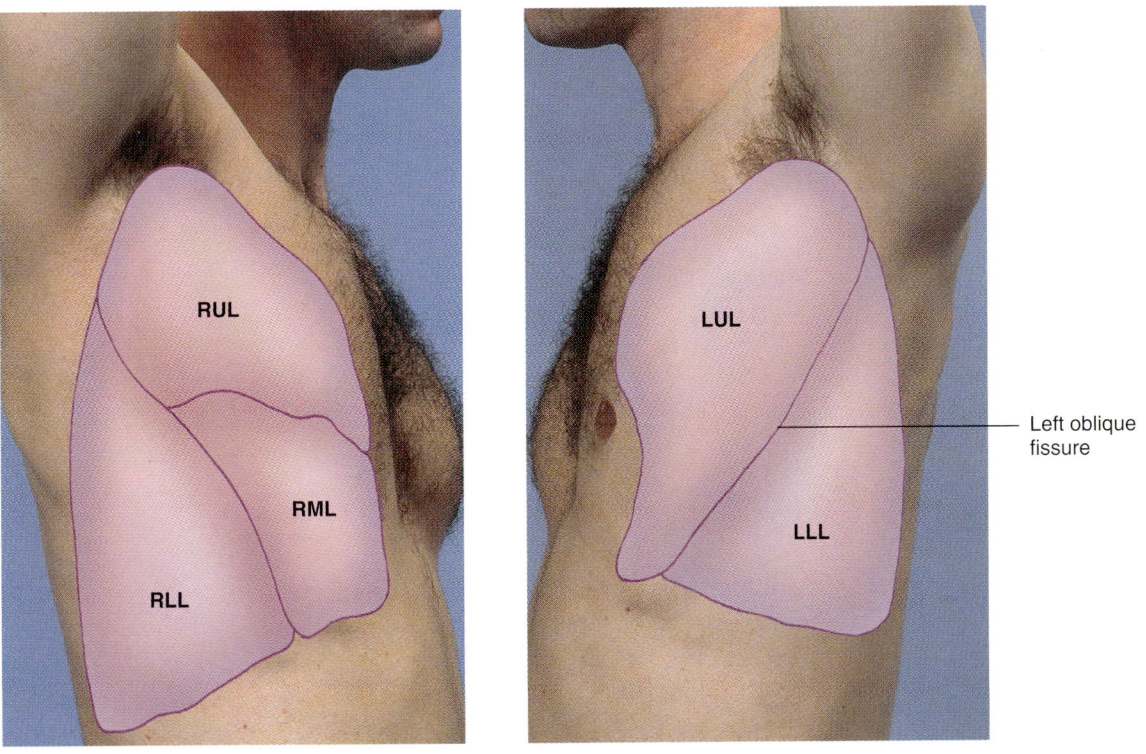

RIGHT AND LEFT LATERAL VIEWS

Locations on the Chest. Be familiar with general anatomic terms used to locate chest findings, such as:

Supraclavicular—above the clavicles
Infraclavicular—below the clavicles
Interscapular—between the scapulae
Infrascapular—below the scapula
Bases of the lungs—the lowermost portions
Upper, middle, and lower lung fields

You may then infer what part(s) of the lung(s) are affected by an abnormal process. Signs in the right upper lung field, for example, almost certainly originate in the right upper lobe. Signs in the right middle lung field laterally, however, could come from any of three different lobes.

The Trachea and Major Bronchi. Breath sounds over the trachea and bronchi have a different quality than breath sounds over the lung parenchyma. Be sure you know the location of these structures. The trachea bifurcates into its mainstem bronchi at the levels of the sternal angle anteriorly and the T4 spinous process posteriorly.

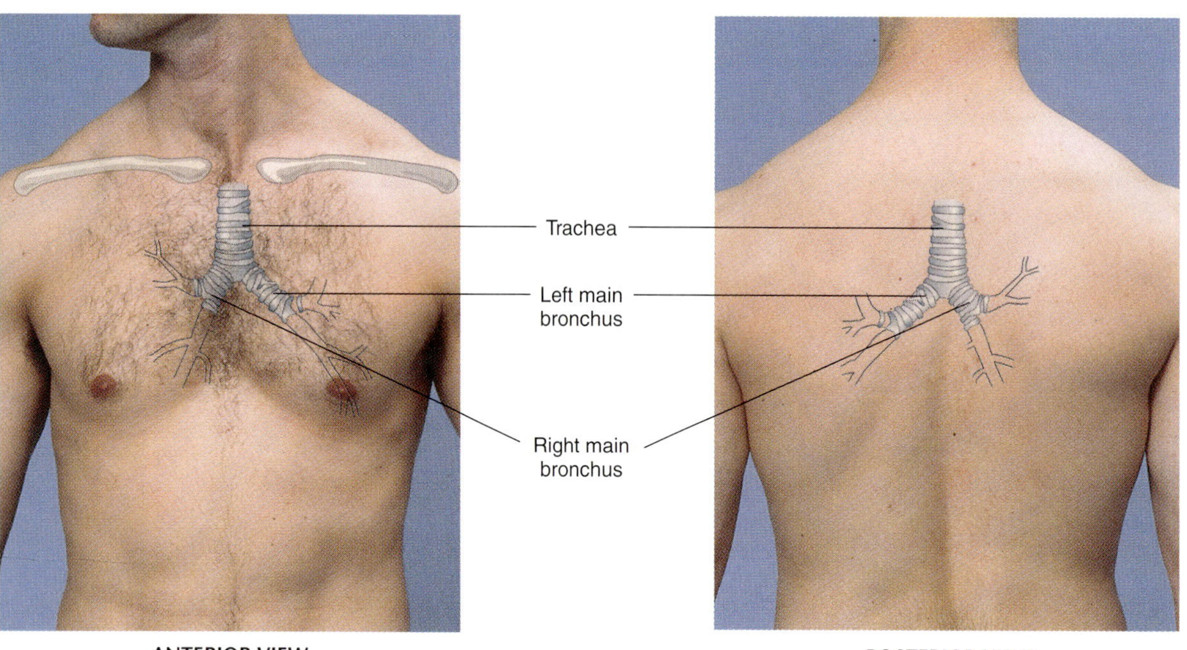

The Pleurae. The pleurae are serous membranes that cover the outer surface of each lung, the *visceral pleura,* and also line the inner rib cage and upper surface of the diaphragm, the *parietal pleura.* Their smooth opposing surfaces, lubricated by pleural fluid, allow the lungs to move easily within the rib cage during inspiration and expiration. The *pleural space* is the potential space between visceral and parietal pleurae.

Breathing. Breathing is largely an automatic act, controlled in the brainstem and mediated by the muscles of respiration. The dome-shaped *diaphragm* is the primary muscle of inspiration. When it contracts, it descends in the chest and enlarges the thoracic cavity. At the same time it compresses the abdominal contents, pushing the abdominal wall outward. Muscles in the rib cage and neck expand the thorax during inspiration, especially the *parasternals,* which run obliquely from sternum to ribs, and the *scalenes,* which run from the cervical vertebrae to the first two ribs.

During inspiration, as these muscles contract, the thorax expands. Intrathoracic pressure decreases, drawing air through the tracheobronchial tree into the *alveoli,* or distal air sacs, and expanding the lungs. Oxygen diffuses into the blood of adjacent pulmonary capillaries, and carbon dioxide diffuses from the blood into the alveoli.

After inspiratory effort stops, the expiratory phase begins. The chest wall and lungs recoil, the diaphragm relaxes and rises passively, air flows outward, and the chest and abdomen return to their resting positions.

Normal breathing is quiet and easy—barely audible near the open mouth as a faint whish. When a healthy person lies supine, the breathing movements of the thorax are relatively slight. In contrast, the abdominal movements are usually easy to see. In the sitting position, movements of the thorax become more prominent.

During exercise and in certain diseases, extra work is required to breathe, and accessory muscles join the inspiratory effort. The sternomastoids are the most important of these, and the scalenes may become visible. Abdominal muscles assist in expiration.

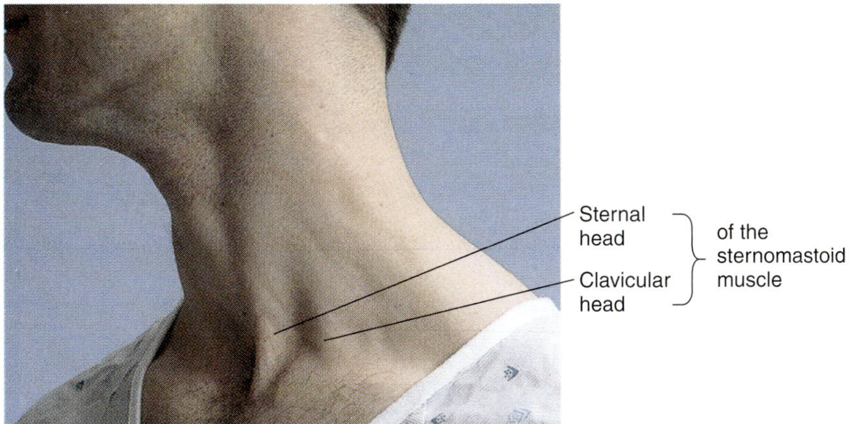

Changes With Aging

As people age, their capacity for exercise decreases. The chest wall becomes stiffer and harder to move, respiratory muscles may weaken, and the lungs lose some of their elastic recoil. The speed of breathing out with maximal effort gradually diminishes. Skeletal changes associated with aging may accentuate the dorsal curve of the thoracic spine, producing kyphosis and increasing the anteroposterior diameter of the chest. The resulting "barrel chest," however, has little effect on function.

THE HEALTH HISTORY

Common or Concerning Symptoms

- Chest pain
- Dyspnea
- Wheezing
- Cough
- Blood-streaked sputum (hemoptysis)

Complaints of *chest pain* or *chest discomfort* raise the specter of heart disease, but often arise from structures in the thorax and lung as well. To assess this symptom, you must pursue a dual investigation of both thoracic and cardiac causes. Sources of chest pain are listed below. For this important symptom, you must keep all of these in mind.

See Table 6-1. Chest Pain, pp. 234–235.

- The myocardium — Angina pectoris, myocardial infarction
- The pericardium — Pericarditis
- The aorta — Dissecting aortic aneurysm
- The trachea and large bronchi — Bronchitis
- The parietal pleura — Pericarditis, pneumonia
- The chest wall, including the musculoskeletal system and skin — Costochondritis, herpes zoster
- The esophagus — Reflux esophagitis, esophageal spasm
- Extrathoracic structures such as the neck, gallbladder, and stomach. — Cervical arthritis, biliary colic, gastritis

This section focuses on *pulmonary complaints*, including general questions about chest symptoms, dyspnea, wheezing, cough, and hemoptysis. For health history questions about exertional chest pain, palpitations, orthopnea, paroxysmal nocturnal dyspnea, and edema, see Chapter 7, The Cardiovascular System.

Your initial questions should be as broad as possible. "Do you have any discomfort or unpleasant feelings in your chest?" As you proceed to the full history, ask the patient to point to where the pain is in the chest. Watch for any gestures as the patient describes the pain. You should elicit all seven attributes of this symptom (see p. 27) to distinguish among the various causes of chest pain.

A clenched fist over the sternum suggests *angina pectoris;* a finger pointing to a tender area on the chest wall suggests musculoskeletal pain; a hand moving from neck to epigastrum suggests heartburn.

Lung tissue itself has no pain fibers. Pain in lung conditions such as pneumonia or pulmonary infarction usually arises from inflammation of the adjacent parietal pleura. Muscle strain from prolonged recurrent coughing may also be responsible. The pericardium also has few pain fibers—the pain of pericarditis stems from inflammation of the adjacent parietal pleura. (Chest pain is commonly associated with anxiety, too, but the mechanism remains obscure.)

Anxiety is the most frequent cause of chest pain in children; costochondritis is also common.

Dyspnea is a nonpainful but uncomfortable awareness of breathing that is inappropriate to the level of exertion. This serious symptom warrants a full explanation and assessment, since dyspnea commonly results from cardiac or pulmonary disease.

See Table 6-2, Dyspnea, pp. 236–237.

Ask "Have you had any difficulty breathing?" Find out when the symptom occurs, at rest or with exercise, and how much effort produces onset. Because of variations in age, body weight, and physical fitness, there is no absolute scale for quantifying dyspnea. Instead, make every effort *to determine its severity based on the patient's daily activities.* How many steps or flights of stairs can the patient climb before pausing for breath? What about work such as carrying bags of groceries, mopping the floor, or making the bed? Has dyspnea altered the patient's lifestyle and daily activities? How? Carefully elicit the timing and setting of dyspnea, any associated symptoms, and relieving or aggravating factors.

Most patients with dyspnea relate shortness of breath to their level of activity. Anxious patients present a different picture. They may describe difficulty taking a deep enough breath, or a smothering sensation with inability to get enough air, along with *paresthesias,* or sensations of tingling or "pins and needles" around the lips or in the extremities.

Anxious patients may have episodic dyspnea during both rest and exercise, and *hyperventilation,* or rapid, shallow breathing. At other times they may have frequent sighs.

Wheezes are musical respiratory sounds that may be audible both to the patient and to others.

Wheezing suggests partial airway obstruction from secretions, tissue inflammation, or a foreign body.

Cough is a common symptom that ranges in significance from trivial to ominous. Typically, cough is a reflex response to stimuli that irritate re-

See Table 6-3, Cough and Hemoptysis, p. 238.

ceptors in the larynx, trachea, or large bronchi. These stimuli include mucus, pus, and blood, as well as external agents such as dusts, foreign bodies, or even extremely hot or cold air. Other causes include inflammation of the respiratory mucosa and pressure or tension in the air passages from a tumor or enlarged peribronchial lymph nodes. Although cough typically signals a problem in the respiratory tract, it may also be cardiovascular in origin.

Cough is an important symptom of left-sided heart failure.

For complaints of cough, a thorough assessment is in order. Ask whether the cough is dry or produces *sputum*, or phlegm. Ask the patient to describe the volume of any sputum and its color, odor, and consistency.

Dry hacking cough in Mycoplasmal pneumonia; productive cough in bronchitis, viral or bacterial pneumonia

Mucoid sputum is translucent, white, or gray; *purulent* sputum is yellowish or greenish.

Foul-smelling sputum in anaerobic lung abscess; tenacious sputum in cystic fibrosis

To help patients quantify volume, a multiple-choice question may be helpful . . . "How much do you think you cough up in 24 hours; a teaspoon, tablespoon, a quarter cup, half cup, cupful?" If possible, ask the patient to cough into a tissue; inspect the phlegm and note its characteristics. The symptoms associated with a cough often lead you to its cause.

Large volumes of purulent sputum in bronchiectasis or lung abscess

Diagnostically helpful symptoms include fever, chest pain, dyspnea, orthopnea, and wheezing.

Hemoptysis is the coughing up of blood from the lungs; it may vary from blood-streaked phlegm to frank blood. For patients reporting hemoptysis, assess the volume of blood produced as well as the other sputum attributes; ask about the related setting and activity and any associated symptoms.

See Table 6-3, Cough and Hemoptysis, p. 238. Hemoptysis is rare in infants, children, and adolescents; it is seen most often in cystic fibrosis.

Before using the term "hemoptysis," try to confirm the source of the bleeding by both history and physical examination. Blood or blood-streaked material may originate in the mouth, pharynx, or gastrointestinal tract and is easily mislabeled. When vomited, it probably originates in the gastrointestinal tract. Occasionally, however, blood from the nasopharynx or the gastrointestinal tract is aspirated and then coughed out.

Blood originating in the stomach is usually darker than blood from the respiratory tract and may be mixed with food particles.

HEALTH PROMOTION AND COUNSELING

Important Topics for Health Promotion and Counseling

- Tobacco cessation

Despite declines in smoking over the past several decades, more than 27% of Americans age 12 and older still smoke.* All adults, pregnant women, parents, and adolescents who smoke should be counseled regularly to stop smoking. Smoking has been definitively linked to significant pulmonary, cardiovascular, and neoplastic disease, and accounts for one out of every five deaths in the United States.† It is considered the leading cause of preventable death. Nonsmokers exposed to smoke are also at increased risk for lung cancer, ear and respiratory infection, asthma, low birthweight, and residential fires. Smoking exposes patients not only to carcinogens, but also to nicotine, an addictive drug. Be especially alert to smoking by teenagers, the age group when tobacco use often begins, and by pregnant women, who may continue smoking during pregnancy.

The disease risks of smoking drop significantly within a year of smoking cessation. Effective interventions include targeted messages by clinicians, group counseling, and use of nicotine-replacement therapies. Clinicians are advised to adopt the four "As":

- **A**sk about smoking at each visit.
- **A**dvise patients regularly to stop smoking in a clear personalized message.
- **A**ssist patients to set stop dates and provide educational materials for self-help.
- **A**rrange for follow-up visits to monitor and support progress.

Preview: Recording the Physical Examination—The Thorax and Lungs

Note that initially you may use sentences to describe your findings; later you will use phrases. The style below contains phrases appropriate for most write-ups. Unfamiliar terms are explained in the next section, Techniques of Examination.

> "Thorax is symmetric with good expansion. Lungs resonant. Breath sounds vesicular; no rales, wheezes, or rhonchi. Diaphragms descend 4 cm bilaterally."
>
> **OR**
>
> "Thorax symmetric with moderate kyphosis and increased anteroposterior (AP) diameter, decreased expansion. Lungs are hyperresonant. Breath sounds distant with delayed expiratory phase and scattered expiratory wheezes. Fremitus decreased; no bronchophony, egophony, or whispered pectoriloquy. Diaphragms descend 2 cm bilaterally."

Suggests chronic obstructive lung disease

* Substance Abuse and Mental Health Services Administration, 1999 National Household Survey. www.samhsa.gov/hhsurvey/content/1999. Accessed 8/13/01.

† Centers for Disease Control and Prevention. Cigarette Smoking: Attributable Mortality and Years of Potential Life Cost—United States. MMWR 42: 645–649, 1993.

Combining clinician and group counseling with nicotine replacement therapy is especially effective for highly addicted patients.

Relapses are common and should be expected. Nicotine withdrawal, weight gain, stress, social pressure, and use of alcohol are often cited as explanations. Help patients to learn from these experiences: work with the patient to pinpoint the precipitating circumstances and develop strategies for alternative responses and health-promoting behaviors.

TECHNIQUES OF EXAMINATION

It is helpful to examine the posterior thorax and lungs while the patient is sitting, and the anterior thorax and lungs with the patient supine. Proceed in an orderly fashion: inspect, palpate, percuss, and auscultate. Try to visualize the underlying lobes, and compare one side with the other, so the patient serves as his or her own control. Arrange the patient's gown so that you can see the chest fully. For women, drape the gown over each half of the anterior chest as you examine the other half. Cover the woman's anterior chest when you examine the back.

With the patient sitting, examine the posterior thorax and lungs. The patient's arms should be folded across the chest with hands resting, if possible, on the opposite shoulders. This position moves the scapulae partly out of the way and increases your access to the lung fields. Then ask the patient to lie down.

With the patient supine, examine the anterior thorax and lungs. The supine position makes it easier to examine women because the breasts can be gently displaced. Furthermore, wheezes, if present, are more likely to be heard. (Some authorities, however, prefer to examine both the back and the front of the chest with the patient sitting. This technique is also satisfactory).

For patients unable to sit up without aid, try to get help so that you can examine the posterior chest in the sitting position. If this is impossible, roll the patient to one side and then to the other. Percuss the upper lung, and auscultate both lungs in each position. Because ventilation is relatively greater in the dependent lung, your chances of hearing wheezes or crackles are greater on the dependent side.

Initial Survey of Respiration and the Thorax

Even though you may have already recorded the respiratory rate when you took the vital signs, it is wise to again *observe the rate, rhythm, depth, and effort of breathing.* A normal resting adult breathes quietly and regularly about

See Table 6-1. Chest Pain, pp. 234–235.

14 to 20 times a minute. An occasional sigh is to be expected. Note whether expiration lasts longer than usual.

Always inspect the patient for any signs of respiratory difficulty.

- *Assess the patient's color* for cyanosis. Recall any relevant findings from earlier parts of your examination, such as the shape of the fingernails.

Cyanosis signals hypoxia. Clubbing of the nails (see p. 110) in chronic obstructive pulmonary disease (COPD) or congenital heart disease

- *Listen to the patient's breathing.* Is there any *audible wheezing?* If so, where does it fall in the respiratory cycle?

Audible *stridor,* a high-pitched wheeze, is an ominous sign of airway obstruction in the larynx or trachea.

- *Inspect the neck.* During inspiration, is there contraction of the sternomastoid or other accessory muscles, or supraclavicular retraction? Is the trachea midline?

Inspiratory contraction of the sternomastoids at rest signals severe difficulty breathing. Lateral displacement of the trachea in pneumothorax, pleural effusion, or atelectasis

Also *observe the shape of the chest.* The anteroposterior (AP) diameter may increase with aging.

The AP diameter also may increase in COPD.

Examination of the Posterior Chest

INSPECTION

From a midline position behind the patient, note the *shape of the chest* and *the way in which it moves,* including:

- Deformities or asymmetry

See Table 6-4, Deformities of the Thorax (p. 239).

- Abnormal retraction of the interspaces during inspiration. Retraction is most apparent in the lower interspaces. Supraclavicular retraction is often associated.

Retraction in severe asthma, COPD, or upper airway obstruction.

- Impaired respiratory movement on one or both sides or a unilateral lag (or delay) in movement.

Unilateral impairment or lagging of respiratory movement suggests disease of the underlying lung or pleura.

PALPATION

As you palpate the chest, focus on areas of tenderness and abnormalities in the overlying skin, respiratory expansion, and fremitus.

Intercostal tenderness over inflamed pleura

Identify tender areas. Carefully palpate any area where pain has been reported or where lesions or bruises are evident.

Bruises over a fractured rib

Assess any observed abnormalities such as masses or sinus tracts (blind, inflammatory, tubelike structures opening onto the skin)

Although rare, sinus tracts usually indicate infection of the underlying pleura and lung (as in tuberculosis, actinomycosis).

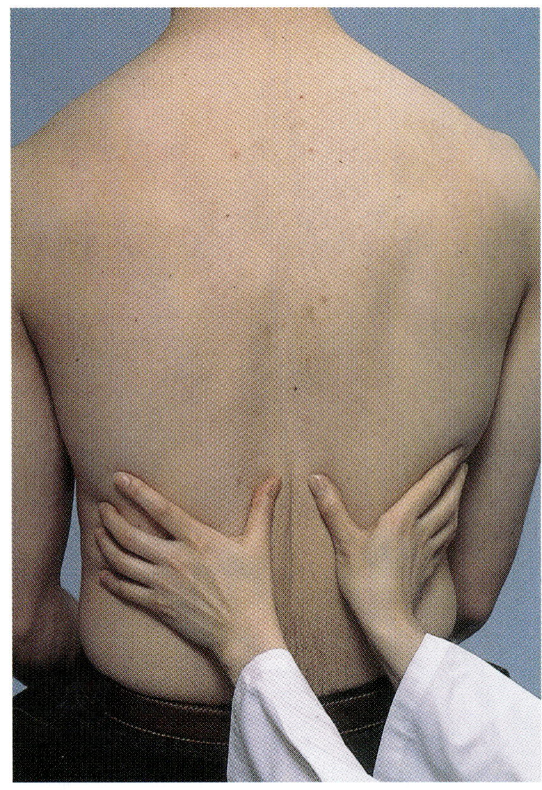

Test chest expansion. Place your thumbs at about the level of the 10th ribs, with your fingers loosely grasping and parallel to the lateral rib cage. As you position your hands, slide them medially just enough to raise a loose fold of skin on each side between your thumb and the spine.

Ask the patient to inhale deeply. Watch the distance between your thumbs as they move apart during inspiration, and feel for the range and symmetry of the rib cage as it expands and contracts.

Causes of unilateral decrease or delay in chest expansion include chronic fibrotic disease of the underlying lung or pleura, pleural effusion, lobar pneumonia, pleural pain with associated splinting, and unilateral bronchial obstruction.

Feel for tactile fremitus. Fremitus refers to the palpable vibrations transmitted through the bronchopulmonary tree to the chest wall when the patient speaks. To detect fremitus, use either the ball (the bony part of the palm at the base of the fingers) or the ulnar surface of your hand to optimize the vibratory sensitivity of the bones in your hand. Ask the patient to repeat the words "ninety-nine" or "one-one-one." If fremitus is faint, ask the patient to speak more loudly or in a deeper voice.

Use one hand until you have learned the feel of fremitus. Some clinicians find using one hand more accurate. The simultaneous use of both hands to compare sides, however, increases your speed and may facilitate detection of differences.

Fremitus is decreased or absent when the voice is soft or when the transmission of vibrations from the larynx to the surface of the chest is impeded. Causes include an obstructed bronchus; COPD; separation of the pleural surfaces by fluid (pleural effusion), fibrosis (pleural thickening), air (pneumothorax), or an infiltrating tumor; and also a very thick chest wall.

Palpate and compare symmetric areas of the lungs in the pattern shown in the photograph. Identify and locate any areas of increased, decreased, or absent fremitus. Fremitus is typically more prominent in the interscapular area than in the lower lung fields, and is often more prominent on the right side than on the left. It disappears below the diaphragm.

Tactile fremitus is a relatively rough assessment tool, but as a scouting technique it directs your attention to possible abnormalities. Later in the examination you will check any suggested findings by listening for breath sounds, voice sounds, and whispered voice sounds. All these attributes tend to increase or decrease together.

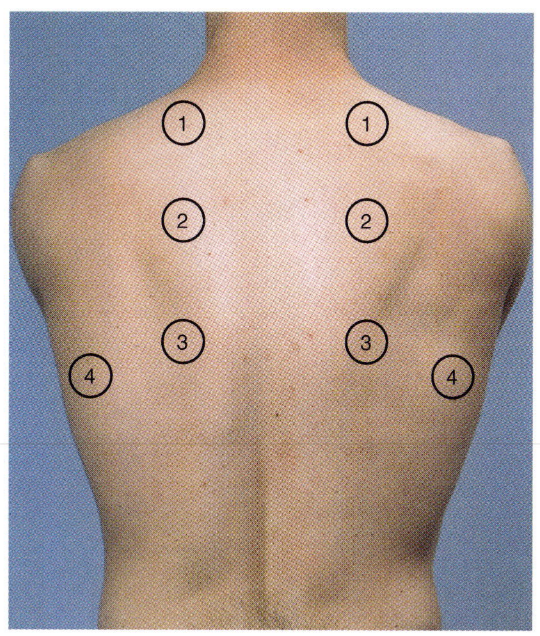

LOCATIONS FOR FEELING FREMITUS

PERCUSSION

Percussion is one of the most important techniques of physical examination. Percussion of the chest sets the chest wall and underlying tissues into motion, producing audible sound and palpable vibrations. Percussion helps you establish whether the underlying tissues are air-filled, fluid-filled, or solid. It penetrates only about 5 cm to 7 cm into the chest, however, and therefore will not help you to detect deep-seated lesions.

The technique of percussion can be practiced on any surface. As you practice, listen for changes in percussion notes over different types of materials or different parts of the body. The key points for good technique, described for a right-handed person, are as follows:

- Hyperextend the middle finger of your left hand, known as the pleximeter finger. Press its distal interphalangeal joint firmly on the surface to be percussed. Avoid surface contact by any other part of the hand, because this dampens out vibrations. Note that the thumb, 2nd, 4th, and 5th fingers are not touching the chest.

- Position your right forearm quite close to the surface, with the hand cocked upward. The middle finger should be partially flexed, relaxed, and poised to strike.

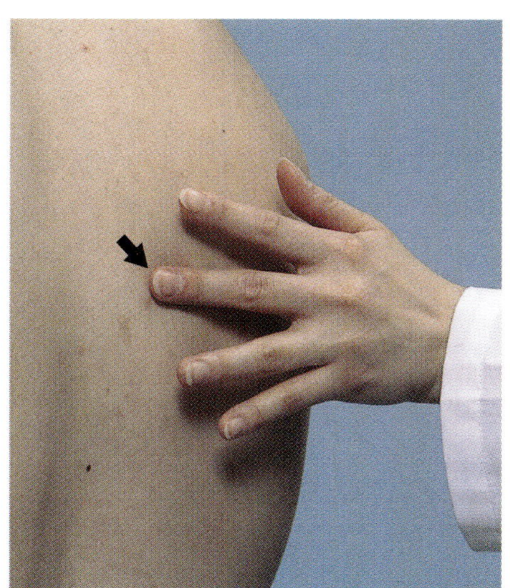

- With a *quick sharp but relaxed wrist motion,* strike the pleximeter finger with the right middle finger, or plexor finger. Aim at your distal interphalangeal joint. You are trying to transmit vibrations through the bones of this joint to the underlying chest wall.

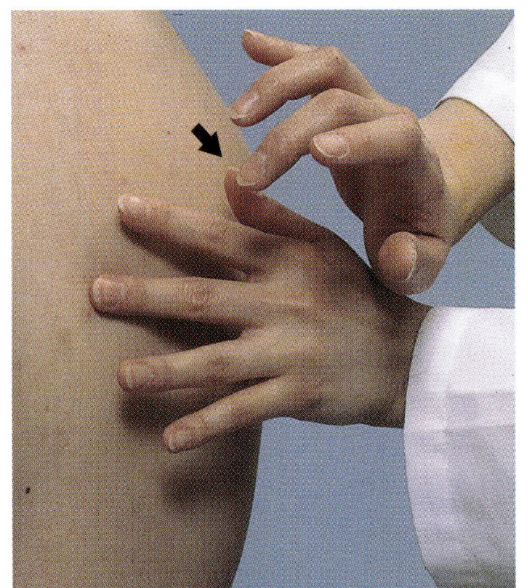

Strike using the *tip of the plexor finger,* not the finger pad. Your finger should be almost at right angles to the pleximeter. A short fingernail is recommended to avoid self-injury.

- Withdraw your striking finger quickly to avoid damping the vibrations you have created.

In summary, the movement is at the wrist. It is directed, brisk yet relaxed, and a bit bouncy.

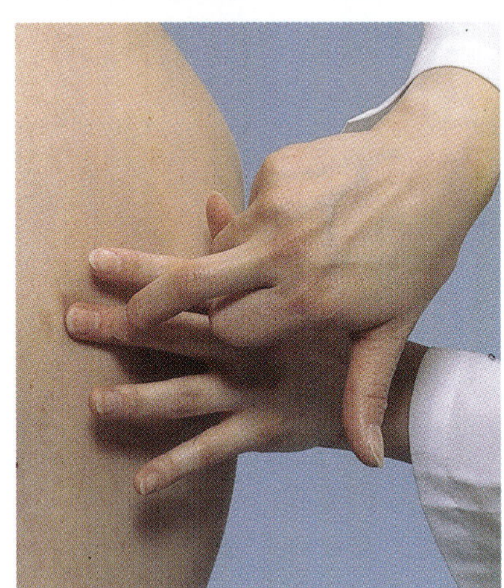

Percussion Notes. With your plexor or tapping finger, use the lightest percussion that produces a clear note. A thick chest wall requires heavier percussion than a thin one. However, if a *louder* note is needed, apply more pressure with the *pleximeter* finger (this is more effective for increasing percussion note volume than tapping harder with the plexor finger).

When percussing the lower posterior chest, stand somewhat to the side rather than directly behind the patient. This allows you to place your pleximeter finger more firmly on the chest and your plexor is more effective, making a better percussion note.

When comparing two areas, use the same percussion technique in both areas. Percuss or strike twice in each location. It is easier to detect differences in percussion notes by comparing one area with another than by striking repetitively in one place.

Learn to identify five percussion notes. You can practice four of them on yourself. These notes differ in their basic qualities of sound: intensity, pitch, and duration. Train your ear to distinguish these differences by concentrating on one quality at a time as you percuss first in one location, then in another. Review the table below. Normal lungs are *resonant.*

Percussion Notes and Their Characteristics

	Relative Intensity	Relative Pitch	Relative Duration	Example of Location	Pathologic Examples
Flatness	Soft	High	Short	Thigh	Large pleural effusion
Dullness	Medium	Medium	Medium	Liver	Lobar pneumonia
Resonance	Loud	Low	Long	Normal lung	Simple chronic bronchitis
Hyperresonance	Very loud	Lower	Longer	None normally	Emphysema, pneumothorax
Tympany	Loud	High*	*	Gastric air bubble or puffed-out cheek	Large pneumothorax

* Distinguished mainly by its musical timbre.

While the patient keeps both arms crossed in front of the chest, percuss the thorax in symmetric locations from the apices to the lung bases.

Percuss one side of the chest and then the other at each level, as shown by the numbers below. Omit the areas over the scapulae—the thickness of muscle and bone alters the percussion notes over the lungs. Identify and locate the area and quality of any abnormal percussion note.

Dullness replaces resonance when fluid or solid tissue replaces air-containing lung or occupies the pleural space beneath your percussing fingers. Examples include: lobar pneumonia, in which the alveoli are filled with fluid and blood cells; and pleural accumulations of serous fluid (pleural effusion), blood (hemothorax), pus (empyema), fibrous tissue, or tumor.

Generalized hyperresonance may be heard over the hyperinflated lungs of emphysema or asthma, but it is not a reliable sign. Unilateral hyperresonance suggests a large pneumothorax or possibly a large air-filled bulla in the lung.

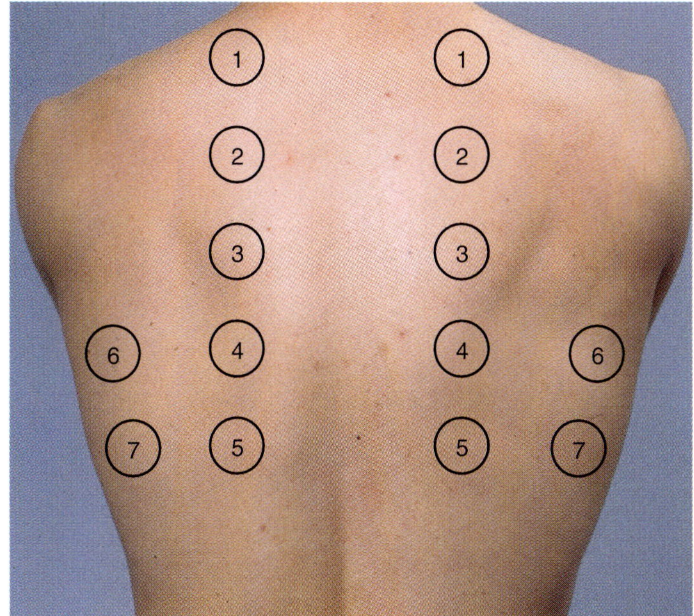

LOCATIONS FOR PERCUSSION AND AUSCULTATION

Identify the descent of the diaphragms, or *diaphragmatic excursion.* First, *determine the level of diaphragmatic dullness* during quiet respiration. Holding the pleximeter finger *above and parallel* to the expected level of dullness, percuss downward in progressive steps until dullness clearly replaces resonance. Confirm this level of change by percussion near the middle of the hemothorax and also more laterally.

An abnormally high level suggests pleural effusion, or a high diaphragm as in atelectasis or diaphragmatic paralysis.

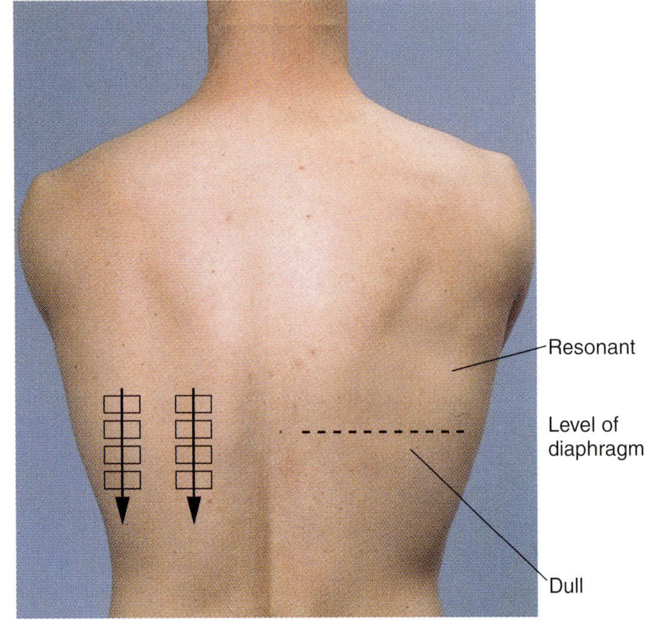

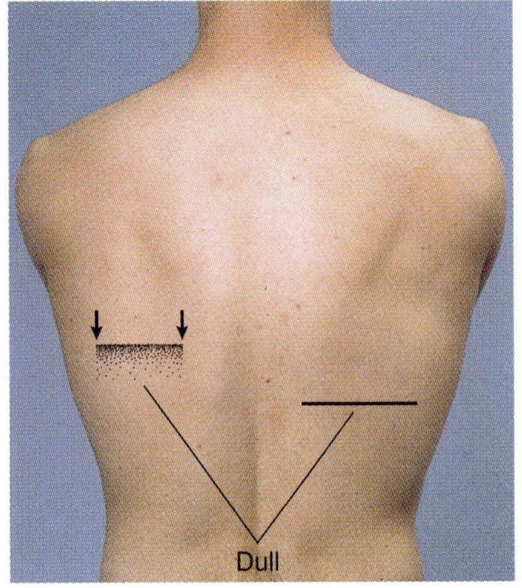

Note that with this technique you are identifying the boundary between the resonant lung tissue and the duller structures below the diaphragm. You are not percussing the diaphragm itself. You can infer the probable location of the diaphragm from the level of dullness.

Now, *estimate the extent of diaphragmatic excursion* by determining the distance between the level of dullness on full expiration and the level of dullness on full inspiration, normally about 5 cm or 6 cm. This estimate does not correlate well, however, with radiologic assessment of diaphragmatic movement.

AUSCULTATION

Auscultation of the lungs is the most important examining technique for assessing air flow through the tracheobronchial tree. Together with percussion, it also helps the clinician to assess the condition of the surrounding lungs and pleural space. Auscultation involves (1) listening to the sounds generated by breathing, (2) listening for any adventitious (added) sounds, and (3) if abnormalities are suspected, listening to the sounds of the patient's spoken or whispered voice as they are transmitted through the chest wall.

Sounds from bedclothes, paper gowns, and the chest itself can generate confusion in auscultation. Hair on the chest may cause crackling sounds. Either press harder or wet the hair. If the patient is cold or tense, you may hear muscle contraction sounds—muffled, low-pitched rumbling or roaring noises. A change in the patient's position may eliminate this noise. You can

Breath Sounds (Lung Sounds). You will learn to identify patterns of breath sounds by their intensity, their pitch, and the relative duration of their inspiratory and expiratory phases. Normal breath sounds are:

- *Vesicular,* or soft and low pitched. They are heard through inspiration, continue without pause through expiration, and then fade away about one third of the way through expiration.
- *Bronchovesicular,* with inspiratory and expiratory sounds about equal in length, at times separated by a silent interval. Differences in pitch and intensity are often more easily detected during expiration.
- *Bronchial,* or louder and higher in pitch, with a short silence between inspiratory and expiratory sounds. Expiratory sounds last longer than inspiratory sounds.

reproduce this sound on yourself by doing a Valsalva maneuver (straining down) as you listen to your own chest.

The characteristics of these three kinds of breath sounds are summarized in the table below. Also shown are the *tracheal* breath sounds—very loud, harsh sounds that are heard by listening over the trachea in the neck.

Characteristics of Breath Sounds

	Duration of Sounds	Intensity of Expiratory Sound	Pitch of Expiratory Sound	Locations Where Heard Normally
Vesicular*	Inspiratory sounds last longer than expiratory ones.	Soft	Relatively low	Over most of both lungs
Broncho-vesicular	Inspiratory and expiratory sounds are about equal.	Intermediate	Intermediate	Often in the 1st and 2nd interspaces anteriorly and between the scapulae
Bronchial	Expiratory sounds last longer than inspiratory ones.	Loud	Relatively high	Over the manubrium, if heard at all
Tracheal	Inspiratory and expiratory sounds are about equal.	Very loud	Relatively high	Over the trachea in the neck

* The thickness of the bars indicates intensity; the steeper their incline, the higher the pitch.

If bronchovesicular or bronchial breath sounds are heard in locations distant from those listed, suspect that air-filled lung has been replaced by fluid-filled or solid lung tissue. See Table 6-5, Normal and Altered Breath and Voice Sounds (p. 240).

Listen to the breath sounds with the diaphragm of a stethoscope after instructing the patient to breathe deeply through an open mouth. Use the pattern suggested for percussion, moving from one side to the other and comparing symmetric areas of the lungs. If you hear or suspect abnormal sounds, auscultate adjacent areas so that you can fully describe the extent of any abnormality. Listen to at least one full breath in each location. Be alert for patient discomfort due to hyperventilation (e.g., light headedness, faintness), and allow the patient to rest as needed.

Note the *intensity* of the breath sounds. Breath sounds are usually louder in the lower posterior lung fields and may also vary from area to area. If the breath sounds seem faint, ask the patient to breathe more deeply. You may then hear them easily. When patients do not breathe deeply enough or when they have a thick chest wall, as in obesity, breath sounds may remain diminished.

Breath sounds may be decreased when air flow is decreased (as by obstructive lung disease or muscular weakness) or when the transmission of sound is poor (as in pleural effusion, pneumothorax, or emphysema).

Is there a *silent gap* between the inspiratory and expiratory sounds?

A gap suggests bronchial breath sounds.

Listen for the *pitch, intensity, and duration of the expiratory and inspiratory sounds*. Are vesicular breath sounds distributed normally over the chest wall? Or are there bronchovesicular or bronchial breath sounds in unexpected places? If so, where are they?

Adventitious (Added) Sounds. Listen for any added, or adventitious, sounds that are superimposed on the usual breath sounds. Detection of adventitious sounds—*crackles* (sometimes called *rales*), *wheezes, and rhonchi*—is an important part of your examination, often leading to diagnosis of cardiac and pulmonary conditions. The most common kinds of these sounds are described below:

For further discussion and other added sounds, see Table 6-6, Adventitious (Added) Lung Sounds: Causes and Qualities (p. 241).

Adventitious Lung Sounds

DISCONTINUOUS SOUNDS (CRACKLES OR RALES) are intermittent, nonmusical, and brief—like dots in time

Fine crackles (• • • • •) are soft, high pitched, and very brief (5–10 msec).

Coarse crackles (● ● ● ● ●) are somewhat louder, lower in pitch, and not quite so brief (20–30 msec).

Crackles may be due to abnormalities of the lungs (pneumonia, fibrosis, early congestive heart failure) or of the airways (bronchitis, bronchiectasis).

CONTINUOUS SOUNDS are > 250 msec, notably longer than crackles—like dashes in time—but do not necessarily persist throughout the respiratory cycle. Unlike crackles, they are musical.

Wheezes (WWWW) are relatively high pitched (around 400 Hz or higher) and have a hissing or shrill quality.

Wheezes suggest narrowed airways, as in asthma, COPD, or bronchitis.

Rhonchi (VWW) are relatively low pitched (around 200 Hz or lower) and have a snoring quality.

Rhonchi suggest secretions in large airways.

If you hear *crackles*, especially those that do not clear after cough, listen carefully for the following characteristics. These are clues to the underlying condition:

- Loudness, pitch, and duration (summarized as fine or coarse crackles)
- Number (few to many)

Fine late inspiratory crackles that persist from breath to breath suggest abnormal lung tissue.

- Timing in the respiratory cycle
- Location on the chest wall
- Persistence of their pattern from breath to breath
- Any change after a cough or a change in the patient's position

Clearing of crackles, wheezes, or rhonchi after cough suggests that secretions caused them, as in bronchitis or atelectasis.

In some normal people, crackles may be heard at the lung bases anteriorly after maximal expiration. Crackles in dependent portions of the lungs may also occur after prolonged recumbency.

If you hear *wheezes or rhonchi,* note their timing and location. Do they change with deep breathing or coughing?

Transmitted Voice Sounds. If you hear abnormally located broncho-vesicular or bronchial breath sounds, continue on to assess transmitted voice sounds. With a stethoscope, listen in symmetric areas over the chest wall as you:

Increased transmission of voice sounds suggests that air-filled lung has become airless. See Table 6-5, Normal and Altered Breath and Voice Sounds (p. 240).

- Ask the patient to say "ninety-nine." Normally the sounds transmitted through the chest wall are muffled and indistinct.

Louder, clearer voice sounds are called *bronchophony.*

- Ask the patient to say "ee." You will normally hear a muffled long E sound.

When "ee" is heard as "ay," an *E-to-A change (egophony)* is present, as in lobar consolidation from pneumonia. The quality sounds nasal.

- Ask the patient to whisper "ninety-nine" or "one-two-three." The whispered voice is normally heard faintly and indistinctly, if at all.

Louder, clearer whispered sounds are called *whispered pectoriloquy.*

Examination of the Anterior Chest

The patient, when examined in the supine position, should lie comfortably with arms somewhat abducted. A patient who is having difficulty breathing should be examined in the sitting position or with the head of the bed elevated to a comfortable level.

Persons with severe COPD may prefer to sit leaning forward, with lips pursed during exhalation and arms supported on their knees or a table.

INSPECTION

Observe *the shape of the patient's chest* and *the movement of the chest wall.* Note:

- Deformities or asymmetry

See Table 6-4, Deformities of the Thorax (p. 239).

- Abnormal retraction of the lower interspaces during inspiration

Severe asthma, COPD, or upper airway obstruction

- Local lag or impairment in respiratory movement

Underlying disease of lung or pleura

PALPATION

Palpation has four potential uses:

- *Identification of tender areas*

Tender pectoral muscles or costal cartilages tend to corroborate, but do not prove, that chest pain has a musculoskeletal origin.

- *Assessment of observed abnormalities*
- *Further assessment of chest expansion.* Place your thumbs along each costal margin, your hands along the lateral rib cage. As you position your hands, slide them medially a bit to raise loose skin folds between your thumbs. Ask the patient to inhale deeply. Observe how far your thumbs diverge as the thorax expands, and feel for the extent and symmetry of respiratory movement.

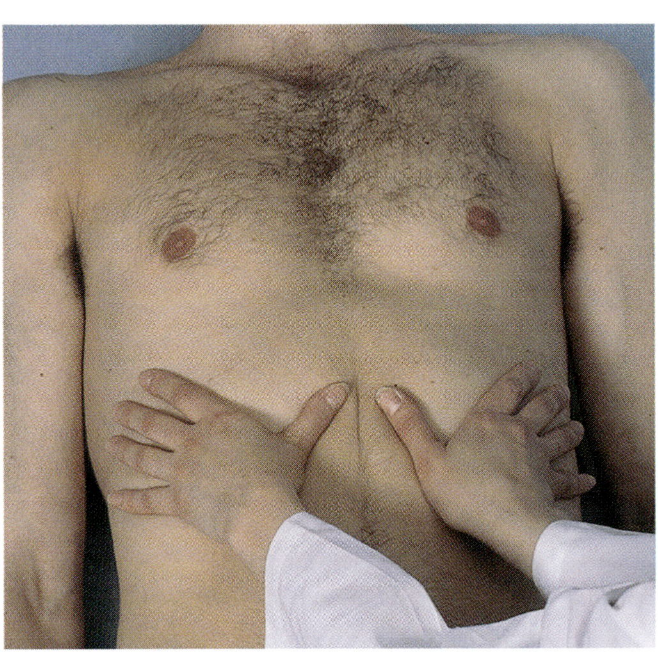

- *Assessment of tactile fremitus.* Compare both sides of the chest, using the ball or ulnar surface of your hand. Fremitus is usually decreased or absent over the precordium. When examining a woman, gently displace the breasts as necessary.

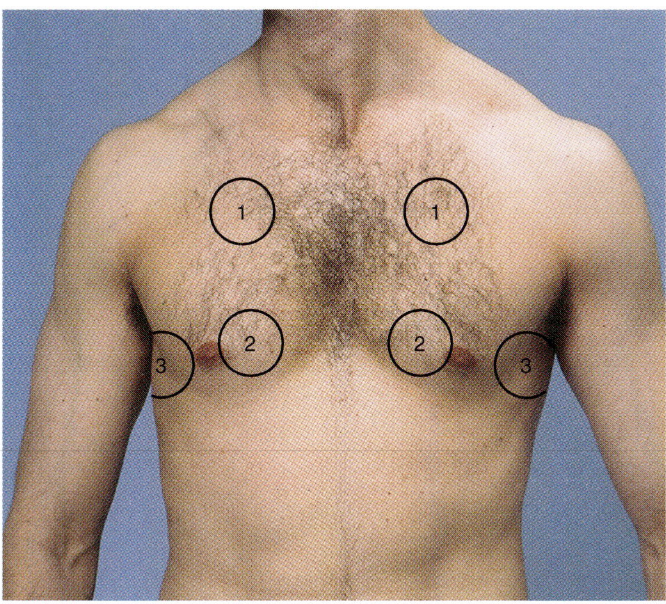

LOCATIONS FOR FEELING FREMITUS

PERCUSSION

Percuss the anterior and lateral chest, again comparing both sides. The heart normally produces an area of dullness to the left of the sternum from the 3rd to the 5th interspaces. Percuss the left lung lateral to it.

Dullness replaces resonance when fluid or solid tissue replaces air-containing lung or occupies the pleural space. Because pleural fluid usually sinks to the lowest part of the pleural space (posteriorly in a supine patient), only a very large effusion can be detected anteriorly.

The hyperresonance of COPD may totally replace cardiac dullness.

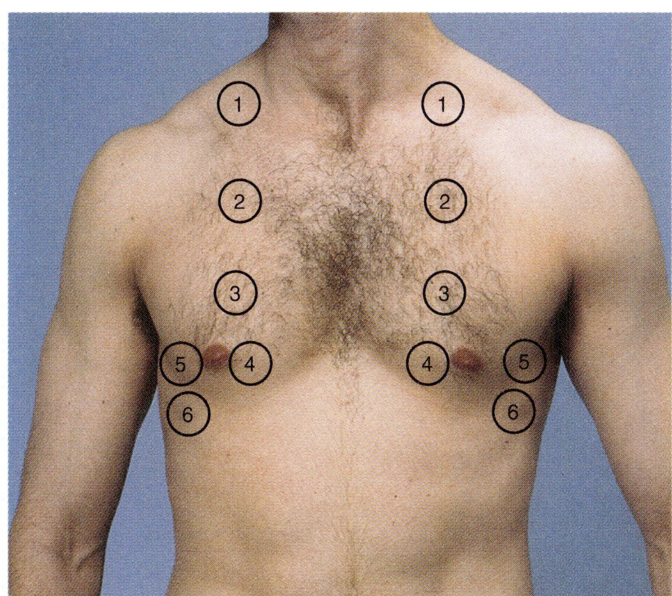

LOCATIONS FOR PERCUSSION AND AUSCULTATION

In a woman, to enhance percussion, gently displace the breast with your left hand while percussing with the right.

The dullness of right middle lobe pneumonia typically occurs behind the right breast. Unless you displace the breast, you may miss the abnormal percussion note.

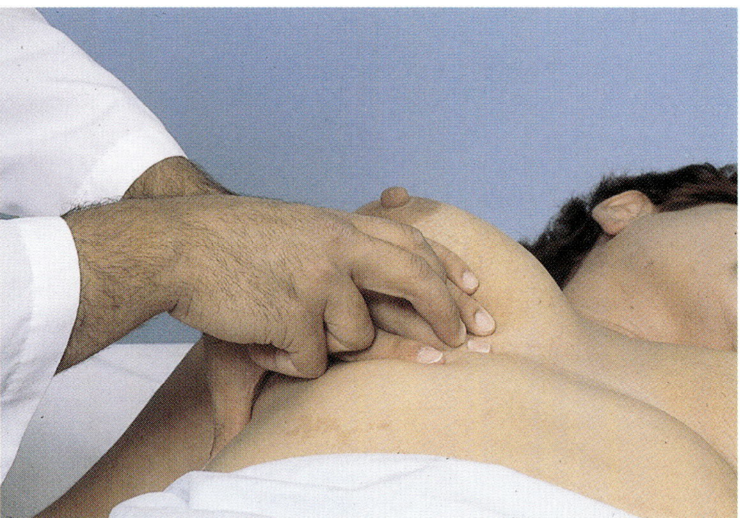

Alternatively, you may ask the patient to move her breast for you.

Identify and locate any area of abnormal percussion note.

With your pleximeter finger above and parallel to the expected upper border of liver dullness, percuss in progressive steps downward in the right midclavicular line. Identify the upper border of liver dullness. Later, during the abdominal examination, you will use this method to estimate the size of the liver. As you percuss down the chest on the left, the resonance of normal lung usually changes to the tympany of the gastric air bubble.

A lung affected by COPD often displaces the upper border of the liver downward. It also lowers the level of diaphragmatic dullness posteriorly.

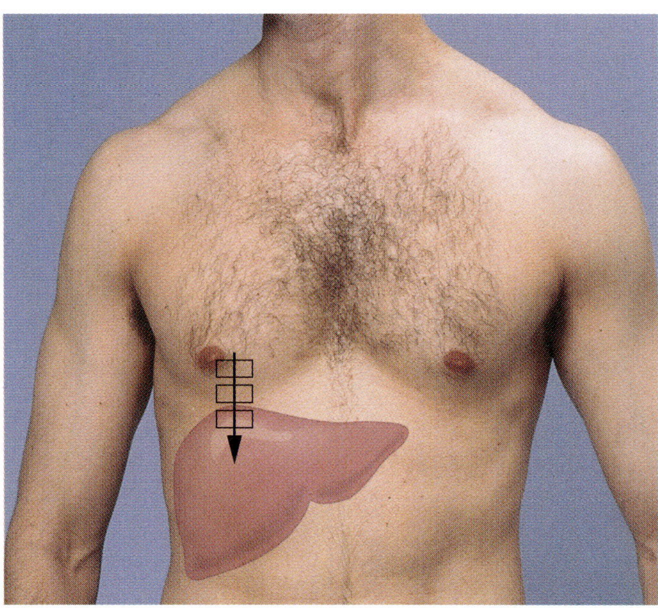

AUSCULTATION

Listen to the chest anteriorly and laterally as the patient breathes with mouth open, somewhat more deeply than normal. Compare symmetric areas of the lungs, using the pattern suggested for percussion and extending it to adjacent areas as indicated.

Listen to the breath sounds, noting their intensity and identifying any variations from normal vesicular breathing. Breath sounds are usually louder in the upper anterior lung fields. Bronchovesicular breath sounds may be heard over the large airways, especially on the right.

Identify any adventitious sounds, time them in the respiratory cycle, and locate them on the chest wall. Do they clear with deep breathing?

If indicated, *listen for transmitted voice sounds.*

See Table 6-6, Adventitious (Added) Lung Sounds: Causes and Qualities (p. 241), and Table 6-7, Physical Findings in Selected Chest Disorders (pp. 242–243).

Special Techniques

Clinical Assessment of Pulmonary Function. A simple but informative way to assess the complaint of breathlessness in an ambulatory patient is to walk with the patient down the hall or climb one flight of stairs. Observe the rate, effort, and sound of the patient's breathing.

Forced Expiratory Time. This test assesses the expiratory phase of breathing, which is typically slowed in obstructive pulmonary disease. Ask the patient to take a deep breath in and then breathe out as quickly and completely as possible with mouth open. Listen over the trachea with the diaphragm of a stethoscope and time the audible expiration. Try to get three consistent readings, allowing a short rest between efforts if necessary.

If the patient understands and cooperates in performing the test, a forced expiration time of 6 or more seconds suggests obstructive pulmonary disease.

Identification of a Fractured Rib. Local pain and tenderness of one or more ribs raise the question of fracture. By anteroposterior compression of the chest, you can help to distinguish a fracture from soft-tissue injury. With one hand on the sternum and the other on the thoracic spine, squeeze the chest. Is this painful, and where?

An increase in the local pain (distant from your hands) suggests rib fracture rather than just soft tissue injury.

TABLE 6-1 ■ Chest Pain

Problem	Process	Location	Quality	Severity
Cardiovascular				
Angina Pectoris	Temporary myocardial ischemia, usually secondary to coronary atherosclerosis	Retrosternal or across the anterior chest, sometimes radiating to the shoulders, arms, neck, lower jaw, or upper abdomen	Pressing, squeezing, tight, heavy, occasionally burning	Mild to moderate, sometimes perceived as discomfort rather than pain
Myocardial Infarction	Prolonged myocardial ischemia, resulting in irreversible muscle damage or necrosis	Same as in angina	Same as in angina	Often but not always a severe pain
Pericarditis	■ Irritation of parietal pleura adjacent to the pericardium	Precordial, may radiate to the tip of the shoulder and to the neck	Sharp, knifelike	Often severe
	■ Mechanism unclear	Retrosternal	Crushing	Severe
Dissecting Aortic Aneurysm	A splitting within the layers of the aortic wall, allowing passage of blood to dissect a channel	Anterior chest, radiating to the neck, back, or abdomen	Ripping, tearing	Very severe
Pulmonary				
Tracheobronchitis	Inflammation of trachea and large bronchi	Upper sternal or on either side of the sternum	Burning	Mild to moderate
Pleural Pain	Inflammation of the parietal pleura, as from pleurisy, pneumonia, pulmonary infarction, or neoplasm	Chest wall overlying the process	Sharp, knifelike	Often severe
Gastrointestinal and other				
Reflex Esophagitis	Inflammation of the esophageal mucosa by reflux of gastric acid	Retrosternal, may radiate to the back	Burning, may be squeezing	Mild to severe
Diffuse Esophageal Spasm	Motor dysfunction of the esophageal muscle	Retrosternal, may radiate to the back, arms, and jaw	Usually squeezing	Mild to severe
Chest Wall Pain	Variable, often unclear	Often below the left breast or along the costal cartilages; also elsewhere	Stabbing, sticking, or dull, aching	Variable
Anxiety	Unclear	Precordial, below the left breast, or across the anterior chest	Stabbing, sticking, or dull, aching	Variable

Note: Remember that chest pain may be referred from extrathoracic structures such as the neck (arthritis) and abdomen (biliary colic, acute cholecystitis). Pleural pain may be due to abdominal conditions such as subdiaphragmatic abscess.

Timing	Factors That Aggravate	Factors That Relieve	Associated Symptoms
Usually 1–3 min but up to 10 min. Prolonged episodes up to 20 min	Exertion, especially in the cold; meals; emotional stress. May occur at rest	Rest, nitroglycerin	Sometimes dyspnea, nausea, sweating
20 min to several hr			Nausea, vomiting, sweating, weakness
Persistent	Breathing, changing position, coughing, lying down, sometimes swallowing	Sitting forward may relieve it.	Of the underlying illness
Persistent			Of the underlying illness
Abrupt onset, early peak, persistent for hours or more	Hypertension		Syncope, hemiplegia, paraplegia
Variable	Coughing		Cough
Persistent	Breathing, coughing, movements of the trunk	Lying on the involved side may relieve it.	Of the underlying illness
Variable	Large meal; bending over, lying down	Antacids, sometimes belching	Sometimes regurgitation, dysphagia
Variable	Swallowing of food or cold liquid; emotional stress	Sometimes nitroglycerin	Dysphagia
Fleeting to hours or days	Movement of chest, trunk, arms		Often local tenderness
Fleeting to hours or day	May follow effort, emotional stress		Breathlessness, palpitations, weakness, anxiety

TABLE 6-2 ■ Dyspnea

Problem	Process	Timing
Left-Sided Heart Failure *(left ventricular failure or mitral stenosis)*	Elevated pressure in pulmonary capillary bed with transudation of fluid into interstitial spaces and alveoli, decreased compliance (increased stiffness) of the lungs, increased work of breathing	Dyspnea may progress slowly, or suddenly as in acute pulmonary edema.
Chronic Bronchitis*	Excessive mucus production in bronchi, followed by chronic obstruction of airways	Chronic productive cough followed by slowly progressive dyspnea
Chronic Obstructive Pulmonary Disease (COPD)*	Overdistention of air spaces distal to terminal bronchioles, with destruction of alveolar septa and chronic obstruction of the airways	Slowly progressive dyspnea; relatively mild cough later
Asthma	Bronchial hyperresponsiveness involving release of inflammatory mediators, increased airway secretions, and bronchoconstriction	Acute episodes, separated by symptom-free periods. Nocturnal episodes are common.
Diffuse Interstitial Lung Diseases *(such as sarcoidosis, widespread neoplasms, asbestosis, and idiopathic pulmonary fibrosis)*	Abnormal and widespread infiltration of cells, fluid, and collagen into interstitial spaces between alveoli. Many causes	Progressive dyspnea, which varies in its rate of development with the cause
Pneumonia	Inflammation of lung parenchyma from the respiratory bronchioles to the alveoli	An acute illness, timing varies with the causative agent
Spontaneous Pneumothorax	Leakage of air into pleural space through blebs on visceral pleura, with resulting partial or complete collapse of the lung	Sudden onset of dyspnea
Acute Pulmonary Embolism	Sudden occlusion of all or part of pulmonary arterial tree by a blood clot that usually originates in deep veins of legs or pelvis	Sudden onset of dyspnea
Anxiety With Hyperventilation	Overbreathing, with resultant respiratory alkalosis and fall in the partial pressure of carbon dioxide in the blood	Episodic, often recurrent

*Chronic bronchitis and *chronic obstructive pulmonary disease (COPD)* may coexist.

Factors That Aggravate	Factors That Relieve	Associated Symptoms	Setting
Exertion, lying down	Rest, sitting up, though dyspnea may become persistent	Often cough, orthopnea, paroxysmal nocturnal dyspnea; sometimes wheezing	History of heart disease or its predisposing factors
Exertion, inhaled irritants, respiratory infections	Expectoration; rest, though dyspnea may become persistent	Chronic productive cough, recurrent respiratory infections; wheezing may develop	History of smoking, air pollutants, recurrent respiratory infections
Exertion	Rest, though dyspnea may become persistent	Cough, with scant mucoid sputum	History of smoking, air pollutants, sometimes a familial deficiency in $alpha_1$-antitrypsin
Variable, including allergens, irritants, respiratory infections, exercise, and emotion	Separation from aggravating factors	Wheezing, cough, tightness in chest	Environmental and emotional conditions
Exertion	Rest, though dyspnea may become persistent	Often weakness, fatigue. Cough less common than in other lung diseases	Varied. Exposure to one of many substances may be causative.
		Pleuritic pain, cough, sputum, fever, though not necessarily present	Varied
		Pleuritic pain, cough	Often a previously healthy young adult
		Often none. Retrosternal oppressive pain if the occlusion is massive. Pleuritic pain, cough, and hemoptysis may follow an embolism if pulmonary infarction ensues. Symptoms of anxiety (see below).	Postpartum or postoperative periods; prolonged bed rest; congestive heart failure, chronic lung disease, and fractures of hip or leg; deep venous thrombosis (often not clinically apparent)
More often occurs at rest than after exercise. An upsetting event may not be evident.	Breathing in and out of a paper or plastic bag sometimes helps the associated symptoms.	Sighing, lightheadedness, numbness or tingling of the hands and feet, palpitations, chest pain	Other manifestations of anxiety may be present.

TABLE 6-3 ■ Cough and Hemoptysis*

Problem	Cough and Sputum	Associated Symptoms and Setting
Acute Inflammation		
Laryngitis	Dry cough (without sputum), may become productive of variable amounts of sputum	An acute, fairly minor illness with hoarseness. Often associated with viral nasopharyngitis
Tracheobronchitis	Dry cough, may become productive (as above)	An acute, often viral illness, with burning retrosternal discomfort
Mycoplasma and Viral Pneumonias	Dry hacking cough, often becoming productive of mucoid sputum	An acute febrile illness, often with malaise, headache, and possibly dyspnea
Bacterial Pneumonias	Pneumococcal: sputum mucoid or purulent; may be blood-streaked, diffusely pinkish, or rusty	An acute illness with chills, high fever, dyspnea, and chest pain. Often is preceded by acute upper respiratory infection.
	Klebsiella: similar; or sticky, red, and jellylike	Typically occurs in older alcoholic men
Chronic Inflammation		
Postnasal Drip	Chronic cough; sputum mucoid or mucopurulent	Repeated attempts to clear the throat. Postnasal discharge may be sensed by patient or seen in posterior pharynx. Associated with chronic rhinitis, with or without sinusitis
Chronic Bronchitis	Chronic cough; sputum mucoid to purulent, may be blood-streaked or even bloody	Often longstanding cigarette smoking. Recurrent superimposed infections. Wheezing and dyspnea may develop.
Bronchiectasis	Chronic cough; sputum purulent, often copious and foul-smelling; may be blood-streaked or bloody	Recurrent bronchopulmonary infections common; sinusitis may coexist
Pulmonary Tuberculosis	Cough dry or sputum that is mucoid or purulent; may be blood-streaked or bloody	Early, no symptoms. Later, anorexia, weight loss, fatigue, fever, and night sweats
Lung Abscess	Sputum purulent and foul-smelling; may be bloody	A febrile illness. Often poor dental hygiene and a prior episode of impaired consciousness
Asthma	Cough, with thick mucoid sputum, especially near end of an attack	Episodic wheezing and dyspnea, but cough may occur alone. Often a history of allergy
Gastroesophageal Reflux	Chronic cough, especially at night or early in the morning	Wheezing, especially at night (often mistaken for asthma), early morning hoarseness, and repeated attempts to clear the throat. Often a history of heartburn and regurgitation
Neoplasm		
Cancer of the Lung	Cough dry to productive; sputum may be blood-streaked or bloody	Usually a long history of cigarette smoking. Associated manifestations are numerous.
Cardiovascular Disorders		
Left Ventricular Failure or Mitral Stenosis	Often dry, especially on exertion or at night; may progress to the pink frothy sputum of pulmonary edema or to frank hemoptysis	Dyspnea, orthopnea, paroxysmal nocturnal dyspnea
Pulmonary Emboli	Dry to productive; may be dark, bright red, or mixed with blood	Dyspnea, anxiety, chest pain, fever; factors that predispose to deep venous thrombosis
Irritating Particles, Chemicals, or Gases	Variable. There may be a latent period between exposure and symptoms.	Exposure to irritants. Eyes, nose, and throat may be affected.

*Characteristics of hemoptysis are printed in red.

TABLE 6-4 ■ Deformities of the Thorax

Cross Section of Thorax

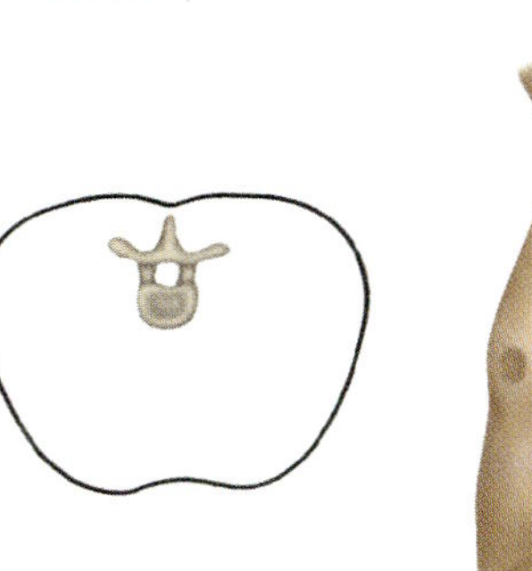

Normal Adult

The thorax in the normal adult is wider than it is deep. Its lateral diameter is larger than its anteroposterior diameter.

Cross Section of Thorax

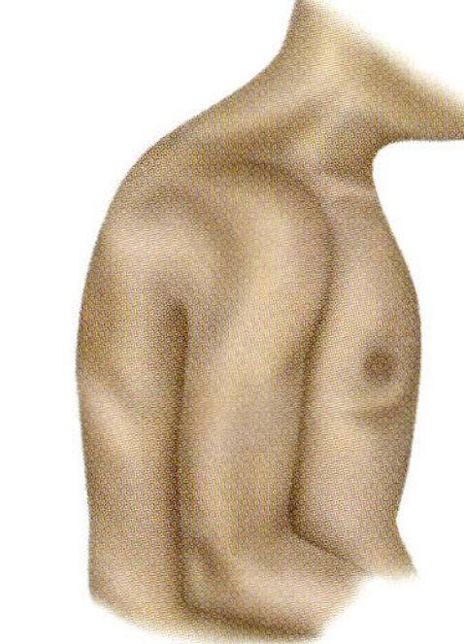

Barrel Chest

A barrel chest has an increased anteroposterior diameter. This shape is normal during infancy, and often accompanies normal aging and chronic obstructive pulmonary disease.

Cross Section of Thorax

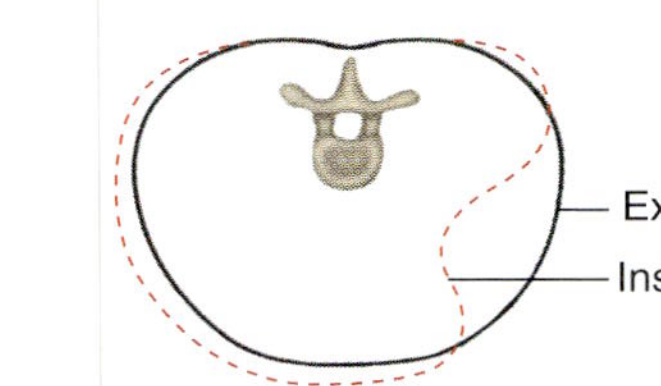

Traumatic Flail Chest

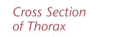

If multiple ribs are fractured, paradoxical movements of the thorax may be seen. As descent of the diaphragm decreases intrathoracic pressure on inspiration, the injured area caves inward; on expiration, it moves outward.

Cross Section of Thorax

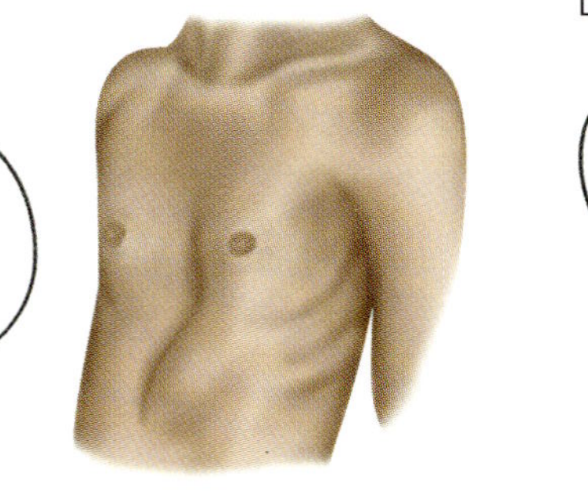

Funnel Chest (*Pectus Excavatum*)

A funnel chest is characterized by a depression in the lower portion of the sternum. Compression of the heart and great vessels may cause murmurs.

Cross Section of Thorax

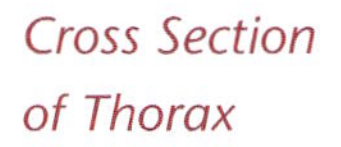
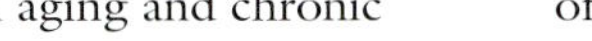
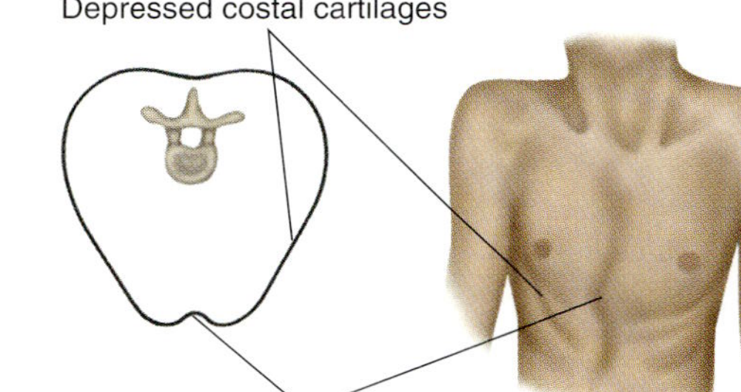

Pigeon Chest (*Pectus Carinatum*)

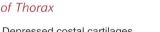

In a pigeon chest, the sternum is displaced anteriorly, increasing the anteroposterior diameter. The costal cartilages adjacent to the protruding sternum are depressed.

Cross Section of Thorax

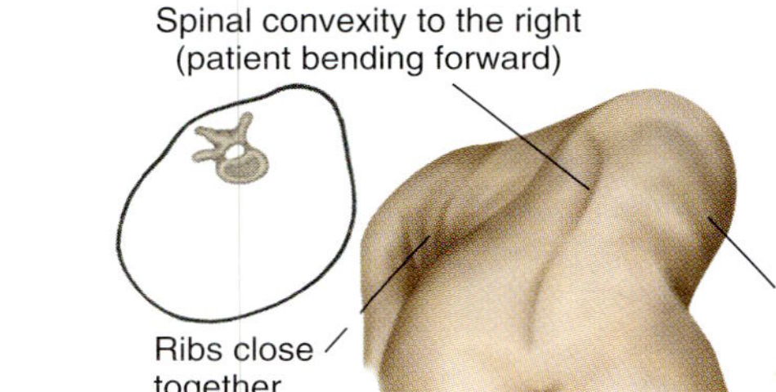

Thoracic Kyphoscoliosis

In thoracic kyphoscoliosis, abnormal spinal curvatures and vertebral rotation deform the chest. Distortion of the underlying lungs may make interpretation of lung findings very difficult.

TABLE 6-5 ■ Normal and Altered Breath and Voice Sounds

The origins of breath sounds are still unclear. According to leading theories, turbulent air flow in the central airways produces the tracheal and bronchial breath sounds. As these sounds pass through the lungs to the periphery, lung tissue filters out their higher-pitched components and only the soft and lower-pitched components reach the chest wall, where they are heard as vesicular breath sounds. Normally, tracheal and bronchial sounds may be heard over the trachea and mainstem bronchi; vesicular breath sounds predominate throughout most of the lungs.

When lung tissue loses its air, it transmits high-pitched sounds much better. If the tracheobronchial tree is open, bronchial breath sounds may replace the normal vesicular sounds over airless areas of the lung. This change is seen in lobar pneumonia when the alveoli fill with fluid, red cells, and white cells—a process called *consolidation*. Other causes include pulmonary edema or hemorrhage. Bronchial breath sounds usually correlate with an increase in tactile fremitus and transmitted voice sounds. These findings are summarized below.

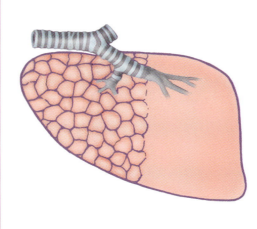

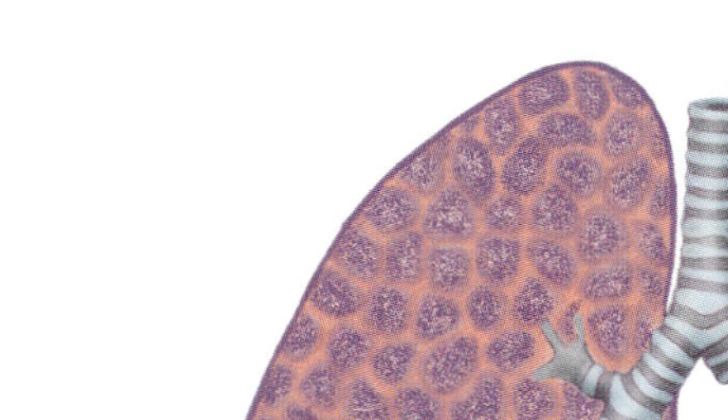

	Normal Air-Filled Lung	Airless Lung, as in Lobar Pneumonia
Breath Sounds	Predominantly vesicular	Bronchial or bronchovesicular over the involved area
Transmitted Voice Sounds	Spoken words muffled and indistinct Spoken "ee" heard as "ee" Whispered words faint and indistinct, if heard at all	Spoken words louder, clearer (*bronchophony*) Spoken "ee" heard as "ay" (*egophony*) Whispered words louder, clearer (*whispered pectoriloquy*)
Tactile Fremitus	Normal	Increased

TABLE 6-6 ■ Adventitious (Added) Lung Sounds: Causes and Qualities

Crackles

Crackles have two leading explanations. (1) They result from a series of tiny explosions when small airways, deflated during expiration, pop open during inspiration. This mechanism probably explains the late inspiratory crackles of interstitial lung disease and early congestive heart failure. (2) Crackles result from air bubbles flowing through secretions or lightly closed airways during respiration. This mechanism probably explains at least some coarse crackles.

Inspiration Expiration

Late inspiratory crackles may begin in the first half of inspiration but must continue into late inspiration. They are usually fine and fairly profuse, and persist from breath to breath. These crackles appear first at the bases of the lungs, spread upward as the condition worsens, and shift to dependent regions with changes in posture. Causes include interstitial lung disease (such as fibrosis) and early congestive heart failure.

Early inspiratory crackles appear soon after the start of inspiration and do not continue into late inspiration. They are often but not always coarse and are relatively few in number. Expiratory crackles are sometimes associated. Causes include chronic bronchitis and asthma.

Midinspiratory and expiratory crackles are heard in bronchiectasis but are not specific for this diagnosis. Wheezes and rhonchi may be associated.

Wheezes and Rhonchi

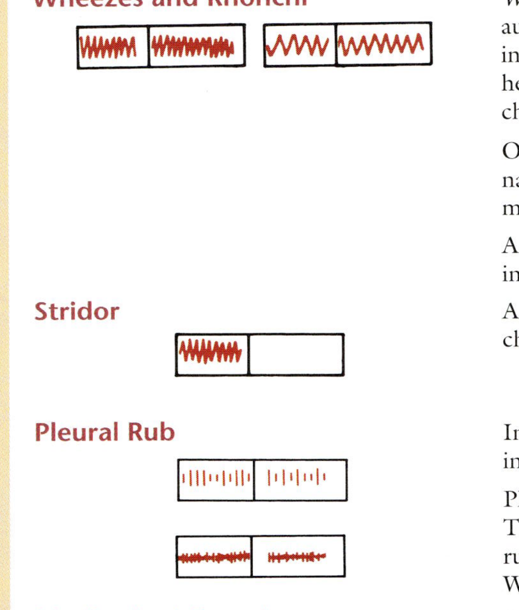

Wheezes occur when air flows rapidly through bronchi that are narrowed nearly to the point of closure. They are often audible at the mouth as well as through the chest wall. Causes of wheezes that are generalized throughout the chest include asthma, chronic bronchitis, COPD, and congestive heart failure (cardiac asthma). In asthma, wheezes may be heard only in expiration or in both phases of the respiratory cycle. Rhonchi suggest secretions in the larger airways. In chronic bronchitis, wheezes and rhonchi often clear with coughing.

Occasionally in severe obstructive pulmonary disease, the patient is no longer able to force enough air through the narrowed bronchi to produce wheezing. The resulting *silent chest* should raise immediate concern and not be mistaken for improvement.

A persistent localized wheeze suggests a partial obstruction of a bronchus, as by a tumor or foreign body. It may be inspiratory, expiratory, or both.

Stridor

A wheeze that is entirely or predominantly inspiratory is called *stridor*. It is often louder in the neck than over the chest wall. It indicates a partial obstruction of the larynx or trachea, and demands immediate attention.

Pleural Rub

Inflamed and roughened pleural surfaces grate against each other as they are momentarily and repeatedly delayed by increased friction. These movements produce creaking sounds known as a *pleural rub* (or pleural friction rub).

Pleural rubs resemble crackles acoustically, although they are produced by different pathologic processes. The sounds may be discrete, but sometimes are so numerous that they merge into a seemingly continuous sound. A rub is usually confined to a relatively small area of the chest wall, and typically is heard in both phases of respiration. When inflamed pleural surfaces are separated by fluid, the rub often disappears.

Mediastinal Crunch (*Hamman's Sign*)

A *mediastinal crunch* is a series of precordial crackles synchronous with the heart beat, not with respiration. Best heard in the left lateral position, it is due to mediastinal emphysema (pneumomediastinum).

TABLE 6-7 ■ Physical Findings in Selected Chest Disorders

The black boxes in this table suggest a framework for clinical assessment. Start with the three boxes under Percussion Note: resonant, dull, and hyperresonant. Then move from each of these to other boxes that emphasize some of the key differences among various conditions. The changes described vary with the extent and severity of the disorder. Abnormalities deep in the chest usually produce fewer signs than superficial ones, and may cause no signs at all. Use the table for the direction of typical changes, not for absolute distinctions.

Condition	Percussion Note	Trachea	Breath Sounds	Adventitious Sounds	Tactile Fremitus and Transmitted Voice Sounds
Normal The tracheobronchial tree and alveoli are clear; pleurae are thin and close together; mobility of the chest wall is unimpaired.	**Resonant**	Midline	Vesicular, except perhaps bronchovesicular and bronchial sounds over the large bronchi and trachea respectively	None, except perhaps a few transient inspiratory crackles at the bases of the lungs	Normal
Chronic Bronchitis The bronchi are chronically inflamed and a productive cough is present. Airway obstruction may develop.	**Resonant**	Midline	Vesicular (normal)	None; or scattered coarse *crackles* in early inspiration and perhaps expiration; or *wheezes* or *rhonchi*	Normal
Left-Sided Heart Failure (*Early*) Increased pressure in the pulmonary veins causes congestion and interstitial edema (around the alveoli); bronchial mucosa may become edematous.	**Resonant**	Midline	Vesicular	*Late inspiratory crackles* in the dependent portions of the lungs; possibly *wheezes*	Normal
Consolidation Alveoli fill with fluid or blood cells, as in pneumonia, pulmonary edema, or pulmonary hemorrhage.	**Dull** over the airless area	Midline	*Bronchial* over the involved area	*Late inspiratory crackles* over the involved area	*Increased* over the involved area, with *bronchophony, egophony,* and *whispered pectoriloquy*

TABLE 6-7 ■ Physical Findings in Selected Chest Disorders

Atelectasis (*Lobar Obstruction*) When a plug in a mainstem bronchus (as from mucus or a foreign object) obstructs air flow, affected lung tissue collapses into an airless state.	**Dull** over the airless area	May be *shifted toward involved side*	*Usually absent* when bronchial plug persists. Exceptions include right upper lobe atelectasis, where adjacent tracheal sounds may be transmitted.	None	*Usually absent* when the bronchial plug persists. In exceptions, e.g., right upper lobe atelectasis, may be increased
Pleural Effusion Fluid accumulates in the pleural space, separates air-filled lung from the chest wall, blocking the transmission of sound.	**Dull** to flat over the fluid	*Shifted toward opposite side* in a large effusion	*Decreased to absent*, but bronchial breath sounds may be heard near top of large effusion.	None, except a *possible pleural* rub	*Decreased to absent, but may be increased* toward the top of a large effusion
Pneumothorax When air leaks into the pleural space, usually unilaterally, the lung recoils from the chest wall. Pleural air blocks transmission of sound.	**Hyperresonant** or tympanitic over the pleural air	*Shifted toward opposite side* if much air	*Decreased to absent* over the pleural air	None, except a *possible pleural* rub	*Decreased to absent* over the pleural air
Chronic Obstructive Pulmonary Disease (COPD) Slowly progressive disorder in which the distal air spaces enlarge and lungs become hyperinflated. Chronic bronchitis is often associated.	Diffusely **hyperresonant**	Midline	*Decreased to absent*	None, or the crackles, wheezes, and rhonchi of associated chronic bronchitis	*Decreased*
Asthma Widespread narrowing of the tracheobronchial tree diminishes airflow to a fluctuating degree. During attacks, airflow decreases further and lungs hyperinflate.	**Resonant** to diffusely **hyperresonant**	Midline	*Often obscured by wheezes*	*Wheezes, possibly crackles*	*Decreased*

CHAPTER

7

The Cardiovascular System

ANATOMY AND PHYSIOLOGY

Surface Projections of the Heart and Great Vessels

Learn to visualize the underlying structures of the heart as you examine the anterior chest. Understanding cardiac anatomy and physiology is particularly important in the examination of the cardiovascular system.

Note that the *right ventricle* occupies most of the anterior cardiac surface. This chamber and the pulmonary artery form a wedgelike structure behind and to the left of the sternum.

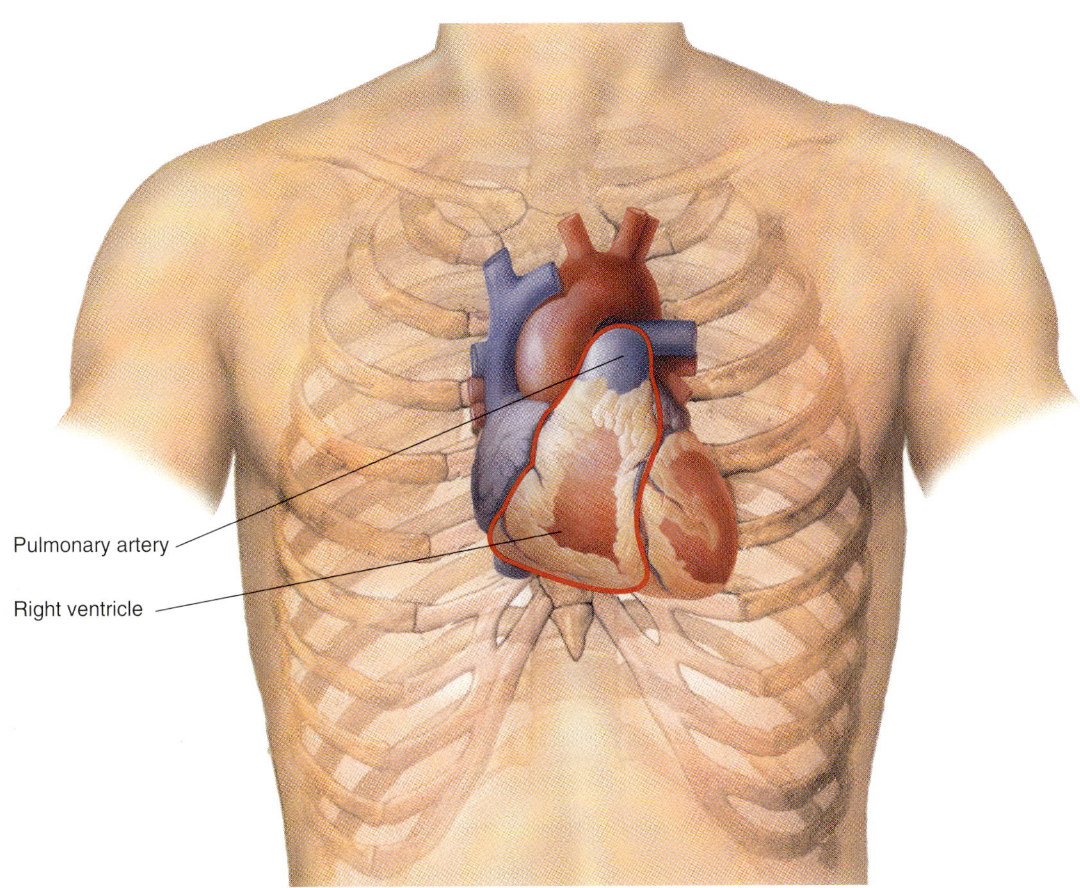

The inferior border of the right ventricle lies below the junction of the sternum and the xiphoid process. The right ventricle narrows superiorly and meets the pulmonary artery at the level of the sternum or "base of the heart"—a clinical term that refers to the right and left 2nd interspaces close to the sternum.

The *left ventricle,* behind the right ventricle and to the left, forms the left lateral margin of the heart. Its tapered inferior tip is often termed the cardiac "apex." It is clinically important because it produces the *apical impulse,* sometimes called the *point of maximal impulse,* or *PMI.** This impulse locates the left border of the heart and is usually found in the 5th interspace 7 cm to 9 cm lateral to the midsternal line. It is about the size of a quarter, roughly 1 to 2.5 cm in diameter.

The right heart border is formed by the *right atrium,* a chamber not usually identifiable on physical examination. The *left atrium* is mostly posterior and cannot be examined directly, although its small atrial appendage may make up a segment of the left heart border between the pulmonary and the left ventricle.

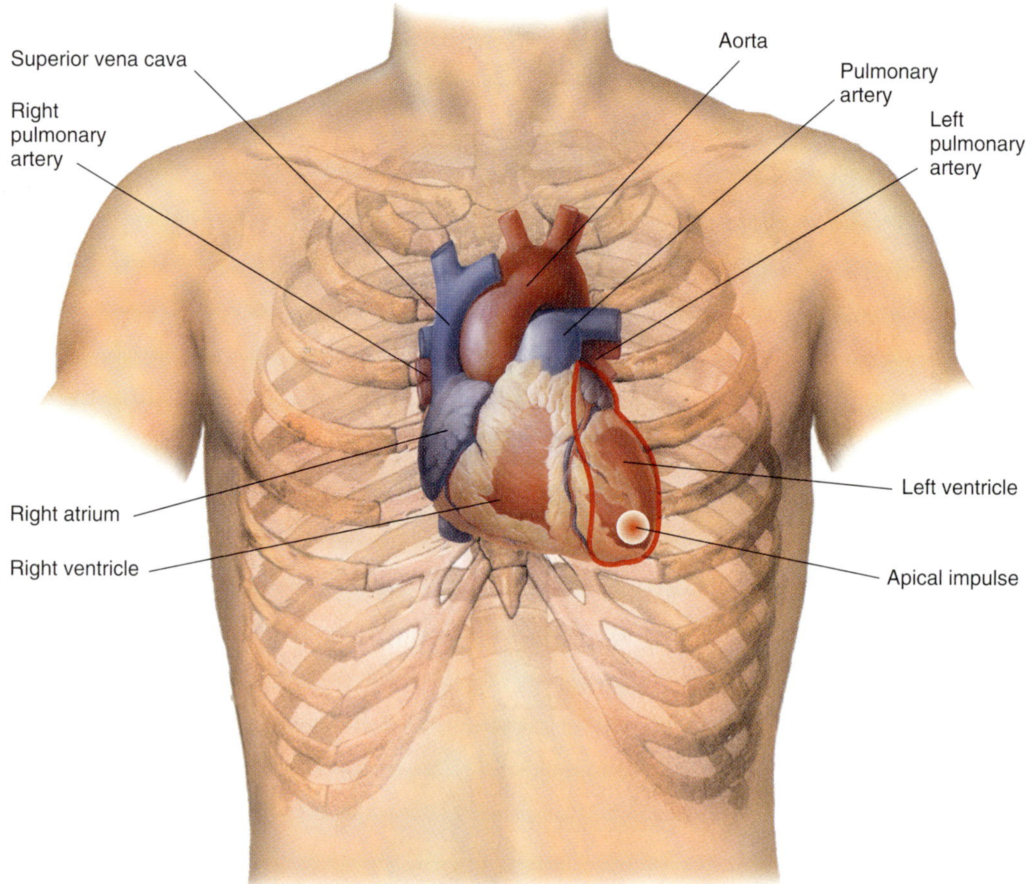

*Because the most prominent cardiac impulse may not be apical, some authorities discourage use of this term.

Above the heart lie the great vessels. The *pulmonary artery*, already mentioned, bifurcates quickly into its left and right branches. The *aorta* curves upward from the left ventricle to the level of the sternal angle, where it arches backward to the left and then down. On the right, the superior vena cava empties into the right atrium.

Although not illustrated, the inferior vena cava also empties into the right atrium. The *superior* and *inferior venae cavae* carry venous blood to the heart from the upper and lower portions of the body.

Cardiac Chambers, Valves, and Circulation

Circulation through the heart is shown in the diagram below, which identifies the cardiac chambers, valves, and direction of blood flow. Because of their positions, the *tricuspid* and *mitral valves* are often called *atrioventricular valves*. The *aortic* and *pulmonic valves* are called *semilunar valves* because each of their leaflets is shaped like a half moon. Although this diagram shows all valves in an open position, they are not all open simultaneously in the living heart.

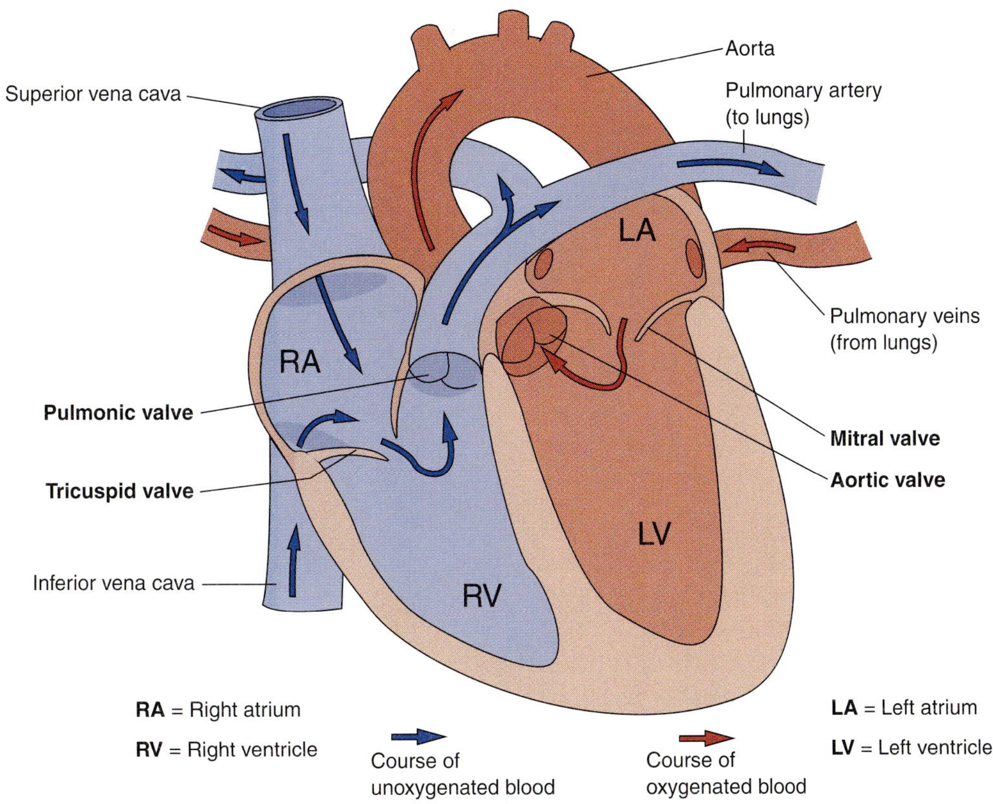

As the heart valves close, the heart sounds arise from vibrations emanating from the leaflets, the adjacent cardiac structures, and the flow of blood. It is essential to understand the positions and movements of the valves in relation to events in the cardiac cycle.

Events in the Cardiac Cycle

The heart serves as a muscular pump that generates varying pressures as its chambers contract and relax. *Systole is the period of ventricular contraction.* In the diagram shown below, pressure in the left ventricle rises from less than 5 mm Hg in its resting state to a normal peak of 120 mm Hg. After the ventricle ejects much of its blood into the aorta, the pressure levels off and starts to fall. *Diastole is the period of ventricular relaxation.* Ventricular pressure falls further to below 5 mm Hg, and blood flows from atrium to ventricle. Late in diastole, ventricular pressure rises slightly during inflow of blood from atrial contraction.

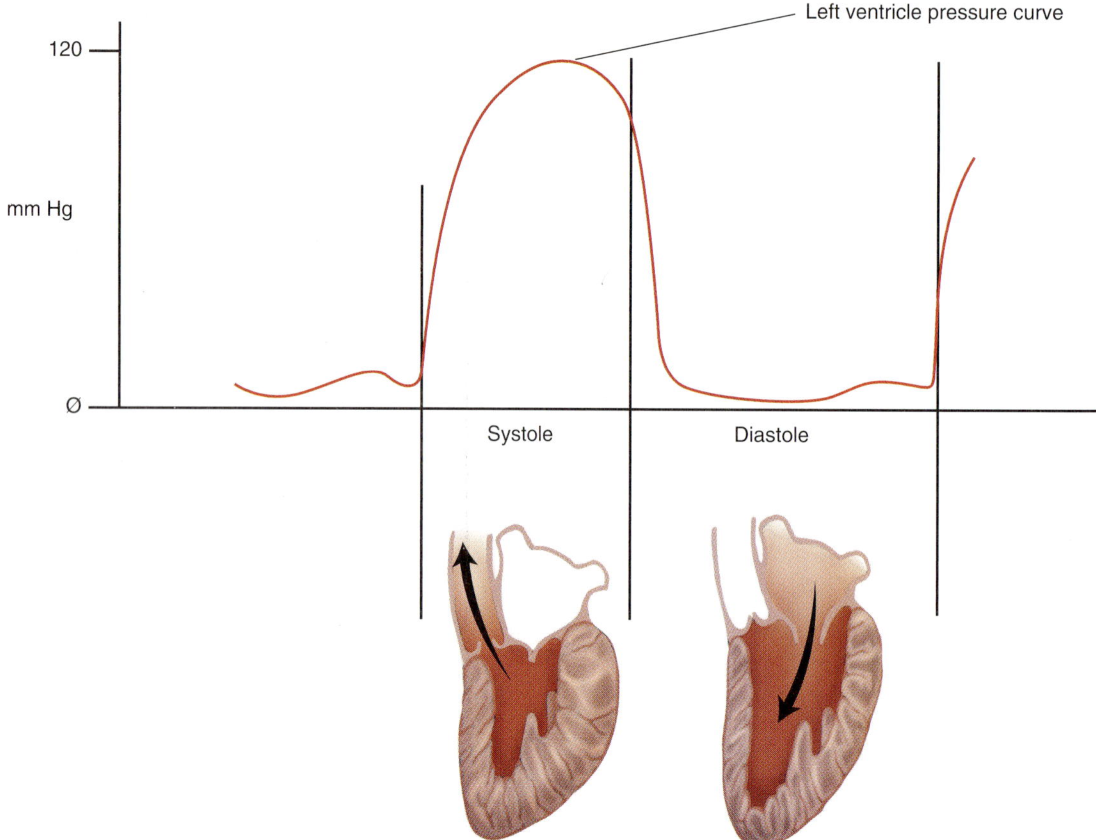

Note that during *systole* the aortic valve is open, allowing ejection of blood from the left ventricle into the aorta. The mitral valve is closed, preventing blood from regurgitating back into the left atrium. In contrast, during *diastole* the aortic valve is closed, preventing regurgitation of blood from the aorta back into the left ventricle. The mitral valve is open, allowing blood to flow from the left atrium into the relaxed left ventricle.

Understanding the interrelationships of the pressures in these three chambers—left atrium, left ventricle, and aorta—together with the position and movement of the valves is fundamental to understanding heart sounds. These changing pressures and the sounds that result are traced here through one cardiac cycle. Note that during auscultation the first and second heart sounds define the duration of *systole* and *diastole*.

During *diastole,* pressure in the blood-filled left atrium slightly exceeds that in the relaxed left ventricle, and blood flows from left atrium to left ventricle across the open mitral valve. Just before the onset of ventricular systole, atrial contraction produces a slight pressure rise in both chambers.

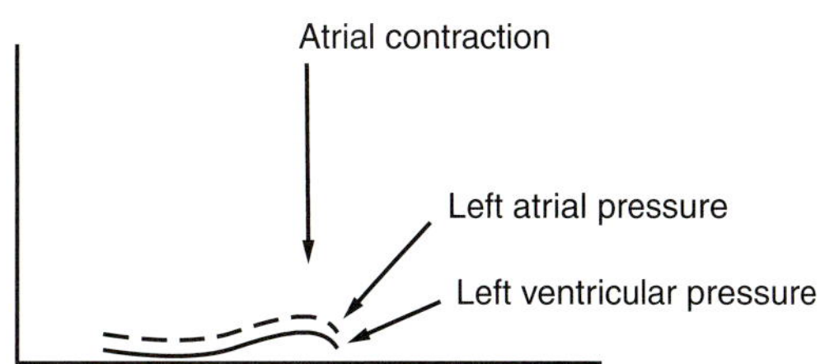

During *systole,* the left ventricle starts to contract and ventricular pressure rapidly exceeds left atrial pressure, thus shutting the mitral valve. *Closure of the mitral valve produces the first heart sound, S_1.*†

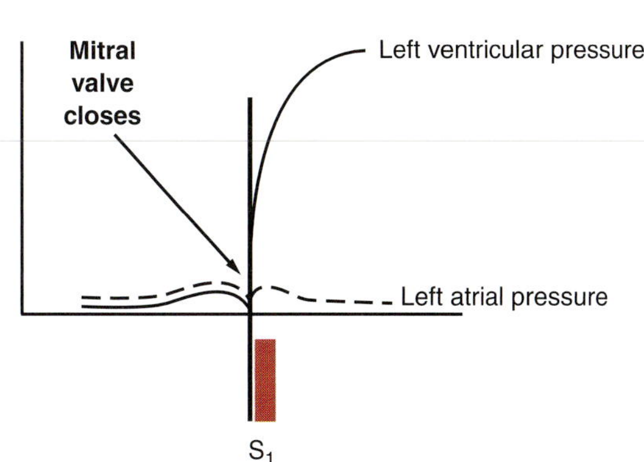

As left ventricular pressure continues to rise, it quickly exceeds the pressure in the aorta and forces the aortic valve open. In some pathologic conditions, opening of the aortic valve is accompanied by an early systolic ejection sound (Ej). Normally, maximal left ventricular pressure corresponds to systolic blood pressure.

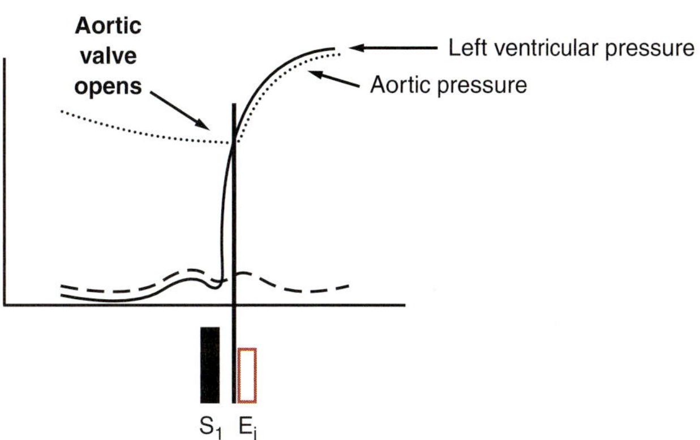

As the left ventricle ejects most of its blood, ventricular pressure begins to fall. When left ventricular pressure drops below aortic pressure, the aortic valve shuts. *Aortic valve closure produces the second heart sound, S_2,* and another diastole begins.

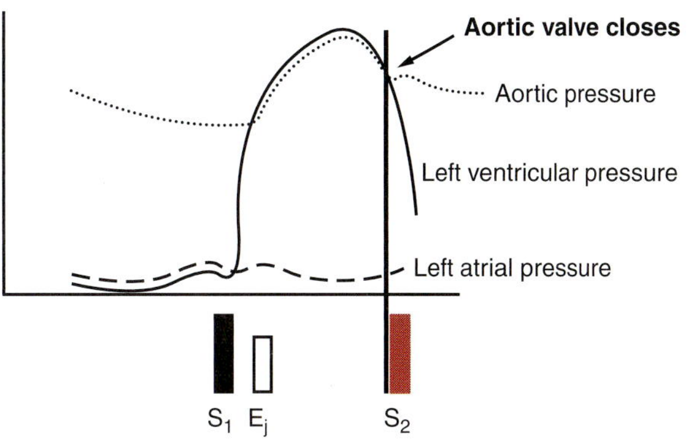

†An extensive literature deals with the exact causes of heart sounds. Possible explanations include actual closure of valve leaflets, tensing of related structures, leaflet positions and pressure gradients at the time of atrial and ventricular systole, and the impact of columns of blood. The explanations given here are oversimplified but retain clinical usefulness.

In *diastole,* left ventricular pressure continues to drop and falls below left atrial pressure. The mitral valve opens. This is usually a silent event, but may be audible as a pathologic opening snap (OS) if valve leaflet motion is restricted, as in mitral stenosis.

After the mitral valve opens, there is a period of rapid ventricular filling as blood flows early in diastole from left atrium to left ventricle. In children and young adults, a third heart sound, S_3, may arise from rapid deceleration of the column of blood against the ventricular wall. In older adults, an S_3, sometimes termed "an S_3 gallop," usually indicates a pathologic change in ventricular compliance.

Finally, although not often heard in normal adults, a fourth heart sound, S_4, marks atrial contraction. It immediately precedes S_1 of the next beat, and also reflects a pathologic change in ventricular compliance.

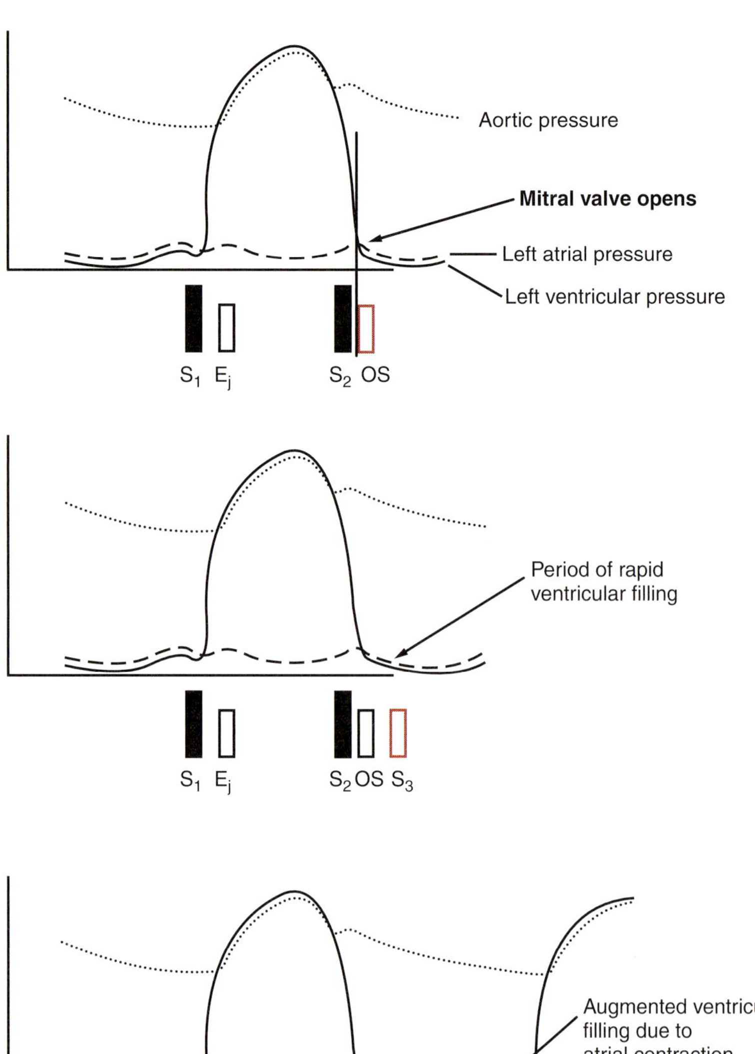

The Splitting of Heart Sounds

While these events are occurring on the left side of the heart, similar changes are occurring on the right, involving the right atrium, right ventricle, tricuspid valve, pulmonic valve, and pulmonary artery. Right ventricular and pulmonary arterial pressures are significantly lower than corresponding pressures on the left side. Furthermore, right-sided events usually occur slightly later than those on the left. Instead of a single heart sound, you may hear two discernible components, the first from left-sided aortic valve closure, or A_2, and the second from right-sided closure of the pulmonic valve, or P_2.

Consider the second heart sound and its two components, A_2 and P_2, which come from closure of the aortic and pulmonic valves respectively. During expiration, these two components are fused into a single sound, S_2. During inspiration, however, A_2 and P_2 separate slightly, and S_2 may split into its two audible components.

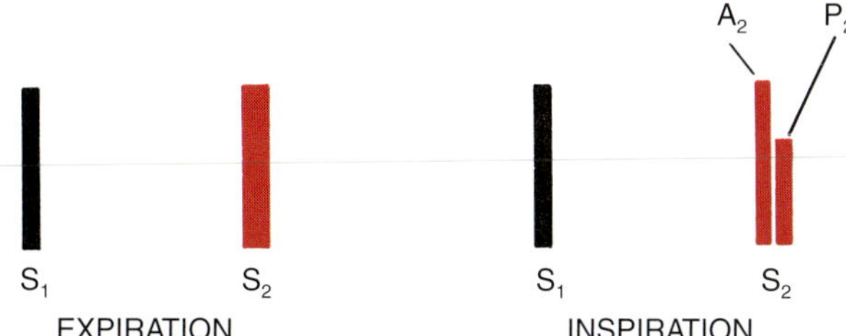

Current explanations of inspiratory splitting cite increased capacitance in the pulmonary vascular bed during inspiration, which prolongs ejection of blood from the right ventricle, delaying closure of the pulmonic valve, or P_2. Ejection of blood from the left ventricle is comparatively shorter, so A_2 occurs slightly earlier.

Of the two components of the second heart sound, A_2 is normally louder, reflecting the high pressure in the aorta. It is heard throughout the precordium. P_2, in contrast, is relatively soft, reflecting the lower pressure in the pulmonary artery. It is heard best in its own area—the 2nd and 3rd left interspaces close to the sternum. It is here that you should search for splitting of the second heart sound.

S_1 also has two components, an earlier mitral and a later tricuspid sound. The mitral sound, its principal component, is much louder, again reflecting the high pressures on the left side of the heart. It can be heard throughout the precordium and is loudest at the cardiac apex. The softer tricuspid component is heard best at the lower left sternal border, and it is here that you may hear a split S_1. The earlier louder mitral component may mask the tricuspid sound, however, and splitting is not always detectable. Splitting of S_1 does not vary with respiration.

Heart Murmurs

Heart murmurs are distinguishable from heart sounds by their longer duration. They are attributed to turbulent blood flow and may be "innocent," as with flow murmurs of young adults, or diagnostic of valvular heart disease. A *stenotic valve* has an abnormally narrowed valvular orifice that obstructs blood flow, as in aortic stenosis, and causes a characteristic murmur. So does a valve that fails to fully close, as in aortic regurgitation or insufficiency. Such a valve allows blood to leak backward in a retrograde direction and produces a *regurgitant* murmur.

To identify murmurs accurately, you must learn to assess the chest wall location where they are best heard, their timing in systole or diastole, and their qualities. In the section on Techniques of Examination, you will learn to integrate several characteristics, including murmur intensity, pitch, duration, and direction of radiation (see pp. 280–283).

Relation of Auscultatory Findings to the Chest Wall

The locations on the chest wall where you hear heart sounds and murmurs help to identify the valve or chamber where they originate. Sounds and murmurs arising from the mitral valve are usually heard best at and around the cardiac apex. Those originating in the tricuspid valve are heard best at or near the lower left sternal border. Murmurs arising from the pulmonic valve are usually heard best in the 2nd and 3rd left interspaces close to the sternum, but at times may also be heard at higher or lower levels, and those originating in the aortic valve may be heard anywhere from the right 2nd interspace to the apex. These areas overlap, as illustrated below, and you will need to correlate auscultatory findings with other portions of the cardiac examination to identify sounds and murmurs accurately.

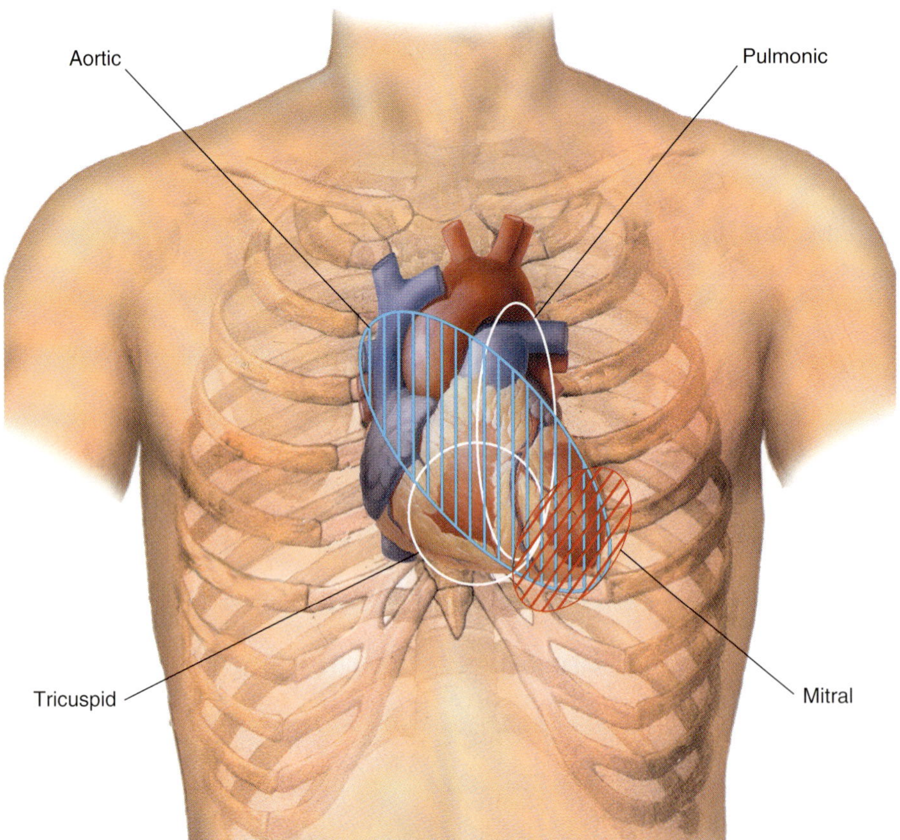

The Conduction System

An electrical conduction system stimulates and coordinates the contraction of cardiac muscle.

Each normal electrical impulse is initiated in the *sinus node*, a group of specialized cardiac cells located in the right atrium near the junction of the vena cava. The sinus node acts as the cardiac pacemaker and automatically discharges an impulse about 60 to 100 times a minute. This impulse travels through both atria to the *atrioventricular node*, a specialized group of cells located low in the atrial septum. Here the impulse is delayed before passing down the bundle of His and its branches to the ventricular myocardium. Muscular contraction follows: first the atria, then the ventricles. The normal conduction pathway is diagrammed in simplified form at the right.

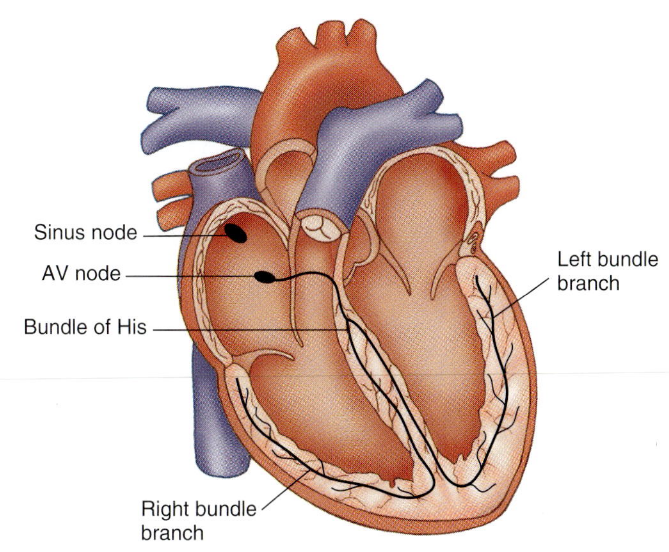

The electrocardiogram, or ECG, records these events. Contraction of cardiac smooth muscle produces electrical activity, resulting in a series of waves on the ECG. The components of the *normal ECG* and their duration are briefly summarized here, but you will need further instruction and practice to interpret recordings from actual patients.

- The small *P wave* of atrial depolarization (duration up to 8 milliseconds; *PR interval* up to 20 milliseconds)
- The larger *QRS complex* of ventricular depolarization (up to 10 milliseconds), consisting of one or more of the following:

  –the *Q wave*, a downward deflection from septal depolarization
  –the *R wave*, an upward deflection from ventricular depolarization
  –the *S wave*, a downward deflection following an R wave

- A *T wave* of ventricular repolarization, or recovery (duration relates to QRS).

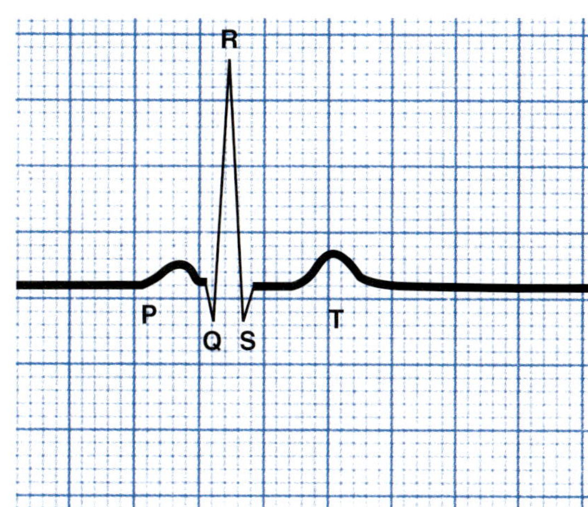

The electrical impulse slightly precedes the myocardial contraction that it stimulates. The relation of electrocardiographic waves to the cardiac cycle is shown below.

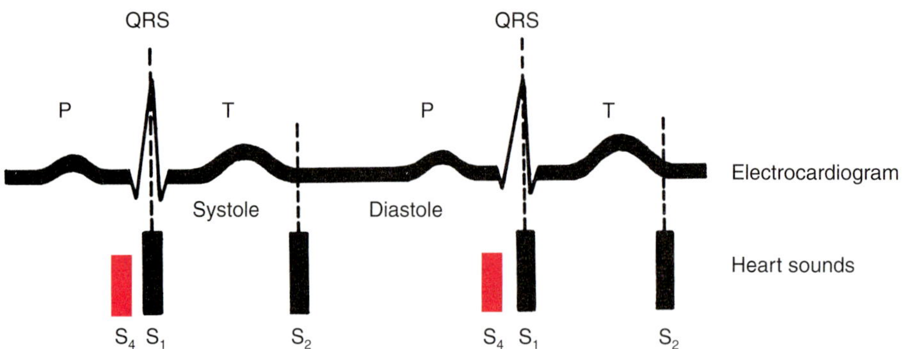

The Heart as a Pump

The left and right ventricles pump blood into the systemic and pulmonary arterial trees, respectively. *Cardiac output,* the volume of blood ejected from each ventricle during 1 minute, is the product of *heart rate* and *stroke volume.* Stroke volume (the volume of blood ejected with each heartbeat) depends in turn on preload, myocardial contractility, and afterload.

Preload refers to the load that stretches the cardiac muscle prior to contraction. The volume of blood in the right ventricle at the end of diastole, then, constitutes its preload for the next beat. Right ventricular preload is increased by increasing venous return to the right heart. Physiologic causes include inspiration and the increased volume of blood that flows from exercising muscles. The increased volume of blood in a dilated ventricle of congestive heart failure also increases preload. Causes of decreased right ventricular preload include exhalation, decreased left ventricular output, and pooling of blood in the capillary bed or the venous system.

Myocardial contractility refers to the ability of the cardiac muscle, when given a load, to shorten. Contractility increases when stimulated by action of the sympathetic nervous system, and decreases when blood flow or oxygen delivery to the myocardium is impaired.

Afterload refers to the vascular resistance against which the ventricle must contract. Sources of resistance to left ventricular contraction include the tone in the walls of the aorta, the large arteries, and the peripheral vascular tree (primarily the small arteries and arterioles), as well as the volume of blood already in the aorta.

Pathologic increases in preload and afterload, called *volume overload* and *pressure overload* respectively, produce changes in ventricular function that may be clinically detectable. These changes include alterations in ventricular impulses, detectable by palpation, and in normal heart sounds. Pathologic heart sounds and murmurs may also develop.

Arterial Pulses and Blood Pressure

With each contraction, the left ventricle ejects a volume of blood into the aorta and on into the arterial tree. The ensuing pressure wave moves rapidly through the arterial system, where it is felt as the *arterial pulse*. Although the pressure wave travels quickly—many times faster than the blood itself—a palpable delay between ventricular contraction and peripheral pulses makes the pulses in the arms and legs unsuitable for timing events in the cardiac cycle.

Blood pressure in the arterial system varies during the cardiac cycle, peaking in systole and falling to its lowest trough in diastole. These are the levels that are measured with the blood pressure cuff, or sphygmomanometer. The difference between systolic and diastolic pressures is known as the *pulse pressure*.

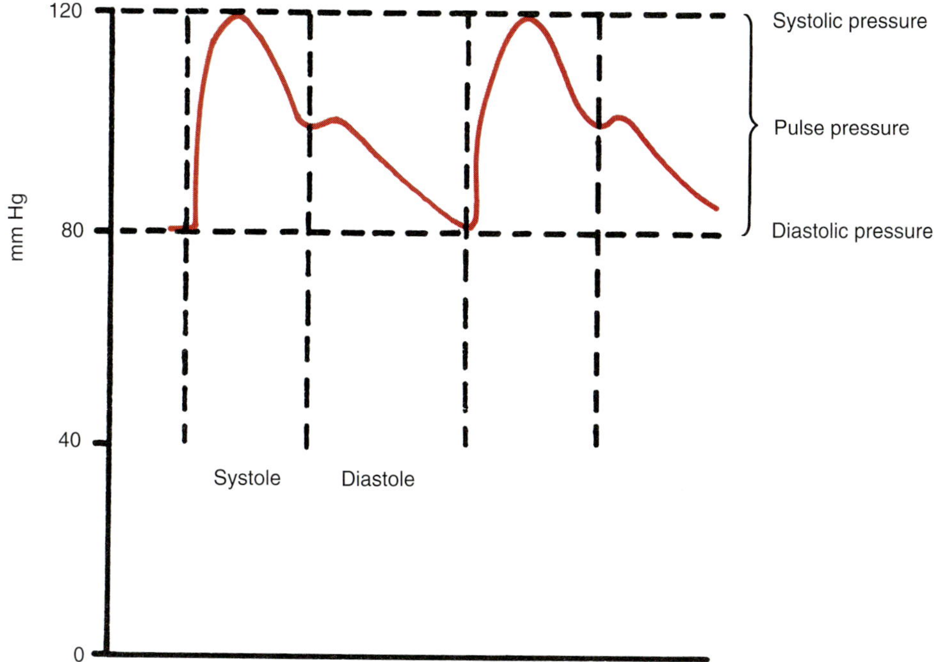

The principal factors influencing arterial pressure are:

- Left ventricular stroke volume
- Distensibility of the aorta and the large arteries
- Peripheral vascular resistance, particularly at the arteriolar level
- Volume of blood in the arterial system.

Changes in any of these four factors alter systolic pressure, diastolic pressure, or both. Blood pressure levels fluctuate strikingly through any 24-hour period, varying with physical activity, emotional state, pain, noise, environmental temperature, the use of coffee, tobacco, and other drugs, and even the time of day.

Jugular Venous Pressure and Pulses

Jugular Venous Pressure (JVP). Systemic venous pressure is much lower than arterial pressure. Although venous pressure ultimately depends on left ventricular contraction, much of this force is dissipated as blood passes through the arterial tree and the capillary bed. Walls of veins contain less smooth muscle than walls of arteries, which reduces venous vascular tone and makes veins more distensible. Other important determinants of venous pressure include blood volume and the capacity of the right heart to eject blood into the pulmonary arterial system. Cardiac disease may alter these variables, producing abnormalities in central venous pressure. For example, venous pressure falls when left ventricular output or blood volume is significantly reduced; it rises when the right heart fails or when increased pressure in the pericardial sac impedes the return of blood to the right atrium. These venous pressure changes are reflected in the height of the venous column of blood in the internal jugular veins, termed the *jugular venous pressure* or *JVP*.

Pressure in the jugular veins reflects right atrial pressure, giving clinicians an important clinical indicator of cardiac function and right heart hemodynamics. Assessing the JVP is an essential, though challenging, clinical skill. The JVP is best estimated from the internal jugular vein, usually on the *right side*, since the right internal jugular vein has a more direct anatomic channel into the right atrium.

The internal jugular veins lie deep to the sternomastoid muscles in the neck and are not directly visible, so the clinician must learn to identify the *pulsa-*

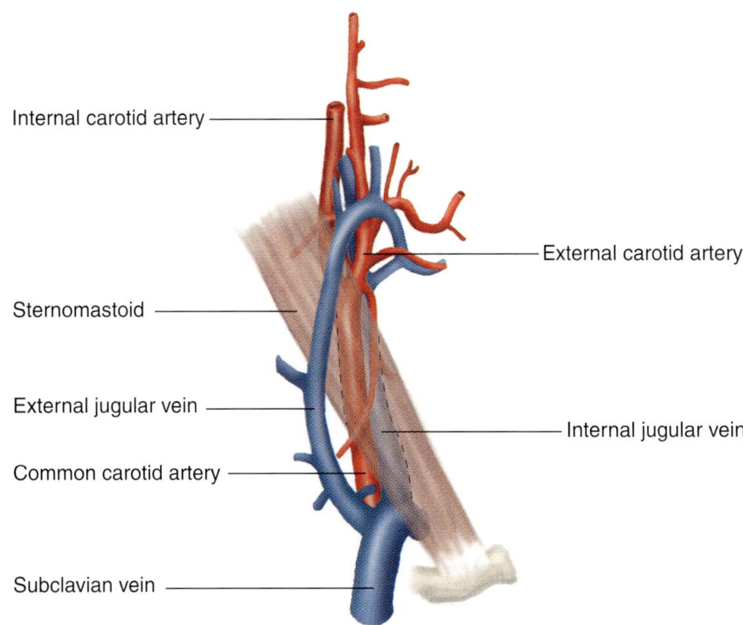

tions of the internal jugular vein that are transmitted to the surface of the neck, making sure to carefully distinguish these venous pulsations from pulsations of the carotid artery. If pulsations from the internal jugular vein cannot be identified, those of the external jugular vein can be used, but they are less reliable.

To estimate the level of the JVP, you will learn to find the *highest point of oscillation in the internal jugular vein* or, if necessary, the point above which the external jugular vein appears collapsed. The JVP is usually measured in vertical distance above the *sternal angle*, the bony ridge adjacent to the second rib where the manubrium joins the body of the sternum.

Study the illustrations below very carefully. Note that regardless of the patient's position, the sternal angle remains roughly 5 cm above the right atrium. In this patient, however, the pressure in the internal jugular vein is somewhat elevated.

- In *Position A,* the head of the bed is raised to the usual level, about 30°, but the JVP cannot be measured because the meniscus, or level of oscillation, is above the jaw and therefore not visible.
- In *Position B,* the head of the bed is raised to 60°. The "top" of the internal jugular vein is now easily visible, so the vertical distance from the sternal angle or right atrium can now be measured.
- In *Position C,* the patient is upright and the veins are barely discernible above the clavicle, making measurement untenable.

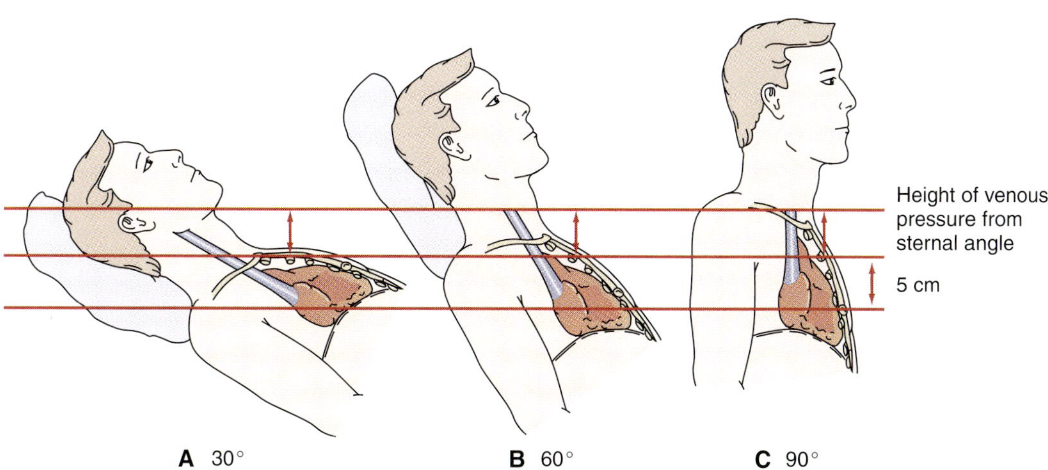

Note that the height of the venous pressure as measured from the sternal angle is the *same* in all three positions, but your ability to *measure* the height of the column of venous blood, or JVP, differs according to how you position the patient. Jugular venous pressure measured at more than 4 cm above the sternal angle, or more than 9 cm above the right atrium, is considered elevated or abnormal. The techniques for measuring the JVP are fully described in Techniques of Examination on pp. 266–268.

Jugular Venous Pulsations. The oscillations that you see in the internal jugular veins (and often in the externals as well) reflect changing pressures within the right atrium. The right internal jugular vein empties more directly into the right atrium and reflects these pressure changes best.

Careful observation reveals that the undulating pulsations of the internal jugular veins (and sometimes the externals) are composed of two quick peaks and two troughs.

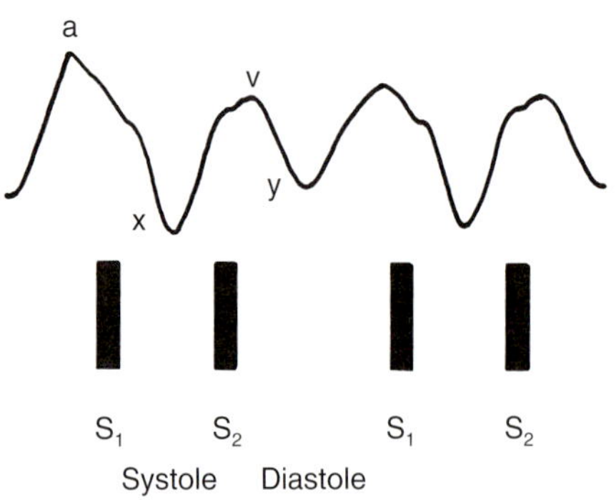

The first elevation, the *a wave,* reflects the slight rise in atrial pressure that accompanies atrial contraction. It occurs just before the first heart sound and before the carotid pulse. The following trough, the *x descent,* starts with atrial relaxation. It continues as the right ventricle, contracting during systole, pulls the floor of the atrium downward. During ventricular systole, blood continues to flow into the right atrium from the venae cavae. The tricuspid valve is closed, the chamber begins to fill, and right atrial pressure begins to rise again, creating the second elevation, the *v wave.* When the tricuspid valve opens early in diastole, blood in the right atrium flows passively into the right ventricle and right atrial pressure falls again, creating the second trough or *y descent.* To remember these four oscillations in a somewhat oversimplified way, think of the following sequence: atrial contraction, atrial relaxation, atrial filling, and atrial emptying. (You can think of the *a* wave as atrial contraction and the *v* wave as venous filling.)

To the naked eye, the two descents are the most obvious events in the normal jugular pulse. Of the two, the sudden collapse of the *x* descent late in systole is the more prominent, occurring just before the second heart sound. The *y* descent follows the second heart sound early in diastole.

Changes With Aging

Cardiovascular findings vary significantly with age. Aging may affect the location of the apical impulse, the pitch of heart sounds and murmurs, the stiffness of the arteries, and blood pressure.

The Apical Impulse and Heart Sounds. The *apical impulse* is usually felt easily in children and young adults; as the chest deepens in its anteroposterior diameter, the impulse gets harder to find. For the same reason, *splitting of the second heart sound* may be harder to hear in older people as its pulmonic component becomes less audible. A physiologic *third heart sound,* commonly heard in children and young adults, may persist as late as the age of 40, especially in women. After approximately age 40, however, an S_3 strongly suggests either ventricular failure or volume overload of the ventricle from valvular heart disease such as mitral regurgitation. In contrast, a *fourth heart sound* is seldom heard in young adults unless they are well conditioned athletes. An S_4 may be heard in apparently healthy older people, but is also frequently associated with decreased ventricular compliance from heart disease. (See Table 7-5, Extra Heart Sounds in Diastole, p. 290.)

Cardiac Murmurs. At some time over the life span, almost everyone has a *heart murmur.* Most murmurs occur without other evidence of cardiovascular abnormality and may therefore be considered innocent normal variants. These common murmurs vary with age, and familiarity with their patterns helps you to distinguish normal from abnormal.

Children, adolescents, and young adults frequently have an innocent systolic murmur, often called a *flow murmur,* that is felt to reflect pulmonic blood flow. It is usually heard best in the 2nd to 4th left interspaces (see p. 291).

Late in pregnancy and during lactation, many women have a so-called *mammary souffle*[‡] secondary to increased blood flow in their breasts. Although this murmur may be noted anywhere in the breasts, it is often heard most easily in the 2nd or 3rd interspace on either side of the sternum. A mammary souffle is typically both systolic and diastolic, but sometimes only the louder systolic component is audible.

Middle-aged and older adults commonly have an *aortic systolic murmur.* This has been heard in about a third of people near the age of 60, and in well over half of those reaching 85. Aging thickens the bases of the aortic cusps with fibrous tissue, calcification follows, and audible vibrations result. Turbulence produced by blood flow into a dilated aorta may contribute to this murmur. In most people, this process of fibrosis and calcification—known as *aortic sclerosis*—does not impede blood flow. In some, however, the valve cusps become progressively calcified and immobile, and true *aortic stenosis,* or obstruction of flow, develops. A normal carotid upstroke may help distinguish aortic sclerosis from aortic stenosis (in which the carotid upstroke is delayed), but clinical differentiation between benign aortic sclerosis and pathologic aortic stenosis may be difficult.

A similar aging process affects the mitral valve, usually about a decade later than aortic sclerosis. Here degenerative changes with calcification of the mitral annulus, or valve ring, impair the ability of the mitral valve to close normally during systole, and cause the *systolic murmur of mitral regurgitation.* Because of the extra load placed on the heart by the leaking mitral valve, a murmur of mitral regurgitation cannot be considered innocent.

Murmurs may originate in large blood vessels as well as in the heart. The *jugular venous hum,* which is very common in children and may still be heard through young adulthood, illustrates this point (see p. 295). A second, more

[‡] Souffle is pronounced soó-fl, not like cheese soufflé. Both words come from a French word meaning puff.

important example is the *cervical systolic murmur* or *bruit*. In older people, systolic bruits heard in the middle or upper portions of the carotid arteries suggest, but do not prove, a partial arterial obstruction secondary to atherosclerosis. In contrast, cervical bruits in younger people are usually innocent. In children and young adults, systolic murmurs (bruits) are frequently heard just above the clavicle. Studies have shown that, while cervical bruits can be heard in almost 9 out of 10 children under the age of 5, their prevalence falls steadily to about 1 out of 3 in adolescence and young adulthood and to less than 1 out of 10 in middle age.

Arteries and Blood Pressure. The aorta and large arteries stiffen with age as they become atherosclerotic. As the aorta becomes less distensible, a given stroke volume causes a greater rise in systolic blood pressure; *systolic hypertension* with a *widened pulse pressure* often ensues. Peripheral arteries tend to lengthen, become tortuous, and feel harder and less resilient. These changes do not necessarily indicate atherosclerosis, however, and you can make no inferences from them as to disease in the coronary or cerebral vessels. Lengthening and tortuosity of the aorta and its branches occasionally result in kinking or buckling of the carotid artery low in the neck, especially on the right. The resulting pulsatile mass, which occurs chiefly in hypertensive women, may be mistaken for a carotid aneurysm—a true dilatation of the artery. A tortuous aorta occasionally raises the pressure in the jugular veins on the left side of the neck by impairing their drainage within the thorax.

In Western societies, systolic blood pressure tends to rise from childhood through old age. Diastolic blood pressure stops rising, however, roughly around the sixth decade. On the other extreme, some elderly people develop an increased tendency toward *postural (orthostatic) hypotension*—a sudden drop in blood pressure when they rise to a sitting or standing position. Elderly people are also more likely to have abnormal heart rhythms. These arrhythmias, like postural hypotension, may cause *syncope,* or temporary loss of consciousness.

THE HEALTH HISTORY

Common or Concerning Symptoms

- Chest pain
- Palpitations
- Shortness of breath, orthopnea, or paroxysmal nocturnal dyspnea
- Swelling or edema

Chest pain or discomfort is one of the most important symptoms you will assess as a clinician. As you listen to the patient's story, you must always keep serious adverse events in mind, such as *angina pectoris, myocardial infarction,* or even a *dissecting aortic aneurysm.* This section approaches chest symp-

See Table 6-1, Chest Pain, pp. 234–235.

toms from the *cardiac standpoint,* including chest pain, palpitations, orthopnea, paroxysmal nocturnal dyspnea (PND), and edema. For this complaint, however, it is wise to think through the range of possible cardiac, pulmonary, and extrathoracic etiologies. You should review the Health History section of Chapter 6, The Thorax and Lungs, which enumerates the various possible sources of chest pain: the myocardium, the pericardium, the aorta, the trachea and large bronchi, the parietal pleura, the esophagus, the chest wall, and extrathoracic structures such as the neck, gallbladder, and stomach. This review is important, since symptoms such as dyspnea, wheezing, cough, and even hemoptysis (see pp. 216–217) can be cardiac as well as pulmonary in origin.

Your initial questions should be broad . . . "Do you have any pain or discomfort in your chest?" Ask the patient to point to the pain and to describe all seven of its attributes. After listening closely to the patient's description, move on to more specific questions such as "Is the pain related to exertion?" and "What kinds of activities bring on the pain?" Also "How intense is the pain, on a scale of 1 to 10?" . . . "Does it radiate into the neck, shoulder, back, or down your arm?" . . . "Are there any associated symptoms like shortness of breath, sweating, palpitations, or nausea?" . . . "Does it ever wake you up at night?" . . . "What do you do to make it better?"

Exertional chest pain with radiation to the left side of the neck and down the left arm in *angina pectoris;* sharp pain radiating into the back or into the neck in *aortic dissection.*

Palpitations are an unpleasant awareness of the heartbeat. When reporting these sensations, patients use various terms such as skipping, racing, fluttering, pounding, or stopping of the heart. Palpitations may result from an irregular heartbeat, from rapid acceleration or slowing of the heart, or from increased forcefulness of cardiac contraction. Such perceptions, however, also depend on the sensitivities of patients to their own body sensations. Palpitations do not necessarily mean heart disease. In contrast, the most serious dysrhythmias, such as ventricular tachycardia, often do not produce palpitations.

See Tables 3-10 and 3-11 for selected heart rates and rhythms (pp. 91–92)

Symptoms or signs of irregular heart action warrant an electrocardiogram. Only *atrial fibrillation,* which is "irregularly irregular," can be reliably identified at the bedside.

You may ask directly about palpitations, but if the patient does not understand your question, reword it. "Are you ever aware of your heartbeat? What is it like?" Ask the patient to tap out the rhythm with a hand or finger. Was it fast or slow? Regular or irregular? How long did it last? If there was an episode of rapid heartbeats, did they start and stop suddenly or gradually? (For this group of symptoms, an electrocardiogram is indicated.)

You may wish to teach selected patients how to make serial measurements of their pulse rates in case they have further episodes.

Clues in the history include transient skips and flipflops (possible premature contractions); rapid regular beating of sudden onset and offset (possible paroxysmal supraventricular tachycardia); a rapid regular rate of less than 120 beats per minute, especially if starting and stopping more gradually (possible sinus tachycardia).

Shortness of breath is a common patient concern and may be reported as dyspnea, orthopnea, or paroxysmal nocturnal dyspnea. *Dyspnea* is an uncomfortable awareness of breathing that is inappropriate to a given level of exertion. This complaint is often made by patients with cardiac and/or pulmonary problems, as discussed in Chapter 6, The Thorax and Lungs, p. 217.

Orthopnea is dyspnea that occurs when the patient is lying down and improves when the patient sits up. Classically, it is quantified according to the

Orthopnea suggests *left ventricular heart failure* or *mitral stenosis;* it number of pillows the patient uses for sleeping, or by the fact that the patient needs to sleep sitting up. (Make sure, however, that the patient uses extra pillows or sleeps upright because of shortness of breath when supine and not for other reasons.)

may also accompany *obstructive lung disease.*

Paroxysmal nocturnal dyspnea, or *PND,* describes episodes of sudden dyspnea and orthopnea that awaken the patient from sleep, usually 1 or 2 hours after going to bed, prompting the patient to sit up, stand up, or go to a window for air. There may be associated wheezing and coughing. The episode usually subsides but may recur at about the same time on subsequent nights.

PND suggests *left ventricular heart failure* or *mitral stenosis* and may be mimicked by *nocturnal asthma* attacks.

Edema refers to the accumulation of excessive fluid in the interstitial tissue spaces and appears as swelling. Questions about edema are typically included in the cardiac history, but edema has many other causes, both local and general. Focus your questions on the location, timing, and setting of the swelling, and on associated symptoms. "Have you had any swelling anywhere? Where? . . . Anywhere else? When does it occur? Is it worse in the morning or at night? Do your shoes get tight?"

Dependent edema appears in the lowest body parts (the feet and lower legs) when sitting or the sacrum when bedridden. Causes may be cardiac (congestive heart failure), nutritional (hypoalbuminemia), or positional.

Continue with "Are the rings tight on your fingers? Are your eyelids puffy or swollen in the morning? Have you had to let out your belt?" Also, "Have your clothes gotten too tight around the middle?" It is useful to ask patients who retain fluid to record daily morning weights, since edema may not be obvious until several liters of extra fluid have accumulated.

Edema occurs in renal and liver disease: periorbital puffiness, tight rings in *nephrotic syndrome;* enlarged waistline from *ascites* and *liver failure.*

HEALTH PROMOTION AND COUNSELING

Important Topics for Health Promotion and Counseling

- Cholesterol level
- Lifestyle management: diet, weight reduction, exercise, smoking
- Screening for hypertension

Despite improvements in risk factor modification, cardiovascular disease remains the leading cause of death for both men and women, accounting for about one third of all U.S. deaths. Both *primary prevention,* in those without evidence of cardiovascular disease, and *secondary prevention,* in those with known cardiovascular events such as angina or myocardial infarction, remain important priorities for the office, the hospital, and the nation's public health. Education and counseling will guide your patients to maintain optimal levels of cholesterol, weight, and exercise.

In May 2001 the National Heart, Lung, and Blood Institute of the National Institutes of Health published the Third Report of the National Cholesterol Education Program Expert Panel, which sets standards for the detection, evaluation, and treatment of high cholesterol levels in adults.[§] Students and clinicians are well-advised to review the Panel's recommended guidelines, which can be summarized only briefly here.

First, obtain a fasting lipid profile in all adults aged 20 years or older once every 5 years. Your counseling and interventions should be based on the patient's levels of low- and high-density lipoproteins, or LDL and HDL, and on the presence of cardiac risk factors. The report notes that the risk of cardiac disease increases continuously as the LDL levels range from low to high. It sets new targets for optimal lipid levels (mg/dL):

- LDL cholesterol <100
- Total cholesterol <200
- HDL cholesterol <40 is low; ≥60 is high

Second, assess additional major risk factors and "risk equivalents." Risk factors are smoking, hypertension if blood pressure is greater than 140/90 mm Hg or the patient is on medication, HDL less than 40 mg/dL, family history of premature coronary heart disease (affected male first-degree relative younger than 55 years; affected female younger than 65 years), and age, namely men 45 years or older and women 55 years or older. *Risk equivalents* include diabetes; other forms of atherosclerotic disease—peripheral vascular disease, abdominal aortic aneurysm, and symptomatic carotid artery disease; and 2 or more risk factors, raising the 10-year risk of coronary heart disease to more than 20%. The report includes tables for assessing 10-year risk for men and for women if multiple risk factors are present.

The desired goal for the patient's LDL level varies according to the number of risk factors, as shown below.

Risk Category	*LDL Level Goal (mg/dL)*
0–1 risk factor	<160
2+ or multiple risk factors	<130
Coronary heart disease (CHD) or CHD risk equivalents	<100

Additional treatment is recommended if the triglyceride level exceeds 200 mg/dL.

Once risk is assessed, your advice about risk reduction should cover lifestyle changes, including diet, weight reduction, and exercise, as well as drug ther-

[§] Third Report of the National Cholesterol Education Program (NCEP) Expert Panel. Detection, Evaluation, and Treatment of High Blood Cholesterol in Adults—Executive Summary. National Cholesterol Education Program, National Heart, Lung, and Blood Institute, National Institutes of Health. NIH Publication No. 01-3670. May 2001. www.nhlbi.nih.gov/guidelines/cholesterol/index.htm. Accessed 8/31/01.

apy when indicated. Dietary recommendations should begin with a dietary history (see pp. 65–66), then target low intake of saturated fats (less than 7% of total calories) and cholesterol (less than 200 mg per day) and high intake of fiber, up to 20 to 30 grams per day. Together with the patient, review the basic principles for all healthy diets: high intake of fruits, vegetables, and grains; use of low-fat dairy products and lean meats, substituting chicken and fish when possible; and minimal intake of processed food and added salt and sugar, both when cooking and at the table. Eggs with yolks, the most concentrated source of cholesterol, should be limited to two to four per week. Sources of fiber include whole-grain breads; pasta; and oat, wheat, corn, or multigrain cereals.

For counseling about weight, apply the principles for assessing *body mass index* enumerated in Chapter 3 (pp. 60–61). To maintain a desirable body weight, energy expended must balance calories consumed. Excess calories are stored as fat. Metabolism of food fat, which contains 9 calories of potential energy per gram, uses up fewer calories than metabolism of foods high in carbohydrate or protein, which provide 4 calories of energy per gram. Patients with high fat intake are more likely to accumulate body fat than patients with increased protein and carbohydrate intake (and patients with low-fat diets may lose weight more quickly). Review the patient's eating habits and weight patterns in the family. Set realistic goals that will help the patient maintain healthy eating patterns *for life*.

Regular exercise is the number one recommendation of the U.S. Public Health Service's *Healthy People 2010*. To reduce risk for coronary artery disease, counsel patients to pursue *aerobic* exercise, or exercise that increases muscle oxygen uptake. (*Anaerobic* exercise relies on energy sources within contracting muscles rather than inhaled oxygen and is usually nonsustained.) Deep breathing, sweating in cool temperatures, and pulse rates exceeding 60% of the maximum normal age-adjusted heart rate (220 minus the person's age) are markers of aerobic exercise. Since the cardiovascular benefits of exercise are long term, to help motivate patients be sure to emphasize that the patient will look and feel better as soon as exercise begins. Before selecting an exercise regimen, do a thorough evaluation of any cardiovascular, pulmonary, or musculoskeletal conditions presenting a risk for exercise. Guiding the patient to make time to exercise as a *regular activity* is often more important than the type of exercise chosen. For cardiovascular benefit, patients should exercise for 20 to 60 minutes at least 3 times a week. For patients losing weight, paradoxically, the metabolic rate may drop when caloric intake declines, known as the starvation response. Regular exercise will counteract this response.

During the physical examination, it is important to screen for hypertension and for lipid-containing nodules on the skin, known as *xanthomas*. Hypertension (see pp. 75–79) contributes significantly to death from CHD and stroke. Recommended blood pressure screening for healthy adults is generally once every 2 years. Search for xanthomas in patients with familial lipoprotein disorders. These may appear around the eyelids, over extensor tendons, and occasionally as small eruptive papules on the extremities, buttocks, and trunk.

Preview: Recording the Physical Examination— The Cardiovascular Examination

Note that initially you may use sentences to describe your findings; later you will use phrases. The style below contains phrases appropriate for most write-ups. Unfamiliar terms are explained in the next section, Techniques of Examination.

> "The jugular venous pulse (JVP) is 3 cm above the sternal angle with the head of bed elevated to 30°. Carotid upstrokes are brisk, without bruits. The point of maximal impulse (PMI) is tapping, 7 cm lateral to the midsternal line in the 5th intercostal space. Good S_1 and S_2. No murmurs or extra sounds."

OR

> "The JVP is 5 cm above the sternal angle with the head of bed elevated to 50°. Carotid upstrokes are brisk; a bruit is heard over the left carotid artery. The PMI is diffuse, 3 cm in diameter, palpated at the anterior axillary line in the 5th and 6th intercostal spaces. S_1 and S_2 are soft. S_3 present. Harsh 2/6 holosystolic murmur best heard at the apex, radiating to the lower left sternal border (LLSB). No S_4 or diastolic murmurs."

Suggests congestive heart failure with possible left carotid occlusion and mitral regurgitation

TECHNIQUES OF EXAMINATION

As you begin the cardiovascular examination, review the blood pressure and heart rate recorded during the General Survey and Vital Signs at the start of the physical examination. If you need to repeat these measurements, or if they have not already been done, take the time to measure the blood pressure and heart rate using optimal technique (see Chapter 3, Beginning the Physical Examination: General Survey and Vital Signs, especially pp. 75–79).

In brief, for *blood pressure,* after letting the patient rest for at least 5 minutes in a quiet setting, choose a correctly sized cuff and position the patient's arm at heart level, either resting on a table if seated or supported at midchest level if standing. Make sure the bladder of the cuff is centered over the brachial artery. Inflate the cuff about 30 mm Hg above the pressure at which the radial pulse disappears. As you deflate the cuff, listen first for the sounds of at least two consecutive heartbeats—these mark the *systolic* pressure. Then listen for the disappearance point of the heartbeats, which marks the *diastolic* pressure. For *heart rate,* measure the radial pulse using the pads of your index and middle fingers, or assess the apical pulse using your stethoscope (see p. 80).

Now you are ready to systematically assess the components of the cardiovascular system:

- The jugular venous pressure
- The carotid upstrokes and presence or absence of bruits
- The point of maximal impulse (PMI) and any heaves, lifts, or thrills
- The first and second heart sounds, S_1 and S_2
- Presence or absence of extra heart sounds such as S_3 or S_4
- Presence or absence of any cardiac murmurs.

Jugular Venous Pressure and Pulsations

Jugular Venous Pressure (JVP). Estimating the JVP is one of the most important and frequently used skills of physical examination. At first it will seem difficult, but with practice and supervision you will find that the JVP provides valuable information about the patient's volume status and cardiac function. As you have learned, the JVP reflects pressure in the right atrium, or central venous pressure, and is best assessed from pulsations in the right internal jugular vein. Note, however, that the jugular veins and pulsations are difficult to see in children younger than 12 years of age, so they are not useful for evaluating the cardiovascular system in this age group (see Chapter 17, p. 66).

To assist you in learning this portion of the cardiac examination, steps for assessing the JVP are outlined on the next page. As you begin your assessment, take a moment to reflect on the patient's volume status and consider how you may need to alter the elevation of the head of the bed or examining table. The usual starting point for assessing the JVP is to elevate the head of the bed to 30°. Identify the external jugular vein on each side, then find the internal jugular venous pulsations transmitted from deep in the neck to the overlying soft tissues. The JVP is the elevation at which the highest oscillation point, or meniscus, of the jugular venous pulsations is usually evident in euvolemic patients. In patients who are *hypovolemic*, you may anticipate that *the JVP will be low*, causing you to subsequently *lower the head of the bed*, sometimes even to 0°, to see the point of oscillation best. Likewise, in volume-overloaded or *hypervolemic* patients, you may anticipate that *the JVP will be high*, causing you to subsequently *raise the head of the bed*.

A hypovolemic patient may have to lie flat before you see the veins. In contrast, when jugular venous pressure is increased, an elevation up to 60° or even 90° may be required. In all these positions, the sternal angle usually remains about 5 cm above the right atrium, as diagrammed on p. 257.

STEPS FOR ASSESSING THE JUGULAR VENOUS PRESSURE (JVP)

- Make the patient comfortable. *Raise the head slightly on a pillow* to relax the sternomastoid muscles.
- *Raise the head of the bed or examining table to about 30°. Turn the patient's head slightly away from the side you are inspecting.*
- Use *tangential lighting* and examine both sides of the neck. Identify the external jugular vein on each side, then find the internal jugular venous pulsations.
- *If necessary, raise or lower the head of the bed* until you can see the oscillation point or meniscus of the internal jugular venous pulsations in the lower half of the neck.
- Focus on the *right internal jugular vein.* Look for pulsations in the suprasternal notch, between the attachments of the sternomastoid muscle on the sternum and clavicle, or just posterior to the sternomastoid. The table below helps you distinguish internal jugular pulsations from those of the carotid artery.
- *Identify the highest point of pulsation in the right internal jugular vein.* Extend a long rectangular object or card horizontally from this point and a centimeter ruler vertically from the sternal angle, making an exact right angle. Measure the vertical distance in centimeters above the sternal angle where the horizontal object crosses the ruler. *This distance, measured in centimeters above the sternal angle or the atrium, is the JVP.*

The following features help to distinguish jugular from carotid artery pulsations:

Internal Jugular Pulsations	Carotid Pulsations
Rarely palpable	Palpable
Soft, rapid, undulating quality, usually with two elevations and two troughs per heart beat	A more vigorous thrust with a single outward component
Pulsations eliminated by light pressure on the vein(s) just above the sternal end of the clavicle	Pulsations not eliminated by this pressure
Level of the pulsations changes with position, dropping as the patient becomes more upright.	Level of the pulsations unchanged by position
Level of the pulsations usually descends with inspiration.	Level of the pulsations not affected by inspiration

Establishing the true vertical and horizontal lines to measure the JVP is difficult, much like the problem of hanging a picture straight when you are close to it. Place your ruler on the sternal angle and line it up with something in the room that you know to be vertical. Then place a card or rectangular object at an exact right angle to the ruler. This constitutes your horizontal line. Move it up or down—still horizontal—so that the lower edge rests at the top of the jugular pulsations, and read the vertical distance on the ruler. Round your measurement off to the nearest centimeter.

Increased pressure suggests right-sided heart failure or, less commonly, constrictive pericarditis, tricuspid stenosis, or superior vena cava obstruction.

In patients with obstructive lung disease, venous pressure may appear elevated on expiration only; the veins collapse on inspiration. This finding does not indicate congestive heart failure.

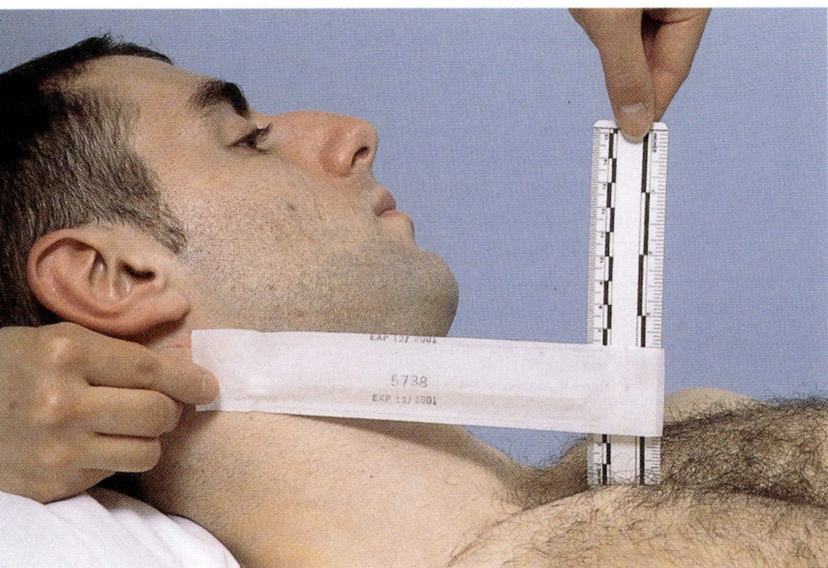

Venous pressure measured at greater than 3 cm or possibly 4 cm above the sternal angle, or more than 8 cm or 9 cm in total distance above the right atrium, is considered elevated above normal.

If you are unable to see pulsations in the internal jugular veins, look for them in the external jugulars, although they may not be visible here. If you see none, use *the point above which the external jugular veins appear to collapse.* Make this observation on each side of the neck. Measure the vertical distance of this point from the sternal angle.

Unilateral distention of the external jugular vein is usually due to local kinking or obstruction. Occasionally, even bilateral distention has a local cause.

The highest point of venous pulsations may lie below the level of the sternal angle. Under these circumstances, venous pressure is not elevated and seldom needs to be measured.

Even though students may not see clinicians making these measurements very frequently in clinical settings, practicing exact techniques for measuring the JVP is important. Eventually, with experience, clinicians and cardiologists come to identify the JVP and estimate its height visually.

Jugular Venous Pulsations. *Observe the amplitude and timing of the jugular venous pulsations.* In order to time these pulsations, feel the left carotid artery with your right thumb or listen to the heart simultaneously.

Prominent *a* waves indicate increased resistance to right atrial contraction, as in tricuspid stenosis

The *a* wave just precedes S_1 and the carotid pulse, the *x* descent can be seen as a systolic collapse, the *v* wave almost coincides with S_2, and the *y* descent follows early in diastole. Look for absent or unusually prominent waves.

or, more commonly, the decreased compliance of a hypertrophied right ventricle. The *a* waves disappear in atrial fibrillation. Larger *v* waves characterize tricuspid regurgitation.

a v x y

S_1 S_2 S_1 S_2

Systole Diastole

Considerable practice and experience are required to master jugular venous pulsations. A beginner is probably well-advised to concentrate primarily on jugular venous pressure.

The Carotid Pulse

After you measure the JVP, move on to assessment of the *carotid pulse.* The carotid pulse provides valuable information about cardiac function and is especially useful for detecting stenosis or insufficiency of the aortic valve. Take the time to assess the quality of the carotid upstroke, its amplitude and contour, and presence or absence of any overlying *thrills* or *bruits.*

For irregular rhythms, see Table 3-10, Selected Heart Rates and Rhythms (p. 91), and Table 3-4, Selected Irregular Rhythms (p. 92).

To assess *amplitude and contour,* the patient should be lying down with the head of the bed still elevated to about 30°. When feeling for the carotid artery, first inspect the neck for carotid pulsations. These may be visible just medial to the sternomastoid muscles. Then place your left index and middle fingers (or left thumb[‖]) on the right carotid artery in the lower third of the neck, press posteriorly, and feel for pulsations.

A tortuous and kinked carotid artery may produce a unilateral pulsatile bulge.

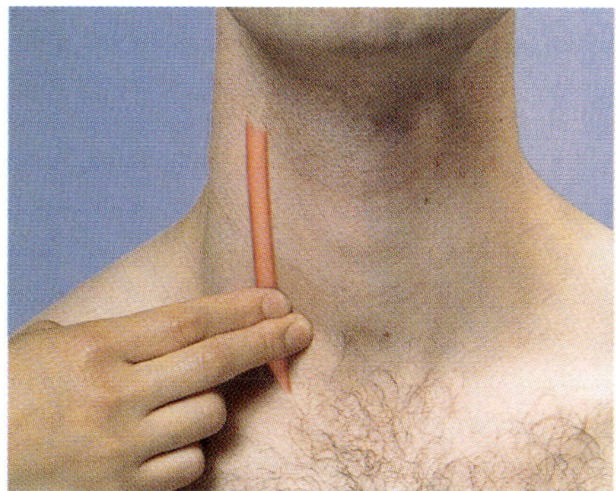

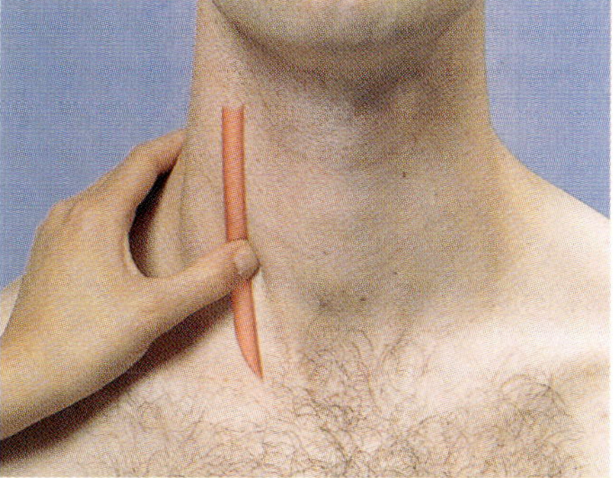

Decreased pulsations may be caused by decreased stroke volume, but may also be due to local factors in the artery such as atherosclerotic narrowing or occlusion.

‖ Although there is a widespread prejudice against using thumbs to assess pulses, they are useful for palpating large arteries.

Press just inside the medial border of a well-relaxed sternomastoid muscle, roughly at the level of the cricoid cartilage. Avoid pressing on the *carotid sinus,* which lies at the level of the top of the thyroid cartilage. For the left carotid artery, use your right fingers or thumb. Never press both carotids at the same time. This may decrease blood flow to the brain and induce syncope.

Pressure on the carotid sinus may cause a reflex drop in pulse rate or blood pressure.

Slowly increase pressure until you feel a maximal pulsation, then slowly decrease pressure until you best sense the arterial pressure and contour. Try to assess:

See Table 3-9, Abnormalities of the Arterial Pulse and Pressure Waves (p. 90).

- The *amplitude of the pulse.* This correlates reasonably well with the pulse pressure.

Small, thready, or weak pulse in cardiogenic shock; *bounding* pulse in aortic insufficiency (see p. 90).

- The *contour of the pulse wave,* namely the speed of the upstroke, the duration of its summit, and the speed of the downstroke. The normal upstroke is *brisk.* It is smooth, rapid, and follows S_1 almost immediately. The summit is smooth, rounded, and roughly midsystolic. The downstroke is less abrupt than the upstroke.

Delayed carotid upstroke in aortic stenosis

- Any *variations in amplitude,* either from beat to beat or with respiration.

Pulsus alternans, bigeminal pulse (beat-to-beat variation); paradoxical pulse (respiratory variation)

Thrills and Bruits. During palpation of the carotid artery, you may detect humming vibrations, or *thrills,* that feel like the throat of a purring cat. Routinely, but especially in the presence of a thrill, you should listen over both carotid arteries with the diaphragm of your stethoscope for a *bruit,* a murmur-like sound of vascular rather than cardiac origin.

You should also listen for bruits over the carotid arteries if the patient is middle-aged or elderly or if you suspect cerebrovascular disease. Ask the patient to hold breathing for a moment so that breath sounds do not obscure the vascular sound. Heart sounds alone do not constitute a bruit.

A carotid bruit with or without a thrill in a middle-aged or older person suggests but does not prove arterial narrowing. An aortic murmur may radiate to the carotid artery and sound like a bruit.

Further examination of arterial pulses is described in Chapter 14, The Peripheral Vascular System.

The Brachial Artery. The carotid arteries reflect aortic pulsations more accurately, but in patients with carotid obstruction, kinking, or thrills, they are unsuitable. If so, assess the pulse in the *brachial artery,* applying the techniques described above for determining amplitude and contour.

Use the index and middle fingers or thumb of your opposite hand. Cup your hand under the patient's elbow and feel for the pulse just medial to the biceps tendon. The patient's arm should rest with the elbow extended, palm up. With your free hand, you may need to flex the elbow to a varying degree to get optimal muscular relaxation.

The Heart

For most of the cardiac examination, the patient should be supine with the upper body raised by elevating the head of the bed or table to about 30°. Two other positions are also needed: (1) turning to the left side, and (2) leaning forward. The examiner should stand at the patient's right side.

The table below summarizes patient positions and a suggested sequence for the examination.

Sequence of the Cardiac Examination

Patient Position	Examination	Accentuated Findings
Supine, with the head elevated 30°	Inspect and palpate the precordium: the 2nd interspaces; the right ventricle; and the left ventricle, including the apical impulse (diameter, location, amplitude, duration).	
Left lateral decubitus	Palpate the apical impulse if not previously detected. Listen at the apex with the bell of the stethoscope.	Low-pitched extra sounds (S_3, opening snap, diastolic rumble of mitral stenosis)
Supine, with the head elevated 30°	Listen at the tricuspid area with the bell.	
	Listen at all the auscultatory areas with the diaphragm.	
Sitting, leaning forward, after full exhalation	Listen along the left sternal border and at the apex.	Soft decrescendo diastolic murmur of aortic insufficiency

During the cardiac examination, remember to correlate your findings with the patient's jugular venous pressure and carotid pulse. It is also important to identify both the anatomic location of your findings and their timing in the cardiac cycle.

- Note the *anatomic location* of sounds in terms of interspaces and their distance from the midsternal, midclavicular, or axillary lines. The midsternal line offers the most reliable zero point for measurement, but some feel that the midclavicular line accommodates the different sizes and shapes of patients.

- Identify the *timing of impulses or sounds* in relation to the cardiac cycle. Timing of sounds is often possible through auscultation alone. In most people with normal or slow heart rates, it is easy to identify the paired heart sounds by listening through a stethoscope. S_1 is the first of these sounds, S_2 is the second, and the relatively long diastolic interval separates one pair from the next.

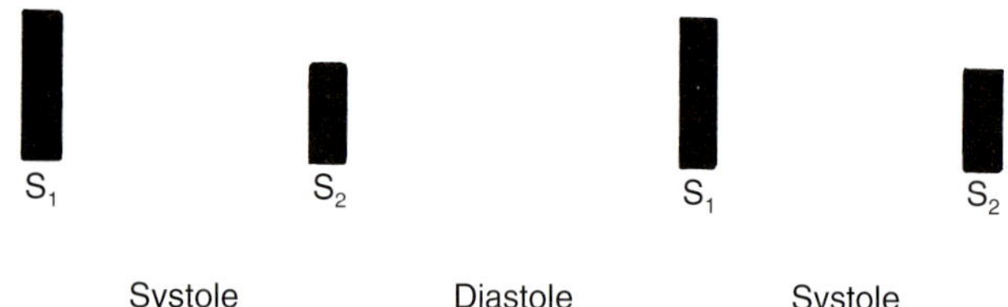

The relative intensity of these sounds may also be helpful. S_1 is usually louder than S_2 at the apex; more reliably, S_2 is usually louder than S_1 at the base.

Even experienced clinicians are sometimes uncertain about the timing of what they hear, especially when they encounter extra heart sounds and murmurs. "Inching" can then be helpful. Return to a place on the chest—most often the base—where it is easy to identify S_1 and S_2. Get their rhythm clearly in mind. Then inch your stethoscope down the chest in steps until you hear the new sound.

Auscultation alone, however, can be misleading. The intensities of S_1 and S_2, for example, may be abnormal. At rapid heart rates, moreover, diastole shortens, and at about a rate of 120 the durations of systole and diastole become indistinguishable. Use *palpation of either the carotid pulse or the apical impulse* to guide the timing of your observations. Both occur in early systole, right after the first heart sound.

For example, S_1 is decreased in first-degree heart block, and S_2 is decreased in aortic stenosis.

INSPECTION AND PALPATION

Careful *inspection* of the anterior chest may reveal the location of the *apical impulse* or *point of maximal impulse (PMI)*, or less commonly, the ventricular movements of a left-sided S_3 or S_4. Tangential light is best for making these observations.

Use *palpation* to confirm the characteristics of the apical impulse. Palpation is also valuable for detecting thrills and the ventricular movements of an S_3 or S_4. Be sure to assess the right ventricle by palpating the right ventricular area at the lower left sternal border and in the subxiphoid area, the pulmonary artery in the left 2nd interspace, and the aortic area in the right 2nd interspace. Review the diagram on the next page. *Note that the "areas" designated for the left and right ventricle, the pulmonary artery, and the aorta pertain to the majority of patients whose hearts are situated in the left chest, with normal anatomy of the great vessels.*

Begin with general palpation of the chest wall. First palpate for impulses using your fingerpads. Hold them flat or obliquely on the body surface, using light pressure for an S_3 or S_4, and firmer pressure for S_1 and S_2. Ventricular impulses may heave or lift your fingers. Then check for *thrills* by pressing the ball of your hand firmly on the chest. If subsequent auscultation reveals a loud murmur, go back and check for thrills over that area again.

Thrills may accompany loud, harsh, or rumbling murmurs as in aortic stenosis, patent ductus arteriosus, ventricular septal defect, and, less commonly, mitral stenosis. They are palpated more easily in patient positions that accentuate the murmur.

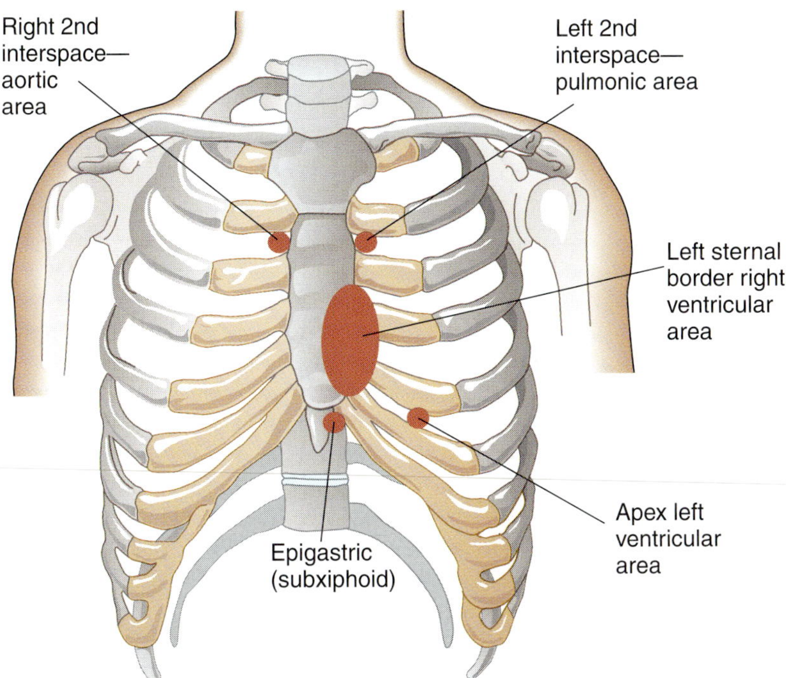

The Apical Impulse or Point of Maximal Impulse (PMI)—Left Ventricular Area. The apical impulse represents the brief early pulsation of the left ventricle as it moves anteriorly during contraction and touches the chest wall. Note that in most examinations the apical impulse is the point of maximal impulse, or PMI; however, some pathologic conditions may produce a pulsation that is more prominent than the apex beat, such as an enlarged right ventricle, a dilated pulmonary artery, or an aneurysm of the aorta.

If you cannot identify the apical impulse with the patient supine, ask the patient to roll partly onto the left side—this is the *left lateral decubitus* position. Palpate again using the palmar surfaces of several fingers. If you cannot find the apical impulse, ask the patient to exhale fully and stop breathing for a few seconds. When examining a woman, it may be helpful to displace the left breast upward or laterally as necessary; alternatively, ask her to do this for you.

On rare occasions, a patient has *dextrocardia*—a heart situated on the right side. The apical impulse will then be found on the right. If you cannot find an apical impulse, percuss for the dullness of heart and liver and for the tympany of the stomach. In *situs inversus,* all three of these structures are on opposite sides from normal. A right-sided heart with a normally placed liver and stomach is usually associated with congenital heart disease.

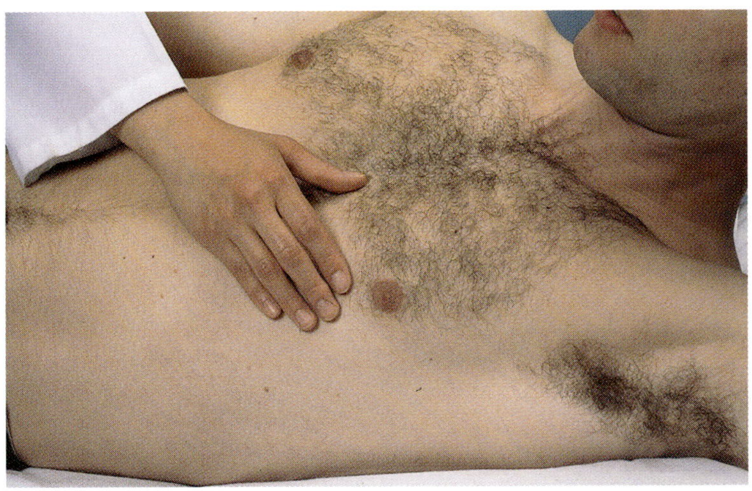

Once you have found the apical impulse, make finer assessments with your fingertips, and then with one finger.

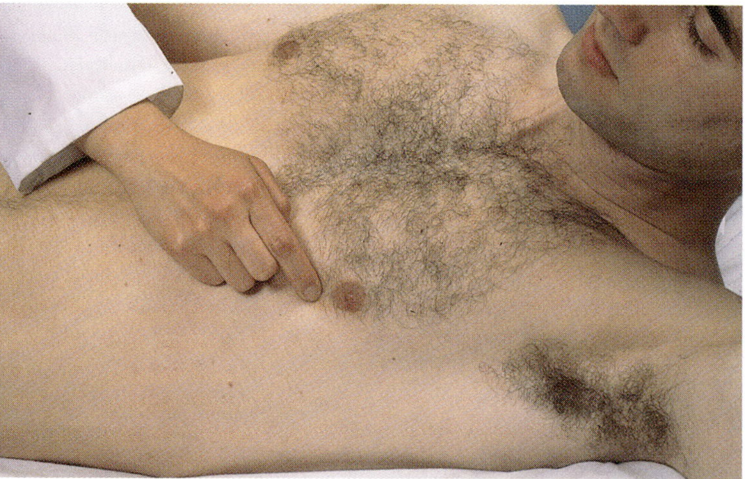

With experience, you will learn to feel the apical impulse in a high percentage of patients, but obesity, a very muscular chest wall, or an increased anteroposterior diameter of the chest may make it undetectable. Some apical impulses hide behind the rib cage, despite positioning.

Now assess the location, diameter, amplitude, and duration of the apical impulse. You may wish to have the patient breathe out and briefly stop breathing to check your findings.

See Table 7-1, Variations and Abnormalities of the Ventricular Impulses (p. 286).

- *Location.* Try to assess location with the patient *supine,* since the left lateral decubitus position displaces the apical impulse to the left. Locate two points: the interspaces, usually the 5th or possibly the 4th, which give the vertical location; and the distance in centimeters from the midsternal line, which gives the horizontal location. (Note that even though the apical impulse normally falls roughly at the midclavicular line, measurements from this line are less reproducible since clinicians vary in their estimates of the midpoint of the clavicle.)

The apical impulse may be displaced upward and to the left by pregnancy or a high left diaphragm.

Lateral displacement from cardiac enlargement in congestive heart failure, cardiomyopathy, ischemic heart disease. Displacement in deformities of the thorax and mediastinal shift.

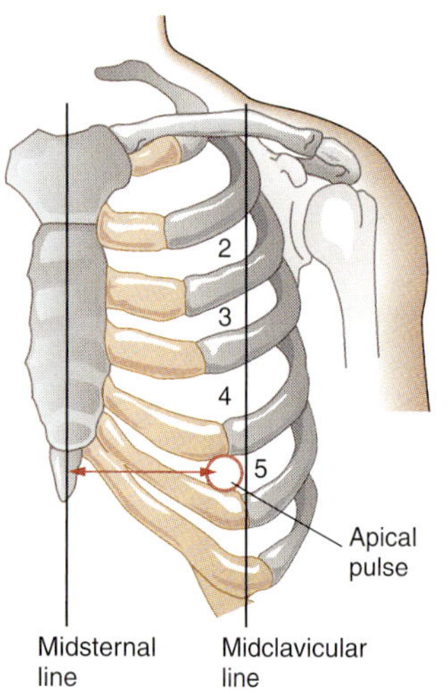

- *Diameter.* Assess the diameter of the apical impulse. In the supine patient, it usually measures less than 2.5 cm and occupies only one interspace. It may be larger in the left lateral decubitus position.

In the left lateral decubitus position, a diameter greater than 3 cm indicates left ventricular enlargement.

- *Amplitude.* Estimate the amplitude of the impulse. It is usually small and feels *brisk* and *tapping*. Some young persons have an increased amplitude, or hyperkinetic impulse, especially when excited or after exercise; its duration, however, is normal.

Increased amplitude may also reflect hyperthyroidism, severe anemia, pressure overload of the left ventricle (e.g., aortic stenosis), or volume overload of the left ventricle (e.g., mitral regurgitation).

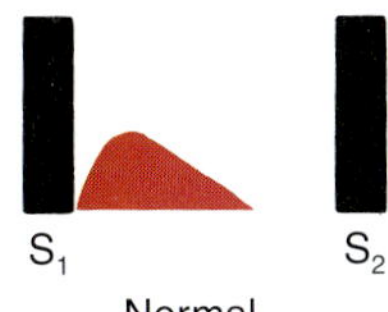

Normal

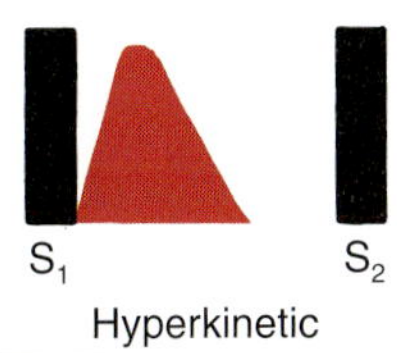

Hyperkinetic

- *Duration.* Duration is the most useful characteristic of the apical impulse for identifying hypertrophy of the left ventricle. To assess duration, listen to the heart sounds as you feel the apical impulse, or watch the movement of your stethoscope as you listen at the apex. Estimate the proportion of systole occupied by the apical impulse. Normally it lasts through the first two thirds of systole, and often less, but does not continue to the second heart sound.

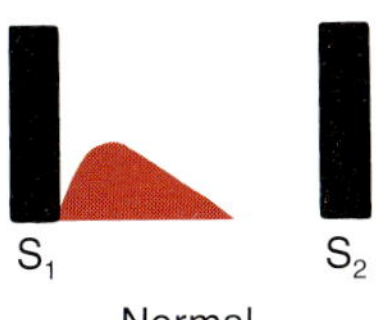

Normal

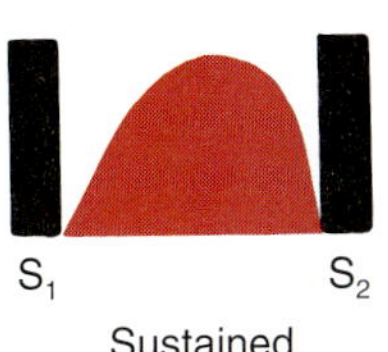

Sustained

A sustained, high-amplitude impulse that is normally located suggests left ventricular hypertrophy from pressure overload (as in hypertension). If such an impulse is displaced laterally, consider volume overload.

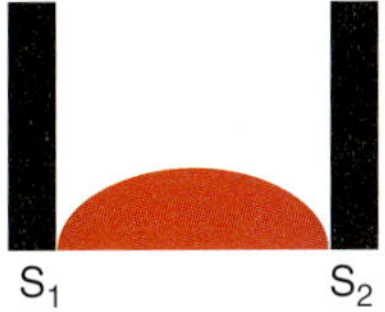

A sustained low-amplitude (hypokinetic) impulse may result from dilated cardiomyopathy.

S3 and S4. By inspection and palpation, you may detect ventricular movements that are synchronous with pathologic third and fourth heart sounds. For the left ventricular impulses, feel the apical beat gently with one finger. The patient should lie partly on the left side, breathe out, and briefly stop breathing. By inking an X on the apex you may be able to see these movements.

A brief middiastolic impulse indicates an S_3; an impulse just before the systolic apical beat itself indicates an S_4.

The Left Sternal Border in the 3rd, 4th, and 5th Interspaces—Right Ventricular Area. The patient should rest supine at 30°. Place the tips of your curved fingers in the 3rd, 4th, and 5th interspaces and try to feel the systolic impulse of the right ventricle. Again, asking the patient to breathe out and then briefly stop breathing improves your observation.

If an impulse is palpable, assess its location, amplitude, and duration. A brief systolic tap of low or slightly increased amplitude is sometimes felt in thin or shallow-chested persons, especially when stroke volume is increased, as by anxiety.

A marked increase in amplitude with little or no change in duration occurs in chronic volume overload of the right ventricle, as from an atrial septal defect.

An impulse with increased amplitude and duration occurs with pressure overload of the right ventricle, as in pulmonic stenosis or pulmonary hypertension.

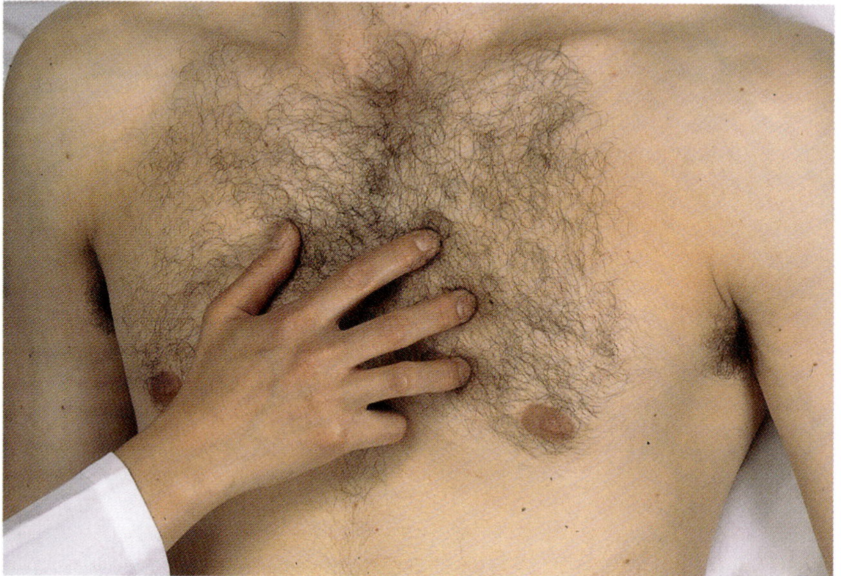

The diastolic movements of right-sided third and fourth heart sounds may be felt occasionally. Feel for them in the 4th and 5th left interspaces. Time them by auscultation or carotid palpation.

In patients with an increased anteroposterior (AP) diameter, palpation of the right ventricle in the *epigastric* or *subxiphoid area* is also useful. With your hand flattened, press your index finger just under the rib cage and up toward the left shoulder and try to feel right ventricular pulsations.

In obstructive pulmonary disease, hyperinflated lung may prevent palpation of an enlarged right ventricle in the left parasternal area. The impulse is felt easily, however, high in the epigastrium and heart sounds are also often heard best here.

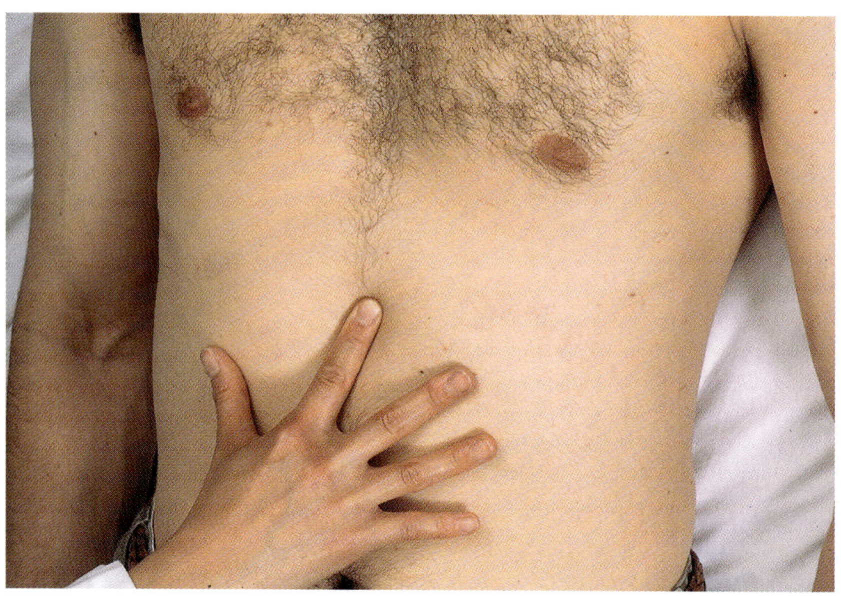

Asking the patient to inhale and briefly stop breathing is helpful. The inspiratory position moves your hand well away from the pulsations of the abdominal aorta, which might otherwise be confusing. The diastolic movements of S_3 and S_4, if present, may also be felt here.

The Left 2nd Interspace—Pulmonic Area. This interspace overlies the *pulmonary artery.* As the patient holds expiration, look and feel for an impulse and feel for possible heart sounds. In thin or shallow-chested patients, the pulsation of a pulmonary artery may sometimes be felt here, especially after exercise or with excitement.

A prominent pulsation here often accompanies dilatation or increased flow in the pulmonary artery. A palpable S_2 suggests increased pressure in the pulmonary artery (pulmonary hypertension).

The Right 2nd Interspace—Aortic Area. This interspace overlies the aortic outflow tract. Search for pulsations and palpable heart sounds.

A palpable S_2 suggests systemic hypertension. A pulsation here suggests a dilated or aneurysmal aorta.

PERCUSSION

In most cases, palpation has replaced percussion in the estimation of cardiac size. When you cannot feel the apical impulse, however, percussion may suggest where to search for it. Occasionally, percussion may be your only tool. Under these circumstances, cardiac dullness often occupies a large area. Starting well to the left on the chest, percuss from resonance toward cardiac dullness in the 3rd, 4th, 5th, and possibly 6th interspaces.

A markedly dilated failing heart may have a hypokinetic apical impulse that is displaced far to the left. A large pericardial effusion may make the impulse undetectable.

AUSCULTATION

Overview. Auscultation of heart sounds and murmurs is a rewarding and important skill of physical examination that leads directly to several clinical diagnoses. In this section, you will learn the techniques for identifying S_1 and S_2, extra sounds in systole and diastole, and systolic and diastolic murmurs. Review the auscultatory areas on the next page with the following caveats: (1) some authorities discourage use of these names since murmurs of more than one origin may occur in a given area; and (2) these areas may not apply to patients with dextrocardia or anomalies of the great vessels. Also, if the heart is enlarged or displaced, your pattern of auscultation should be altered accordingly.

Listen to the heart with your stethoscope *in the right 2nd interspace* close to the sternum, *along the left sternal border* in each interspace from the 2nd through the 5th, and *at the apex.* Recall that the upper margins of the heart are sometimes termed the "base" of the heart. Some clinicians begin auscultation at the apex, others at the base. Either pattern is satisfactory. The room should be quiet. You should also listen in any area where you detect an abnormality and in areas adjacent to murmurs to determine where they are loudest and where they radiate.

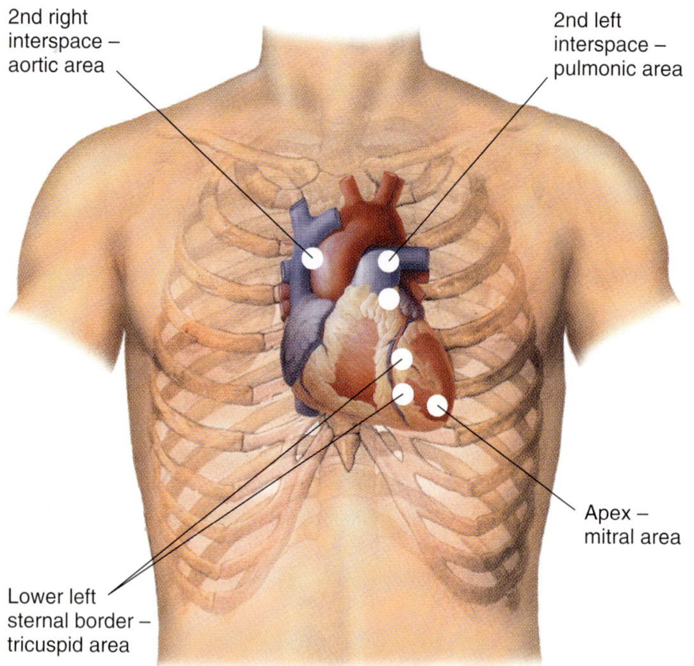

Heart sounds and murmurs that originate in the four valves are illustrated in the diagram below. Pulmonic sounds are usually heard best in the 2nd and 3rd left interspaces, but may extend further.

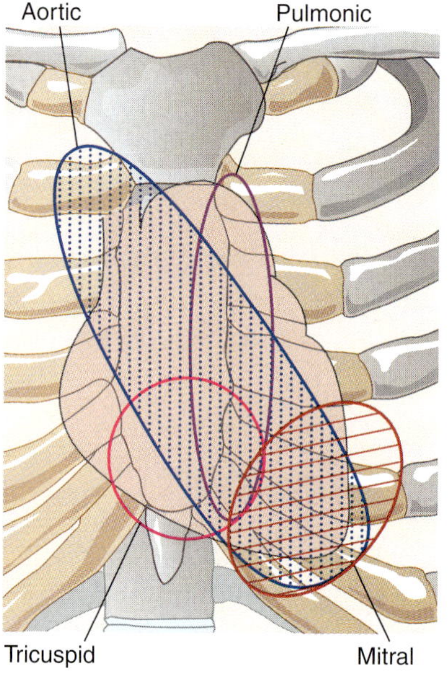

(Redrawn from Leatham A: Introduction to the Examination of the Cardiovascular System, 2nd ed. Oxford, Oxford University Press, 1979)

Know your stethoscope! It is important to understand the uses of both the diaphragm and the bell.

- *The diaphragm.* The diaphragm is better for picking up the relatively high-pitched sounds of S_1 and S_2, the murmurs of aortic and mitral regurgitation, and pericardial friction rubs. *Listen throughout the precordium* with the diaphragm, pressing it firmly against the chest.

- *The bell.* The bell is more sensitive to the low-pitched sounds of S_3 and S_4 and the murmur of mitral stenosis. Apply the bell lightly, with just enough pressure to produce an air seal with its full rim. *Use the bell at the apex, then move medially along the lower sternal border.* Resting the heel of your hand on the chest like a fulcrum may help you to maintain light pressure.

  Pressing the bell firmly on the chest makes it function more like the diaphragm by stretching the underlying skin. Low-pitched sounds such as S_3 and S_4 may disappear with this technique—an observation that may help to identify them. In contrast, high-pitched sounds such as a midsystolic click, an ejection sound, or an opening snap, will persist or get louder.

  Listen to the entire precordium with the patient supine. For new patients and patients needing a complete cardiac examination, use two other important positions to listen for mitral stenosis and aortic regurgitation.

- Ask the patient to *roll partly onto the left side into the left lateral decubitus position,* bringing the left ventricle close to the chest wall. Place the bell of your stethoscope lightly on the apical impulse.

This position accentuates or brings out a left-sided S_3 and S_4 and mitral murmurs, especially mitral stenosis. You may otherwise miss these important findings.

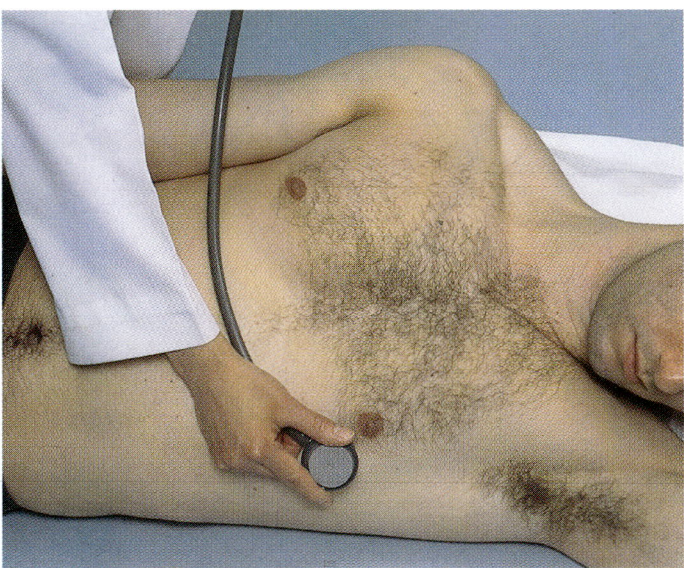

- Ask the patient to *sit up, lean forward, exhale completely, and stop breathing in expiration.* Pressing the diaphragm of your stethoscope on the chest, listen along the left sternal border and at the apex, pausing periodically so the patient may breathe.

This position accentuates or brings out aortic murmurs. You may easily miss the soft diastolic murmur of aortic regurgitation unless you use this position.

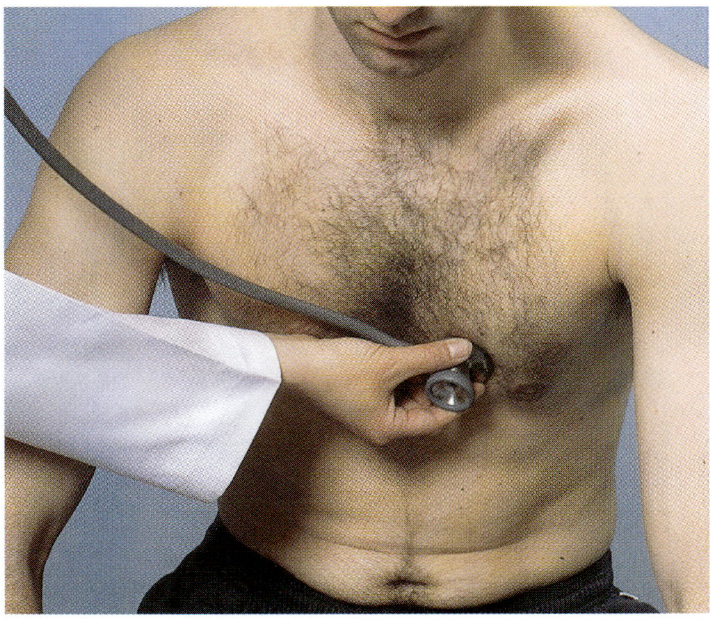

Listening for Heart Sounds. Throughout your examination, take your time at each auscultatory area. Concentrate on each of the events in the cardiac cycle listed on the next page and sounds you may hear in systole and diastole.

Auscultatory Sounds

Heart Sounds	Guides to Auscultation	Examples of Abnormalities
S_1	Note its intensity and any apparent splitting. Normal splitting is detectable along the lower left sternal border.	See Table 7-2, Variations in the First Heart Sound (p. 287).
S_2	Note its intensity.	
Split S_3	Listen for splitting of this sound in the 2nd and 3rd left interspaces. Ask the patient to breathe quietly, and then slightly more deeply than normal. Does S_2 split into its two components, as it normally does? If not, ask the patient to (1) breathe a little more deeply, or (2) sit up. Listen again. A thick chest wall may make the pulmonic component of S_1 inaudible.	See Table 7-3, Variations in the Second Heart Sound (p. 288). When either A_2 or P_2 is absent, as in disease of the respective valves, S_2 is persistently single.
	Width of split. How wide is the split? It is normally quite narrow.	
	Timing of split. When in the respiratory cycle do you hear the split? It is normally heard late in inspiration.	Expiratory splitting suggests an abnormality (p. 288).
	Does the split disappear as it should, during exhalation? If not, listen again with the patient sitting up.	Persistent splitting results from delayed closure of the pulmonic valve or early closure of the aortic valve.
	Intensity of A_2 and P_2. Compare the intensity of the two components, A_2 and P_2. A_2 is usually louder.	A loud P_2 suggests pulmonary hypertension.
Extra Sounds in Systole	Such as ejection sounds or systolic clicks Note their location, timing, intensity, and pitch, and the effects of respiration on the sounds.	The systolic click of mitral valve prolapse is the most common of these sounds. See Table 7-4, Extra Heart Sounds in Systole (p. 289).
Extra Sounds in Diastole	Such as S_3, S_4, or an opening snap Note the location, timing, intensity, and pitch, and the effects of respiration on the sounds. (An S_3 or S_4 in athletes is a normal finding.)	See Table 7-5, Extra Heart Sounds in Diastole (p. 290).
Systolic and Diastolic Murmurs	Murmurs are differentiated from heart sounds by their longer duration.	See Table 7-6, Midsystolic Murmurs (pp. 291–292), Table 7-7, Pansystolic (Holosystolic) Murmurs (p. 293), and Table 7-8, Diastolic Murmurs (p. 294).

Attributes of Heart Murmurs. If you detect a heart murmur, you must learn to identify and describe its *timing, shape, location of maximal intensity, radiation* or transmission from this location, *intensity, pitch,* and *quality.*

- *Timing.* First decide if you are hearing a *systolic murmur,* falling between S_1 and S_2, or a *diastolic murmur,* falling between S_2 and S_1. Palpating the carotid pulse as you listen can help you with timing. Murmurs that coincide with the carotid upstroke are systolic.

  Diastolic murmurs usually indicate valvular heart disease. Systolic murmurs may indicate valvular disease, but often occur when the heart is entirely normal.

  Systolic murmurs are usually *midsystolic* or *pansystolic.* Late systolic murmurs may also be heard.

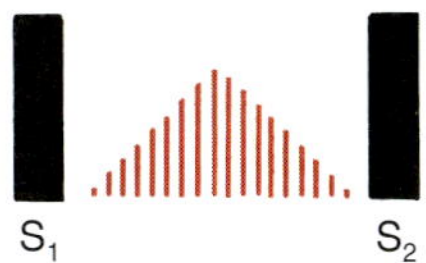

A *midsystolic murmur* begins after S_1 and stops before S_2. Brief gaps are audible between the murmur and the heart sounds. Listen carefully for the gap just before S_2. It is heard more easily and, if present, usually confirms the murmur as midsystolic, not pansystolic.

Midsystolic murmurs most often are related to blood flow across the semilunar (aortic and pulmonic) valves. See Table 7-6, Midsystolic Murmurs (pp. 291–292).

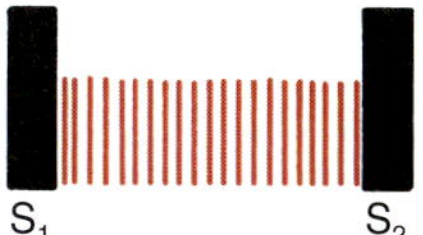

A *pansystolic (holosystolic) murmur* starts with S_1 and stops at S_2, without a gap between murmur and heart sounds.

Pansystolic murmurs often occur with regurgitant (backward) flow across the atrioventricular valves. See Table 7-7, Pansystolic (Holosystolic) Murmurs (p. 293).

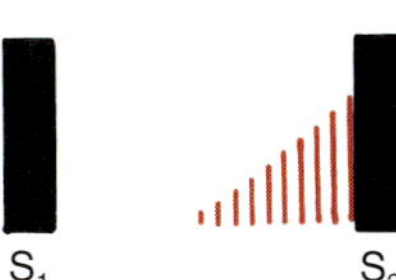

A *late systolic murmur* usually starts in mid- or late systole and persists up to S_2.

This is the murmur of mitral valve prolapse and is often, but not always, preceded by a systolic click (see p. 289).

Diastolic murmurs may be *early diastolic, middiastolic*, or *late diastolic.*

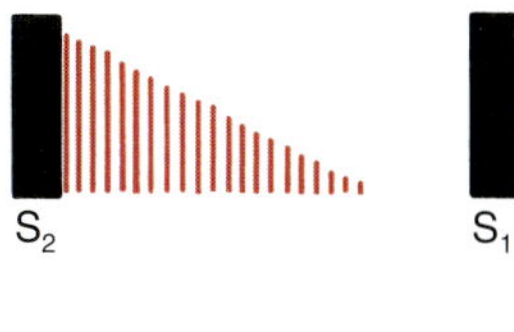

An *early diastolic murmur* starts right after S_2, without a discernible gap, and then usually fades into silence before the next S_1.

Early diastolic murmurs typically accompany regurgitant flow across incompetent semilunar valves.

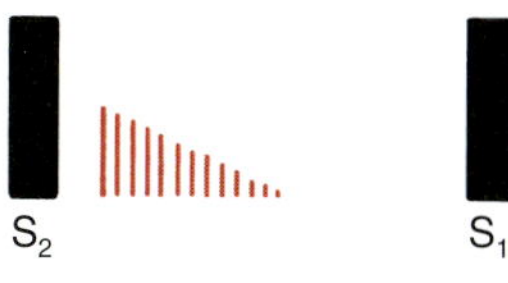

A *middiastolic murmur* starts a short time after S_2. It may fade away, as illustrated, or merge into a late diastolic murmur.

Middiastolic and presystolic murmurs reflect turbulent flow across the atrioventricular valves. See Table 7-8, Diastolic Murmurs (p. 294).

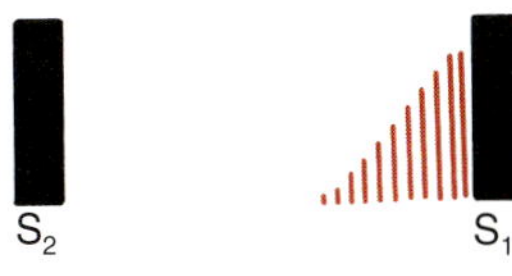

A *late diastolic (presystolic) murmur* starts late in diastole and typically continues up to S_1.

An occasional murmur, such as the murmur of a patent ductus arteriosus, starts in systole and continues without pause through S_2 into but not necessarily throughout diastole. It is then called a *continuous murmur.* Other cardiovascular sounds, such as pericardial friction rubs or venous hums, have *both systolic and diastolic components.* Observe and describe these sounds according to the characteristics used for systolic and diastolic murmurs.

The combination of systolic and diastolic murmurs, each with its own characteristics, may have similar timing. See Table 7-9, Cardiovascular Sounds With Both Systolic and Diastolic Components (p. 295).

- *Shape.* The shape or configuration of a murmur is determined by its intensity over time.

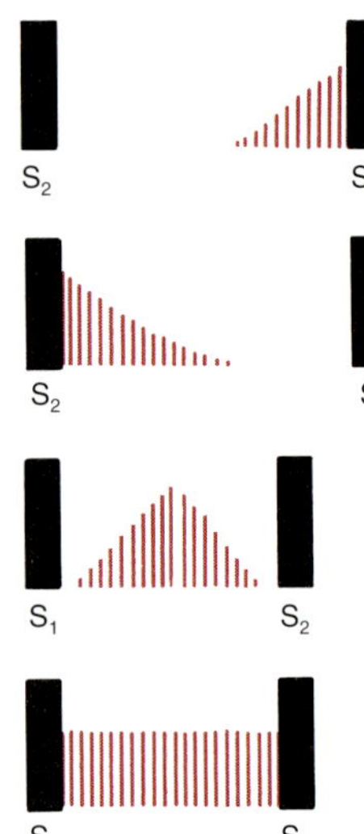

A *crescendo murmur* grows louder.

The presystolic murmur of mitral stenosis in normal sinus rhythm

A *decrescendo murmur* grows softer.

The early diastolic murmur of aortic regurgitation

A *crescendo–descrescendo murmur* first rises in intensity, then falls.

The midsystolic murmur of aortic stenosis and innocent flow murmurs

A *plateau murmur* has the same intensity throughout.

The pansystolic murmur of mitral regurgitation

- *Location of Maximal Intensity.* This is determined by the site where the murmur originates. Find the location by exploring the area where you hear the murmur. Describe where you hear it best in terms of the interspace and its relation to the sternum, the apex, or the midsternal, the midclavicular, or one of the axillary lines.

For example, a murmur best heard in the 2nd right interspace usually originates at or near the aortic valve.

- *Radiation or Transmission from the Point of Maximal Intensity.* This reflects not only the site of origin but also the intensity of the murmur and the direction of blood flow. Explore the area around a murmur and determine where else you can hear it.

A loud murmur of aortic stenosis often radiates into the neck (in the direction of arterial flow).

- *Intensity.* This is usually graded on a 6-point scale and expressed as a fraction. The numerator describes the intensity of the murmur wherever it is loudest, and the denominator indicates the scale you are using. Intensity is influenced by the thickness of the chest wall and the presence of intervening tissue.

An identical degree of turbulence would cause a louder murmur in a thin person than in a very muscular or obese one. Emphysematous lungs may diminish the intensity of murmurs.

Learn to grade murmurs using the 6-point scale below. Note that grades 4 through 6 require the added presence of a palpable thrill.

Gradations of Murmurs

Grade	Description
Grade 1	Very faint, heard only after listener has "tuned in"; may not be heard in all positions
Grade 2	Quiet, but heard immediately after placing the stethoscope on the chest
Grade 3	Moderately loud
Grade 4	Loud, with palpable thrill
Grade 5	Very loud, with thrill. May be heard when the stethoscope is partly off the chest
Grade 6	Very loud, with thrill. May be heard with stethoscope entirely off the chest

- *Pitch*. This is categorized as high, medium, or low.
- *Quality*. This is described in terms such as blowing, harsh, rumbling, and musical.

A fully described murmur might be: a "medium-pitched, grade 2/6, blowing decrescendo murmur, heard best in the 4th left interspace, with radiation to the apex" (aortic regurgitation).

Other useful characteristics of murmurs—and heart sounds too—include variation with respiration, with the position of the patient, or with other special maneuvers.

Murmurs originating in the right side of the heart tend to change more with respiration than left-sided murmurs.

A Note on Cardiovascular Assessment

A good cardiovascular examination requires more than observation. You need to think about the possible meanings of your individual observations, fit them together in a logical pattern, and correlate your cardiac findings with the patient's blood pressure, arterial pulses, venous pulsations, jugular venous pressure, the remainder of your physical examination, and the patient's history.

Evaluating the common systolic murmur illustrates this point. In examining an asymptomatic teenager, for example, you might hear a grade 2/6 midsystolic murmur in the 2nd and 3rd left interspaces. Since this suggests a murmur of pulmonic origin, you should assess the size of the right ventricle by carefully palpating the left parasternal area. Because pulmonic stenosis and atrial septal defects can occasionally cause such murmurs, listen carefully to the splitting of the second heart sound and try to hear any ejection sounds. Listen to the murmur after the patient sits up. Look for evidence of anemia, hyperthyroidism, or pregnancy that could produce such a murmur by increasing the flow across the aortic or the pulmonic valve. If all your findings are normal, your patient probably has an *innocent murmur*—one with no pathologic significance.

In a 60-year-old person with angina, you might hear a harsh 3/6 midsystolic crescendo–decrescendo murmur in the right 2nd interspace radiating to the neck. These findings suggest *aortic stenosis,* but could arise from *aortic sclerosis* (leaflets sclerotic but not stenotic), a dilated aorta, or increased flow across a normal valve. Check the apical impulse for left ventricular enlargement. Listen for *aortic regurgitation* as the patient leans forward and exhales.

Assess any delay in the carotid upstroke and the blood pressure for evidence of aortic stenosis. Put all this information together to make a tentative hypothesis about the origin of the murmur.

Special Techniques

Aids to Identify Systolic Murmurs. Elsewhere in this chapter you have learned how to improve your auscultation of heart sounds and murmurs by placing the patient in different positions. Two additional techniques will help you distinguish the murmurs of mitral valve prolapse and hypertrophic cardiomyopathy from aortic stenosis.

(1) Standing and Squatting. When a person stands, venous return to the heart decreases as does peripheral vascular resistance. Arterial blood pressure, stroke volume, and the volume of blood in the left ventricle all decline. On squatting, changes occur in the opposite direction. These changes help (1) to identify a prolapsed mitral valve, and (2) to distinguish hypertrophic cardiomyopathy from aortic stenosis.

Secure the patient's gown so that it will not interfere with your examination, and ready yourself for prompt auscultation. Instruct the patient to squat next to the examining table and hold on to it for balance. Listen to the heart with the patient in the squatting position and again in the standing position.

(2) Valsalva Maneuver. When a person strains down against a closed glottis, venous return to the right heart is decreased and after a few seconds left ventricular volume and arterial blood pressure both fall. Release of the effort has the opposite effects. These changes help to distinguish prolapse of the mitral valve and hypertrophic cardiomyopathy from aortic stenosis.

The patient should be lying down. Ask the patient to "bear down," or place one hand on the midabdomen and instruct the patient to strain against it. By adjusting the pressure of your hand you can alter the patient's effort to the desired level. Use your other hand to place your stethoscope on the patient's chest.

Maneuvers to Identify Systolic Murmurs

		Effect on Systolic Sounds and Murmurs		
Maneuver	**Cardiovascular Effect**	*Mitral Valve Prolapse*	*Hypertrophic Cardiomyopathy*	*Aortic Stenosis*
Standing; Strain Phase of Valsalva	**Decreased left ventricular volume** from ↓ venous return to heart **Decreased vascular tone:** ↓ arterial blood pressure; ↓ peripheral vascular resistance	↑ prolapse of mitral valve Click moves earlier in systole and murmur lengthens **↑ intensity of murmur**	↑ outflow obstruction **↑ intensity of murmur**	↓ blood volume ejected into aorta **↓ intensity of murmur**
Squatting; Release of Valsalva	**Increased left ventricular volume** from ↑ venous return to heart **Increased vascular tone:** ↑ arterial blood pressure; ↑ peripheral vascular resistance	↓ prolapse of mitral valve Delay of click and murmur shortens **↓ intensity of murmur**	↓ outflow obstruction **↓ intensity of murmur**	↑ blood volume ejected into aorta **↑ intensity of murmur**

Pulsus Alternans. If you suspect left-sided heart failure, feel the pulse specifically for alternating amplitudes. These are usually felt best in the radial or the femoral arteries. A blood-pressure cuff gives you a more sensitive method. After raising the cuff pressure, lower it slowly to the systolic level and then below it. While you do this, the patient should breathe quietly or stop breathing in the respiratory midposition. If dyspnea prevents this, help the patient to sit up and dangle both legs over the side of the bed.

Alternately loud and soft Korotkoff sounds or a sudden doubling of the apparent heart rate as the cuff pressure declines indicates a pulsus alternans (see p. 90).

The upright position may accentuate the alternation.

Paradoxical Pulse. If you have noted that the pulse varies in amplitude with respiration or if you suspect pericardial tamponade (because of increased jugular venous pressure, a rapid and diminished pulse, and dyspnea, for example), use a blood-pressure cuff to check for a paradoxical pulse. This is a greater than normal drop in systolic pressure during inspiration. As the patient breathes, quietly if possible, lower the cuff pressure slowly to the systolic level. Note the pressure level at which the first sounds can be heard. Then drop the pressure very slowly until sounds can be heard throughout the respiratory cycle. Again note the pressure level. The difference between these two levels is normally no greater than 3 or 4 mm Hg.

The level identified by first hearing Korotkoff sounds is the highest systolic pressure during the respiratory cycle. The level identified by hearing sounds throughout the cycle is the lowest systolic pressure. A difference between these levels of more than 10 mm Hg indicates a paradoxical pulse and suggests pericardial tamponade, possibly constrictive pericarditis, but most commonly obstructive airway disease (see p. 90).

TABLE 7-1 ■ Variations and Abnormalities of the Ventricular Impulses

When a ventricle works under conditions of chronic pressure overload or *increased afterload*, its walls gradually thicken or *hypertrophy*. Volume overload (*increased preload*), in contrast, produces dilatation of the ventricle as well as thickening of its walls. A hyperkinetic impulse results from increased stroke volume and does not necessarily signify heart disease. An impulse may feel hyperkinetic when the chest wall is unusually thin.

	Left Ventricle				Right Ventricle			
	Normal	*Hyperkinetic*	*Pressure Overload*	*Volume Overload*	*Normal*	*Hyperkinetic*	*Pressure Overload*	*Volume Overload*
The Impulse								
Location	5th or possibly 4th left interspace, medial to the midclavicular line	Normal	Normal	Displaced to the left and possibly downward	Indeterminate	3rd, 4th, or 5th left interspaces	3rd, 4th, or 5th left interspaces, also subxiphoid	Left sternal border, extending toward the left cardiac border, also subxiphoid
Diameter	Little more than 2 cm in adults (1 cm in children); 3 cm or less in left-sided position	Normal, though increased amplitude may make it seem larger	Increased	Increased	Indeterminate	Not useful	Not useful	Not useful
Amplitude	Small, gentle	Increased	Increased	Increased	Not palpable beyond infancy	Slightly increased	Increased	Slightly to markedly increased
Duration	Usually less than ⅔ of systole; the impulse stops before S_2	Normal	Prolonged, may be sustained up to S_2	Often slightly prolonged	Indeterminate	Normal	Prolonged	Normal to slightly prolonged
Examples of Causes		Anxiety, hyperthyroidism, severe anemia	Aortic stenosis, hypertension	Aortic or mitral regurgitation		Anxiety, hyperthyroidism, severe anemia	Pulmonic stenosis, pulmonary hypertension	Atrial septal defect

TABLE 7-2 ■ Variations in the First Heart Sound

Normal Variations	S_1 S_2	S_1 is softer than S_2 at the *base* (right and left 2nd interspaces).
	S_1 S_2	S_1 is often but not always louder than S_2 at the *apex*.
Accentuated S_1	S_1 S_2	S_1 is accentuated in (1) tachycardia, rhythms with a short PR interval, and high cardiac output states (e.g., exercise, anemia, hyperthyroidism), and (2) mitral stenosis. In these conditions, the mitral valve is still open wide at the onset of ventricular systole, and then closes quickly.
Diminished S_1	S_1 S_2	S_1 is diminished in first-degree heart block (delayed conduction from atria to ventricles). Here the mitral valve has had time after atrial contraction to float back into an almost closed position before ventricular contraction shuts it. It closes less loudly. S_1 is also diminished (1) when the mitral valve is calcified and relatively immobile, as in mitral regurgitation, and (2) when left ventricular contractility is markedly reduced, as in congestive heart failure or coronary heart disease.
Varying S_1	S_1 S_2 S_1 S_2	S_1 varies in intensity (1) in complete heart block, when atria and ventricles are beating independently of each other, and (2) in any totally irregular rhythm (e.g., atrial fibrillation). In these situations, the mitral valve is in varying positions before being shut by ventricular contraction. Its closure sound, therefore, varies in loudness.
Split S_1	S_1 S_2	S_1 may be split normally along the lower left sternal border where the tricuspid component, often too faint to be heard, becomes audible. This split may sometimes be heard at the apex, but consider also an S_4, an aortic ejection sound, and an early systolic click. Abnormal splitting of both heart sounds may be heard in right bundle branch block and in premature ventricular contractions.

TABLE 7-3 ■ Variations in the Second Heart Sound

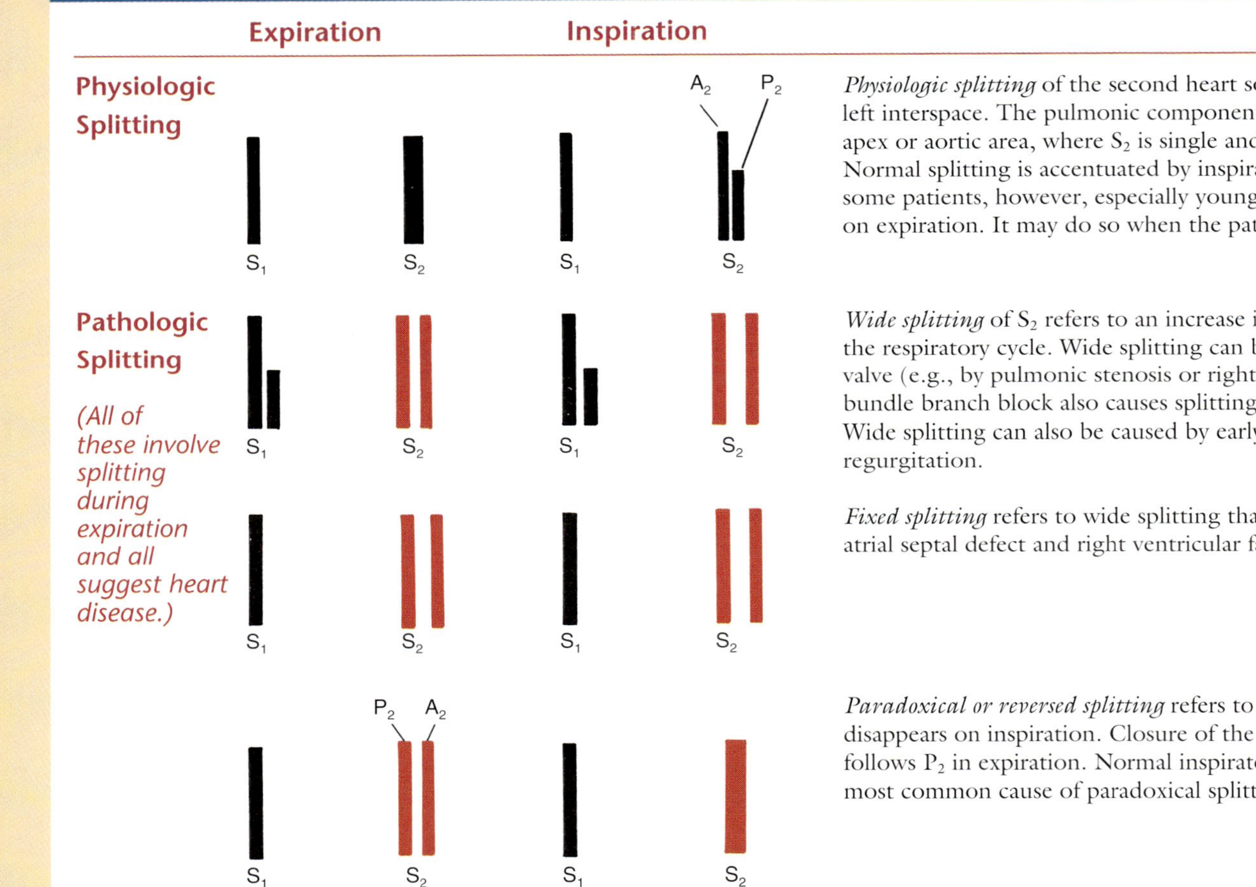

Physiologic splitting of the second heart sound can usually be detected in the 2nd or 3rd left interspace. The pulmonic component of S_2 is usually too faint to be heard at the apex or aortic area, where S_2 is single and derived from aortic valve closure alone. Normal splitting is accentuated by inspiration and usually disappears on expiration. In some patients, however, especially younger ones, S_2 may not become completely single on expiration. It may do so when the patient sits up.

Wide splitting of S_2 refers to an increase in the usual splitting that persists throughout the respiratory cycle. Wide splitting can be caused by delayed closure of the pulmonic valve (e.g., by pulmonic stenosis or right bundle branch block). As illustrated here, right bundle branch block also causes splitting of S_1 into its mitral and tricuspid components. Wide splitting can also be caused by early closure of the aortic valve, as in mitral regurgitation.

Fixed splitting refers to wide splitting that does not vary with respiration. It occurs in atrial septal defect and right ventricular failure.

Paradoxical or reversed splitting refers to splitting that appears on expiration and disappears on inspiration. Closure of the aortic valve is abnormally delayed so that A_2 follows P_2 in expiration. Normal inspiratory delay of P_2 makes the split disappear. The most common cause of paradoxical splitting is left bundle branch block.

Increased Intensity of A_2 in the Right Second Interspace (where only A_2 can usually be heard) occurs in systemic hypertension because of the increased pressure. It also occurs when the aortic root is dilated, probably because the aortic valve is then closer to the chest wall.

A Decreased or Absent A_2 in the Right Second Interspace is noted in calcific aortic stenosis because of immobility of the valve. If A_2 is inaudible, no splitting is heard.

Increased Intensity of P_2. When P_2 is equal to or louder than A_2, pulmonary hypertension may be suspected. Other causes include a dilated pulmonary artery and an atrial septal defect. Splitting of the second heart sound that is heard widely, even at the apex and the right base, indicates an accentuated P_2.

A Decreased or Absent P_2 is most commonly due to the increased anteroposterior diameter of the chest associated with aging. It can also result from pulmonic stenosis. If P_2 is inaudible, no splitting is heard.

TABLE 7-4 ■ Extra Heart Sounds in Systole

Extra heart sounds in systole are of two kinds: (1) early ejection sounds, and (2) clicks, most commonly heard in mid- and late systole.

Early Systolic Ejection Sounds

S_1 E_j S_2

Early systolic ejection sounds occur shortly after the first heart sound, coincident with the opening of the aortic and pulmonic valves. They are relatively high in pitch, have a sharp, clicking quality, and are heard better with the diaphragm of the stethoscope. An ejection sound indicates cardiovascular disease.

An *aortic ejection sound* is heard at both base and apex and may be louder at the apex. It does not usually vary with respiration. An aortic ejection sound may accompany a dilated aorta or aortic valve disease, such as congenital stenosis or a bicuspid valve.

A *pulmonic ejection sound* is heard best in the 2nd and 3rd left interspaces. When the first heart sound, usually relatively soft in this area, appears to be loud, you may instead be hearing a pulmonic ejection sound. Its intensity often decreases with inspiration. Causes include dilatation of the pulmonary artery, pulmonary hypertension, and pulmonic stenosis.

Systolic Clicks

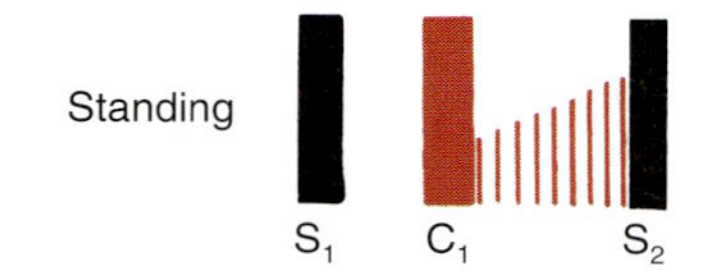

Systolic clicks are usually due to *mitral valve prolapse*—an abnormal systolic ballooning of part of the mitral valve into the left atrium. The clicks are usually mid- or late systolic. Prolapse of the mitral valve is a common cardiac condition, affecting about 5% of the general population. It is now felt to have equal prevalence in men and women. The click is usually single, but more than one may be heard. A click is heard best at or medial to the apex but may also be heard at the lower left sternal border. It is high-pitched and heard better with the diaphragm. The click is often followed by a late systolic murmur, which usually represents mitral regurgitation—a flow of blood from left ventricle to left atrium. The murmur usually crescendos up to S_2. Systolic clicks may also be of extracardial or mediastinal origin.

Auscultatory findings are notably variable. Most patients have only a click, some have only a murmur, and some have both. Findings vary from time to time and often change with body position. Several positions are recommended to identify the syndrome: supine, seated, squatting, and standing. Squatting delays the click and murmur; standing moves them closer to S_1.

TABLE 7-5 ■ Extra Heart Sounds in Diastole

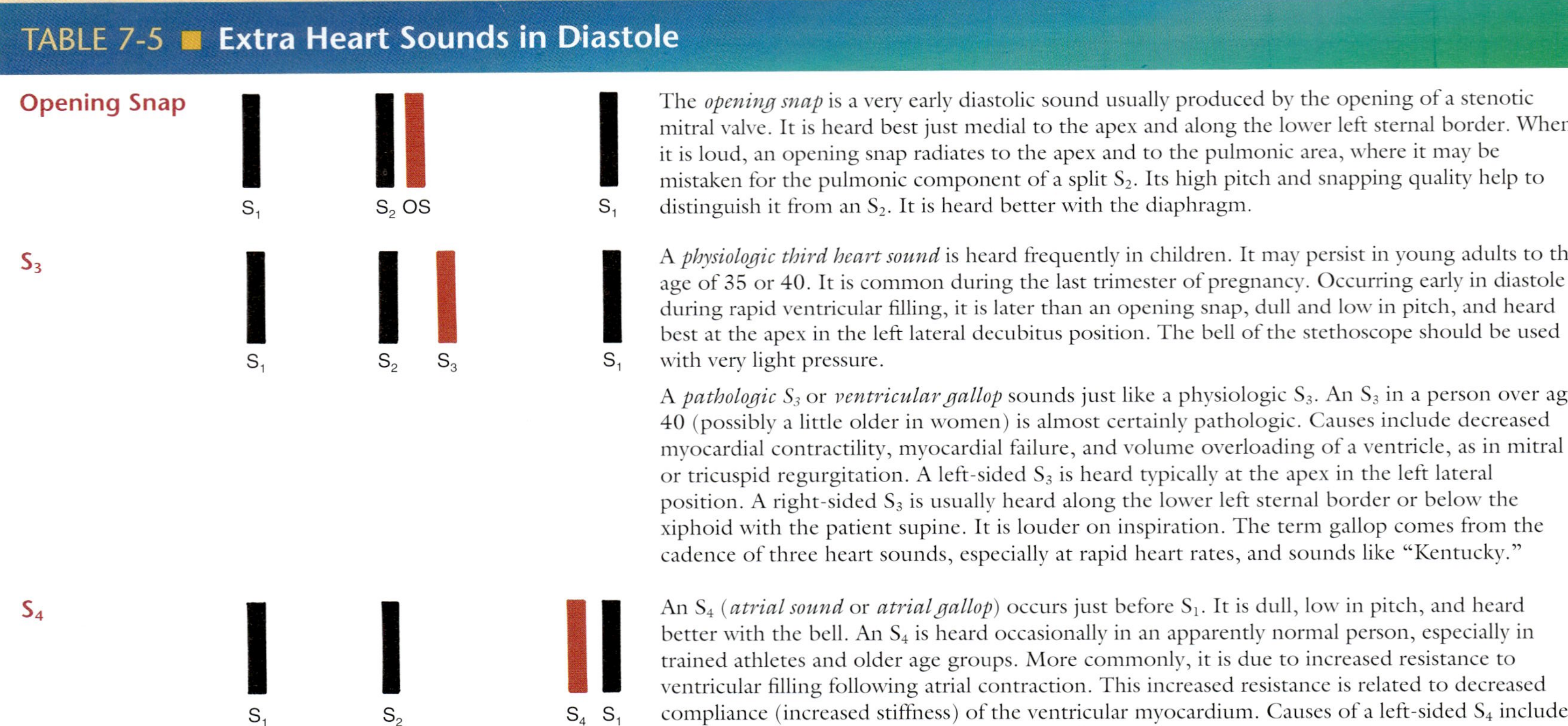

Opening Snap

The *opening snap* is a very early diastolic sound usually produced by the opening of a stenotic mitral valve. It is heard best just medial to the apex and along the lower left sternal border. When it is loud, an opening snap radiates to the apex and to the pulmonic area, where it may be mistaken for the pulmonic component of a split S_2. Its high pitch and snapping quality help to distinguish it from an S_2. It is heard better with the diaphragm.

S_3

A *physiologic third heart sound* is heard frequently in children. It may persist in young adults to the age of 35 or 40. It is common during the last trimester of pregnancy. Occurring early in diastole during rapid ventricular filling, it is later than an opening snap, dull and low in pitch, and heard best at the apex in the left lateral decubitus position. The bell of the stethoscope should be used with very light pressure.

A *pathologic S_3* or *ventricular gallop* sounds just like a physiologic S_3. An S_3 in a person over age 40 (possibly a little older in women) is almost certainly pathologic. Causes include decreased myocardial contractility, myocardial failure, and volume overloading of a ventricle, as in mitral or tricuspid regurgitation. A left-sided S_3 is heard typically at the apex in the left lateral position. A right-sided S_3 is usually heard along the lower left sternal border or below the xiphoid with the patient supine. It is louder on inspiration. The term gallop comes from the cadence of three heart sounds, especially at rapid heart rates, and sounds like "Kentucky."

S_4

An S_4 (*atrial sound* or *atrial gallop*) occurs just before S_1. It is dull, low in pitch, and heard better with the bell. An S_4 is heard occasionally in an apparently normal person, especially in trained athletes and older age groups. More commonly, it is due to increased resistance to ventricular filling following atrial contraction. This increased resistance is related to decreased compliance (increased stiffness) of the ventricular myocardium. Causes of a left-sided S_4 include hypertensive heart disease, coronary artery disease, aortic stenosis, and cardiomyopathy. A left-sided S_4 is heard best at the apex in the left lateral position; it may sound like "Tennessee." The less common right-sided S_4 is heard along the lower left sternal border or below the xiphoid. It often gets louder with inspiration. Causes of a right-sided S_4 include pulmonary hypertension and pulmonic stenosis.

An S_4 may also be associated with delayed conduction between atria and ventricles. This delay separates the normally faint atrial sound from the louder S_1 and makes it audible. An S_4 is never heard in the absence of atrial contraction, as occurs with atrial fibrillation.

Occasionally, a patient has both an S_3 and an S_4, producing a *quadruple rhythm* of four heart sounds. At rapid heart rates the S_3 and S_4 may merge into one loud extra heart sound, called a *summation gallop*.

TABLE 7-6 ■ Midsystolic Murmurs

Midsystolic ejection murmurs are the most common kind of heart murmur. They may be (1) *innocent*—without any detectable physiologic or structural abnormality; (2) *physiologic*—from physiologic changes in body metabolism; or (3) *pathologic*—arising from a structural abnormality in the heart or great vessels. Midsystolic murmurs tend to peak near midsystole and usually stop before S_2. The crescendo–decrescendo or "diamond" shape is not always audible, but the gap between the murmur and S_2 helps to distinguish midsystolic from pansystolic murmurs.

	Mechanism	Murmur	Associated Findings
Innocent Murmurs S_1 S_2	Innocent murmurs result from turbulent blood flow, probably generated by left ventricular ejection of blood into the aorta. Occasionally, turbulence from right ventricular ejection may also cause them. There is no evidence of cardiovascular disease. Innocent murmurs—very common in children and young adults—may also be heard in older people.	*Location.* 2nd to 4th left interspaces between the left sternal border and the apex *Radiation.* Little *Intensity.* Grade 1 to 2, possibly 3 *Pitch.* Medium *Quality.* Variable *Aids.* Usually decreases or disappears on sitting	None: normal splitting, no ejection sounds, no diastolic murmurs, and no palpable evidence of ventricular enlargement. Occasionally, a patient has both an innocent murmur and another kind of murmur.
Physiologic Murmurs S_1 S_2	Turbulence due to a temporary increase in blood flow causes this murmur. Predisposing conditions include anemia, pregnancy, fever, and hyperthyroidism.	Similar to innocent murmurs	Possible signs of a likely cause
Pathologic Murmurs *Pulmonic Stenosis* S_1 E_j A_2 P_2	Stenosis of the pulmonic valve impairs flow across the valve, increasing afterload on the right ventricle. It is congenital and most often found in children. *Pathologically increased flow across the pulmonic valve* may mimic the murmur of pulmonic stenosis. The systolic murmur of an atrial septal defect originates from this flow, not the defect itself.	*Location.* 2nd and 3rd left interspaces *Radiation.* If loud, toward the left shoulder and neck *Intensity.* Soft to loud; if loud, associated with a thrill *Pitch.* Medium *Quality.* Often harsh	In severe stenosis, S_2 is widely split and P_2 is diminished. When P_2 is inaudible, no splitting is heard. An early pulmonic ejection sound is common. A right-sided S_4 may be present. The right ventricular impulse is often increased in amplitude and may be prolonged.

(table continues on next page)

TABLE 7-6 ■ Midsystolic Murmurs *(Continued)*

	Mechanism	Murmur	Associated Findings
Aortic Stenosis May be decreased S_1 S_2	Significant stenosis of the aortic valve impairs blood flow across the valve, causing turbulence, and increases the afterload on the left ventricle. Causes are congenital, rheumatic, and degenerative, and findings may differ with each cause. Other conditions may mimic the murmur of aortic stenosis without obstructing flow: ■ *Aortic sclerosis,* a stiffening of aortic valve leaflets associated with aging ■ A *bicuspid aortic valve,* a congenital condition, which may not be recognized until adulthood ■ A *dilated aorta,* as from arteriosclerosis, syphilis, or Marfan's syndrome ■ A *pathologically increased flow across the aortic valve* during systole, as in aortic regurgitation	*Location.* Right 2nd interspace *Radiation.* Often to the neck and down the left sternal border, even to the apex *Intensity.* Sometimes soft but often loud, with a thrill *Pitch.* Medium; at the apex, it may be higher *Quality.* Often harsh; at the apex it may be more musical *Aids.* Heard best with the patient sitting and leaning forward	A_2 decreases as the stenosis worsens. A_2 may be delayed, merging with P_2 to form a single expiratory sound or causing paradoxical splitting. An S_4, reflecting the decreased compliance of the hypertrophied left ventricle, may be present at the apex. An aortic ejection sound, if present, suggests a congenital cause. A sustained apical impulse often reveals left ventricular hypertrophy. The carotid artery impulse may rise slowly and feel small in amplitude.
Hypertrophic Cardiomyopathy S_1 S_2	Massive hypertrophy of ventricular muscle is associated with unusually rapid ejection of blood from the left ventricle during systole. Obstruction to flow may coexist. Accompanying distortion of the mitral valve may cause mitral regurgitation.	*Location.* 3rd and 4th left interspaces *Radiation.* Down the left sternal border to the apex, possibly to the base, but not to the neck *Intensity.* Variable *Pitch.* Medium *Quality.* Harsh *Aids.* Decreases with squatting, increases with straining down	An S_3 may be present. An S_4 is often present at the apex (unlike mitral regurgitation). The apical impulse may be sustained and have two palpable components. The carotid pulse rises quickly (unlike the pulse in aortic stenosis).

TABLE 7-7 ■ Pansystolic (Holosystolic) Murmurs

Pansystolic (holosystolic) murmurs are pathologic. They are heard when blood flows from a chamber of high pressure to one of lower pressure through a valve or other structure that should be closed. The murmur begins immediately with S_1 and continues up to S_2.

	Mechanism	Murmur	Associated Findings
Mitral Regurgitation Decreased S_1 S_2 S_3	When the mitral valve fails to close fully in systole, blood regurgitates from left ventricle to left atrium, causing a murmur. This leakage creates a volume overload on the left ventricle, with subsequent dilatation and hypertrophy. Several structural abnormalities cause this condition, and findings may vary accordingly.	*Location.* Apex *Radiation.* To the left axilla, less often to the left sternal border *Intensity.* Soft to loud; if loud, associated with an apical thrill *Pitch.* Medium to high *Quality.* Blowing *Aids.* Unlike tricuspid regurgitation, it does not become louder in inspiration.	S_1 is often decreased. An apical S_3 reflects volume overload on the left ventricle. The apical impulse is increased in amplitude and may be prolonged.
Tricuspid Regurgitation S_1 S_2 S_3	When the tricuspid valve fails to close fully in systole, blood regurgitates from right ventricle to right atrium, producing a murmur. The most common cause is right ventricular failure and dilatation, with resulting enlargement of the tricuspid orifice. Either pulmonary hypertension or left ventricular failure is the usual initiating cause.	*Location.* Lower left sternal border *Radiation.* To the right of the sternum, to the xiphoid area, and perhaps to the left midclavicular line, but not into the axilla *Intensity.* Variable *Pitch.* Medium *Quality.* Blowing *Aids.* Unlike mitral regurgitation, the intensity may increase slightly with inspiration.	The right ventricular impulse is increased in amplitude and may be prolonged. An S_3 may be audible along the lower left sternal border. The jugular venous pressure is often elevated, and large *v* waves may be seen in the jugular veins.
Ventricular Septal Defect S_1 S_2	A ventricular septal defect is a congenital abnormality in which blood flows from the relatively high-pressure left ventricle into the low-pressure right ventricle through a hole. The defect may be accompanied by other abnormalities, but an uncomplicated lesion is described here.	*Location.* 3rd, 4th, and 5th left interspaces *Radiation.* Often wide *Intensity.* Often very loud, with a thrill *Pitch.* High *Quality.* Often harsh	A_2 may be obscured by the loud murmur. Findings vary with the severity of the defect and with associated lesions.

TABLE 7-8 ■ Diastolic Murmurs

Diastolic murmurs almost always indicate heart disease. There are two basic types. *Early decrescendo diastolic murmurs* signify regurgitant flow through an incompetent semilunar valve, more commonly the aortic. *Rumbling diastolic murmurs in mid- or late diastole* suggest stenosis of an atrioventricular valve, more often the mitral.

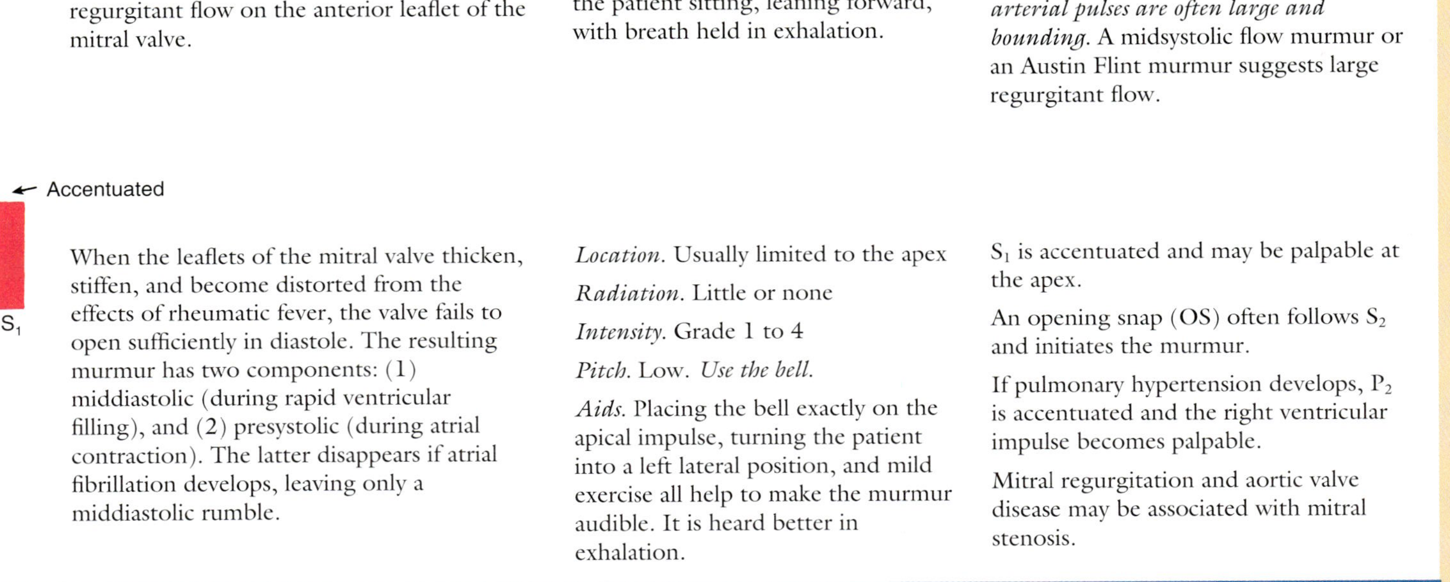

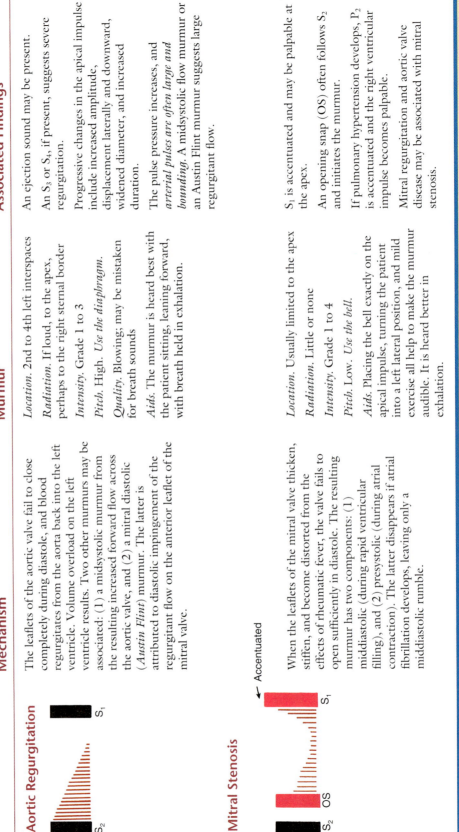

	Mechanism	Murmur	Associated Findings
Aortic Regurgitation	The leaflets of the aortic valve fail to close completely during diastole, and blood regurgitates from the aorta back into the left ventricle. Volume overload on the left ventricle results. Two other murmurs may be associated: (1) a midsystolic murmur from the resulting increased forward flow across the aortic valve, and (2) a mitral diastolic (*Austin Flint*) murmur. The latter is attributed to diastolic impingement of the regurgitant flow on the anterior leaflet of the mitral valve.	*Location.* 2nd to 4th left interspaces *Radiation.* If loud, to the apex, perhaps to the right sternal border *Intensity.* Grade 1 to 3 *Pitch.* High. *Use the diaphragm.* *Quality.* Blowing; may be mistaken for breath sounds *Aids.* The murmur is heard best with the patient sitting, leaning forward, with breath held in exhalation.	An ejection sound may be present. An S_3 or S_4, if present, suggests severe regurgitation. Progressive changes in the apical impulse include increased amplitude, displacement laterally and downward, widened diameter, and increased duration. The pulse pressure increases, and *arterial pulses are often large and bounding*. A midsystolic flow murmur or an Austin Flint murmur suggests large regurgitant flow.
Mitral Stenosis	When the leaflets of the mitral valve thicken, stiffen, and become distorted from the effects of rheumatic fever, the valve fails to open sufficiently in diastole. The resulting murmur has two components: (1) middiastolic (during rapid ventricular filling), and (2) presystolic (during atrial contraction). The latter disappears if atrial fibrillation develops, leaving only a middiastolic rumble.	*Location.* Usually limited to the apex *Radiation.* Little or none *Intensity.* Grade 1 to 4 *Pitch.* Low. *Use the bell.* *Aids.* Placing the bell exactly on the apical impulse, turning the patient into a left lateral position, and mild exercise all help to make the murmur audible. It is heard better in exhalation.	S_1 is accentuated and may be palpable at the apex. An opening snap (OS) often follows S_2 and initiates the murmur. If pulmonary hypertension develops, P_2 is accentuated and the right ventricular impulse becomes palpable. Mitral regurgitation and aortic valve disease may be associated with mitral stenosis.

TABLE 7-9 ■ Cardiovascular Sounds With Both Systolic and Diastolic Components

Some cardiovascular sounds are not confined to one portion of the cardiac cycle. Three examples are: (1) a *pericardial friction rub,* produced by inflammation of the pericardial sac; (2) *patent ductus arteriosus,* a congenital abnormality in which an open channel persists between aorta and pulmonary artery; and (3) a *venous hum,* a benign sound produced by turbulence of blood in the jugular veins (common in children). Their characteristics are contrasted below. *Continuous murmurs* begin in systole and continue through the second sound into all or part of diastole. Therefore the murmur of patent ductus arteriosus may be classified as continuous.

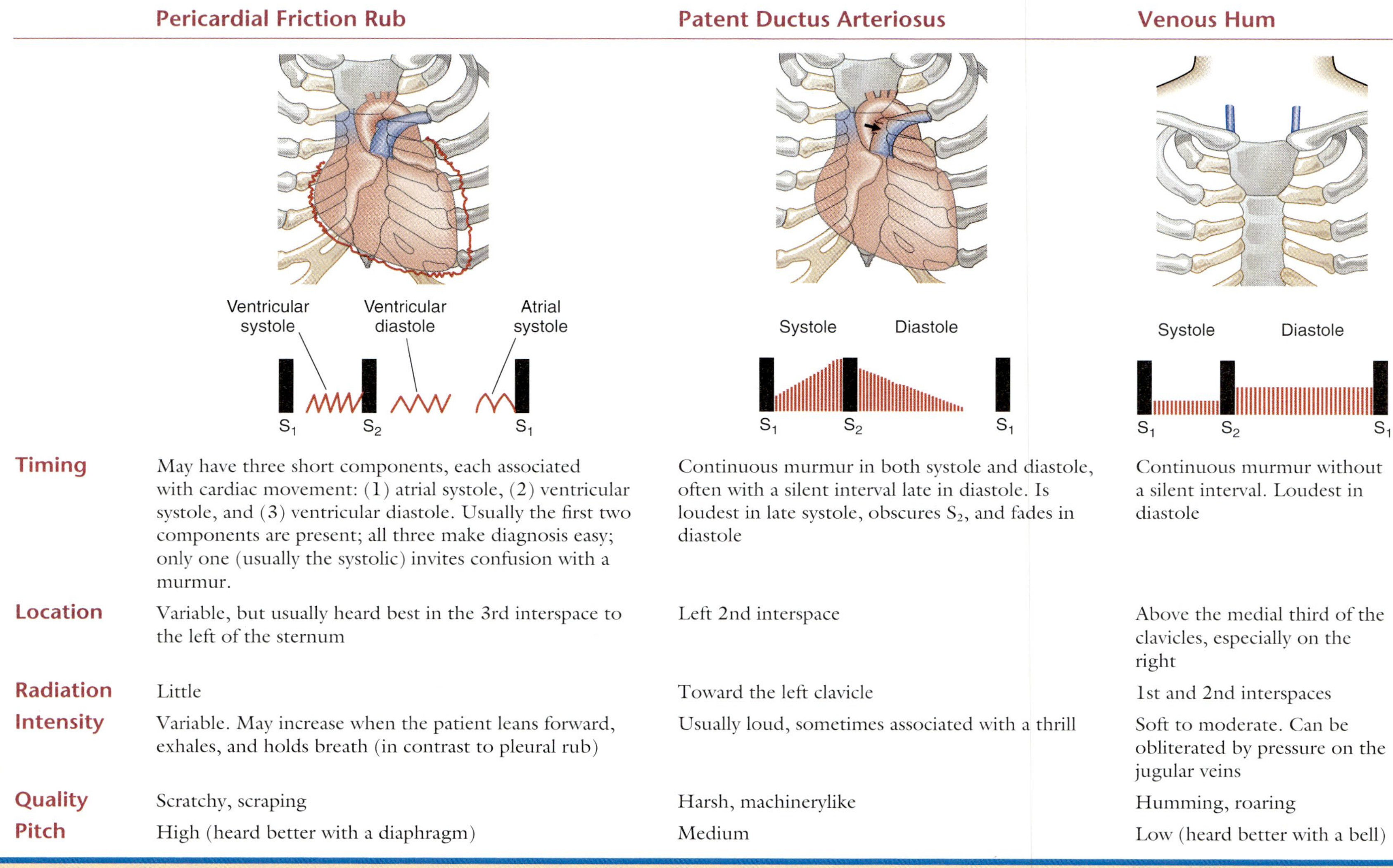

	Pericardial Friction Rub	Patent Ductus Arteriosus	Venous Hum
Timing	May have three short components, each associated with cardiac movement: (1) atrial systole, (2) ventricular systole, and (3) ventricular diastole. Usually the first two components are present; all three make diagnosis easy; only one (usually the systolic) invites confusion with a murmur.	Continuous murmur in both systole and diastole, often with a silent interval late in diastole. Is loudest in late systole, obscures S_2, and fades in diastole	Continuous murmur without a silent interval. Loudest in diastole
Location	Variable, but usually heard best in the 3rd interspace to the left of the sternum	Left 2nd interspace	Above the medial third of the clavicles, especially on the right
Radiation	Little	Toward the left clavicle	1st and 2nd interspaces
Intensity	Variable. May increase when the patient leans forward, exhales, and holds breath (in contrast to pleural rub)	Usually loud, sometimes associated with a thrill	Soft to moderate. Can be obliterated by pressure on the jugular veins
Quality	Scratchy, scraping	Harsh, machinerylike	Humming, roaring
Pitch	High (heard better with a diaphragm)	Medium	Low (heard better with a bell)

CHAPTER

8

The Breasts and Axillae

ANATOMY AND PHYSIOLOGY

The female breast lies against the anterior thoracic wall, extending from the clavicle and 2nd rib down to the 6th rib, and from the sternum across to the midaxillary line. Its surface area is generally rectangular rather than round. The breast overlies the pectoralis major and at its inferior margin, the serratus anterior.

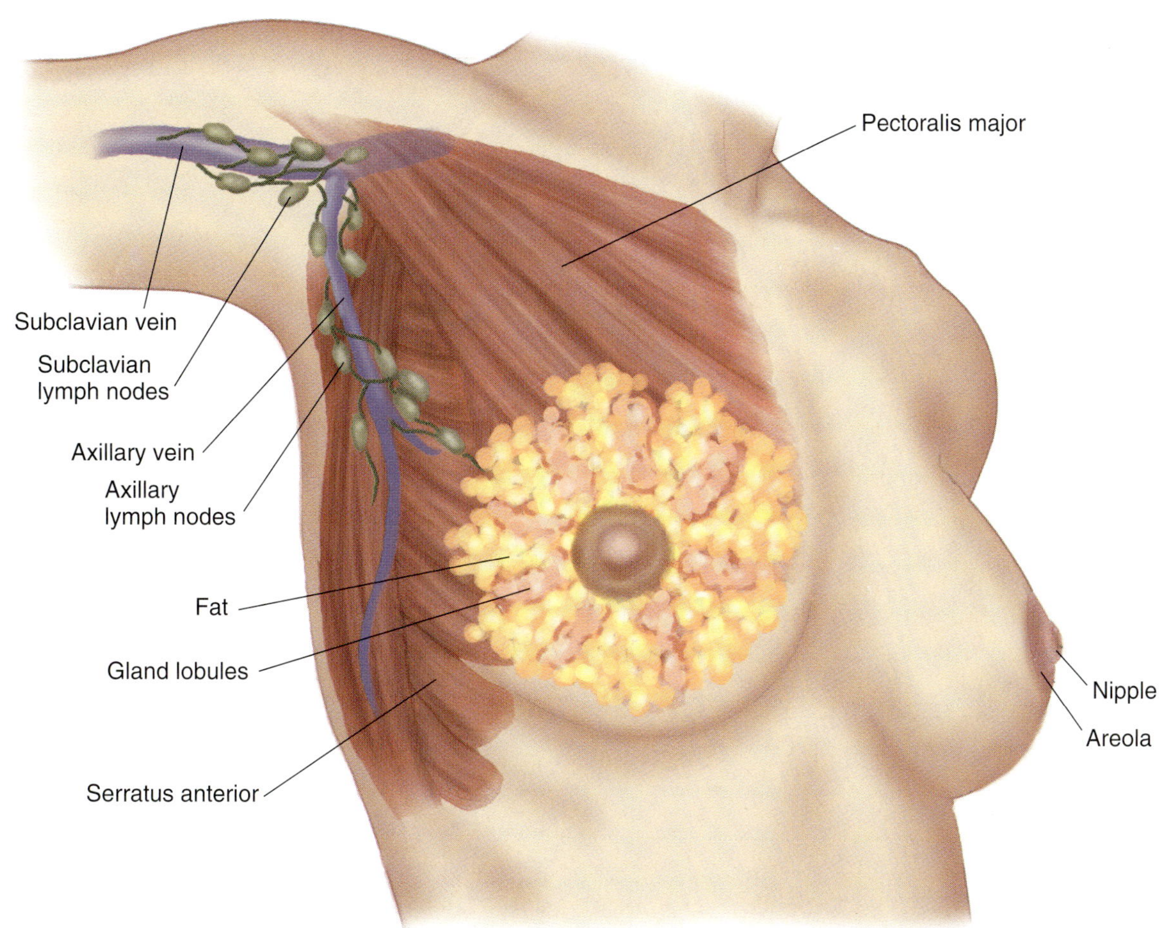

To describe clinical findings, the breast is often divided into four quadrants based on horizontal and vertical lines crossing at the nipple. An axillary tail of breast tissue extends toward the anterior axillary fold. Alternatively, findings can be localized as the time on the face of a clock (e.g., 3 o'clock) and the distance in centimeters from the nipple.

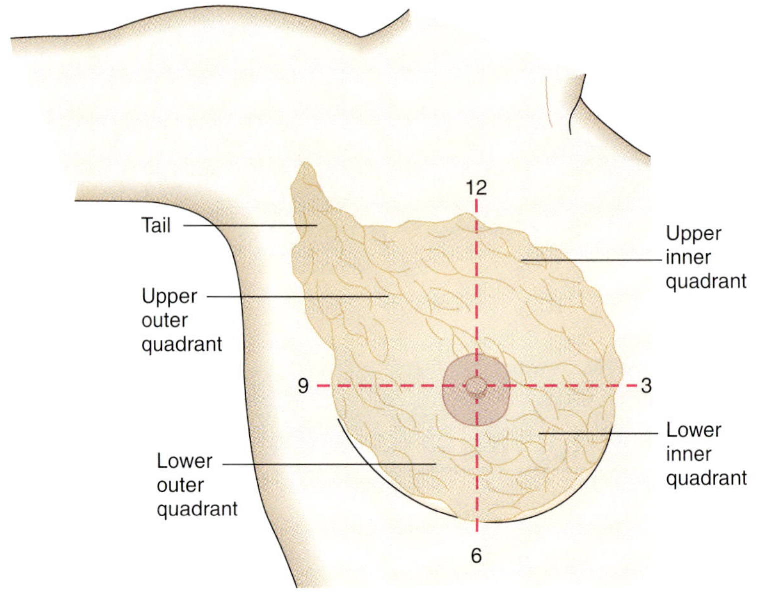

The breast is hormonally sensitive tissue, responsive to the changes of monthly cycling and aging. *Glandular tissue,* namely secretory tubuloalveolar glands and ducts, forms 15 to 20 septated *lobes* radiating around the nipple. Within each lobe are many smaller *lobules.* These drain into milk-producing ducts and sinuses that open onto the surface of the *areola,* or nipple. *Fibrous connective tissue* provides structural support in the form of fibrous bands or suspensory ligaments connected to both the skin and the underlying fascia. *Adipose tissue,* or fat, surrounds the breast, predominantly in the superficial and peripheral areas. The proportions of these components vary with age, the general state of nutrition, pregnancy, exogenous hormone use, and other factors.

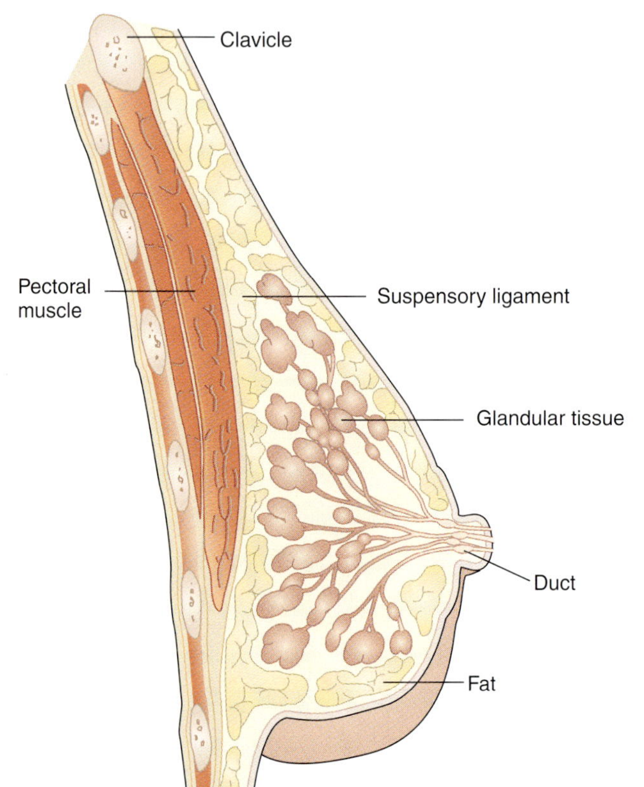

The surface of the areola has small, rounded elevations formed by sebaceous glands, sweat glands, and accessory areolar glands. A few hairs are often seen on the areola.

Both the nipple and the areola are well supplied with smooth muscle that contracts to express milk from the ductal system during breast-feeding. Rich sensory innervation, especially in the nipple, triggers "milk letdown" following neurohormonal stimulation from infant sucking. Tactile stimulation of the area, including the breast examination, makes the nipple smaller, firmer, and more erect, while the areola puckers and wrinkles. These normal smooth muscle reflexes should not be mistaken for signs of breast disease.

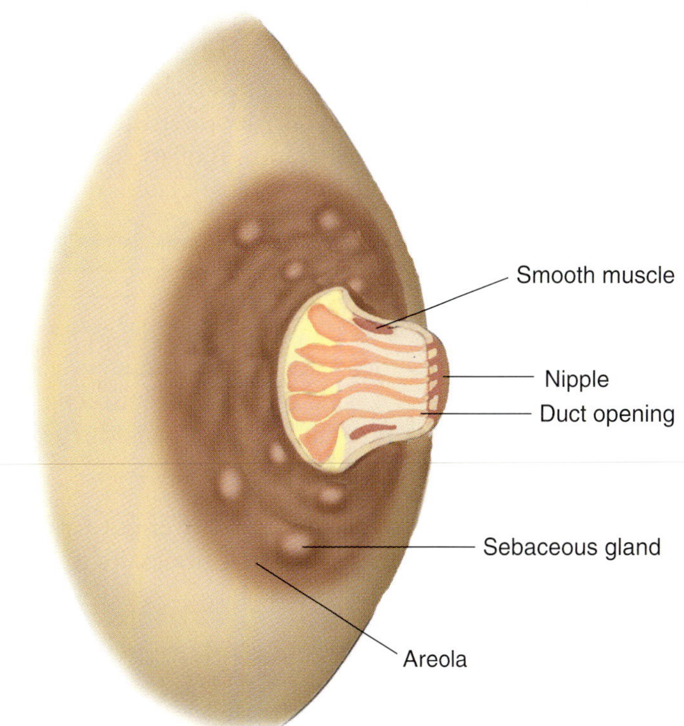

Occasionally, one or more extra or supernumerary nipples are located along the "milk line," illustrated on the right. Only a small nipple and areola are usually present, often mistaken for a common mole. There may be underlying glandular tissue. An extra nipple has no pathologic significance.

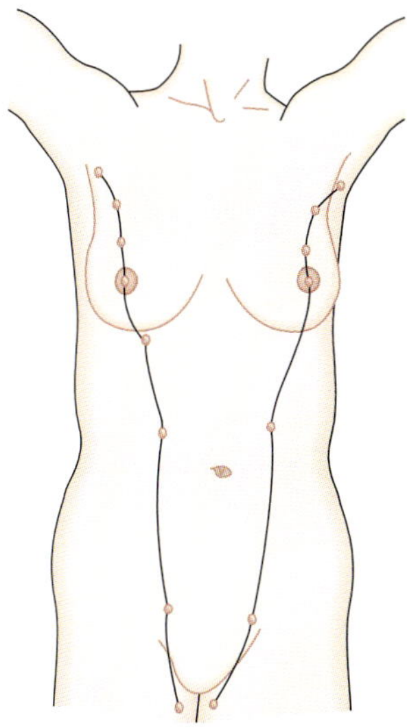

The *male breast* consists chiefly of a small nipple and areola. These overlie a thin disc of undeveloped breast tissue that may not be distinguishable clinically from the surrounding tissues. A firm button of breast tissue 2 cm or more in diameter has been described in roughly one out of three adult men. The limits of normal have not yet been clearly established.

Changes With Aging

Adulthood. The normal adult breast may be soft, but it often feels granular, nodular, or lumpy. This uneven texture is normal and may be termed *physiologic nodularity*. It is often bilateral. It may be evident throughout the breast or only in parts of it. The nodularity may increase premenstrually—a time when breasts often enlarge and become tender or even painful. For breast changes during adolescence and pregnancy, see p. 409 and pp. 699–700.

Aging. The breasts of an aging woman tend to diminish in size as glandular tissue atrophies and is replaced by fat. Although the proportion of fat increases, its total amount may also decrease. The breasts often become flaccid and more pendulous. The ducts surrounding the nipple may become more easily palpable as firm, stringy strands. Axillary hair diminishes.

Lymphatics

Lymphatics from most of the breast drain toward the axilla. Of the axillary lymph nodes, the *central nodes* are palpable most frequently. They lie along the chest wall, usually high in the axilla and midway between the anterior and posterior axillary folds. Into them drain channels from three other groups of lymph nodes, which are seldom palpable:

- *Pectoral nodes—anterior*, located along the lower border of the pectoralis major inside the anterior axillary fold. These nodes drain the anterior chest wall and much of the breast.
- *Subscapular nodes—posterior*, located along the lateral border of the scapula; palpated deep in the posterior axillary fold. They drain the posterior chest wall and a portion of the arm.
- *Lateral nodes*—located *along the upper humerus*. They drain most of the arm.

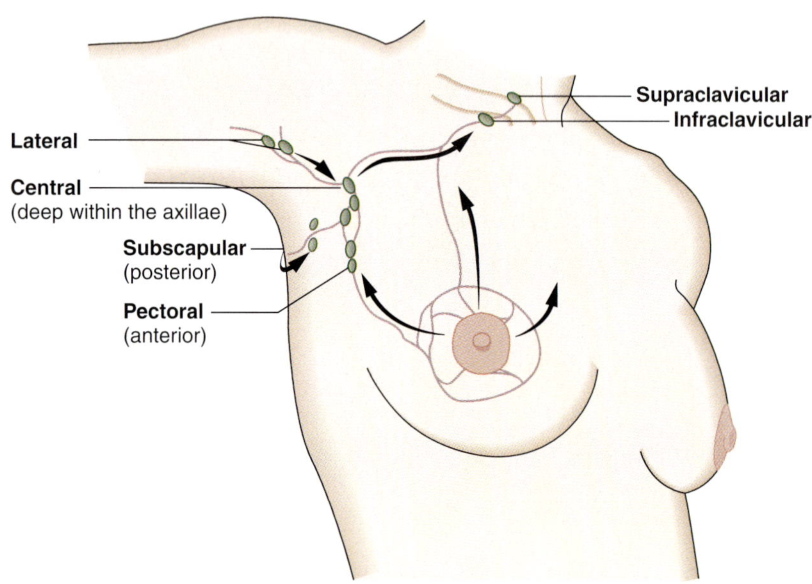

ARROWS INDICATE DIRECTION OF LYMPH FLOW

Lymph drains from the central axillary nodes to the *infraclavicular* and *supraclavicular* nodes.

Not all the lymphatics of the breast drain into the axilla. Malignant cells from a breast cancer may spread directly to the infraclavicular nodes or into deep channels within the chest.

THE HEALTH HISTORY

Common or Concerning Symptoms

- Breast lump or mass
- Breast pain or discomfort
- Nipple discharge

Questions about a woman's breasts may be included in the history or deferred to the physical examination. Ask "Do you examine your breasts?" . . . "How often?" In menstruating women, inquire "When during your monthly cycle?" Ask if she has any *lumps, pain,* or *discomfort* in her breasts. Approximately 50% of women have palpable lumps or nodularity in their breasts. Premenstrual enlargement and tenderness are common.

Lumps may be physiologic or pathologic, ranging from cysts and fibroadenomas to breast cancer. See Table 8-1, Visible Signs of Breast Cancer (p. 314), and Table 8-2, Common Breast Masses, (p. 315).

Also ask about any *discharge from the nipples* and when it occurs. If it appears only after squeezing the nipple, it is considered physiologic. If the discharge is spontaneous and seen on the underwear or nightclothes without local stimulation, ask about its color, consistency, and quantity. Is it unilateral or bilateral?

A milky bilateral discharge, or *galactorrhea,* may reflect pregnancy or prolactin or other hormonal imbalance.

A nonmilky unilateral discharge suggests local breast disease.

HEALTH PROMOTION AND COUNSELING

Important Topics for Health Promotion and Counseling

- Risk factors for breast cancer
- Breast cancer screening
- Breast self-examination (BSE)

Women may experience a wide range of changes in breast tissue and sensation, from cyclic swelling and nodularity to a distinct lump or mass. The examination of the breast provides a meaningful opportunity for the clinician and the woman patient to explore concerns important to women's health—what to do if a lump or mass is detected, risk factors for breast cancer, and screening measures such as breast self-examination, the clinical breast examination (CBE) by a skilled clinician, and mammography.

Breast masses show marked variation in etiology, from fibroadenomas and cysts seen in younger women, to abscess or mastitis, to primary breast cancer. All breast masses warrant careful evaluation. On initial assessment, the woman's age and physical characteristics of the mass provide clues to its origin, but definitive diagnostic measures should be pursued.

Palpable Masses of the Breast

Age	Common Lesion	Characteristics
15–25	Fibroadenoma	Usually fine, round, mobile, nontender
25–50	Cysts	Usually soft to firm, round, mobile; often tender
	Fibrocystic changes	Nodular, ropelike
	Cancer	Irregular, stellate, firm, not clearly delineated from surrounding tissue
Over 50	Cancer until proven otherwise	As above
Pregnancy/lactation	Lactating adenomas, cysts, mastitis, and cancer	As above

Adapted from Schultz MZ, Ward BA, Reiss M: Ch. 149. Breast Diseases. In Noble J, Greene HL, Levinson W, Modest GA, Young MJ (eds): Primary Care Medicine, 2nd ed. St. Louis, Mosby, 1996.

Risk Factors for Breast Cancer. Breast cancer is the most common cause of cancer in women worldwide, accounting for 18% of all female malignancies. In the United States, a woman has more than a 12% lifetime risk of developing breast cancer and an approximately 22% risk of dying from the disease.* Although 70% of affected women have no known predisposing factors, definite risk factors are well-established. The clinician and the inquiring patient should understand and review factors such as age, family history, reproductive history, and previous history of benign breast disease, especially if a previous biopsy showed atypical hyperplasia or lobular carcinoma in situ.

To calculate an individual woman's risk of breast cancer, you may wish to make use of the Breast Cancer Risk Assessment Tool of the National Cancer Institute (www.brca.nci.gov) or other available clinical models such as the Gail model (see Bibliography). Advise your patients that more than two thirds of new cases of breast cancer localized to the breast are attributed to earlier detection.

Age. Although one in eight women will eventually develop breast cancer, it is important to note that this is a cumulative lifetime risk that increases with age. More than three fourths of breast cancer cases occur in women 50 years or older; more than half in women older than age 65. For women between the ages of 35 and 55 without major risk factors, the chance of developing breast cancer is approximately 2.5%.

Family History. The relative risk (or risk relative to an individual without a given risk factor) of breast cancer associated with menstrual history, preg-

*Harris JR, Morrow M, Bonadonna G: Cancer of the breast. In DeVita VT, Hellman S, Rosenberg SA (eds): Cancer Principles & Practice of Oncology, 5th ed. Philadelphia, Lippincott-Raven, 1997.

Summary of Breast Cancer Risk Factors

Factor	Relative Risk (%)
Family History	
First-degree relative with breast cancer	1.2–3.0
Premenopausal	3.1
Premenopausal and bilateral	8.5–9.0
Postmenopausal	1.5
Postmenopausal and bilateral	4.0–5.4
Menstrual History	
Age at menarche <12	1.3
Age at menopause >55	1.5–2.0
Pregnancy	
First live birth from ages 25–29	1.5
First live birth after age 30	1.9
First live birth after age 35	2.0–3.0
Nulliparous	3.0
Breast Conditions and Diseases	
Nonproliferative disease	1.0
Proliferative disease	1.9
Proliferative with atypical hyperplasia	4.4
Lobular carcinoma in situ	6.9–12.0

Adapted from Bilmoria MM and Morrow M: The woman at increased risk for breast cancer: evaluation and management strategies. Ca 45(5):263, 1995. See also American Cancer Society, www.cancer.org.

nancy, and breast conditions and diseases is summarized in the table above. Risk from familial breast cancer falls into two patterns: family history of breast cancer and genetic predisposition. First-degree relatives, namely a mother or sister with breast cancer, establish a "positive family history." Within this group, menopausal status and extent of disease play a key role. Having first-degree relatives with breast cancer who are premenopausal with bilateral disease confers the highest risk. Even when a mother and a sister have bilateral breast cancer, however, the probability of breast cancer is only 25%.

Inherited disease in women carrying mutations in the breast cancer susceptibility genes BRCA1 and BRCA2 accounts for only 5% to 10% of breast cancers. However, these genes confer a 50% risk of the disease in women under 50, and an 80% risk by age 65. Red flags for possible inherited disease include multiple relatives (maternal or paternal) with breast cancer, a family history of combined breast cancer and ovarian cancer, and a family history of bilateral and/or early onset of breast cancer.

Menstrual History and Pregnancy. Early menarche, delayed menopause, and first live birth after age 35 or no pregnancy all raise the risk of breast cancer two- to three-fold.

Breast Conditions and Diseases. Benign breast disease with biopsy findings of atypical hyperplasia or lobular carcinoma in situ carry significantly increased relative risks—4.4 and 6.9 to 12.0, respectively.

Breast Cancer Screening. Although not yet confirmed as a method for increasing detection, it is wise to teach all women the *breast self-examination* to promote health awareness (see pp. 312–313). To enhance early detection, the American Cancer Society recommends monthly breast self-examination beginning at age 20, *clinical breast examination* (CBE) by a health care professional every 3 years for women between the ages of 20 and 39, and annually after age 40, and yearly *mammography* for women 40 and older.* For women at increased risk, many clinicians advise a screening mammogram at age 35 or 40, then every 2 to 3 years until age 50. Mammography is less accurate when breast tissue is more glandular and dense, especially before menopause, resulting in different recommendations about the benefits of mammography for women in the 40-to-50 age group.† For women aged 50 to 69, mammography and CBE are widely recommended every 1 to 2 years. After age 70, the benefits of mammography are less well studied, and testing should be considered on an individual basis.

Preview: Recording the Physical Examination—Breasts and Axillae

Note that initially you may use sentences to describe your findings; later you will use phrases. The style below contains phrases appropriate for most write-ups. Unfamiliar terms are explained in the next section, Techniques of Examination.

"Breasts symmetric and without masses. Nipples without discharge." (Axillary adenopathy usually included after Neck in section on Lymph Nodes, see p. 143.)

OR

"Breasts pendulous with diffuse fibrocystic changes. Single firm 1 × 1 cm mass, mobile and nontender, with overlying peau d'orange appearance in right breast, upper outer quadrant at 11 o'clock."

Suggests possible breast cancer

*American Cancer Society. www.cancer.org. Accessed 9/1/01.

†U.S. Preventive Services Task Force: "Screening for Breast Cancer" in *Guide to Clinical Preventive Services,* 2nd ed. Baltimore: Williams & Wilkins, pp. 73–87, 1996.

TECHNIQUES OF EXAMINATION

The Female Breast

The clinical breast examination is an important component of women's health care: it enhances detection of breast cancers that mammography may miss and provides an opportunity to demonstrate techniques for self-examination to the patient. Clinical investigation has shown, however, that variations in examiner experience and technique affect the value of the clinical breast examination. Clinicians are advised to adopt a more standardized approach, especially for palpation, and to use a systemic and thorough search pattern, varying palpation pressure, and a circular motion with the fingerpads.* These techniques will be discussed in more detail in the following pages. Inspection is routinely recommended, but its value in breast cancer detection is less well studied.

Risk factors for breast cancer include previous breast cancer, an affected mother or sister, biopsy showing atypical hyperplasia, increasing age, early menarche, late menopause, late or no pregnancies, and previous radiation to the chest wall.

As you begin the examination of the breasts, be aware that women and girls may feel apprehensive. Be reassuring and adopt a courteous and gentle approach. Before you begin, let the patient know that you are about to examine her breasts. This may be a good time to ask if she has noticed any lumps or other problems and if she performs a monthly breast self-examination. If she does not, teach her good technique and watch as she repeats the steps of examination after you, giving helpful correction as needed.

See Patient Instructions for the Breast Self-Examination, p. 313.

An adequate inspection requires full exposure of the chest, but later in the examination you may find it helpful to cover one breast while you are palpating the other. Because breasts tend to swell and become more nodular before menses as a result of increasing estrogen stimulation, the best time for examination is 5 to 7 days *after* the onset of menstruation. Nodules appearing during the premenstrual phase should be reevaluated at this later time.

INSPECTION

Inspect the breasts and nipples with the patient in the sitting position and disrobed to the waist. A thorough examination of the breast includes careful inspection for skin changes, symmetry, contours, and retraction in four views—arms at sides, arms over head, arms pressed against hips, and leaning forward. When examining an adolescent girl, assess her breast development according to Tanner's sex maturity ratings described on page 700.

*Barton MB, Harris R, and Fletcher S: Does This Patient Have Breast Cancer? The Screening Clinical Breast Examination: Should It be Done? How? *JAMA* 282 (13); 1270–1280, 1999.

Arms at Sides. Note the clinical features listed below.

- The *appearance of the skin,* including

  Color

  Redness from local infection or inflammatory carcinoma

  Thickening of the skin and unusually prominent pores, which may accompany lymphatic obstruction

  Thickening and prominent pores suggest a breast cancer.

- The *size and symmetry of the breasts.* Some difference in the size of the breasts, including the areolae, is common and is usually normal, as shown in the photograph below.

- The *contour of the breasts.* Look for changes such as masses, dimpling, or flattening. Compare one side with the other.

Flattening of the normally convex breast suggests cancer. See Table 8-1, Visible Signs of Breast Cancer (p. 314).

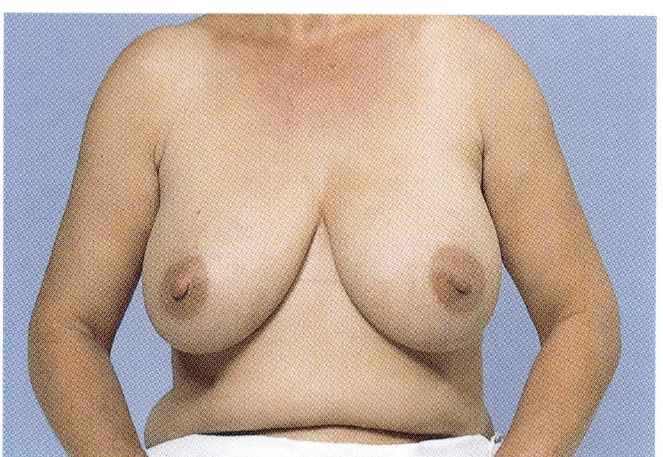

ARMS AT SIDES

- The *characteristics of the nipples,* including *size and shape, direction* in which they point, any *rashes* or *ulceration,* or any *discharge.*

Asymmetry of directions in which nipples point suggests an underlying cancer. Rash or ulceration in Paget's disease of the breast (see p. 314).

Occasionally, the shape of the nipple in *inverted,* or depressed below the areolar surface. It may be enveloped by folds of areolar skin, as illustrated. Long-standing inversion is usually a normal variant of no clinical consequence, except for possible difficulty when breast-feeding.

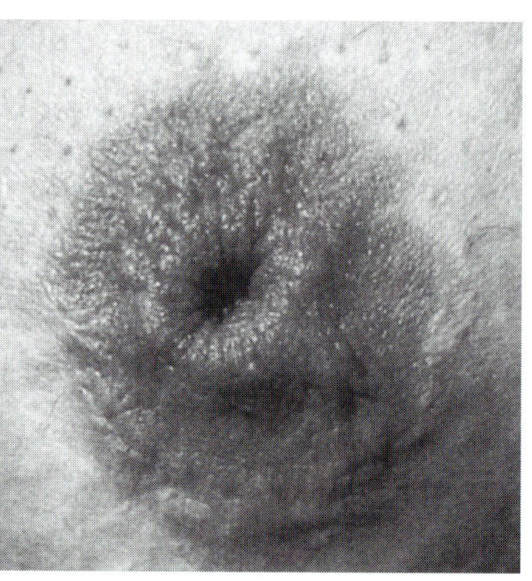

Recent or fixed flattening or depression of the nipple suggests nipple retraction. A retracted nipple may also be broadened and thickened, suggesting an underlying cancer.

Arms Over Head; Hands Pressed Against Hips; Leaning Forward. To bring out dimpling or retraction that may otherwise be invisible, ask the patient to raise her arms over her head, then press her hands against her hips to contract the pectoral muscles. Inspect the breast contours carefully in each position. If the breasts are large or pendulous, it may be useful to have the patient stand and lean forward, supported by the back of the chair or the examiner's hands.

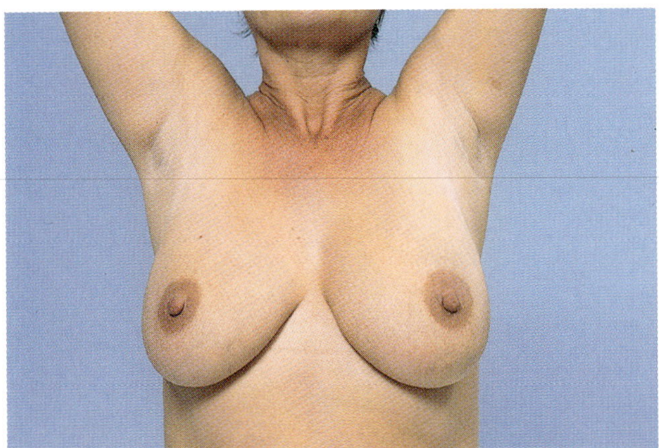

ARMS OVER HEAD

Dimpling or retraction of the breasts in these positions suggests an underlying cancer. When a cancer or its associated fibrous strands are attached to both the skin and the fascia overlying the pectoral muscles, pectoral contraction can draw the skin inward, causing dimpling.

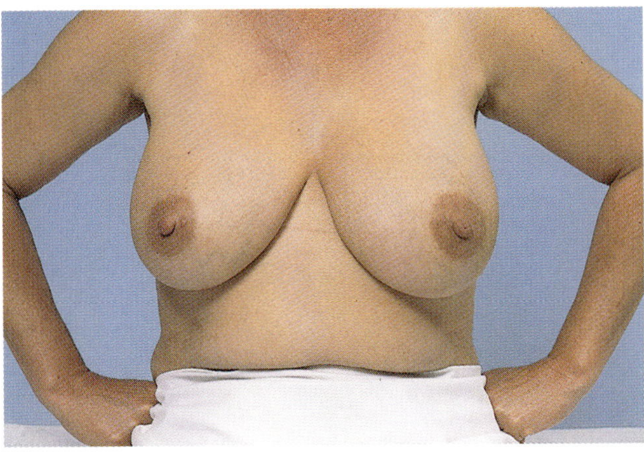

HANDS PRESSED AGAINST HIPS

Occasionally, these signs may be associated with benign lesions such as posttraumatic fat necrosis or mammary duct ectasia, but they must always be evaluated with great care.

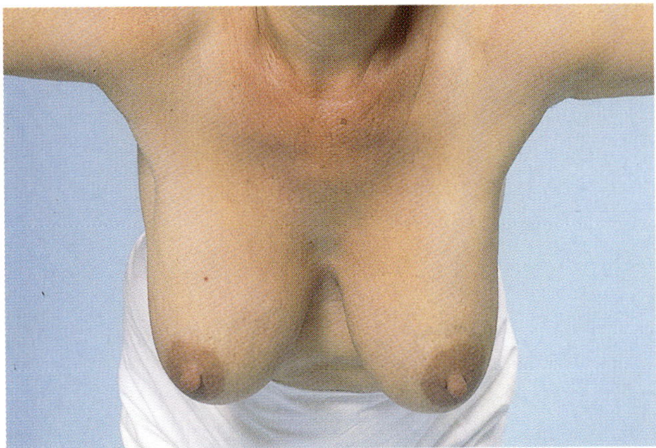

LEANING FORWARD

This position may reveal an asymmetry of the breast or nipple not otherwise visible. Retraction of the nipple and areola suggests an underlying cancer. See Table 8-1, Visible Signs of Breast Cancer (p. 314).

PALPATION

The Breast. Palpation is best performed when the breast tissue is flattened. The patient should be supine. Plan to palpate a rectangular area extending from the clavicle to the inframammary fold or bra line, and from the midsternal line to the posterior axillary line and well into the axilla for the tail of the breast.

A thorough examination will take 3 minutes for each breast. Use the *fingerpads* of the 2nd, 3rd, and 4th fingers, keeping the fingers slightly flexed. It is important to be *systematic.* Although a circular or wedge pattern can be used, the *vertical strip pattern* is currently the best validated technique for detecting breast masses. Palpate in *small, concentric circles* at each examining point, if possible applying light, medium, and deep pressure. You will need to press more firmly to reach the deeper tissues of a large breast. Your examination should cover the entire breast, including the periphery, tail, and axilla.

When pressing deeply on the breast, you may mistake a normal rib for a hard breast mass.

- To examine *the lateral portion of the breast,* ask the patient to roll onto the opposite hip, placing her hand on her forehead but keeping the shoulders pressed against the bed or examining table. This flattens the lateral breast tissue. Begin palpation in the axilla, moving in a straight line down to the bra line, then move the fingers medially and palpate in a vertical strip up the chest to the clavicle. Continue in vertical overlapping strips until you reach the nipple, then reposition the patient to flatten the medial portion of the breast.

Nodules in the tail of the breast are sometimes mistaken for enlarged axillary lymph nodes (and vice versa).

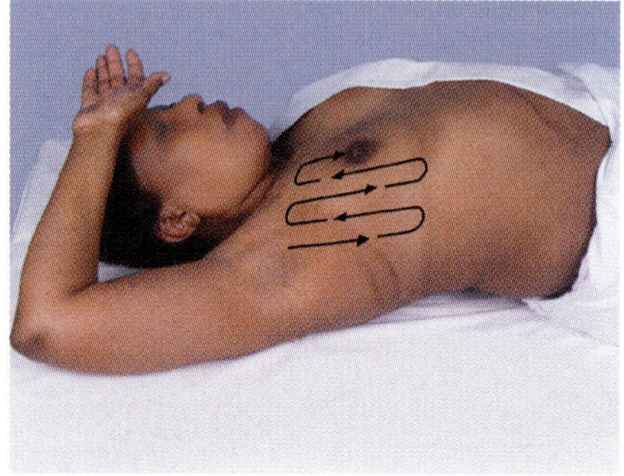

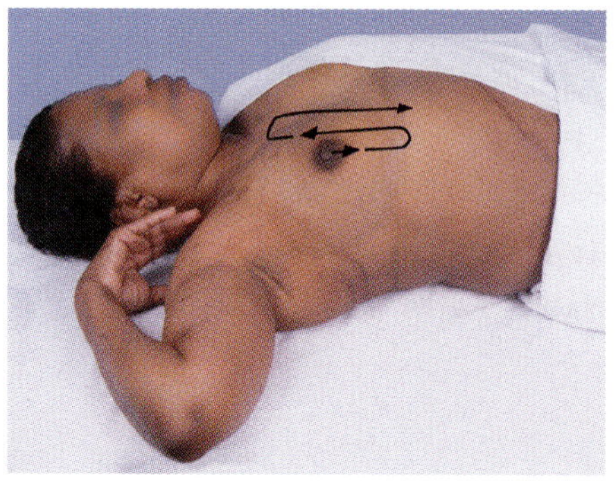

- To examine *the medial portion of the breast,* ask the patient to lie with her shoulders flat against the bed or examining table, placing her hand at her neck and lifting up her elbow until it is even with her shoulder. Palpate in a straight line down from the nipple to the bra line, then back to the clavicle, continuing in vertical overlapping strips to the midsternum.

Examine the breast tissue carefully for:

- *Consistency* of the tissues. Normal consistency varies widely, depending in part on the relative proportions of firmer glandular tissue and soft fat. Physiologic nodularity may be present, increasing before menses. There may be a firm transverse ridge of compressed tissue along the lower mar-

Tender cords suggest *mammary duct ectasia,* a benign but sometimes painful condition of dilated ducts with surrounding inflamma-

gin of the breast, especially in large breasts. This is the normal inframammary ridge, not a tumor.

tion, sometimes with associated masses.

- *Tenderness,* as in premenstrual fullness
- *Nodules.* Palpate carefully for any lump or mass that is qualitatively different from or larger than the rest of the breast tissue. This is sometimes called a dominant mass and may reflect a pathologic change that requires evaluation by mammogram, aspiration, or biopsy. Assess and describe the characteristics of any nodule:

See Table 8-2, Common Breast Masses (p. 315).

Location—by quadrant or clock, with centimeters from the nipple

Size—in centimeters

Shape—round or cystic, disclike, or irregular in contour

Consistency—soft, firm, or hard

Hard, irregular, poorly circumscribed nodules, fixed to the skin or underlying tissues, strongly suggest cancer.

Delimitation—well circumscribed or not

Tenderness

Cysts, inflamed areas, some cancers may be tender

Mobility—in relation to the skin, pectoral fascia, and chest wall. Gently move the breast near the mass and watch for dimpling.

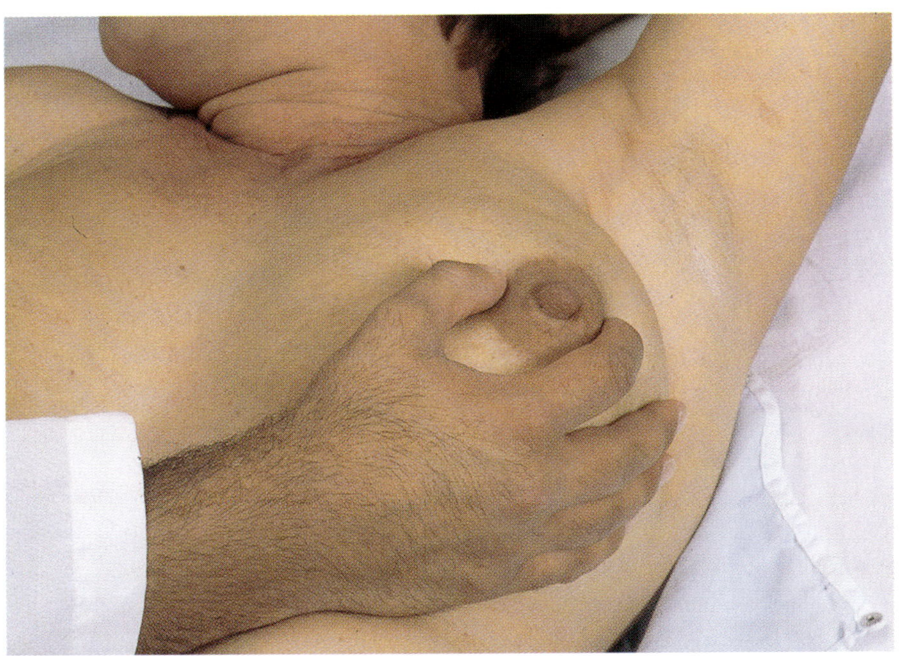

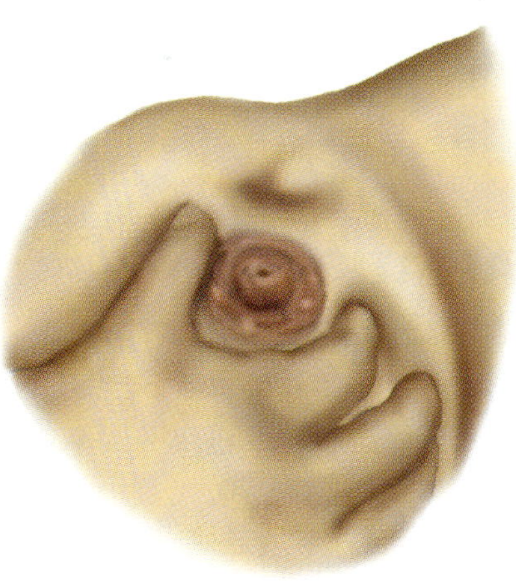

Next, try to move the mass itself while the patient relaxes her arm and then while she presses her hand against her hip.

A mobile mass that becomes fixed when the arm relaxes is attached to the ribs and intercostal muscles; if fixed when the hand is pressed against the hip, it is attached to the pectoral fascia.

The Nipple. Palpate each nipple, noting its elasticity.

Thickening of the nipple and loss of elasticity suggest an underlying cancer.

The Male Breast

Examination of the male breast may be brief but is sometimes important. *Inspect the nipple and areola* for nodules, swelling, or ulceration. *Palpate the areola and breast tissue* for nodules. If the breast appears enlarged, distinguish between the soft fatty enlargement of obesity and the firm disc of glandular enlargement, called *gynecomastia*.

Gynecomastia is attributed to an imbalance of estrogens and androgens, sometimes drug-related. A hard, irregular, eccentric, or ulcerating nodule is not gynecomastia and suggests breast cancer.

The Axillae

Although the axillae may be examined with the patient lying down, a sitting position is preferable.

INSPECTION

Inspect the skin of each axilla, noting evidence of:

- Rash

Deodorant and other rashes

- Infection

Sweat gland infection (*hidradenitis suppurativa*)

- Unusual pigmentation

Deeply pigmented, velvety axillary skin suggests *acanthosis nigricans,* one form of which is associated with internal malignancy.

PALPATION

To examine the left axilla, ask the patient to relax with the left arm down. Help by supporting the left wrist or hand with your left hand. Cup together the fingers of your right hand and reach as high as you can toward the apex of the axilla. Warn the patient that this may feel uncomfortable. Your fingers should lie directly behind the pectoral muscles, pointing toward the midclavicle. Now press your fingers in toward the chest wall and slide them downward, trying to feel the central nodes against the chest wall. Of the axillary nodes, these are the most often palpable. One or more soft, small (<1 cm), nontender nodes are frequently felt.

Enlarged axillary nodes from infection of the hand or arm, recent immunizations or skin tests in the arm, or part of a generalized lymphadenopathy. Check the epitrochlear nodes and other groups of lymph nodes.

Nodes that are large (≥1 cm) and firm or hard, matted together, or fixed to the skin or to underlying tissues suggest malignant involvement.

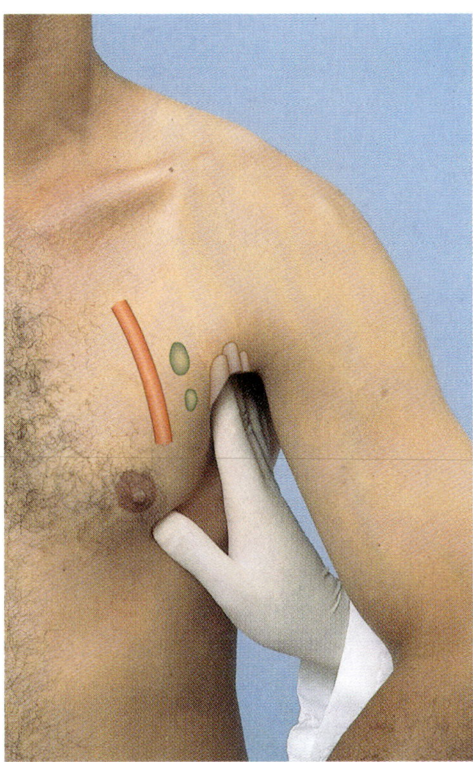

Use your left hand to examine the right axilla.

If the central nodes feel large, hard, or tender, or if there is a suspicious lesion in the drainage areas for the axillary nodes, feel for the other groups of axillary lymph nodes:

- *Pectoral nodes*—grasp the anterior axillary fold between your thumb and fingers, and with your fingers palpate inside the border of the pectoral muscle.
- *Lateral nodes*—from high in the axilla, feel along the upper humerus.
- *Subscapular nodes*—step behind the patient and with your fingers feel inside the muscle of the posterior axillary fold.

Also, feel for infraclavicular nodes and reexamine the supraclavicular nodes.

Special Techniques

Assessment of Spontaneous Nipple Discharge. If there is a history of spontaneous nipple discharge, try to determine its origin by compressing the areola with your index finger, placed in radial positions around the nipple. Watch for discharge appearing through one of the duct openings on the nipple's surface. Note the color, consistency, and quantity of any discharge and the exact location where it appears.

Milky discharge unrelated to a prior pregnancy and lactation is called *nonpuerperal galactorrhea.* Leading causes are hormonal and pharmacologic.

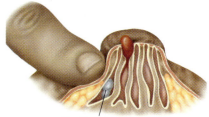

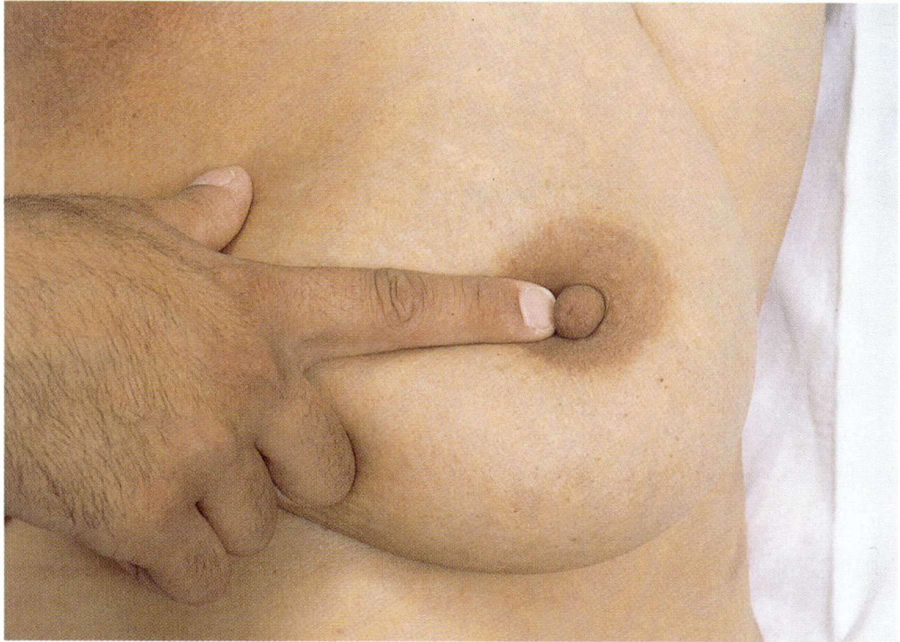

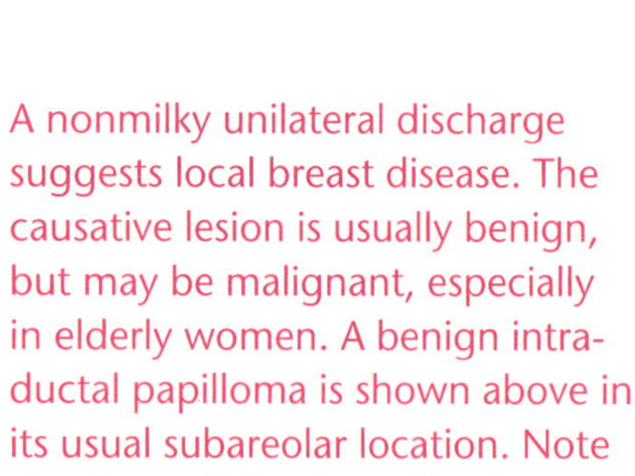

A nonmilky unilateral discharge suggests local breast disease. The causative lesion is usually benign, but may be malignant, especially in elderly women. A benign intraductal papilloma is shown above in its usual subareolar location. Note the drop of blood exuding from a duct opening.

Examination of The Mastectomy Patient. The woman with a mastectomy warrants special care on examination. Inspect the mastectomy scar and axilla carefully for any masses or unusual nodularity. Note any change in color or signs of inflammation. Lymphedema may be present in the axilla and upper arm from impaired lymph drainage after surgery. Palpate gently along the scar—these tissues may be unusually sensitive. Use a circular motion with two or three fingers. Pay special attention to the upper outer quadrant and axilla. Note any enlargement of the lymph nodes or signs of inflammation or infection.

Masses, nodularity, change in color or inflammation, especially in the incision line, suggest recurrence of breast cancer.

It is especially important to carefully palpate the breast tissue and incision lines of women with breast augmentation or reconstruction.

Instructions for The Breast Self-Examination. The office or hospital visit is an important time to teach the patient how to perform the breast self-examination (BSE). A high proportion of breast masses are detected by women examining their own breasts. Although BSE has not been shown to reduce breast cancer mortality, monthly BSE is inexpensive and may promote stronger health awareness and more active self-care. For early detection of breast cancer, the BSE is most useful when coupled with regular breast examination by an experienced clinician and mammography. The BSE is best timed just after menses, when hormonal stimulation of breast tissue is low.

PATIENT INSTRUCTIONS FOR THE BREAST SELF-EXAMINATION (BSE)

Lying Supine

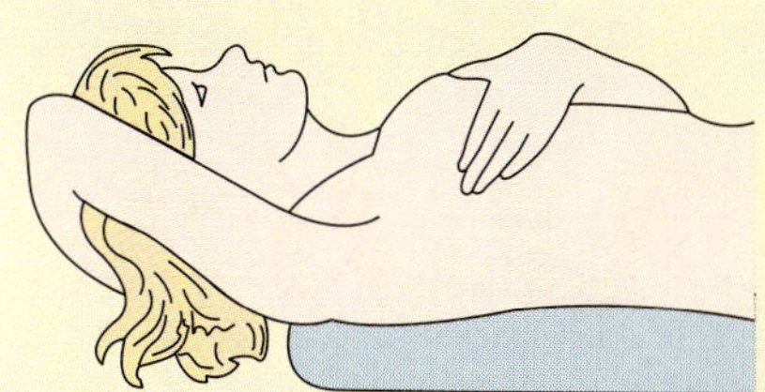

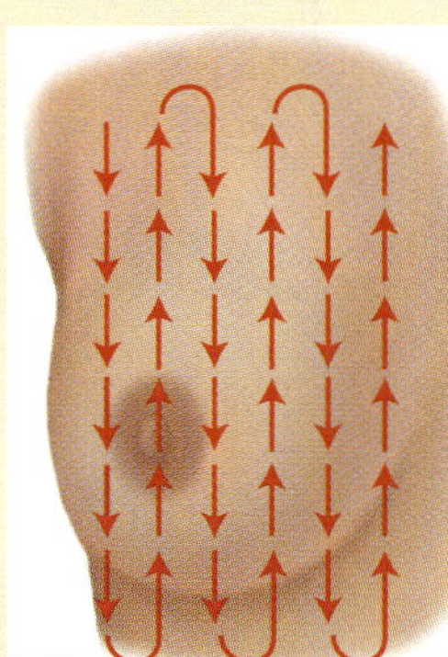

1. Lie down with a pillow under your right shoulder. Place your right arm behind your head.
2. Use the finger pads of the three middle fingers on your left hand to feel for lumps in the right breast. The finger pads are the top third of each finger.
3. Press firmly enough to know how your breast feels. A firm ridge in the lower curve of each breast is normal. If you're not sure how hard to press, talk with your health care provider, or try to copy the way the doctor or nurse does it.
4. Press firmly on the breast in an up-and-down or "strip" pattern. You can also use a circular or wedge pattern, but be sure to use the same pattern every time. Check the entire breast area, and remember how your breast feels from month to month.
5. Repeat the examination on your left breast, using the finger pads of the right hand.
6. If you find any changes, see your doctor right away.

Standing

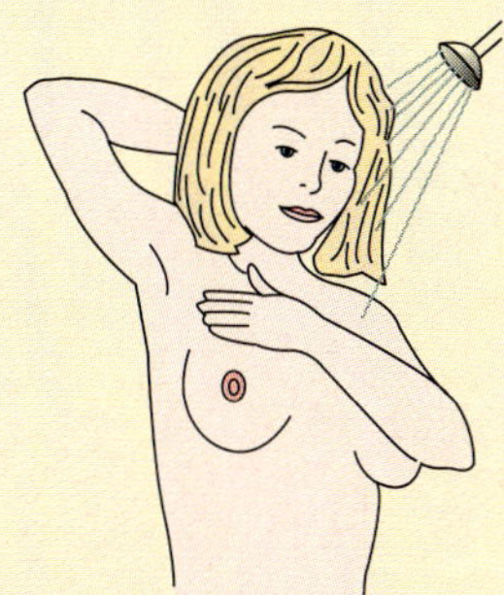

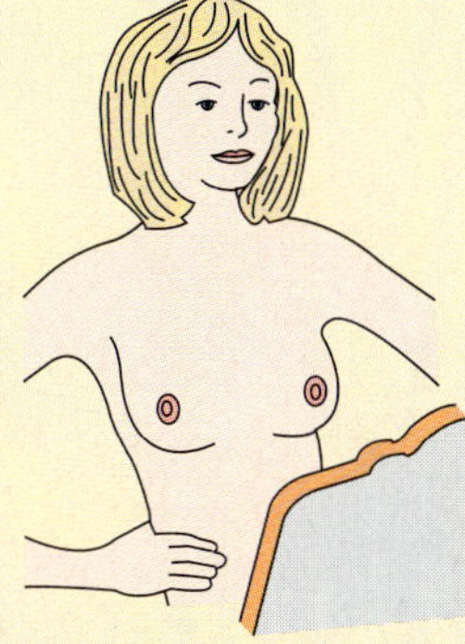

1. Repeat the examination of both breasts while standing, with one arm behind your head. The upright position makes it easier to check the upper outer part of the breasts (toward your armpit). This is where about half of breast cancers are found. You may want to do the upright part of the BSE while you are in the shower. Your soapy hands will make it easy to check how your breasts feel as they glide over the wet skin.
2. For added safety, you might want to check your breasts by standing in front of a mirror right after your BSE each month. See if there are any changes in the way your breasts look, such as dimpling of the skin, changes in the nipple, redness, or swelling.
3. If you find any changes, see your doctor right away.

Adapted from the American Cancer Society, www.cancer.org. Accessed 9/1/01.

TABLE 8-1 ■ Visible Signs of Breast Cancer

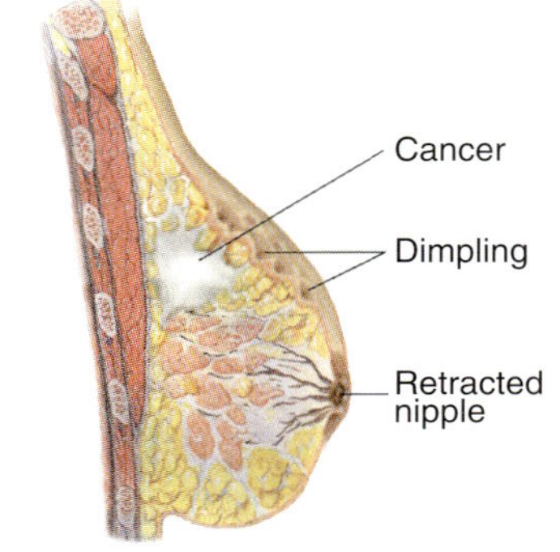

Retraction Signs

Mechanism

As breast cancer advances, it causes fibrosis (scar tissue). Shortening of this fibrotic tissue produces retraction signs, including dimpling, changes in contour, and retraction or deviation of the nipple. Other causes of retraction include fat necrosis and mammary duct ectasia.

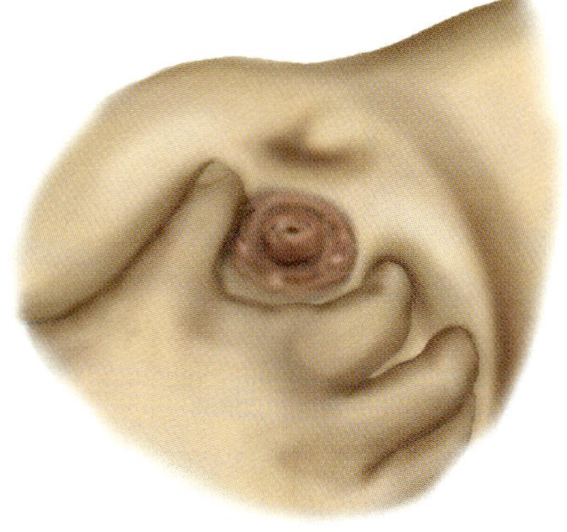

Skin Dimpling

Look for this sign with the patient's arm at rest, during special positioning, and on moving or compressing the breast, as illustrated here.

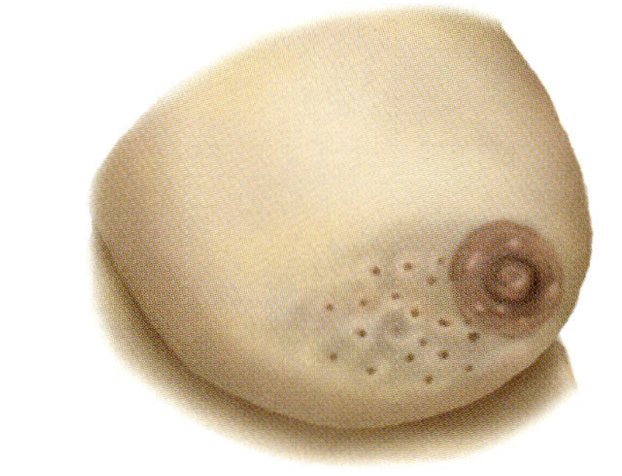

Edema of the Skin

Edema of the skin is produced by lymphatic blockade. It appears as thickened skin with enlarged pores—the so-called *peau d'orange* (orange peel) *sign*. It is often seen first in the lower portion of the breast or areola.

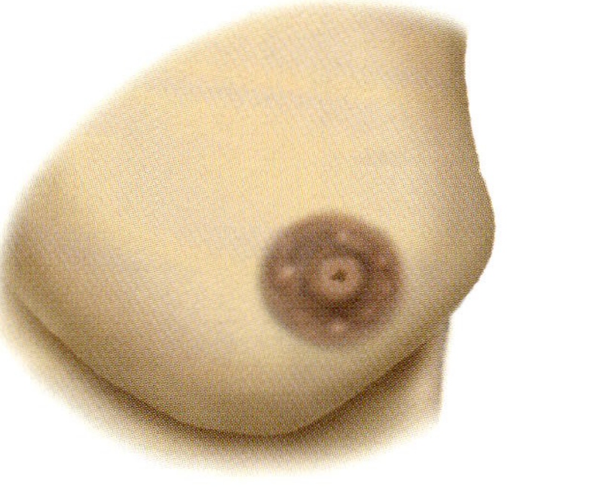

Abnormal Contours

Look for any variation in the normal convexity of each breast, and compare one side with the other. Special positioning may again be useful. Shown here is marked flattening of the lower outer quadrant of the left breast.

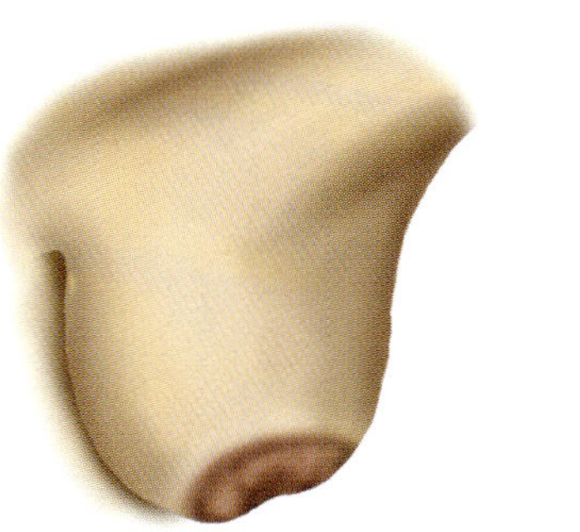

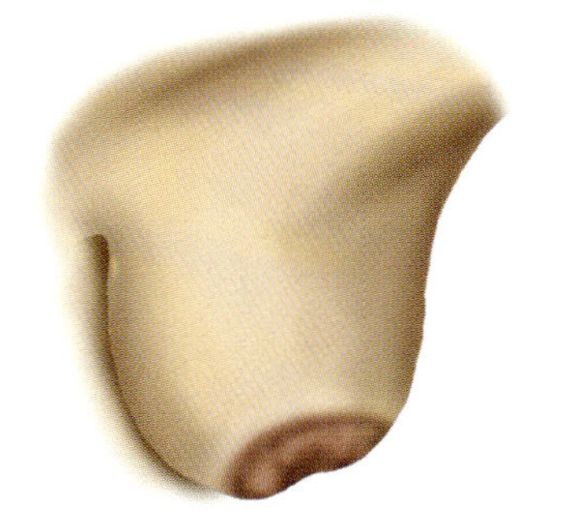

Nipple Retraction and Deviation

A retracted nipple is flattened or pulled inward, as illustrated here. It may also be broadened, and feels thickened. When involvement is radially asymmetric, the nipple may deviate, i.e., point in a different direction from its normal counterpart, typically toward the underlying cancer.

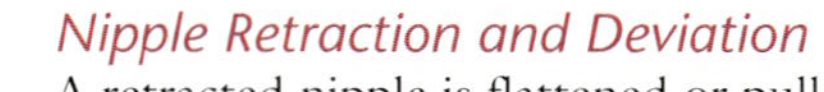

Paget's Disease of the Nipple

This is an uncommon form of breast cancer that usually starts as a scaly, eczemalike lesion. The skin may also weep, crust, or erode. A breast mass may be present. Suspect Paget's disease in any persisting dermatitis of the nipple and areola.

TABLE 8-2 ■ Common Breast Masses

The three most common kinds of breast masses are *fibroadenoma* (a benign tumor), *cysts,* and *breast cancer*. The clinical characteristics of these masses are listed below. However, any breast mass should be carefully evaluated and usually warrants further investigation by ultrasound, aspiration, mammography, or biopsy. The masses depicted below are rather large, for purposes of illustration. Ideally, breast cancer should be identified early, when the mass is small. *Fibrocystic changes,* not illustrated, are also commonly palpable as nodular, ropelike densities in women ages 25–50. They may be tender or painful. They are considered benign and are not considered a risk factor for breast cancer.

	Fibroadenoma	Cysts	Cancer
Usual Age	15–25, usually puberty and young adulthood, but up to age 55	30–50, regress after menopause except with estrogen therapy	30–90, most common over 50 in middle-aged and elderly women
Number	Usually single, may be multiple	Single or multiple	Usually single, although may coexist with other nodules
Shape	Round, disclike, or lobular	Round	Irregular or stellate
Consistency	May be soft, usually firm	Soft to firm, usually elastic	Firm or hard
Delimitation	Well delineated	Well delineated	Not clearly delineated from surrounding tissues
Mobility	Very mobile	Mobile	May be fixed to skin or underlying tissues
Tenderness	Usually nontender	Often tender	Usually nontender
Retraction Signs	Absent	Absent	May be present

CHAPTER

9

The Abdomen

ANATOMY AND PHYSIOLOGY

Inspect the abdominal wall and pelvis, and visualize or palpate the landmarks illustrated. The rectus abdominis muscles become more prominent when the patient raises the head and shoulders from the supine position.

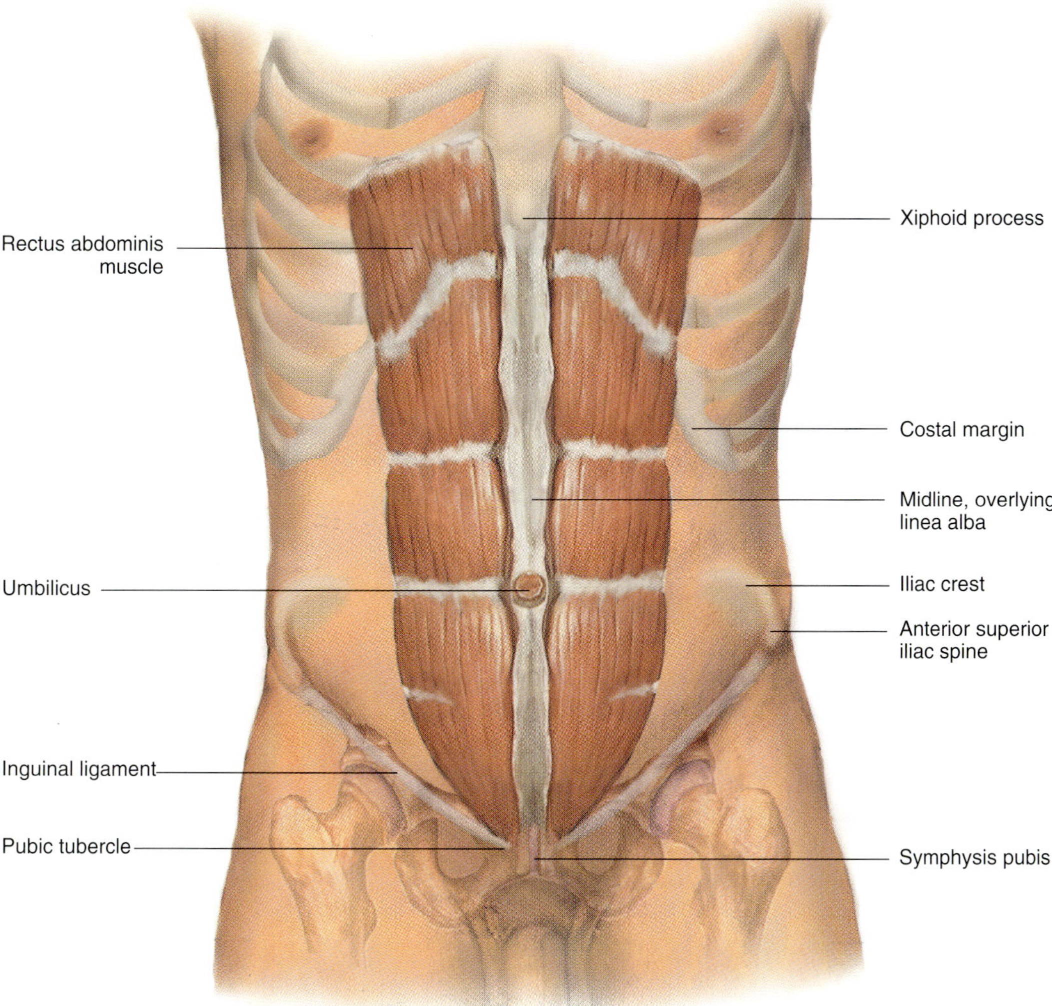

For descriptive purposes, the abdomen is often divided by imaginary lines crossing at the umbilicus, forming the right upper, right lower, left upper, and left lower quadrants. Another system divides the abdomen into nine sections. Terms for three of them are commonly used: epigastric, umbilical, and hypogastric, or suprapubic.

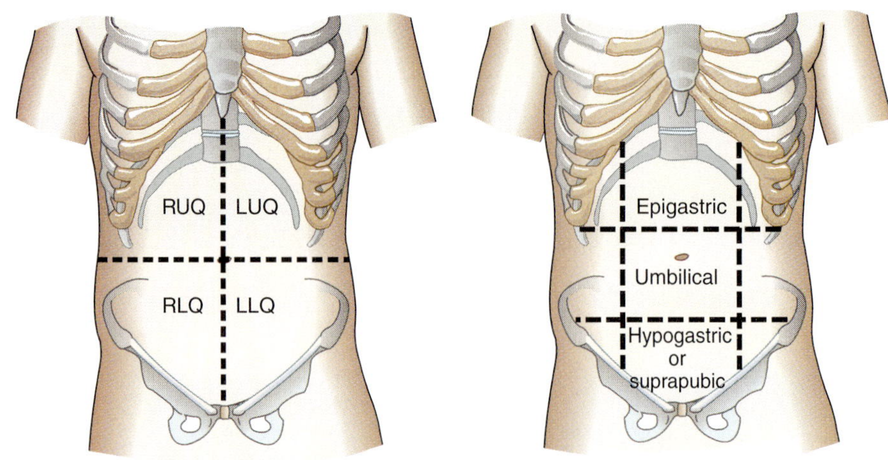

When examining the abdomen, you may be able to feel several normal structures. The sigmoid *colon* is frequently palpable as a firm, narrow tube in the left lower quadrant, while the cecum and part of the ascending colon form a softer, wider tube in the right lower quadrant. Portions of the transverse and descending colon may also be palpable. None of these structures should be mistaken for a tumor. Although the normal *liver* often extends down just below the right costal margin, its soft consistency makes it difficult to feel through the abdominal wall. The lower margin of the liver, the liver edge, is often palpable. Also in the right upper quadrant, but usually at a deeper level, lies the lower pole of the right kidney. It is occasionally palpable, especially in thin individuals with relaxed abdominal muscles. Pulsations of the *abdominal aorta* are frequently visible and usually palpable in the upper abdomen, while the pulsations of the *iliac arteries* may sometimes be felt in the lower quadrants.

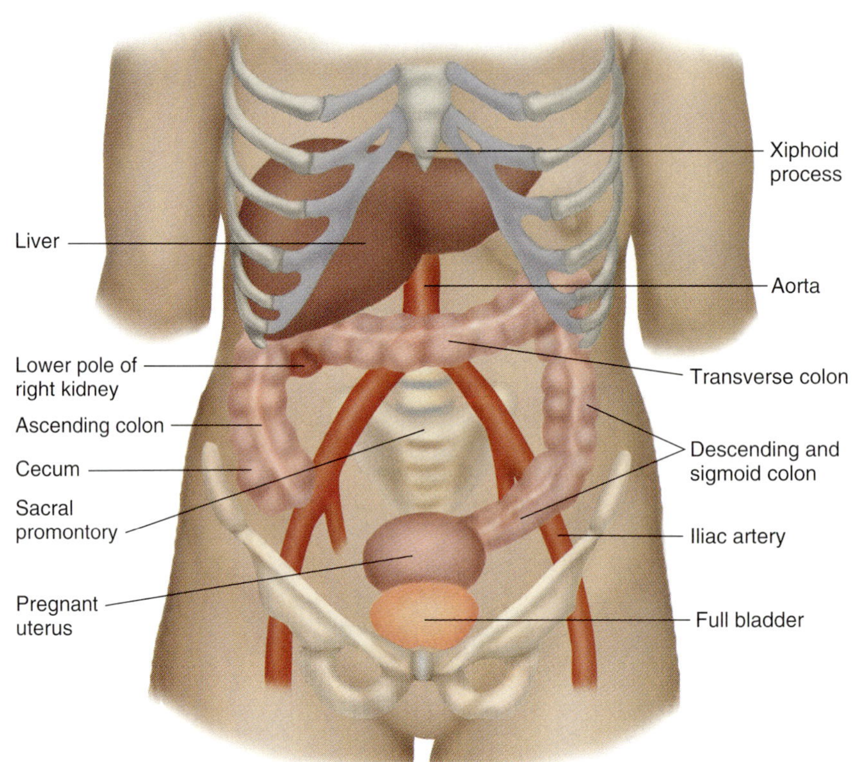

The abdominal cavity extends up under the rib cage to the dome of the diaphragm. In this protected location, beyond the reach of the palpating hand, are much of the liver and *stomach* and all of the usual normal spleen. The *spleen* lies against the diaphragm at the level of the 9th, 10th, and 11th ribs, mostly posterior to the left midaxillary line. It is lateral to and behind the stomach, and just above the left kidney. The tip of a normal spleen is palpable below the left costal margin in a small percentage of adults.

Most of the normal *gallbladder* lies deep to the liver and cannot be distinguished from it clinically. The *duodenum* and *pancreas* lie deep in the upper abdomen, where they are not normally palpable.

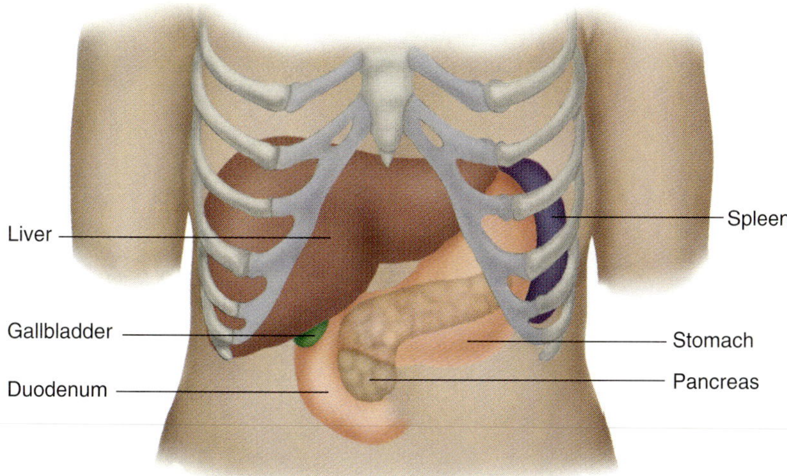

ANTERIOR VIEW

A distended *bladder* may be palpable above the symphysis pubis. The bladder accommodates roughly 300 ml of urine filtered by the kidneys into the renal pelvis and the ureters. Bladder expansion stimulates contraction of bladder smooth muscle, the *detrusor muscle,* at relatively low pressures. Rising pressure in the bladder triggers the conscious urge to void.

Increased intraurethral pressure can overcome rising pressures in the bladder and prevent incontinence. Intraurethral pressure is related to such factors as smooth muscle tone in the internal urethral sphincter, the thickness of the urethral mucosa, and in women, sufficient support to the bladder and proximal urethra from pelvic muscles and ligaments to maintain proper anatomic relationships. Striated muscle around the urethra can also contract voluntarily to interrupt voiding.

Neuroregulatory control of the bladder functions at several levels. In infants, the bladder empties by reflex mechanisms in the sacral spinal cord. Voluntary control of the bladder depends on higher centers in the brain and on motor and sensory pathways between the brain and the reflex arcs of the sacral spinal cord. When voiding is inconvenient, higher centers in the brain can inhibit detrusor contractions until the capacity of the bladder, about 400 to 500 ml, is exceeded. The integrity of the sacral nerves that innervate the bladder can be tested by assessing perirectal and perineal sensation in the S2, S3, and S4 dermatomes (see p. 546).

Other structures sometimes palpable in the lower abdomen include the *uterus* enlarged by pregnancy or fibroids, which may also rise above the symphysis pubis, and the *sacral promontory,* the anterior edge of the first sacral vertebra. Until you are familiar with this normal structure, you may mistake its stony hard outlines for a tumor. Another stony hard lump that can sometimes mislead you, and may occasionally alarm a patient, is a normal *xiphoid process.*

The *kidneys* are posterior organs. Their upper portions are protected by the ribs. The *costovertebral angle*—the angle formed by the lower border of the

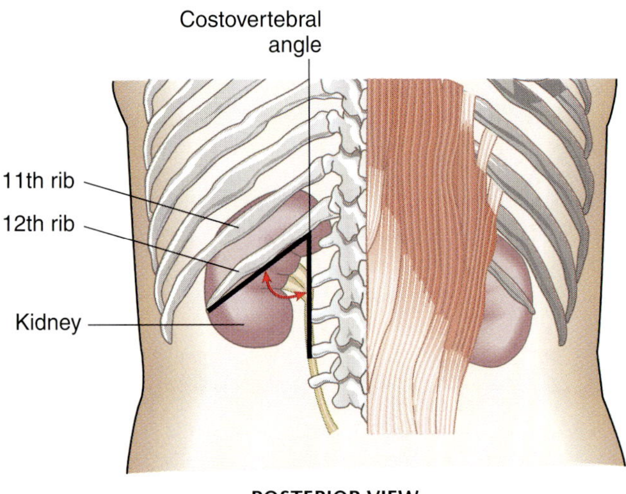

POSTERIOR VIEW

12th rib and the transverse processes of the upper lumbar vertebrae—defines the region to assess for kidney tenderness.

Changes With Aging

During the middle and later years, fat tends to accumulate in the lower abdomen and near the hips, even when total body weight is stable. This accumulation, together with weakening of the abdominal muscles, often produces a potbelly. Occasionally a person notes this change with alarm and interprets it as fluid or evidence of disease.

Old age may blunt the manifestations of acute abdominal disease. Pain may be less severe, fever is often less pronounced, and signs of peritoneal inflammation, such as muscular guarding and rebound tenderness (p. 335), may be diminished or even absent.

THE HEALTH HISTORY

Common or Concerning Symptoms

Gastrointestinal Disorders

- Indigestion or anorexia
- Nausea, vomiting, or hematemesis
- Abdominal pain
- Dysphagia and/or odynophagia
- Change in bowel function
- Constipation or diarrhea
- Jaundice

Urinary and Renal Disorders

- Suprapubic pain
- Dysuria, urgency, or frequency
- Hesitancy, decreased stream in males
- Polyuria or nocturia
- Urinary incontinence
- Hematuria
- Kidney or flank pain
- Ureteral colic

You will encounter a wide variety of gastrointestinal and urinary complaints in clinical practice. Careful interviewing will often lead you to the underlying disorder. This section addresses such gastrointestinal concerns as *indigestion, anorexia, nausea* or *vomiting, hematemesis, abdominal pain, dysphagia* or *odynophagia, change in bowel function, constipation* and *diarrhea,* and *jaundice.* There is also health history information on disorders of the urinary tract, including complaints of *suprapubic pain, dysuria, urgency, frequency, hesitancy* or *decreased stream* in males, *polyuria, nocturia, incontinence, hematuria, kidney pain,* and *ureteral colic.*

The Gastrointestinal Tract

"How is your *appetite*?" is a good starting question and may lead into other important areas such as *indigestion, nausea, vomiting,* and *anorexia.* Patients often complain of *indigestion,* a common complaint that refers to distress associated with eating, but patients use the term for many different symptoms. Find out just what your patient means. Possibilities include:

Anorexia, nausea, vomiting in many gastrointestinal disorders; also in pregnancy, diabetic ketoacidosis, adrenal insufficiency, hypercalcemia, uremia, liver disease, emotional states, adverse drug reactions, and other conditions. Induced but without nausea in anorexia/bulimia.

- *Heartburn,* or a sense of burning or warmth that is retrosternal and may radiate from the epigastrium to the neck. It usually originates in the esophagus. If persistent, especially in the epigastric area, it may raise the question of heart disease. Some patients with coronary artery disease describe their pain as burning, "like indigestion." Pay special attention to what brings on the discomfort and what relieves it. Is it precipitated by exertion and relieved by rest, suggesting angina, or is it related to meals and made worse during or after eating, suggesting gastroesophageal reflux?

Heartburn suggests gastric acid reflux into the esophagus; often precipitated by a heavy meal, lying down, or bending forward, also by ingested alcohol, citrus juices, or aspirin. If chronic, consider reflux esophagitis. See Table 6-1, Chest Pain, pp. 234–235.

- *Excessive gas,* especially with frequent belching, abdominal bloating or distention, or *flatus,* the passage of gas by rectum, normally about 600 ml per day. Find out if these symptoms are associated with eating specific foods. Ask if symptoms are related to ingestion of milk or milk products.

Belching, but not bloating or excess flatus, normally seen in *aerophagia,* or swallowing air. Also consider legumes and other gas-producing foods, intestinal lactase deficiency, irritable bowel syndrome.

- Unpleasant *abdominal fullness* after meals of normal size, or *early satiety,* the inability to eat a full meal.

Consider diabetic gastroparesis, anticholinergic drugs, gastric outlet obstruction, gastric cancer; early satiety in hepatitis.

- *Nausea and vomiting*
- *Abdominal pain*

Anorexia is a loss or lack of appetite. Find out if it arises from intolerance to certain foods or reluctance to eat due to anticipated discomfort. *Nausea*, often described as "feeling sick to my stomach," may progress to retching or vomiting. *Retching* describes the spasmodic movements of the chest and diaphragm that precede and culminate in *vomiting*, the forceful expulsion of gastric contents out through the mouth.

Anorexia, nausea, vomiting in many gastrointestinal disorders; also in pregnancy, diabetic ketoacidosis, adrenal insufficiency, hypercalcemia, uremia, liver disease, emotional states, adverse drug reactions. Induced but without nausea in anorexia/bulimia nervosa.

Some patients may not actually vomit but raise esophageal or gastric contents in the absence of nausea or retching, called *regurgitation*.

Regurgitation in esophageal narrowing from stricture or cancer; also with incompetent gastroesophageal sphincter

Ask about any vomitus or regurgitated material and inspect it yourself if possible. What color is it? What does the vomitus smell like? How much has there been? Ask specifically if it contains any blood and try to determine how much. You may have to help the patient with the amount . . . a teaspoon? Two teaspoons? A cupful?

Fecal odor in small bowel obstruction or gastrocolic fistula

Gastric juice is clear or mucoid. Small amounts of yellowish or greenish bile are common and have no special significance. Brownish or blackish vomitus with a "coffee-grounds" appearance suggests blood altered by gastric acid. Coffee-grounds emesis or red blood are termed *hematemesis.*

Hematemesis in duodenal or peptic ulcer, esophageal or gastric varices, gastritis

Do the patient's symptoms suggest any complications of vomiting such as *aspiration* into the lungs, seen in elderly, debilitated, or obtunded patients? Is there dehydration or electrolyte imbalance from prolonged vomiting, or significant loss of blood?

Symptoms of blood loss such as light-headedness or syncope depend on the rate and volume of bleeding, and rarely appear until blood loss ≥ 500 ml.

Abdominal pain has several possible mechanisms and clinical patterns and warrants careful clinical assessment. Be familiar with three broad categories of abdominal pain:

See Table 9-1, Abdominal Pain (pp. 350–351).

- *Visceral pain* occurs when hollow abdominal organs such as the intestine or biliary tree contract unusually forcefully or when they are distended or stretched. Solid organs such as the liver can also become painful when their capsules are stretched. Visceral pain may be difficult to localize. It is typically, though not necessarily, palpable near the midline, at levels that vary according to the structure involved, as illustrated on the next page.

  Visceral pain in the right upper quadrant from liver distention against its capsule in alcoholic hepatitis

  Visceral pain varies in quality and may be gnawing, burning, cramping, or aching. When it becomes severe, it may be associated with sweating, pallor, nausea, vomiting, and restlessness.

  Visceral periumbilical pain in early acute appendicitis from distention of inflamed appendix, gradually changing to parietal pain in the right lower quadrant from inflammation of the adjacent parietal peritoneum

- *Parietal pain* originates in the parietal peritoneum and is caused by inflammation. It is a steady aching pain that is usually more severe than visceral pain and more precisely localized over the involved structure. It is typically aggravated by movement or coughing. Patients with this type of pain usually prefer to lie still.

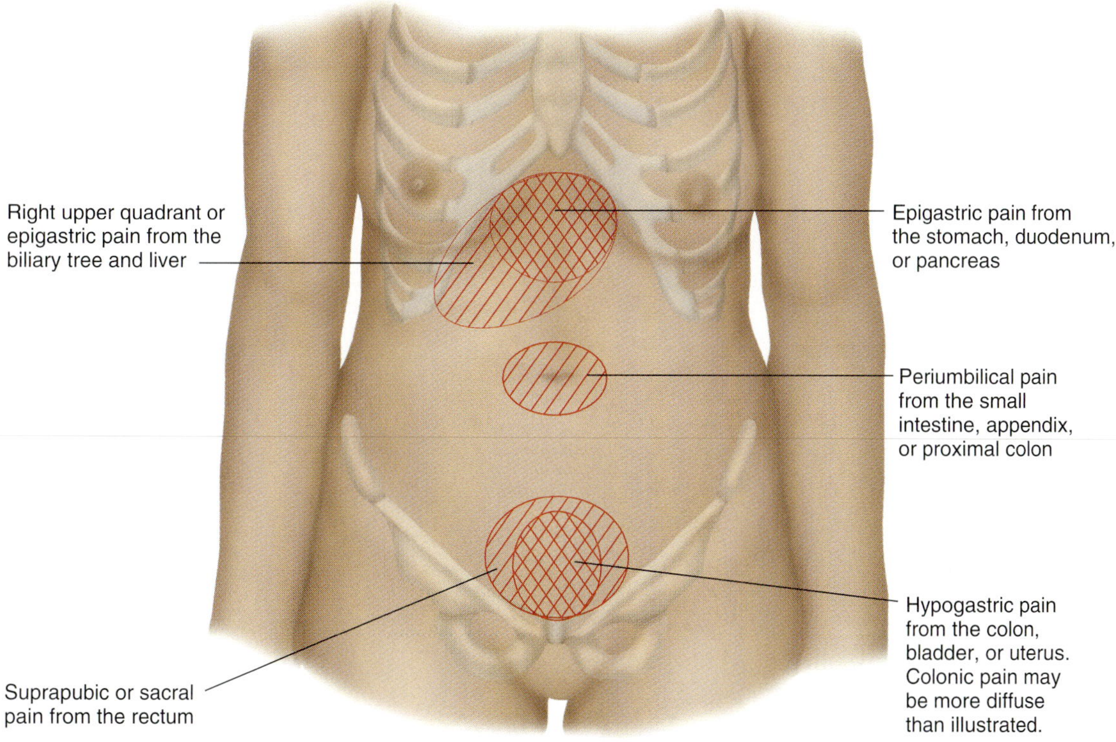
Right upper quadrant or epigastric pain from the biliary tree and liver
Epigastric pain from the stomach, duodenum, or pancreas
Periumbilical pain from the small intestine, appendix, or proximal colon
Hypogastric pain from the colon, bladder, or uterus. Colonic pain may be more diffuse than illustrated.
Suprapubic or sacral pain from the rectum

- *Referred pain* is felt in more distant sites, which are innervated at approximately the same spinal levels as the disordered structure. Referred pain often develops as the initial pain becomes more intense and thus seems to radiate or travel from the initial site. It may be felt superficially or deeply but is usually well localized.

  Pain may also be referred to the abdomen from the chest, spine, or pelvis, thus complicating the assessment of abdominal pain.

Pain of duodenal or pancreatic origin may be referred to the back; pain from the biliary tree, to the right shoulder or the right posterior chest.

Pain from pleurisy or acute myocardial infarction may be referred to the upper abdomen.

Ask patients to *describe the abdominal pain in their own words,* then ask them to *point to the pain.* If clothes interfere, repeat the question during the physical examination. You may need to pursue important details: "Where does the pain start?" "Does it radiate or travel anywhere?" "What is the pain like?" If the patient has trouble describing the pain, try a multiple-choice question such as "Is it aching, burning, gnawing, or what?"

Cramping colicky pain often is related to peristalsis.

You need to ask "How severe is the pain?" "How about on a scale of 1 to 10?" Find out if it is bearable and if it interferes with the patient's usual activities. Does it make the patient lie down?

The description of the *severity of the pain* may tell you something about the patient's responses to pain and its impact on the patient's life, but it is not consistently helpful in assessing the pain's cause. Sensitivity to abdominal pain varies widely and tends to diminish over the later years, masking acute abdominal problems in older people, especially those in or beyond their 70s.

Careful *timing of the pain*, on the other hand, is particularly helpful. Did it start suddenly or gradually? When did the pain begin? How long does it last? What is its pattern over a 24-hour period? Over weeks and months? Are you dealing with an acute illness or a chronic or recurring one?

Determine *what factors aggravate or relieve the pain*, with special reference to meals, antacids, alcohol, medications (including aspirin and aspirinlike drugs and any over-the-counter drugs), emotional factors, and body position. Also, is the pain related to defecation, urination, or menstruation? You also need to elicit any *symptoms that are associated with the pain*, such as fever or chills, and ask in what sequence they occur.

Citrus fruits may aggravate the pain of reflux esophagitis; possible lactase deficiency if abdominal discomfort from milk ingestion

Less commonly, patients may report difficulty swallowing, or *dysphagia*, the sense that food or liquid is sticking, hesitating, or "won't go down right." Dysphagia may result from esophageal disorders or from difficulty transferring food from the mouth to the esophagus. The sensation of a lump in the throat or in the retrosternal area, unassociated with swallowing, is not true dysphagia.

For types of dysphagia, see Table 9-2, Dysphagia, p. 352.

Ask the patient to point to where the dysphagia occurs and describe with what types of food. Does it occur with relatively solid foods such as meat, with softer foods such as ground meat and mashed potatoes, or with hot or cold liquids? Has the pattern changed?

Pointing to the throat suggests a transfer or esophageal disorder; pointing to the chest suggests an esophageal disorder.

Establish the timing. When did it start? Is it intermittent or persistent? Is it progressing? If so, over what period of time? What are the associated symptoms and medical conditions?

Dysphagia with solid food in mechanical narrowing of the esophagus; dysphagia related to both solids and liquids suggests a disorder of esophageal motility.

Odynophagia, or pain on swallowing, may occur in two forms. A sharp, burning pain suggests mucosal inflammation, while a squeezing, cramping pain suggests a muscular cause. Odynophagia may accompany dysphagia, but either symptom may occur independently.

Mucosal inflammation in reflux esophagitis or infection from *Candida*, herpesvirus, or cytomegalovirus.

With respect to the lower gastrointestinal tract, you will frequently need to assess *bowel function*. Start with open-ended questions: "How are your bowel movements?" "How frequent are they?" "Do you have any difficulties?" "Have you noticed any change in your bowel habits?" Frequency of bowel movements normally ranges from about three times a day to twice a week. A change in pattern within these limits, however, may be significant for an individual patient.

Patients vary widely in their views of constipation and diarrhea. Be sure to clarify what the patient means by these terms. For example, is *constipation* . . . a decrease in frequency of bowel movements? . . . The passage of hard and perhaps painful stools? . . . The need to strain unusually hard? . . . A sense of incomplete defecation or pressure in the rectum? Ask if the patient actually looks at the stool. If yes, what does the stool look like in terms of color and bulk? What remedies has the patient tried? Do medications, stress, unrealistic ideas

See Table 9-3, Constipation (p. 353).

Thin pencil-like stool in an obstructing "apple-core" lesion of the sigmoid colon

about normal bowel habits, or time and setting allotted for defecation play a role? Occasionally there is complete constipation with no passage of either feces or gas, or *obstipation*.

Obstipation in intestinal obstruction

Inquire about the color of the stools and ask about any *black tarry stools*, suggesting *melena*, or *red blood in the stools*, known as *hematochezia*. If either condition is present, find out how long and how often. If the blood is red, how much is there? Is it pure blood mixed in with stool or on the surface of the stool? Is there blood on the toilet paper?

See Table 9-5, Black and Bloody Stools, p. 356.

Blood on the stool surface and on toilet paper in *hemorrhoids*

Diarrhea is an excessive frequency in the passage of stools that are usually unformed or watery. Ask about size, frequency, and volume. Are the stools bulky or small? How many episodes of diarrhea occur each day?

Consistently large diarrheal stools often in small bowel or proximal colon disorders; small frequent stools with urgency of defecation in left colon or rectal disorders

Ask for descriptive terms. Are the stools greasy or oily? Frothy? Foul smelling? Floating on the surface because of excessive gas, making them difficult to flush? Accompanied by mucus, pus, or blood?

Large yellowish or gray greasy foul smelling, sometimes frothy or floating stools in *steatorrhea*, or fatty stools—seen in malabsorption

Assess the course of diarrhea over time. Is it acute, chronic, or recurrent? Or is your patient experiencing the first acute episode of a chronic or recurrent illness?

See Table 9-4, Diarrhea (pp. 354–355).

Look into other factors as well. Does the diarrhea awaken the patient at night? What seem to be the aggravating or relieving factors? Does the patient get relief from a bowel movement, or is there an intense urge with straining but little or no result, known as *tenesmus*. What is the setting? Does it entail travel, stress, or a new medication? Do family members or companions have similar symptoms? Are there associated symptoms?

Nocturnal diarrhea suggests a pathophysiologic cause.

Relief after passing feces or gas suggests left colon or rectal disorders; tenesmus in rectal conditions near the anal sphincter

In some patients, you will be struck by *jaundice* or *icterus*, the yellowish discoloration of the skin and sclerae from increased levels of bilirubin, a bile pigment derived chiefly from the breakdown of hemoglobin. Normally the hepatocytes conjugate, or combine, unconjugated bilirubin with other substances, making the bile water soluble, and then excrete it into the bile. The bile passes through the cystic duct into the common bile duct, which also drains the extrahepatic ducts from the liver. More distally the common bile duct and the pancreatic ducts empty into the duodenum at the ampulla of Vater. Mechanisms of jaundice include:

- Increased production of bilirubin
- Decreased uptake of bilirubin by the hepatocytes
- Decreased ability of the liver to conjugate bilirubin

Predominantly unconjugated bilirubin from the first three mechanisms, as in hemolytic anemia (increased production) and Gilbert's syndrome

- Decreased excretion of bilirubin into the bile, resulting in absorption of *conjugated* bilirubin back into the blood.

Impaired excretion of conjugated bilirubin in viral hepatitis, cirrhosis, primary biliary cirrhosis, drug-induced cholestasis, as with oral contraceptives, methyl testosterone, chlorpromazine

Intrahepatic jaundice can be *hepatocellular*, from damage to the hepatocytes, or *cholestatic*, from impaired excretion due to damaged hepatocytes or intrahepatic bile ducts. *Extrahepatic* jaundice arises from obstruction of the extrahepatic bile ducts, most commonly the cystic and common bile ducts.

Obstruction of the common bile duct by gallstones or pancreatic carcinoma

As you assess the jaundiced patient, pay special attention to the associated symptoms and the setting in which the illness occurred. What was the *color of the urine* as the patient became ill? When the level of conjugated bilirubin increases in the blood, it may be excreted into the urine, turning the urine a dark yellowish brown or tea color. Unconjugated bilirubin is not water-soluble so is not excreted into urine.

Dark urine from bilirubin indicates impaired excretion of bilirubin into the gastrointestinal tract.

Ask also about the *color of the stools.* When excretion of bile into the intestine is completely obstructed, the stools become gray or light-colored, or *acholic*, without bile.

Acholic stools briefly in viral hepatitis, common in obstructive jaundice

Does the skin itch without other obvious explanation? Is there associated pain? What is its pattern? Has it been recurrent in the past?

Itching in cholestatic or obstructive jaundice; pain from a distended liver capsule, biliary cholic, pancreatic cancer

Are there risk factors for liver diseases such as:

- *Hepatitis:* Travel or meals in areas of poor sanitation, ingestion of contaminated water or foodstuffs (hepatitis A); parenteral or mucous membrane exposure to infectious body fluids such as blood, serum, semen, and saliva, especially through sexual contact with an infected partner or use of shared needles for injection drug use (hepatitis B); intravenous illicit drug use or blood transfusion (hepatitis C)
- *Alcoholic hepatitis* or *alcoholic cirrhosis* (interview the patient carefully about alcohol use)
- *Toxic liver damage* from medications, industrial solvents, or environmental toxins
- *Gallbladder disease or surgery* that may result in extrahepatic biliary obstruction
- *Hereditary disorders* in the Family History

The Urinary Tract

General questions for a urinary history include: "Do you have any difficulty passing your urine?" "How often do you go?" "Do you have to get up at night? How often?" "How much urine do you pass at a time?" "Is there any pain or burning?" "Do you ever have trouble getting to the toilet in time?" "Do you ever leak any urine? Or wet yourself involuntarily?" Does the patient sense when the bladder is full and when voiding occurs?

See Table 9-6, Frequency, Nocturia, and Polyuria (p. 357).

Involuntary voiding or lack of awareness suggests cognitive or neurosensory deficits.

Ask women if sudden coughing, sneezing, or laughing makes them lose urine. Roughly half of young women report this experience even before bearing children. Occasional leakage is not necessarily significant. Ask older men "Do you have trouble starting your stream?" "Do you have to stand close to the toilet to void?" "Is there a change in the force or size of your stream, or straining to void?" "Do you hesitate or stop in the middle of voiding?" "Is there dribbling when you're through?"

Stress incontinence from decreased intraurethral pressure (see below)

Common in men with partial bladder outlet obstruction from benign prostatic hyperplasia; also seen with urethral stricture

What color is the urine? Has it ever been reddish or brown?

Hematuria, or blood in the urine

Disorders in the urinary tract may cause pain in either the abdomen or the back. Bladder disorders may cause *suprapubic pain*. In *bladder infection*, pain in the lower abdomen is typically dull and pressurelike. In sudden overdistention of the bladder, pain is often agonizing; in contrast, chronic bladder distention is usually painless.

Pain of sudden overdistention in acute urinary retention

Infection or irritation of either the bladder or urethra often provokes several symptoms. Frequently there is *pain on urination*, usually felt as a burning sensation. Some clinicians refer to this as *dysuria*, while others reserve the term dysuria for difficulty voiding. Women may report internal urethral discomfort, sometimes described as a pressure, or an external burning from the flow of urine across irritated or inflamed labia. Men typically feel a burning sensation proximal to the glans penis. In contrast, *prostatic pain* is felt in the perineum and occasionally in the rectum.

Painful urination with cystitis or urethritis

Also consider bladder stones, foreign bodies, tumors; also acute prostatitis. In women, internal burning in urethritis, external burning in vulvovaginitis

Commonly, there are other associated symptoms. Urinary *urgency* is an unusually intense and immediate desire to void, sometimes leading to involuntary voiding or *urge incontinence*. Urinary *frequency*, or abnormally frequent voiding, may occur. Ask about any related fever or chills, blood in the urine, or any pain in the abdomen, flank, or back (see the next page). Men with partial obstruction to urinary outflow often report *hesitancy* in starting the urine stream, *straining to void, reduced caliber and force of the urinary stream*, or *dribbling* as voiding is completed.

Urgency in bladder infection or irritation. In men, painful urination without frequency or urgency suggests urethritis.

Three additional terms describe important alterations in the pattern of urination. *Polyuria* refers to a significant increase in 24-hour urine volume,

Abnormally high renal production of urine in polyuria. Frequency

roughly defined as exceeding 3 liters. It should be distinguished from urinary frequency, which can involve voiding in high amounts, seen in polyuria, or in small amounts, as in infection. *Nocturia* refers to urinary frequency at night, sometimes defined as awakening the patient more than once; urine volumes may be large or small. Clarify any change in nocturnal voiding patterns and the number of trips to the bathroom.

without polyuria during the day or night in bladder disorder or impairment to flow at or below the bladder neck

Up to 30% of older patients are concerned about *urinary incontinence*, an involuntary loss of urine that may become socially embarrassing or cause problems with hygiene. If the patient reports incontinence, ask when it happens and how often. Find out if the patient has leaking of small amounts of urine with increased intra-abdominal pressure from coughing, sneezing, laughing, or lifting. Or is it difficult for the patient to hold the urine once there is an urge to void, and loss of large amounts of urine? Is there a sensation of bladder fullness, frequent leakage or voiding of small amounts but difficulty emptying the bladder?

See Table 9-7, Urinary Incontinence (pp. 358–359).

Stress incontinence with increased intra-abdominal pressure from decreased contractility of urethral sphincter or poor support of bladder neck; *urge incontinence* if unable to hold the urine, from detrusor overactivity; *overflow incontinence* when the bladder cannot be emptied until bladder pressure exceeds urethral pressure, from anatomic obstruction by prostatic hypertrophy or stricture, also neurogenic abnormalities

As described earlier, bladder control involves complex neuroregulatory and motor mechanisms (see p. 319). A number of central or peripheral nerve lesions may affect normal voiding. Can the patient sense when the bladder is full? And when voiding occurs? Although there are four broad categories of incontinence, a patient may have a combination of causes.

In addition, the patient's functional status may have a significant impact on voiding behaviors even when the urinary tract is intact. Is the patient mobile? Alert? Able to respond to voiding cues and reach the bathroom? Is alertness or voiding affected by medications?

Functional incontinence from impaired cognition, musculoskeletal problems, immobility

Blood is the urine, or *hematuria*, is an important cause for concern. When visible to the naked eye, it is called *gross hematuria*. The urine may appear

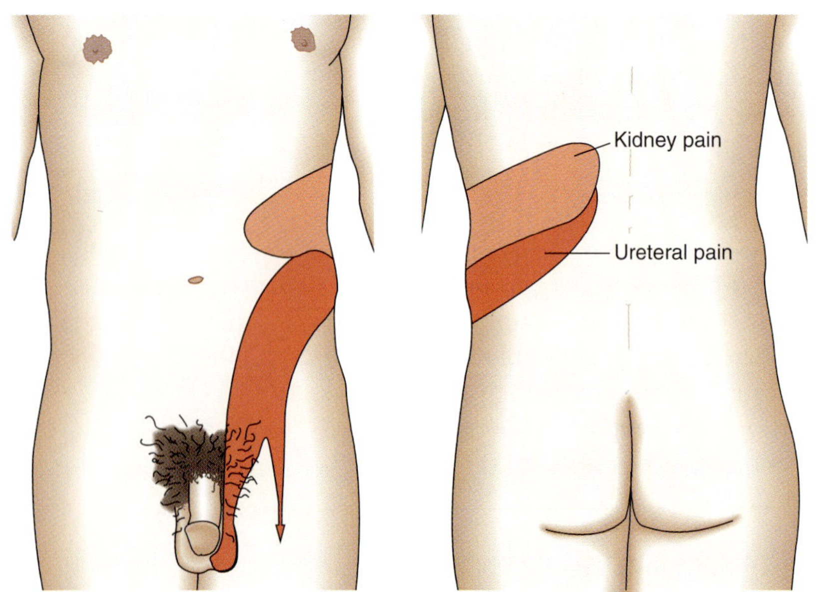

frankly bloody. Blood may be detected only during microscopic urinalysis, known as *microscopic hematuria.* Smaller amounts of blood may tinge the urine with a pinkish or brownish cast. In women, be sure to distinguish menstrual blood from hematuria. If the urine is reddish, ask about ingestion of beets or medications that might discolor the urine. Test the urine with a dipstick and microscopic examination before you settle on the term hematuria.

Disorders of the urinary tract may also cause *kidney pain,* often reported as *flank pain* at or below the posterior costal margin near the costovertebral angle. It may radiate anteriorly toward the umbilicus. Kidney pain is a visceral pain usually produced by distention of the renal capsule and typically dull, aching, and steady. *Ureteral pain* is dramatically different. It is usually severe and colicky, originating at the costovertebral angle and radiating around the trunk into the lower quadrant of the abdomen, or possibly into the upper thigh and testicle or labium. Ureteral pain results from sudden distention of the ureter and associated distention of the renal pelvis. Ask about any associated fever or chills, or hematuria.

Kidney pain occurs in acute pyelonephritis.

Renal or ureteral colic is caused by sudden obstruction of a ureter, as by urinary stones or blood clots.

HEALTH PROMOTION AND COUNSELING

Important Topics for Health Promotion and Counseling

- Screening for alcohol and substance abuse
- Risk factors for hepatitis A, B, and C
- Screening for colon cancer

Health promotion and counseling relevant to the abdomen include screening for alcoholism, risk of infectious hepatitis, and risk of colon cancer. Clues from social patterns and behavioral problems in the history and findings of liver enlargement or tenderness on physical examination often alert the clinician to possible alcoholism or risk of infectious hepatitis. Past medical history and family history are important when assessing risk of colon cancer.

The impact of alcohol and substance abuse on public health may be even greater than that of illicit drugs. Assessing patients for use of alcohol and other substances is a primary responsibility of all clinicians. The clinician should focus on detection, counseling, and, for significant impairment, specific recommendations for treatment. These interventions need not be time-consuming. Use the four CAGE questions, validated across many studies, to screen for alcohol dependence or abuse in all adolescents and adults, including pregnant women (see p. 413). Brief counseling interventions have been shown to reduce alcohol consumption by up to 25%.*

*U.S. Preventive Services Task Force: Guide to Clinical Preventive Services (2nd ed.). Baltimore, Williams & Wilkins, p. 572, 1996.

Focus on (1) sharing concern about the adverse effects of alcohol and education about harmful consequences, and (2) setting goals for behavioral change and follow-up. Tailor recommendations for treatment to the severity of the problem, ranging from support groups to inpatient detoxification to more extended rehabilitation.

Protective measures against infectious hepatitis include counseling about how the viruses are spread and the need for immunization. Transmission of hepatitis A is fecal–oral: fecal shedding in food handlers leads to contamination of water and foods. Illness occurs approximately 30 days after exposure. Hepatitis A vaccine is recommended for travelers to endemic areas, food handlers, military personnel, caretakers of children, Native Americans and Alaskan natives, and selected health care, sanitation, and laboratory workers. Vaccination is also recommended for homosexual contacts and injection drug users. For immediate protection and prophylaxis for household contacts and travelers, consider administering immune serum globulin.

Hepatitis B poses more serious threats to patients' health, including risk of fulminant hepatitis as well as chronic infection and subsequent cirrhosis and hepatocellular carcinoma. Transmission occurs during contact with infected body fluids, such as blood, semen, saliva, and vaginal secretions. Adults between the ages of 20 and 39 are most affected, especially injection drug users and sex workers. Up to a tenth of infected adults become chronically infected asymptomatic carriers. Behavioral counseling and serologic screening are advised for patients at risk. Because up to 30% of patients have no identifiable risk factors, hepatitis B vaccine is recommended for all young adults not previously immunized, injection drug users and their sexual partners, persons at risk for sexually transmitted disease, travelers to endemic areas, recipients of blood products as in hemodialysis, and health care workers with frequent exposure to blood products. Many of these groups should also be screened for HIV infection.

It is also important to screen patients for colorectal cancer, second highest of the malignancies in both prevalence and mortality. Risk factors include family history of colonic polyps, history of colorectal cancer or adenoma in a first-degree relative, and a personal history of ulcerative colitis, adenomatous polyps, or prior diagnosis of endometrial, ovarian, or breast cancer. The U.S. Preventive Services Task Force recommends annual testing of all persons over age 50 with the fecal occult blood test (FOBT), sigmoidoscopy, or both, but details several caveats.** The FOBT has a highly variable sensitivity (26%–92%), but good specificity (90%–99%). It produces many false positives related to diet, selected medications, and gastrointestinal conditions such as ulcer disease, diverticulosis, and hemorrhoids. The benefits of sigmoidoscopy are linked to the length of the sigmoidoscope and its depth of insertion. Detection rates for colorectal cancer and insertion depths are roughly as follows: 25%–30% at 20 cm; 50%–55% at 35 cm; 40%–65% at

** U.S. Preventive Services Task Force: Guide to Clinical Preventive Services (2nd ed.). Baltimore, Williams & Wilkins, pp. 89–103, 1996.

40–50 cm. Full colonoscopy or air contrast barium enema detects 80%–95% of colorectal cancers, but these procedures are more uncomfortable and colonoscopy is more expensive. When counseling patients about prevention, there is preliminary but inconsistent evidence that diets high in fiber may reduce risk of colorectal malignancy.

Preview: Recording the Physical Examination—The Abdomen

Note that initially you may use sentences to describe your findings; later you will use phrases. The style below contains phrases appropriate for most write-ups. Unfamiliar terms are explained in the next section, Techniques of Examination.

"Abdomen is protuberant with active bowel sounds. It is soft and nontender; no masses or hepatosplenomegaly. Liver span is 7 cm in the right midclavicular line; edge is smooth and palpable 1 cm below the right costal margin. Spleen and kidneys not felt. No costovertebral angle (CVA) tenderness."

OR

"Abdomen is flat. No bowel sounds heard. It is firm and boardlike, with increased tenderness, guarding, and rebound in the right midquadrant. Liver percusses to 7 cm in the midclavicular line; edge not felt. Spleen and kidneys not felt. No CVA tenderness.

Suggests peritonitis from possible appendicitis (see pp. 347–348 and pp. 363–364)

TECHNIQUES OF EXAMINATION

For a good abdominal examination you need (1) good light, (2) a relaxed patient, and (3) full exposure of the abdomen from above the xiphoid process to the symphysis pubis. The groin should be visible. The genitalia should remain draped. The abdominal muscles should be relaxed to enhance all aspects of the examination, but especially palpation.

Steps for Enhancing Examination of the Abdomen

- The patient should have an empty bladder.
- Make the patient comfortable in a supine position, with a pillow for the head and perhaps another under the knees. Slide your hand under the low back to see if the patient is relaxed and flat on the table.
- Have the patient keep arms at the sides or folded across the chest. Often patients raise their arms over their heads, but this stretches and tightens the abdominal wall, making palpation difficult.
- Before you begin palpation, ask the patient to point to any areas of pain and examine these areas last.
- Warm your hands and stethoscope, and avoid long fingernails. You may need to rub your hands together or warm them up with hot water; you can also begin palpation through the patient's gown to absorb warmth from the patient's body before exposing the abdomen properly. Anxiety may make the hands cool, a problem that decreases over time.
- Approach slowly and avoid quick unexpected movements. Watch the patient's face closely for any signs of pain or discomfort.
- Distract the patient if necessary with conversation or questions. If the patient is frightened or ticklish, begin palpation with the patient's hand under yours. After a few moments, slip your hand underneath to palpate directly.

An arched back thrusts the abdomen forward, thus tightening the abdominal muscles.

Visualize each organ in the region you are examining. Stand at the patient's right side and proceed in an orderly fashion with inspection, auscultation, percussion, and palpation. Assess the liver, spleen, kidneys, and aorta.

The Abdomen

INSPECTION

Starting from your usual standing position at the right side of the bed, inspect the abdomen. As you look at the contour of the abdomen and watch for peristalsis, it is helpful to sit or bend down so that you can view the abdomen tangentially.

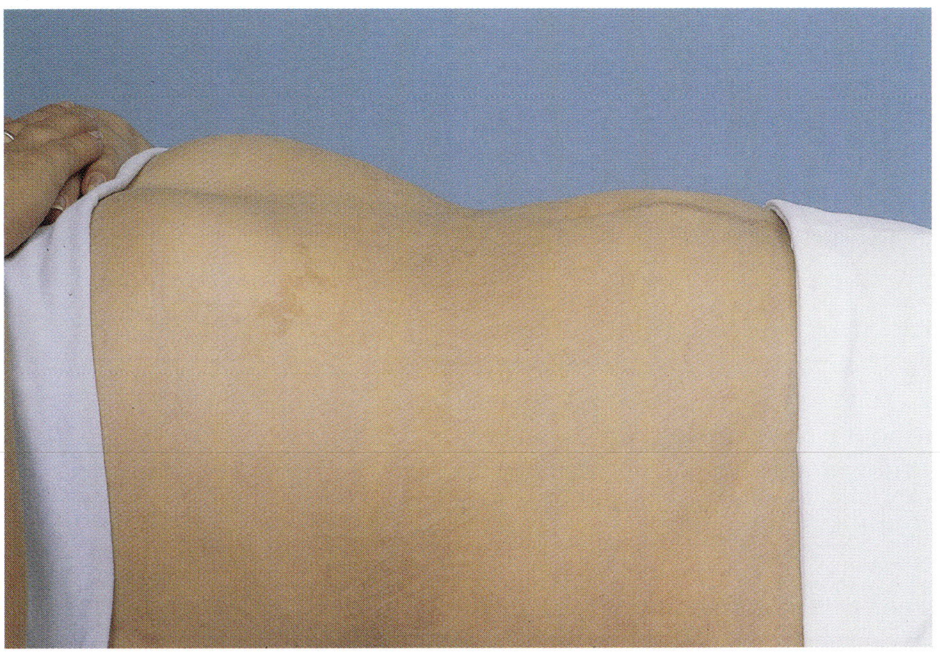

Note:

- *The skin,* including:

Scars. Describe or diagram their location.

Striae. Old silver striae or stretch marks, as illustrated above, are normal.

Pink–purple striae of Cushing's syndrome

Dilated veins. A few small veins may be visible normally.

Dilated veins of hepatic cirrhosis or of inferior vena cava obstruction

Rashes and lesions

- *The umbilicus.* Observe its contour and location, and any signs of inflammation or hernia

See Table 9-8, Localized Bulges in the Abdominal Wall (p. 360).

- *The contour of the abdomen*

Is it flat, rounded, protuberant, or scaphoid (markedly concave or hollowed)?

See Table 9-9, Protuberant Abdomens (p. 361).

Do the flanks bulge or are there any local bulges? Include in this survey the inguinal and femoral areas.

Bulging flanks of ascites; suprapubic bulge of a distended bladder or pregnant uterus; hernias

Is the abdomen symmetric?

Asymmetry due to an enlarged organ or mass

Are there visible organs or masses? Look for an enlarged liver or spleen that has descended below the rib cage.

Lower abdominal mass of an ovarian or a uterine tumor

- *Peristalsis.* Observe for several minutes if you suspect intestinal obstruction. Peristalsis may be visible normally in very thin people.

Increased peristaltic waves of intestinal obstruction

- *Pulsations.* The normal aortic pulsation is frequently visible in the epigastrium.

Increased pulsation of an aortic aneurysm or of increased pulse pressure

AUSCULTATION

Auscultation provides important information about bowel motility. *Listen to the abdomen before performing percussion or palpation, since these maneuvers may alter the frequency of bowel sounds.* You should practice auscultation until you are thoroughly familiar with variations in normal bowel sounds and can detect changes suggestive of inflammation or obstruction. Auscultation may also reveal *bruits*, vascular sounds resembling heart murmurs, over the aorta or other arteries in the abdomen, which suggest vascular occlusive disease.

Place the diaphragm of your stethoscope gently on the abdomen. Listen for bowel sounds and note their frequency and character. Normal sounds consist of clicks and gurgles, occurring at an estimated frequency of 5 to 34 per minute. Occasionally you may hear *borborygmi*—long prolonged gurgles of hyperperistalsis—the familiar "stomach growling." Because bowel sounds are widely transmitted through the abdomen, listening in one spot, such as the right lower quadrant, is usually sufficient.

Bowel sounds may be altered in diarrhea, intestinal obstruction, paralytic ileus, and peritonitis. See Table 9-10, Sounds in the Abdomen (p. 362).

If the patient has high blood pressure, listen in the epigastrium and in each upper quadrant for *bruits.* Later in the examination, when the patient sits up, listen also in the costovertebral angles. Epigastric bruits confined to systole may be heard in normal persons.

A bruit in one of these areas that has both systolic and diastolic components strongly suggests renal artery stenosis as the cause of hypertension.

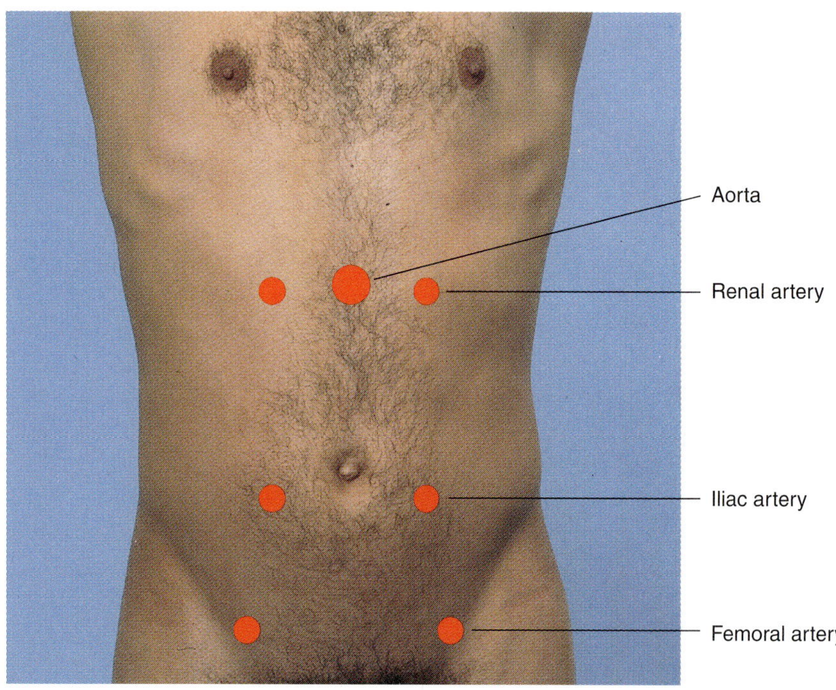

If you suspect arterial insufficiency in the legs, listen for bruits over the aorta, the iliac arteries, and the femoral arteries. Bruits confined to systole are relatively common, however, and do not necessarily signify occlusive disease.

Bruits with both systolic and diastolic components suggest the turbulent blood flow of partial arterial occlusion. See Table 9-10, Sounds in the Abdomen (p. 362).

Listening points for bruits in these vessels are illustrated on p. 334.

If you suspect a liver tumor, gonococcal infection around the liver, or splenic infarction, listen over the liver and spleen for *friction rubs*.

See Table 9-10, Sounds in the Abdomen (p. 362).

PERCUSSION

Percussion helps you to assess the amount and distribution of gas in the abdomen and to identify possible masses that are solid or fluid filled. Its use in estimating the size of the liver and spleen will be described in later sections.

Percuss the abdomen lightly in all four quadrants to assess the distribution of *tympany* and *dullness*. Tympany usually predominates because of gas in the gastrointestinal tract, but scattered areas of dullness due to fluid and feces there are also typical.

A protuberant abdomen that is tympanitic throughout suggests intestinal obstruction. See Table 9-9, Protuberant Abdomens (p. 361).

- Note any large dull areas that might indicate an underlying mass or enlarged organ. This observation will guide your palpation.

Pregnant uterus, ovarian tumor, distended bladder, large liver or spleen

- On each side of a protuberant abdomen, note where abdominal tympany changes to the dullness of solid posterior structures.

Dullness in both flanks indicates further assessment for ascites (see pp. 345–347).

Briefly percuss the lower anterior chest, between lungs above and costal margins below. On the right, you will usually find the dullness of liver; on the left, the tympany that overlies the gastric air bubble and the splenic flexure of the colon.

In situs inversus (rare), organs are reversed: air bubble on the right, liver dullness on the left.

PALPATION

Light Palpation. Feeling the abdomen gently is especially helpful in identifying abdominal tenderness, muscular resistance, and some superficial organs and masses. It also serves to reassure and relax the patient.

Keeping your hand and forearm on a horizontal plane, with fingers together and flat on the abdominal surface, palpate the abdomen with a light, gentle, dipping motion. When moving your hand from place to place, raise it just off the skin. Moving smoothly, feel in all quadrants.

Identify any superficial organs or masses and any area of tenderness or increased resistance to your hand. If resistance is present, try to distinguish voluntary guarding from involuntary muscular spasm. To do this:

- Try all the relaxing methods you know (see p. 332).

Involuntary rigidity (muscular spasm) typically persists despite these maneuvers. It indicates peritoneal inflammation.

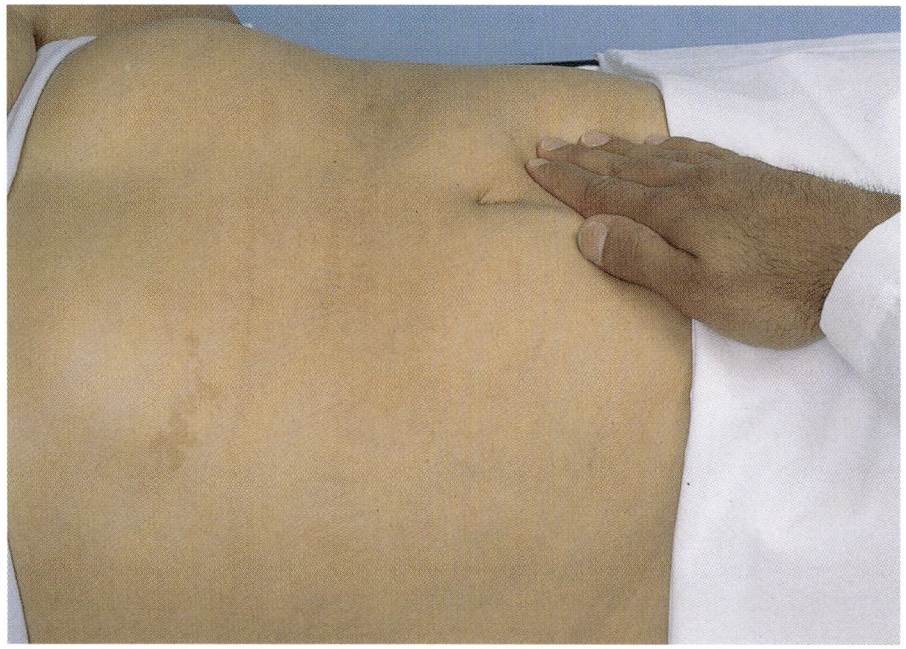

- Feel for the relaxation of abdominal muscles that normally accompanies exhalation.
- Ask the patient to mouth-breathe with jaw dropped open.

Voluntary guarding usually decreases with these maneuvers.

Deep Palpation. This is usually required to delineate abdominal masses. Again using the palmar surfaces of your fingers, feel in all four quadrants. Identify any masses and note their location, size, shape, consistency, tenderness, pulsations, and any mobility with respiration or with the examining hand. Correlate your palpable findings with their percussion notes.

Abdominal masses may be categorized in several ways: physiologic (pregnant uterus), inflammatory (diverticulitis of the colon), vascular (an aneurysm of the abdominal aorta), neoplastic (carcinoma of the colon), or obstructive (a distended bladder or dilated loop of bowel).

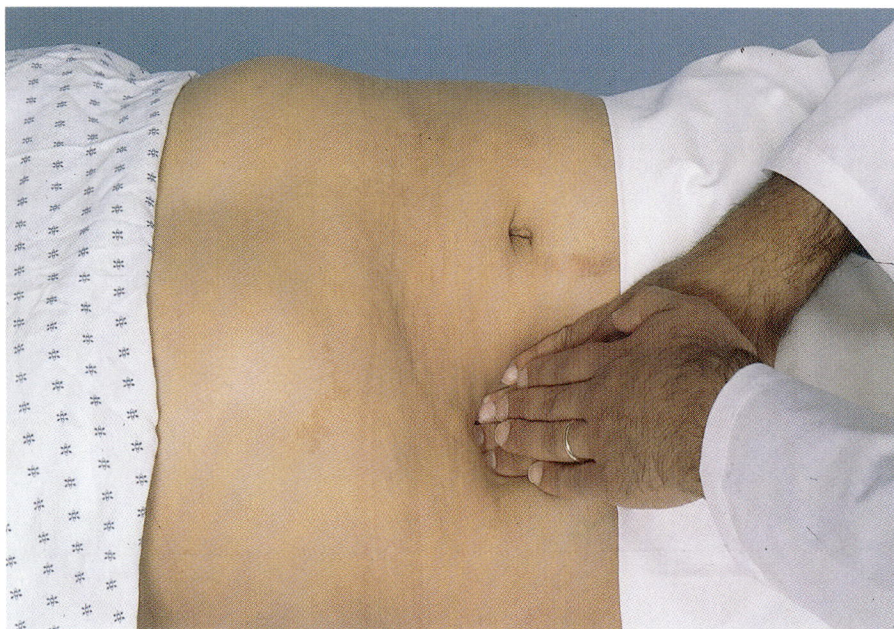

TWO-HANDED DEEP PALPATION

Assessment for Peritoneal Inflammation. Abdominal pain and tenderness, especially when associated with muscular spasm, suggest inflammation of the parietal peritoneum. Localize the pain as accurately as possible. First, even before palpation, *ask the patient to cough* and determine where the cough produced pain. Then, *palpate gently with one finger* to map the tender area. Pain produced by light percussion has similar localizing value. These gentle maneuvers may be all you need to establish an area of peritoneal inflammation.

Abdominal pain on coughing or with light percussion suggests peritoneal inflammation. See Table 9-11, Tender Abdomens (pp. 363–364).

If not, *look for rebound tenderness.* Press your fingers in firmly and slowly, and then quickly withdraw them. Watch and listen to the patient for signs of pain. Ask the patient (1) to compare which hurt more, the pressing or the letting go, and (2) to show you exactly where it hurt. Pain induced or increased by quick withdrawal constitutes rebound tenderness. It results from the rapid movement of an inflamed peritoneum.

Rebound tenderness suggests peritoneal inflammation. If tenderness is felt elsewhere than where you were trying to elicit rebound, that area may be the real source of the problem.

The Liver

Because most of the liver is sheltered by the rib cage, assessing it is difficult. Its size and shape can be estimated by percussion and perhaps palpation, however, and the palpating hand may enable you to evaluate its surface, consistency, and tenderness.

PERCUSSION

Measure the vertical span of liver dullness in the right midclavicular line. Starting at a level below the umbilicus (in an area of tympany, not dullness), lightly percuss upward toward the liver. Ascertain the lower border of liver dullness in the midclavicular line.

Next, identify the upper border of liver dullness in the midclavicular line. Lightly percuss from lung resonance down toward liver dullness. Gently displace a woman's breast as necessary to be sure that you start in a resonant area. The course of percussion is shown below.

The span of liver dullness is *increased* when the liver is enlarged.

The span of liver dullness is *decreased* when the liver is small, or when free air is present below the diaphragm, as from a perforated hollow viscus. Serial observations may show a decreasing span of dullness with resolution of hepatitis or congestive heart failure or, less commonly, with progression of fulminant hepatitis.

Liver dullness may be displaced downward by the low diaphragm of chronic obstructive lung disease. Span, however, remains normal.

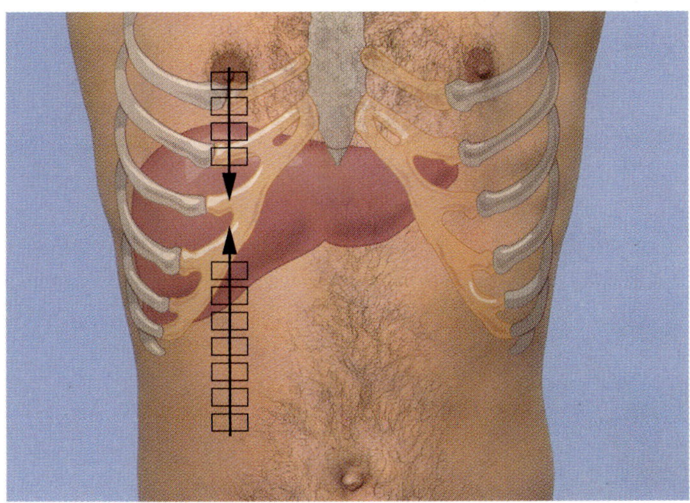

PERCUSSING LIVER SPAN

Now measure in centimeters the distance between your two points—the vertical span of liver dullness. Normal liver spans, shown below, are generally greater in men than in women, in tall people than in short. If the liver seems to be enlarged, outline the lower edge by percussing in other areas.

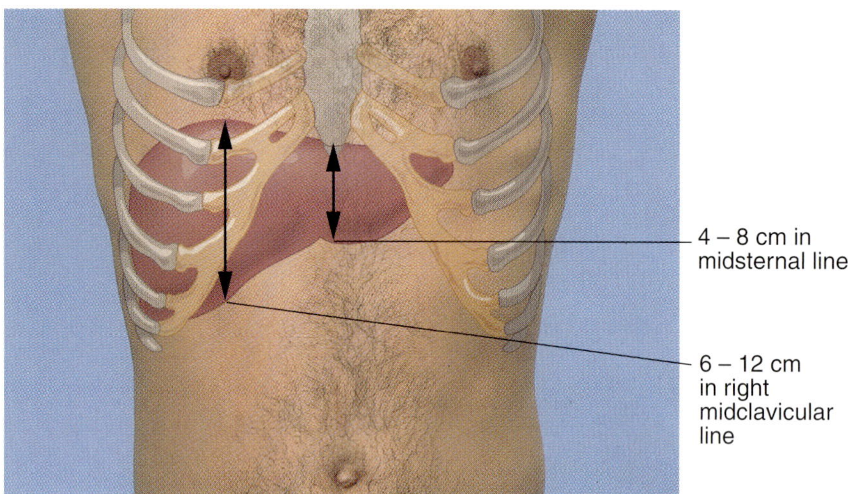

NORMAL LIVER SPANS

Dullness of a right pleural effusion or consolidated lung, if adjacent to liver dullness, may falsely increase the estimate of liver size.

Gas in the colon may produce tympany in the right upper quadrant, obscure liver dullness, and falsely decrease the estimate of liver size.

Although percussion is probably the most accurate clinical method for estimating the vertical size of the liver, it typically leads to underestimation.

PALPATION

Place your left hand behind the patient, parallel to and supporting the right 11th and 12th ribs and adjacent soft tissues below. Remind the patient to relax on your hand if necessary. By pressing your left hand forward, the patient's liver may be felt more easily by your other hand.

Place your right hand on the patient's right abdomen lateral to the rectus muscle, with your fingertips well below the lower border of liver dullness. Some examiners like to point their fingers up toward the patient's head, while others prefer a somewhat more oblique position, as shown on the next page. In either case, press gently in and up.

Ask the patient to take a deep breath. Try to feel the liver edge as it comes down to meet your fingertips. If you feel it, lighten the pressure of your palpating hand slightly so that the liver can slip under your finger pads and you can feel its anterior surface. Note any tenderness. If palpable at all, the edge of a normal liver is soft, sharp, and regular, its surface smooth. The normal liver may be slightly tender.

Firmness or hardness of the liver, bluntness or rounding of its edge, and irregularity of its contour suggest an abnormality of the liver.

On inspiration, the liver (on the following page) is palpable about 3 cm below the right costal margin in the midclavicular line.

An obstructed, distended gallbladder may form an oval mass below the edge of the liver and merging with it. It is dull to percussion.

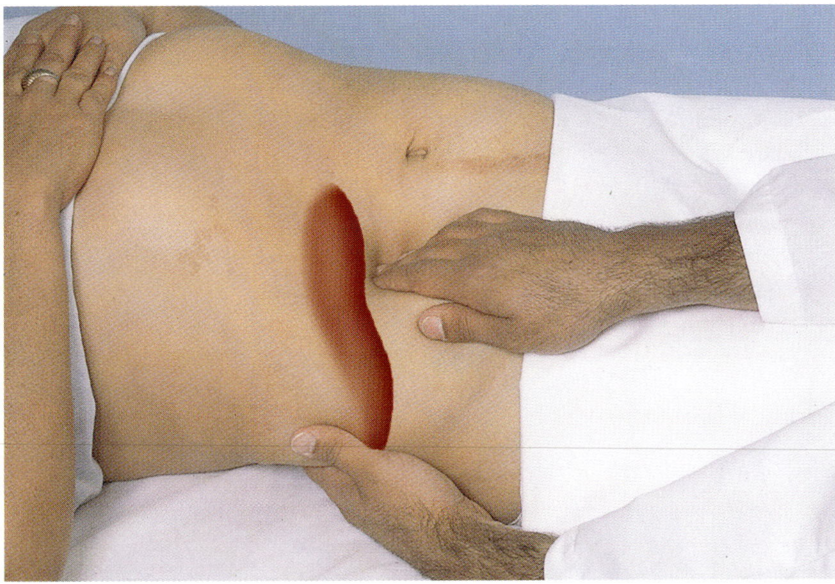

Some people breathe more with their chests than with their diaphragms. It may be helpful to train such a patient to "breathe with the abdomen," thus bringing the liver, as well as the spleen and kidneys, into a palpable position during inspiration.

Try to trace the liver edge both laterally and medially. Palpation through the rectus muscles, however, is especially difficult. Describe or sketch the liver edge, and measure its distance from the right costal margin in the midclavicular line.

See Table 9-12, Liver Enlargement: Apparent and Real (pp. 365–366).

In order to feel the liver, you may have to alter your pressure according to the thickness and resistance of the abdominal wall. If you cannot feel it, move your palpating hand closer to the costal margin and try again.

The edge of an enlarged liver may be missed by starting palpation too high in the abdomen, as shown below.

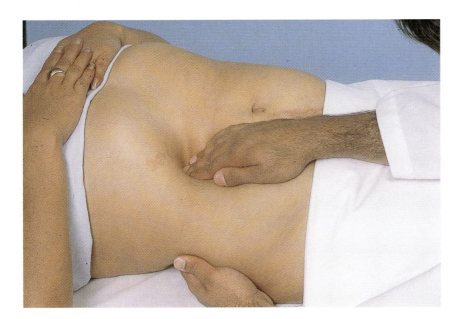

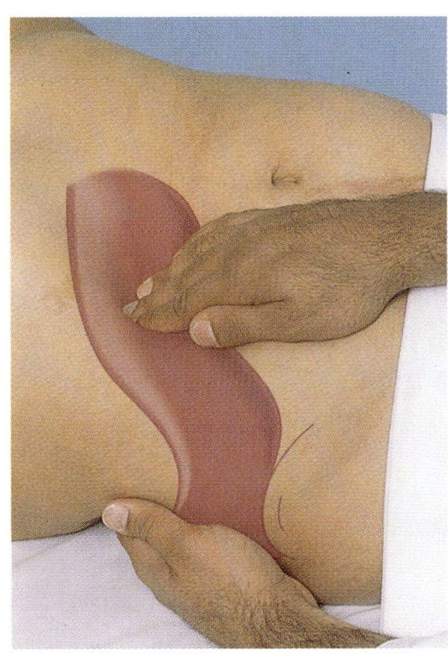

The "hooking technique" may be helpful, especially when the patient is obese. Stand to the right of the patient's chest. Place both hands, side by side, on the right abdomen below the border of liver dullness. Press in with your fingers and up toward the costal margin. Ask the patient to take a deep breath. The liver edge shown below is palpable with the fingerpads of both hands.

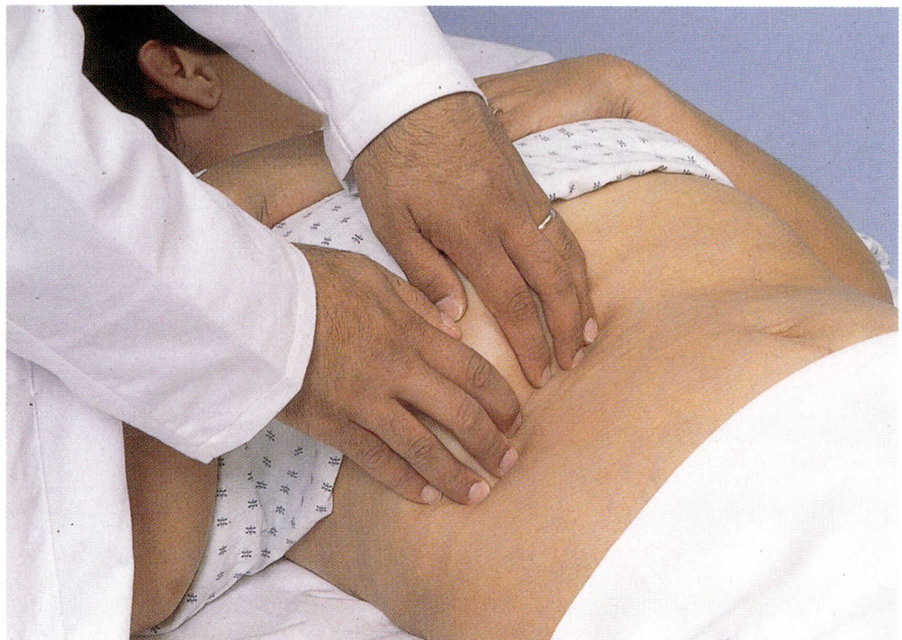

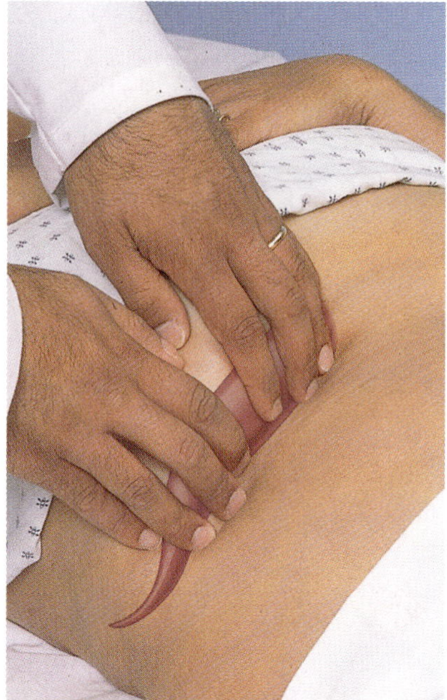

Assessing Tenderness of a Nonpalpable Liver. Place your left hand flat on the lower right rib cage and then gently strike your hand with the ulnar surface of your right fist. Ask the patient to compare the sensation with that produced by a similar strike on the left side.

Tenderness over the liver suggests inflammation, as in hepatitis, or congestion, as in heart failure.

The Spleen

When a spleen enlarges, it expands anteriorly, downward, and medially, often replacing the tympany of stomach and colon with the dullness of a solid organ. It then becomes palpable below the costal margin. Percussion cannot confirm splenic enlargement but can raise your suspicions of it. Palpation can confirm the enlargement, but often misses large spleens that do not descend below the costal margin.

PERCUSSION

Two techniques may help you to detect *splenomegaly,* an enlarged spleen:

- *Percuss the left lower anterior chest wall* between lung resonance above and the costal margin (an area termed *Traube's space*). As you percuss along the routes suggested by the arrows in the following figures, note the lateral extent of tympany.

Dullness, as shown on the following page, raises the question of splenomegaly.

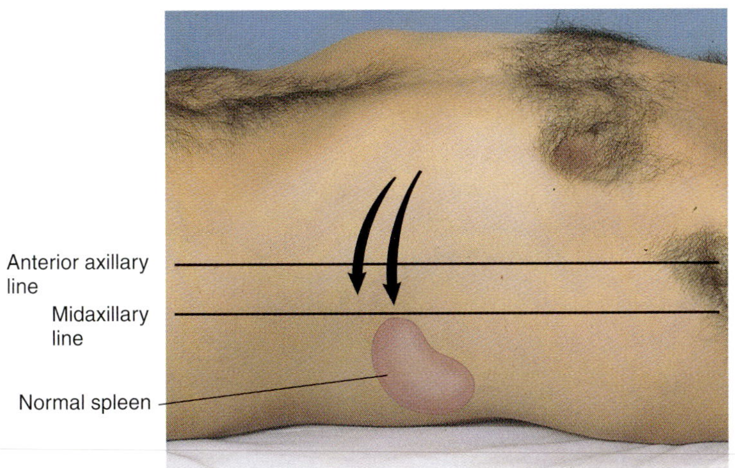

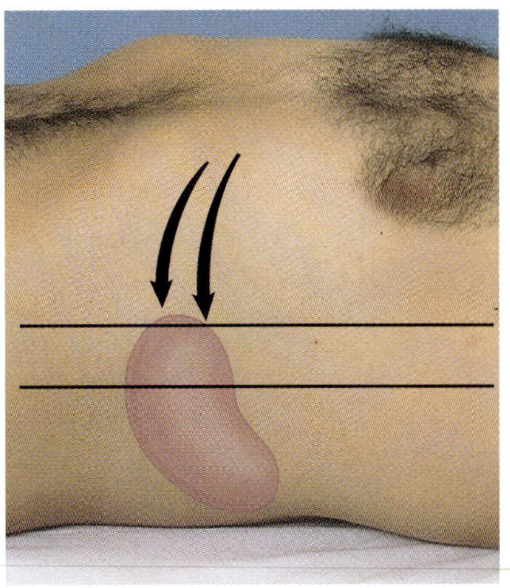

This is variable, but if tympany is prominent, especially laterally, splenomegaly is not likely. The dullness of a normal spleen is usually hidden within the dullness of other posterior tissues.

Fluid or solids in the stomach or colon may also cause dullness in Traube's space.

- *Check for a splenic percussion sign.* Percuss the lowest interspace in the left anterior axillary line, as shown below. This area is usually tympanitic. Then ask the patient to take a deep breath, and percuss again. When spleen size is normal, the percussion note usually remains tympanitic.

A change in percussion note from tympany to dullness on inspiration suggests splenic enlargement. This is a *positive splenic percussion sign.*

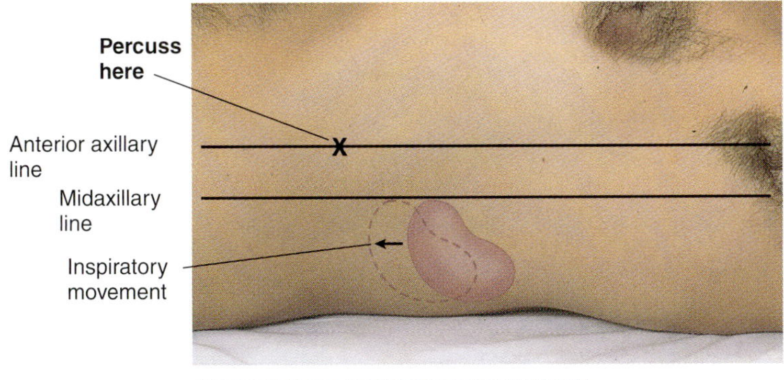

NEGATIVE SPLENIC PERCUSSION SIGN

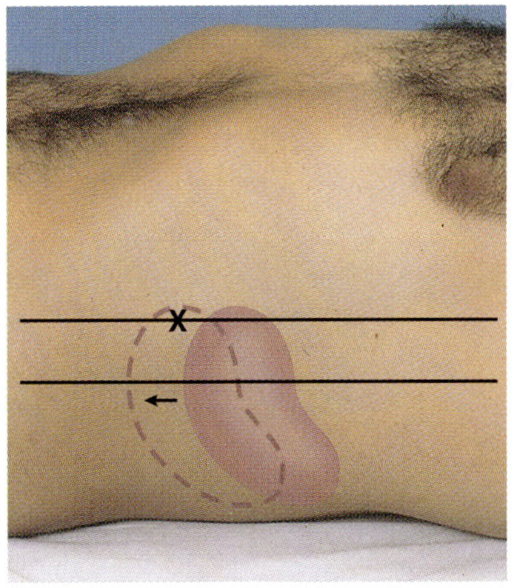

POSITIVE SPLENIC PERCUSSION SIGN

If either or both of these tests is positive, pay extra attention to palpating the spleen.

The splenic percussion sign may also be positive when spleen size is normal.

PALPATION

With your left hand, reach over and around the patient to support and press forward the lower left rib cage and adjacent soft tissue. With your right hand below the left costal margin, press in toward the spleen. Begin palpation low

An enlarged spleen may be missed if the examiner starts too high in the abdomen to feel the lower edge.

enough so that you are below a possibly enlarged spleen. (If your hand is close to the costal margin, moreover, it is not sufficiently mobile to reach up under the rib cage.) Ask the patient to take a deep breath. Try to feel the tip or edge of the spleen as it comes down to meet your fingertips. Note any tenderness, assess the splenic contour, and measure the distance between the spleen's lowest point and the left costal margin. In a small percentage of normal adults, the tip of the spleen is palpable. Causes include a low, flat diaphragm, as in chronic obstructive pulmonary disease, and a deep inspiratory descent of the diaphragm.

A palpable spleen tip, though not necessarily abnormal, may indicate splenic enlargement. The spleen tip below is just palpable deep to the left costal margin.

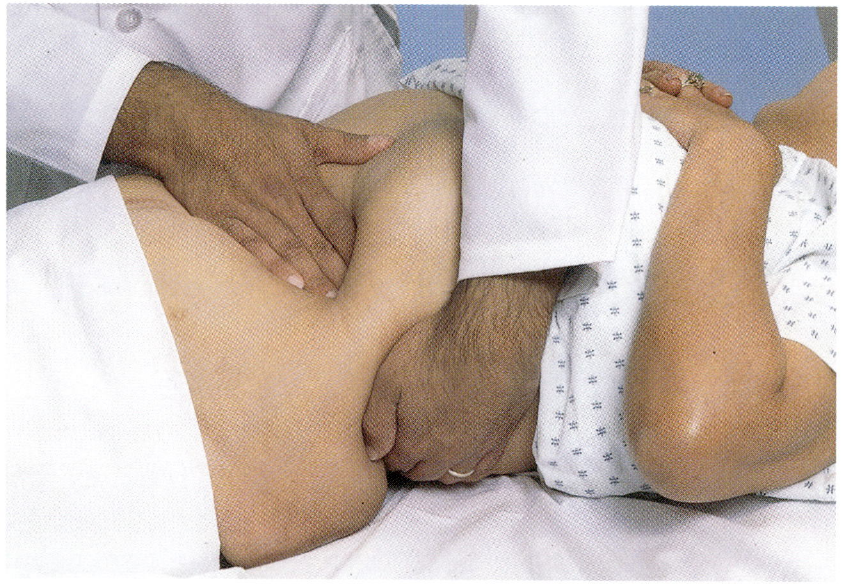

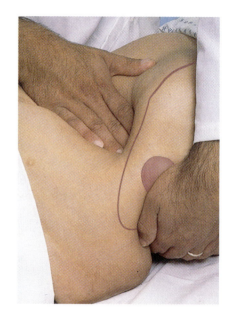

Repeat with the patient lying on the right side with legs somewhat flexed at hips and knees. In this position, gravity may bring the spleen forward and to the right into a palpable location.

The enlarged spleen shown below is palpable about 2 cm below the left costal margin on deep inspiration.

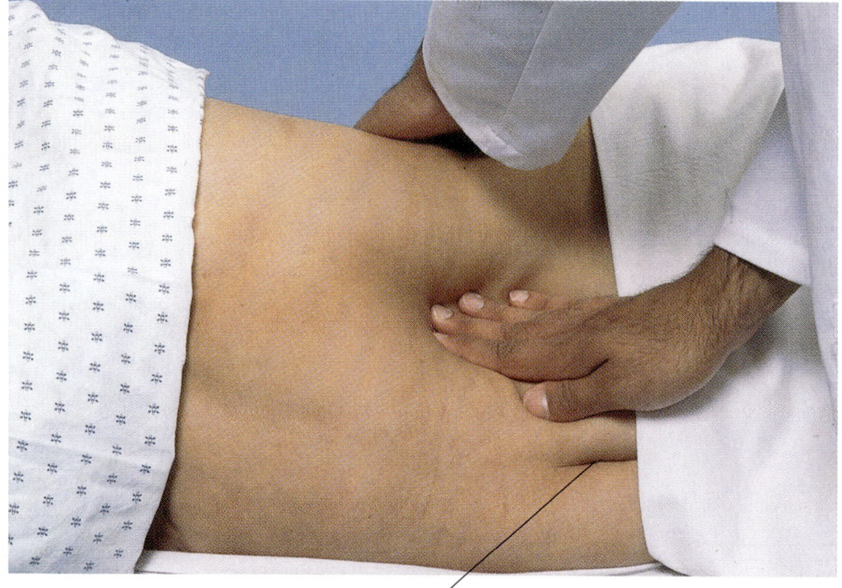

PALPATING THE SPLEEN—PATIENT LYING ON RIGHT SIDE

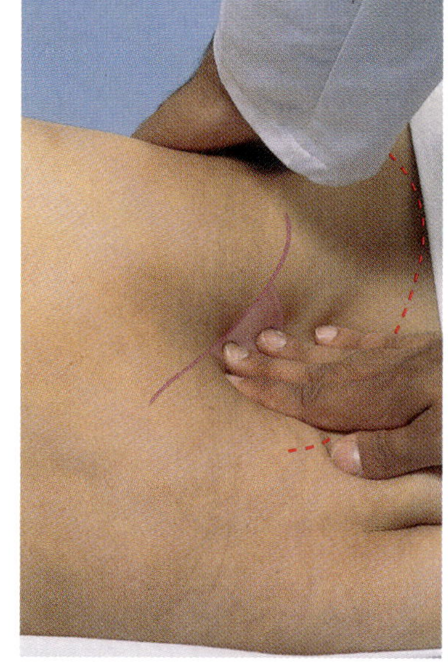

The Kidneys

PALPATION

Although kidneys are not usually palpable, you should learn and practice the techniques. Detecting an enlarged kidney may prove to be very important.

A left flank mass (see the solid line on photo on previous page) may represent marked splenomegaly or an enlarged left kidney. Suspect splenomegaly if notch palpated on medial border, edge extends beyond the midline, percussion is dull, and your fingers can probe deep to the medial and lateral borders but not between the mass and the costal margin. Confirm findings with further evaluation.

Palpation of the Left Kidney. Move to the patient's left side. Place your right hand behind the patient just below and parallel to the 12th rib, with your fingertips just reaching the costovertebral angle. Lift, trying to displace the kidney anteriorly. Place your left hand gently in the left upper quadrant, lateral and parallel to the rectus muscle. Ask the patient to take a deep breath. At the peak of inspiration, press your left hand firmly and deeply into the left upper quadrant, just below the costal margin, and try to "capture" the kidney between your two hands. Ask the patient to breathe out and then to stop breathing briefly. Slowly release the pressure of your left hand, feeling at the same time for the kidney to slide back into its expiratory position. If the kidney is palpable, describe its size, contour, and any tenderness.

Attributes favoring an enlarged kidney over an enlarged spleen include preservation of normal tympany in the left upper quadrant and the ability to probe with your fingers between the mass and the costal margin but not deep to its medial and lower borders.

Alternatively, try to feel for the left kidney by a method similar to feeling for the spleen. With your left hand, reach over and around the patient to lift the left loin, and with your right hand feel deep in the left upper quadrant. Ask the patient to take a deep breath, and feel for a mass. A normal left kidney is rarely palpable.

Palpation of the Right Kidney. To capture the right kidney, return to the patient's right side. Use your left hand to lift from in back, and your right hand to feel deep in the left upper quadrant. Proceed as before.

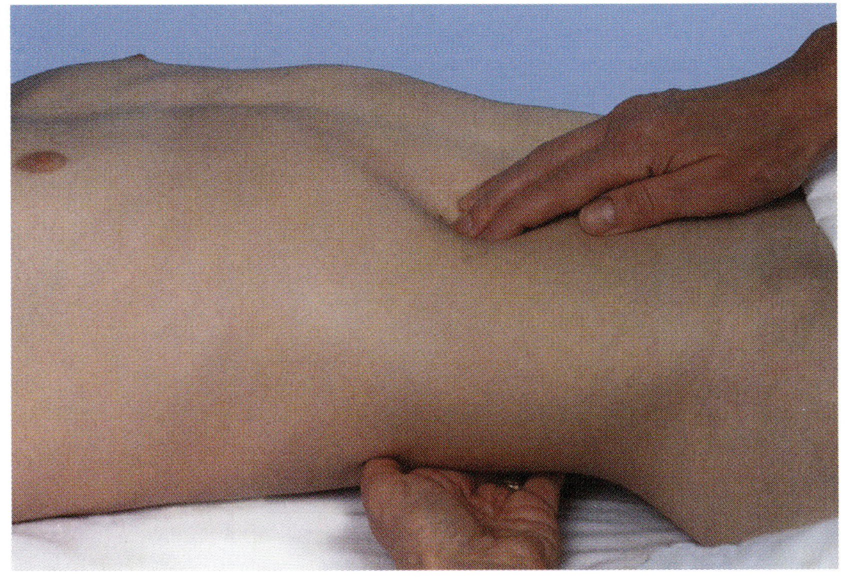

A normal right kidney may be palpable, especially in thin, well-relaxed women. It may or may not be slightly tender. The patient is usually aware of a capture and release. Occasionally, a right kidney is located more anteriorly than usual and then must be distinguished from the liver. The edge of the liver, if palpable, tends to be sharper and to extend farther medially and laterally. It cannot be captured. The lower pole of the kidney is rounded.

Causes of kidney enlargement include hydronephrosis, cysts, and tumors. Bilateral enlargement suggests polycystic disease.

Assessing Kidney Tenderness. You may note tenderness when examining the abdomen, but also search for it at each costovertebral angle. Pressure from your fingertips may be enough to elicit tenderness, but if not, use fist percussion. Place the ball of one hand in the costovertebral angle and strike it with the ulnar surface of your fist. Use enough force to cause a perceptible but painless jar or thud in a normal person.

Pain with pressure or fist percussion suggests *pyelonephritis*, but may also have a musculoskeletal cause.

To save the patient needless exertion, integrate this assessment with your examination of the back (see p. 10).

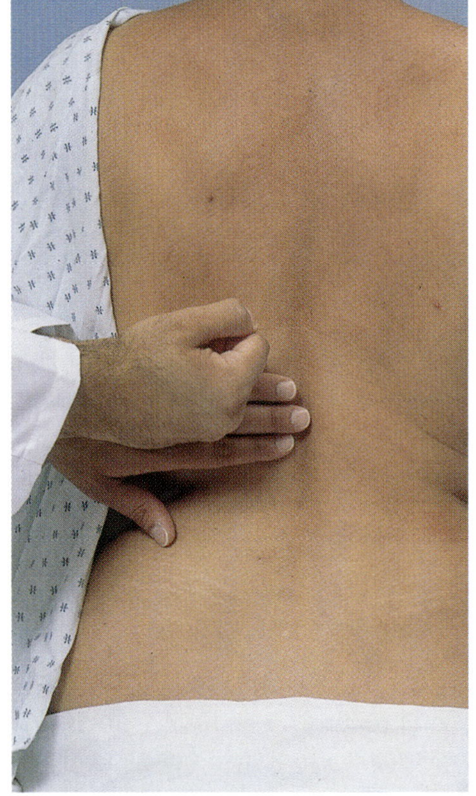

ASSESSING COSTOVERTEBRAL ANGLE TENDERNESS

The Bladder

The bladder normally cannot be examined unless it is distended above the symphysis pubis. On palpation, the dome of the distended bladder feels smooth and round. Check for tenderness. Use percussion to check for dullness and to determine how high the bladder rises above the symphysis pubis.

Bladder distention from outlet obstruction due to urethral stricture, prostatic hyperplasia; also from medications and neurologic disorders such as stroke, multiple sclerosis.

Suprapubic tenderness in bladder infection

The Aorta

Press firmly deep in the upper abdomen, slightly to the left of the midline, and identify the aortic pulsations. In persons over age 50, try to assess the width of the aorta by pressing deeply in the upper abdomen with one hand on each side of the aorta, as illustrated. In this age group, a normal aorta is

In an older person, a periumbilical or upper abdominal mass with expansile pulsations suggests an *aortic aneurysm.*

not more than 3.0 cm wide (average 2.5 cm). This measurement does not include the thickness of the abdominal wall. The ease of feeling aortic pulsations varies greatly with the thickness of the abdominal wall and with the anteroposterior diameter of the abdomen.

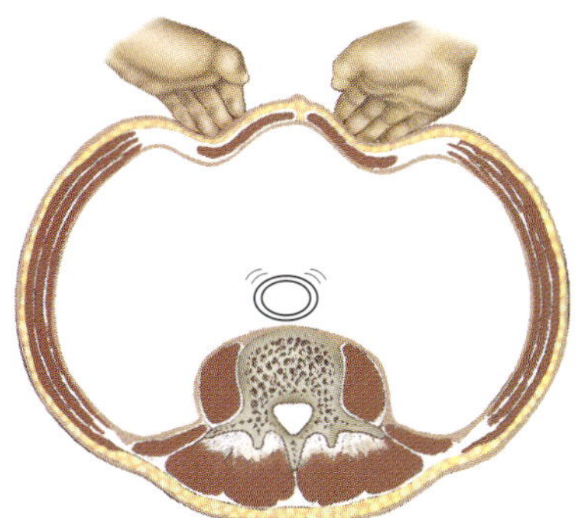

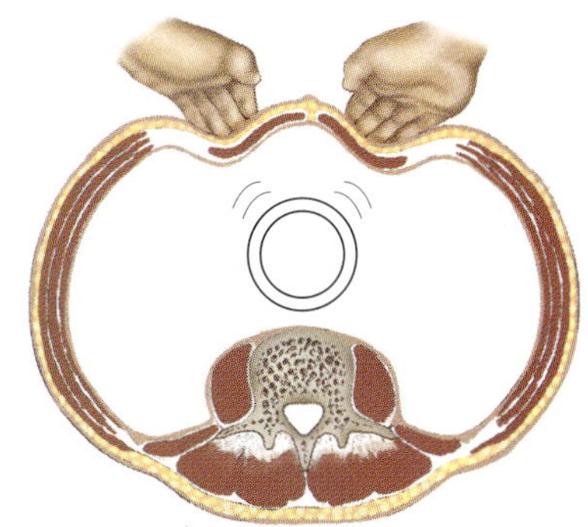

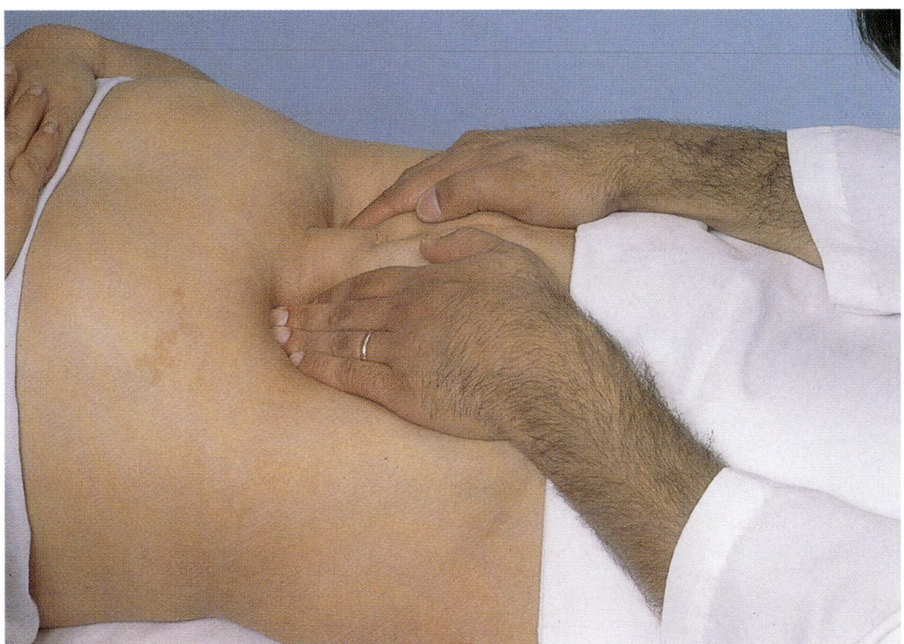

An aortic aneurysm is a pathologic dilatation of the aorta, usually due to arteriosclerosis. A merely tortuous abdominal aorta, however, may be difficult to distinguish from an aneurysm on clinical grounds.

Although an aneurysm is usually painless, pain may herald its most dreaded and frequent complication—rupture of the aorta.

Apparent enlargement of the aorta indicates assessment by ultrasound.

Special Techniques

Assessment Techniques for:

- Ascites
- Appendicitis
- Acute cholecystitis
- Ventral hernia
- Mass in abdominal wall

ASSESSING POSSIBLE ASCITES

A protuberant abdomen with bulging flanks suggests the possibility of ascitic fluid. Because ascitic fluid characteristically sinks with gravity, while gas-filled loops of bowel float to the top, percussion gives a dull note in dependent areas of the abdomen. Look for such a pattern by percussing outward in several directions from the central area of tympany. Map the border between tympany and dullness.

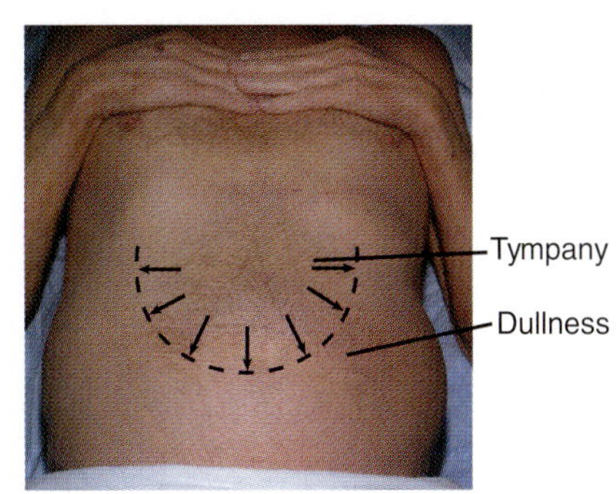

Two further techniques help to confirm the presence of ascites, although both signs may be misleading.

- *Test for shifting dullness.* After mapping the borders of tympany and dullness, ask the patient to turn onto one side. Percuss and mark the borders again. In a person without ascites, the borders between tympany and dullness usually stay relatively constant.

In ascites, dullness shifts to the more dependent side, while tympany shifts to the top.

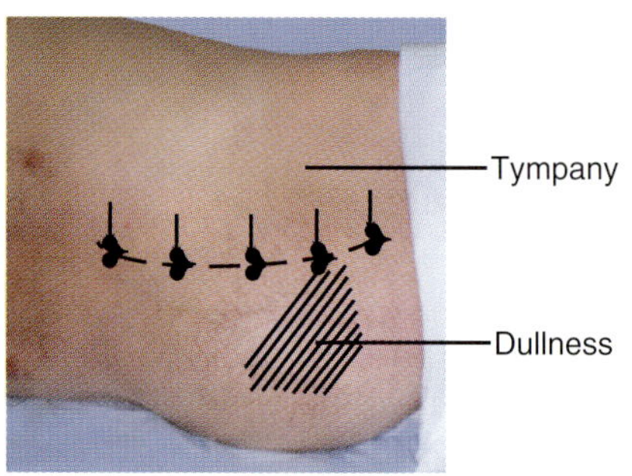

- *Test for a fluid wave.* Ask the patient or an assistant to press the edges of both hands firmly down the midline of the abdomen. This pressure helps to stop the transmission of a wave through fat. While you tap one flank sharply with your fingertips, feel on the opposite flank for an impulse transmitted through the fluid. Unfortunately, this sign is often negative until ascites is obvious, and it is sometimes positive in people without ascites.

An easily palpable impulse suggests ascites.

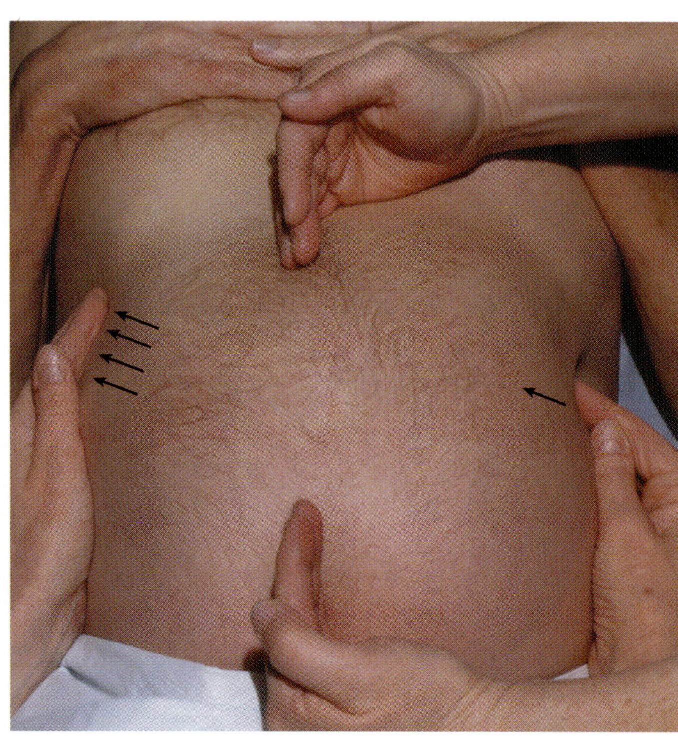

Identifying an Organ or a Mass in an Ascitic Abdomen. Try to *ballotte* the organ or mass, exemplified here by an enlarged liver. Straighten and stiffen the fingers of one hand together, place them on the abdominal surface, and make a brief jabbing movement directly toward the anticipated structure. This quick movement often displaces the fluid so that your fingertips can briefly touch the surface of the structure through the abdominal wall.

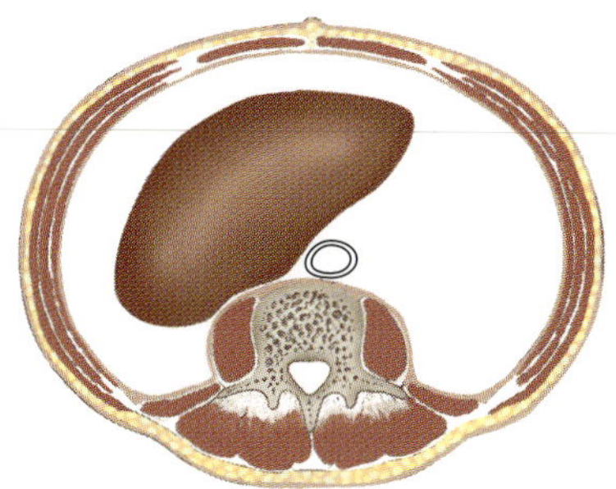

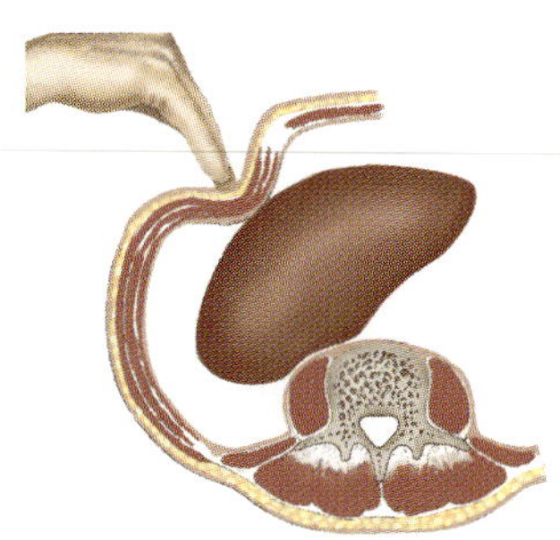

ASSESSING POSSIBLE APPENDICITIS

- Ask the patient to point to where the pain began and where it is now. Ask the patient to cough. Determine whether and where pain results.

The pain of appendicitis classically begins near the umbilicus, then shifts to the right lower quadrant, where coughing increases it. Elderly patients report this pattern less frequently than younger ones.

- Search carefully for an area of local tenderness.

Localized tenderness anywhere in the right lower quadrant, even in the right flank, may indicate appendicitis.

- Feel for muscular rigidity.

Early voluntary guarding may be replaced by involuntary muscular rigidity.

- *Perform a rectal examination and, in women, a pelvic examination.* These maneuvers may not help you to discriminate well between a normal and an inflamed appendix, but they may help to identify an inflamed appendix atypically located within the pelvic cavity. They may also suggest other causes of the abdominal pain.

Right-sided rectal tenderness may be caused by, for example, inflamed adnexa or an inflamed seminal vesicle, as well as by an inflamed appendix.

Some additional techniques are sometimes helpful.

- Check the tender area for rebound tenderness. (If other signs are typically positive, you can save the patient unnecessary pain by omitting this test.)

Rebound tenderness suggests peritoneal inflammation, as from appendicitis.

- Check for *Rovsing's sign* and for referred rebound tenderness. Press deeply and evenly in the *left* lower quadrant. Then quickly withdraw your fingers.

Pain in the *right* lower quadrant during *left*-sided pressure suggests appendicitis (a positive Rovsing's sign). So does right lower quadrant pain on quick withdrawal (*referred rebound tenderness*).

- Look for a *psoas sign*. Place your hand just above the patient's right knee and ask the patient to raise that thigh against your hand. Alternatively, ask the patient to turn onto the left side. Then extend the patient's right leg at the hip. Flexion of the leg at the hip makes the psoas muscle contract; extension stretches it.

Increased abdominal pain on either maneuver constitutes a positive psoas sign, suggesting irritation of the psoas muscle by an inflamed appendix.

- Look for an *obturator sign*. Flex the patient's right thigh at the hip, with the knee bent, and rotate the leg internally at the hip. This maneuver stretches the internal obturator muscle. (Internal rotation of the hip is described on p. 510.)

Right hypogastric pain constitutes a positive obturator sign, suggesting irritation of the obturator muscle by an inflamed appendix.

- Test for *cutaneous hyperesthesia*. At a series of points down the abdominal wall, gently pick up a fold of skin between your thumb and index finger, without pinching it. This maneuver should not normally be painful.

Localized pain with this maneuver, in all or part of the right lower quadrant, may accompany appendicitis.

ASSESSING POSSIBLE ACUTE CHOLECYSTITIS

When right upper quadrant pain and tenderness suggest acute cholecystitis, look for *Murphy's sign*. Hook your left thumb or the fingers of your right hand under the costal margin at the point where the lateral border of the rectus muscle intersects with the costal margin. Alternatively, if the liver is enlarged, hook your thumb or fingers under the liver edge at a comparable point below. Ask the patient to take a deep breath. Watch the patient's breathing and note the degree of tenderness.

A sharp increase in tenderness with a sudden stop in inspiratory effort constitutes a positive Murphy's sign of acute cholecystitis. Hepatic tenderness may also increase with this maneuver, but is usually less well localized.

ASSESSING VENTRAL HERNIAS

Ventral hernias are hernias in the abdominal wall exclusive of groin hernias. If you suspect but do not see an umbilical or incisional hernia, ask the patient to raise both head and shoulders off the table.

The bulge of a hernia will usually appear with this action (see p. 360).

Inguinal and femoral hernias are discussed in the next chapter. They can give rise to important abdominal problems and must not be overlooked.

The cause of intestinal obstruction or peritonitis may be missed by overlooking a strangulated femoral hernia.

MASS IN THE ABDOMINAL WALL

To Distinguish an Abdominal Mass From a Mass in the Abdominal Wall. An occasional mass is in the abdominal wall rather than inside the abdominal cavity. Ask the patient either to raise the head and shoulders or to strain down, thus tightening the abdominal muscles. Feel for the mass again.

A mass in the abdominal wall remains palpable; an intra-abdominal mass is obscured by muscular contraction.

TABLE 9-1 ■ Abdominal Pain

Problem	Process	Location	Quality
Peptic Ulcer and Dyspepsia *(These disorders cannot be reliably differentiated by symptoms and signs.)*	Peptic ulcer refers to a demonstrable ulcer, usually in the duodenum or stomach. Dyspepsia causes similar symptoms but no ulceration. Infection by *Helicobacter pylori* is often present.	Epigastric, may radiate to the back	Variable: gnawing burning, boring, aching, pressing, or hungerlike
Cancer of the Stomach	A malignant neoplasm	Epigastric	Variable
Acute Pancreatitis	An acute inflammation of the pancreas	Epigastric, may radiate to the back or other parts of the abdomen; may be poorly localized	Usually steady
Chronic Pancreatitis	Fibrosis of the pancreas secondary to recurrent inflammation	Epigastric, radiating through to the back	Steady, deep
Cancer of the Pancreas	A malignant neoplasm	Epigastric and in either upper quadrant; often radiates to the back	Steady, deep
Biliary Colic	Sudden obstruction of the cystic duct or common bile duct by a gallstone	Epigastric or right upper quadrant; may radiate to the right scapula and shoulder	Steady, aching; *not* colicky
Acute Cholecystitis	Inflammation of the gallbladder, usually from obstruction of the cystic duct by a gallstone	Right upper quadrant or upper abdominal; may radiate to the right scapular area	Steady, aching
Acute Diverticulitis	Acute inflammation of a colonic diverticulum, a saclike mucosal outpouching through the colonic muscle	Left lower quadrant	May be cramping at first, but becomes steady
Acute Appendicitis	Acute inflammation of the appendix with distention or obstruction	■ Poorly localized *periumbilical pain*, followed usually by ■ *Right lower quadrant pain*	■ Mild but increasing, possibly cramping ■ Steady and more severe
Acute Mechanical Intestinal Obstruction	Obstruction of the bowel lumen, most commonly caused by (1) adhesions or hernias (small bowel), or (2) cancer or diverticulitis (colon)	■ *Small bowel:* periumbilical or upper abdominal ■ *Colon:* lower abdominal or generalized	■ Cramping ■ Cramping
Mesenteric Ischemia	Blood supply to the bowel and mesentery blocked from thrombosis or embolus (acute arterial occlusion), or reduced from hypoperfusion	May be periumbilical at first, then diffuse	Cramping at first, then steady

Timing	Factors That May Aggravate	Factors That May Relieve	Associated Symptoms and Setting
Intermittent. Duodenal ulcer is more likely than gastric ulcer or dyspepsia to cause pain that (1) wakes the patient at night, and (2) occurs intermittently over a few weeks, then disappears for months, and then recurs.	Variable	Food and antacids may bring relief, but not necessarily in any of these disorders and least commonly in gastric ulcer.	Nausea, vomiting, belching, bloating; heartburn (more common in duodenal ulcer); weight loss (more common in gastric ulcer). Dyspepsia is more common in the young (20–29 yr), gastric ulcer in those over 50 yr, and duodenal ulcer in those from 30–60 yr.
The history of pain is typically shorter than in peptic ulcer. The pain is persistent and slowly progressive.	Often food	*Not* relieved by food or antacids	Anorexia, nausea, early satiety, weight loss, and sometimes bleeding. Most common in ages 50–70
Acute onset, persistent pain	Lying supine	Leaning forward with trunk flexed	Nausea, vomiting, abdominal distention, fever. Often a history of previous attacks and alcohol abuse or gallstones
Chronic or recurrent course	Alcohol, heavy or fatty meals	Possibly leaning forward with trunk flexed; often intractable	Symptoms of decreased pancreatic function may appear: diarrhea with fatty stools (steatorrhea) and diabetes mellitus.
Persistent pain; relentlessly progressive illness		Possibly leaning forward with trunk flexed; often intractable	Anorexia, nausea, vomiting, weight loss, and jaundice. Emotional symptoms, including depression
Rapid onset over a few minutes, lasts one to several hours and subsides gradually. Often recurrent			Anorexia, nausea, vomiting, restlessness
Gradual onset; course longer than in biliary colic	Jarring, deep breathing		Anorexia, nausea, vomiting, and fever
Often a gradual onset			Fever, constipation. There may be initial brief diarrhea.
▪ Lasts roughly 4–6 hr ▪ Depends on intervention	▪ Movement or cough	▪ If it subsides temporarily, suspect perforation of the appendix.	Anorexia, nausea, possibly vomiting, which typically follow the onset of pain; low fever
▪ Paroxysmal; may decrease as bowel mobility is impaired			▪ Vomiting of bile and mucus (high obstruction) or fecal material (low obstruction). Obstipation develops.
▪ Paroxysmal, though typically milder			▪ Obstipation early. Vomiting late if at all. Prior symptoms of underlying cause.
Usually abrupt in onset, then persistent			Vomiting, diarrhea (sometimes bloody), constipation, shock

TABLE 9-2 ■ Dysphagia

Process and Problem	Timing	Factors That Aggravate	Factors That Relieve	Associated Symptoms and Conditions
Transfer Dysphagia, *due to motor disorders affecting the pharyngeal muscles*	Acute or gradual onset and a variable course, depending on the underlying disorder	Attempts to start the swallowing process		Aspiration into the lungs or regurgitation into the nose with attempts to swallow. Neurologic evidence of stroke, bulbar palsy, or other neuromuscular conditions
Esophageal Dysphagia				
Mechanical Narrowing				
■ Mucosal rings and webs	Intermittent	Solid foods	Regurgitation of the bolus of food	Usually none
■ Esophageal stricture	Intermittent, may become slowly progressive	Solid foods	Regurgitation of the bolus of food	A long history of heartburn and regurgitation
■ Esophageal cancer	May be intermittent at first; progressive over months	Solid foods, with progression to liquids	Regurgitation of the bolus of food	Pain in the chest and back and weight loss, especially late in the course of illness
Motor Disorders				
■ Diffuse esophageal spasm	Intermittent	Solids or liquids	Maneuvers described below; sometimes nitroglycerin	Chest pain that mimics angina pectoris or myocardial infarction and lasts minutes to hours; possibly heartburn
■ Scleroderma	Intermittent, may progress slowly	Solids or liquids	Repeated swallowing, movements such as straightening the back, raising the arms, or a Valsalva maneuver (straining down against a closed glottis)	Heartburn. Other manifestations of scleroderma
■ Achalasia	Intermittent, may progress	Solids or liquids		Regurgitation, often at night when lying down, with nocturnal cough; possibly chest pain precipitated by eating

TABLE 9-3 ■ Constipation

Problem	Process	Associated Symptoms and Setting
Life Activities and Habits		
Inadequate Time or Setting for the Defecation Reflex	Ignoring the sensation of a full rectum inhibits the defecation reflex.	Hectic schedules, unfamiliar surroundings, bed rest
False Expectations of Bowel Habits	Expectations of "regularity" or more frequent stools than a person's norm	Beliefs, treatments, and advertisements that promote the use of laxatives
Diet Deficient in Fiber	Decreased fecal bulk	Other factors such as debilitation and constipating drugs may contribute.
Irritable Bowel Syndrome	A common disorder of bowel motility	Small, hard stools, often with mucus. Periods of diarrhea. Cramping abdominal pain. Stress may aggravate.
Mechanical Obstruction		
Cancer of the Rectum or Sigmoid Colon	Progressive narrowing of the bowel lumen	Change in bowel habits; often diarrhea, abdominal pain, and bleeding. In rectal cancer, tenesmus and pencil-shaped stools
Fecal Impaction	A large, firm, immovable fecal mass, most often in the rectum	Rectal fullness, abdominal pain, and diarrhea around the impaction. Common in debilitated, bedridden, and often elderly patients
Other Obstructing Lesions (such as diverticulitis, volvulus, intussusception, or hernia)	Narrowing or complete obstruction of the bowel	Colicky abdominal pain, abdominal distention, and in intussusception, often "currant jelly" stools (red blood and mucus)
Painful Anal Lesions	Pain may cause spasm of the external sphincter and voluntary inhibition of the defecation reflex.	Anal fissures, painful hemorrhoids, perirectal abscesses
Drugs	A variety of mechanisms	Opiates, anticholinergics, antacids containing calcium or aluminum, and many others
Depression	A disorder of mood. See Table 16-1, Disorders of Mood.	Fatigue, feelings of depression, and other somatic symptoms
Neurologic Disorders	Interference with the autonomic innervation of the bowel	Spinal cord injuries, multiple sclerosis, Hirschsprung's disease, and other conditions
Metabolic Conditions	Interference with bowel motility	Pregnancy, hypothyroidism, hypercalcemia

TABLE 9-4 ■ Diarrhea

Problem	Process	Characteristics of Stool
Acute Diarrhea		
Secretory Infections	Infection by viruses, preformed bacterial toxins (such as *Staphylococcus aureus, Clostridium perfringens,* toxigenic *Escherichia coli, Vibrio cholerae*), cryptosporidium, *Giardia lamblia*	Watery, without blood, pus, or mucus
Inflammatory Infections	Colonization or invasion of intestinal mucosa (nontyphoid *Salmonella, Shigella, Yersinia, Campylobacter,* enteropathic *E. coli, Entamoeba histolytica)*	Loose to watery, often with blood, pus, or mucus
Drug-Induced Diarrhea	Action of many drugs, such as magnesium-containing antacids, antibiotics, antineoplastic agents, and laxatives	Loose to watery
Chronic Diarrhea		
Diarrheal Syndromes		
■ Irritable bowel syndrome	A disorder of bowel motility with alternating diarrhea and constipation	Loose; may show mucus but no blood. Small, hard stools with constipation
■ Cancer of the sigmoid colon	Partial obstruction by a malignant neoplasm	May be blood-streaked
Inflammatory Bowel Disease		
■ Ulcerative colitis	Inflammation of the mucosa and submucosa of the rectum and colon with ulceration; cause unknown	From soft to watery, often containing blood
■ Crohn's disease of the small bowel (regional enteritis) or colon (granulomatous colitis)	Chronic inflammation of the bowel wall, typically involving the terminal ileum and/or proximal colon	Small, soft to loose or watery, usually free of gross blood (enteritis) or with less bleeding than ulcerative colitis (colitis)
Voluminous Diarrheas		
■ Malabsorption syndromes	Defective absorption of fat, including fat-soluble vitamins, with steatorrhea (excessive excretion of fat) as in pancreatic insufficiency, bile salt deficiency, bacterial overgrowth	Typically bulky, soft, light yellow to gray, mushy, greasy or oily, and sometimes frothy; particularly foul-smelling; usually floats in the toilet
■ Osmotic diarrheas		
Lactose intolerance	Deficiency in intestinal lactase	Watery diarrhea of large volume
Abuse of osmotic purgatives	Laxative habit, often surreptitious	Watery diarrhea of large volume
■ Secretory diarrheas from bacterial infection, secreting villous adenoma, fat or bile salt malabsorption, hormone-mediated conditions (gastrin in Zollinger–Ellison syndrome, vasoactive intestinal peptide [VIP])	Variable	Watery diarrhea of large volume

Timing	Associated Symptoms	Setting, Persons at Risk
Duration of a few days, possibly longer. Lactase deficiency may lead to a longer course.	Nausea, vomiting, periumbilical cramping pain. Temperature normal or slightly elevated	Often travel, a common food source, or an epidemic
An acute illness of varying duration	Lower abdominal cramping pain and often rectal urgency, tenesmus; fever	Travel, contaminated food or water. Men and women who have had frequent anal intercourse.
Acute, recurrent, or chronic	Possibly nausea; usually little if any pain	Prescribed or over-the-counter medications
Often worse in the morning. Diarrhea rarely wakes the patient at night.	Crampy lower abdominal pain, abdominal distention, flatulence, nausea, constipation	Young and middle-aged adults, especially women
Variable	Change in usual bowel habits, crampy lower abdominal pain, constipation	Middle-aged and older adults, especially over 55 yr
Onset ranges from insidious to acute. Typically recurrent, may be persistent. Diarrhea may wake the patient at night.	Crampy lower or generalized abdominal pain, anorexia, weakness, fever	Often young people
Insidious onset, chronic or recurrent. Diarrhea may wake the patient at night.	Crampy periumbilical or right lower quadrant (enteritis) or diffuse (colitis) pain, with anorexia, low fever, and/or weight loss. Perianal or perirectal abscesses and fistulas	Often young people, especially in the late teens, but also in the middle years. More common in people of Jewish descent
Onset of illness typically insidious	Anorexia, weight loss, fatigue, abdominal distention, often crampy lower abdominal pain. Symptoms of nutritional deficiencies such as bleeding (vitamin K), bone pain and fractures (vitamin D), glossitis (vitamin B), and edema (protein)	Variable, depending on cause
Follows the ingestion of milk and milk products; is relieved by fasting	Crampy abdominal pain, abdominal distention, flatulence	African Americans, Asians, Native Americans
Variable	Often none	Persons with anorexia nervosa or bulimia nervosa
Variable	Weight loss, dehydration, nausea, vomiting, and cramping abdominal pain	Variable depending on cause

TABLE 9-5 ■ Black and Bloody Stools

Problem	Selected Causes	Associated Symptoms and Setting
Melena Melena refers to the passage of black, tarry (sticky and shiny) stools. Tests for occult blood are positive. Melena signifies the loss of at least 60 ml of blood into the gastrointestinal tract (less in infants and children), usually from the esophagus, stomach, or duodenum. Less commonly, when intestinal transit is slow, the blood may originate in the jejunum, ileum, or ascending colon. In infants, melena may result from swallowing blood during the birth process.	Peptic ulcer	Often, but not necessarily, a history of epigastric pain
	Gastritis or stress ulcers	Recent ingestion of alcohol, aspirin, or other anti-inflammatory drugs; recent bodily trauma, severe burns, surgery, or increased intracranial pressure
	Esophageal or gastric varices	Cirrhosis of the liver or other cause of portal hypertension
	Reflux esophagitis	History of heartburn
	Mallory–Weiss tear, a mucosal tear in the esophagus due to retching and vomiting	Retching, vomiting, often recent ingestion of alcohol
Black, Nonsticky Stools Black stools may result from other causes and then usually give negative results when tested for occult blood. (Ingestion of iron or other substances, however, may cause a positive test result in the absence of blood.) These stools have no pathologic significance.	Ingestion of iron, bismuth salts as in Pepto-Bismol, licorice, or even commercial chocolate cookies	
Red Blood in the Stools Red blood usually originates in the colon, rectum, or anus, and much less frequently in the jejunum or ileum. Upper gastrointestinal hemorrhage, however, may also cause red stools. The amount of blood lost is then usually large (more than a liter). Transit time through the intestinal tract is accordingly rapid, giving insufficient time for the blood to turn black.	Cancer of the colon	Often a change in bowel habits
	Benign polyps of the colon	Often no other symptoms
	Diverticula of the colon	Often no other symptoms
	Inflammatory conditions of the colon and rectum	
	■ Ulcerative colitis	See Table 9-5, Diarrhea.
	■ Infectious dysenteries	See Table 9-5, Diarrhea.
	■ Proctitis (various causes) in men or women who have had frequent anal intercourse	Rectal urgency, tenesmus
	Ischemic colitis	Lower abdominal pain and sometimes fever or shock in persons over age 50 yr
	Hemorrhoids	Blood on the toilet paper, on the surface of the stool, or dripping into the toilet
	Anal fissure	Blood on the toilet paper or on the surface of the stool; anal pain
Reddish But Nonbloody Stools	The ingestion of beets	Pink urine, which usually precedes the reddish stool

TABLE 9-6 ■ Frequency, Nocturia, and Polyuria

Problem	Mechanisms	Selected Causes	Associated Symptoms
Frequency	Decreased capacity of the bladder		
	■ Increased bladder sensitivity to stretch because of inflammation	*Infection*, stones, tumor, or foreign body in the bladder	Burning on urination, urinary urgency, sometimes gross hematuria
	■ Decreased elasticity of the bladder wall	Infiltration by scar tissue or tumor	Symptoms of associated inflammation (see above) are common.
	■ Decreased cortical inhibition of bladder contractions	Motor disorders of the central nervous system, such as a stroke	Urinary urgency; neurologic symptoms such as weakness and paralysis
	Impaired emptying of the bladder, with residual urine in the bladder		
	■ Partial mechanical obstruction of the bladder neck or proximal urethra	Most commonly, benign prostatic hyperplasia; also urethral stricture and other obstructive lesions of the bladder or prostate	Prior obstructive symptoms: hesitancy in starting the urinary stream, straining to void, reduced size and force of the stream, and dribbling during or at the end of urination
	■ Loss of peripheral nerve supply to the bladder	Neurologic disease affecting the sacral nerves or nerve roots, e.g., diabetic neuropathy	Weakness or sensory defects
Nocturia *With High Volumes*	Most types of polyuria (see pp. 327–328)		
	Decreased concentrating ability of the kidney with loss of the normal decrease in nocturnal urinary output	Chronic renal insufficiency due to a number of diseases	Possibly other symptoms of renal insufficiency
	Excessive fluid intake before bedtime	Habit, especially involving alcohol and coffee	
	Fluid-retaining, edematous states. Dependent edema accumulates during the day and is excreted when the patient lies down at night.	Congestive heart failure, nephrotic syndrome, hepatic cirrhosis with ascites, chronic venous insufficiency	Edema and other symptoms of the underlying disorder. Urinary output during the day may be reduced as fluid reaccumulates in the body. See Table 14-4, Some Peripheral Causes of Edema.
With Low Volumes	Frequency		
	Voiding while up at night without a real urge, a "pseudo-frequency"	Insomnia	Variable
Polyuria	Deficiency of antidiuretic hormone (diabetes insipidus)	A disorder of the posterior pituitary and hypothalamus	Thirst and polydipsia, often severe and persistent; nocturia
	Renal unresponsiveness to antidiuretic hormone (nephrogenic diabetes insipidus)	A number of kidney diseases, including hypercalcemic and hypokalemic nephropathy; drug toxicity, e.g., from lithium	Thirst and polydipsia, often severe and persistent; nocturia
	Solute diuresis		
	■ Electrolytes, such as sodium salts	Large saline infusions, potent diuretics, certain kidney diseases	Variable
	■ Nonelectrolytes, such as glucose	Uncontrolled diabetes mellitus	Thirst, polydipsia, and nocturia
	Excessive water intake	Primary polydipsia	Polydipsia tends to be episodic. Thirst may not be present. Nocturia is usually absent.

TABLE 9-7 ■ Urinary Incontinence*

Problem	Mechanisms
Stress Incontinence The urethral sphincter is weakened so that transient increases in intraabdominal pressure raise the bladder pressure to levels that exceed urethral resistance.	In women, most often a weakness of the pelvic floor with inadequate muscular support of the bladder and proximal urethra and a change in the angle between the bladder and the urethra. Suggested causes include childbirth and surgery. Local conditions affecting the internal urethral sphincter, such as postmenopausal atrophy of the mucosa and urethral infection, may also contribute. In men, stress incontinence may follow prostatic surgery.
Urge Incontinence Detrusor contractions are stronger than normal and overcome the normal urethral resistance. The bladder is typically small.	■ Decreased cortical inhibition of detrusor contractions, as by strokes, brain tumors, dementia, and lesions of the spinal cord above the sacral level ■ Hyperexcitability of sensory pathways, caused by, for example, bladder infections, tumors, and fecal impaction ■ Deconditioning of voiding reflexes, caused by, for example, frequent voluntary voiding at low bladder volumes
Overflow Incontinence Detrusor contractions are insufficient to overcome urethral resistance. The bladder is typically large, even after an effort to void.	■ Obstruction of the bladder outlet, as by benign prostatic hyperplasia or tumor ■ Weakness of the detrusor muscle associated with peripheral nerve disease at the sacral level ■ Impaired bladder sensation that interrupts the reflex arc, as from diabetic neuropathy
Functional Incontinence This is a functional inability to get to the toilet in time because of impaired health or environmental conditions.	Problems in mobility resulting from weakness, arthritis, poor vision, or other conditions. Environmental factors such as an unfamiliar setting, distant bathroom facilities, bedrails, or physical restraints
Incontinence Secondary to Medications Drugs may contribute to any type of incontinence listed.	Sedatives, tranquilizers, anticholinergics, sympathetic blockers, and potent diuretics

*Patients may have more than one kind of incontinence.

Symptoms	Physical Signs
Momentary leakage of small amounts of urine concurrent with stresses such as coughing, laughing, and sneezing while the person is in an upright position. A desire to urinate is not associated with pure stress incontinence.	The bladder is not detected on abdominal examination. Stress incontinence may be demonstrable, especially if the patient is examined before voiding and in a standing position. Atrophic vaginitis may be evident.
Incontinence preceded by an urge to void. The volume tends to be moderate. Urgency Frequency and nocturia with small to moderate volumes If acute inflammation is present, pain on urination Possibly "pseudo-stress incontinence"—voiding 10–20 sec after stresses such as a change of position, going up or down stairs, and possibly coughing, laughing, or sneezing	The bladder is not detectable on abdominal examination. When cortical inhibition is decreased, mental deficits or motor signs of central nervous system disease are often, though not necessarily, present. When sensory pathways are hyperexcitable, signs of local pelvic problems or a fecal impaction may be present.
A continuous dripping or dribbling incontinence Decreased force of the urinary stream Prior symptoms of partial urinary obstruction or other symptoms of peripheral nerve disease may be present.	An enlarged bladder is often found on abdominal examination and may be tender. Other possible signs include prostatic enlargement, motor signs of peripheral nerve disease, a decrease in sensation including perineal sensation, and diminished to absent reflexes.
Incontinence on the way to the toilet or only in the early morning	The bladder is not detectable on physical examination. Look for physical or environmental clues to the likely cause.
Variable. A careful history and chart review are important.	Variable

TABLE 9-8 ■ Localized Bulges in the Abdominal Wall

Localized bulges in the abdominal wall include ventral hernias (defects in the wall through which tissue protrudes) and subcutaneous tumors such as lipomas. The more common ventral hernias are umbilical, incisional, and epigastric. Hernias and a rectus diastasis usually become more evident when the patient raises head and shoulders from a supine position.

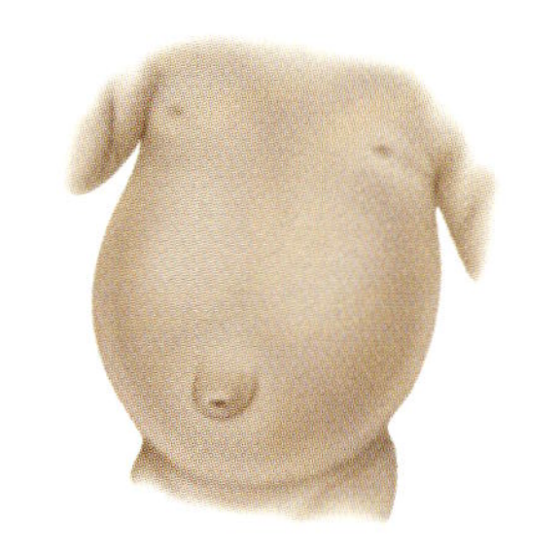

INFANT

Umbilical Hernia

Umbilical hernias protrude through a defective umbilical ring. They are most common in infants but also occur in adults. In infants, but not in adults, they usually close spontaneously within a year or two.

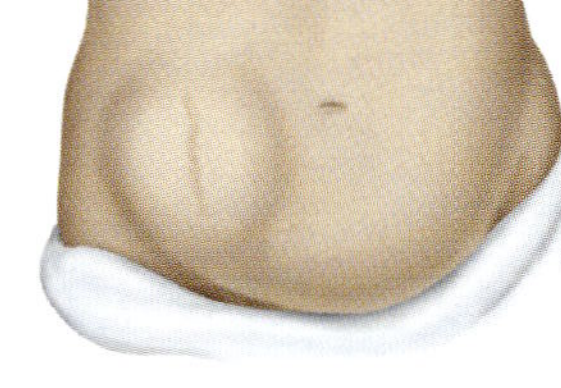

Incisional Hernia

An incisional hernia protrudes through an operative scar. By palpation, note the length and width of the defect in the abdominal wall. A small defect, through which a large hernia has passed, has a greater risk of complications than a large defect.

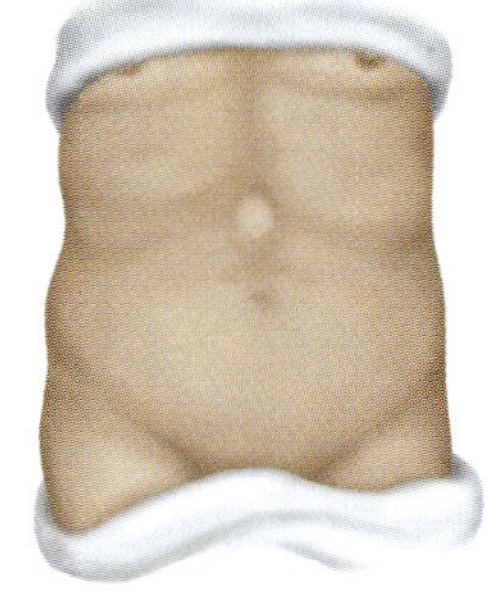

Epigastric Hernia

An epigastric hernia is a small midline protrusion through a defect in the linea alba, somewhere between the xiphoid process and the umbilicus. With the patient's head and shoulders raised (or with the patient standing), look for it, and run your fingerpad down the linea alba to feel it.

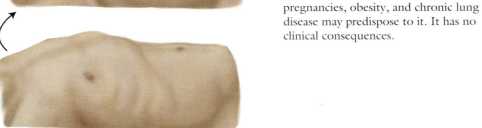

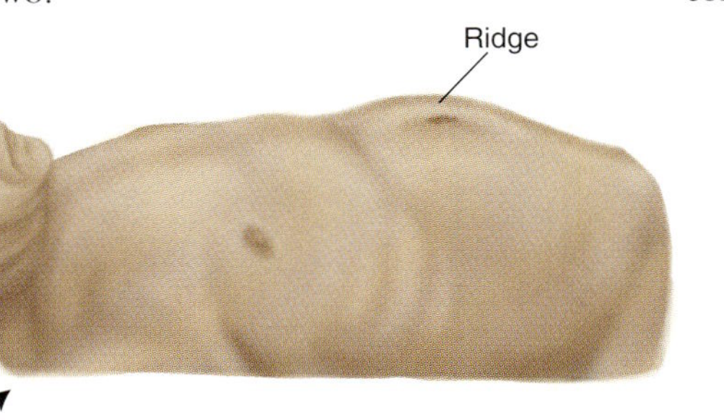

Diastasis Recti

A rectus diastasis is a separation of the two rectus abdominis muscles, through which abdominal contents bulge to form a midline ridge when the patient raises head and shoulders. Repeated pregnancies, obesity, and chronic lung disease may predispose to it. It has no clinical consequences.

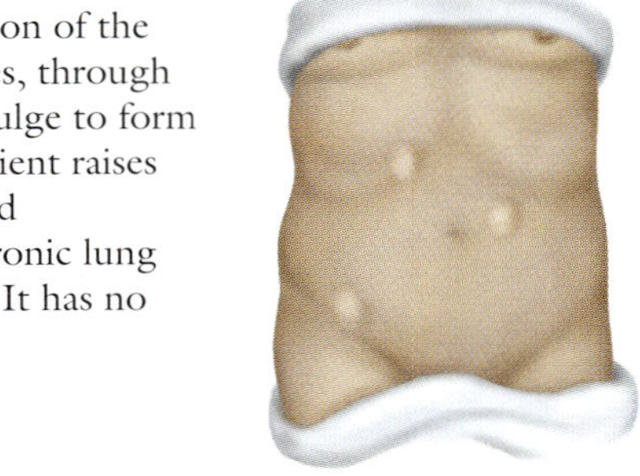

Lipoma

Lipomas are common, benign, fatty tumors usually located in the subcutaneous tissues almost anywhere in the body, including the abdominal wall. Small or large, they are usually soft and often lobulated. When your finger presses down on the edge of a lipoma, the tumor typically slips out from under it.

TABLE 9-9 ■ Protuberant Abdomens

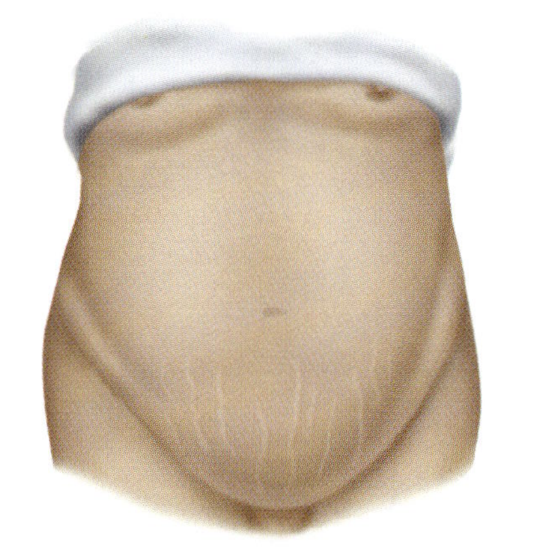

Fat

Fat is the most common cause of a protuberant abdomen and is associated with generalized obesity. The abdominal wall is thick. Fat in the mesentery and omentum also contributes to abdominal size. The umbilicus may appear sunken. The percussion note is normal. A pannus, or apron of fatty tissue, may extend below the inguinal ligaments. Lift it to look for inflammation in the skin fold or even for a hidden hernia.

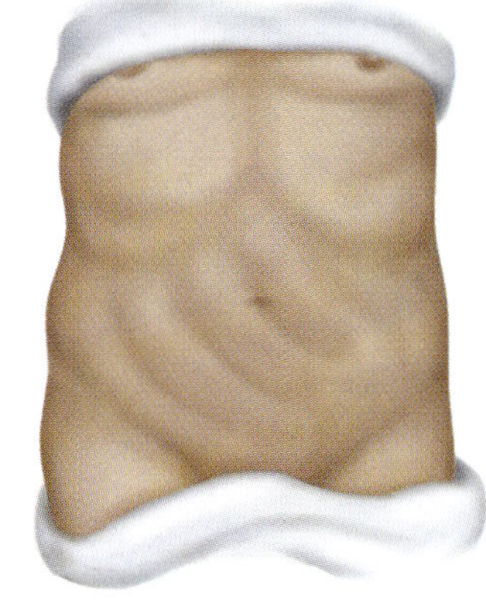

Gas

Gaseous distention may be localized or generalized. It causes a tympanitic percussion note. Increased intestinal gas production due to certain foods may cause mild distention. More serious are intestinal obstruction and adynamic (paralytic) ileus. Note the location of the distention. Distention becomes more marked in colonic than in small bowel obstruction.

Tumor

A large, solid tumor, usually rising out of the pelvis, is dull to percussion. Air-filled bowel is displaced to the periphery. Causes include ovarian tumors and uterine myomata. Occasionally, a markedly distended bladder may be mistaken for such a tumor.

Pregnancy

Pregnancy is a common cause of a pelvic "mass." Listen for the fetal heart (see pp. 421–422).

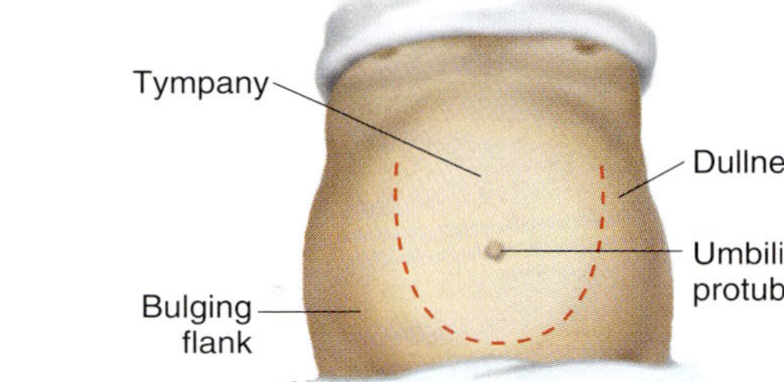

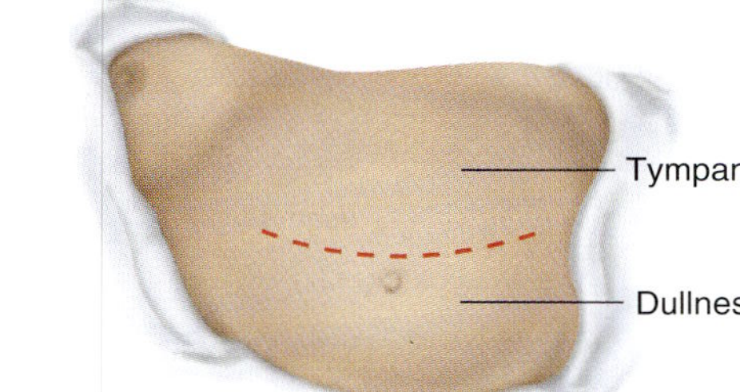

Ascitic Fluid

Ascitic fluid seeks the lowest point in the abdomen, producing bulging flanks that are dull to percussion. The umbilicus may protrude. Turn the patient onto one side to detect the shift in position of the fluid level (shifting dullness). (See pp. 345–347 for the assessment of ascites.)

TABLE 9-10 ■ Sounds in the Abdomen

Bowel Sounds

Bowel sounds may be:

- *Increased*, as from diarrhea or *early intestinal obstruction*
- *Decreased*, then absent, as in *adynamic ileus and peritonitis.* Before deciding that bowel sounds are absent, sit down and listen where shown for 2 min or even longer.

High-pitched tinkling sounds suggest intestinal fluid and air under tension in a dilated bowel. Rushes of high-pitched sounds coinciding with an abdominal cramp indicate intestinal obstruction.

Bruits

A *hepatic bruit* suggests carcinoma of the liver or alcoholic hepatitis. *Arterial bruits* with both systolic and diastolic components suggest partial occlusion of the aorta or large arteries. Partial occlusion of a renal artery may cause and explain hypertension.

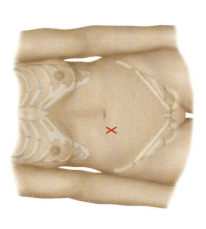

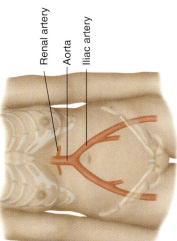

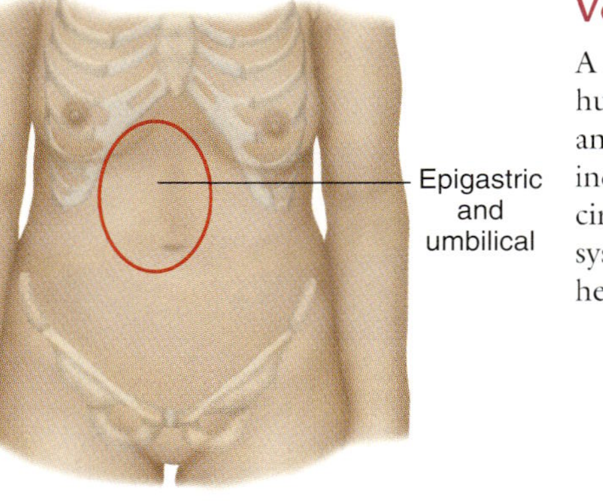

Venous Hum

A venous hum is rare. It is a soft humming noise with both systolic and diastolic components. It indicates increased collateral circulation between portal and systemic venous systems, as in hepatic cirrhosis.

Friction Rubs

Friction rubs are rare. They are grating sounds with respiratory variation. They indicate inflammation of the peritoneal surface of an organ, as from a liver tumor, chlamydial or gonococcal perihepatitis, recent liver biopsy, or splenic infarct. When a systolic bruit accompanies a hepatic friction rub, suspect carcinoma of the liver.

TABLE 9-11 ■ Tender Abdomens

Abdominal Wall Tenderness

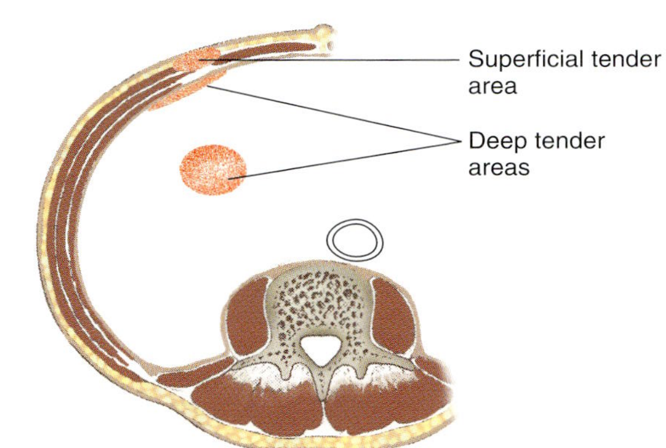

Tenderness may originate in the abdominal wall. When the patient raises head and shoulders, this tenderness persists, whereas tenderness from a deeper lesion (protected by the tightened muscles) decreases.

Visceral Tenderness

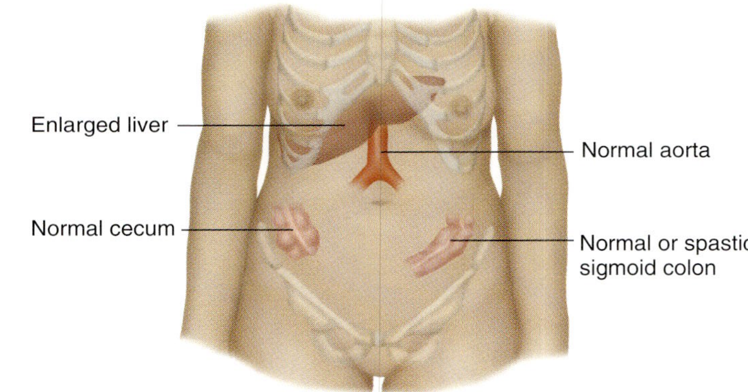

The structures shown may be tender to deep palpation. Usually the discomfort is dull and there is no muscular rigidity or rebound tenderness. A reassuring explanation to the patient may prove quite helpful.

Tenderness From Disease in the Chest and Pelvis

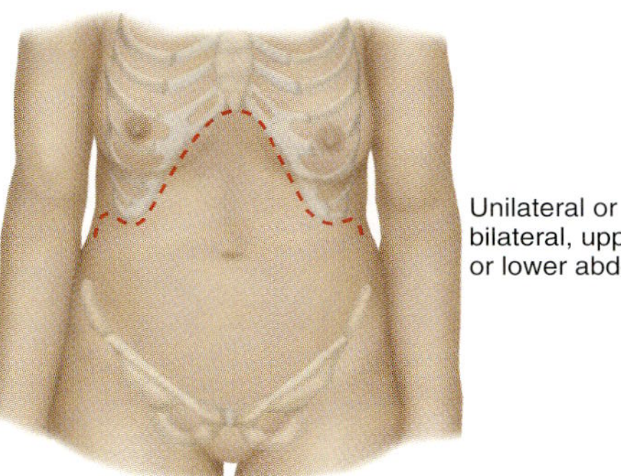

Acute Pleurisy

Abdominal pain and tenderness may be due to acute pleural inflammation. When unilateral, it may mimic acute cholecystitis or appendicitis. Rebound tenderness and rigidity are less common; chest signs are usually present.

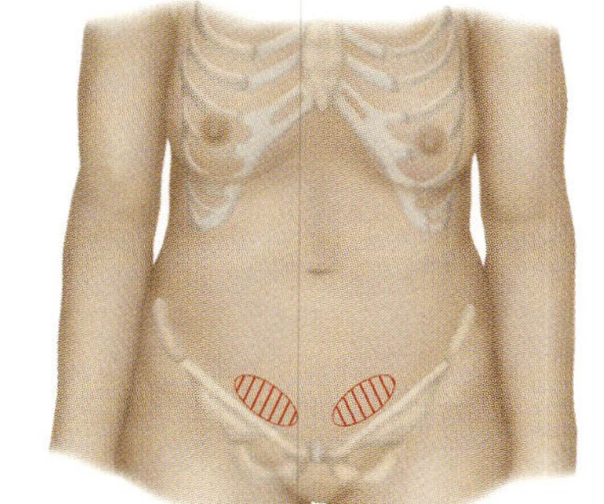

Acute Salpingitis

Frequently bilateral, the tenderness of acute salpingitis (inflammation of the fallopian tubes) is usually maximal just above the inguinal ligaments. Rebound tenderness and rigidity may be present. On pelvic examination, motion of the uterus causes pain.

(table continues next page)

TABLE 9-11 ■ Tender Abdomens *(Continued)*

Tenderness of Peritoneal Inflammation

Tenderness associated with peritoneal inflammation is more severe than visceral tenderness. Muscular rigidity and rebound tenderness are frequently but not necessarily present. Generalized peritonitis causes exquisite tenderness throughout the abdomen, together with boardlike muscular rigidity. Local causes of peritoneal inflammation include:

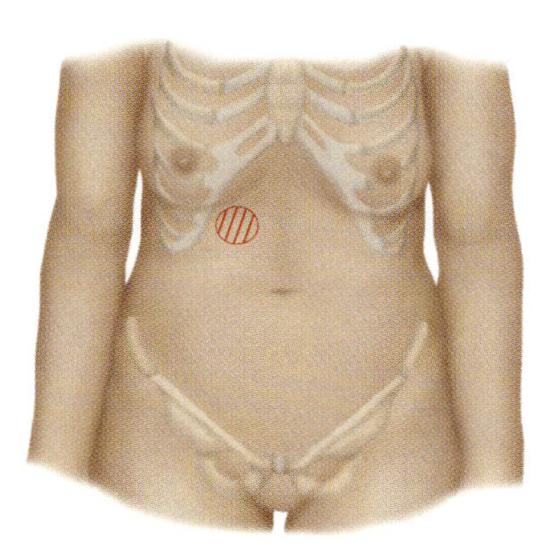

Acute Cholecystitis

Signs are maximal in the right upper quadrant. Check for Murphy's sign (see p. 348).

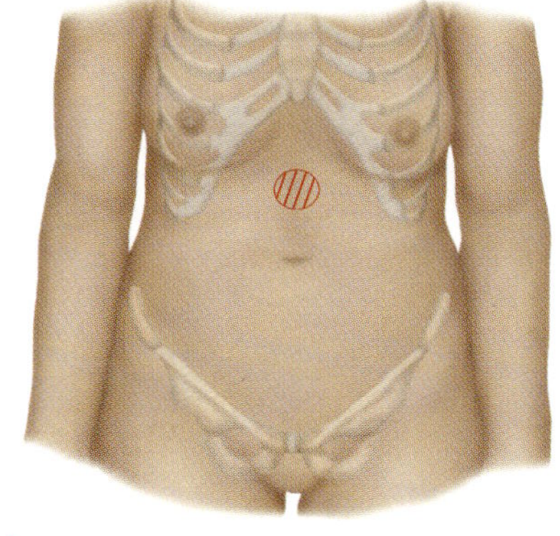

Acute Pancreatitis

In acute pancreatitis, epigastric tenderness and rebound tenderness are usually present, but the abdominal wall may be soft.

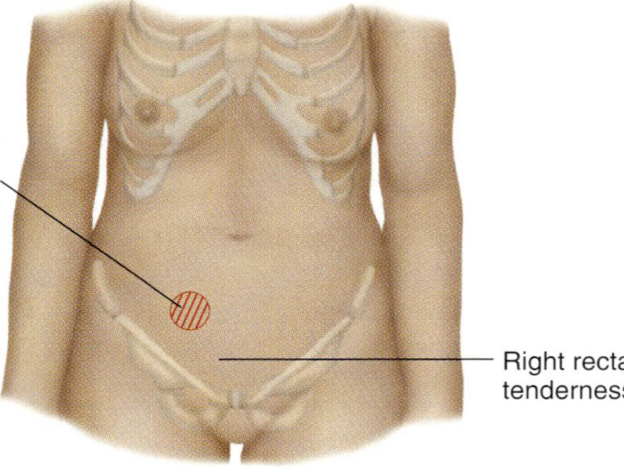

Acute Appendicitis

Right lower quadrant signs are typical of acute appendicitis, but may be absent early in the course. The typical area of tenderness is illustrated. Explore other portions of the right lower quadrant as well as the right flank.

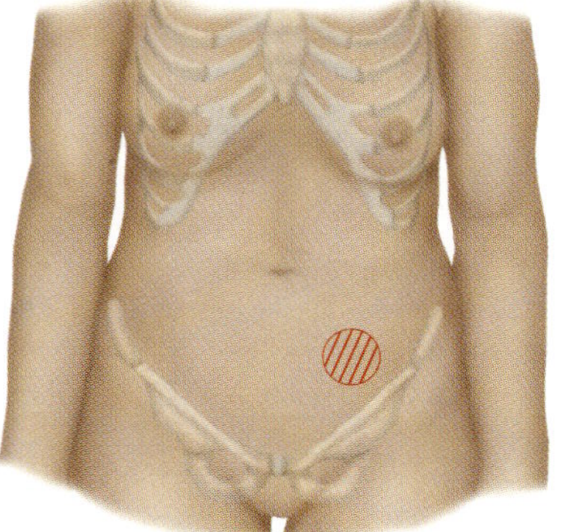

Acute Diverticulitis

Acute diverticulitis most often involves the sigmoid colon and then resembles a left-sided appendicitis.

TABLE 9-12 ■ Liver Enlargement: Apparent and Real

A palpable liver does not necessarily indicate hepatomegaly (an enlarged liver), but more often results from a change in consistency—from the normal softness to an abnormal firmness or hardness, as in cirrhosis. Clinical estimates of liver size should be based on both percussion and palpation, although even then they are far from perfect.

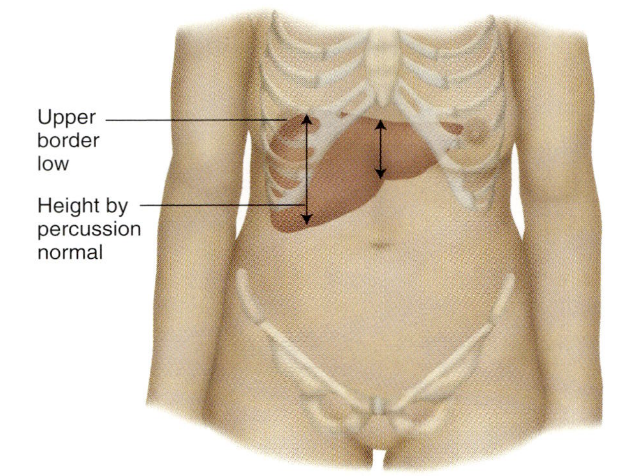

Downward Displacement of the Liver by a Low Diaphragm

This is a common finding (e.g., in emphysema) when the diaphragm is low. The liver edge may be readily palpable well below the costal margin. Percussion, however, reveals a low upper edge also, and the vertical span of the liver is normal.

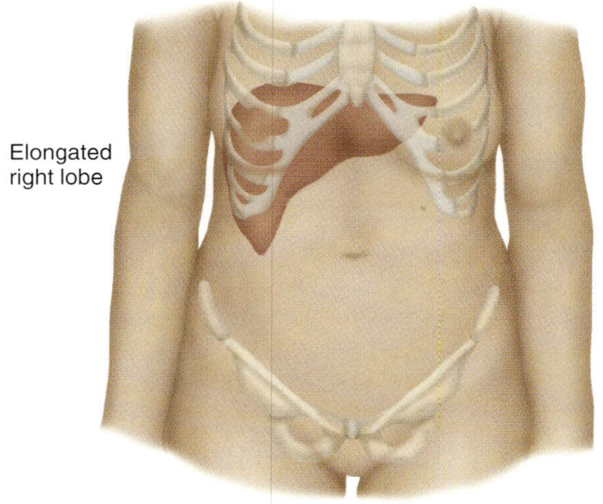

Normal Variations in Liver Shape

In some persons, especially those with a lanky build, the liver tends to be somewhat elongated so that its right lobe is easily palpable as it projects downward toward the iliac crest. Such an elongation, sometimes called *Riedel's* lobe, represents a variation in shape, not an increase in liver volume or size. This variant illustrates the basic limitations of assessing liver size. We can only estimate the upper and lower borders of an organ that has three dimensions and differing shapes. Some error is unavoidable.

(table continues next page)

TABLE 9-12 ■ Liver Enlargement: Apparent and Real *(Continued)*

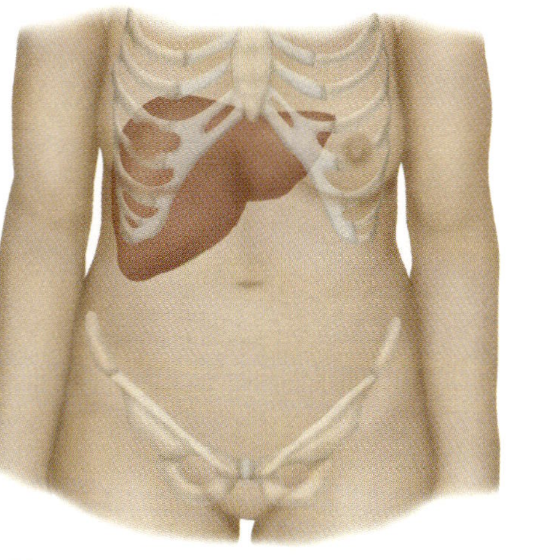

Smooth Large Nontender Liver

Cirrhosis may produce an enlarged liver with a firm nontender edge. The liver is not always enlarged in this condition, however, and many other diseases may produce similar findings.

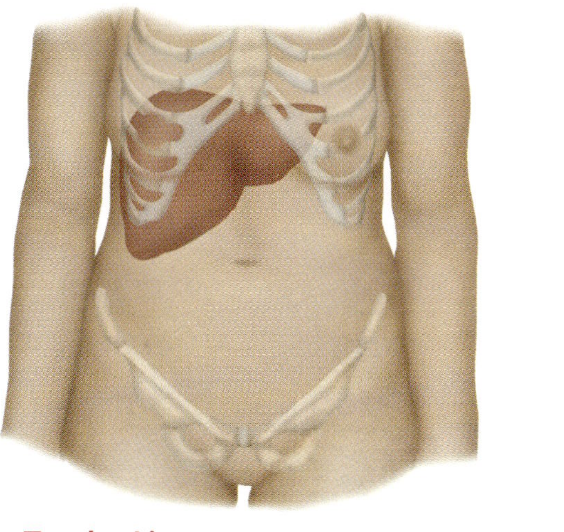

Smooth Large Tender Liver

An enlarged liver with a smooth tender edge suggests inflammation, as in hepatitis, or venous congestion, as in right-sided heart failure.

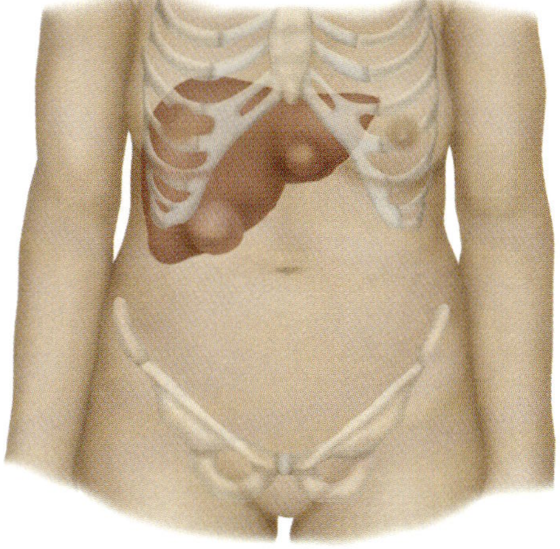

Large Irregular Liver

An enlarged liver that is firm or hard and has an irregular edge or surface suggests malignancy. There may be one or more nodules. The liver may or may not be tender.

CHAPTER

10

Male Genitalia and Hernias

ANATOMY AND PHYSIOLOGY

Review the anatomy of the male genitalia.

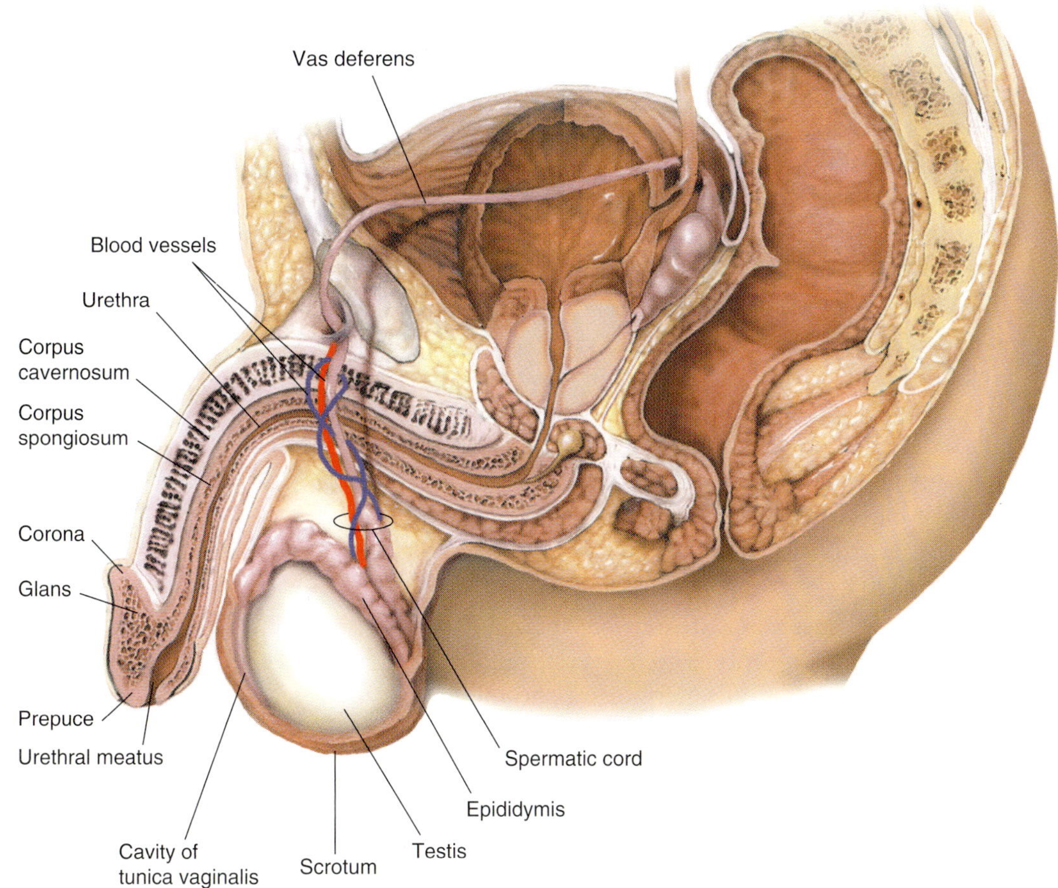

The *shaft of the penis* is formed by three columns of vascular erectile tissue: the *corpus spongiosum,* containing the urethra, and two *corpora cavernosa.* The corpus spongiosum forms the bulb of the penis, ending in the cone-shaped *glans* with its expanded base, or *corona.* In uncircumsized men, the glans is covered by a loose, hoodlike fold of skin called the *prepuce* or *foreskin* where *smegma,* or secretions of the glans, may collect. The urethra is located ventrally in the shaft of the penis; urethral abnormalities may sometimes be felt there. The urethra opens into the vertical, slitlike *urethral meatus,* located somewhat ventrally at the tip of the glans.

The *scrotum* is a loose, wrinkled pouch divided into two compartments, each of which contains a testis or testicle. The *testes* are ovoid, somewhat rubbery structures, about 4.5 cm long in the adult, with a range from 3.5 cm to 5.5 cm. The left usually lies somewhat lower than the right. On the posterolateral surface of each testis is the softer, comma-shaped *epididymis.* It is most prominent along the superior margin of the testis. The epididymis may be located anteriorly in 6% to 7% of males. Surrounding the testis, except posteriorly, is the *tunica vaginalis,* a serous membrane enclosing a potential cavity.

The testes produce spermatozoa and testosterone. Testosterone stimulates the pubertal growth of the male genitalia, prostate, and seminal vesicles. It also stimulates the development of masculine secondary sex characteristics, including the beard, body hair, musculoskeletal development, and enlarged larynx with the associated low-pitched voice.

The *vas deferens,* a cordlike structure, begins at the tail of the epididymis, ascends within the scrotal sac, and passes through the external inguinal ring on its way to the abdomen and pelvis. Behind the bladder it is joined by the duct from the seminal vesicle and enters the urethra within the prostate gland. Sperm thus pass from the testis and the epididymis through the vas deferens into the urethra. Secretions from the vasa deferentia, the seminal vesicles, and the prostate all contribute to the semen. Within the scrotum each vas is closely associated with blood vessels, nerves, and muscle fibers. These structures make up the *spermatic cord.*

Male sexual function depends on normal levels of testosterone, adequate arterial blood flow to the inferior epigastric artery and its cremasteric and pubic branches, and intact neural innervation from α-adrenergic and cholinergic pathways. Erection from venous engorgement of the corpora cavernosa results from two types of stimuli. Visual, auditory, or erotic cues trigger sympathetic outflow from higher brain centers to the T11 through L2 levels of the spinal cord. Tactile stimulation initiates sensory impulses from the genitalia to S_2–S_4 reflex arcs and parasympathetic pathways via the pudendal nerve. Both sets of stimuli appear to increase levels of nitric oxide and cyclic GMP, resulting in local vasodilation.

Lymphatics. Lymphatics from the penile and scrotal surfaces drain into the inguinal nodes. *When you find an inflammatory or possibly malignant lesion* on these surfaces, *assess the inguinal nodes especially carefully* for enlargement or tenderness. The lymphatics of the testes, however, drain into the abdomen, where enlarged nodes are clinically undetectable. See page 452 for further discussion of the inguinal nodes.

Anatomy of the Groin. Because hernias are relatively common, it is important to understand the anatomy of the groin. The basic landmarks are the anterior superior iliac spine, the pubic tubercle, and the inguinal ligament that runs between them. Find these on yourself or a colleague.

The *inguinal canal,* which lies above and approximately parallel to the inguinal ligament, forms a tunnel for the vas deferens as it passes through the abdominal muscles. The exterior opening of the tunnel—the *external inguinal ring*—is a triangular slitlike structure palpable just above and lateral to the pubic tubercle. The internal opening of the canal—or internal inguinal ring—is about 1 cm above the midpoint of the inguinal ligament. Neither canal nor internal ring is palpable through the abdominal wall. When loops of bowel force their way through weak areas of the inguinal canal they produce inguinal hernias, as illustrated on pp. 381–382.

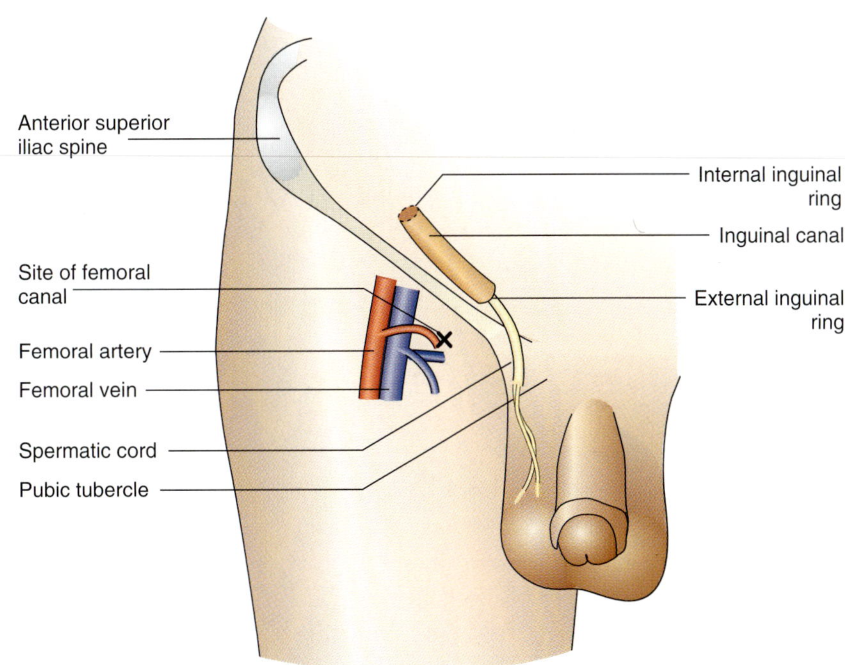

Another potential route for a herniating mass is the *femoral canal.* This lies below the inguinal ligament. Although you cannot see it, you can estimate its location by placing your right index finger, from below, on the right femoral artery. Your middle finger will then overlie the femoral vein; your ring finger, the femoral canal. Femoral hernias protrude here.

Changes With Aging

Note that in about 80% of men, pubic hair spreads farther up the abdomen in a triangular pattern pointing toward the umbilicus. Because this kind of spread, known as stage 6, is not completed until the mid-20s or later, it is not considered a pubertal change.

Testosterone levels decline with aging and may affect both libido and sexual function. Erection becomes more dependent on tactile stimulation and less responsive to erotic cues. Pubic hair may decrease and become gray. The penis decreases in size and the testicles drop lower in the scrotum. Although the testes often decrease in size with protracted illnesses, they do not necessarily change size with aging *per se.*

THE HEALTH HISTORY

Common or Concerning Symptoms

- Sexual function, sexual preference
- Sexual response: libido, arousal, orgasm, ejaculation
- Penile discharge or lesions
- Scrotal pain, swelling, or lesions

For men, questions about the genital system follow naturally after those dealing with the urinary system. You will need to review sexual function and screen for symptoms of infection. Begin with general questions such as "How is sexual function for you?" "Are you satisfied with your sexual life?" "What about your ability to perform sexually?" If the patient reports a sexual problem, ask him to tell you about it. Ask if there has been any change in desire or level of sexual activity in recent years. What does he think has caused it, what has he tried to do about it, and what are his hopes? Identify the patient's sexual preference as to partners (male, female, or both). Find out if the patient's partner has any concerns.

Direct questions help you to assess each phase of the sexual response. To assess *libido,* or desire, ask "Have you maintained an interest in sex?" For the *arousal phase,* ask "Are you able to achieve and maintain an erection?" Explore the timing, severity, setting, and any other factors that may be contributing. Have any changes in the relationship with his partner or in his life circumstances coincided with onset of the problem? Are there circumstances when erection is normal? On awakening in the early morning or during the night? With other partners? With masturbation?

Lack of libido may arise from psychogenic causes such as depression, endocrine dysfunction, or side effects of medications.

Erectile dysfunction from psychogenic causes, especially if early morning erection preserved; also from decreased testosterone, decreased blood flow in hypogastric arterial system, impaired neural innervation

Other questions relate to the phase of *orgasm* and *ejaculation* of semen. If ejaculation is premature, or early and out of control, ask "About how long does intercourse last?" "Do you climax too soon?" "Do you feel like you have any control over climaxing?" "Do you think your partner would like intercourse to last longer?" For reduced or absent ejaculation, "Do you find that you cannot have orgasm even though you can have an erection?" Try to determine if the problem involves the pleasurable sensation of orgasm, the ejaculation of seminal fluid, or both. Review the frequency and setting of the problem, medications, surgery, and neurologic symptoms.

Premature ejaculation is common, especially in young men. Less common is reduced or absent ejaculation affecting middle-aged or older men. Possible causes are medications, surgery, neurologic deficits, or lack of androgen. Lack of orgasm with ejaculation is usually psychogenic.

To assess the possibility of genital infection from sexually transmitted diseases (STDs), ask about any *discharge from the penis,* dripping, or staining of underwear. If penile discharge is present, assess the amount, its color and consistency, and any fever, chills, rash, or associated symptoms.

Penile discharge in gonococcal (usually yellow) and nongonococcal urethritis (may be clear or white)

Inquire about *sores or growths on the penis,* and any *pain or swelling in the scrotum.* Ask about previous genital symptoms or a past history of diseases such as herpes, gonorrhea, or syphilis. A patient who has multiple partners, is homosexual, uses illicit drugs, or has a prior history of STDs is at increased risk for STDs.

See Table 10-1, Abnormalities of the Penis (p. 378) and Table 10-2, Abnormalities of the Male Genitalia (pp. 379–380). In addition to STDs, many skin conditions affect the genitalia; likewise some STDs have minimal symptoms or signs.

Because STDs may involve other parts of the body, additional questions are often indicated. An introductory explanation may be useful. "Sexually transmitted diseases can involve any body opening where you have sex. It's important for you to tell me which openings you use." And further, as needed, "Do you have oral sex? Anal sex?" If the patient's answers are affirmative, ask about symptoms such as sore throat, diarrhea, rectal bleeding, and anal itching or pain.

Infections from oral–penile transmission include gonorrhea, *Chlamydia*, syphilis, and herpes. Symptomatic or asymptomatic proctitis may follow anal intercourse.

For the many patients without symptoms or known risk factors, it is wise to ask, "Do you have any concerns about HIV infection?" and to continue with the more general questions suggested on pp. 45–46.

HEALTH PROMOTION AND COUNSELING

Important Topics for Health Promotion and Counseling

- Prevention of STDs and HIV
- Testicular self-examination

Health promotion and counseling should address patient education about STDs and HIV, early detection of infection during history taking and physical examination, and identification and treatment of infected partners. Discussion of risk factors for STDs and HIV is especially important for adolescents and younger patients, the age groups that are most adversely affected. Clinicians must be comfortable with eliciting the sexual history and with asking frank but tactful questions about sexual practices. A minimal history includes identifying the patient's sexual orientation, the number of sexual partners in the past month, and any history of STDs (see Chap. 2, p. 45). Questions should be clear and nonjudgmental. You should also identify use of alcohol and drugs, particularly injection drugs. Counsel patients at risk about limiting the number of partners, using condoms, and establishing regular medical care for treatment of STDs and HIV. It is important for men to seek prompt attention for any genital lesions or penile discharge.

The U.S. Preventive Services Task Force recommends counseling and testing for HIV infection in the following groups: all persons at increased risk for infection with HIV, STDs, or both; men with male partners; past or present injection drug users; any past or present partners of individuals with HIV infection, bisexual practices, or injection drug use; and patients with a history of transfusion between 1978 and 1985.

In addition, encourage men, especially those between the ages of 15 and 35, to perform monthly testicular self-examinations and to seek physician evaluation for the following findings: any painless lump, swelling, or enlargement in either testicle; pain or discomfort in a testicle or the scrotum; a feeling of heaviness or a sudden fluid collection in the scrotum; or a dull ache in the lower abdomen or the groin. (See p. 377 for instructions to patients.)

Preview: Recording the Physical Examination—Male Genitalia and Hernias

Note that initially you may use sentences to describe your findings; later you will use phrases. The style below contains phrases appropriate for most write-ups. Unfamiliar terms are explained in the next section, Techniques of Examination.

"Circumsized male. No penile discharge or lesions. No scrotal swelling or discoloration. Testes descended bilaterally, smooth, without masses. Epididymis nontender. No inguinal or femoral hernias."

OR

"Uncircumsized male; prepuce easily retractible. No penile discharge or lesions. No scrotal swelling or discoloration. Testes descended bilaterally; right testicle smooth; 1 × 1 cm firm nodule on left lateral testicle. It is fixed and nontender. Epididymis nontender. No inguinal or femoral hernias."

Suspicious for testicular carcinoma, the most common form of cancer in men between the ages of 15 and 35

TECHNIQUES OF EXAMINATION

Many students feel uneasy about examining a man's genitalia. "How will the patient react?" "Will he have an erection?" "Will he let me examine him?" It may be reassuring to explain each step of the examination so the patient knows what to expect. A male patient may occasionally have an erection. If so, you should explain that this is a normal response, finish your examination, and proceed with an unruffled demeanor. If the man refuses to be examined, you should respect his wishes.

A good genital examination can be done with the patient either standing or supine. To check for hernias or varicoceles, however, the patient should stand, and you should sit comfortably on a chair or stool. A gown conveniently covers the patient's chest and abdomen. Wear gloves throughout the examination. Expose the genitalia and inguinal areas. For younger patients, review the sexual maturity ratings on p. 707.

The Penis

INSPECTION

Inspect the penis, including:

See Table 10-1, Abnormalities of the Penis (p. 378).

- The *skin*
- The *prepuce* (foreskin). If it is present, retract it or ask the patient to retract it. This step is essential for the detection of many chancres and carcinomas. Smegma, a cheesy, whitish material, may accumulate normally under the foreskin.

Phimosis is a tight prepuce that cannot be retracted over the glans. *Paraphimosis* is a tight prepuce that, once retracted, cannot be returned. Edema ensues.

- The *glans*. Look for any ulcers, scars, nodules, or signs of inflammation.

Balanitis (inflammation of the glans); *balanoposthitis* (inflammation of the glans and prepuce)

Check the skin around the base of the penis for excoriations or inflammation. Look for nits or lice at the bases of the pubic hairs.

Pubic or genital excoriations suggest the possibility of lice (crabs) or sometimes scabies.

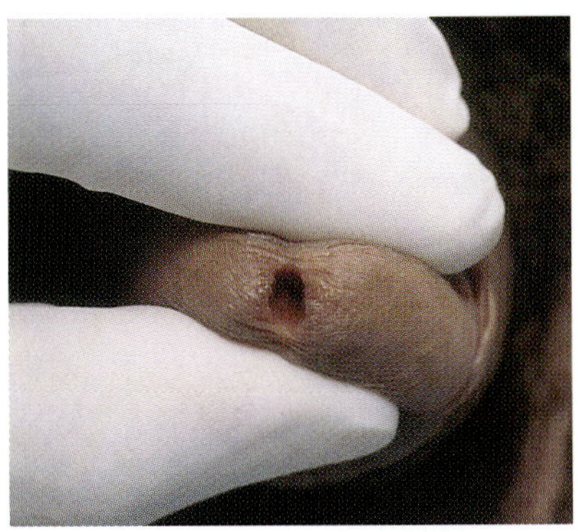

Note the location of the urethral meatus.

Hypospadias is a congenital, ventral displacement of the meatus on the penis (p. 378).

Compress the glans gently between your index finger above and your thumb below. This maneuver should open the urethral meatus and allow you to inspect it for discharge. Normally there is none.

Profuse yellow discharge in gonococcal urethritis; scanty white or clear discharge in nongonococcal urethritis. Definitive diagnosis requires Gram stain and culture.

If the patient has reported a discharge but you do not see any, ask him to strip, or milk, the shaft of the penis from its base to the glans. Alternatively, do it yourself. This maneuver may bring some discharge out of the urethral meatus for appropriate examination. Have a glass slide and culture materials ready.

PALPATION

Palpate any abnormality of the penis, noting any tenderness or induration. Palpate the shaft of the penis between your thumb and first two fingers, noting any induration. Palpation of the shaft may be omitted in a young, asymptomatic male patient.

Induration along the ventral surface of the penis suggests a urethral stricture or possibly a carcinoma. Tenderness of such an indurated area suggests periurethral inflammation secondary to a urethral stricture.

If you retract the foreskin, replace it before proceeding on to examine the scrotum.

The Scrotum and Its Contents

INSPECTION

See Table 10-2, Abnormalities of the Male Genitalia (pp. 379–380).

Inspect the scrotum, including:

- The *skin*. Lift up the scrotum so that you can see its posterior surface.

Rashes, epidermoid cysts, rarely skin cancer

- The *scrotal contours*. Note any swelling, lumps, or veins.

A poorly developed scrotum on one or both sides suggests *cryptorchidism* (an undescended testicle). Common scrotal swellings include indirect inguinal hernias, hydroceles, and scrotal edema. Tender, painful scrotal swelling in acute epididymitis, acute orchitis, torsion of the spermatic cord, or a strangulated inguinal hernia.

PALPATION

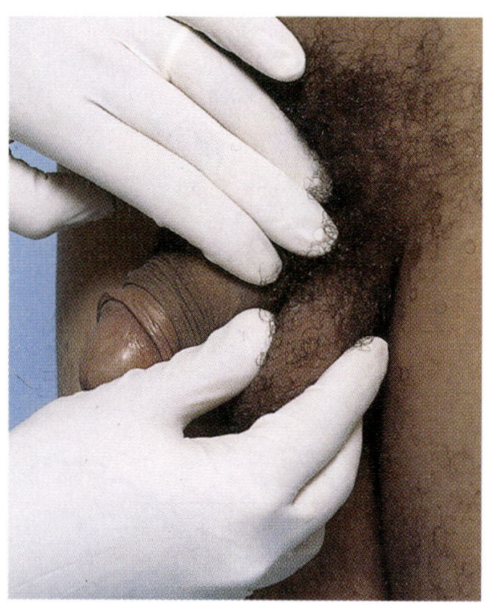

Palpate each testis and epididymis between your thumb and first two fingers.

Note size, shape, consistency, and tenderness; feel for any nodules. Pressure on the testis normally produces a deep visceral pain.

Any painless nodule in the testis must raise the possibility of testicular cancer, a potentially curable cancer with a peak incidence between the ages of 15 and 35 years.

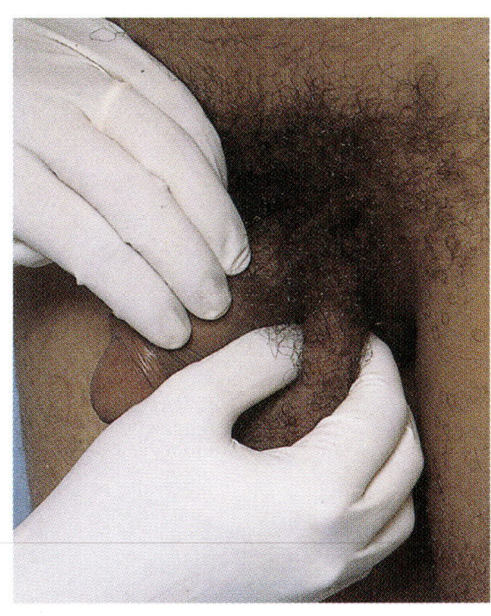

Palpate each spermatic cord, including the vas deferens, between your thumb and fingers from the epididymis to the superficial inguinal ring.

Note any nodules or swellings.

Multiple tortuous veins in this area, usually on the left, may be palpable and even visible. They indicate a varicocele (p. 380).

The vas deferens, if chronically infected, may feel thickened or beaded. A cystic structure in the spermatic cord suggests a hydrocele of the cord.

Swelling in the scrotum other than the testicles can be evaluated by transillumination. After darkening the room, shine the beam of a strong flashlight from behind the scrotum through the mass. Look for transmission of the light as a red glow.

Swellings containing serous fluid, as in hydroceles, light up with a red glow, or transilluminate. Those containing blood or tissue, such as a normal testis, a tumor, or most hernias, do not.

Hernias

INSPECTION

Inspect the inguinal and femoral areas carefully for bulges. While you continue your observation, ask the patient to strain down.

A bulge that appears on straining suggests a hernia.

PALPATION

Palpate for an inguinal hernia. Using in turn your right hand for the patient's right side and your left hand for the patient's left side, invaginate loose scrotal skin with your index finger. Start at a point low enough to be sure that your finger will have enough mobility to reach as far as the internal inguinal ring if this proves possible. Follow the spermatic cord upward to above the inguinal ligament and find the triangular slitlike opening of the external inguinal ring. This is just above and lateral to the pubic tubercle. If the ring is somewhat enlarged, it may admit your index finger. If possible, gently follow the inguinal canal laterally in its oblique course. With your finger located either at the external ring or within the canal, ask the patient to strain down or cough. Note any palpable herniating mass as it touches your finger.

See Table 10-3, Course and Presentation of Hernias in the Groin (p. 381).

See Table 10-4, Differentiation of Hernias in the Groin (p. 382).

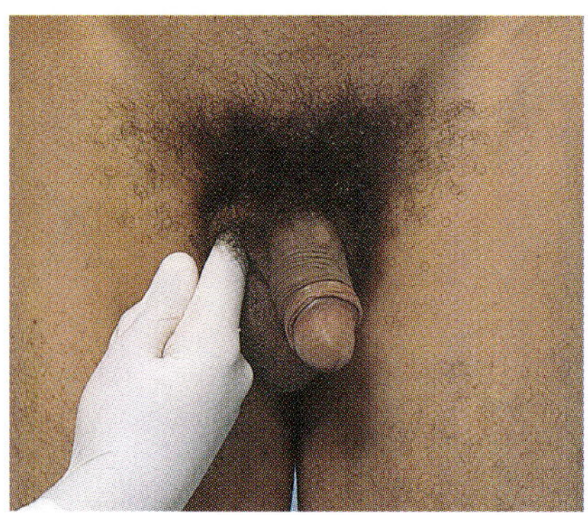

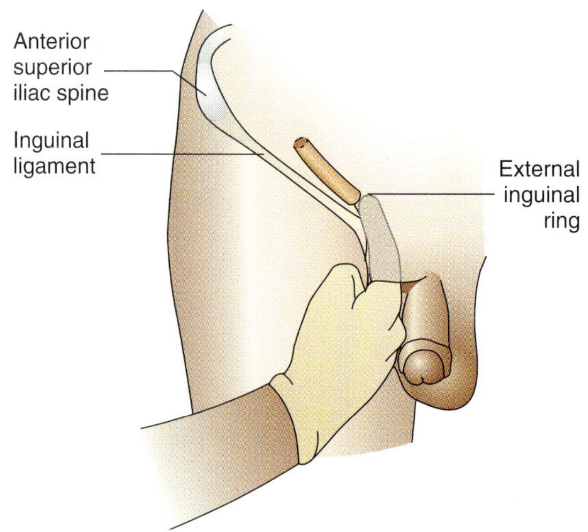

Palpate for a femoral hernia by placing your fingers on the anterior thigh in the region of the femoral canal. Ask the patient to strain down again or cough. Note any swelling or tenderness.

Evaluating a Possible Scrotal Hernia. If you find a large scrotal mass and suspect that it may be a hernia, ask the patient to lie down. The mass may return to the abdomen by itself. If so, it is a hernia. If not:

- Can you get your fingers above the mass in the scrotum?

If you can, suspect a hydrocele.

- Listen to the mass with a stethoscope for bowel sounds.

Bowel sounds may be heard over a hernia, but not over a hydrocele.

If the findings suggest a hernia, gently try to reduce it (return it to the abdominal cavity) by sustained pressure with your fingers. Do not attempt this maneuver if the mass is tender or the patient reports nausea and vomiting.

A hernia is *incarcerated* when its contents cannot be returned to the abdominal cavity. A hernia is *strangulated* when the blood supply to the entrapped contents is compromised. Suspect strangulation in the presence of tenderness, nausea, and vomiting, and consider surgical intervention.

History may be helpful here. The patient can usually tell you what happens to his swelling on lying down and may be able to demonstrate how he reduces it himself. Remember to ask him.

Special Techniques

THE TESTICULAR SELF-EXAMINATION

The incidence of testicular cancer is low, about 4 per 100,000 men, but it is the most common cancer of young men between ages 15 and 35. Although the testicular self-examination (TSE) has not been formally endorsed as a screen for testicular carcinoma, you may wish to teach your patient the TSE to enhance health awareness and self-care. When detected early, testicular carcinoma has an excellent prognosis. Risk factors include: cryptorchidism, which confers a high risk of testicular carcinoma in the undescended testicle; a history of carcinoma in the contralateral testicle; mumps orchitis; an inguinal hernia; and a hydrocele in childhood.

PATIENT INSTRUCTIONS FOR THE TESTICULAR SELF-EXAMINATION

This examination is best performed after a warm bath or shower. The heat relaxes the scrotum and makes it easier to find anything unusual.

- Standing in front of a mirror, check for any swelling on the skin of the scrotum.
- Examine each testicle with both hands. Cup the index and middle fingers under the testicle and place the thumbs on top.
- Roll the testicle gently between the thumbs and fingers. One testicle may be larger than the other . . . that's normal, but be concerned about any lump or area of pain.
- Find the epididymis. This is a soft, tubelike structure at the back of the testicle that collects and carries sperm, not an abnormal lump.
- If you find any lump, don't wait. See your doctor. The lump may just be an infection, but if it is cancer, it will spread unless stopped by treatment.

*Adapted from the National Cancer Institute. Rex.nih.gov/WTNK_PUBS/testicular/testexam.htm. Accessed 9/27/01.

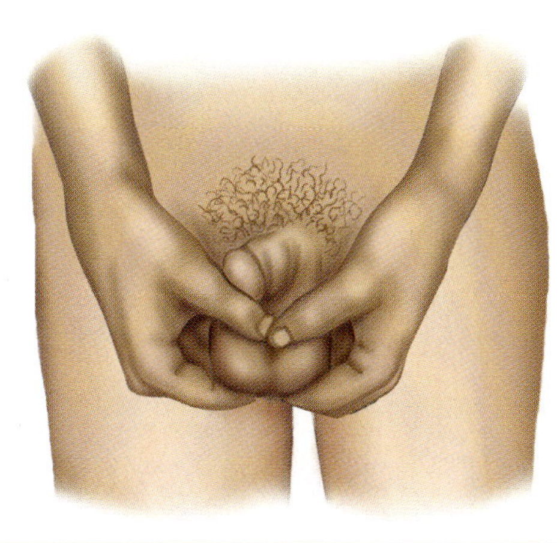

TABLE 10-1 ■ Abnormalities of the Penis

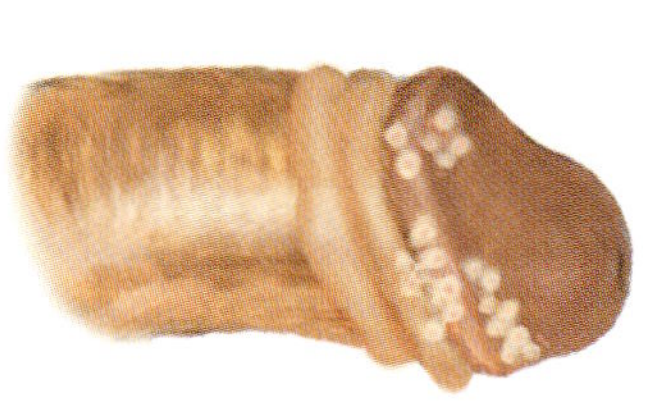

Venereal Wart
(Condyloma acuminatum)

Venereal warts are rapidly growing excrescences that are moist and often malodorous. They result from infection by human papillomavirus.

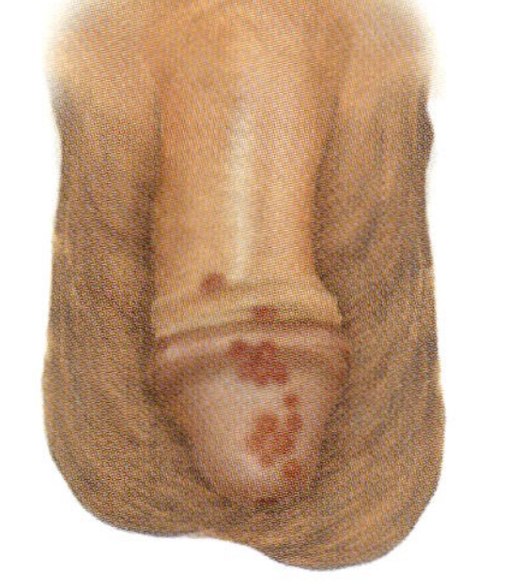

Genital Herpes

A cluster of small vesicles, followed by shallow, painful, nonindurated ulcers on red bases, suggests a herpes simplex infection. The lesions may occur anywhere on the penis. Usually there are fewer lesions when the infection recurs.

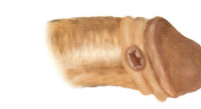

Syphilitic Chancre

A syphilitic chancre usually appears as an oval or round, dark red, painless erosion or ulcer with an indurated base. Nontender enlarged inguinal lymph nodes are typically associated. Chancres may be multiple, and when secondarily infected may be painful. They may then be mistaken for the lesions of herpes. Chancres are infectious.

Hypospadias

Hypospadias is a congenital displacement of the urethral meatus to the inferior surface of the penis. A groove extends from the actual urethral meatus to its normal location on the tip of the glans.

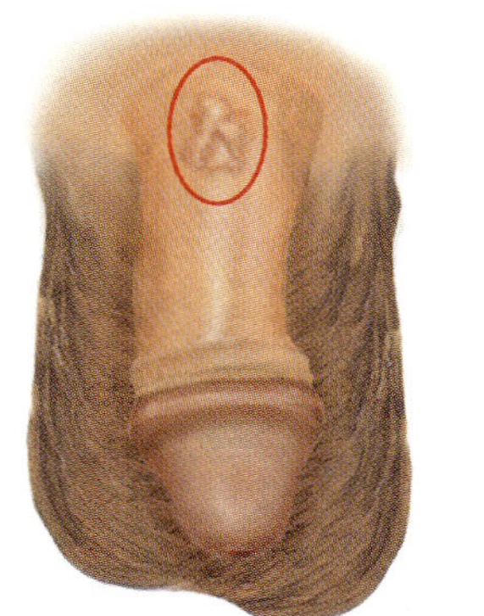

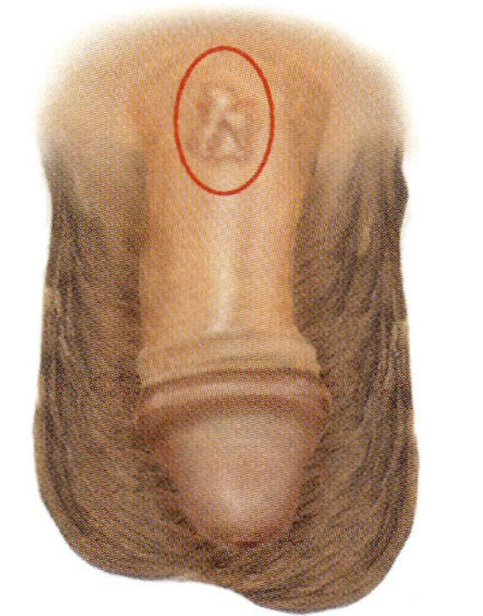

Peyronie's Disease

In Peyronie's disease, there are palpable nontender hard plaques just beneath the skin, usually along the dorsum of the penis. The patient complains of crooked, painful erections.

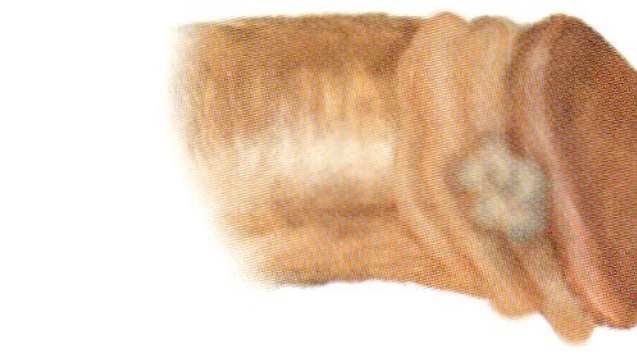

Carcinoma of the Penis

Carcinoma may appear as an indurated nodule or ulcer that is usually nontender. Limited almost completely to men who are not circumcised in childhood, it may be masked by the prepuce. Any persistent penile sore must be considered suspicious.

TABLE 10-2 ■ Abnormalities of the Male Genitalia

Hydrocele

A hydrocele is a nontender, fluid-filled mass within the tunica vaginalis. It transilluminates and the examining fingers can get above the mass within the scrotum.

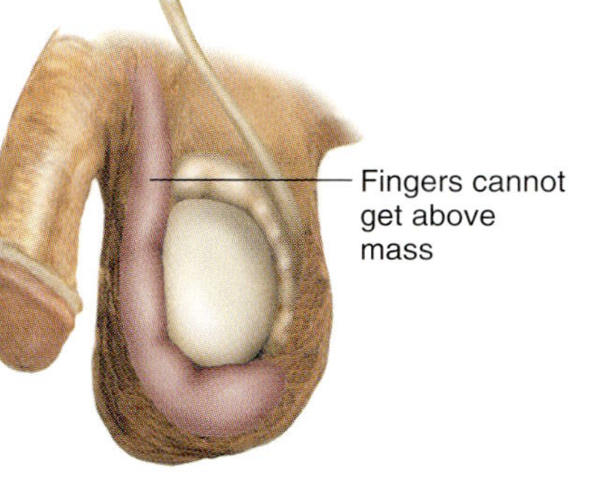

Scrotal Hernia

A hernia within the scrotum is usually an *indirect inguinal hernia*. It comes through the external inguinal ring, so the examining fingers cannot get above it in the scrotum.

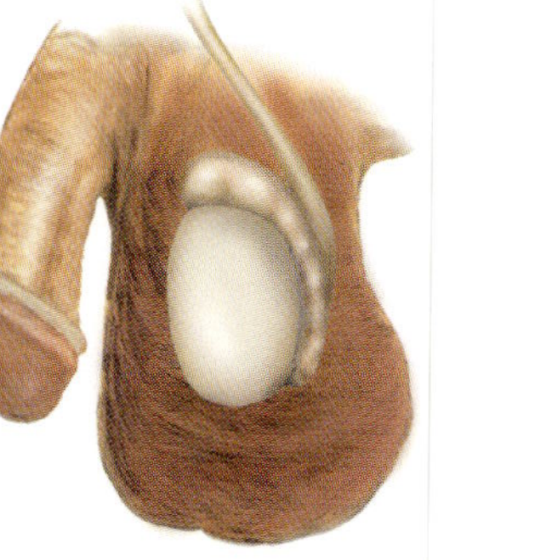

Scrotal Edema

Pitting edema may make the scrotal skin taut. This may accompany the generalized edema of congestive heart failure or nephrotic syndrome.

Cryptorchidism

In cryptorchidism, the testis is atrophied and may lie in the inguinal canal or the abdomen, resulting in an undeveloped scrotum as above. There is no palpable left testis or epididymis. Cryptorchidism markedly raises the risk of testicular cancer.

Acute Orchitis

The testis is acutely inflamed, painful, tender, and swollen. It may be difficult to distinguish from the epididymis. The scrotum may be reddened. Seen in mumps and other viral infections; usually unilateral.

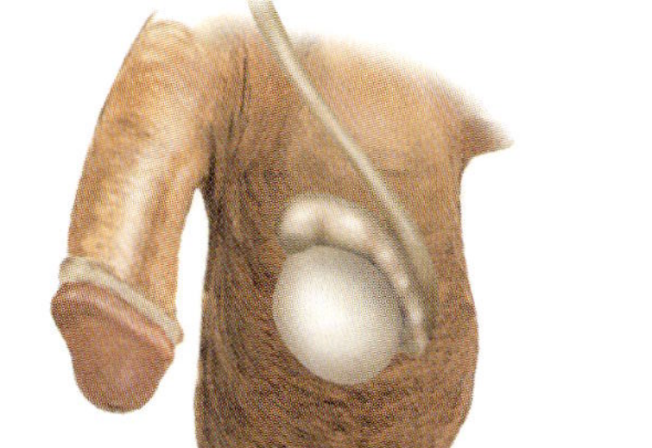
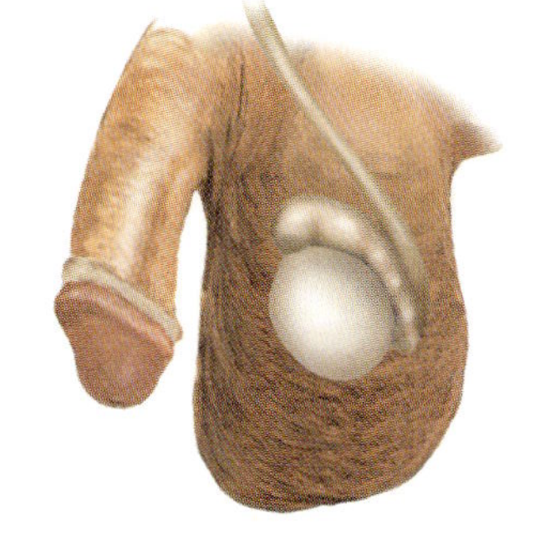
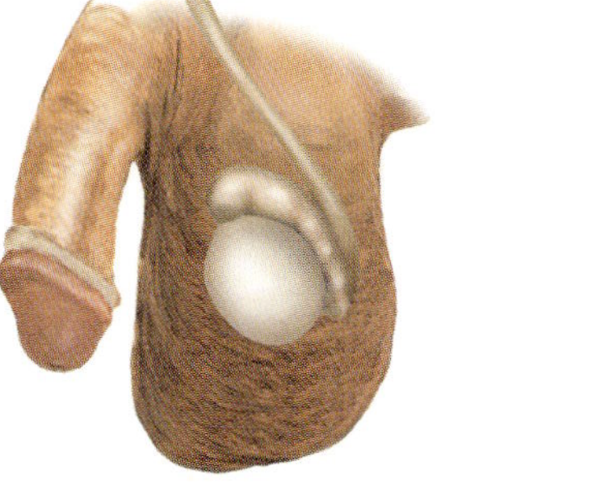

Small Testis

In adults, the length is usually ≤ 3.5 cm. Small firm testes in *Klinefelter's syndrome*, usually ≤ 2 cm. Small soft testes suggesting atrophy seen in cirrhosis, mytonic dystrophy, use of estrogens, hypopituitarism; may also follow orchitis.

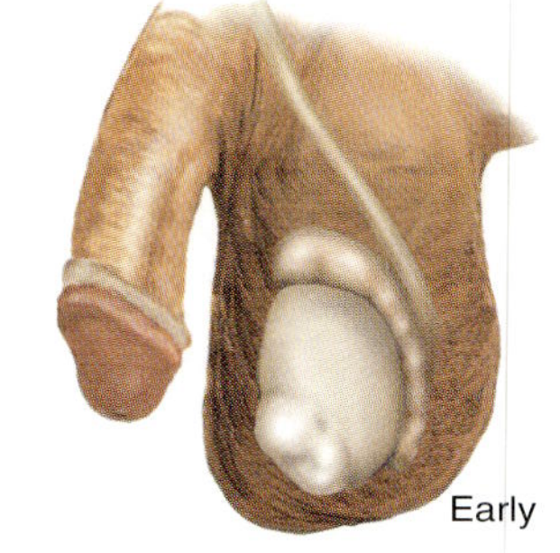

Tumor of the Testis

Usually appears as a painless nodule. Any nodule within the testis warrants investigation for malignancy.

As a testicular neoplasm grows and spreads, it may seem to replace the entire organ. The testicle characteristically feels heavier than normal.

(table continues next page)

TABLE 10-2 ■ Abnormalities of the Male Genitalia *(Continued)*

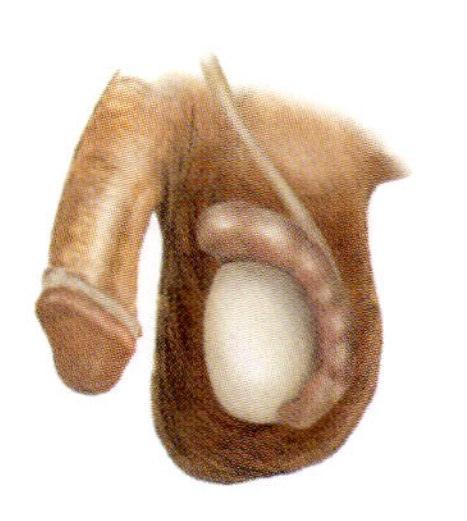

Acute Epididymitis

An acutely inflamed epididymis is tender and swollen and may be difficult to distinguish from the testis. The scrotum may be reddened, and the vas deferens inflamed. It occurs chiefly in adults. Coexisting urinary tract infection or prostatitis supports the diagnosis.

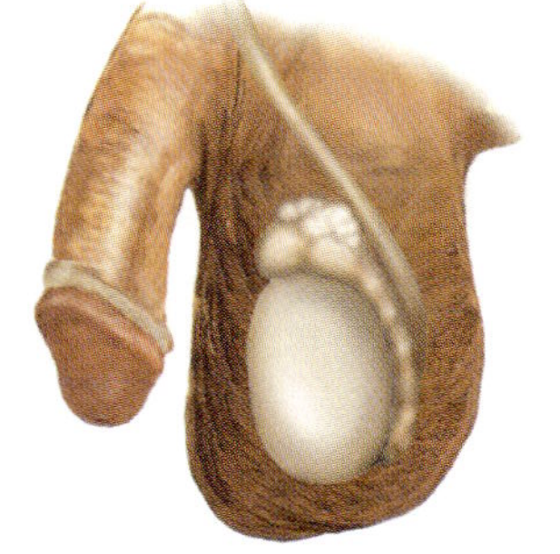

Spermatocele and Cyst of the Epididymis

A painless, movable cystic mass just above the testis suggests a spermatocele or an epididymal cyst. Both transilluminate. The former contains sperm and the latter does not, but they are clinically indistinguishable.

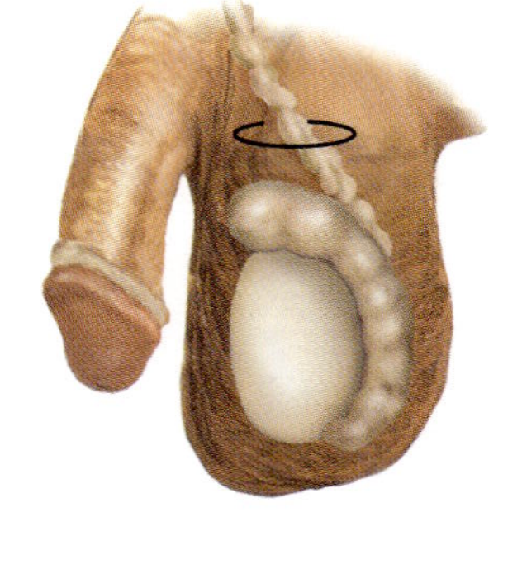

Tuberculous Epididymitis

The chronic inflammation of tuberculosis produces a firm enlargement of the epididymis, which is sometimes tender, with thickening or beading of the vas deferens.

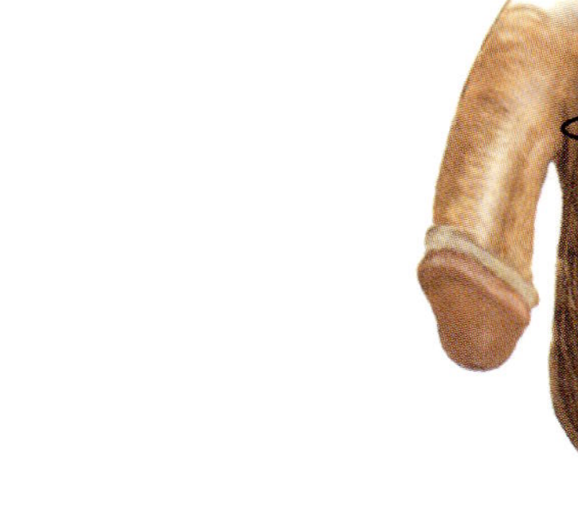

Varicocele

Varicocele refers to varicose veins of the spermatic cord, usually found on the left. It feels like a soft "bag of worms" separate from the testis, and slowly collapses when the scrotum is elevated in the supine patient. Infertility may be associated.

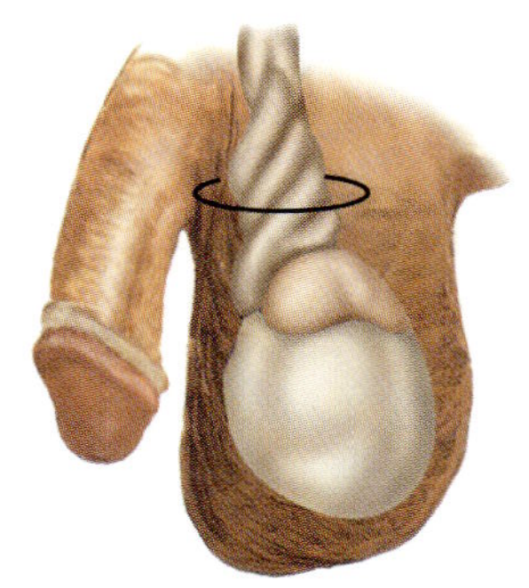
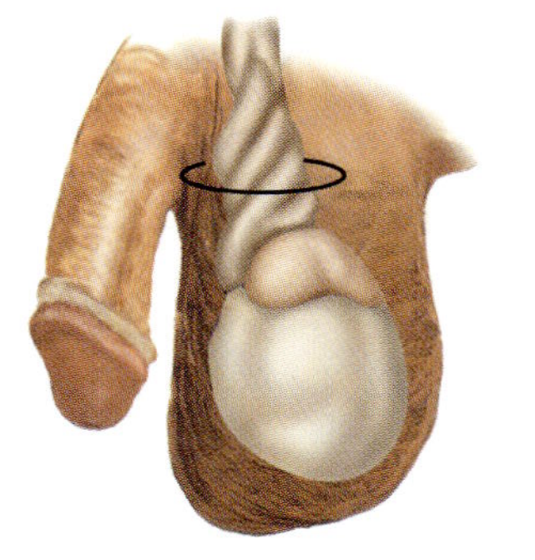

Torsion of the Spermatic Cord

Torsion, or twisting, of the testicle on its spermatic cord produces an acutely painful, tender, and swollen organ that is retracted upward in the scrotum. The scrotum becomes red and edematous. There is no associated urinary infection. Torsion, most common in adolescents, is a surgical emergency because of obstructed circulation.

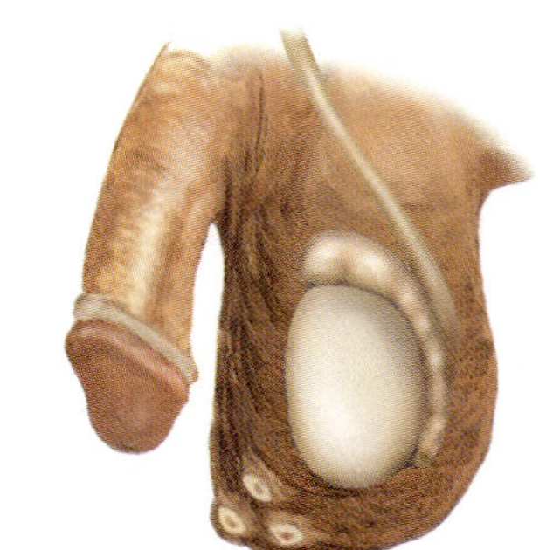

Epidermoid Cysts

These are firm, yellowish, nontender, cutaneous cysts up to about 1 cm in diameter. They are common and frequently multiple.

TABLE 10-3 ■ Course and Presentation of Hernias in the Groin

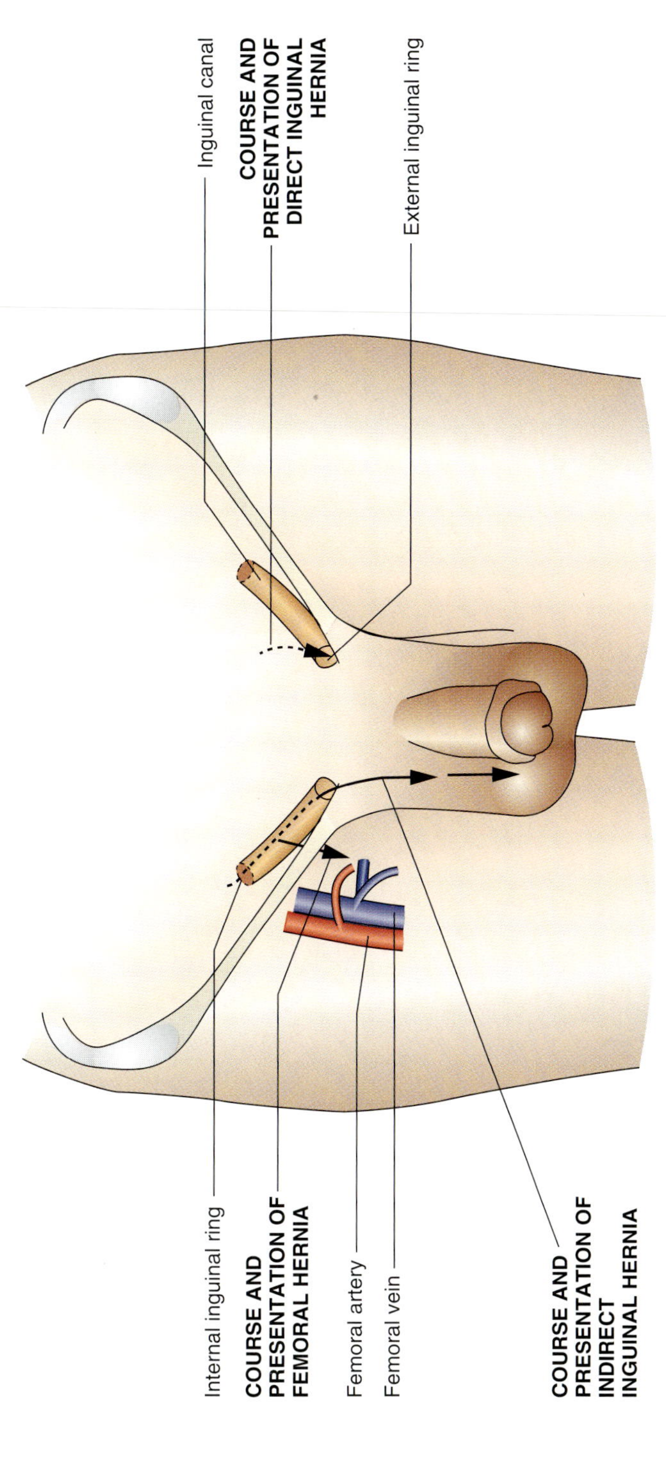

TABLE 10-4 ■ Differentiation of Hernias in the Groin

Differentiation among these hernias is not always clinically possible. Understanding their features, however, improves your observation.

	Inguinal		
	Indirect	*Direct*	**Femoral**
Frequency	Most common, all ages, both sexes	Less common	Least common
Age and Sex	Often in children, may be in adults	Usually in men over age 40, rare in women	More common in women than in men
Point of Origin	Above inguinal ligament, near its midpoint (the internal inguinal ring)	Above inguinal ligament, close to the pubic tubercle (near the external inguinal ring)	Below the inguinal ligament; appears more lateral than an inguinal hernia and may be hard to differentiate from lymph nodes
Course	Often into the scrotum	Rarely into the scrotum	Never into the scrotum
With the examining finger in the inguinal canal during straining or cough	The hernia comes down the inguinal canal and touches the fingertip.	The hernia bulges anteriorly and pushes the side of the finger forward.	The inguinal canal is empty.

CHAPTER

11

Female Genitalia

ANATOMY AND PHYSIOLOGY

Review the anatomy of the external female genitalia (vulva), including the *mons pubis,* a hair-covered fat pad overlying the symphysis pubis; the *labia majora,* rounded folds of adipose tissue; the *labia minora,* thinner pinkish red folds that extend anteriorly to form the *prepuce;* and the *clitoris.* The *vestibule* is the boat-shaped fossa between the labia minora. In its posterior portion lies the vaginal opening (*introitus*), which in virgins may be hidden by the *hymen*. The term *perineum,* as commonly used clinically, refers to the tissue between the introitus and the anus.

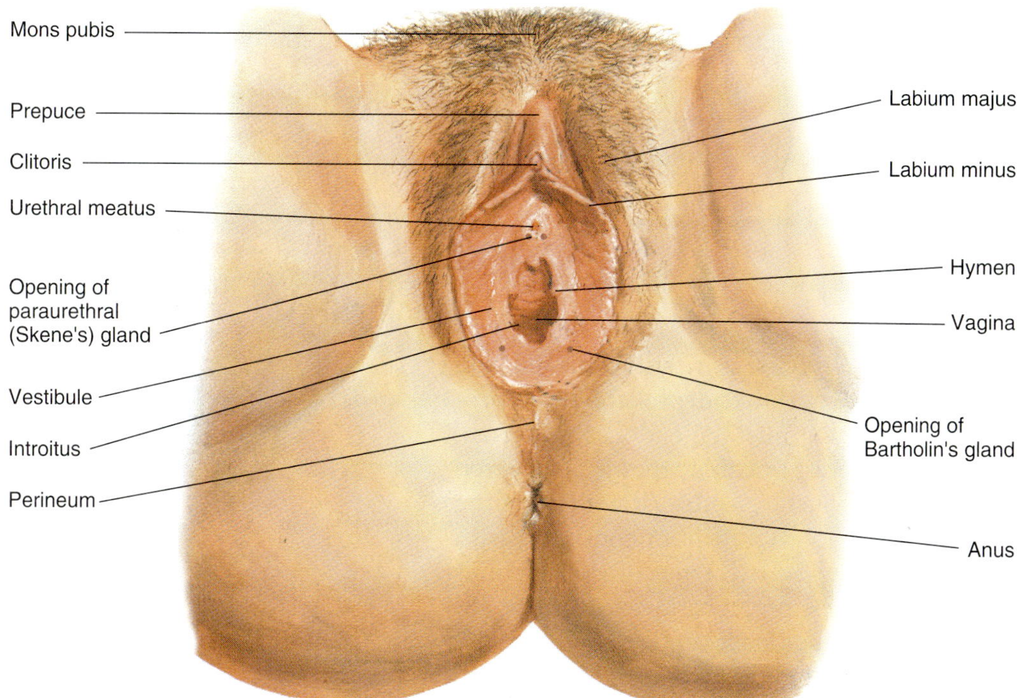

The *urethral meatus* opens into the vestibule between the clitoris and the vagina. Just posterior to it on either side lie the openings of the *paraurethral* (Skene's) *glands.*

The openings of *Bartholin's glands* are located posteriorly on either side of the vaginal opening, but are not usually visible. Bartholin's glands themselves are situated more deeply.

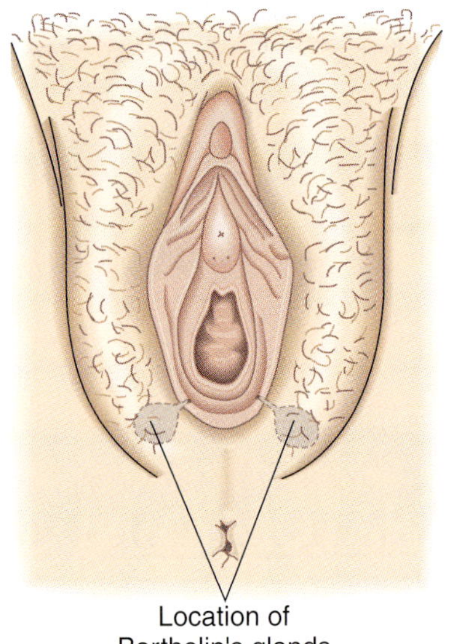

The *vagina* is a hollow tube extending upward and posteriorly between the urethra and the rectum. Its upper third takes a horizontal plane and terminates in the cup-shaped *fornix*. The vaginal mucosa lies in transverse folds, or rugae.

At almost right angles to the vagina sits the *uterus*, a flattened fibromuscular structure shaped like an inverted pear. The uterus has two parts: the body (corpus) and the cervix, which are joined together by the isthmus. The convex upper surface of the body is called the *fundus* of the uterus. The lower part of the uterus, the *cervix*, protrudes into the vagina, dividing the fornix into anterior, posterior, and lateral fornices.

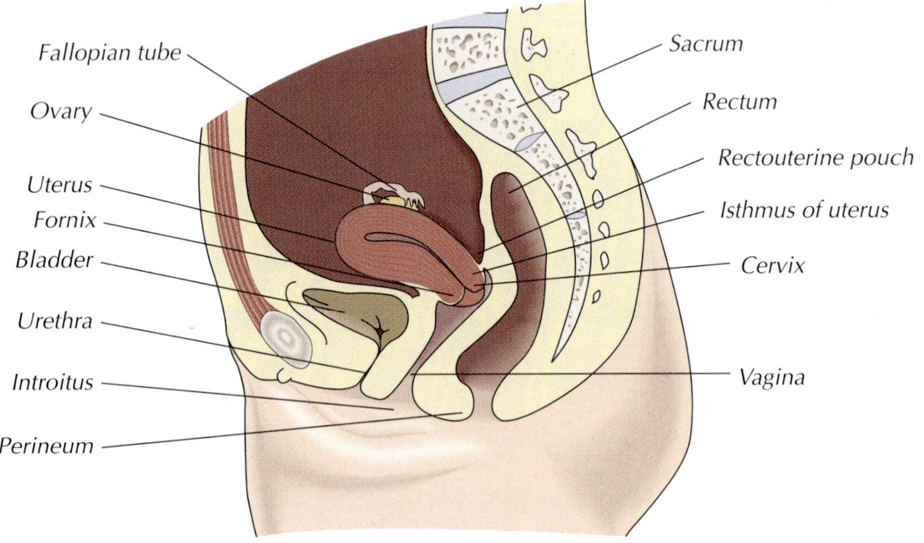

The vaginal surface of the cervix, the *ectocervix*, is seen easily with the help of a speculum. At its center is a round, oval, or slitlike depression, the *external os* of the cervix, which marks the opening into the endocervical canal. The ectocervix is covered by epithelium of two possible types: a plushy, red columnar epithelium surrounding the os, which resembles the lining of the endocervical canal; and a shiny pink squamous epithelium continous with the vaginal lining. The boundary between these two types of epithelium is the *squamocolumnar junction*. In puberty, the broad band of columnar epithelium encircling the os, called *ectropion*, is gradually replaced by columnar epithelium. The squamocolumnar junction migrates toward the os, creating the *transformation zone*. (This is the area at risk for later dysplasia, which is sampled by the Papanicolaou, or Pap, smear.)

A *fallopian tube* with a fanlike tip extends from each side of the uterus toward the ovary. The two ovaries are almond-shaped structures that vary con-

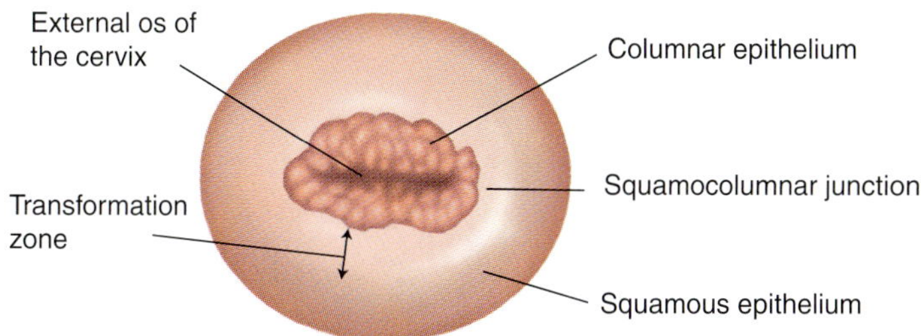

siderably in size but average about 3.5 × 2 × 1.5 cm from adulthood through menopause. The ovaries are palpable on pelvic examination in roughly half of women during the reproductive years. Normally, fallopian tubes cannot be felt. The term *adnexa* (a plural Latin word meaning appendages) refers to the ovaries, tubes, and supporting tissues.

The ovaries have two primary functions: the production of ova and the secretion of hormones, including estrogen, progesterone, and testosterone. Increased hormonal secretions during puberty stimulate the growth of the uterus and its endometrial lining. They enlarge the vagina and thicken its epithelium. They also stimulate the development of secondary sex characteristics, including the breasts and pubic hair.

The parietal peritoneum extends downward behind the uterus into a cul de sac called the *rectouterine pouch* (pouch of Douglas). You can just reach this area on rectovaginal examination.

The pelvic organs are supported by a sling of tissues composed of muscle, ligaments, and fascia, through which the urethra, vagina, and rectum all pass.

Lymphatics. Lymph from the vulva and the lower vagina drains into the inguinal nodes. Lymph from the internal genitalia, including the upper vagina, flows into the pelvic and abdominal lymph nodes, which are not palpable clinically.

Changes With Aging

During the pubertal years, the vulva and the internal genitalia grow and change to their adult proportions. Assessment of sexual maturity in girls, as classified by Tanner, depends not on internal examination, however, but on the growth of pubic hair and the development of breasts. Tanner's stages, or sexual maturity ratings, as they relate to pubic hair and breasts are shown in Chapter 17, Assessing Children: Infancy Through Adolescence.

In most women, pubic hair spreads downward in a triangular pattern, pointing toward the vagina. In 10% of women, it may form an inverted triangle, pointing toward the umbilicus. This growth is usually not completed until the middle 20s or later.

Just before menarche there is a physiologic increase in vaginal secretions—a normal change that sometimes worries a girl or her mother. As menses become established, increased secretions (*leukorrhea*) coincide with ovulation. They also accompany sexual arousal. These normal kinds of discharges must be differentiated from those of infectious processes.

Ovarian function usually starts to diminish during a woman's 40s, and menstrual periods cease on the average between the ages of 45 and 52, sometimes earlier and sometimes later. Pubic hair becomes sparse as well as gray. As estrogen stimulation falls, the labia and the clitoris become smaller. The vagina narrows and shortens and its mucosa becomes thin, pale, and dry. The uterus and ovaries diminish in size. Once menopause has occurred, the ovaries may no longer be palpable. The suspensory ligaments of the adnexa, uterus, and bladder may also relax.

THE HEALTH HISTORY

Common or Concerning Symptoms

- Menarche, menstruation, menopause
- Pregnancy
- Vulvovaginal symptoms
- Sexual activity

Questions in this section focus on menstruation, pregnancy and related topics, vulvovaginal symptoms, and sexual function.

Menarche, Menstruation, Menopause. For the menstrual history, ask the patient how old she was when her monthly, or menstrual, periods began (age at *menarche*). When did her last period start, and, if possible, the one before that? How often do the periods come (as measured by the intervals between the first days of successive periods)? How regular or irregular are they? How long do they last? How heavy is the flow? What color is it? Flow can be assessed roughly by the number of pads or tampons used daily. Because women vary in their practices for sanitary measures, however, ask the patient whether she usually soaks a pad or tampon, spots it lightly, etc. Further, does she use more than one at a time? Does she have any bleeding between periods? Any bleeding after intercourse or after douching?

The dates of previous periods may alert you to possible pregnancy or menstrual irregularities.

Unlike the normal dark red menstrual discharge, excessive flow tends to be bright red and may include "clots" (not true fibrin clots).

Does the patient have any discomfort or pain before or during her periods? If so, what is it like, how long does it last, and does it interfere with her usual activities? Are there other associated symptoms? Ask a middle-aged or older woman if she has stopped menstruating. When? Did any symptoms accompany her change? Has she had any bleeding since?

Questions about *menarche, menstruation,* and *menopause* often give you an opportunity to explore the patient's need for information and her attitude toward her body. When talking with an adolescent girl, for example, opening questions might include: "How did you first learn about monthly periods? How did you feel when they started? Many girls worry when their periods aren't regular or come late. Has anything like that bothered you?" You can explain that girls in the United States usually begin to menstruate between the ages of 9 and 16 years, and often take a year or more before they settle into a reasonable, regular pattern. Age at menarche is variable, depending on genetic endowment, socioeconomic status, and nutrition. The interval between periods ranges roughly from 24 to 32 days; the flow lasts from 3 to 7 days.

Menopause, the absence of menses for 12 consecutive months, usually occurs between the ages of 45 and 52 years. Associated symptoms include hot flashes, flushing, sweating, and disturbances of sleep. Often you will ask, "How do (did) you feel about not having your periods anymore? Has it affected your life in any way?" *Postmenopausal bleeding* is defined as bleeding that occurs after 6 months without periods and warrants further investigation.

Postmenopausal bleeding raises the question of endometrial cancer, although it also has other causes.

Amenorrhea refers to the absence of periods. Failure to initiate periods is called *primary amenorrhea,* while the cessation of periods after they have been established is termed *secondary amenorrhea.* Pregnancy, lactation, and menopause are physiologic forms of the secondary type. *Oligomenorrhea* refers to infrequent periods, which may also be irregular. This pattern is common for as long as 2 years after menarche, and it also occurs before menopause.

Other causes of secondary amenorrhea include low body weight from any cause, including malnutrition and anorexia nervosa, stress, chronic illness, and hypothalamic–pituitary–ovarian dysfunction.

Dysmenorrhea is pain with menstruation, and is usually felt as a bearing down, aching, or cramping sensation in the lower abdomen and pelvis. Women may report *premenstrual syndrome (PMS),* a complex of symptoms occurring 4 to 10 days before a period. PMS symptoms include tension, nervousness, irritability, depression, and mood swings; weight gain, abdominal bloating, edema, and tenderness of the breasts; and headaches. Though usually mild, PMS symptoms may be severe and disabling.

Polymenorrhea means abnormally frequent periods, and *menorrhagia* refers to an increased amount or duration of flow. Bleeding may also occur between periods, termed *metrorrhagia* or *intermenstrual bleeding,* after intercourse (*postcoital bleeding*), or after other vaginal contact from practices such as douching.

Increased frequency, increased flow, or bleeding between periods may have systemic causes or may be dysfunctional. Postcoital bleeding suggests cervical disease (e.g., polyps, cancer) or, in an older woman, atrophic vaginitis.

Pregnancy. Questions relating to pregnancy include: "Have you ever been (or how often have you been) pregnant? Have you ever had a miscarriage or an abortion? How often? How many living children do you have?" Inquire about any difficulties with the pregnancies and the timing and the circumstances of any abortion (spontaneous or induced). What kind of birth control methods, if any, have the patient and her partner used, and how satisfied is she with them?

If amenorrhea suggests a *current pregnancy,* inquire about the history of intercourse and *common early symptoms:* tenderness, tingling, or increased size of the breasts; urinary frequency; nausea and vomiting; easy fatigability; and feelings that the baby is moving (the last usually noted at about 20 weeks).

Amenorrhea followed by heavy bleeding suggests a threatened abortion or dysfunctional uterine bleeding related to lack of ovulation.

Be alert to the patient's feelings in discussing all these topics and explore them as seems indicated. (See also Chapter 12, The Pregnant Woman).

Vulvovaginal Symptoms. The most common vulvovaginal symptoms are *vaginal discharge* and local *itching*. Follow your usual approach. If the patient reports a discharge, inquire about its amount, color, consistency, and odor. Ask about any local *sores* or *lumps* in the vulvar area. Are they painful or not? Because patients vary in their understanding of anatomic terms, be prepared to try alternative phrasing such as "Any itching (or other symptoms) near your vagina? . . . between your legs? . . . where you urinate?"

See Table 11-1, Lesions of the Vulva, p. 401; also Table 11-5, Vaginitis, p. 405.

Sexual Activity. Start with general questions such as "How is sex for you?" Or "Are you having any problems with sex?" You can also ask, "Are you satisfied with your sex life as it is now? Has there been any significant change in the last few years? Are you satisfied with you ability to perform sexually? How satisfied do you think your partner is? Do you feel that your partner is satisfied with the frequency of sexual activity?"

If the patient seems to have a sexual problem, ask her to tell you about it. Direct questions help you assess each phase of the sexual response: desire, arousal, and orgasm. "Do you have an interest in (appetite for) sex?" inquires about the desire phase. For the orgasmic phase, "Are you able to reach climax (reach an orgasm or 'come')?" "Is it important for you to reach climax?" For arousal, "Do you get sexually aroused? Do you lubricate easily (get wet or slippery)? Do you stay too dry?"

Sexual dysfunctions are classified by the phase of sexual response. A woman may lack desire, she may fail to become aroused and to attain adequate vaginal lubrication, or, despite adequate arousal, she may be unable to reach orgasm much or all of the time. Causes include lack of estrogen, medical illness, and psychiatric conditions.

Ask also about *dyspareunia*, or discomfort or pain during intercourse. If present, try to localize the symptom. Is it near the outside, occurring at the start of intercourse, or does she feel it farther in, when her partner is pushing deeper? *Vaginismus* refers to an involuntary spasm of the muscles surrounding the vaginal orifice that makes penetration during intercourse painful or impossible.

Superficial pain suggests local inflammation, atrophic vaginitis, or inadequate lubrication; deeper pain may be due to pelvic disorders or pressure on a normal ovary. The cause of vaginismus may be physical or psychological.

In addition to ascertaining the nature of a sexual problem, ask about its onset, severity (persistent or sporadic), setting, and factors, if any, that make it better or worse. What does the patient think is the cause of the problem, what has she tried to do about it, and what does she hope for? The setting of sexual dysfunction is an important but complicated topic, involving the patient's general health, medications and drugs, including use of alcohol, her partner's and her own knowledge of sexual practices and techniques, her attitudes, values, and fears, the relationship and communication between her and her partner(s), and the setting in which sexual activity takes place.

More commonly, however, a sexual problem is related to situational or psychosocial factors.

Local symptoms or findings on physical examination may raise the possibility of *sexually transmitted diseases* (STDs). After establishing the usual attributes of any symptoms, identify the sexual preference as to partners (male, female, or both). Inquire about sexual contacts and establish the number of sexual partners in the prior month. Ask if the patient has concerns about HIV infection, desires HIV testing, or has current or past partners at risk. Also ask about oral and anal sex and, if indicated, about symptoms involving the mouth, throat, anus, and rectum. Review the past history of venereal disease. "Have you ever had herpes? . . . any other problems such as gonorrhea? . . . syphilis? . . . pelvic infections?" Continue with the more general questions suggested on pp. 45–46.

HEALTH PROMOTION AND COUNSELING

Important Topics for Health Promotion and Counseling

- The Pap smear
- Options for family planning
- Sexually transmitted diseases and HIV
- Changes in menopause

The Pap Smear. Widespread testing by Papanicolaou (Pap) smear has contributed to a significant drop in the incidence of invasive cervical cancer. Careful technique to ensure sampling of endocervical cells at the squamocolumnar junction and use of accredited laboratories to interpret smears improve accuracy of the test. Screening should begin at age 18 or with onset of sexual activity. Recommendations about frequency of testing are undergoing revision. Annual testing until age 65 has been common, but does not appear to improve detection compared to longer intervals. A number of professional organizations recommend annual Pap smears for 3 years and then, if these are normal, less frequent testing based on clinician discretion. The U.S. Preventive Health Services Task Force recommends a 3-year interval beginning with onset of sexual activity. More frequent testing is warranted for women at increased risk—those with early onset of sexual activity, multiple partners, infection with human papillomavirus or HIV, or limited access to regular medical care. The upper age limit for the Pap smear testing is not well established. For women over 65, continued testing is indicated if recent tests have been abnormal or screening over the prior 10 years has been incomplete. Women who have never had sexual intercourse or with complete hysterectomies (cervix removed) do not require screening.

Options for Family Planning. It is important to counsel women, particularly adolescents, about the timing of ovulation in the menstrual cycle and how to plan or prevent pregnancy. Survey data indicate that more than half of U.S. pregnancies are unintended, affecting up to 80% of the one million teen pregnancies each year.* Clinicians should be familiar with the numerous op-

*U.S. Preventive Health Services Task Force: Guide to Clinical Preventive Services, 2nd ed. Baltimore, Williams & Wilkins, 1996, pp. 739–740.

tions for family planning and their effectiveness. These include: natural methods (periodic abstinence, withdrawal, lactation); barrier methods (condom, diaphragm, cervical cap); implantable methods (intrauterine device, subdermal implant); pharmacologic interventions (spermicide, birth control pill, subdermal implant of levonorgestrel, estrogen/progesterone injectables); and surgery (tubal ligation). The clinician must take the time to understand the patient or couple's concerns and preferences and respect these preferences whenever possible. Continued use of a preferred method is superior to a more effective method that is abandoned. For teenagers, providing a confidential setting eases discussion of topics that may seem private and difficult to explore.

STDs and HIV. As with men, the clinician should assess risk factors for infection with STDs and HIV by taking a careful sexual history and counseling patients about spread of disease and ways to reduce high-risk practices (see Chap. 2, pp. 45–46). Women with STDs are at higher risk for asymptomatic infection and loss of fertility. Learn to assess women for genital and pelvic infections through careful examination and collection of appropriate cultures and to apply recommended guidelines for serologic testing for infection with HIV (see Chap. 10, pp. 371–373).

Changes in Menopause. For middle-aged and older women, the clinician should be familiar with the psychological and physiologic changes of menopause—mood shifts and changes in self-concept, vasomotor changes ("hot flashes"), accelerated bone loss, increases in total and LDL cholesterol, and vulvo-vaginal atrophy leading to symptoms of vaginal drying, dysuria, and sometimes dyspareunia. The clinician must be knowledgeable about estrogen and progesterone replacement therapy and help the patient to weigh the benefits and risks of treatment, taking into account the personal and family history of cardiovascular disease and osteoporosis (risk of developing these conditions decreases with hormone treatment) and breast cancer and endometrial cancer (treatment increases risk). Counseling patients about these decisions may extend over several visits.

Preview: Recording the Pelvic Examination—Female Genitalia

Note that initially you may use sentences to describe your findings; later you will use phrases. The style below contains phrases appropriate for most write-ups. Unfamiliar terms are explained in the next section, "Techniques of Examination."

"No inguinal adenopathy. External genitalia without erythema or lesions; no lesions or masses. Vaginal mucosa pink. Cervix parous, pink, and without discharge. Uterus anterior, midline, smooth, and not enlarged. No adnexal tenderness. Pap smear obtained. Rectovaginal wall intact."

OR

"Bilateral spotty inguinal adenopathy. External genitalia without erythema or lesions. Vaginal mucosa and cervix coated with thin white homogeneous discharge with mild fishy odor. After swabbing cervix, no discharge visible in cervical os. Uterus midline; no adnexal masses. Rectal vault without masses. Stool brown and hemoccult negative."

Suggests bacterial vaginosis.

TECHNIQUES OF EXAMINATION

Important Areas of Examination

External Examination

- Mons pubis
- Labia majora and minora
- Urethral meatus, clitoris
- Vaginal introitus
- Perineum

Internal Examination

- Vagina, vaginal walls
- Cervix
- Uterus, ovaries
- Pelvic muscles
- Rectovaginal wall

Many students feel anxious or uncomfortable when first examining the genitalia of another person. At the same time, patients have their own concerns. Some women have had painful, embarrassing, or even demeaning experiences during previous pelvic examinations, while others may be facing their first examination. Patients may fear what the clinician will find and how these findings may affect their lives.

The woman's reactions and behavior give important clues to her feelings and to attitudes toward sexuality. If she adducts her thighs, pulls away, or expresses negative feelings during the examination, you can gently confront her as you would during the interview. "I notice you are having some trouble relaxing. Is it just being here, or are you troubled by the examination? . . . is anything worrying you?" Behaviors that seem to present an obstacle to your examination may become the key to understanding your patient's concerns. Adverse reactions may be a sign of prior abuse, and these issues should be explored.

A patient who has never had a pelvic examination is often unsure of what to expect. Try to shape the experience so that she learns about her body and the steps of the pelvic examination, and becomes more comfortable with them. Before she undresses, explain the relevant anatomy with the help of three-dimensional models. Show her the speculum and other equipment and encourage her to handle them during the examination so that she can better understand your explanations and procedures. It is especially important to avoid hurting the patient during her first encounter.

Indications for a pelvic examination during adolescence include menstrual abnormalities such as amenorrhea, excessive bleeding, or dysmenorrhea, unexplained abdominal pain, vaginal discharge, the prescription of contraceptives, bacteriologic and cytologic studies in a sexually active girl, and the patient's own desire for assessment.

Regardless of age, rape merits special evaluation, usually requiring gynecologic consultation and documentation.

TIPS FOR THE SUCCESSFUL PELVIC EXAMINATION

The Patient	*The Examiner*
■ Avoids intercourse, douching, or use of vaginal suppositories for 24 to 48 hours before examination ■ Empties bladder before examination ■ Lies supine, with head and shoulders slightly elevated, arms at sides or folded across chest to reduce tightening of abdominal muscles	■ Explains each step of the examination in advance ■ Drapes patient from mid-abdomen to knees; depresses drape between knees to provide eye contact with patient ■ Avoids unexpected or sudden movements ■ Warms speculum with tap water ■ Monitors comfort of the examination by watching the patient's face ■ Uses excellent but gentle technique, especially when inserting the speculum (see below).

Be sure always to wear gloves, both during the examination and when handling equipment and specimens. Plan ahead, so that any needed equipment or culture media are readily at hand.

Helping the patient to relax is essential for an adequate examination. Be sensitive to her feelings. Adopting the tips above will help ensure the patient's comfort.

Choosing Equipment. You should have within reach a good light, a vaginal speculum of appropriate size, water-soluble lubricant, and equipment for taking Papanicolaou smears, bacteriologic cultures, or other diagnostic tests. Review the supplies and procedures of your own facility before taking cultures and other samples.

Specula are made of metal or plastic, and come in two basic shapes, named for Pedersen and Graves. Both are available in small, medium, and large sizes. The medium Pedersen speculum is usually most comfortable for sexually active women. The narrow-bladed Pedersen speculum is best for the patient with a relatively small introitus, such as a virgin or an elderly woman. The Graves specula are best suited for parous women with vaginal prolapse.

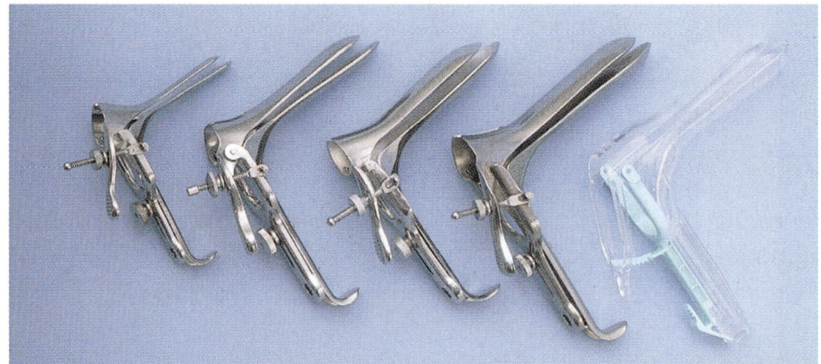

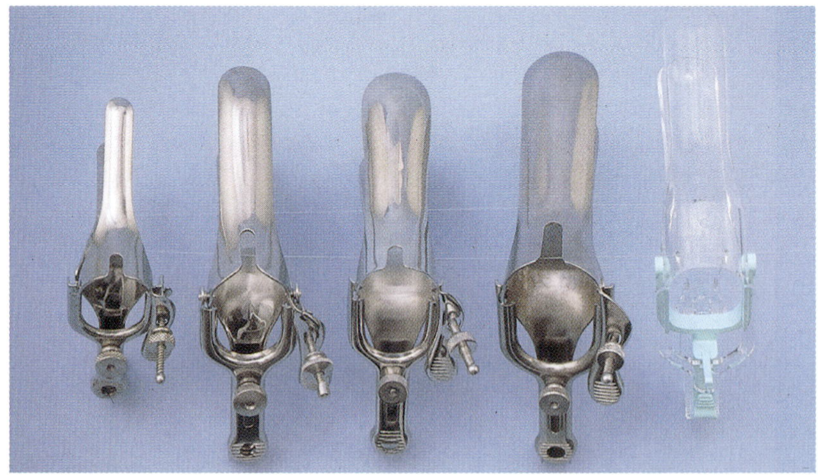

Speculae, from left to right: small metal Pedersen, medium metal Pedersen, medium metal Graves, large metal Graves, and large plastic Pedersen

Before using a speculum, become thoroughly familiar with how to open and close its blades, lock the blades in an open position, and release them again. Although the instructions in this chapter refer to a metal speculum, you can easily adapt them to a plastic one by handling the speculum before using it.

Plastic specula typically make a loud click or may pinch when locked or released. Forewarning the patient helps to avoid unnecessary surprise.

Male examiners should be accompanied by female assistants. Female examiners should also be assisted if the patient is physically or emotionally disturbed.

Positioning the Patient. Drape the patient appropriately and then assist her into the lithotomy position. Help her to place first one heel and then the other into the stirrups. She may be more comfortable with shoes on than with bare feet. Then ask her to slide all the way down the examining table until her buttocks extend slightly beyond the edge. Her thighs should be flexed, abducted, and externally rotated at the hips. A pillow should support her head.

EXTERNAL EXAMINATION

Assess the Sexual Maturity of an Adolescent Patient. You can assess pubic hair during either the abdominal or the pelvic examination. Note its character and distribution, and rate it according to Tanner's stages described on p. 714.

Delayed puberty is often familial or related to chronic illness. It may also be due to abnormalities in the hypothalamus, anterior pituitary gland, or ovaries.

Inspect the Patient's External Genitalia. Seat yourself comfortably and inspect the mons pubis, labia, and perineum. Separate the labia and inspect:

Excoriations or itchy, small, red maculopapules suggest pediculosis pubis (lice or "crabs"). Look for nits or lice at the bases of the pubic hairs.

- The labia minora
- The clitoris

Enlarged clitoris in masculinizing conditions

- The urethral meatus

Urethral caruncle, prolapse of the urethral mucosa (p. 402)

- The vaginal opening, or introitus

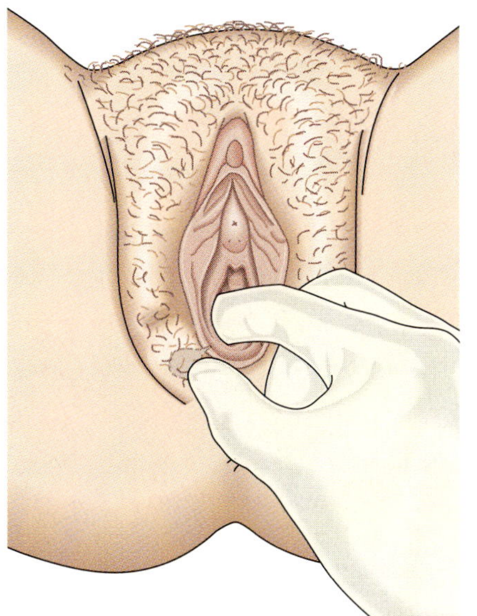

PALPATING BARTHOLIN'S GLAND

Note any inflammation, ulceration, discharge, swelling, or nodules. If there are any lesions, palpate them.

Syphilitic chancre, epidermoid cyst. See Table 11-1, Lesions of the Vulva (p. 401).

If there is a history or an appearance of labial swelling, check Bartholin's glands. Insert your index finger into the vagina near the posterior end of the introitus. Place your thumb outside the posterior part of the labium

A Bartholin's gland may become acutely or chronically infected and then produce a swelling. See Table 11-2, Bulges and Swelling of Vulva, Vagina, and Urethra (p. 402).

majus. On each side in turn, palpate between your finger and thumb for swelling or tenderness. Note any discharge exuding from the duct opening of the gland. If any is present, culture it.

INTERNAL EXAMINATION

Assess the Support of the Vaginal Walls. With the labia separated by your middle and index fingers, ask the patient to strain down. Note any bulging of the vaginal walls.

Bulging from a cystocele or rectocele. See Table 11-2, Bulges and Swelling of Vulva, Vagina, and Urethra (p. 402).

Insert the Speculum. Select a speculum of appropriate size and shape, and lubricate it with warm water. (Other lubricants may interfere with cytologic studies and bacterial or viral cultures.) You can enlarge the vaginal introitus by lubricating one finger with water and applying downward pressure at its lower margin. (You may also wish to check the location of the cervix to help angle the speculum more accurately.) Enlarging the introitus greatly eases insertion of the speculum and the patient's comfort. With your other hand (usually the left), introduce the closed speculum past your fingers at a somewhat downward slope. Be careful not to pull on the pubic hair or pinch the labia with the speculum. Separating the labia majora with your other hand can help to avoid this.

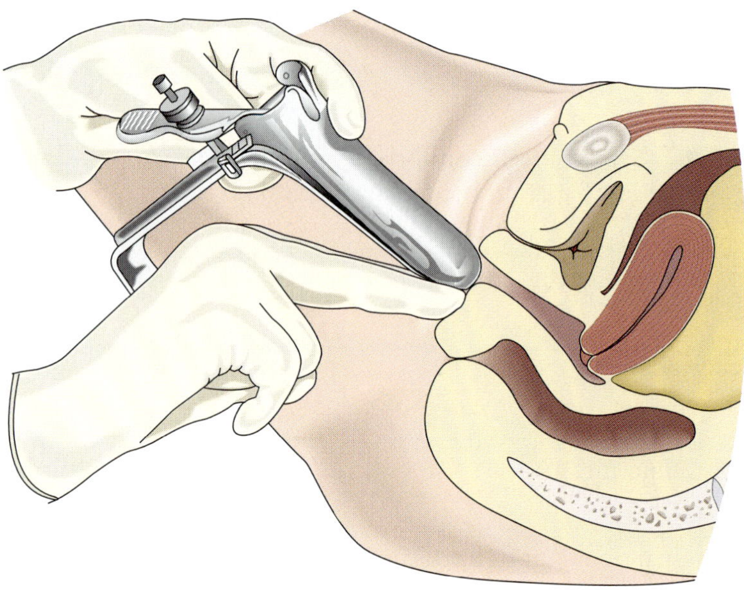

THE SMALL INTROITUS

Many virginal vaginal orifices admit a single examining finger. Modify your technique so as to use your index finger only. A small Pedersen speculum may make inspection possible. When the vaginal orifice is even smaller, a fairly good bimanual examination can be performed by placing one finger in the rectum rather than in the vagina.

Similar techniques may be indicated in elderly women in whom the introitus has become atrophied and tight.

An imperforate hymen occasionally delays menarche. Be sure to check for this possibility when menarche seems unduly late in relation to the development of a girl's breasts and pubic hair.

Two methods help you to avoid placing pressure on the sensitive urethra. (1) When inserting the speculum, hold it at an angle (shown below on the left), and then (2) slide the speculum inward along the posterior wall of the vagina.

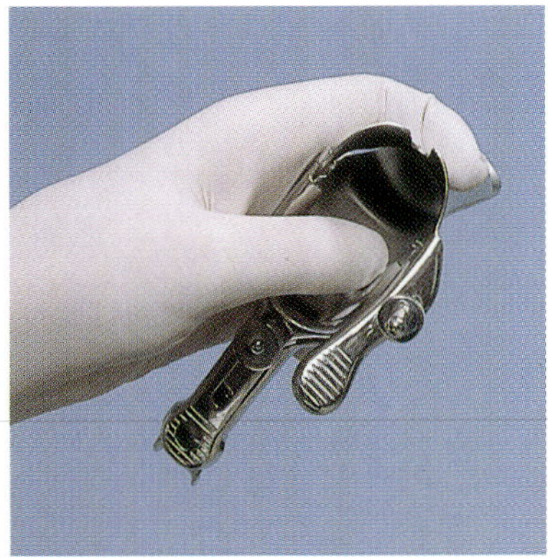

ENTRY ANGLE

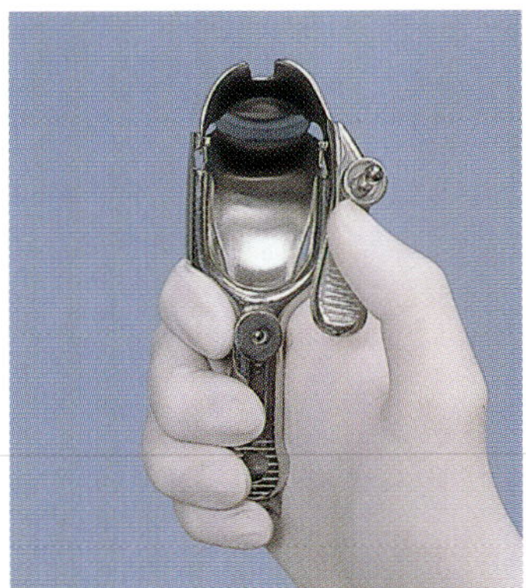

ANGLE AT FULL INSERTION

After the speculum has entered the vagina, remove your fingers from the introitus. You may wish to switch the speculum to the right hand to enhance maneuverability of the speculum and subsequent collection of specimens. Rotate the speculum into a horizontal position, maintaining the pressure posteriorly, and insert it to its full length. Be careful not to open the blades of the speculum prematurely.

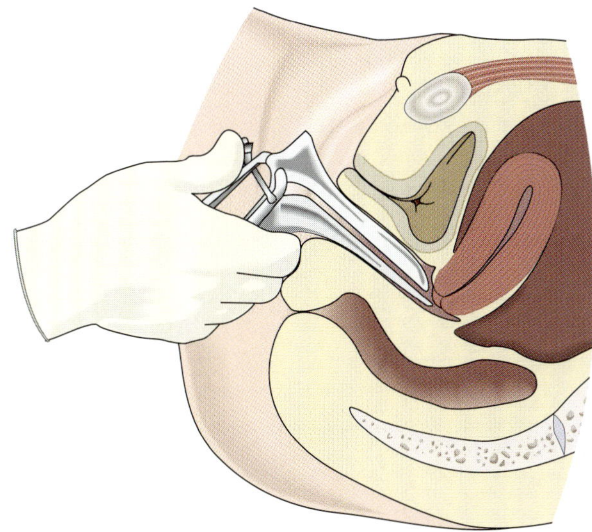

Inspect the Cervix. Open the speculum carefully. Rotate and adjust the speculum until it cups the cervix and brings it into full view. Position the light until you can visualize the cervix well. When the uterus is retroverted, the cervix points more anteriorly than illustrated. If you have difficulty finding the cervix, withdraw the speculum slightly and reposition it on a different slope. If discharge obscures your view, wipe it away gently with a large cotton swab.

See retroversion of the uterus, p. 407.

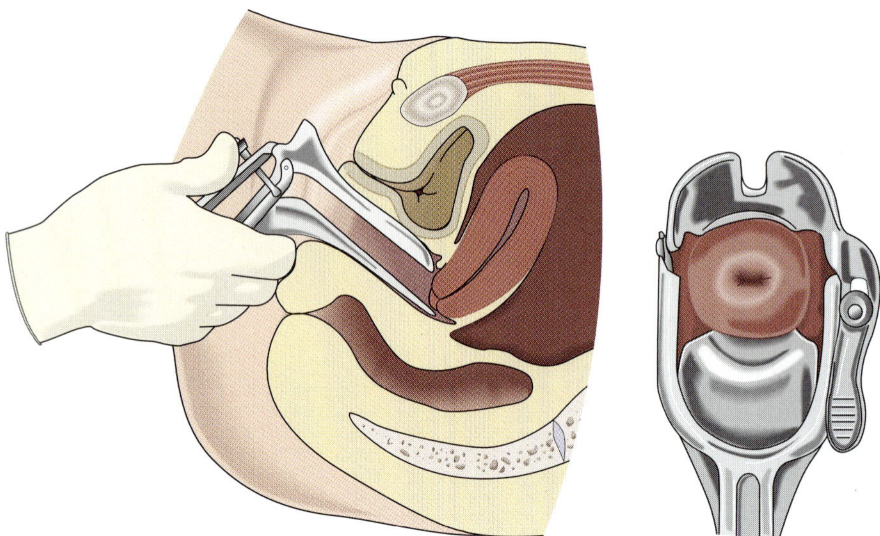

Inspect the cervix and its os. Note the color of the cervix, its position, the characteristics of its surface, and any ulcerations, nodules, masses, bleeding, or discharge.

See Table 11-3, Variations in the Cervix (p. 403), and Table 11-4, Abnormalities of the Cervix (p. 404).

Maintain the open position of the speculum by tightening the thumb screw.

Obtain Specimens for Cervical Cytology (Papanicolaou Smears). Obtain one specimen from the endocervix and another from the ectocervix, or a combination specimen using the cervical brush ("broom"). For best results the patient should not be menstruating. She should avoid intercourse and use of douches or vaginal suppositories for 24 to 48 hours before the examination.

A yellowish discharge on the endocervical swab suggests a mucopurulent cervicitis, commonly caused by *Chlamydia trachomatis, Neisseria gonorrhoeae,* or herpes simplex (p. 404).

OBTAINING THE PAP SMEAR: OPTIONS FOR SPECIMEN COLLECTION

Cervical Scrape and Endocervical Brush

Cervical Scrape. Place the longer end of the scraper in the cervical os. Press, turn, and scrape in a full circle, making sure to include the *transformation zone* and the *squamocolumnar junction.* Smear the specimen on a glass slide. Set the slide in a safe spot that is easy to reach. Note that doing the cervical scrape first reduces obscuring cells with blood, which sometimes appears with use of the endocervical brush.

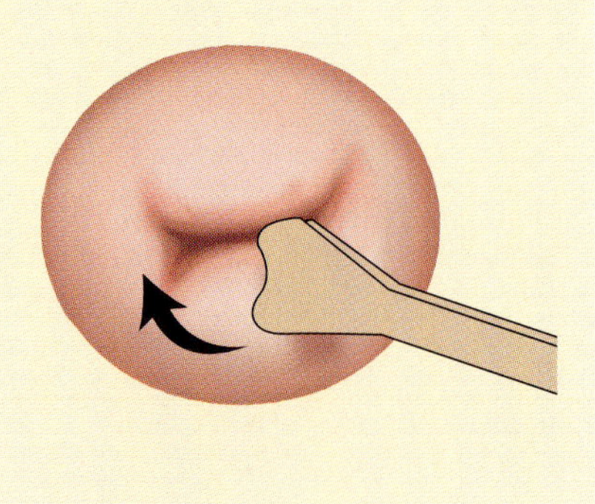

Endocervical Brush. Now take the endocervical brush and place it in the cervical os. Roll it between your thumb and index finger, clockwise and counterclockwise. Remove the brush and pick up the slide you have set aside. Smear the slide with the brush, using a gentle painting motion to avoid destroying any cells. Place the slide into an ether–alcohol solution at once, or spray it promptly with a special fixative.

Note that for pregnant women, a cotton-tip applicator, moistened with saline, is advised in place of the endocervical brush.

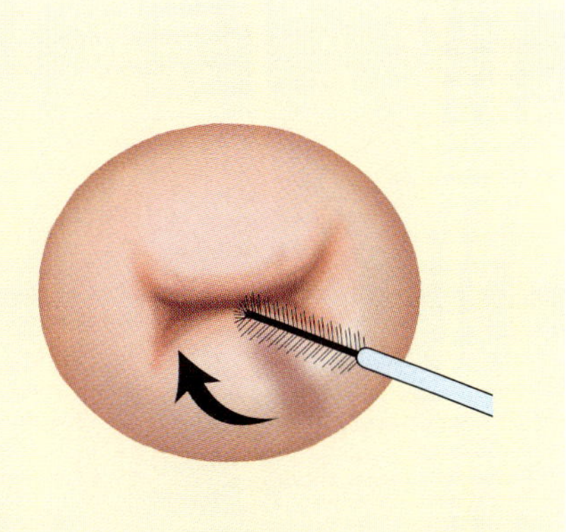

Cervical Broom

Many clinicians now use a plastic brush tipped with a broomlike fringe for collection of a single specimen containing both squamous and columnar epithelial cells. Rotate the tip of the brush in the cervical os, in a full clockwise direction, then stroke each side of the brush on the glass slide. Promptly place the slide in solution or spray with a fixative as described above.

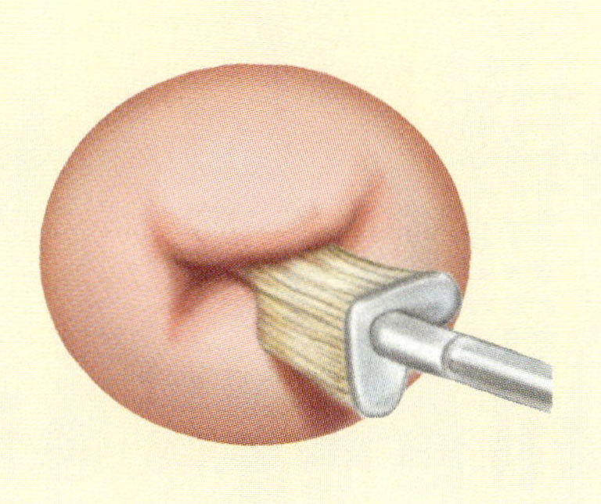

Inspect the Vagina. Withdraw the speculum slowly while observing the vagina. As the speculum clears the cervix, release the thumb screw and maintain the open position of the speculum with your thumb. Close the speculum as it emerges from the introitus, avoiding both excessive stretching and pinching of the mucosa. During withdrawal inspect the vaginal mucosa, noting its color and any inflammation, discharge, ulcers, or masses.

See Table 11-5, Vaginitis (p. 405).

Cancer of the vagina

Perform a Bimanual Examination. Lubricate the index and middle fingers of one of your gloved hands, and *from a standing position* insert them into the vagina, again exerting pressure primarily posteriorly. Your thumb should be abducted, your ring and little fingers flexed into your palm. Pressing inward on the perineum with your flexed fingers causes little if any discomfort and allows you to position your palpating fingers correctly. Note any nodularity or tenderness in the vaginal wall, including the region of the urethra and the bladder anteriorly.

Stool in the rectum may simulate a rectovaginal mass, but unlike a tumor mass can usually be dented by digital pressure. Rectovaginal examination confirms the distinction.

Palpate the cervix, noting its position, shape, consistency, regularity, mobility, and tenderness. Normally the cervix can be moved somewhat without pain. Feel the fornices around the cervix.

Pain on movement of the cervix, together with adnexal tenderness, suggests pelvic inflammatory disease.

Palpate the uterus. Place your other hand on the abdomen about midway between the umbilicus and the symphysis pubis. While you elevate the cervix and uterus with your pelvic hand, press your abdominal hand in and down, trying to grasp the uterus between your two hands. Note its size, shape, consistency, and mobility, and identify any tenderness or masses.

See Table 11-6, Abnormalities and Positions of the Uterus (pp. 406–407).

Uterine enlargement suggests pregnancy or benign or malignant tumors.

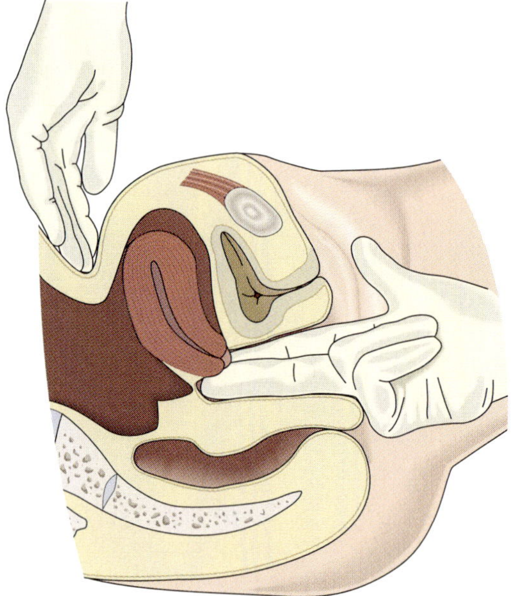

Now slide the fingers of your pelvic hand into the anterior fornix and palpate the body of the uterus between your hands. In this position your pelvic fingers can feel the anterior surface of the uterus, and your abdominal hand can feel part of the posterior surface.

Nodules on the uterine surfaces suggest myomas (see p. 406).

If you cannot feel the uterus with either of these maneuvers, it may be tipped posteriorly (retrodisplaced). Slide your pelvic fingers into the posterior fornix and feel for the uterus butting against your fingertips. An obese or poorly relaxed abdominal wall may also prevent you from feeling the uterus even when it is located anteriorly.

See retroversion and retroflexion of the uterus (p. 407).

Palpate each ovary. Place your abdominal hand on the right lower quadrant, your pelvic hand in the right lateral fornix. Press your abdominal hand in and down, trying to push the adnexal structures toward your pelvic hand. Try to identify the right ovary or any adjacent adnexal masses. By moving your hands slightly, slide the adnexal structures between your fingers, if possible, and note their size, shape, consistency, mobility, and tenderness. Repeat the procedure on the left side.

Three to five years after menopause, the ovaries have usually atrophied and are no longer palpable. If you can feel an ovary in a postmenopausal woman, consider an abnormality such as a cyst or a tumor.

Normal ovaries are somewhat tender. They are usually palpable in slender, relaxed women but are difficult or impossible to feel in others who are obese or poorly relaxed.

Adnexal masses include ovarian cysts, tumors, and abscesses, also the swollen fallopian tube(s) of pelvic inflammatory disease, and a tubal pregnancy. A uterine myoma may simulate an adnexal mass. See Table 11-7, Adnexal Masses (p. 408).

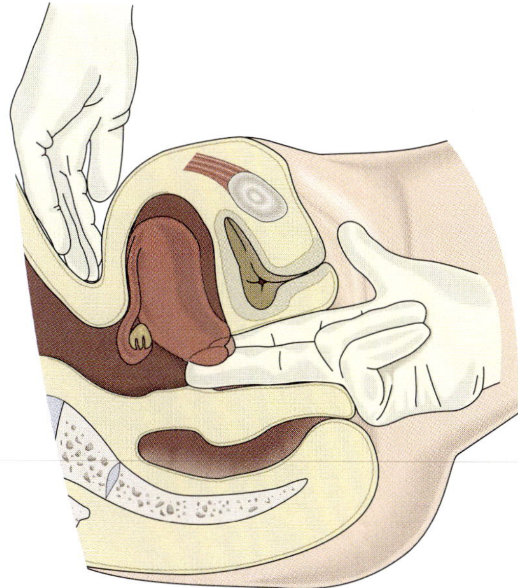

Assess the Strength of the Pelvic Muscles. Withdraw your two fingers slightly, just clear of the cervix, and spread them to touch the sides of the vaginal walls. Ask the patient to squeeze her muscles around them as hard and long as she can. A squeeze that compresses your fingers snugly, moves them upward and inward, and lasts 3 seconds or more is full strength.

Impaired strength may be due to age, vaginal deliveries, or neurologic deficits. Weakness may be associated with urinary stress incontinence.

Do a Rectovaginal Examination. Withdraw your fingers. Lubricate your gloves again if necessary. (See note on using lubricant p. 400.) Then slowly reintroduce your index finger into the vagina, your middle finger into the rectum. Ask the patient to strain down as you do this so that her anal sphincter will relax. Tell her that this examination may make her feel as if she has to move her bowels but that she will not do so. Repeat the maneuvers of the bimanual examination, giving special attention to the region behind the cervix that may be accessible only to the rectal finger.

Rectovaginal palpation is especially valuable in assessing a retrodisplaced uterus, as illustrated.

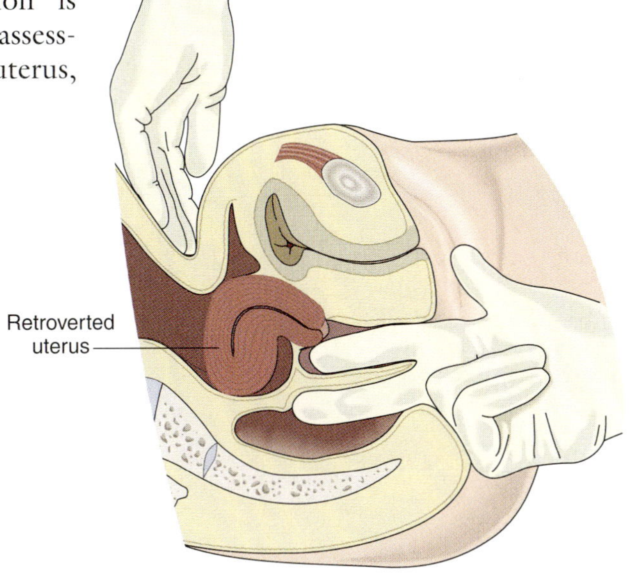

Proceed to the rectal examination (see Chapter 13). If a hemoccult test is planned, you should change gloves to avoid contaminating fecal material with any blood provoked by the Pap smear. After the examination, wipe off the external genitalia and rectum, or offer the patient some tissue so she can do it herself.

USING LUBRICANTS

If you use a large tube of lubricant during a pelvic or rectal examination, you may inadvertently contaminate it by touching the tube with your gloved fingers after touching the patient. To avoid this problem, let the lubricant drop onto your gloved fingers without allowing contact between the tube and the gloves. If you or your assistant should inadvertently contaminate the tube, discard it. Small disposable tubes for use with one patient circumvent this problem.

HERNIAS

Hernias of the groin occur in women as well as in men, but they are much less common. The examination techniques (see pp. 375–376) are basically the same as for men. A woman too should stand up to be examined. To feel an indirect inguinal hernia, however, palpate in the labia majora and upward to just lateral to the pubic tubercles.

An indirect inguinal hernia is the most common hernia that occurs in the female groin. A femoral hernia ranks next in frequency.

SPECIAL TECHNIQUES

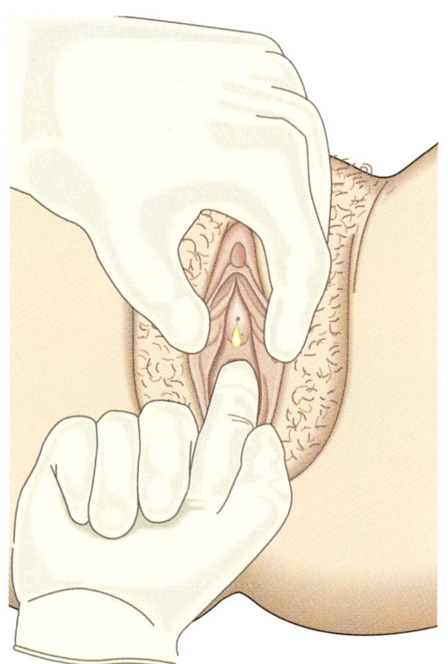

MILKING THE URETHRA

If you suspect urethritis or inflammation of the paraurethral glands, insert your index finger into the vagina and milk the urethra gently from inside outward. Note any discharge from or about the urethral meatus. If present, culture it.

Urethritis may arise from infection with *Chlamydia trachomatis* or *Neisseria gonorrhoeae.*

TABLE 11-1 ■ Lesions of the Vulva

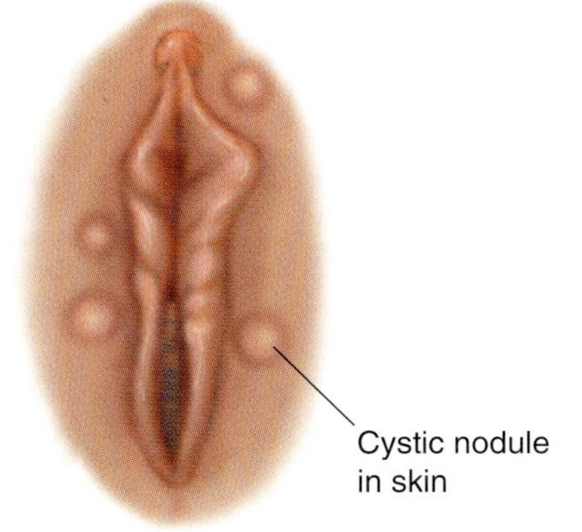

Epidermoid Cyst

Small, firm, round cystic nodules in the labia suggest epidermoid cysts. They are sometimes yellowish in color. Look for the dark punctum marking the blocked opening of the gland.

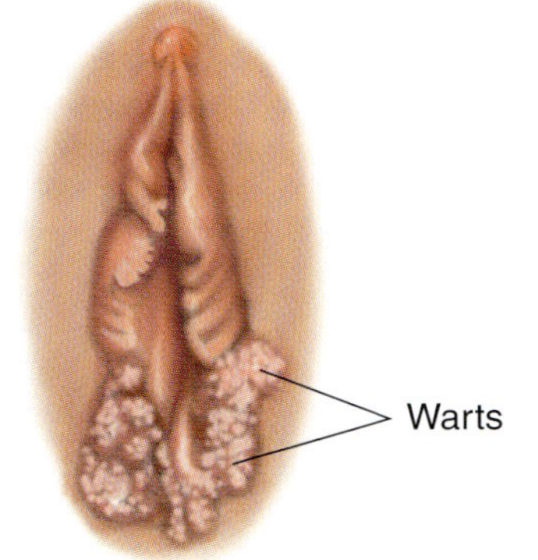

Venereal Wart
(Condyloma Acuminatum)

Warty lesions on the labia and within the vestibule suggest condylomata acuminata. They are due to infection with human papillomavirus.

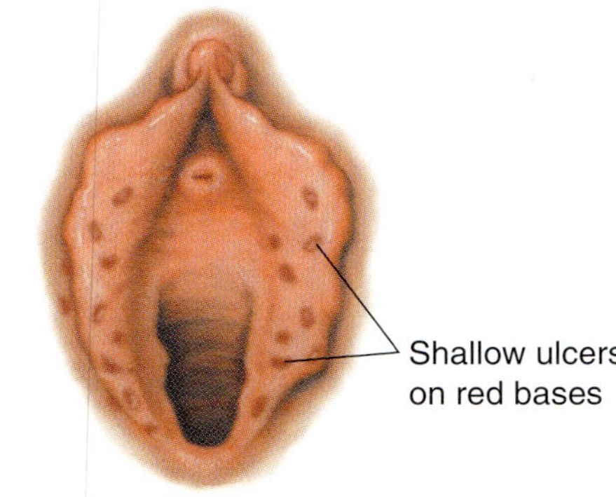

Genital Herpes

Shallow, small, painful ulcers on red bases suggest a herpes infection. Initial infection may be extensive, as illustrated here. Recurrent infections are usually confined to a small local patch.

Syphilitic Chancre

A firm, painless ulcer suggests the chancre of primary syphilis. Since most chancres in women develop internally, they often go undetected.

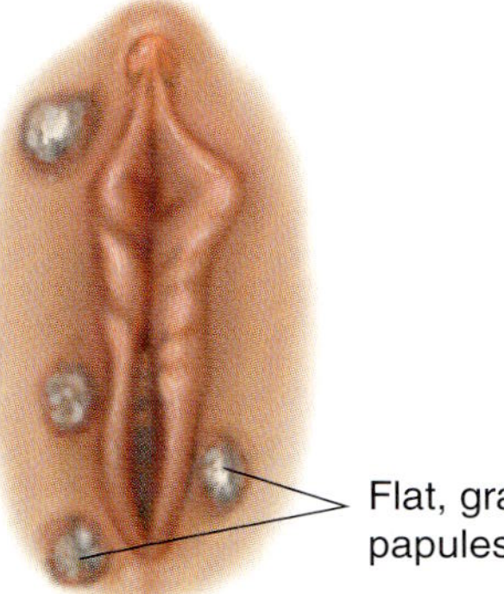
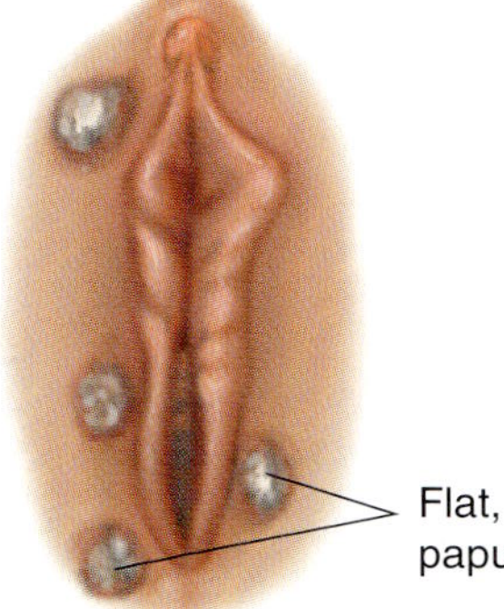

Secondary Syphilis
(Condyloma Latum)

Slightly raised, flat, round or oval papules covered by a gray exudate suggest condylomata lata. These constitute one manifestation of secondary syphilis and are contagious.

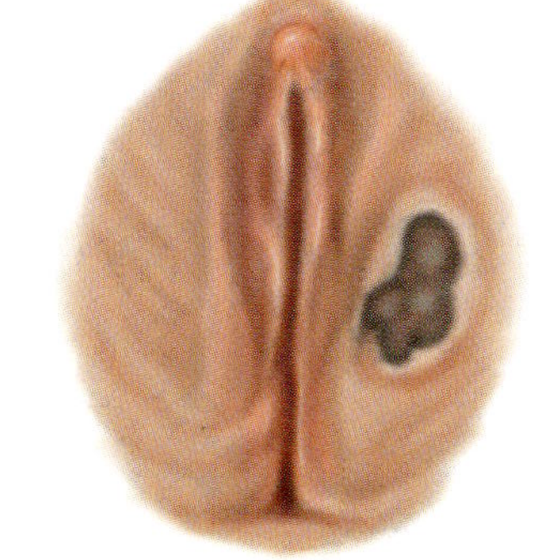

Carcinoma of the Vulva

An ulcerated or raised red vulvar lesion in an elderly woman may indicate vulvar carcinoma.

TABLE 11-2 ■ Bulges and Swelling of the Vulva, Vagina, and Urethra

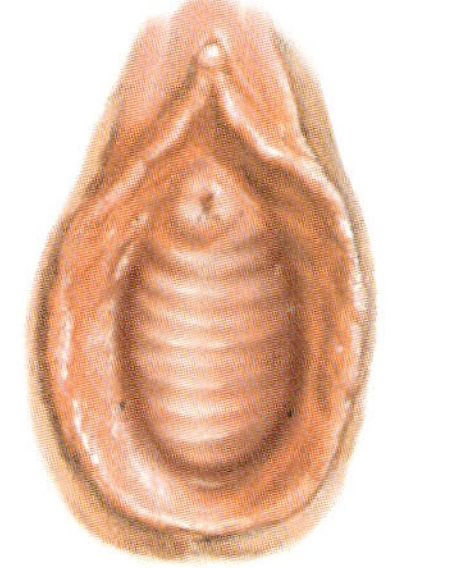

Cystocele

A cystocele is a bulge of the anterior vaginal wall, together with the bladder above it, that results from weakened supporting tissues. The upper two thirds of the vaginal wall are involved.

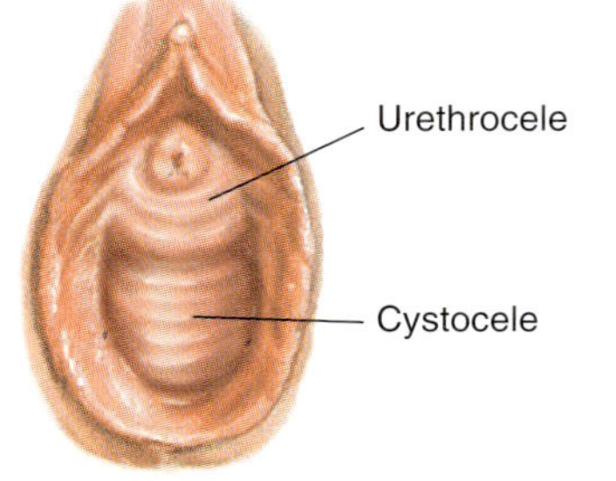

Cystourethrocele

When the entire anterior vaginal wall, together with the bladder and the urethra, is involved in the bulge, a cystourethrocele is present. A groove sometimes defines the border between urethrocele and cystocele, but is not always present.

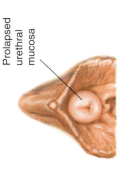

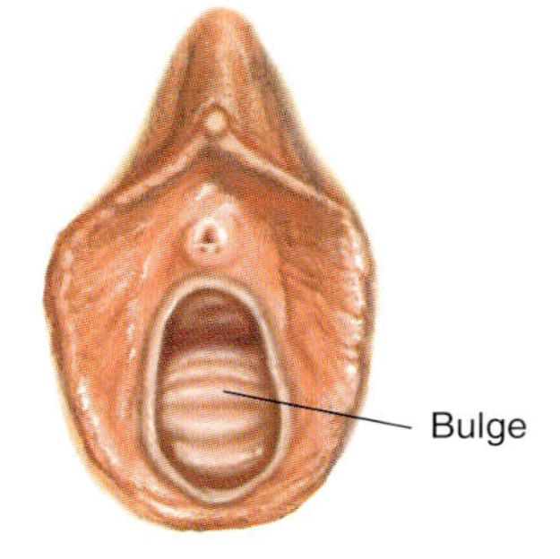

Rectocele

A rectocele is a herniation of the rectum into the posterior wall of the vagina, resulting from a weakness or defect in the endopelvic fascia.

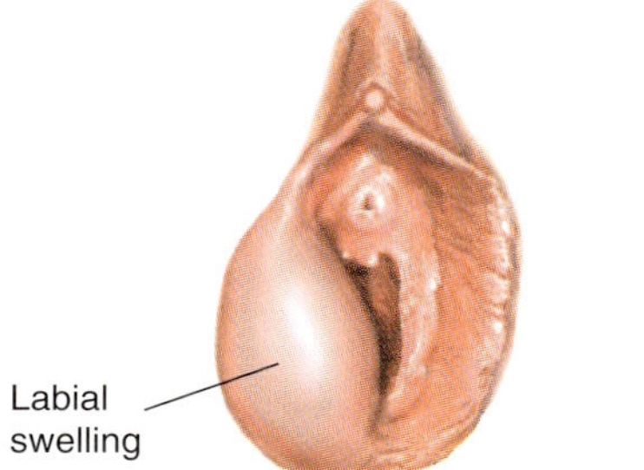

Bartholin's Gland Infection

Causes of a Bartholin's gland infection include gonococci, *Chlamydia trachomatis,* and other organisms. Acutely, it appears as a tense, hot, very tender abscess. Look for pus coming out of the duct or erythema around the duct opening. Chronically, a nontender cyst is felt. It may be large or small.

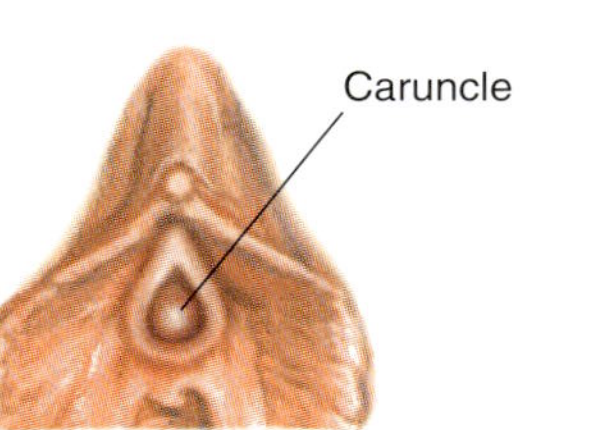

Urethral Caruncle

A urethral caruncle is a small, red, benign tumor visible at the posterior part of the urethral meatus. It occurs chiefly in postmenopausal women, and usually causes no symptoms. Occasionally, a carcinoma of the urethra is mistaken for a caruncle. To check for this, palpate the urethra through the vagina for thickening, nodularity, or tenderness, and feel for inguinal lymphadenopathy.

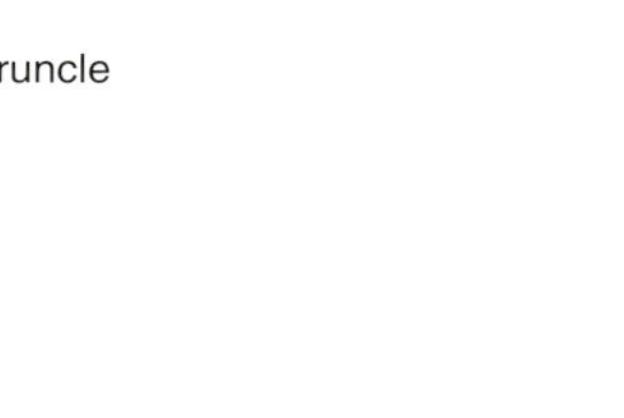

Prolapse of the Urethral Mucosa

Prolapsed urethral mucosa forms a swollen red ring around the urethral meatus. It usually occurs before menarche or after menopause. Identify the urethral meatus at the center of the swelling to make this diagnosis.

TABLE 11-3 ■ Variations in the Cervix

Shapes of the Cervical Os

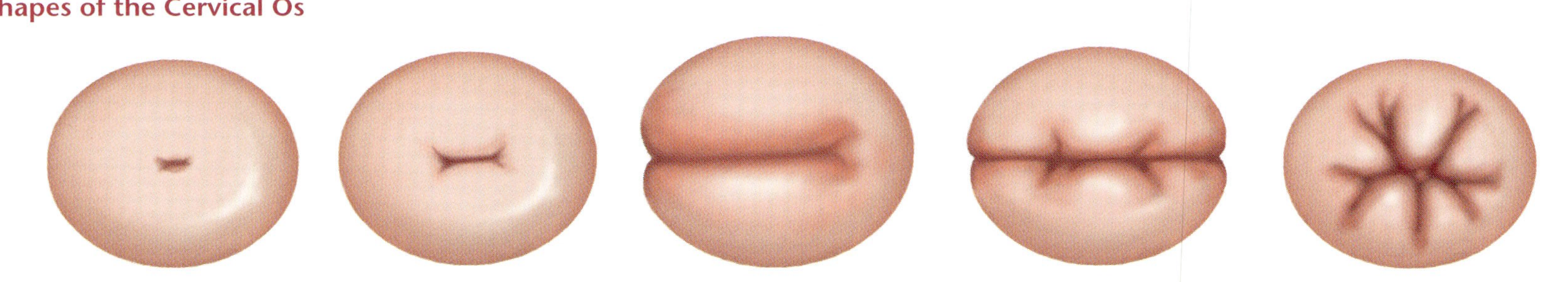

The normal cervical os may be round, oval, or slitlike. The trauma of one or more vaginal deliveries may tear the cervix, producing lacerations. Illustrated here, from left to right, are an oval os, a slitlike os, and lacerations described as unilateral transverse, bilateral transverse, and stellate.

Variations in the Cervical Surface

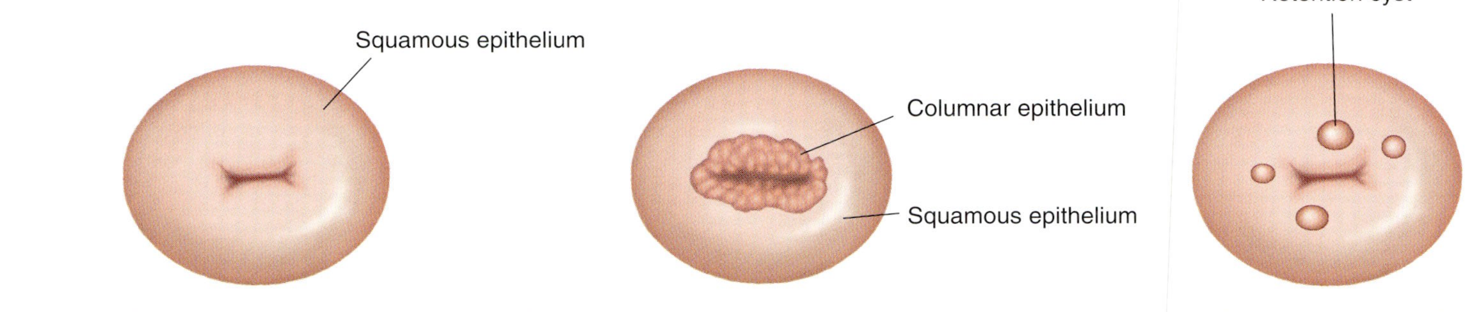

Two kinds of epithelia may cover the cervix: (1) shiny pink *squamous epithelium*, which resembles the vaginal epithelium, and (2) deep red, plushy *columnar epithelium*, which is continuous with the endocervical lining. These two meet at the *squamocolumnar junction*. When this junction is at or inside the cervical os, only squamous epithelium is seen. A ring of columnar epithelium is often visible to a varying extent around the os—the result of a normal process that accompanies fetal development, menarche, and the first pregnancy.*

With increasing estrogen stimulation during adolescence, all or part of this columnar epithelium is transformed into squamous epithelium by a process termed *metaplasia*. This change may block the secretions of columnar epithelium and cause *retention cysts* (sometimes called nabothian cysts). These appear as one or more translucent nodules on the cervical surface and have no pathologic significance.

*Terminology is in flux. Other terms for the columnar epithelium that is visible on the ectocervix are ectropion, ectopy, and eversion.

TABLE 11-4 ■ Abnormalities of the Cervix

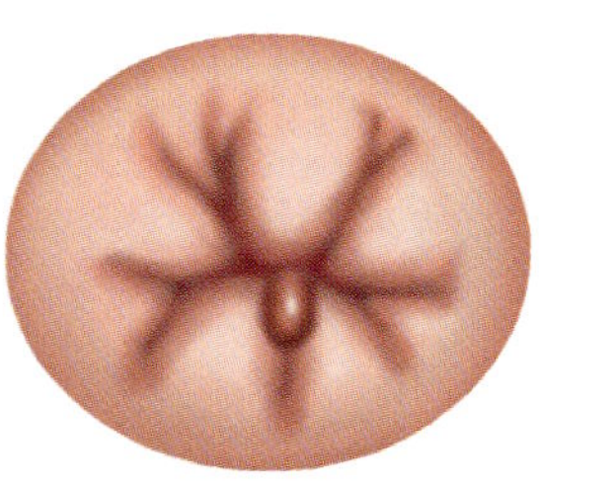

Cervical Polyp

A cervical polyp usually arises from the endocervical canal, becoming visible when it protrudes through the cervical os. It is bright red, soft, and rather fragile. When only the tip is seen, it cannot be differentiated clinically from a polyp originating in the endometrium. Polyps are benign but may bleed.

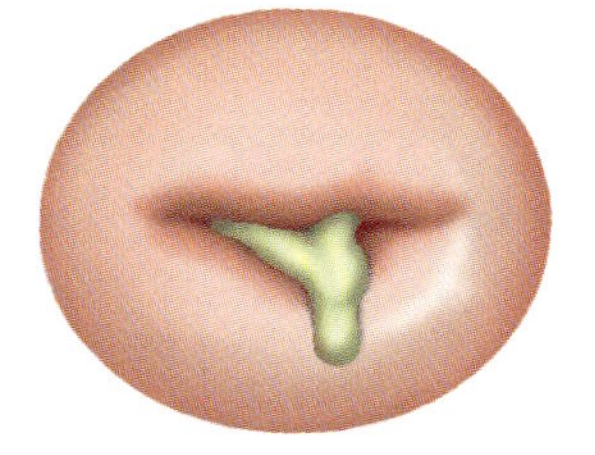

Mucopurulent Cervicitis

Mucopurulent cervicitis produces purulent yellow drainage from the cervical os, usually due to infection from *Chlamydia trachomatis, Neisseria gonorrhoeae,* or herpes. These infections are sexually transmitted, and may occur without symptoms or signs.

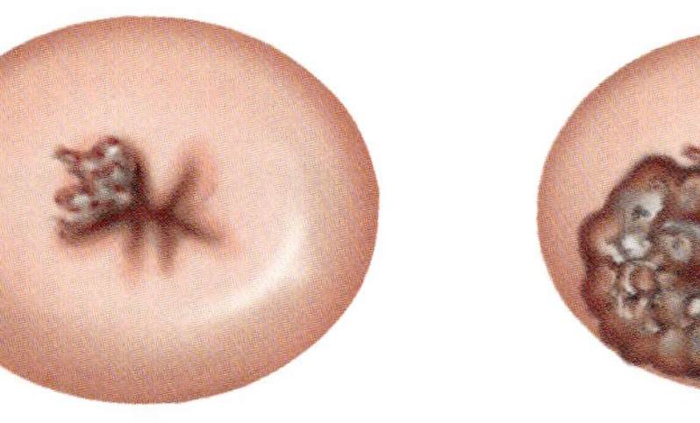

Carcinoma of the Cervix

Carcinoma of the cervix begins in an area of metaplasia. In its earliest stages, it cannot be distinguished from a normal cervix. In a late stage, an extensive, irregular, cauliflowerlike growth may develop. Early frequent intercourse, multiple partners, smoking, and infection with human papillomavirus increase the risk for cervical cancer.

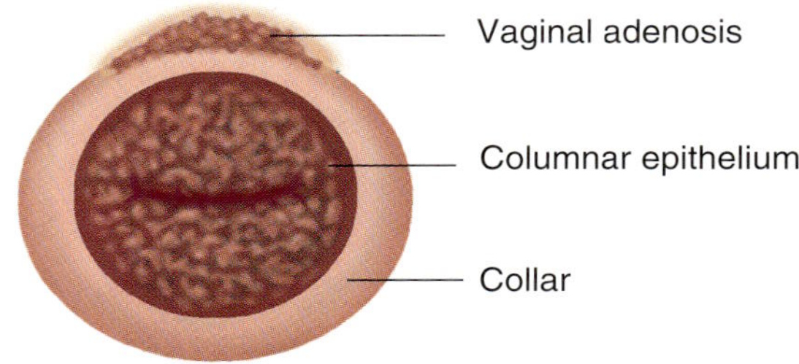

Fetal Exposure to Diethylstilbestrol (DES)*

Daughters of women who took DES during pregnancy are at much higher risk for a number of abnormalities, including (1) columnar epithelium that covers most or all of the cervix, (2) vaginal adenosis, i.e., extension of this epithelium to the vaginal wall, and (3) a circular collar or ridge of tissue, of varying shapes, between cervix and vagina. Much less common is an otherwise rare carcinoma of the upper vagina.

*In the United States, exposure to DES diminished in the late 1960s and stopped in 1971 when the drug was banned.

TABLE 11-5 ■ Vaginitis

The vaginal discharge that often accompanies vaginitis must be distinguished from a physiologic discharge. The latter is clear or white and may contain white clumps of epithelial cells; it is not malodorous. It is also important to distinguish vaginal from cervical discharges. Use a large cotton swab to wipe off the cervix. If no cervical discharge is present in the os, suspect a vaginal origin and consider the causes below. Remember that diagnosis of cervicitis or vaginitis hinges on careful collection and analysis of the appropriate laboratory specimens.

	Trichomonas Vaginitis	Candida Vaginitis	Bacterial Vaginosis*	Atrophic Vaginitis
Cause	*Trichomonas vaginalis,* a protozoa. Often but not always acquired sexually.	*Candida albicans,* a yeast (a normal vaginal inhabitant). Many factors predispose.	Unknown; probably anaerobic bacteria. May be transmitted sexually	Decreased estrogen production after menopause
Discharge	Yellowish green or gray, possibly frothy; often profuse and pooled in the vaginal fornix; may be malodorous	White and curdy; may be thin but typically thick; not as profuse as in *Trichomonas* infection; not malodorous	Gray or white, thin, homogeneous, malodorous; coats the vaginal walls. Usually not profuse, may be minimal	Variable in color, consistency, and amount; may be blood-tinged; rarely profuse
Other Symptoms	Pruritus (though not usually as severe as with *Candida* infection), pain on urination (from skin inflammation or possibly urethritis), and dyspareunia	Pruritus, vaginal soreness, pain on urination (from skin inflammation), and dyspareunia	Unpleasant fishy or musty genital odor	Pruritus, vaginal soreness, or burning and dyspareunia
Vulva	The vestibule and labia minora may be reddened.	The vulva and even the surrounding skin are often inflamed and sometimes swollen to a variable extent.	Usually normal	Atrophic
Vaginal Mucosa	May be diffusively reddened, with small red granular spots or petechiae in the posterior fornix. In mild cases, the mucosa looks normal.	Often reddened, with white, often tenacious patches of discharge. The mucosa may bleed when these patches are scraped off. In mild cases, the mucosa looks normal.	Usually normal	Atrophic, dry, pale; may be red, petechial, or ecchymotic; bleeds easily; may show erosions or filmy adhesions
Laboratory Evaluation	Scan saline wet mount for trichomonads.	Scan potassium hydroxide (KOH) preparation for branching hyphae of *Candida.*	Scan saline wet mount for clue cells (epithelial cells with stippled borders); sniff for fishy odor after applying KOH ("whiff test").	

* Previously termed *Gardnerella* vaginitis.

TABLE 11-6 ■ Abnormalities and Positions of the Uterus

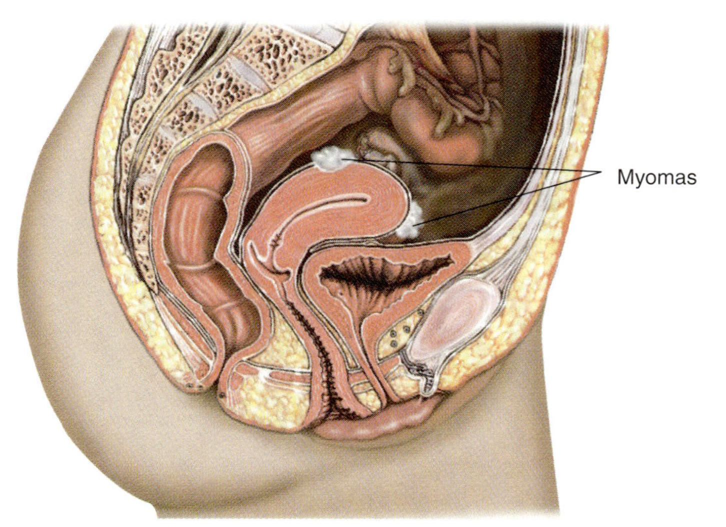

Myomas of the Uterus (Fibroids)

Myomas are very common benign uterine tumors. They may be single or multiple and vary greatly in size, occasionally reaching massive proportions. They feel like firm, irregular nodules in continuity with the uterine surface. Occasionally, a myoma projecting laterally can be confused with an ovarian mass; a nodule projecting posteriorly can be mistaken for a retroflexed uterus. Submucous myomas project toward the endometrial cavity and are not themselves palpable, although they may be suspected because of an enlarged uterus.

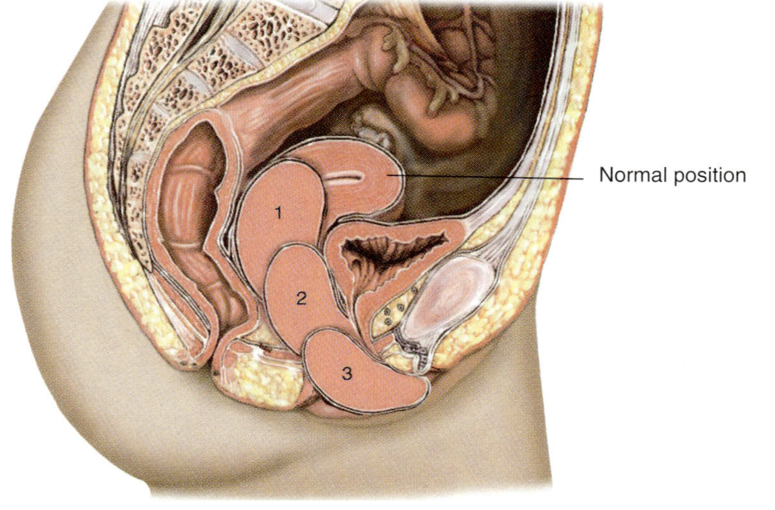

Prolapse of the Uterus

Prolapse of the uterus results from weakness of the supporting structures of the pelvic floor, and is often associated with a cystocele and rectocele. In progressive stages, the uterus becomes retroverted and descends down the vaginal canal to the outside. In first-degree prolapse, the cervix is still well within the vagina. In second-degree prolapse, it is at the introitus. In third-degree prolapse (procidentia), the cervix and vagina are outside the introitus.

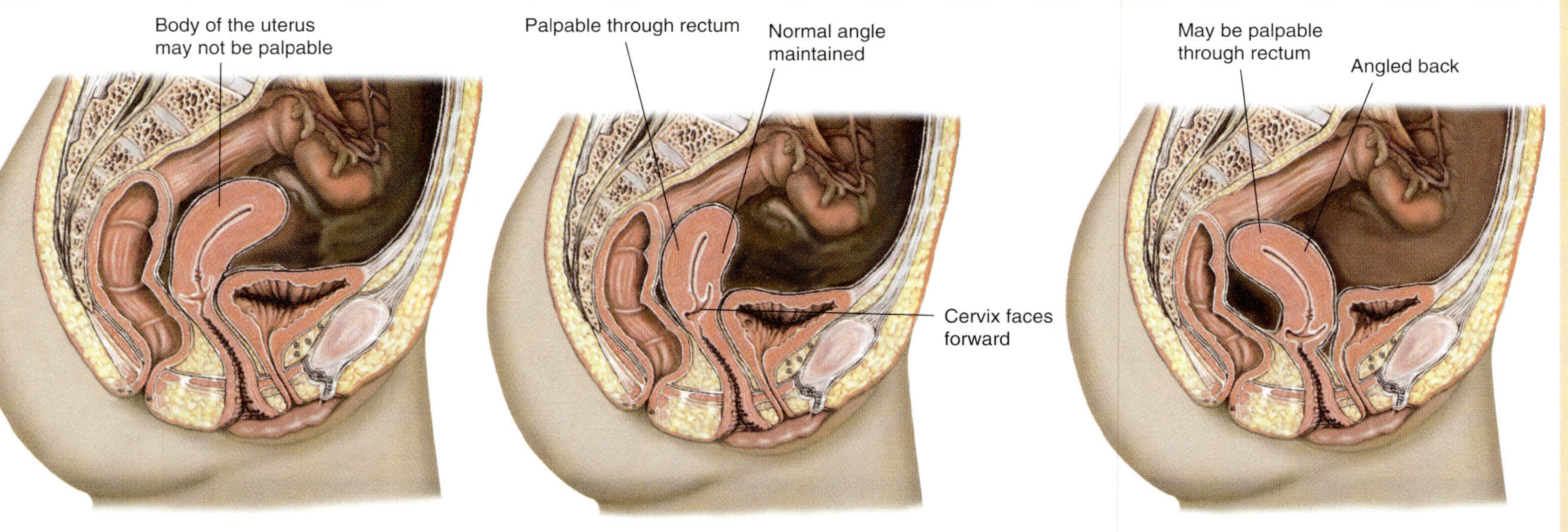

Retroversion of the Uterus

Retroversion of the uterus refers to a tilting backward of the entire uterus, including both body and cervix. It is a common variant occurring in about 1 out of 5 women. Early clues on pelvic examination are a cervix that faces forward and a uterine body that cannot be felt by the abdominal hand. In moderate retroversion, shown on the left, the body may not be palpable with either hand. In marked retroversion, shown on the right, the body can be felt posteriorly, either through the posterior fornix or through the rectum. A retroverted uterus is usually both mobile and asymptomatic. Occasionally, such a uterus is fixed and immobile, held in place by conditions such as endometriosis or pelvic inflammatory disease.

Retroflexion of the Uterus

Retroflexion of the uterus refers to a backward angulation of the body of the uterus in relation to the cervix. The cervix maintains its usual position. The body of the uterus is often palpable through the posterior fornix or through the rectum.

Both retroversion and retroflexion are usually normal variants.

TABLE 11-7 ■ Adnexal Masses

Adnexal masses most commonly result from disorders of the fallopian tubes or ovaries. Three examples—often hard to differentiate—are described. In addition, inflammatory disease of the bowel (such as diverticulitis), carcinoma of the colon, and a pedunculated myoma of the uterus may simulate an adnexal mass.

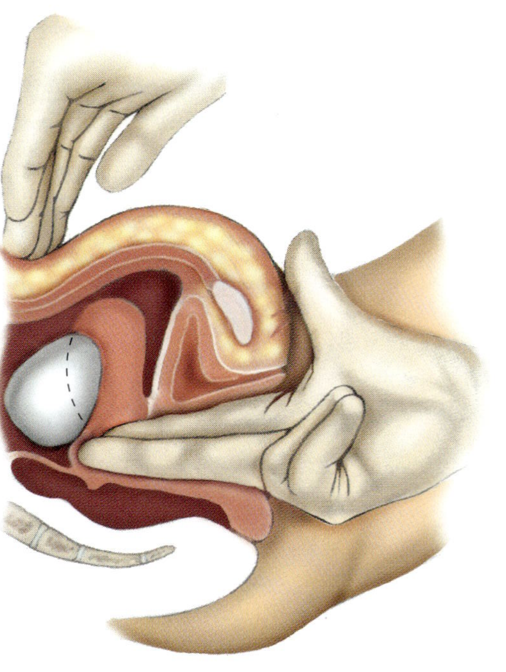

Ovarian Cysts and Tumors

Ovarian cysts and tumors may be detected as adnexal masses on one or both sides. Later, they may extend out of the pelvis. Cysts tend to be smooth and compressible, tumors more solid and often nodular. Uncomplicated cysts and tumors are not usually tender.

Small (≤6 cm in diameter), mobile, cystic masses in a young woman are usually benign and often disappear after the next menstrual period.

Ruptured Tubal Pregnancy

A ruptured tubal pregnancy spills blood into the peritoneal cavity, causing severe abdominal pain and tenderness. Guarding and rebound tenderness are sometimes associated. A unilateral adnexal mass may be palpable, but tenderness often prevents its detection. Faintness, syncope, nausea, vomiting, tachycardia, and shock may be present, reflecting the hemorrhage. There may be a prior history of amenorrhea or other symptoms of a pregnancy.

Pelvic Inflammatory Disease

Pelvic inflammatory disease (PID) is most often a result of sexually transmitted infection of the fallopian tubes (salpingitis) or of the tubes and ovaries (salpingo-oophoritis). It is caused by *Neisseria gonorrhoeae*, *Chlamydia trachomatis*, and other organisms. *Acute* disease is associated with very tender, bilateral adnexal masses, although pain and muscle spasm usually make it impossible to delineate them. Movement of the cervix produces pain. If not treated, a *tuboovarian abscess* or infertility may ensue.

Infection of the fallopian tubes and ovaries may also follow delivery of a baby or gynecologic surgery.

CHAPTER

12

The Pregnant Woman

Joyce E. (Beebe) Thompson

This chapter focuses on the evaluation of the healthy adult woman who is pregnant. The techniques of history-taking and examination for pregnant and nonpregnant women are similar. However, it is important to recognize the changes in anatomy and physiology that are related to pregnancy rather than an abnormality. This chapter emphasizes the common changes in anatomy and physiology that evolve throughout pregnancy, special concerns for the health history, and recommendations for nutrition and exercise. There is also information on screening pregnant women for domestic violence. Next are the techniques of examination for initial and follow-up care. Ideally, the pregnant woman begins her prenatal visits 6 to 8 weeks after conception. For those women seeking initial care in the second or third trimesters, the modified Leopold's maneuvers are reviewed to help you assess the woman presenting late in pregnancy.

ANATOMY AND PHYSIOLOGY

As you begin thinking about the pregnant woman, you may wish to review the sections on anatomy and physiology in Chapter 8, The Breasts and Axillae, and in Chapter 11, Female Genitalia. During pregnancy, there are changes in the thyroid gland, breasts, abdomen, and pelvis. You may also detect minor skin changes such as the mask of pregnancy and abdominal striae.

During pregnancy, the thyroid gland and the breasts undergo moderate enlargement due to hormonal stimulation and increased vascularity and hyperplasia of glandular tissue. There may be tenderness and tingling in the breasts that makes them more sensitive during examination. By the third month of gestation, the breasts become more nodular, requiring careful palpation to avoid discomfort as you examine for any breast masses. The nipples become larger and more erectile. From mid to late pregnancy, *colostrum*, a thick, yellowish secretion rich in nutrients, may be expressed from the nipples. The areolae darken, and Montgomery's glands are more prominent. The venous pattern over the breasts becomes increasingly visible as pregnancy progresses.

The abdomen's most notable change is distention, primarily from the increasing size of the growing uterus and fetus. Early distention from fluid retention and relaxation of abdominal muscles may be noted before the uterus becomes an abdominal organ (12–14 weeks of gestation). The expected growth patterns of the normal uterus and fetus are illustrated on the right, and the standing contours of the primigravid abdomen in each trimester of pregnancy are illustrated below.

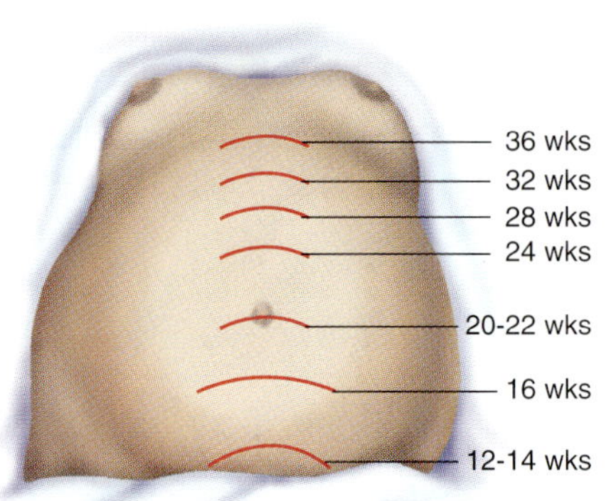

EXPECTED HEIGHT OF THE UTERINE FUNDUS BY MONTH OF PREGNANCY

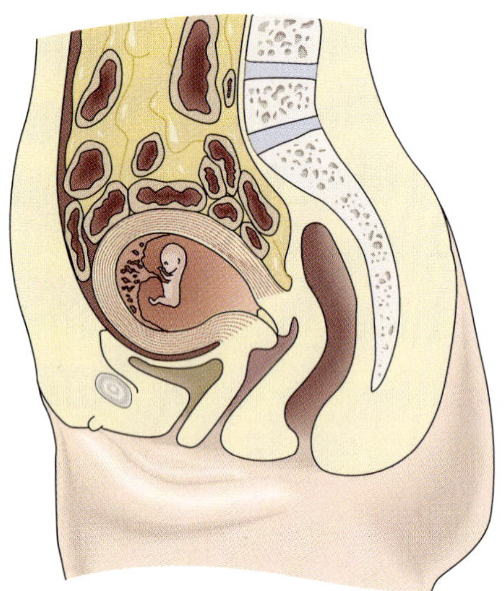

First Trimester

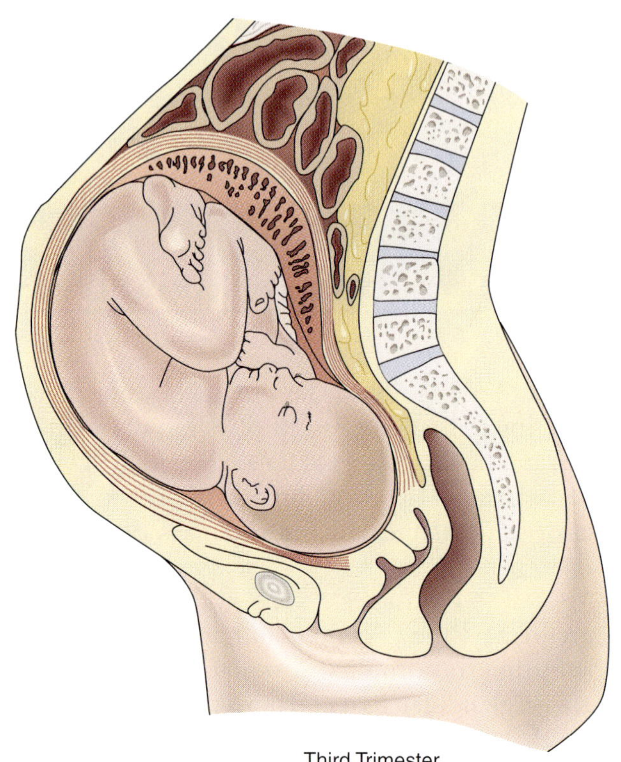

Third Trimester

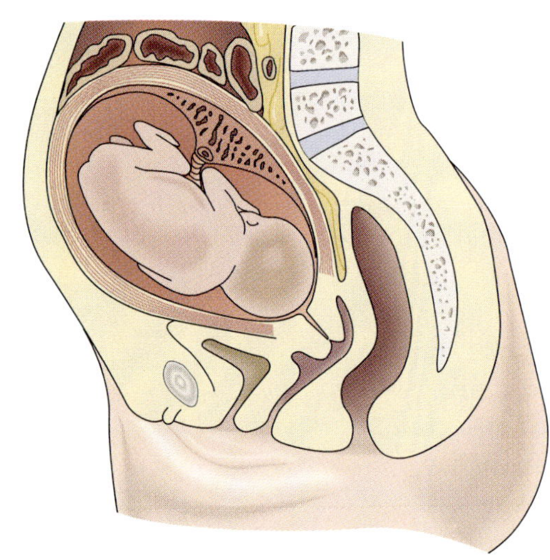

Second Trimester

CHANGING CONTOURS OF THE PRIMIGRAVID ABDOMEN

As the skin stretches to accommodate the growth of the fetus, purplish striae may appear. The *linea nigra,* a brownish black pigmented line following the midline of the abdomen, may become evident. Muscle tone is diminished as pregnancy advances, and *diastasis recti,* or separation of the rectus muscles at the midline of the abdomen, may be noticeable in the later trimesters of pregnancy. If diastasis is severe, as it may be in multiparous women, only a layer of skin, fascia, and peritoneum covers most of the anterior uterine wall. The fetus is felt easily through this muscular gap.

Many anatomical changes take place in the pelvis through the course of pregnancy. The early diagnosis of pregnancy is based in part on changes in the vagina and the uterus. With the increased vascularity throughout the pelvic region, the vagina takes on a bluish or violet color. The vaginal walls appear thicker and deeply rugated because of increased thickness of the mucosa, loosening of the connective tissue, and hypertrophy of smooth muscle cells. Vaginal secretions are thick, white, and more profuse. Vaginal pH becomes more acidic due to the action of *Lactobacillus acidophilus* on the increased levels of glycogen stored in the vaginal epithelium. This change in pH helps protect the woman against some vaginal infections, but increased glycogen may contribute to higher rates of vaginal candidiasis (see p. 405).

The uterus is the organ most affected. Early in pregnancy, it loses the firmness and resistance of the nonpregnant organ. The palpable softening at the isthmus, called *Hegar's sign,* is an early diagnostic sign of pregnancy, and is illustrated on the right.

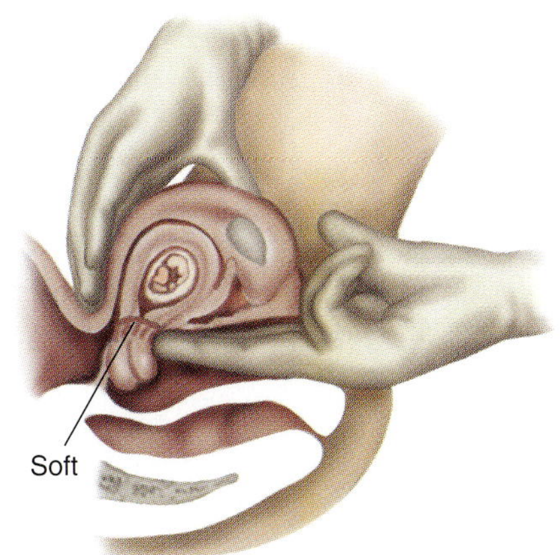

HEGAR'S SIGN

Over the course of 9 months, the uterus increases in both weight and size. Its weight grows from 2 ounces to 2 pounds, chiefly due to larger muscle cells, more extensive fibrous and elastic tissue, and the considerable increase in the size and number of blood vessels and lymphatics. The size of the uterus increases 500- to 1000-fold, with a capacity of approximately 10 liters by the end of the pregnancy.

As the uterus grows, it changes shape and position. The nongravid uterus may be anteverted, retroverted, or retroflexed. Up to 12 weeks of gestation, the gravid uterus is still a pelvic organ. Regardless of its initial positioning, the enlarging uterus becomes anteverted and quickly fills space usually occupied by the bladder, triggering frequent voiding. By 12 weeks' gestation, the uterus straightens and rises out of the pelvis and can be felt when palpating the abdomen.

The enlarging uterus pushes the intestinal contents laterally and superiorly and stretches its supporting ligaments, sometimes causing pain in the lower quadrants. It adapts to fetal growth and positions and tends to rotate to the right to accommodate to the rectosigmoid structures in the left side of the pelvis.

The cervix also looks and feels quite different. Pronounced softening and cyanosis appear very early after conception and continue throughout pregnancy (*Chadwick's sign*). The cervical canal is filled with a tenacious *mucous plug* that protects the developing fetus from infection. Red, velvety mucosa around the os is common on the cervix during pregnancy and is considered normal.

Common Concerns During Pregnancy and Their Explanations

Common Concerns	Time in Pregnancy	Explanation and Effects on Woman's Body
No menses (*amenorrhea*)	Throughout	Continued high levels of estrogen, progesterone, and human chorionic gonadotropin following fertilization of the ovum build up the endometrium to support the developing pregnancy, averting menses and shedding of the endometrial lining.
Nausea with or without vomiting	1st trimester	Possible causes include hormonal changes of pregnancy leading to slowed peristalsis throughout the GI tract, changes in taste and smell, the growing uterus, or emotional factors. Women may have a modest (2–5 lb) weight loss in the first trimester.
Breast tenderness, tingling	1st trimester	The hormones of pregnancy stimulate the growth of breast tissue. As the breasts enlarge throughout pregnancy, women may experience upper backache from their increased weight. There is also increased blood flow throughout the breasts, increasing pressure on the tissue.
Weight loss	1st trimester	If a woman experiences nausea and vomiting, she may not be eating normally in early pregnancy (see nausea above).
Groin/lower abdominal pain	2nd trimester: 14–20 weeks	Rapid uterine growth early in second trimester causes tension and stretching of round ligaments, causing spasm with sudden movement or change of position.
Urinary frequency (nonpathologic)	1st/3rd trimesters	There is increased blood volume and increased filtration rate in the kidneys with increased urine production. Due to less space for the bladder from pressure from the growing uterus (first trimester) or from the descent of the fetal head (third trimester), the woman needs to empty her bladder more frequently.
Fatigue	1st/3rd trimesters	Rapid change in energy requirements; hormonal changes (progesterone has a sedative effect); in third trimester, weight gain, changes in mechanics of movement, and sleep disturbances contribute.
Edema	3rd trimester	There is increased venous pressure in the legs, obstruction of lymphatic flow, and reduced plasma colloid osmotic pressure.
Heartburn, constipation	Throughout	Relaxation of the lower esophageal sphincter allows stomach contents to back up into the lower esophagus. The decreased GI motility caused by pregnancy hormones slows peristalsis and causes constipation. Constipation may cause or aggravate existing hemorrhoids.
Backache (nonpathologic)	Throughout	Hormonally induced relaxation of joints and ligaments and the minor lordosis required to balance the growing uterus sometimes result in a lower backache. Pathologic causes must be ruled out.
Leukorrhea	Throughout	Increased secretions from the cervix and the vaginal epithelium, due to the hormones and vasocongestion of pregnancy, result in an asymptomatic milky white vaginal discharge.

The ovaries and fallopian tubes undergo changes as well, but few are noticeable during physical examination. Early in pregnancy, the *corpus luteum,* the ovarian follicle that has discharged its ovum, may be sufficiently prominent to be felt on the affected ovary as a small nodule, but it disappears by midpregnancy. It is important to examine the fallopian tubes to rule out a tubal pregnancy (see p. 408).

THE HEALTH HISTORY

Common or Concerning Symptoms

- Symptoms of pregnancy
- Toxic exposures, use of illicit drugs, domestic violence
- Prior complications of pregnancy
- Chronic illnesses in patient or family members

An accurate history is essential for assessing the pregnant woman's health. It also shapes the order and content of the physical examination, which is directed primarily to confirming the woman's suspicion of pregnancy. The woman will usually have many questions for you about her pregnancy and seek understanding of her symptoms.

During the initial visit, focus the history on the woman's *current state of health* and on risk factors for any conditions that could adversely affect her or the developing fetus. Ask about symptoms of pregnancy such as breast tenderness, nausea or vomiting, urinary frequency, change in bowel habits, and fatigue (see table on p. 412). Review her attitude toward the pregnancy, and if she plans to continue to term. Look into her eating patterns and quality of nutrition. Does she smoke or drink alcohol? What about her income and her social support network?

Although best identified and addressed before conception, are there any sources of high-level stress? If she works, has there been any exposure to teratogenic drugs or toxic substances? What about any use of illicit drugs? Is there any history of domestic violence that may escalate during pregnancy?

What about *prior pregnancies,* since past obstetrical problems tend to recur? Has she had any major complications of pregnancy or problems with labor or delivery? Has she had a premature or growth-retarded infant? Ask also about her *past medical history,* especially any chronic diseases like hypertension, diabetes, or cardiac conditions. You should also review her *family history* for these conditions.

In addition, the clinician should get information needed for calculating the *expected weeks of gestation by dates.* This is currently counted in weeks from either (1) the first day of the last menstrual period (*LMP*), known as *men-*

strual age, or (2) the date of conception, if this is known (*conception age*). Menstrual age is used most frequently to express the weeks of gestation calculated by dates. The first day of the LMP is also used to calculate the *expected date of confinement* (*EDC*) or projected time of term labor and birth for women with regular 28- to 30-day cycles. The EDC can be determined by adding 7 days to the first day of the LMP, subtracting 3 months, and adding one year (*Naegele's rule*). This information is often one of the first questions the pregnant woman asks when seeking confirmation of pregnancy.

The weeks of gestation at the time of examination tell you the expected size of the uterus if the LMP was normal, the dates were remembered accurately, and conception actually occurred. You should estimate this size before examining the woman. You can then compare the expected size by dates with what you actually palpate during the bimanual examination, or abdominally, if pregnancy is beyond 14 weeks of gestation. Uterine size is measured by the palpable size of the uterus if still within the pelvic cavity, or by the height of the fundus if above the symphysis pubis. If there is a discrepancy, you need to look for the causes. Accurately dating the pregnancy is best done early, and contributes to good decision-making later in pregnancy if the fetus is not growing well, if preterm labor is suspected, or if the pregnancy goes beyond 42 weeks of gestation. If the woman does not remember her LMP or has irregular menstrual cycles, dating the pregnancy is done by palpation and subsequent monitoring of the growth curve (see p. 410) along with the time of first fetal movements. In some cases, ultrasound is an appropriate adjunct for dating an early pregnancy.

As you begin preparing the patient for the physical examination, ask the woman if she has ever had a complete pelvic examination. If not, take the time to explain what is involved and seek her cooperation for each of its components. Explaining what you do and what you find is important if you are to strengthen rapport and help her to understand the changes in her body and its response to pregnancy, and how she can best maintain her health. Be sure to ask in a sensitive and confidential manner if she has ever experienced a sexual assault, since this may cause her to resist any examination of the pelvis.

HEALTH PROMOTION AND COUNSELING

Important Topics for Health Promotion and Counseling

- Nutrition
- Weight gain
- Exercise
- Screening for domestic violence

Counseling about nutrition and exercise is important to the health of the pregnant woman and baby. Evaluate the nutritional status of the woman at the first prenatal visit, including a diet history, measurement of height and weight, and screening for anemia by checking the hematocrit. Be sure to explore the woman's habits and attitudes about eating and weight gain, as well as her use of needed vitamin and mineral supplements. Develop a nutrition plan that is appropriate to the woman's cultural preferences. Be sure there is a balanced increase in calories and protein, since protein will be used for energy, rather than growth, unless sufficient calories are consumed. Women with low incomes should be helped to obtain additional food. At each visit, monitor weight gain and review nutritional goals for women at risk.

Ideal weight gain during pregnancy follows a pattern: very little gain the first trimester, rapid increase in the second, and a mild slowing of the increase in the third trimester. Women should be weighed at each visit, with the results plotted on a graph for the woman and health care provider to review and discuss.

Recommended Total Weight Gain Ranges for Pregnant Women

Prepregnancy Weight-for-Height Category	**Recommended Total Gain**	
	lb	*kg*
Low (BMI <19.8)	28–40	12.5–18
Normal (BMI 19.8 to 26.0)	25–35	11.5–16
High (BMI 26.0 to 29.0)	15–25	7.0–11.5
Obese (BMI >29.0)	≥15	≥7.0

Figures are for single pregnancies. The range for women carrying twins is 35 to 45 lb (16 to 20 kg). Young adolescents (<2 years after menarche) should strive for gains at the upper end of the range. Short women (<62 in. or <157 cm) should strive for gains at the lower end of the range.

Institute of Medicine. Nutrition During Pregnancy. Part I, Weight Gain. Committee on Nutritional Status During Pregnancy and Lactation, Food and Nutrition Board, National Academy Press, Washington, DC, 1990.

Exercise is an important part of the lifestyle of many women. Guidelines are contradictory, but the recommendations of the American College of Obstetrics and Gynecology (1994) suggest that in the absence of either obstetric or medical complications, most women can perform moderate exercise to maintain cardiorespiratory and muscular fitness throughout pregnancy and the postpartum period. Women exercising regularly prior to pregnancy can continue mild to moderate exercise, preferably for short periods three times a week. Women initiating exercise during pregnancy should be more cautious, and consider programs developed specifically for pregnant women. After the first trimester, women should avoid exercise in the supine position, which can compress the inferior vena cava and decrease blood flow to the placenta. The pregnant woman should stop exercise when she feels fatigued or uncomfortable and avoid overheating and dehydration. Since the center of gravity shifts in the third trimester, advise her that exercises that could cause loss of balance are unwise.

Pregnancy may be a time when women are more likely to be abused by an intimate partner or when patterns of abuse may intensify, increasing the risk of miscarriage and low-birthweight babies, as well as late prenatal care. Abuse in pregnancy ranges from 8% to 22%, and may result in femicide. Because violence survivors often disclose their experiences to their health care provider before confiding in their family, clergy, or friends, many experts consider universal screening an ethical imperative. No woman deserves to be hurt. Safety and legal concerns also surround domestic violence, but the woman needs to be supported and offered multiple opportunities to talk about any form of abuse or violence in the safety and privacy of a prenatal visit. When to ask, how to bring up the subject, and how to respond when the woman reveals that she is or has been abused are important questions to consider before screening for violence and abuse. Direct questioning in a nonjudgmental manner in a private setting is recommended at each prenatal visit. Validation of positive responses and marking the area of any injury on a body map is suggested. Above all, in situations of admitted abuse, ask the woman how you might help her. Offer information on safe shelters, counseling centers, hotline telephone numbers to call*, and other sources of help when she is ready to take advantage of these. Clues to physical violence may also arise from behavior during the interview or from frequent changes in appointments at the last minute to avoid detection of bruises or other signs of injury.

Preview: Recording the Physical Examination — The Pregnant Woman

Note that initially you may use sentences to describe your findings; later you will use phrases. The style below contains phrases appropriate for most write-ups. Unfamiliar terms are explained in the next section, Techniques of Examination.

"Abdomen: No surgical scars. Active bowel sounds. Soft, nontender; no palpable hepatosplenomegaly or masses. Fundus palpable 2 fingerbreadths below the umbilicus; shape is ovoid and smooth. Fetal heart rate 144. No inguinal adenopathy. External genitalia: midline episiotomy scar present. No lesions, discharge, or signs of infection. Bimanual examination: cervix midline, soft; external os admits fingertip, internal os closed. No pain elicited on movement of cervix; no adnexal masses. Fundus enlarged to 20 weeks' size, midline, smooth; vaginal tone reduced."

Describes examination of healthy pregnant woman at 20 weeks' gestation, third pregnancy

OR

"Abdomen: Low transverse surgical scar. Active bowel sounds. Soft, nontender; no palpable hepatosplenomegaly or masses. Fundus: barely palpable above symphysis pubis. Fetal heart rate not heard. No inguinal adenopathy. Bimanual examination: cervix midline, soft, internal os closed. No pain on movement of cervix. Right ovary palpable, left nonpalpable; no other adnexal masses. Fundus anteverted, enlarged to 14–16 weeks' size; moderate vaginal tone."

Describes examination of healthy pregnant woman reporting dates of 20-week gestation but with examination consistent with 16-week gestation

*National Domestic Violence Hotline: 1-800-799-SAFE (7233)
National Domestic Violence Resource Center: 1-800-537-2238

TECHNIQUES OF EXAMINATION

As with all patients, as you begin your examination of the pregnant woman show consideration for her comfort and sense of privacy, as well as for her individual needs and sensitivities. Have the needed equipment readily at hand. If you have not met the woman before, taking the history before asking her to gown shows respect for her right to be treated with dignity. Ask the woman to put on the gown with the opening in front to ease the examination of both the breasts and the pregnant abdomen. Draping for the abdominal and pelvic examinations is similar to that discussed in earlier chapters.

Positioning. Positioning is important when examining the abdomen of a pregnant woman given the added time and attention needed to palpate the uterus and listen to the fetal heart. The semi-sitting position with the knees bent, as shown below, affords the greatest comfort, as well as protection from the negative effects of the weight of the gravid uterus on abdominal organs and vessels.

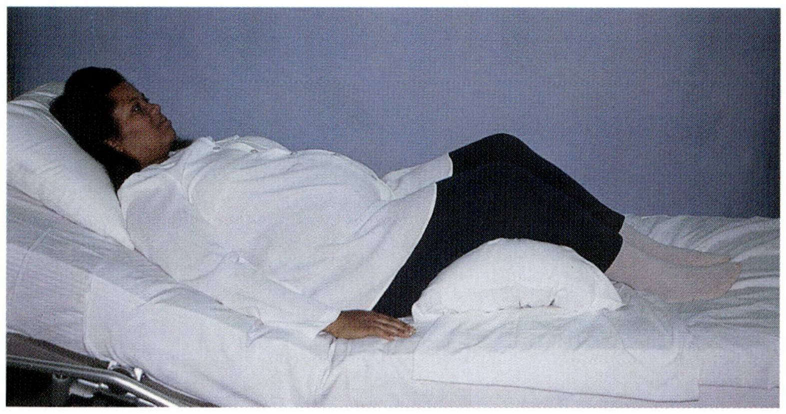

This position is especially important when examining a woman with an advanced pregnancy. Prolonged periods of lying on the back should be avoided because the uterus then lies directly on the woman's vertebral column and may compress the descending aorta and inferior vena cava, interfering with return of venous blood from the lower extremities and the pelvic vessels. Therefore, abdominal palpation should be efficient in time and results.

Supine hypotension is a severe form of this diminished circulation and may lead the woman to feel dizzy and faint, especially when lying down.

Encourage the woman to sit again briefly before proceeding to the pelvic evaluation. This pause also provides time for the woman to empty her bladder again. Make sure, however, that she is acclimated to sitting before allowing her to stand up. The pelvic examination should likewise be relatively quick. All other examination procedures should be done in the sitting or left-side–lying position.

Equipment. The examiner's hands are the primary "equipment" for examination of the pregnant woman; they should be warm and firm yet gentle in palpation. Whenever possible the fingers should be together and flat against the abdominal or pelvic tissue to minimize discomfort. Likewise, all touching and palpation should be done with smooth continuous contact against the skin rather than kneading or abrupt motion. The more sensitive palmar surfaces of the ends of the fingers yield the greatest amount of information. Avoid tender areas on the woman's body until the end of the examination.

The gynecologic speculum is used for inspecting the cervix and the vagina and for taking specimens for cytologic or bacteriologic study. Because the vaginal walls are relaxed during pregnancy and may fall medially, obscuring your view, a speculum of larger than expected size may be needed. The relaxation of perineal and vulvar structures allows you to use it with minimal discomfort for the woman. Because of the increased vascularity of the vaginal and cervical structures, insert and open the speculum gently. You will thus avoid tissue trauma and bleeding, which interfere with the interpretation of Pap smears.

The cervical brush is not recommended for Pap smears in pregnant women because it often causes bleeding. The Ayre wooden spatula and/or cotton-tipped applicator is appropriate.

Review Chapter 11 for instruments and techniques used to take cervical smears.

General Inspection

Inspect the overall health, nutritional status, neuromuscular coordination, and emotional state as the woman walks into the exam room and climbs on the examination table. Discussion of the woman's priorities for the examination, her responses to pregnancy, and her general health provide useful information and help to put the woman at ease.

Vital Signs and Weight

Take the blood pressure. A baseline reading helps to determine the woman's usual range. In midpregnancy, blood pressure is normally lower than in the nonpregnant state.

High blood pressure prior to 24 weeks indicates chronic hypertension. After 24 weeks, further evaluation is required to diagnose and treat *pregnancy-induced hypertension (PIH).*

Measure the weight. First-trimester weight loss related to nausea and vomiting is common but should not exceed 5 pounds.

Weight loss of more than 5 pounds during the first trimester may be due to excessive vomiting or *hyperemesis.*

Head and Neck

Stand facing the seated woman and observe the head and neck, including the following features:

- *Face*. The mask of pregnancy, *chloasma,* is normal. It consists of irregular brownish patches around the eyes or across the bridge of the nose.

Facial edema after 24 weeks of gestation suggests PIH.

- *Hair,* including texture, moisture, and distribution. Dryness, oiliness, and sometimes minor generalized hair loss may be noted.

Localized patches of hair loss should not be attributed to pregnancy.

- *Eyes*. Note the conjunctival color.

Anemia of pregnancy may cause pallor.

- *Nose,* including the mucous membranes and the septum. Nasal congestion is common during pregnancy.

Nosebleeds are more common during pregnancy. Signs of cocaine use may be present.

- *Mouth,* especially the gums and teeth.

Gingival enlargement with bleeding (p. 203) is common during pregnancy.

- *Thyroid gland*. Inspect and palpate the gland. Symmetric enlargement is expected.

Marked or asymmetric enlargement is not due to pregnancy.

Thorax and Lungs

Inspect the thorax for the pattern of breathing. Although women late in pregnancy sometimes report difficulty in breathing, there are usually no abnormal physical signs.

If signs of respiratory distress are noted, examine the lungs thoroughly. Expect respiratory alkalosis in later trimesters.

Heart

Palpate the apical impulse. In advanced pregnancy, it may be slightly higher than normal because of dextrorotation of the heart due to the higher diaphragm.

Auscultate the heart. Soft, blowing murmurs are common during pregnancy, reflecting increased blood flow in normal vessels.

These murmurs may also accompany anemia.

Breasts

Inspect the breasts and nipples for symmetry and color. The venous pattern may be marked, the nipples and areolae are dark, and Montgomery's glands are prominent.

An inverted nipple needs attention if breast-feeding is planned.

Palpate for masses. During pregnancy, breasts are tender and nodular.

A pathologic mass may be difficult to isolate.

Compress each nipple between your index finger and thumb. This maneuver may express colostrum from the nipples.

A bloody or purulent discharge should not be attributed to pregnancy.

Abdomen

Position the pregnant woman in a semi-sitting position with her knees flexed (see p. 417).

Inspect any scars or striae, the shape and contour of the abdomen, and the fundal height. Purplish striae and linea nigra are normal in pregnancy. The shape and contour may indicate pregnancy size (see figures on p. 410).

Scars may confirm the type of prior surgery, especially cesarean section.

Palpate the abdomen for:

- *Organs or masses.* The mass of pregnancy is expected.
- *Fetal movements.* These can usually be felt by the examiner after 24 weeks (and by the mother at 18–20 weeks).

If movements cannot be felt after 24 weeks, consider error in calculating gestation, fetal death or morbidity, or false pregnancy.

- *Uterine contractility.* The uterus contracts irregularly after 12 weeks and often in response to palpation during the third trimester. The abdomen then feels tense or firm to the examiner, and it is difficult to feel fetal parts. If the hand is left resting on the fundal portion of the uterus, the fingers will sense the relaxation of the uterine muscle.

Prior to 37 weeks, regular uterine contractions with or without pain or bleeding are abnormal, suggesting preterm labor.

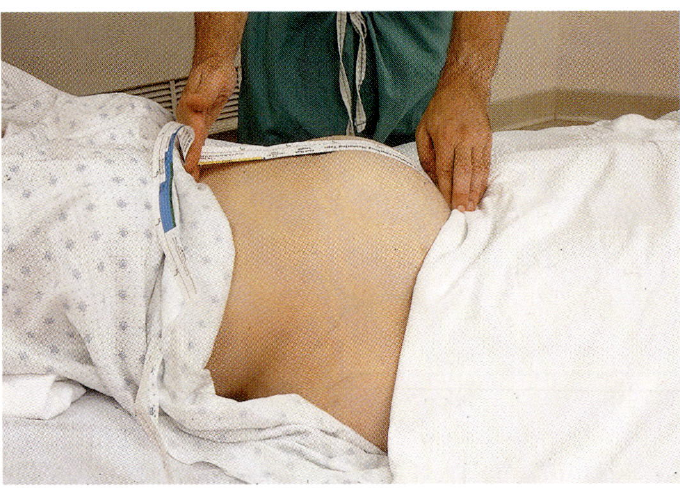

Measure the fundal height with a tape measure if the woman is more than 20 weeks' pregnant. Holding the tape as illustrated and following the midline of the abdomen, measure from the top of the symphysis pubis to the top of the uterine fundus. After 20 weeks, measurement in centimeters should roughly equal the weeks of gestation. For estimating fetal height between 12 and 20 weeks, see p. 410.

If fundal height is more than 2 cm higher than expected, consider multiple gestation, a big baby, extra amniotic fluid, or uterine myomata. If it is lower than expected by more than 2 cm, consider missed abortion, transverse lie, growth retardation, or false pregnancy.

Auscultate the fetal heart, noting its rate (FHR), location, and rhythm. Use either:

- A doptone, with which the FHR is audible after 12 weeks, or
- A fetoscope, with which it is audible after 18 weeks.

Lack of an audible fetal heart may indicate pregnancy of fewer weeks than expected, fetal demise, or false pregnancy.

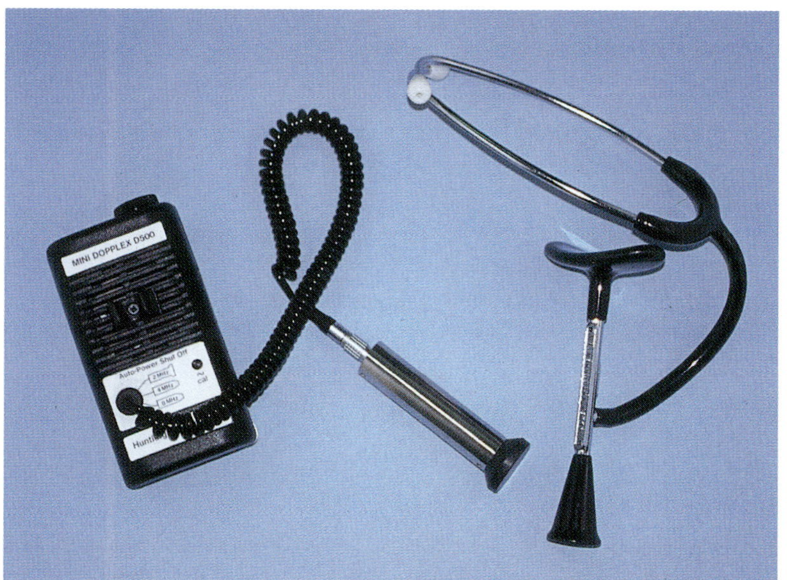

DOPTONE (LEFT) AND FETOSCOPE (RIGHT)

The *rate* is usually in the 160s during early pregnancy, and then slows to the 120s to 140s near term. After 32 to 34 weeks, the FHR should increase with fetal movement.

An FHR that drops noticeably near term with fetal movement could indicate poor placental circulation.

The *location* of the audible FHR is in the midline of the lower abdomen from 12 to 18 weeks of gestation. After 28 weeks, the fetal heart is heard best over the fetal back or chest. The location of the FHR then depends on how the fetus is positioned. Palpating the fetal head and back helps you identify where to listen. (See Modified Leopold's Maneuvers, pp. 424–426.) If the fetus is head down with the back on the woman's left side, the FHR is heard best in the lower left quadrant. If the fetal head is under the xiphoid process (*breech presentation*) with the back on the right, the FHR is heard in the upper right quadrant.

After 24 weeks, auscultation of more than one FHR with varying rates in different locations suggests more than one fetus.

Rhythm becomes important in the third trimester. Expect a variance of 10 to 15 beats per minute (BPM) over 1 to 2 minutes.

Lack of beat-to-beat variability late in pregnancy suggests fetal compromise.

Genitalia, Anus, and Rectum

Inspect the *external genitalia,* noting the hair distribution, the color, and any scars. Parous relaxation of the introitus and noticeable enlargement of the labia and clitoris are normal. Scars from an *episiotomy,* a perineal incision to facilitate delivery of an infant, or from perineal lacerations may be present in multiparous women.

Some women have labial varicosities that become tortuous and painful.

Inspect the *anus* for *hemorrhoids.* If these are present, note their size and location.

Varicosities often engorge later in pregnancy. They may be painful and bleed.

Palpate *Bartholin's* and *Skene's glands.* No discharge or tenderness should be present.

Check for a *cystocele* or *rectocele.*

May be pronounced due to the muscle relaxation of pregnancy

Speculum Examination. Inspect the *cervix* for color, shape, and healed lacerations. A parous cervix may look irregular because of lacerations (see p. 403).

A pink cervix suggests a nonpregnant state.

Take *Pap smears* and, if indicated, other vaginal or cervical specimens. The cervix may bleed more easily when touched due to the vasocongestion of pregnancy.

Vaginal infections are more common during pregnancy, and specimens may be needed for diagnosis.

Inspect the *vaginal walls* for color, discharge, rugae, and relaxation. A bluish or violet color, deep rugae, and an increased milky white discharge, *leukorrhea,* are normal.

A pink vagina suggests a nonpregnant state. Vaginal irritation and itching with discharge suggest infection.

Bimanual Examination. Insert two lubricated fingers into the introitus, palmar side down, with slight pressure downward on the perineum. Slide the fingers into the posterior vaginal vault. Maintaining downward pressure, gently turn the fingers palmar side up. Avoid the sensitive urethral structures at all times. With the relaxation of pregnancy, the bimanual examination is usually easier to accomplish. Tissues are soft and the vaginal walls usually close in on the examining fingers, giving the sensation of being immersed in a bowl of oatmeal. It may be difficult to distinguish the cervix at first because of its softer texture.

Place your finger gently in the os, then sweep it around the *surface of the cervix.* A nulliparous cervix should be closed, while a multiparous cervix may admit a fingertip through the external os. The internal os—the narrow passage between the endocervical canal and the uterine cavity—should be closed in both situations. The surface of a normal multiparous cervix may feel irregular due to the healed lacerations from a previous birth.

A shortened effaced cervix prior to 32 weeks may indicate preterm labor.

Estimate the *length of the cervix* by palpating the lateral surface of the cervix from the cervical tip to the lateral fornix. Prior to 34 to 36 weeks, the cervix should retain its normal length of about 1.5 to 2 cm.

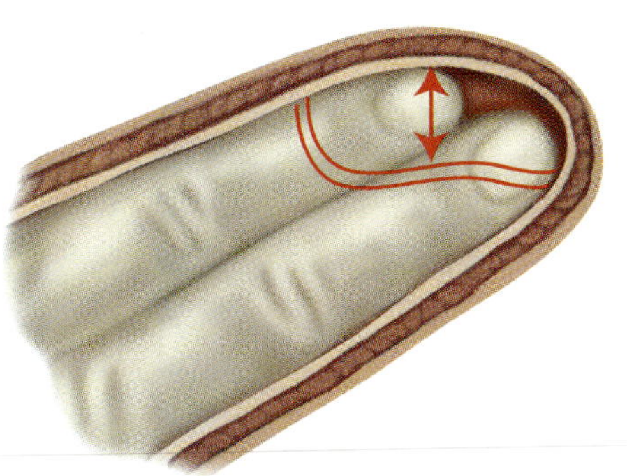

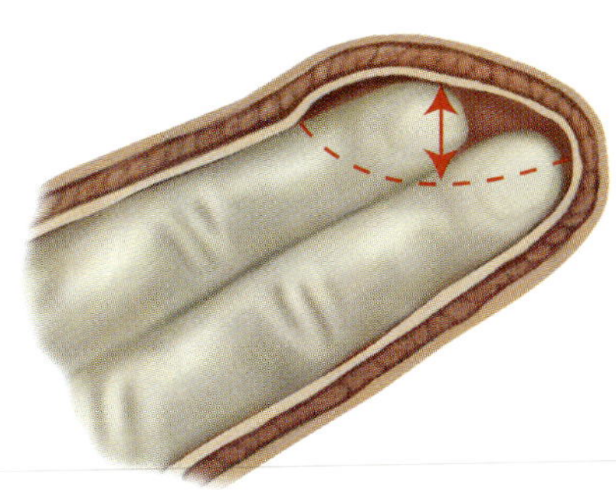

Palpate the *uterus* for size, shape, consistency, and position. These depend on the weeks of gestation. Early softening of the isthmus, *Hegar's sign,* is characteristic of pregnancy. The uterus is shaped like an inverted pear until 8 weeks, with slight enlargement in the fundal portion. The uterus becomes globular by 10 to 12 weeks. Anteflexion or retroflexion is lost by 12 weeks, with the fundal portion measuring about 8 cm in diameter.

With your internal fingers placed at either side of the cervix, palmar surfaces upward, gently lift the uterus toward the abdominal hand. Capture the fundal portion of the uterus between your two hands and gently estimate uterine size.

An irregularly shaped uterus suggests uterine myomata or a *bicornuate uterus,* which has two distinct uterine cavities separated by a septum.

Palpate the *left and right adnexa*. The corpus luteum may feel like a small nodule on the affected ovary during the first few weeks after conception. Late in pregnancy, adnexal masses may be difficult to feel.

Early in pregnancy, it is important to rule out a tubal (*ectopic*) pregnancy. See Table 11-7 Adnexal Masses, p. 408.

Palpate for *pelvic muscle strength* as you withdraw your examining fingers.

A *rectovaginal examination* may be done if you need to confirm uterine size or the integrity of the rectovaginal septum. A pregnancy of less than 10 weeks in a retroverted and retroflexed uterus lies totally in the posterior pelvis. Its size can be confirmed only by this examination.

Extremities

General inspection may be done with the woman seated or lying on her left side.

Inspect the legs for *varicose veins.*

Varicose veins may begin or worsen during pregnancy.

Inspect the hands and legs for *edema*. Palpate for pretibial, ankle, and pedal edema. Edema is rated on a 0 to 4+ scale. Physiologic edema is more common in advanced pregnancy, during hot weather, and in women who stand a lot.

Pathologic edema associated with PIH is often 3+ or more pretibially; it also affects the hands and face.

Obtain knee and ankle *reflexes.*

After 24 weeks, reflexes greater than 2+ may indicate PIH.

Special Techniques

MODIFIED LEOPOLD'S MANEUVERS

These maneuvers are important adjuncts to palpation of the pregnant abdomen beginning at 28 weeks of gestation. They help determine where the fetus is lying in relation to the woman's back (longitudinal or transverse), what end of the fetus is presenting at the pelvic inlet (head or buttocks), where the fetal back is located, how far the presenting part of the fetus has descended into the maternal pelvis, and the estimated weight of the fetus. This information is necessary to assess the adequacy of fetal growth and the probability of successful vaginal birth.

Interpretation

Common deviations include *breech presentation* (the fetal buttocks presenting at the outlet of the maternal pelvis) and absence of the presenting part well down into the maternal pelvis at term. Neither situation necessarily precludes vaginal birth. The most serious findings are a *transverse lie* close to term and slowed fetal growth that could represent *intrauterine growth retardation (IUGR).*

First Maneuver (Upper Pole). Stand at the woman's side facing her head. Keeping the fingers of both examining hands together, palpate gently with the fingertips to determine what part of the fetus is in the upper pole of the uterine fundus.

Most commonly, the fetal buttocks are at the upper pole. They feel firm but irregular, and less globular than the head. The fetal head feels firm, round, and smooth.

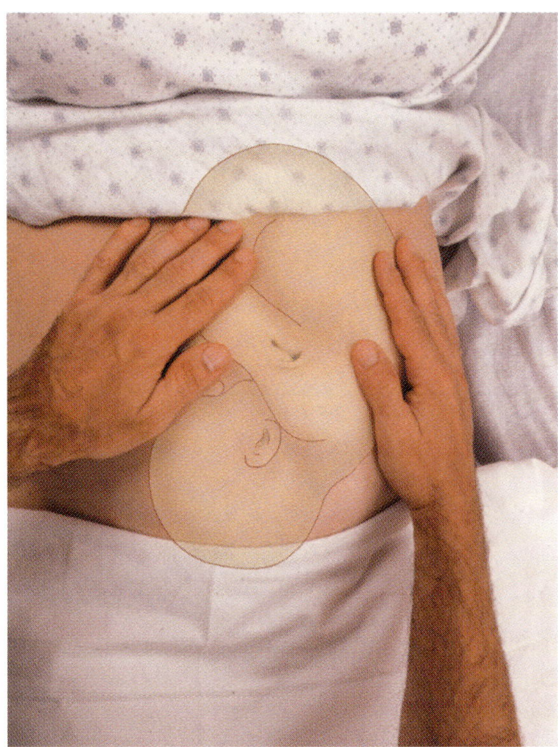

© B. Proud (photograph).

Second Maneuver (Sides of the Maternal Abdomen). Place one hand on each side of the woman's abdomen, aiming to capture the body of the fetus between them. Use one hand to steady the uterus and the other to palpate the fetus.

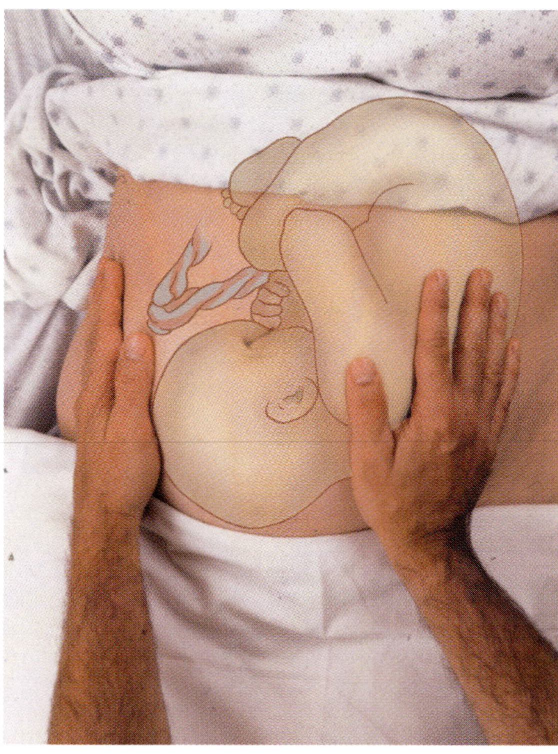

© B. Proud (photograph).

The hand on the fetal back feels a smooth, firm surface the length of the hand (or longer) by 32 weeks of gestation. The hand on the fetal arms and legs feels irregular bumps, and also perhaps kicking if the fetus is awake and active.

Third Maneuver (Lower Pole). Turn and face the woman's feet. Using the flat palmar surfaces of the fingers of both hands and, at the start, touching the fingertips together, palpate the area just above the symphysis pubis. Note whether the hands diverge with downward pressure or stay together. This tells you whether or not the presenting part of the fetus, head or buttocks, is descending into the pelvic inlet.

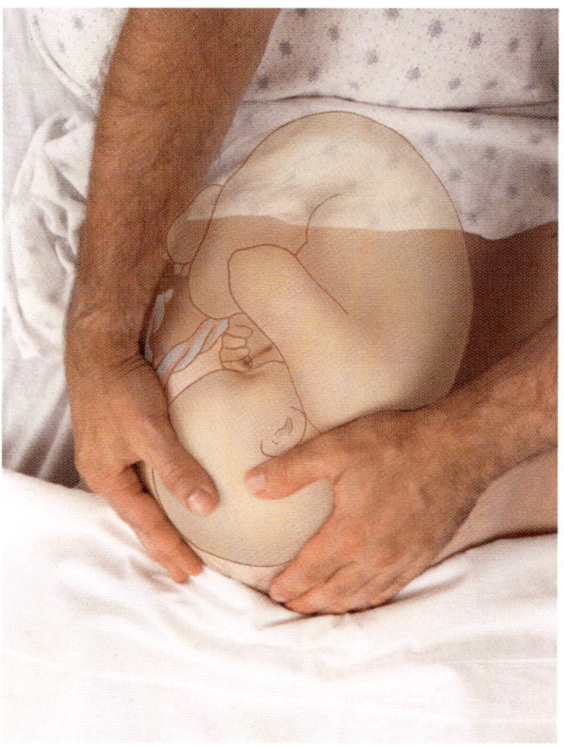

© B. Proud (photograph).

If the fetal head is presenting, the fingers feel a smooth, firm, rounded surface on both sides.

If the hands diverge, the presenting part is descending into the pelvic inlet, as illustrated.

If the hands stay together and you can gently depress the tissue over the bladder without touching the fetus, the presenting part is above your hands.

If the presenting fetal part is descending, palpate its texture and firmness. If not, gently move your hands up the lower abdomen and capture the presenting part between your hands.

The fetal head feels smooth, firm, and rounded; the buttocks, firm but irregular.

Fourth Maneuver (Confirmation of the Presenting Part). With your dominant hand grasp the part of the fetus in the lower pole, and with your nondominant hand, the part of the fetus in the upper pole. With this maneuver, you may be able to distinguish between the head and the buttocks.

Most commonly, the head is in the lower pole and the fetal buttocks are in the upper pole. If the head is above the pelvic inlet, it moves somewhat independently of the rest of the fetal body.

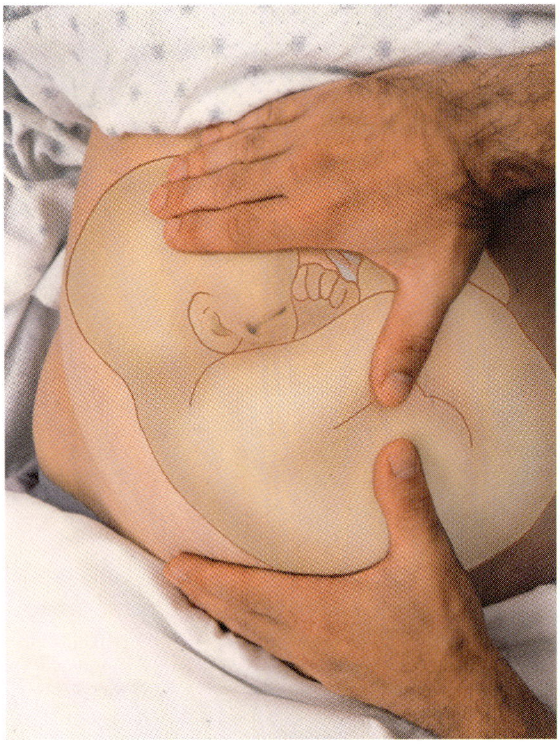

Concluding the Visit

Once the examination is completed and the woman is dressed, review the findings with her. If further data are necessary to confirm pregnancy, discuss how these may be obtained. Reinforce the importance of regular prenatal care. Record all your findings on the prenatal record.

CHAPTER

13

The Anus, Rectum, and Prostate

ANATOMY AND PHYSIOLOGY

The gastrointestinal tract terminates in a short segment, the *anal canal.* Its external margin is poorly demarcated, but the skin of the anal canal can usually be distinguished from the surrounding perianal skin by its moist, hairless appearance. The anal canal is normally held in a closed position by the muscle action of the voluntary *external anal sphincter* and involuntary *internal anal sphincter,* the latter an extension of the muscular coat of the rectal wall.

The direction of the anal canal on a line roughly between anus and umbilicus should be noted carefully. Unlike the rectum above it, the canal is liberally supplied by somatic sensory nerves, and a poorly directed finger or instrument will produce pain.

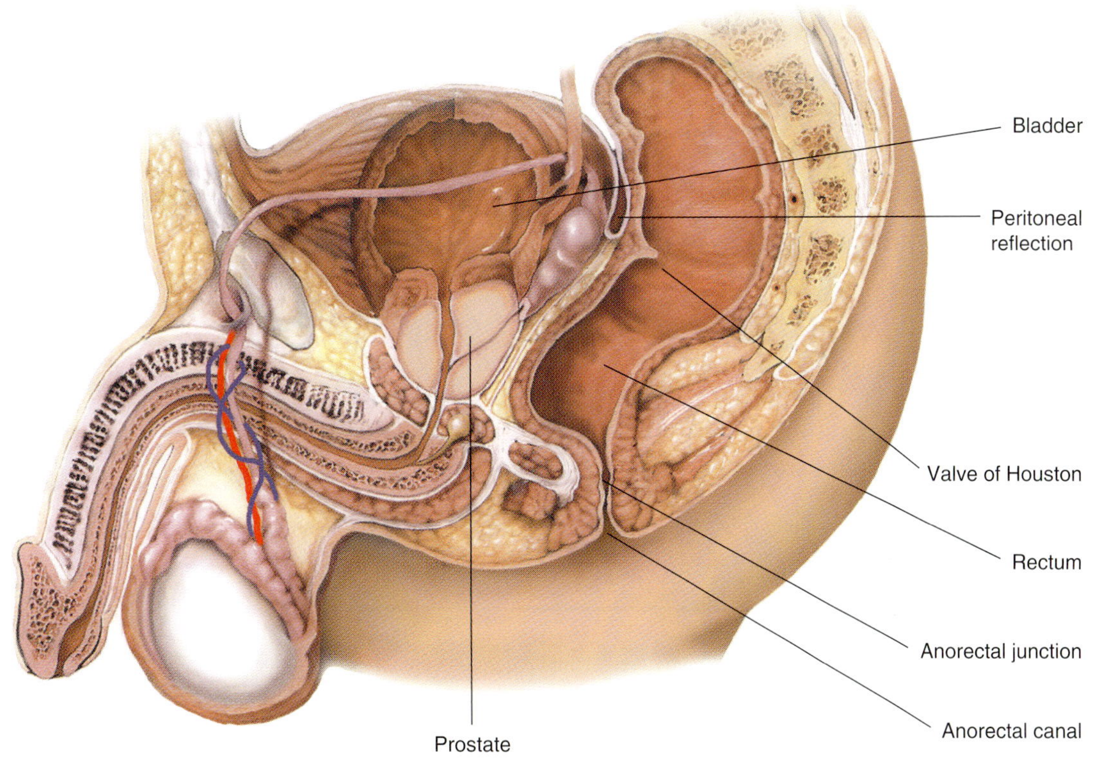

MEDIAN SECTION—VIEW FROM THE LEFT SIDE

The anal canal is demarcated from the rectum superiorly by a serrated line marking the change from skin to mucous membrane. This anorectal junction, often called the *pectinate* or *dentate line*, also denotes the boundary between somatic and visceral nerve supplies. It is readily visible on proctoscopic examination, but is not palpable.

Above the anorectal junction, the rectum balloons out and turns posteriorly into the hollow of the coccyx and the sacrum. In the male, the three lobes of the *prostate gland* surround the urethra. The two lateral lobes lie against the anterior rectal wall, where they are readily palpable as a rounded, heart-shaped structure about 2.5 cm in length. They are separated by a shallow median sulcus or groove, also palpable. The third, or median, lobe is anterior to the urethra and cannot be examined. The *seminal vesicles*, shaped like rabbit ears above the prostate, are also not normally palpable.

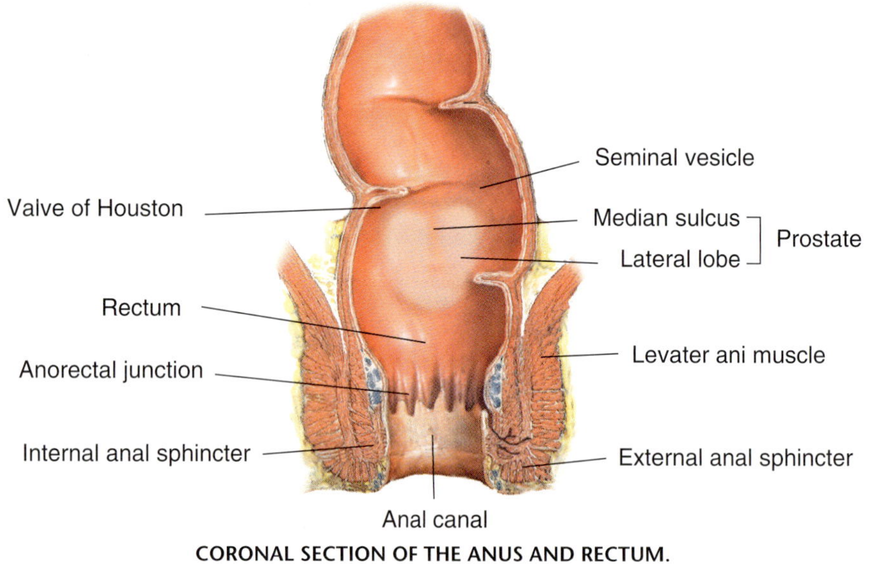

CORONAL SECTION OF THE ANUS AND RECTUM. VIEW FROM BEHIND, SHOWING THE ANTERIOR WALL

In the female, the uterine *cervix* can usually be felt through the anterior wall of the rectum.

The rectal wall contains three inward foldings, called *valves of Houston*. The lowest of these can sometimes be felt, usually on the patient's left. Most of the rectum that is accessible to digital examination does not have a peritoneal surface. The anterior rectum usually does, however, and you may reach it with the tip of your examining finger. You may thus be able to identify the tenderness of peritoneal inflammation or the nodularity of peritoneal metastases.

Changes With Aging

The prostate gland is small during boyhood, but between puberty and the age of about 20 years it increases roughly five-fold in size. Starting in about the 5th decade, further enlargement is increasingly common as the gland becomes hyperplastic (see p. 439).

THE HEALTH HISTORY

Common or Concerning Symptoms

- Change in bowel habits
- Blood in the stool
- Pain with defecation, rectal bleeding, or tenderness
- Anal warts or fissures
- Weak stream of urine
- Burning with urination

Many questions concerning symptoms related to the anorectal area and the prostate have been addressed in other chapters. For example, you will need to ask if there has been any change in the pattern of bowel function or the size or caliber of the stools. What about diarrhea or constipation? You will need to ask about the color of the stools. Turn to pp. 324–326 and review the health history regarding these symptoms, as well as queries about *blood in the stool*, ranging from black stools, suggesting *melena*, to the red blood of *hematochezia* to *bright red blood per rectum*. Has there been any mucus present in the stool?

See Table 9-5, Black and Bloody Stools, and Table 9-3, Constipation.

Change in bowel pattern, especially stools of thin pencil-like caliber, may warn of cancer. Blood in the stool from polyps or cancer, also from gastrointestinal bleeding, local hemorrhoids, mucus in villous adenoma.

Is there any pain on defecation? Any itching? Any extreme tenderness in the anus or rectum? Is there any mucopurulent discharge or bleeding? Any ulcerations? Does the patient have anal intercourse?

Proctitis with anorectal pain, pruritus, tenesmus, discharge or bleeding in anorectal infection from gonorrhea, *Chlamydia,* lymphogranuloma venereum; ulcerations in herpes simplex, chancre in primary syphilis. May arise from receptive anal intercourse. Itching in younger patients from pinworms.

Is there any history of anal warts, or anal fissures?

Genital warts from *human papillomavirus, condylomata lata* in secondary syphilis. Anal fissures in proctitis, Crohn's disease

In men, review the pattern of urination (see pp. 327–328). Does the patient have any difficulty starting the urine stream or holding back urine? Is the flow weak? What about frequent urination, especially at night? Or pain or burning as urine is passed? Any blood in the urine or semen or pain with ejaculation? Is there frequent pain or stiffness in the lower back, hips, or upper thighs?

These symptoms suggest urethral obstruction as in benign prostatic hyperplasia or prostate cancer, especially in men older than age 70.

Also in men, is there any feeling of discomfort or heaviness in the prostate area at the base of the penis? Any associated malaise, fever, or chills?

Suggests possible prostatitis

HEALTH PROMOTION AND COUNSELING

Important Topics for Health Promotion and Counseling

- Screening for prostate cancer
- Screening for polyps and colorectal cancer.

Clinicians should discuss screening issues related to prostate cancer to promote health for men, and provide screening recommendations to both men and women for detection of colorectal cancer and adenomatous colonic polyps.

Prostate cancer is the leading cancer diagnosed in men in the United States, and the second leading cause of death in North American men. Ethnicity and age strongly influence risk. African American men have the highest incidence rate of prostate cancer in the world, and Asian and native American men have the lowest rates. Sixty percent of all new cases and approximately 80% of deaths occur in men age 70 or older. Also at risk are men with a family history of prostate cancer.

To educate patients about prostate cancer, clinicians must be knowledgeable about several issues related to general screening of patients *without symptoms.* Prognosis is most favorable when the cancer is confined to the prostate, and worsens with extracapsular or metastatic spread. Autopsy studies show that many men over 50, and even some who are younger, have nests of cancerous prostate cells that never cause disease. Since many of these tumors are quiescent, early detection may increase unnecessary testing and treatment without affecting survival. A further complication in decisions about screening is that currently available screening tests are not highly accurate, which heightens patient concern and leads to additional noninvasive and invasive testing.

The two principal screening tests for prostate cancer are the digital rectal examination (DRE) and the prostate-specific antigen test (PSA). Each of these tests has distinct limitations that warrant careful review with the patient.* The DRE reaches only the posterior and lateral surfaces of the prostate, missing 25% to 35% of tumors in other areas. Sensitivity of the DRE for prostate

*U.S. Preventive Health Services Task Force. Guide to Clinical Preventive Services, 2nd ed. Baltimore, Williams & Wilkins, pp. 119–134, 1996.

cancer is low, ranging from 20% to 68%. In addition, because the DRE has a high rate of false positives, further testing by transrectal ultrasound or even biopsy is common. Many professional societies recommend annual DRE between the ages of 40 or 50 and 70. In contrast, the U.S. Preventive Health Services Task Force currently recommends against routine screening by DRE until there is more definitive evidence of increased survival from early detection and of decreased adverse effects from testing and even surgery (prostatectomy carries up to a 20% risk of impotence and a 5% risk of urinary incontinence). Instead, the Task Force advises clinicians to counsel all men requesting screening about the utility of testing and "the benefits and harms of early detection and treatment."

The benefits of PSA testing are equally unclear. The PSA can be elevated in benign conditions like hyperplasia and prostatitis, and its detection rate for prostate cancer is low, about 28% to 35% in asymptomatic men. Several groups recommend annual combined screening with PSA and DRE for men over 50 and for African Americans and men over age 40 with a positive family history. Other groups, including the U.S. Preventive Health Services Task Force, do not recommend routine PSA screening until its benefits are more firmly established.

For men *with symptoms* of prostate disorders, the clinician's role is more straightforward. As men approach 50, risk of prostate cancer begins to increase. Review the symptoms of prostate disorders—incomplete emptying of the bladder, urinary frequency or urgency, weak or intermittent stream or straining to initiate flow, hematuria, nocturia, or even bony pains in the pelvis. Men may be reluctant to report such symptoms, but should be encouraged to seek evaluation and treatment early.

To increase detection of colorectal cancer, clinicians can make use of three screening tests that are currently available: the DRE, the fecal occult blood test (FOBT), and sigmoidoscopy. Both the DRE and the FOBT have significant limitations. The DRE permits the clinician to examine only 7 to 8 cm of the rectum (usually about 11 cm long)—only about 10% of colorectal cancers arise in this zone. The FOBT (see discussion on p. 330) detects only 2% to 11% of colorectal cancers and 20% to 30% of adenomas in individuals over age 50, and results in a high rate of false positives. Among advocates, the DRE and FOBT are usually performed annually after age 40 to 50. Flexible sigmoidoscopy (also discussed on p. 330) permits good surveillance of the distal third of the colon. It is generally recommended every 3 to 5 years for patients over 50. Patients over 40 with familial polyposis, inflammatory bowel disease, or history of colon cancer in a first-degree relative should be advised to obtain a colonoscopy or air contrast barium enema every 3 to 5 years.

Preview: Recording the Physical Examination—The Anus, Rectum, and Prostate

Note that initially you may use sentences to describe your findings; later you will use phrases. The style below contains phrases appropriate for most write-ups. Unfamiliar terms are explained in the next section, Techniques of Examination.

"No perirectal lesions or fissures. External sphincter tone intact. Rectal vault without masses. Prostate smooth and nontender with palpable median sulcus. (Or in a female, uterine cervix nontender). Stool brown and hemoccult negative."

OR

"Perirectal area inflamed; no ulcerations, warts, or discharge. Unable to examine external sphincter, rectal vault, or prostate because of spasm of external sphincter and marked inflammation and tenderness of anal canal."

Raises concern of proctitis from infectious cause

OR

"No perirectal lesions or fissures. External sphincter tone intact. Rectal vault without masses. Left lateral prostate lobe with 1 × 1 cm firm hard nodule; right lateral lobe smooth; median sulcus is obscured. Stool brown and hemoccult negative."

Raises concern of prostate cancer

TECHNIQUES OF EXAMINATION

For many patients, the rectal examination is probably the least popular segment of the physical examination. It may cause discomfort for the patient, perhaps embarrassment, but, if skillfully done, should not be truly painful in most circumstances. Although you may choose to omit a rectal examination in adolescents who have no relevant complaints, you should do one in adult patients. In middle-aged and older persons, omission risks missing an asymptomatic carcinoma. A successful examination requires gentleness, slow movement of your finger, a calm demeanor, and an explanation to the patient of what he or she may feel.

Male

The anus and rectum may be examined with the patient in one of several positions. For most purposes, the side-lying position is satisfactory and allows good views of the perianal and sacrococcygeal areas. This is the position described below. The lithotomy position may help you to reach a cancer high in the rectum. It also permits a bimanual examination, enabling you to delineate a pelvic mass. Some clinicians prefer to examine a patient while he stands with his hips flexed and his upper body resting across the examining table.

No matter how you position the patient, your examining finger cannot reach the full length of the rectum. If a rectosigmoid cancer is suspected or screening is warranted, inspection by sigmoidoscopy is necessary.

Ask the patient to lie on his left side with his buttocks close to the edge of the examining table near you. Flexing the patient's hips and knees, especially in the top leg, stabilizes his position and improves visibility. Drape the patient appropriately and adjust the light for the best view. Glove your hands and spread the buttocks apart.

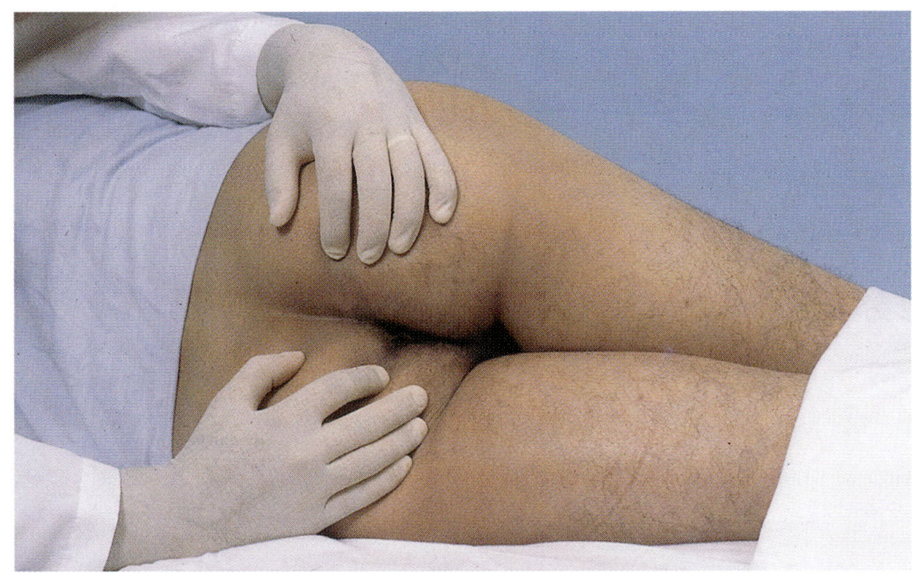

- *Inspect the sacrococcygeal and perianal areas* for lumps, ulcers, inflammation, rashes, or excoriations. Adult perianal skin is normally more pigmented and somewhat coarser than the skin over the buttocks. Palpate any abnormal areas, noting lumps or tenderness.

Anal and perianal lesions include hemorrhoids, venereal warts, herpes, syphilitic chancre, and carcinoma. A perianal abscess produces a painful, tender, indurated, and reddened mass. Pruritus ani causes swollen, thickened, fissured skin with excoriations.

- *Examine the anus and rectum.* Lubricate your gloved index finger, explain to the patient what you are going to do, and tell him that the examination may make him feel as if he were moving his bowels but that he will not do so. Ask him to strain down. Inspect the anus, noting any lesions.

As the patient strains, place the pad of your lubricated and gloved index finger over the anus. As the sphincter relaxes, gently insert your fingertip into the anal canal, in a direction pointing toward the umbilicus.

Soft, pliable tags of redundant skin at the anal margin are common. Though sometimes due to past anal surgery or previously thrombosed hemorrhoids, they are often unexplained.

See Table 13-1, Abnormalities of the Anus, Surrounding Skin, and Rectum (pp. 437–438).

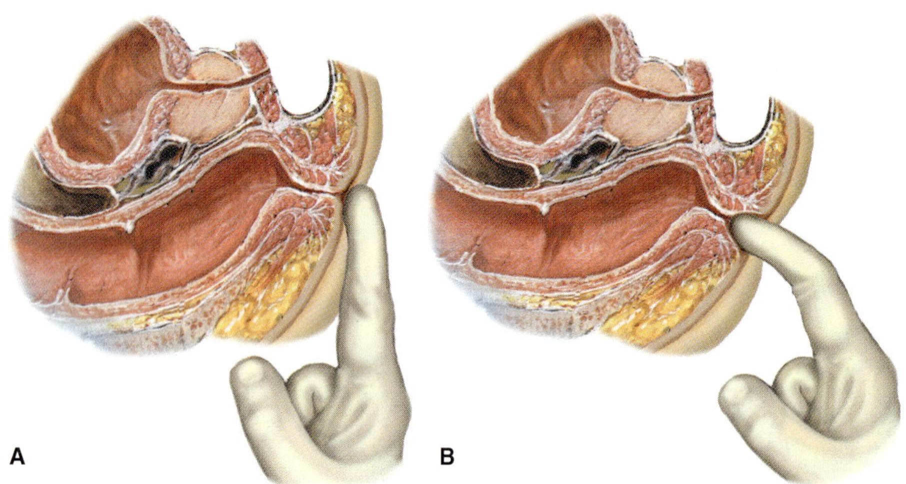

MEDIAN SECTIONS—VIEW FROM THE PATIENT'S RIGHT SIDE. PATIENT LYING ON HIS LEFT SIDE

If you feel the sphincter tighten, pause and reassure the patient. When in a moment the sphincter relaxes, proceed. Occasionally, severe tenderness prevents you from examining the anus. Do not try to force it. Instead, place your fingers on both sides of the anus, gently spread the orifice, and ask the patient to strain down. Look for a lesion, such as an anal fissure, that might explain the tenderness.

If you can proceed without undue discomfort, note:

- The sphincter tone of the anus. Normally, the muscles of the anal sphincter close snugly around your finger.

Sphincter tightness in anxiety, inflammation, or scarring; laxity in some neurologic diseases

- Tenderness, if any

- Induration

Induration may be due to inflammation, scarring, or malignancy.

- Irregularities or nodules

Insert your finger into the rectum as far as possible. Rotate your hand clockwise to palpate as much of the rectal surface as possible on the patient's right side, then counterclockwise to palpate the surface posteriorly and on the patient's left side.

Note any nodules, irregularities, or induration. To bring a possible lesion into reach, take your finger off the rectal surface, ask the patient to strain down, and palpate again.

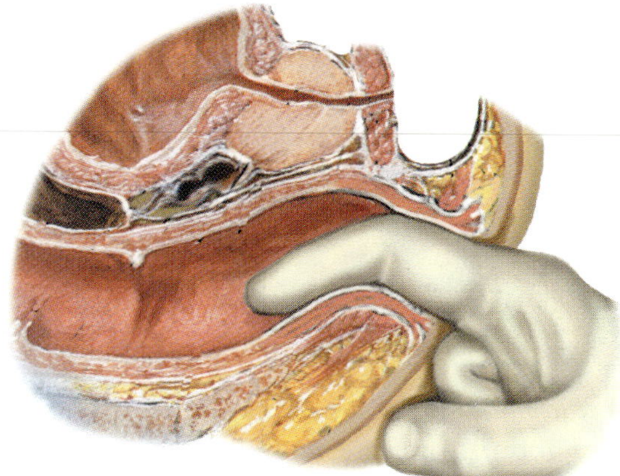

The irregular border of a rectal cancer is shown below.

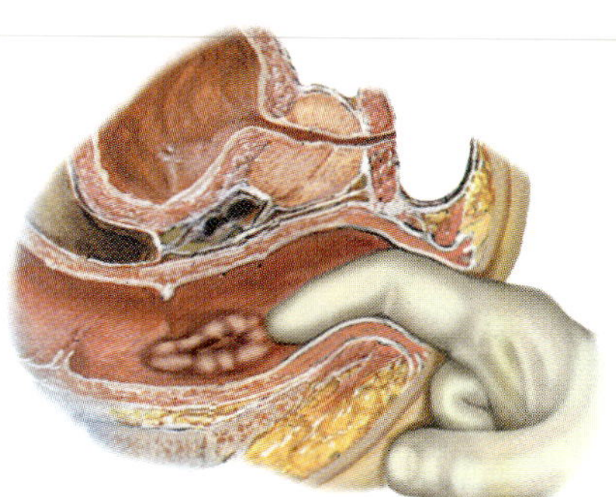

Then rotate your hand further counterclockwise so that your finger can *examine the posterior surface of the prostate gland*. By turning your body somewhat away from the patient, you can feel this area more easily. Tell the patient that you are going to feel his prostate gland, and that it may make him want to urinate but he will not do so.

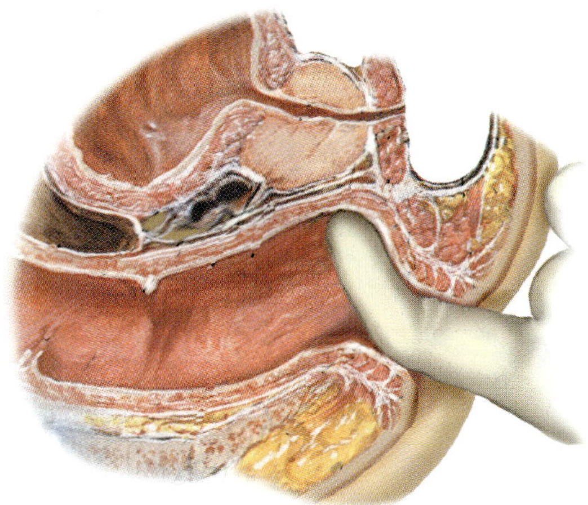

Sweep your finger carefully over the prostate gland, identifying its lateral lobes and the median sulcus between them. Note the size, shape, and consistency of the prostate, and identify any nodules or tenderness. The normal prostate is rubbery and nontender.

See Table 13-2, Abnormalities of the Prostate (p. 439).

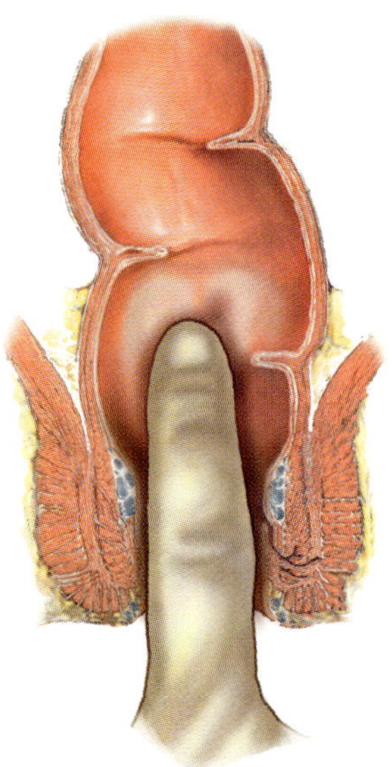

**PALPATING THE PROSTATE—
VIEW FROM BELOW**

If possible, *extend your finger above the prostate* to the region of the seminal vesicles and the peritoneal cavity. Note nodules or tenderness.

A rectal "shelf" of peritoneal metastases (see p. 438) or the tenderness of peritoneal inflammation

Gently withdraw your finger, and wipe the patient's anus or give him tissues to do it himself. Note the color of any fecal matter on your glove, and test it for occult blood.

Female

The rectum is usually examined after the female genitalia, while the patient is in the lithotomy position. If a rectal examination alone is indicated, the lateral position offers a satisfactory alternative. It affords a much better view of the perianal and sacrococcygeal areas.

The technique is basically similar to that described for males. The cervix is usually felt readily through the anterior rectal wall. Sometimes, a retroverted uterus is also palpable. Neither of these, nor a vaginal tampon, should be mistaken for a tumor.

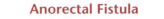

TABLE 13-1 ■ Abnormalities of the Anus, Surrounding Skin, and Rectum

Pilonidal Cyst and Sinus

A pilonidal cyst is a fairly common, probably congenital abnormality located in the midline superficial to the coccyx or the lower sacrum. It is clinically identified by the opening of a sinus tract. This opening may exhibit a small tuft of hair and be surrounded by a halo of erythema. Although pilonidal cysts are generally asymptomatic except perhaps for slight drainage, abscess formation and secondary sinus tracts may complicate the picture.

Anorectal Fistula

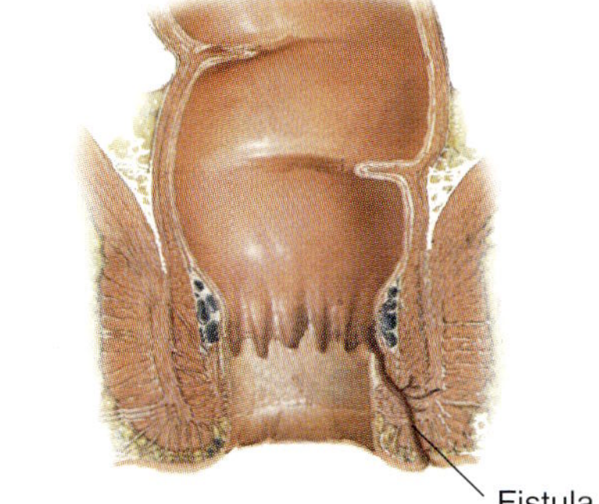
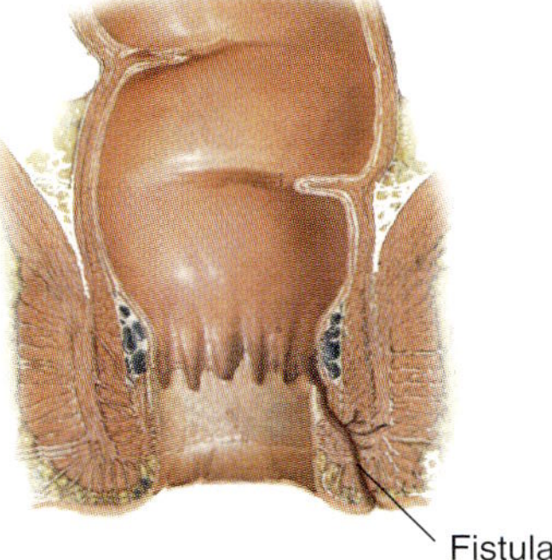

An anorectal fistula is an inflammatory tract or tube that opens at one end into the anus or rectum and at the other end onto the skin surface (as shown here) or into another viscus. An abscess usually antedates such a fistula. Look for the fistulous opening or openings anywhere in the skin around the anus.

Anal Fissure

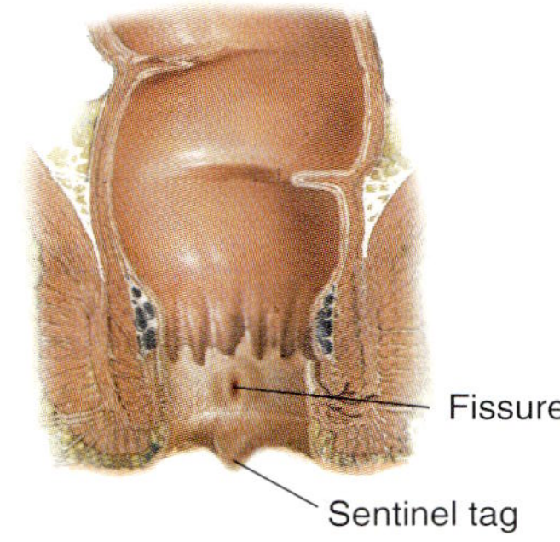

An anal fissure is a very painful oval ulceration of the anal canal, found most commonly in the midline posteriorly, less commonly in the midline anteriorly. Its long axis lies longitudinally. Inspection may show a swollen "sentinel" skin tag just below it, and gentle separation of the anal margins may reveal the lower edge of the fissure. The sphincter is spastic; the examination painful. Local anesthesia may be required.

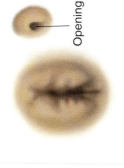

(table continues next page)

TABLE 13-1 ■ Abnormalities of the Anus, Surrounding Skin, and Rectum *(Continued)*

External Hemorrhoids *(Thrombosed)*

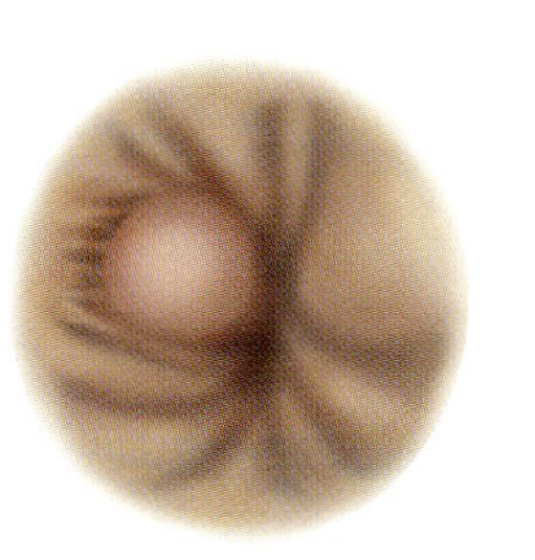

External hemorrhoids are dilated hemorrhoidal veins that originate below the pectinate line and are covered with skin. They seldom produce symptoms unless thrombosis occurs. This causes acute local pain that is increased by defecation and by sitting. A tender, swollen, bluish, ovoid mass is visible at the anal margin.

Internal Hemorrhoids *(Prolapsed)*

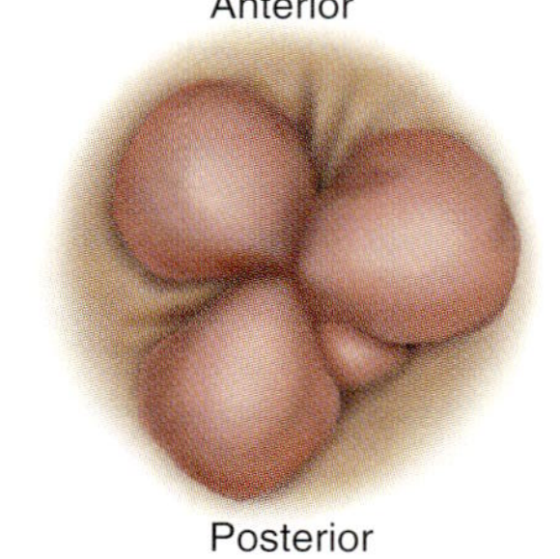

Internal hemorrhoids are an enlargement of the normal vascular cushions that are located above the pectinate line. Here they are not usually palpable. Sometimes, especially during defecation, internal hemorrhoids may cause bright red bleeding. They may also prolapse through the anal canal and appear as reddish, moist, protruding masses, typically located in one or more of the positions illustrated.

Prolapse of the Rectum

On straining for a bowel movement the rectal mucosa, with or without its muscular wall, may prolapse through the anus, appearing as a doughnut or rosette of red tissue. A prolapse involving only mucosa is relatively small and shows radiating folds, as illustrated. When the entire bowel wall is involved, the prolapse is larger and covered by concentrically circular folds.

Polyps of the Rectum

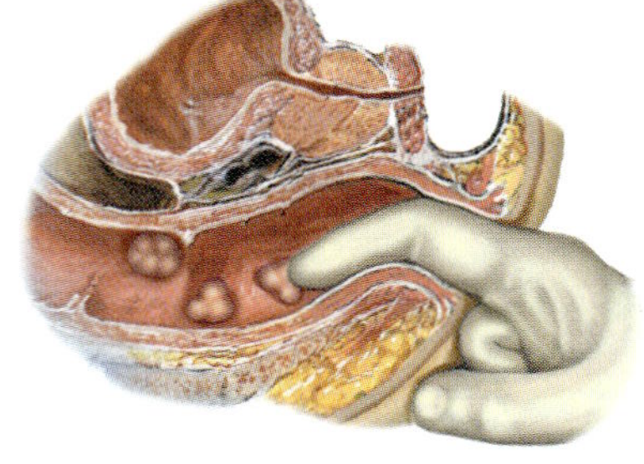

Polyps of the rectum are fairly common. Variable in size and number, they can develop on a stalk (*pedunculated*) or lie on the mucosal surface (*sessile*). They are soft and may be difficult or impossible to feel even when in reach of the examining finger. Proctoscopy is usually required for diagnosis, as is biopsy for the differentiation of benign from malignant lesions.

Cancer of the Rectum

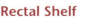

Asymptomatic carcinoma of the rectum makes routine rectal examination important for adults. Illustrated here is the firm, nodular, rolled edge of an ulcerated cancer. Polyps, as noted above, may also be malignant.

Rectal Shelf

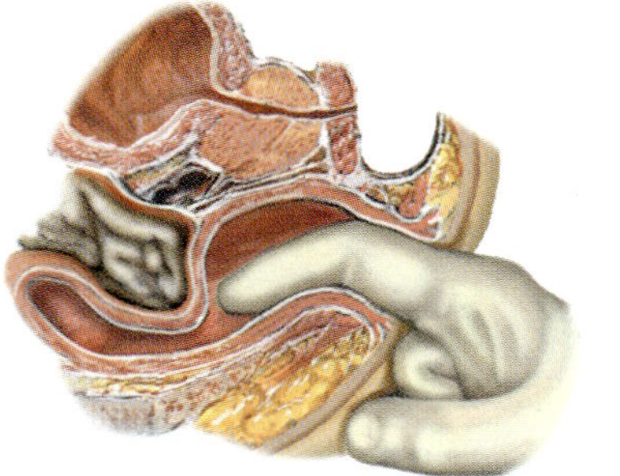

Widespread peritoneal metastases from any source may develop in the area of the peritoneal reflection anterior to the rectum. A firm to hard nodular rectal "shelf" may be just palpable with the tip of the examining finger. In a woman, this shelf of metastatic tissue develops in the rectouterine pouch, behind the cervix and the uterus.

TABLE 13-2 ■ Abnormalities of the Prostate

Normal Prostate Gland

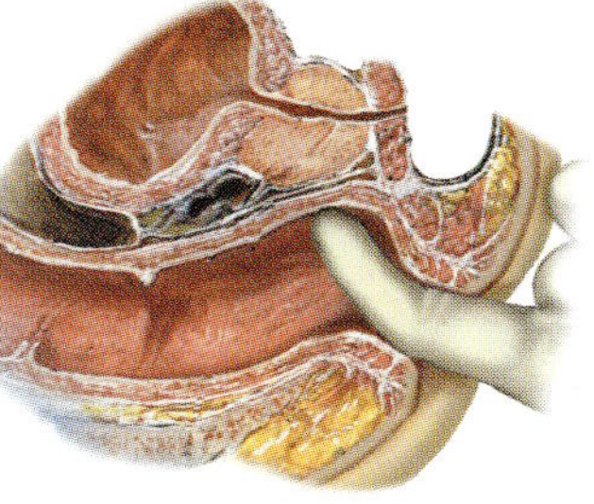

As palpated through the anterior rectal wall, the normal prostate is a rounded, heart-shaped structure about 2.5 cm in length. The median sulcus can be felt between the two lateral lobes. Only the posterior surface of the prostate is palpable. Anterior lesions, including those that may obstruct the urethra, are not detectable by physical examination.

Cancer of the Prostate

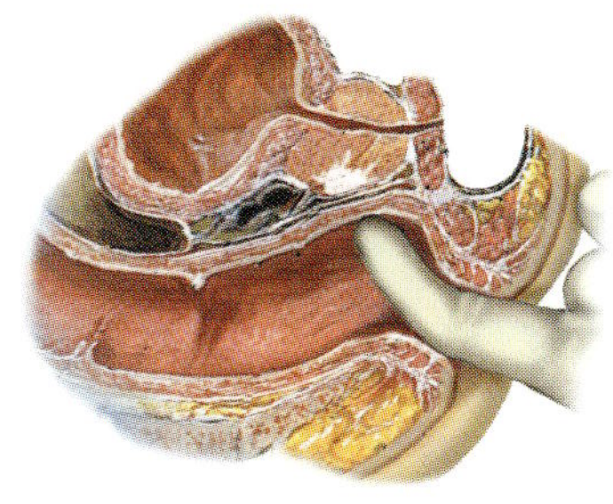

Cancer of the prostate is suggested by an area of hardness in the gland. A distinct hard nodule that alters the contour of the gland may or may not be palpable. As the cancer enlarges, it feels irregular and may extend beyond the confines of the gland. The median sulcus may be obscured. Hard areas in the prostate are not always malignant. They may also result from prostatic stones, chronic inflammation, and other conditions.

Benign Prostatic Hyperplasia

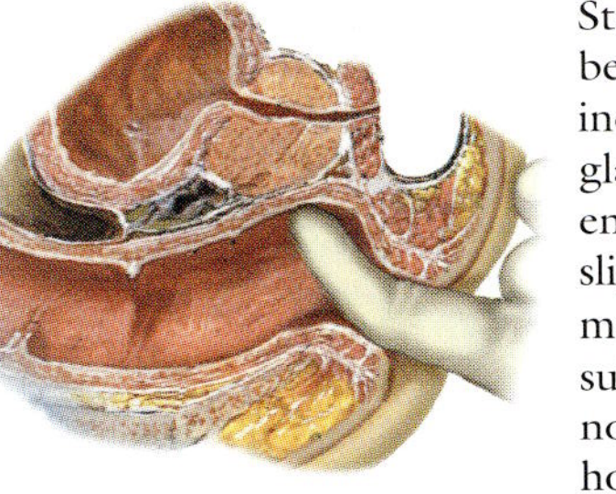

Starting in the 5th decade of life, benign prostatic hyperplasia becomes increasingly prevalent. The affected gland usually feels symmetrically enlarged, smooth, and firm though slightly elastic. It seems to protrude more into the rectal lumen. The median sulcus may be obliterated. Finding a normal-sized gland by palpation, however, does not rule out this diagnosis. Prostatic hyperplasia may obstruct urinary flow, causing symptoms, yet not be palpable.

Prostatitis

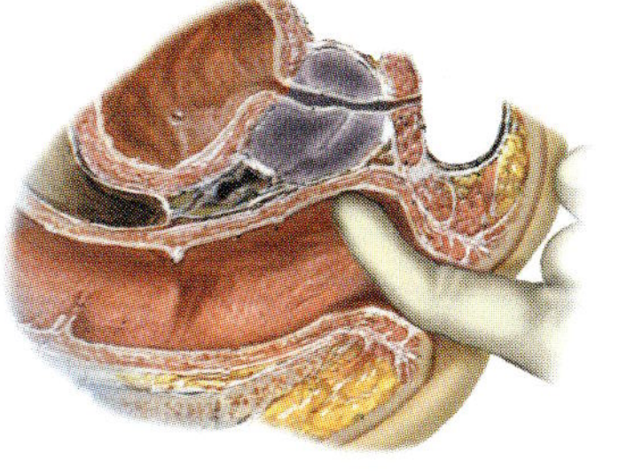

Acute prostatitis (illustrated here) is an acute, febrile condition caused by bacterial infection. The gland is very tender, swollen, firm, and warm. Examine it gently.

Chronic prostatitis does not produce consistent physical findings and must be evaluated by other methods.

CHAPTER

The Peripheral Vascular System

14

ANATOMY AND PHYSIOLOGY

This chapter focuses on circulation to the arms and legs. It includes the arteries, the veins, the capillary bed that connects them, and the lymphatic system with its lymph nodes.

Arteries

Arterial pulses are palpable when an artery lies close to the body surface. In the arms, there are two or sometimes three such locations. Pulsations of the *brachial artery* can be felt in and above the bend of the elbow, just medial to the biceps tendon and muscle. The brachial artery divides into the radial and ulnar arteries. *Radial artery* pulsations can be felt on the flexor surface of the wrist laterally. Medially, pulsations of the *ulnar artery* may be palpable, but overlying tissues frequently obscure them.

The radial and ulnar arteries are interconnected by two vascular arches within the hand. Circulation to the hand and fingers is thereby doubly protected against possible arterial occlusion.

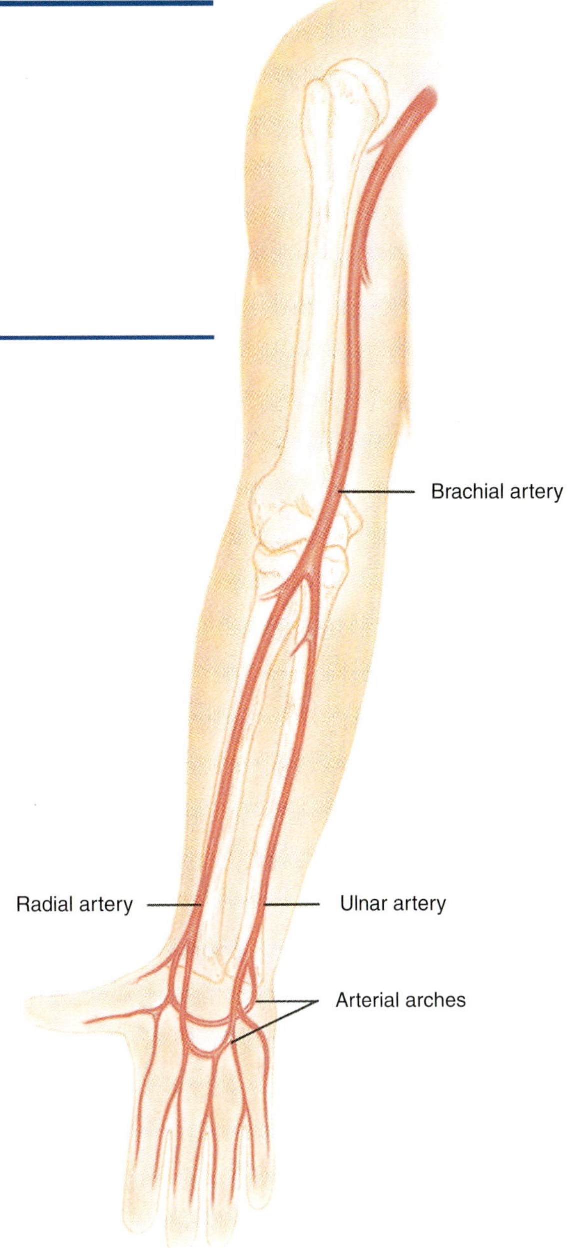

In the legs, arterial pulsations can usually be felt in four places. Those of the *femoral artery* are palpable below the inguinal ligament, midway between the anterior superior iliac spine and the symphysis pubis. The femoral artery travels downward deep within the thigh, passes medially behind the femur, and becomes the *popliteal artery*. Popliteal pulsations can be felt in the tissues behind the knee. Below the knee, the popliteal artery divides into two branches, both of which continue to the foot. There the anterior branch becomes the *dorsalis pedis artery*. Its pulsations are palpable on the dorsum of the foot just lateral to the extensor tendon of the big toe. The posterior branch, the *posterior tibial artery*, can be felt as it passes behind the medial malleolus of the ankle.

Like the hand, the foot is protected by an interconnecting arch between its two chief arterial branches.

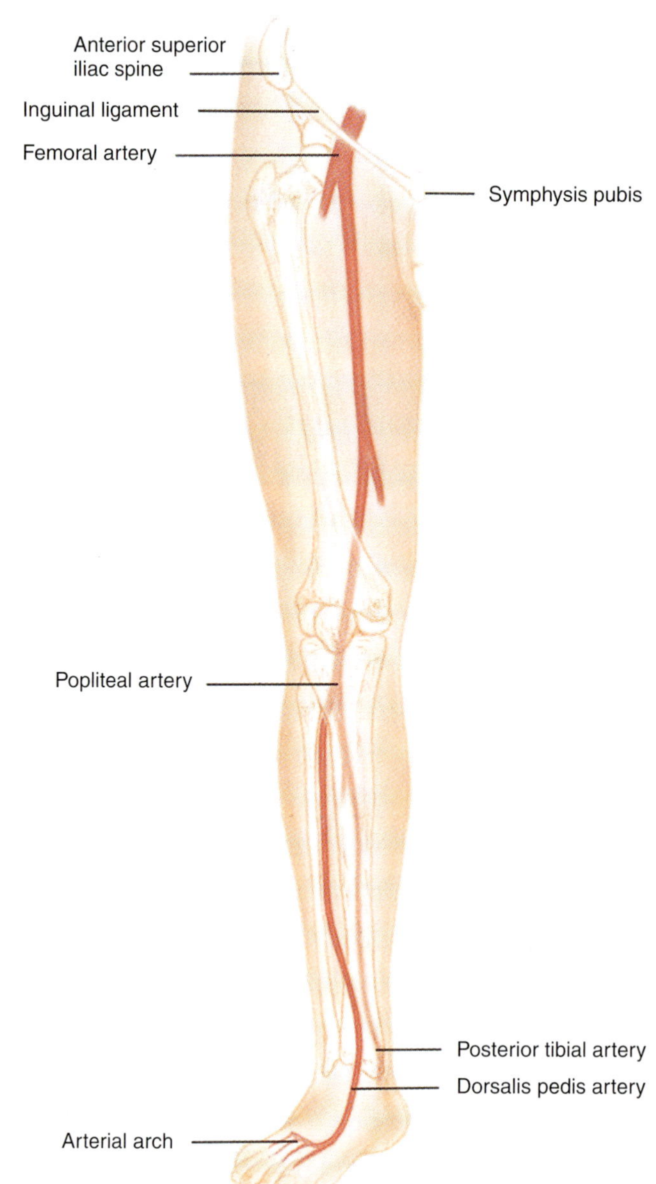

Veins

The veins from the arms, together with those from the upper trunk and the head and neck, drain into the superior vena cava and on into the right atrium. Veins from the legs and the lower trunk drain upward into the inferior vena cava. Because the leg veins are especially susceptible to dysfunction, they warrant special attention.

The *deep veins* of the legs carry about 90% of the venous return from the lower extremities. They are well supported by surrounding tissues.

In contrast, the *superficial veins* are located subcutaneously, and are supported relatively poorly. The superficial veins include (1) the *great saphenous vein,* which originates on the dorsum of the foot, passes just in front of the medial malleolus, and then continues up the medial aspect of the leg to join the deep venous system (the femoral vein) below the inguinal ligament; and (2) the *small saphenous vein,* which begins at the side of the foot and passes upward along the back of the leg to join the deep system in the popliteal space. Anastomotic veins connect the two saphenous veins superficially and, when dilated, are readily visible. In addition, *communicating (or perforating) veins* connect the saphenous system with the deep venous system.

Deep, superficial, and communicating veins all have one-way valves. These allow venous blood to flow from the superficial to the deep system and toward the heart, but not in the opposite directions. Muscular activity contributes importantly to venous blood flow. As calf muscles contract in walking, for example, blood is squeezed upward against gravity, and competent valves keep it from falling back again.

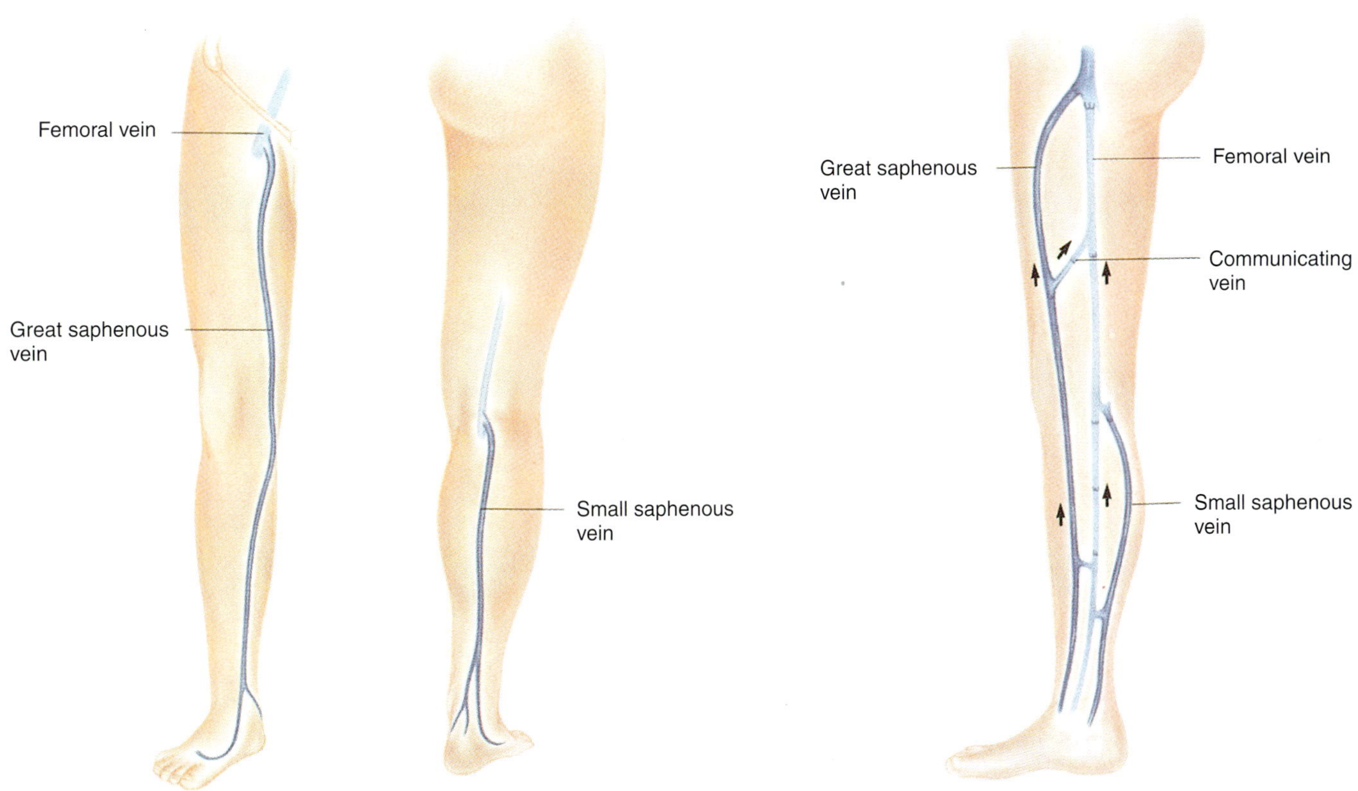

The Lymphatic System and Lymph Nodes

The lymphatic system comprises an extensive vascular network that drains fluid, called lymph, from bodily tissues and returns it to the venous circulation. The system starts peripherally as blind lymphatic capillaries, and continues centrally as thin vascular vessels and then collecting ducts that finally empty into major veins at the root of the neck. The lymph transported in these channels is filtered through lymph nodes that are interposed along the way.

Lymph nodes are round, oval, or bean-shaped structures that vary in size according to their location. Some lymph nodes, such as the preauriculars, if palpable at all, are typically very small. The inguinal nodes, in contrast, are relatively larger—often 1 cm in diameter and occasionally even 2 cm in an adult.

In addition to its vascular functions, the lymphatic system plays an important role in the body's immune system. Cells within the lymph nodes engulf cellular debris and bacteria and produce antibodies.

Only the superficial lymph nodes are accessible to physical examination. These include the cervical nodes (p. 133), the axillary nodes (p. 300), and nodes in the arms and legs.

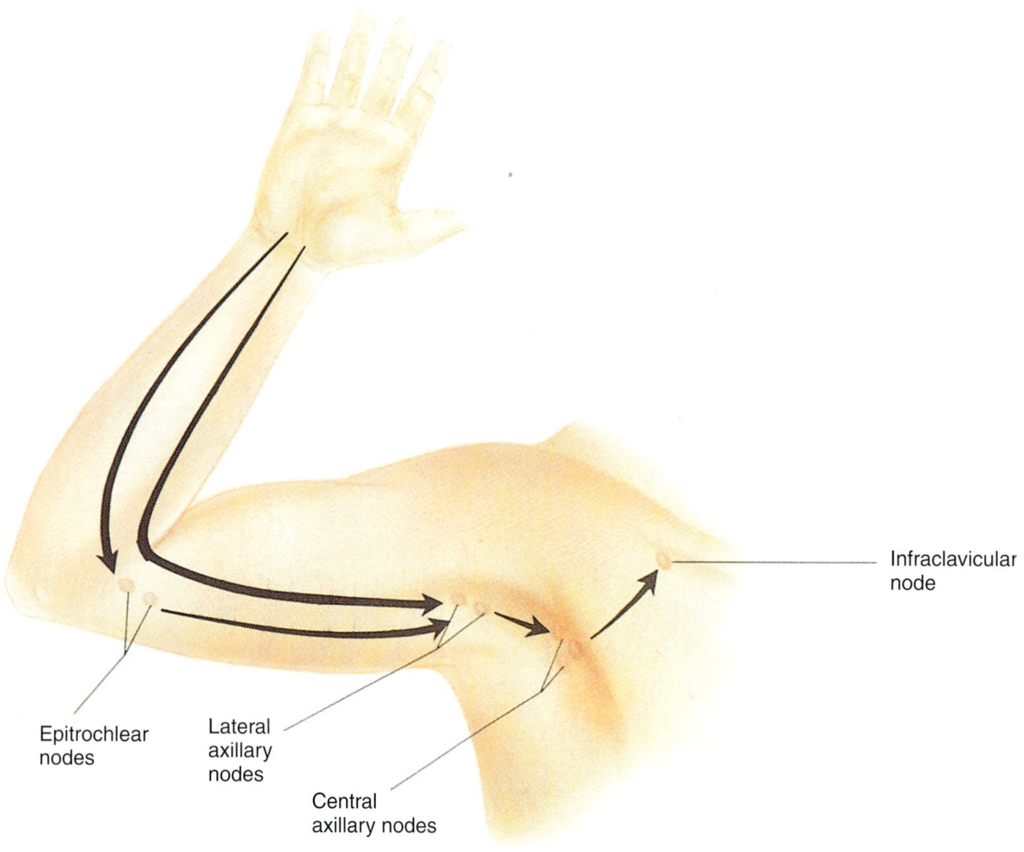

Recall that the axillary lymph nodes drain most of the arm. Lymphatics from the ulnar surface of the forearm and hand, the little and ring fingers, and the adjacent surface of the middle finger, however, drain first into the *epitrochlear nodes.* These are located on the medial surface of the arm about 3 cm above the elbow. Lymphatics from the rest of the arm drain mostly into the axillary nodes. A few may go directly to the infraclaviculars.

The lymphatics of the lower limb, following the venous supply, consist of both deep and superficial systems. Only the superficial nodes are palpable. The *superficial inguinal nodes* include two groups. The *horizontal group* lies in a chain high in the anterior thigh below the inguinal ligament. It drains the superficial portions of the lower abdomen and buttock, the external genitalia (but not the testes), the anal canal and perianal area, and the lower vagina.

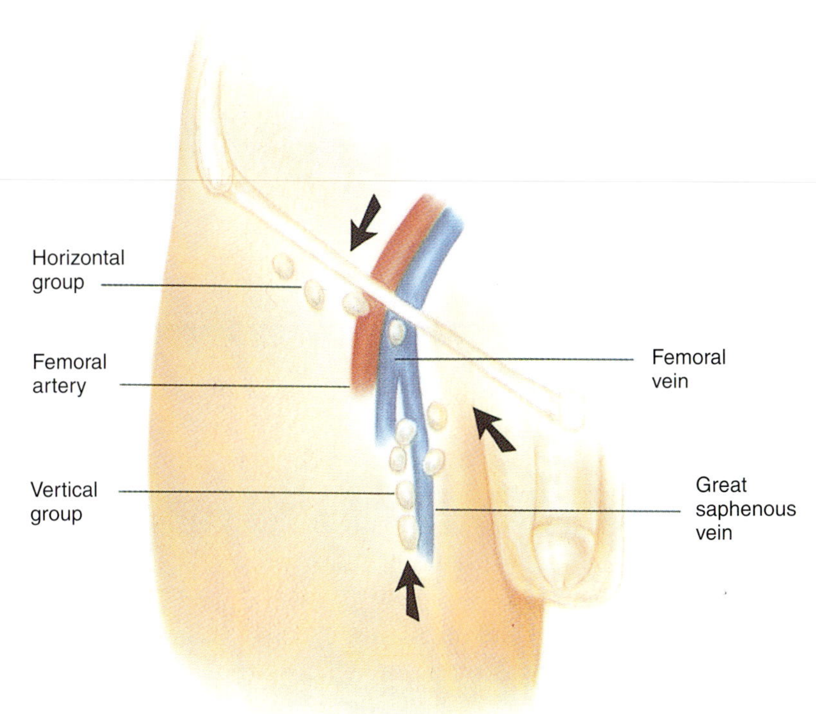

The *vertical group* clusters near the upper part of the saphenous vein and drains a corresponding region of the leg. In contrast, lymphatics from the portion of leg drained by the small saphenous vein (the heel and outer aspect of the foot) join the deep system at the level of the popliteal space. Lesions in this area, therefore, are not usually associated with palpable inguinal lymph nodes.

Fluid Exchange and the Capillary Bed

Blood circulates from arteries to veins through the capillary bed. Here fluids diffuse across the capillary membrane, maintaining a dynamic equilibrium between the vascular and interstitial spaces. Blood pressure (*hydrostatic pressure*) within the capillary bed, especially near the arteriolar end, forces fluid out into the tissue spaces. In effecting this movement, it is aided by the relatively weak osmotic attraction of proteins within the tissues (*interstitial colloid oncotic pressure*) and is opposed by the hydrostatic pressure of the tissues.

As blood continues through the capillary bed toward the venous end its hydrostatic pressure falls, and another force gains dominance. This is the *colloid oncotic pressure of plasma proteins,* which pulls fluid back into the vascular tree. Net flow of fluid, which was directed outward on the arteriolar side of the capillary bed, reverses itself and turns inward on the venous side. Lymphatic capillaries, which also play an important role in this equilibrium, remove excessive fluid, including protein, from the interstitial space.

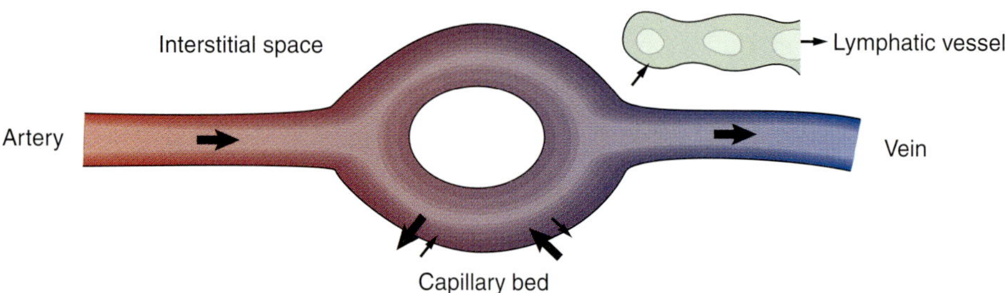

Lymphatic dysfunction or disturbances in hydrostatic or osmotic forces can all disrupt this equilibrium. The most common clinical result is the increased interstitial fluid known as edema (see Table 14-4, Some Peripheral Causes of Edema, p. 464).

Changes With Aging

Aging itself brings relatively few clinically important changes to the peripheral vascular system. Although arterial and venous disorders, especially atherosclerosis, do afflict older people more frequently, they probably cannot be considered part of the aging process. Age lengthens the arteries, makes them tortuous, and typically stiffens their walls, but these changes develop with or without atherosclerosis and therefore lack diagnostic specificity. Loss of arterial pulsations is not a part of normal aging, however, and demands careful evaluation. Skin may get thin and dry with age, nails may grow more slowly, and hair on the legs often becomes scant. Because these changes are common, they are not specific for arterial insufficiency, although they are classically associated with it.

THE HEALTH HISTORY

Common or Concerning Symptoms

- Pain in the arms or legs
- Intermittent claudication
- Cold, numbness, pallor in the legs, hair loss
- Color change in fingertips or toes in cold weather
- Swelling in calves, legs, or feet
- Swelling with redness or tenderness

To assess possible peripheral vascular disease, begin by asking patients about any *pain in the arms and legs.* Be aware that pain in the extremities may arise from the skin, the peripheral vascular system, the musculoskeletal system, or the nervous system. In addition, visceral pain may be referred to the ex-

See Table 14-1, Painful Peripheral Vascular Disorders and Their Mimics, pp. 460–461.

tremities, like the pain of myocardial infarction that radiates to the left arm or cervical arthritis that radiates to the shoulder.

To elicit symptoms of *arterial peripheral vascular disease* in the legs, inquire about *intermittent claudication,* which is exercise-induced pain that is absent at rest, makes the patient stop exertion, and remits within about 10 minutes. Ask "Have you ever had any pain or cramping in your legs when you walk or exercise?" and "How far can you walk without stopping to rest?" Also, "Does the pain get better with rest?" These questions clarify what makes the patient stop and how quickly the pain is relieved. Ask also about *coldness, numbness,* or *pallor* in the legs or feet or *loss of hair* over the anterior tibial surfaces.

Atherosclerosis can cause symptomatic limb ischemia with exertion; distinguish this from *spinal stenosis,* which produces leg pain with exertion that may be reduced by leaning forward (stretching the spinal cord in the narrowed vertebral canal) and less readily relieved by rest.

Hair loss over the anterior tibiae in decreased arterial perfusion. "Dry" or brown-black ulcers from gangrene may ensue.

Many patients with arterial peripheral vascular disease have few symptoms, so it is important to identify background risk factors. Assess the patient's history of tobacco abuse. Ask if the patient has had hypertension, diabetes, or hyperlipidemia. Further, is there any history of myocardial infarction or stroke? Such patients warrant further evaluation, even if without symptoms in the extremities (see p. 448).

Only about 10% of affected patients have the classic symptoms of exertional calf pain relieved by rest.

To elicit symptoms of arterial spasm in the fingers or toes, ask "Do your fingertips ever change color in cold weather or when you handle cold objects?" . . . "What color changes do you notice?" . . . "What about your toes?"

Digital ischemic changes of blanching, followed by cyanosis, then rubor with cold exposure and rewarming in Raynaud's phenomenon or disease

There may be symptoms of *venous peripheral vascular disease,* such as *swelling of the feet and legs.* Ask about any ulcers on the lower legs, often the near ankles.

Hyperpigmentation, edema, and possible cyanosis, especially when legs are dependent, in *venous stasis ulcers*

The redness, swelling, and tenderness of local inflammation are seen in some vascular disorders and in other conditions that mimic them. In contrast, relatively brief leg cramps that commonly occur at night in otherwise healthy people do not indicate a circulatory problem, and cold hands and feet are so common in healthy people that they have relatively little predictive value.

Inflammation in *cellulitis, superficial thrombophlebitis,* and *erythema nodosum*

Etiology of common leg cramps and "restless legs" not well understood. Leg cramps sometimes from diuretic use with hypokalemia

HEALTH PROMOTION AND COUNSELING

Important Topics for Health Promotion and Counseling

- Detection of peripheral arterial disease (PAD)
- Risk factors for PAD
- Screening for PAD: the ankle–brachial index (ABI)

Peripheral arterial disease (PAD) generally refers to atherosclerotic occlusion of arteries in the lower extremities. The femoral and popliteal arteries are involved most commonly, followed by the tibial and peroneal arteries. PAD affects from 12% to 25% of community populations; however, recent studies* have shown that despite significant associations with cardiovascular and cerebrovascular disease, PAD often is underdiagnosed in office practices. Most patients with PAD have either no symptoms or a range of nonspecific leg symptoms, such as aching, cramping, numbness, or fatigue. The classic triad for vascular claudication, exercise-induced calf pain that causes stopping of exercise and results in relief of pain in 10 minutes or less, may be present in only about 10% of affected patients.*

Patients with current or past tobacco use, diabetes, hypertension, hyperlipidemia, or cardiovascular or cerebrovascular disease are at increased risk of atherosclerotic PAD. Such patients should be screened for subclinical PAD and targeted for aggressive risk factor intervention. For screening, clinicians should consider use of the ankle–brachial index (ABI), a highly accurate test for detecting 50% or greater stenoses of 50% or more in major vessels of the legs. The ABI is readily performed by clinicians or office staff, and consists of measuring the systolic blood pressure with Doppler ultrasonography in each arm and in the dorsalis pedis and posterior tibial pulses. The ABI is calculated on both the right and left by dividing the higher right ankle pressure by the higher right arm pressure, and the higher left ankle pressure by the higher left arm pressure. ABI values are as follows: 0.90–1.30 is considered normal; 0.41–0.90—mild to moderate peripheral arterial disease, usually with symptoms of claudication; and 0.00–0.40—severe peripheral vascular disease with critical leg ischemia.

The severity of peripheral vascular disease closely parallels the risk of myocardial infarction, ischemic stroke, and death from vascular causes. Patients with ABIs in the lowest category have a 20% to 25% annual risk of death.* A wide range of interventions is available to reduce both onset and progres-

*Hirsh AT, Criqui MH, Treat-Jacobson D, et al: Peripheral Arterial Disease: Detection, Awareness, and Treatment in Primary Care. JAMA 286 (11):1317–1324, 2001; Hiatt WR: Medical Treatment of Peripheral Arterial Disease and Claudication. NEJM 344 (21):1608–1620, 2001.

sion of subclinical PAD, including meticulous foot care and well-fitting shoes, tobacco cessation, treatment of hyperlipidemia, optimal control and treatment of diabetes and hypertension, use of antiplatelet agents, and, if needed, surgical revascularization.

(Students should consult specialty texts for less common forms of vascular occlusion from arterial or venous thrombosis or endarteritis from infection, inflammation, or autoimmune disease.)

Preview: Recording the Physical Examination— The Peripheral Vascular System

Note that initially you may use sentences to describe your findings; later you will use phrases. The style below contains phrases appropriate for most write-ups. Unfamiliar terms are explained in the next section, Techniques of Examination. Recall that the written description of lymph nodes appears after the Head and Neck section (see p.143). Likewise, assessment of the carotid pulse is recorded in the Cardiovascular section (see p. 265).

> "Extremities are warm and without edema. No varicosities or stasis changes. Calves are supple and nontender. No femoral or abdominal bruits. Brachial, radial, femoral, popliteal, dorsalis pedis (DP), and posterior tibial (PT) pulses are 2+ and symmetric."

OR

> "Extremities are pale below the midcalf, with notable hair loss. Rubor noted when legs dependent but no edema or ulceration. Bilateral femoral bruits; no abdominal bruits heard. Brachial and radial pulses 2+; femoral, popliteal, DP and PT pulses 1+." (Alternatively, pulses can be recorded as below.)

Suggests atherosclerotic peripheral arterial disease

	Radial	Brachial	Femoral	Popliteal	Dorsalis Pedis	Posterior Tibial
RT	2+	2+	1+	1+	1+	1+
LT	2+	2+	1+	1+	1+	1+

TECHNIQUES OF EXAMINATION

Important Areas of Examination

The Arms

- Size, symmetry, skin color
- Radial pulse, brachial pulse
- Epitrochlear lymph nodes

The Legs

- Size, symmetry, skin color
- Femoral pulse and inguinal lymph nodes
- Popliteal, dorsalis pedis, and posterior tibial pulses
- Peripheral edema

Assessment of the peripheral vascular system relies primarily on inspection of the arms and legs, palpation of the pulses, and a search for edema. See Chapter 3 for a method of integrating these techniques into your examination of the limbs. Additional techniques may be useful when you suspect an abnormality.

Arms

Inspect both arms from the fingertips to the shoulders. Note:

- Their size, symmetry, and any swelling

Lymphedema of arm and hand may follow axillary node dissection and radiation therapy.

- The venous pattern

Prominent veins in an edematous arm suggest venous obstruction.

- The color of the skin and nail beds and the texture of the skin

Palpate the radial pulse with the pads of your fingers on the flexor surface of the wrist laterally. Partially flexing the patient's wrist may help you feel this pulse. Compare the pulses in both arms.

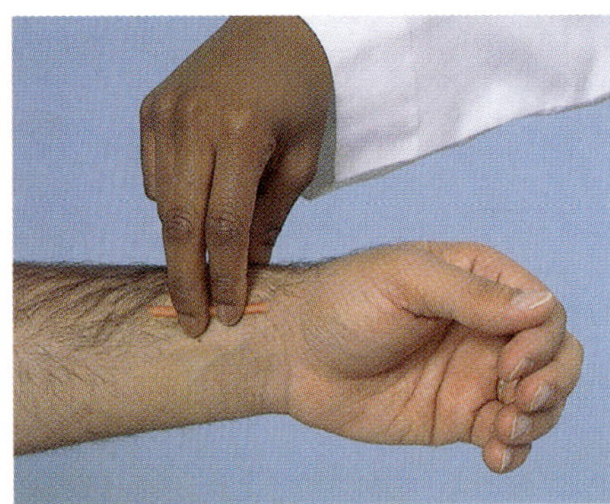

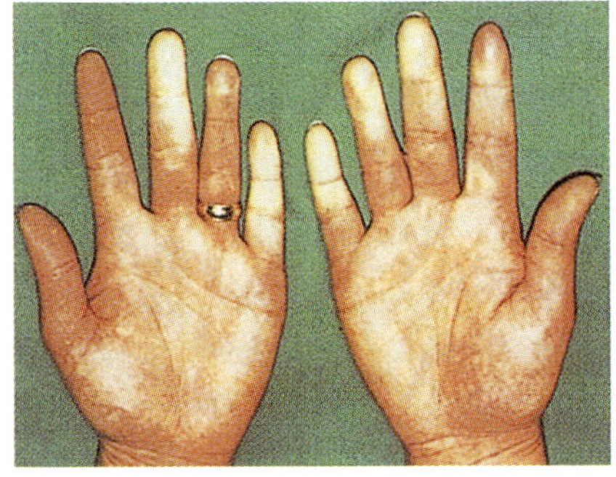

(Source of photo above: Marks R: Skin Disease in Old Age. Philadelphia, JB Lippincott, 1987)

In Raynaud's disease, wrist pulses are typically normal but spasm of more distal arteries causes episodes of sharply demarcated pallor of the fingers (see Table 14-1, Painful Peripheral Vascular Disorders and Their Mimics, pp. 460–461).

There are several systems for grading the amplitude of the arterial pulses. One system is to use a scale of 0 to 4, as below; however, you should check to see what scale is used in your institution.

Note that if an artery is widely dilated, it is *aneurysmal.*

4+	Bounding
3+	Increased
2+	Brisk, expected
1+	Diminished, weaker than expected
0	Absent, unable to palpate

Bounding carotid, radial, and femoral pulses in aortic insufficiency; asymmetric diminished pulses in arterial occlusion from atherosclerosis or embolism

If you suspect arterial insufficiency, feel for the *brachial pulse.* Flex the patient's elbow slightly, and with the thumb of your opposite hand palpate the artery just medial to the biceps tendon at the antecubital crease. The brachial artery can also be felt higher in the arm in the groove between the biceps and triceps muscles.

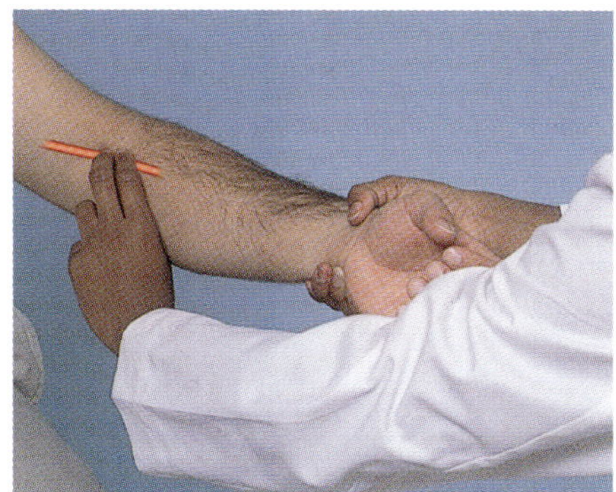

Feel for one or more *epitrochlear nodes.* With the patient's elbow flexed to about 90° and the forearm supported by your hand, reach around behind the arm and feel in the groove between the biceps and triceps muscles, about 3 cm above the medial epicondyle. If a node is present, note its size, consistency, and tenderness.

Epitrochlear nodes are difficult or impossible to identify in most normal people.

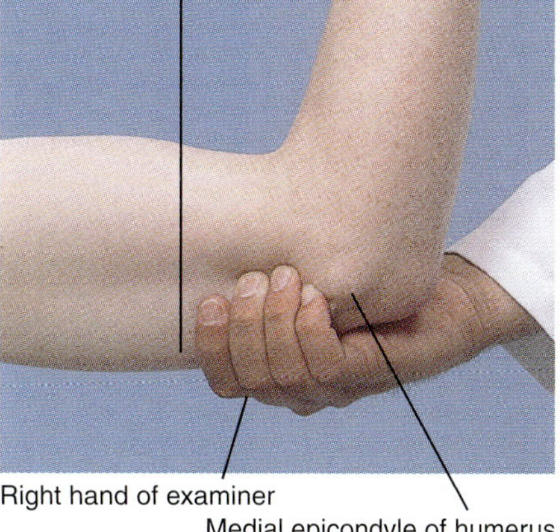

An enlarged epitrochlear node may be secondary to a lesion in its drainage area or may be associated with generalized lymphadenopathy.

Legs

The patient should be lying down and draped so that the external genitalia are covered and the legs fully exposed. A good examination is impossible through stockings or socks!

Inspect both legs from the groin and buttocks to the feet. Note:

- Their size, symmetry, and any swelling
- The venous pattern and any venous enlargement
- Any pigmentation, rashes, scars, or ulcers
- The color and texture of the skin, the color of the nail beds, and the distribution of hair on the lower legs, feet, and toes.

See Table 14-2, Chronic Insufficiency of Arteries and Veins (p. 462).

See Table 14-3, Common Ulcers of the Feet and Ankles (p. 463).

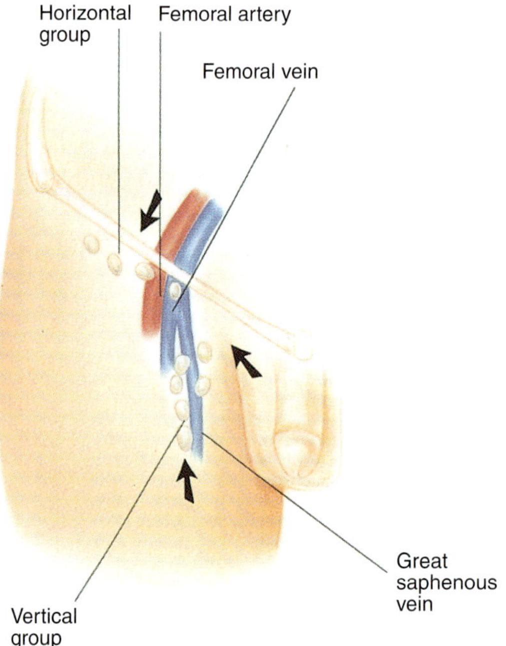

Palpate the *superficial inguinal nodes,* including both the horizontal and the vertical groups. Note their size, consistency, and discreteness, and note any tenderness. Nontender, discrete inguinal nodes up to 1 cm or even 2 cm in diameter are frequently palpable in normal people.

Lymphadenopathy refers to enlargement of the nodes, with or without tenderness. Try to distinguish between local and generalized lymphadenopathy, respectively, by finding either (1) a causative lesion in the drainage area, or (2) enlarged nodes in at least two other noncontiguous lymph node regions.

Palpate the pulses in order to assess the arterial circulation.

- *The femoral pulse.* Press deeply, below the inguinal ligament and about midway between the anterior superior iliac spine and the symphysis pubis. As in deep abdominal palpation, the use of two hands, one on top of the other, may facilitate this examination, especially in obese patients.

A diminished or absent pulse indicates partial or complete occlusion proximally; for example, at the aortic or iliac level, all pulses distal to the occlusion are typically affected. Chronic arterial occlusion, usually from atherosclerosis, causes *intermittent claudication,* (pp. 460–461), postural color changes (p. 458), and trophic changes in the skin (p. 462)

An exaggerated, widened femoral pulse suggests a femoral aneurysm, a pathologic dilatation of the artery.

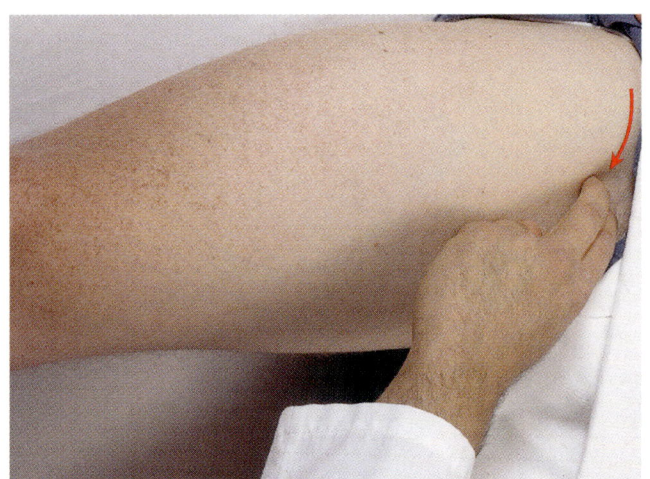

- *The popliteal pulse.* The patient's knee should be somewhat flexed, the leg relaxed. Place the fingertips of both hands so that they just meet in the midline behind the knee and press them deeply into the popliteal fossa. The popliteal pulse is often more difficult to find than other pulses. It is deeper and feels more diffuse.

An exaggerated, widened popliteal pulse suggests an aneurysm of the popliteal artery. Neither popliteal nor femoral aneurysms are common. They are usually due to atherosclerosis, and occur primarily in men over age 50.

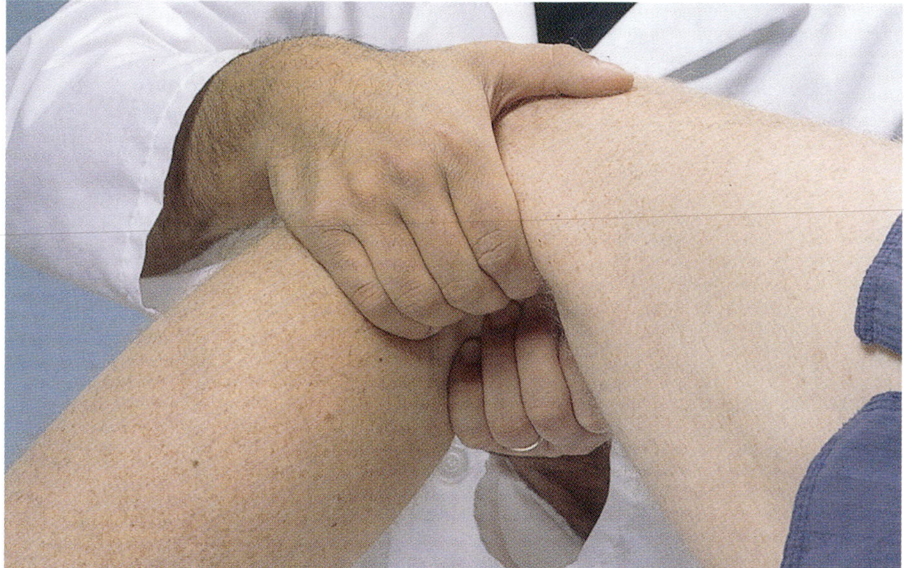

If you cannot feel the popliteal pulse with this approach, try with the patient prone. Flex the patient's knee to about 90°, let the lower leg relax against your shoulder or upper arm, and press your two thumbs deeply into the popliteal fossa.

Atherosclerosis (arteriosclerosis obliterans) most commonly obstructs arterial circulation in the thigh. The femoral pulse is then normal, the popliteal decreased or absent.

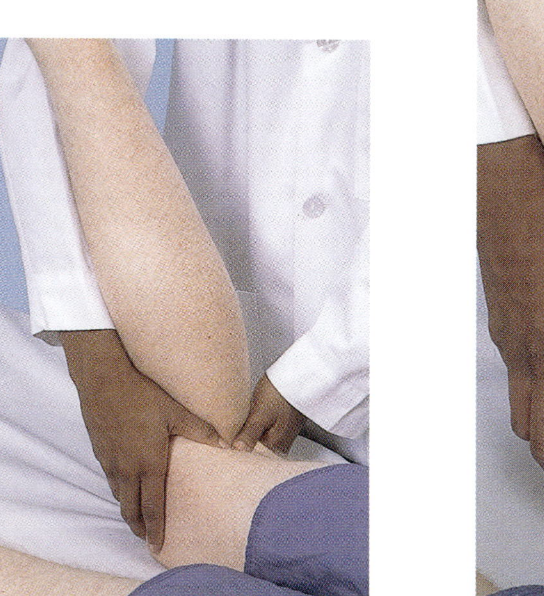

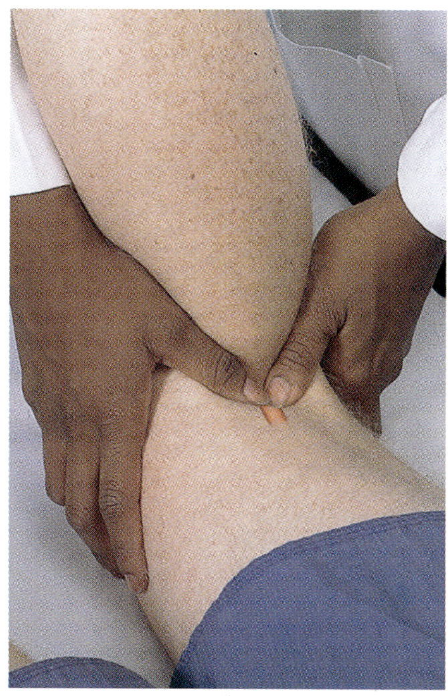

- *The dorsalis pedis pulse.* Feel the dorsum of the foot (not the ankle) just lateral to the extensor tendon of the great toe. If you cannot feel a pulse, explore the dorsum of the foot more laterally.

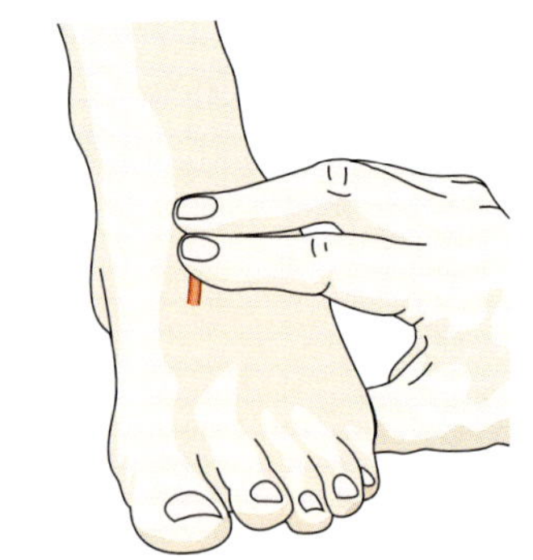

The dorsalis pedis artery may be congenitally absent or may branch higher in the ankle. Search for a pulse more laterally.

Decreased or absent foot pulses (assuming a warm environment) with normal femoral and popliteal pulses suggest occlusive disease in the lower popliteal artery or its branches—a pattern often associated with diabetes mellitus.

- *The posterior tibial pulse.* Curve your fingers behind and slightly below the medial malleolus of the ankle. (This pulse may be hard to feel in a fat or edematous ankle.)

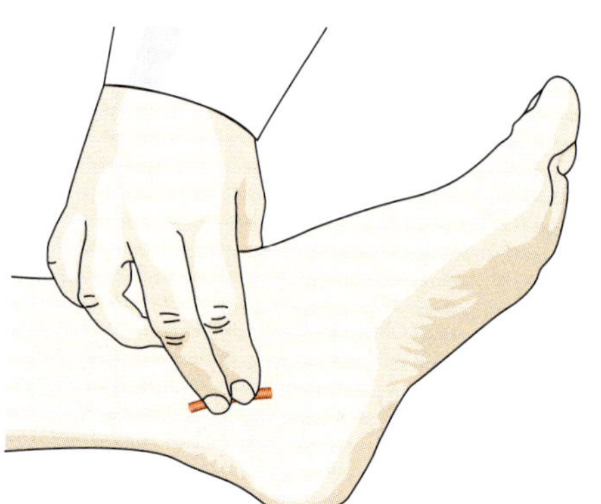

Sudden arterial occlusion, as by embolism or thrombosis, causes pain and numbness or tingling. The limb distal to the occlusion becomes cold, pale, and pulseless. Emergency treatment is required. If collateral circulation is good, only numbness and coolness may result.

Tips on feeling difficult pulses: (1) Position your own body and examining hand comfortably; awkward positions decrease your tactile sensitivity. (2) Place your hand properly and linger there, varying the pressure of your fingers to pick up a weak pulsation. If unsuccessful, then explore the area deliberately. (3) Do not confuse the patient's pulse with your own pulsating fingertips. If you are unsure, count your own heart rate and compare it with the patient's. The rates are usually different. Your carotid pulse is convenient for this comparison.

Note the temperature of the feet and legs with the backs of your fingers. Compare one side with the other. Bilateral coldness is most often due to a cold environment or anxiety.

Coldness, especially when unilateral or associated with other signs, suggests arterial insufficiency from inadequate arterial circulation.

Look for edema. Compare one foot and leg with the other, noting their relative size and the prominence of veins, tendons, and bones.

Edema causes swelling that may obscure the veins, tendons, and bony prominences.

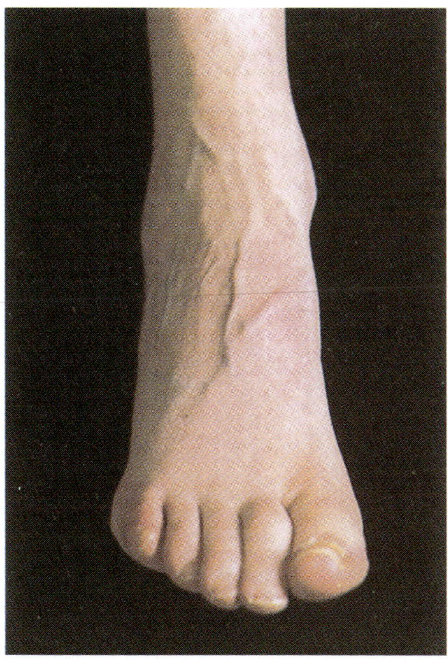

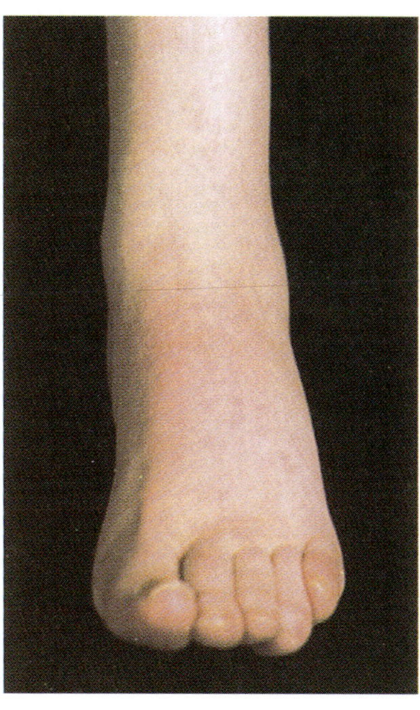

Check for pitting edema. Press firmly but gently with your thumb for at least 5 seconds (1) over the dorsum of each foot, (2) behind each medial malleolus, and (3) over the shins. Look for *pitting*—a depression caused by pressure from your thumb. Normally there is none. The severity of edema is graded on a four-point scale, from slight to very marked.

See Table 14-4, Some Peripheral Causes of Edema (p. 464).

Shown below is 3+ pitting edema.

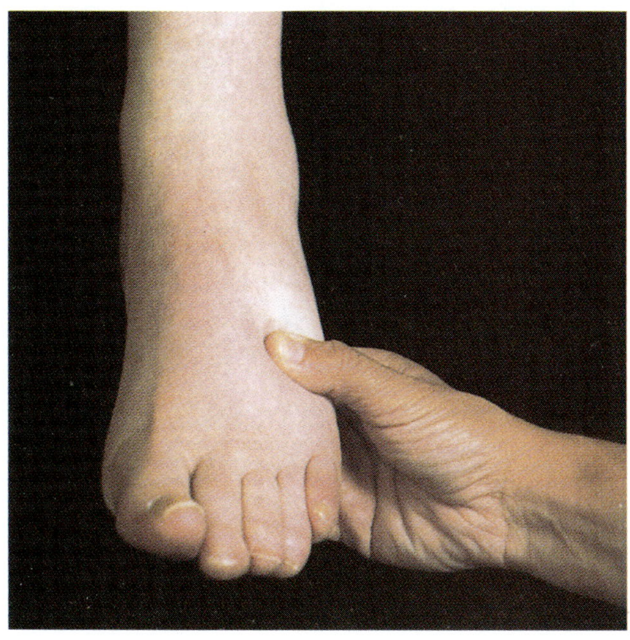

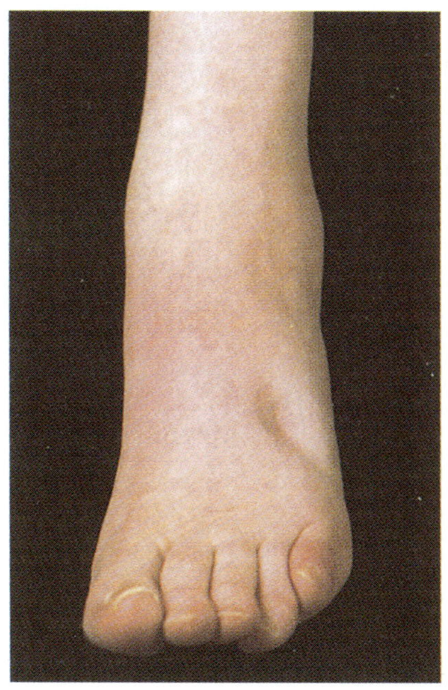

If you suspect edema, *measurement of the legs* may help you to identify it and to follow its course. With a flexible tape, measure (1) the forefoot, (2) the smallest possible circumference above the ankle, (3) the largest circumference at the calf, and (4) the midthigh a measured distance above the patella with the knee extended. Compare one side with the other. A difference of more than 1 cm just above the ankle or 2 cm at the calf is unusual in normal people and suggests edema.

Conditions such as muscular atrophy can also cause different circumferences in the legs.

If edema is present, look for possible causes in the peripheral vascular system. These include (1) recent deep venous thrombosis, (2) chronic venous insufficiency due to previous deep venous thrombosis or to incompetence of the venous valves, and (3) lymphedema. Note the extent of the swelling. How far up the leg does it go?

In deep venous thrombosis, the extent of edema suggests the location of the occlusion: the calf when the lower leg or the ankle is swollen, the iliofemoral veins when the entire leg is swollen.

Is the swelling unilateral or bilateral? Are the veins unusually prominent?

Venous distention suggests a venous cause of edema.

Try to identify any venous tenderness that may accompany deep venous thrombosis. Palpate the groin just medial to the femoral pulse for tenderness of the femoral vein. Next, with the patient's leg flexed at the knee and relaxed, palpate the calf. With your fingerpads, gently compress the calf muscles against the tibia, and search for any tenderness or cords. Deep venous thrombosis, however, may have no demonstrable signs, and diagnosis often depends on high clinical suspicion and other testing.

A painful, pale swollen leg, together with tenderness in the groin over the femoral vein, suggests deep *iliofemoral thrombosis.* Approximately half of patients with *deep venous thrombosis* in the calf have tenderness and cords deep in the calf. Calf tenderness is nonspecific, however, and may be present without thrombosis.

Note the *color of the skin.*

- Is there a local area of redness? If so, note its temperature, and gently try to feel the firm cord of a thrombosed vein in the area. The calf is most often involved.

Local swelling, redness, warmth, and a subcutaneous cord suggest *superficial thrombophlebitis.*

- Are there brownish areas near the ankles?
- Note any ulcers in the skin. Where are they?

A brownish color or ulcers just above the ankle suggest chronic venous insufficiency.

- Feel the thickness of the skin.

Thickened brawny skin occurs in lymphedema and advanced venous insufficiency.

Ask the patient to stand, and *inspect the saphenous system for varicosities.* The standing posture allows any varicosities to fill with blood and makes them visible. You can easily miss them when the patient is in a supine position. Feel for any varicosities, noting any signs of thrombophlebitis.

Varicose veins are dilated and tortuous. Their walls may feel somewhat thickened. Many varicose veins can be seen in the leg on p. 459.

Special Techniques

Evaluating the Arterial Supply to the Hand. If you suspect arterial insufficiency in the arm or hand, try to feel the *ulnar pulse* as well as the radial and brachial pulses. Feel for it deeply on the flexor surface of the wrist medially. Partially flexing the patient's wrist may help you. The pulse of a normal ulnar artery, however, may not be palpable.

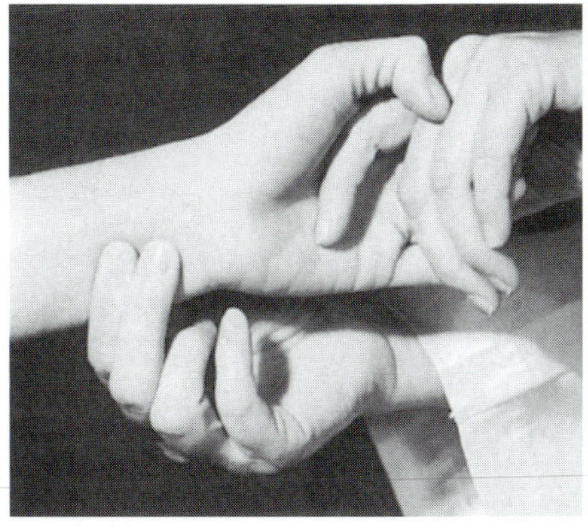

Arterial occlusive disease is much less common in the arms than in the legs. Absent or diminished pulses at the wrist in acute embolic occlusion and in *Buerger's disease,* or thromboangiitis obliterans.

The *Allen test* gives further information. This test is also useful to assure the patency of the ulnar artery before puncturing the radial artery for blood samples. The patient should rest with hands in lap, palms up.

Ask the patient to make a tight fist with one hand; then compress both radial and ulnar arteries firmly between your thumbs and fingers. Next, ask the patient to open the hand into a relaxed, slightly flexed position. The palm is pale.

Extending the hand fully may cause pallor and a falsely positive test.

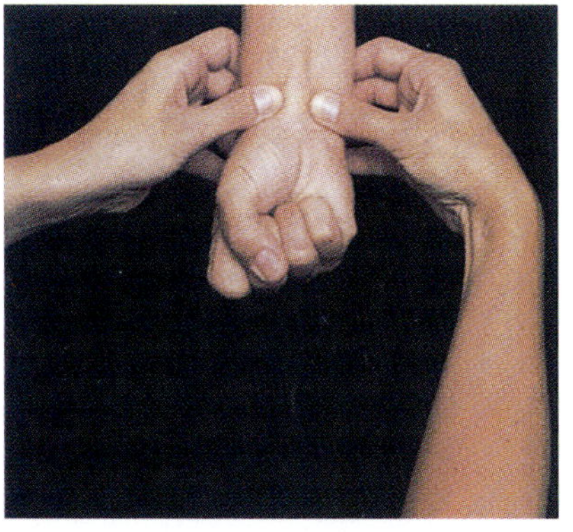

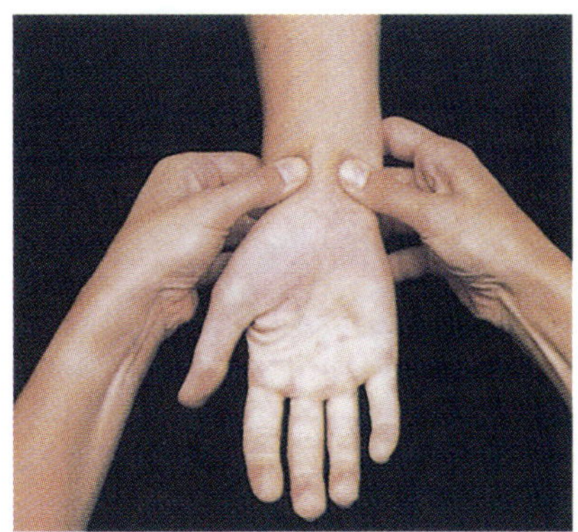

Release your pressure over the ulnar artery. If the ulnar artery is patent, the palm flushes within about 3 to 5 seconds.

Persisting pallor indicates occlusion of the ulnar artery or its distal branches.

Patency of the radial artery may be tested by releasing the radial artery while still compressing the ulnar.

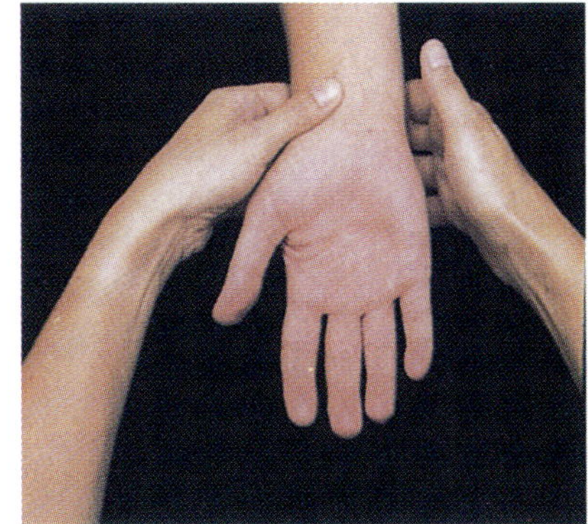

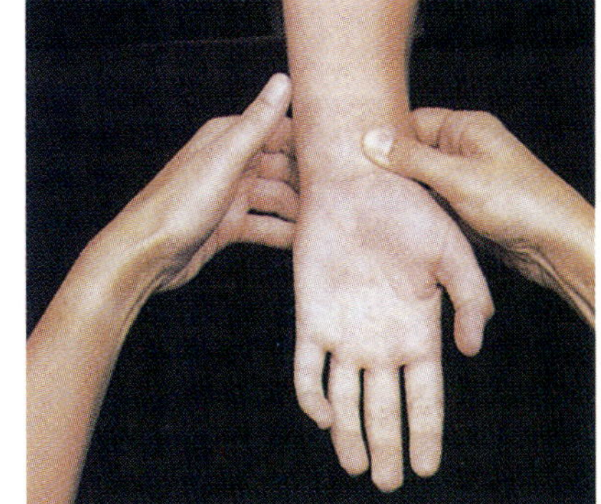

Postural Color Changes of Chronic Arterial Insufficiency.

If pain or diminished pulses suggest arterial insufficiency, look for postural color changes. Raise both legs, as shown at the right, to about 60° until maximal pallor of the feet develops—usually within a minute. In light-skinned persons, either maintenance of normal color, as seen in this right foot, or slight pallor is normal.

Marked pallor on elevation suggests arterial insufficiency.

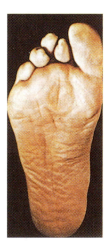

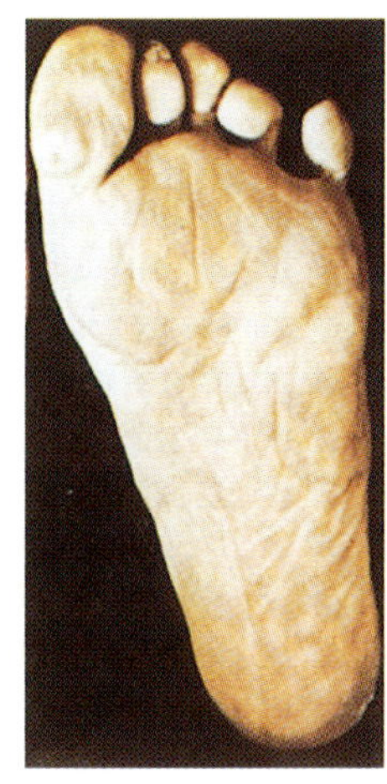

Then ask the patient to sit up with legs dangling down. Compare both feet, noting the time required for:

- Return of pinkness to the skin, normally about 10 seconds or less
- Filling of the veins of the feet and ankles, normally about 15 seconds.

This right foot has normal color and the veins on the foot have filled. These normal responses suggest an adequate circulation.

The foot below is still pale and the veins are just starting to fill—signs of arterial insufficiency.

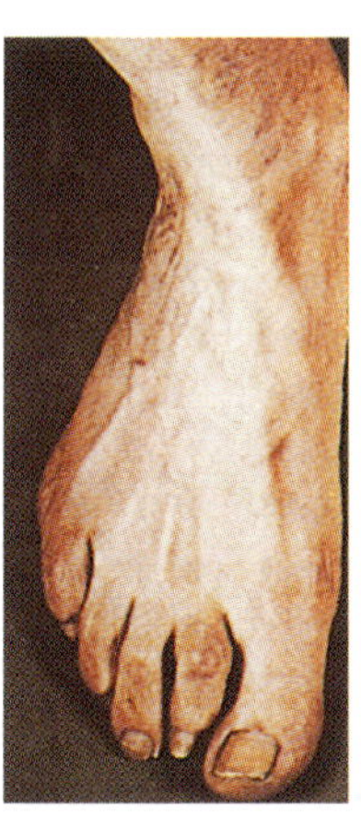

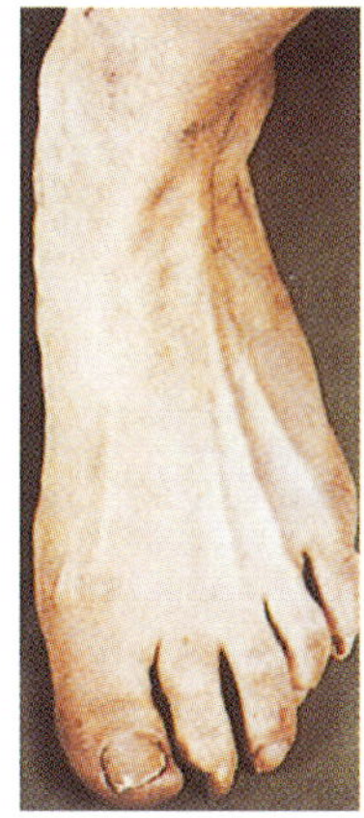

Look for any unusual *rubor* (dusky redness) to replace the pallor of the dependent foot. Rubor may take a minute or more to appear.

Normal responses accompanied by diminished arterial pulses suggest that a good collateral circulation has developed around an arterial occlusion.

Color changes may be difficult to see in darker-skinned persons. Inspect the soles of the feet for these changes, and use tangential lighting to see the veins.

Persisting rubor on dependency suggests arterial insufficiency (see p. 462). When veins are incompetent, dependent rubor and the timing of color return and venous filling are not reliable tests of arterial insufficiency.

(Source of foot photos: Kappert A, Winsor T: Diagnosis of Peripheral Vascular Disease. Philadelphia, FA Davis, 1972).

Mapping Varicose Veins. You can map out the course and connections of varicose veins by transmitting pressure waves along the blood-filled veins. With the patient standing, place your palpating fingers gently on a vein and, with your other hand below it, compress the vein sharply. Feel for a pressure wave transmitted to the fingers of your upper hand. A palpable pressure wave indicates that the two parts of the vein are connected.

A wave may also be transmitted downward, but not as easily.

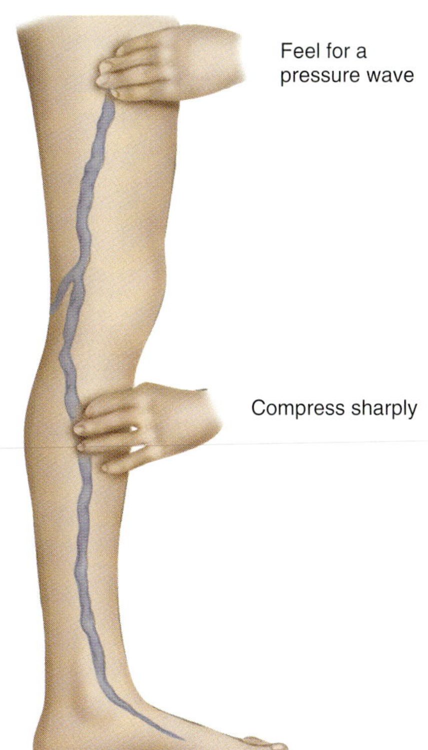

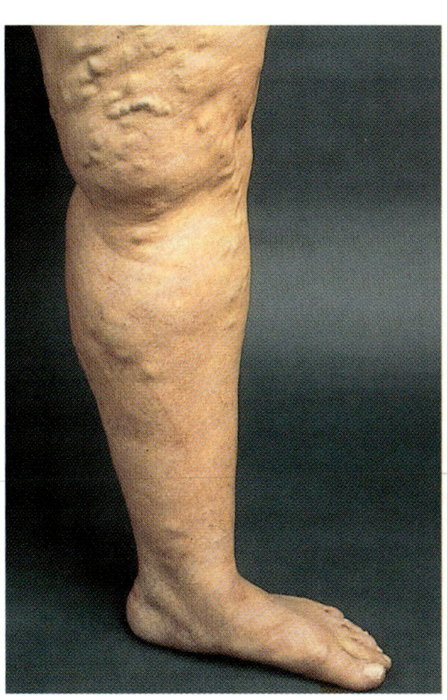

Evaluating the Competency of Venous Valves. By the *retrograde filling (Trendelenburg) test,* you can assess the valvular competency in both the communicating veins and the saphenous system. Start with the patient supine. Elevate one leg to about 90° to empty it of venous blood.

Next, occlude the great saphenous vein in the upper thigh by manual compression, using enough pressure to occlude this vein but not the deeper vessels. Ask the patient to stand. While you keep the vein occluded, watch for venous filling in the leg. Normally the saphenous vein fills from below, taking about 35 seconds as blood flows through the capillary bed into the venous system.

Rapid filling of the superficial veins while the saphenous vein is occluded indicates incompetent valves in the communicating veins. Blood flows quickly in a retrograde direction from the deep to the saphenous system.

After the patient has stood for 20 seconds, release the compression and look for any sudden additional venous filling. Normally there is none: competent valves in the saphenous vein block retrograde flow. Slow venous filling continues.

Sudden additional filling of superficial veins after release of compression indicates incompetent valves in the saphenous vein.

When both steps of this test are normal, the response is termed negative–negative. Negative–positive and positive–negative responses may also occur.

When both steps are abnormal, the test is positive–positive.

TABLE 14-1 ■ Painful Peripheral Vascular Disorders and Their Mimics

Problem	Process	Location of Pain
Arterial Disorders		
Atherosclerosis (arteriosclerosis obliterans)		
■ Intermittent claudication	Episodic muscular ischemia induced by exercise, due to obstruction of large or middle-sized arteries by atherosclerosis	Usually the calf, but also may be in the buttock, hip, thigh, or foot, depending on the level of obstruction
■ Rest pain	Ischemia even at rest	Distal pain, in the toes or forefoot
Acute Arterial Occlusion	Embolism or thrombosis, possibly superimposed on arteriosclerosis obliterans	Distal pain, usually involving the foot and leg
Raynaud's Disease and Phenomenon	*Raynaud's disease:* Episodic spasm of the small arteries and arterioles; no vascular occlusion. *Raynaud's phenomenon:* Syndrome is secondary to other conditions such as collagen vascular disease, arterial occlusion, trauma, drugs	Distal portions of one or more fingers. Pain is usually not prominent unless fingertip ulcers develop. Numbness and tingling are common.
Venous Disorders		
Superficial Thrombophlebitis	Clot formation and acute inflammation in a superficial vein	Pain in a local area along the course of a superficial vein, most often in the saphenous system
Deep Venous Thrombosis	Clot formation in a deep vein	Pain, if present, is usually in the calf, but the process more often is painless.
Chronic Venous Insufficiency (deep)	Chronic venous engorgement secondary to venous occlusion or incompetency of venous valves	Diffuse aching of the leg(s)
Thromboangiitis Obliterans *(Buerger's disease)*	Inflammatory and thrombotic occlusions of small arteries and also of veins, occurring in smokers	■ Intermittent claudication, particularly in the arch of the foot ■ Rest pain in the fingers or toes
Acute Lymphangitis	Acute bacterial infection (usually streptococcal) spreading up the lymphatic channels from a portal of entry such as an injured area or an ulcer	An arm or a leg
Mimics*		
Acute Cellulitis	Acute bacterial infection of the skin and subcutaneous tissues	Arms, legs, or elsewhere
Erythema Nodosum	Subcutaneous inflammatory lesions associated with a variety of systemic conditions such as pregnancy, sarcoidosis, tuberculosis, and streptococcal infections	Anterior surfaces of both lower legs

* Mistaken primarily for acute superficial thrombophlebitis.

Timing	Factors That Aggravate	Factors That Relieve	Associated Manifestations
Fairly brief; pain usually forces the patient to rest.	Exercise such as walking	Rest usually stops the pain in 1–3 min.	Local fatigue, numbness, diminished pulses, often signs of arterial insufficiency (see p. 462)
Persistent, often worse at night	Elevation of the feet, as in bed	Sitting with legs dependent	Numbness, tingling, trophic signs and color changes of arterial insufficiency (see p. 462)
Sudden onset; associated symptoms may occur without pain.			Coldness, numbness, weakness, absent distal pulses
Relatively brief (minutes) but recurrent	Exposure to cold, emotional upset	Warm environment	Color changes in the distal fingers: severe pallor (essential for the diagnosis) followed by cyanosis and then redness
An acute episode lasting days or longer			Local redness, swelling, tenderness, a palpable cord, possibly fever
Often hard to determine because of lack of symptoms			Possibly swelling of the foot and calf and local calf tenderness; often nothing
Chronic, increasing as the day wears on	Prolonged standing	Elevation of the leg(s)	Chronic edema, pigmentation, possibly ulceration (see pp. 462, 463)
■ Fairly brief but recurrent ■ Chronic, persistent, may be worse at night	■ Exercise	■ Rest ■ Permanent cessation of smoking helps both kinds of pain (but patients seldom stop)	Distal coldness, sweating, numbness, and cyanosis; ulceration and gangrene at the tips of fingers or toes; migratory thrombophlebitis
An acute episode lasting days or longer			Red streak(s) on the skin, with tenderness, enlarged, tender lymph nodes, and fever
An acute episode lasting days or longer			A local area of diffuse swelling, redness, and tenderness with enlarged, tender lymph nodes and fever; no palpable cord
Pain associated with a series of lesions over several weeks			Raised, red, tender swellings recurring in crops; often malaise, joint pains, and fever

TABLE 14-2 ■ Chronic Insufficiency of Arteries and Veins

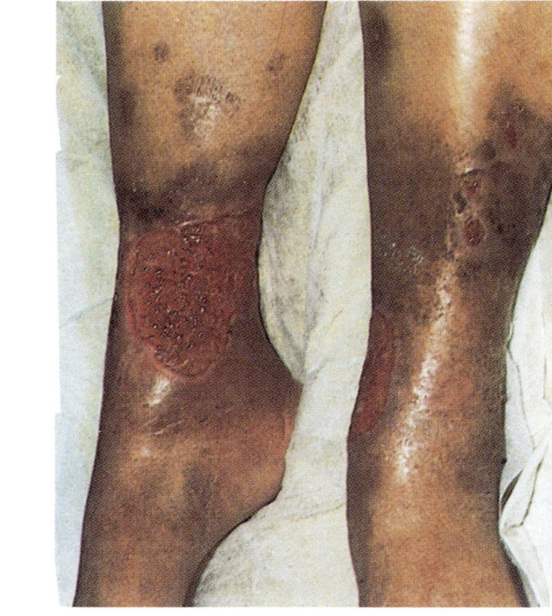

	Chronic Arterial Insufficiency *(Advanced)*	Chronic Venous Insufficiency *(Advanced)*
Pain	Intermittent claudication, progressing to pain at rest	None to an aching pain on dependency
Pulses	Decreased or absent	Normal, though may be difficult to feel through edema
Color	Pale, especially on elevation; dusky red on dependency	Normal, or cyanotic on dependency. Petechiae and then brown pigmentation appear with chronicity.
Temperature	Cool	Normal
Edema	Absent or mild; may develop as the patient tries to relieve rest pain by lowering the leg	Present, often marked
Skin Changes	Trophic changes: thin, shiny, atrophic skin; loss of hair over the foot and toes; nails thickened and ridged	Often brown pigmentation around the ankle, stasis dermatitis, and possible thickening of the skin and narrowing of the leg as scarring develops
Ulceration	If present, involves toes or points of trauma on feet	If present, develops at sides of ankle, especially medially
Gangrene	May develop	Does not develop

(Sources of photos: *Arterial Insufficiency*—Kappert A, Winsor T: Diagnosis of Peripheral Vascular Disease. Philadelphia, FA Davis, 1972; *Venous Insufficiency*—Marks R: Skin Disease in Old Age. Philadelphia, JB Lippincott, 1987)

TABLE 14-3 ■ Common Ulcers of the Feet and Ankles

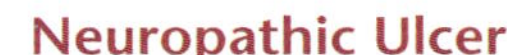

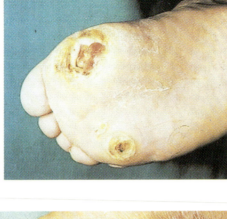

	Arterial Insufficiency	Chronic Venous Insufficiency	Neuropathic Ulcer
	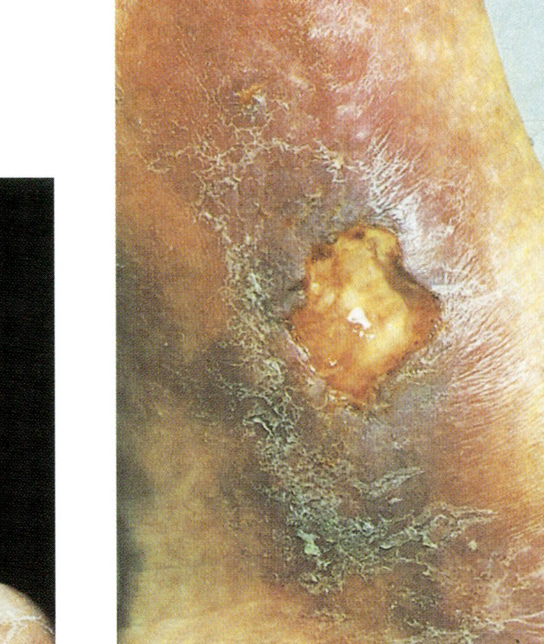	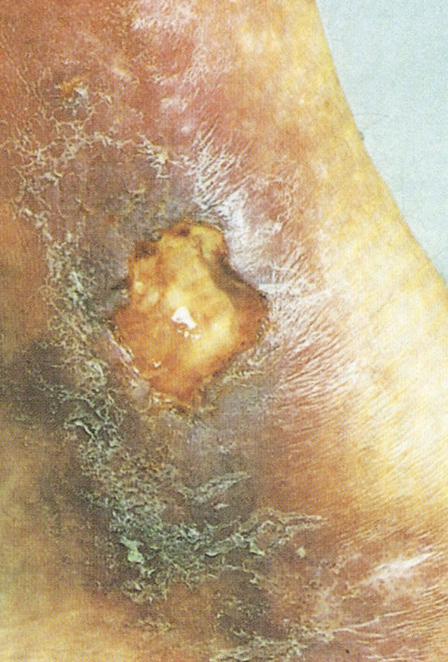	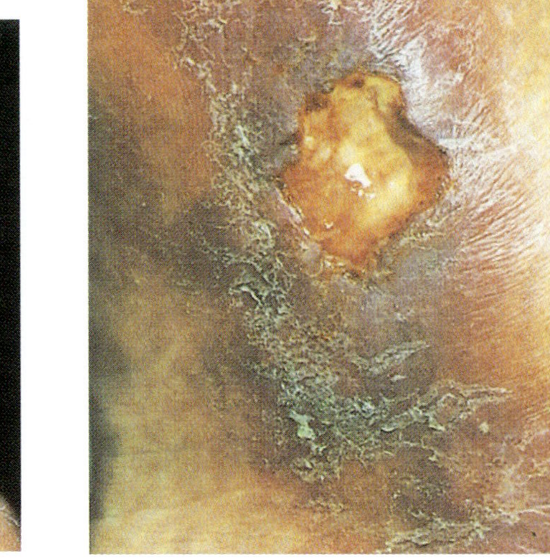
Location	Toes, feet, or possibly in areas of trauma (e.g., the shin)	Inner or sometimes outer ankle	Pressure points in areas with diminished sensation, as in diabetic polyneuropathy
Skin Around the Ulcer	No callus or excess of pigment; may be atrophic	Pigmented, sometimes fibrotic	Calloused
Pain	Often severe, unless neuropathy masks it	Not severe	Absent (and therefore the ulcer may go unnoticed)
Associated Gangrene	May be present	Absent	In uncomplicated neuropathic ulcer, absent
Associated Signs	Decreased pulses, trophic changes, pallor of the foot on elevation, dusky rubor on dependency	Edema, pigmentation, stasis dermatitis, and possibly cyanosis of the foot on dependency	Decreased sensation, absent ankle jerks

(Source of photos: Marks R: Skin Disease in Old Age. Philadelphia, JB Lippincott, 1987)

TABLE 14-4 ■ Some Peripheral Causes of Edema

About one third of total body water is extracellular, or outside the body's cells. About 25% of extracellular fluid is plasma and the remainder is interstitial fluid. At the arteriolar end of the capillaries, *hydrostatic pressure* in the blood vessels and the *colloid oncotic pressure* in the interstitium cause fluid to move into the tissues; at the venous end of the capillaries and in the lymphatics, hydrostatic pressure in the interstitium and the colloid oncotic pressure of plasma proteins cause fluid to return to the vascular compartment. A number of clinical conditions disrupt this balance, resulting in *edema*, or a clinically evident accumulation of interstitial fluid. Not depicted below is capillary leak syndrome, where protein leaks into the interstitial space, seen in burns, angioedema, snake bites, and allergic reactions.

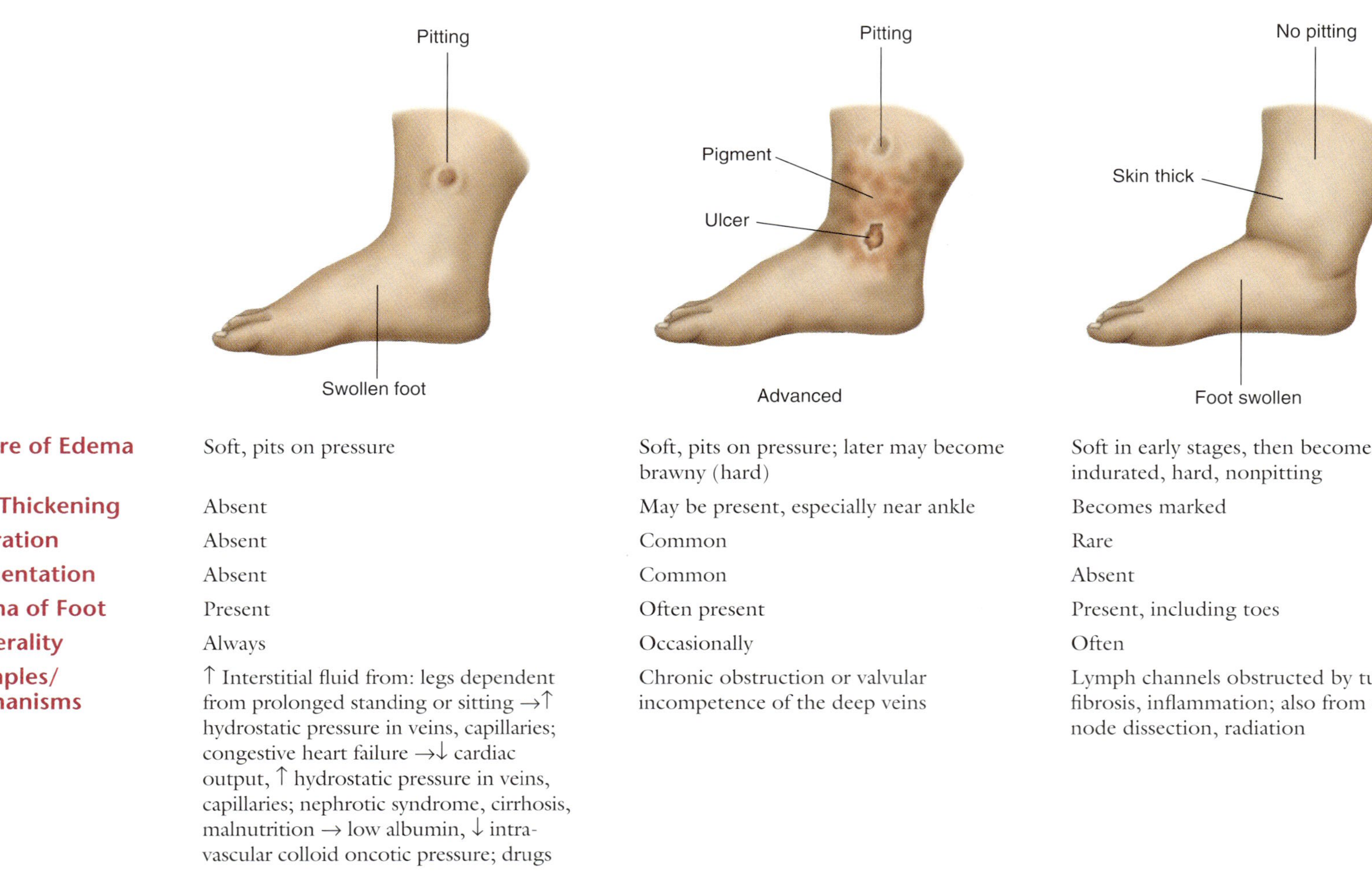

	Pitting Edema	Chronic Venous Insufficiency	Lymphedema
Nature of Edema	Soft, pits on pressure	Soft, pits on pressure; later may become brawny (hard)	Soft in early stages, then becomes indurated, hard, nonpitting
Skin Thickening	Absent	May be present, especially near ankle	Becomes marked
Ulceration	Absent	Common	Rare
Pigmentation	Absent	Common	Absent
Edema of Foot	Present	Often present	Present, including toes
Bilaterality	Always	Occasionally	Often
Examples/ Mechanisms	↑ Interstitial fluid from: legs dependent from prolonged standing or sitting →↑ hydrostatic pressure in veins, capillaries; congestive heart failure →↓ cardiac output, ↑ hydrostatic pressure in veins, capillaries; nephrotic syndrome, cirrhosis, malnutrition → low albumin, ↓ intravascular colloid oncotic pressure; drugs	Chronic obstruction or valvular incompetence of the deep veins	Lymph channels obstructed by tumor, fibrosis, inflammation; also from axillary node dissection, radiation

CHAPTER

15 The Musculoskeletal System

ANATOMY AND PHYSIOLOGY

This section reviews the structure and function of the major joints and their connecting bony structures, muscles, and soft tissues. To lay the foundation for skilled assessment of the musculoskeletal system, it is essential for you to learn both the surface landmarks and underlying anatomy of each of the major joints. ***Anatomy and Physiology*** follows a "head to toe" sequence, beginning with the jaw and joints of the upper extremities, then proceeding to the spine and hip and the joints of the lower extremities. For each joint there are subsections on *Overview, Bony Structures and Joints,* and *Muscle Groups and Additional Structures.* The Overview should help orient you to the distinguishing anatomic and functional features of each joint. As you study Anatomy and Physiology, practice identifying the important surface landmarks on yourself or a fellow student. Then turn to ***Techniques of Examination,*** also "head to toe," to learn the fundamental steps for examining the joints—inspection; palpation of bony landmarks and soft-tissue structures; assessment of range of motion, or the directions of joint movement; and maneuvers to test joint function.

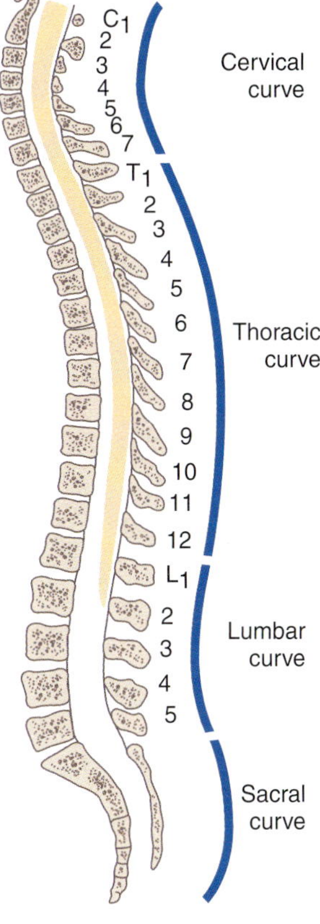

It is helpful to begin by reviewing some anatomic terminology. *Articular structures* include the joint capsule and articular cartilage, the synovium and synovial fluid, intra-articular ligaments, and juxta-articular bone. *Nonarticular structures* include periarticular ligaments, tendons, bursae, muscle, fascia, bone, nerve, and overlying skin. You will need to visualize and assess all these structures to care for your patients with joint complaints. Note that *ligaments* are ropelike bundles of collagen fibrils that connect bone to bone. *Tendons* are collagen fibers connecting muscle to bone. Another type of collagen matrix forms the *cartilage* that overlies bony surfaces. *Bursae* are pouches of synovial fluid that cushion the movement of tendons and muscles over bone or other joint structures.

Structure and Function of Joints

To understand joint function, begin by reviewing the various types of joints and how they articulate, or interconnect, and the role of bursae in easing joint movement.

Types of Joints. There are three primary types of joint articulation—synovial, cartilaginous, and fibrous—allowing varying degrees of joint movement.

Type of Joint	Extent of Movement	Example
Synovial	Freely movable	Knee, shoulder
Cartilaginous	Slightly movable	Vertebral bodies of the spine
Fibrous	Immovable	Skull sutures

In *synovial joints,* the bones do not touch each other, and the joint articulations are *freely moveable.* The bones are covered by *articular cartilage* and separated by a *synovial cavity* that cushions joint movement, as shown. A *synovial membrane* lines the synovial cavity and secretes a small amount of viscous lubricating fluid—the *synovial fluid.* The membrane is attached at the margins of the articular cartilage and pouched or folded to accommodate joint movement. Surrounding the synovial membrane is a fibrous *joint capsule,* which is strengthened by ligaments extending from bone to bone.

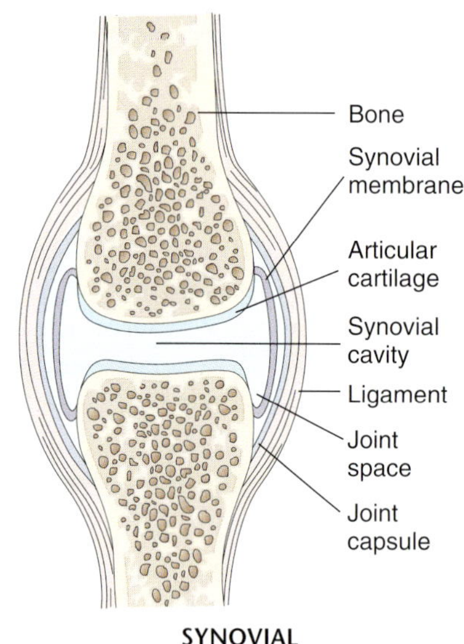

SYNOVIAL

Cartilaginous joints, such as those between vertebrae and the symphysis pubis, are *slightly moveable.* Fibrocartilaginous discs separate the bony surfaces. At the center of each disc is the *nucleus pulposus,* fibrocartilaginous material that serves as a cushion or shock absorber between bony surfaces.

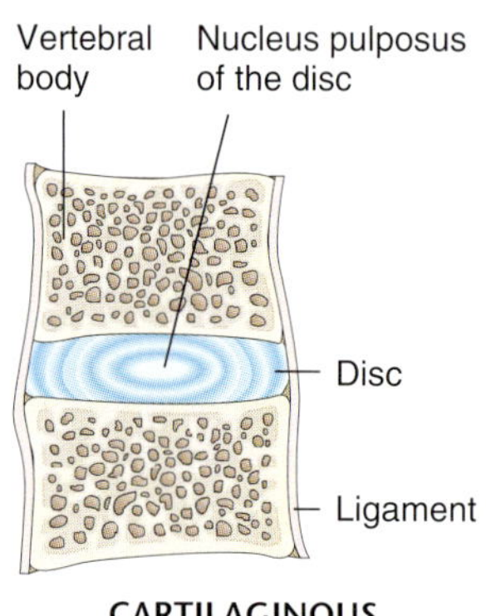

CARTILAGINOUS

In *fibrous joints,* such as the sutures of the skull, intervening layers of fibrous tissue or cartilage hold the bones together. The bones are almost in direct contact, which allows *no appreciable movement.*

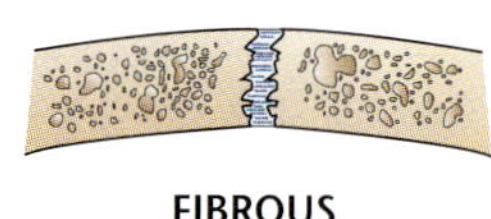

FIBROUS

As you learn about the examination of the musculoskeletal system, think about how the anatomy of the joint relates to its movement. Many of the joints we examine are *synovial,* or movable, *joints.* The shape of the articulating surfaces of synovial joints determines the type of motion in the joint. *Spheroidal joints* have a ball-and-socket configuration—a rounded convex surface articulating with a cuplike cavity, allowing a wide range of rotatory movement as in the shoulder and hip. *Hinge joints* are flat, planar, or slightly curved, allowing a gliding motion in one plane only, as in flexion and extension of the digits. In *condylar joints,* such as the knee, the articulating surfaces are convex or concave, and referred to as condyles.

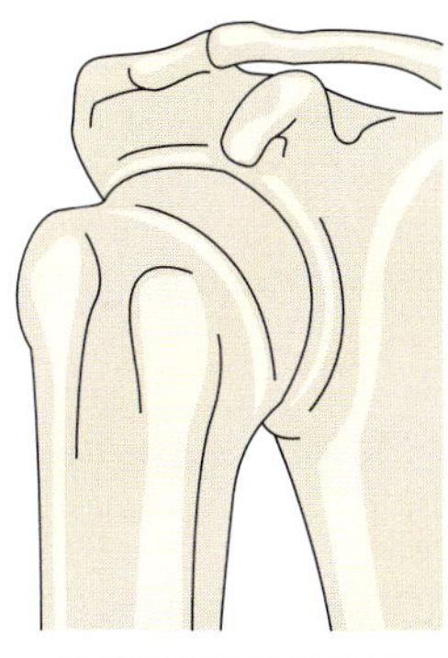
SPHEROIDAL JOINT (BALL AND SOCKET)

Synovial Joints

Type of Joint	Articular Shape	Movement	Example
Spheroidal (ball and socket)	Convex surface in concave cavity	Wide-ranging flexion, extension, abduction, adduction, rotation, circumduction	Shoulder, hip
Hinge	Flat, planar	Motion in one plane; flexion, extension	Interphalangeal joints of hand and foot; elbow
Condylar	Convex or concave	Movement of two articulating surfaces not dissociable	Knee; temporomandibular joint

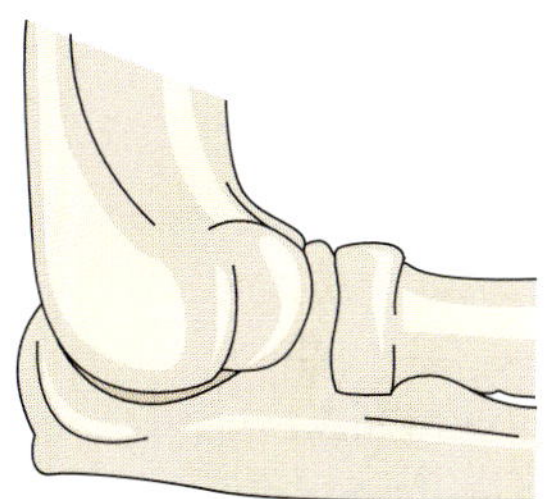
HINGE JOINT

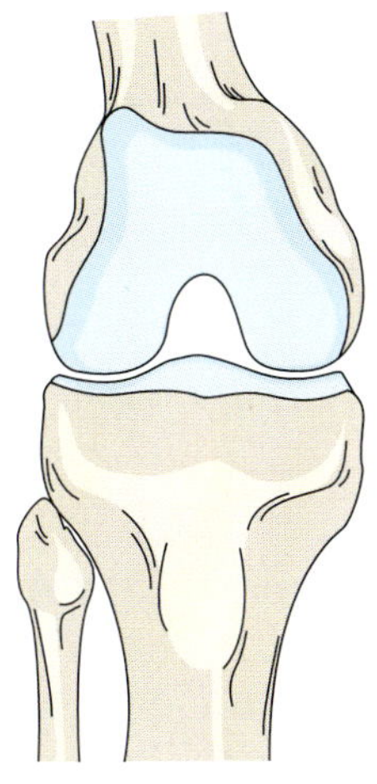
CONDYLAR JOINT

Bursae. Easing joint action are *bursae,* roughly disc-shaped synovial sacs that allow adjacent muscles or muscles and tendons to glide over each other during movement. They lie between the skin and the convex surface of a bone or joint (as in the prepatellar bursa of the knee, p. 481) or in areas where tendons or muscles rub against bone, ligaments, or other tendons or muscles (as in the subacromial bursa of the shoulder, p. 472).

Knowledge of the underlying joint anatomy and movement will help you assess joints subjected to trauma. Your knowledge of the soft-tissue structures, ligaments, tendons, and bursae will help you evaluate the changes of aging, as well as arthritis.

Temporomandibular Joint

Overview, Bony Structures, and Joints. The temporomandibular joint is the most active joint in the body, opening and closing up to 2000 times a day. It is formed by the fossa and articular tubercle of the temporal bone and the condyle of the mandible. It lies midway between the external acoustic meatus and the zygomatic arch.

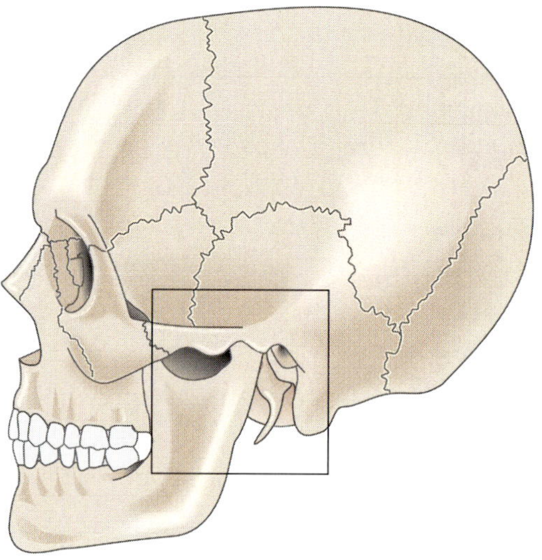

A fibrocartilaginous disc cushions the action of the condyle of the mandible against the synovial membrane and capsule of the articulating surfaces of the temporal bone. Hence, it is a condylar synovial joint.

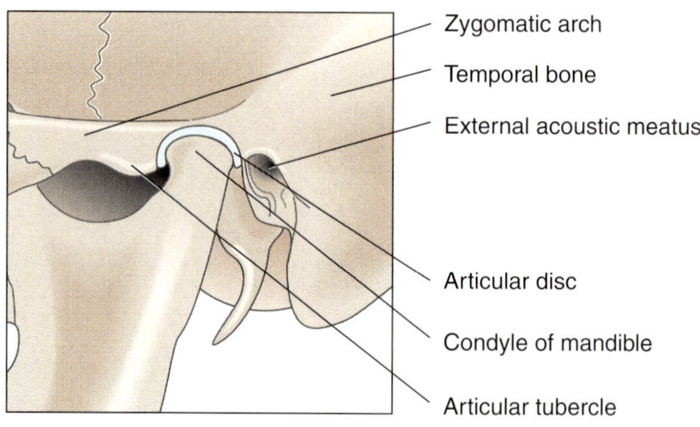

Muscle Groups and Additional Structures. The principal muscles opening the mouth are the *external pterygoids.* Closing the mouth are the muscles innervated by Cranial Nerve V, the trigeminal nerve (see p. 538)—the *masseter,* the *temporalis,* and the *internal pterygoids.*

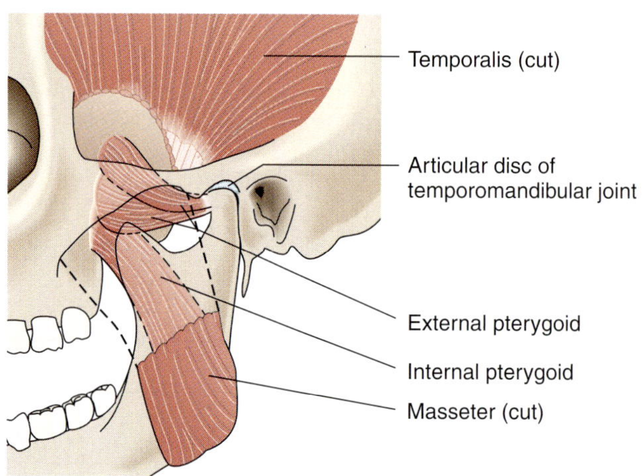

The Shoulder

Overview. The shoulder is distinguished by wide-ranging movement in all directions. The humerus virtually dangles from the scapula, suspended from the shallow glenoid fossa by the joint capsule, the intra-articular capsular ligaments, the glenoid labrum, and a meshwork of muscles and tendons. The shoulder derives its mobility from a complex interconnected structure of four joints, three large bones, and three principal muscle groups, often referred to as the *shoulder girdle*. The clavicle and acromion stabilize the shoulder girdle, allowing the humerus to swing out and away from the body, giving the shoulder its remarkable range of motion.

Bony Structures. The bony structures of the shoulder include the humerus, the clavicle, and the scapula. The scapula is anchored to the axial skeleton only by the sternoclavicular joint and inserting muscles, often called the *scapulothoracic articulation* since it is not a true joint.

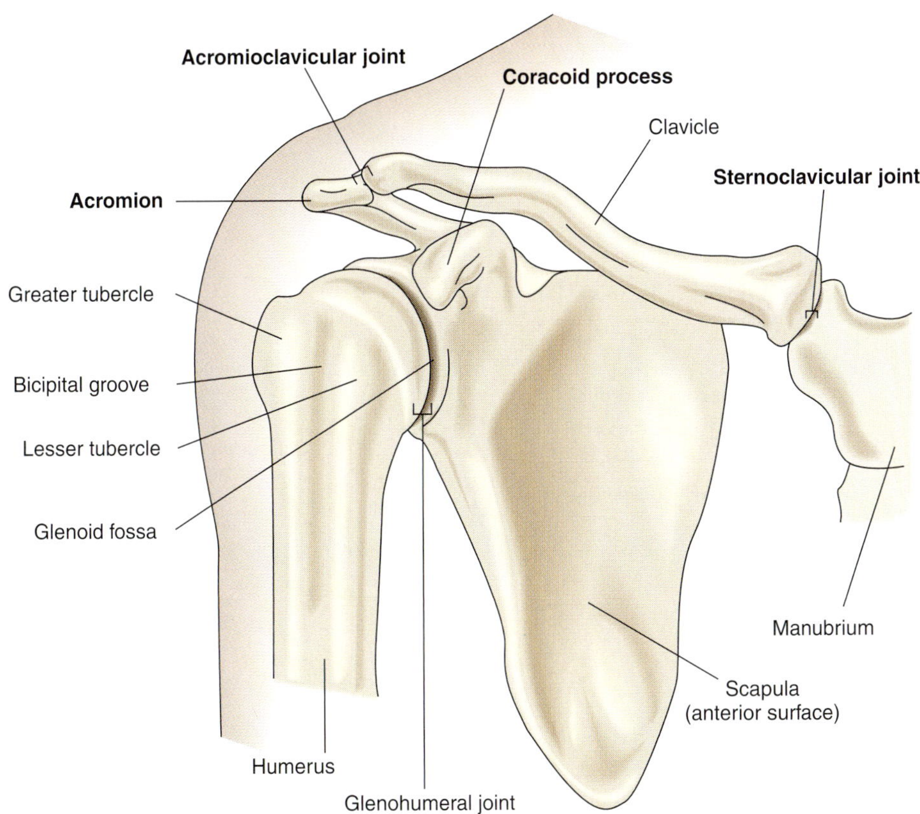

Identify the manubrium, the sternoclavicular joint, and the clavicle. With your fingers, trace the clavicle laterally. Now, from behind, follow the bony spine of the scapula laterally and upward until it becomes the *acromion*, the summit of the shoulder. Its upper surface is rough and slightly convex. Identify the anterior tip of the acromion (**A**) and mark it with ink. With your index finger on top of the acromion, just behind its tip, press medially to find the slightly elevated ridge that marks the distal end of the clavicle at the *acromioclavicular joint* (shown by the arrow). Move your finger laterally and down a short step to the next bony prominence, the *greater tubercle of the humerus* (**B**). Mark this with ink. Now sweep your finger medially until you feel a large bony prominence, the *coracoid process* of the scapula (**C**). Mark this also. These three points—the tip of the acromion, the greater tubercle of the humerus, and the coracoid process—orient you to the anatomy of the shoulder.

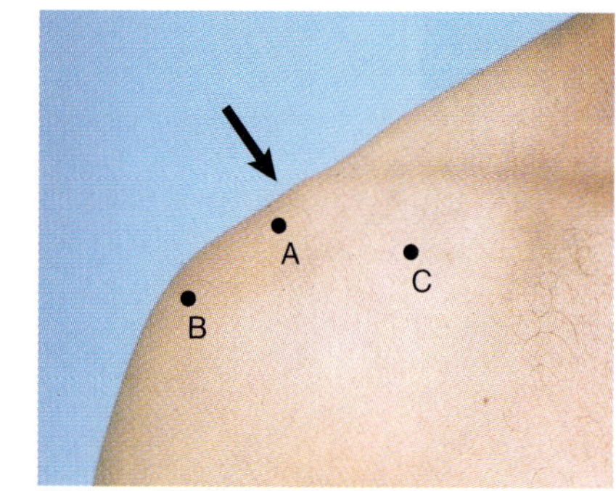

Joints. Three different joints articulate at the shoulder:

- The *glenohumeral joint.* In this joint, the head of the humerus articulates with the shallow glenoid fossa of the scapula. This joint is deeply situated and not normally palpable. It is a ball-and-socket joint, allowing the arm its wide arc of movement—flexion, extension, abduction (movement away from the trunk), adduction (movement toward the trunk), rotation, and circumduction.
- The *sternoclavicular joint.* The convex medial end of the clavicle articulates with the concave hollow in the upper sternum.
- The *acromioclavicular joint.* The lateral end of the clavicle articulates with the acromion process of the scapula.

Muscle Groups. Three groups of muscles attach at the shoulder:

The Scapulohumeral Group. This group extends from the scapula to the humerus and includes the muscles inserting directly on the humerus, known as *"SITS muscles"* of the *rotator cuff:*

- *Supraspinatus*—runs above the glenohumeral joint; inserts on the greater tubercle
- *Infraspinatus* and *teres minor*—cross the glenohumeral joint posteriorly; insert on the greater tubercle
- *Subscapularis* (not illustrated)—originates on the anterior surface of the scapula and crosses the joint anteriorly; inserts on the lesser tubercle.

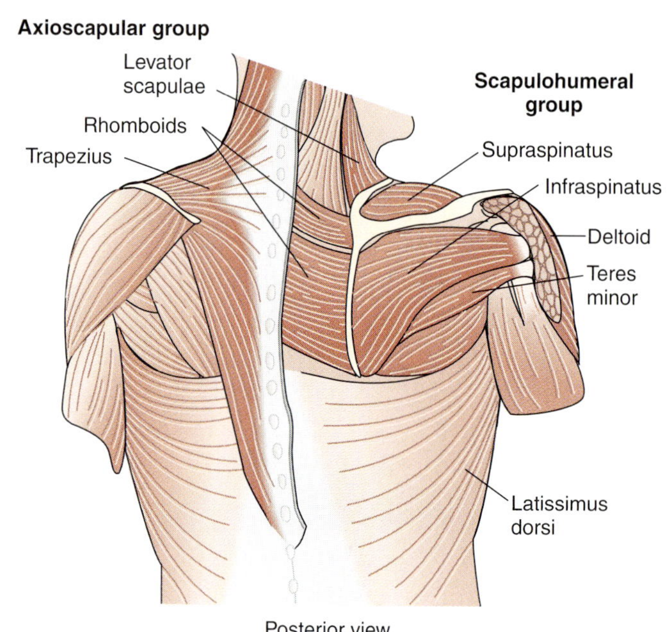

Axioscapular group (pulls shoulder backward)
Scapulohumeral group (rotates shoulder laterally; includes rotator cuff)

The scapulohumeral group rotates the shoulder laterally (the rotator cuff) and depresses and rotates the head of the humerus. (See pp. 526–527 for discussion of rotator cuff injuries.)

The Axioscapular Group. This group attaches the trunk to the scapula and includes the trapezius, rhomboids, serratus anterior, and levator scapulae. These muscles rotate the scapula.

The Axiohumeral Group. This group attaches the trunk to the humerus and includes the pectoralis major and minor and the latissimus dorsi. These muscles produce internal rotation of the shoulder.

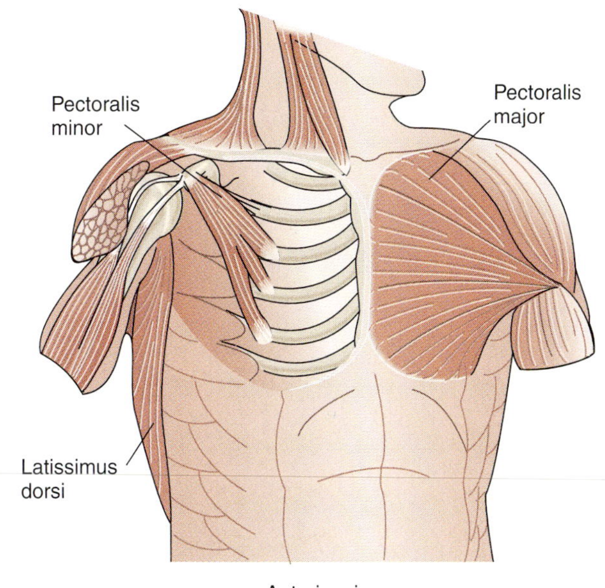

Axiohumeral group (rotates shoulder internally)

The biceps and triceps, which connect the scapula to the bones of the forearm, are also involved in shoulder movement, particularly abduction.

Additional Structures. Also important to shoulder movement are the *articular capsule and bursae.* Surrounding the glenohumeral joint is a fibrous articular capsule formed by the tendon insertions of the rotator cuff and other capsular muscles. The loose fit of the capsule allows the shoulder bones to separate, and contributes to the shoulder's wide range of movement. The capsule is lined by a synovial membrane with two outpouchings—the subscapular bursa and the synovial sheath of the tendon of the long head of the biceps.

To locate the biceps tendon, rotate the arm externally and find the tendinous cord that runs just medial to the greater tubercle. Roll it under your fingers. This is the tendon of the *long head of the biceps.* It runs in the bicipital groove between the greater and lesser tubercles.

The principal bursa of the shoulder is the *subacromial bursa,* positioned between the acromion and the head of the humerus and overlying the supraspinatus tendon. Abduction of the shoulder compresses this bursa. Normally, the supraspinatus tendon and the subacromial bursa are not palpable. However, if the bursal surfaces are inflamed (subacromial bursitis), there may be tenderness just below the tip of the acromion, pain with abduction and rotation, and loss of smooth movement.

The Elbow

Overview, Bony Structures, and Joints. The elbow helps position the hand in space and stabilizes the lever action of the forearm. The elbow

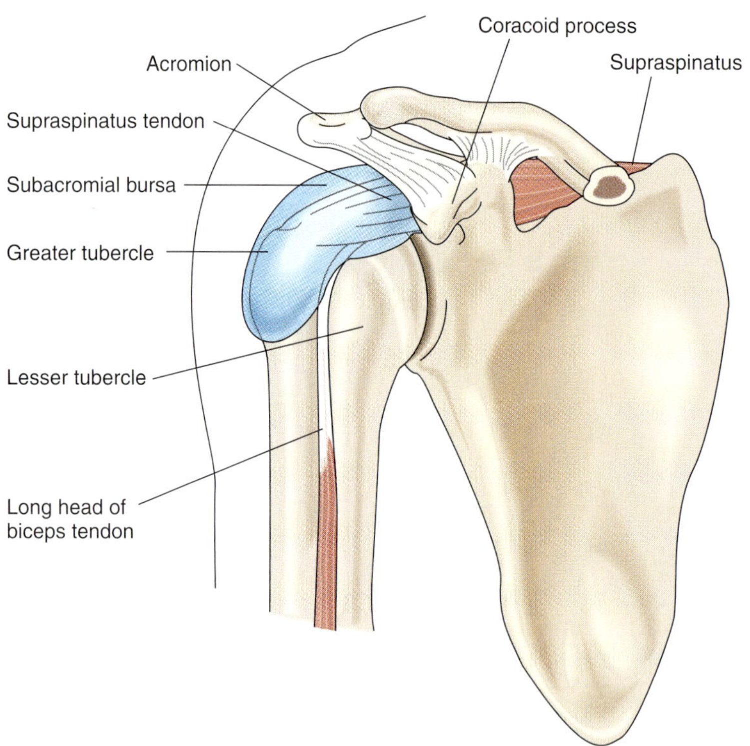

joint is formed by the humerus and the two bones of the forearm, the radius and the ulna. Identify the medial and lateral epicondyles of the humerus and the olecranon process of the ulna.

These bones have three articulations: the *humeroulnar joint*, the *radiohumeral joint*, and the *radioulnar joint*. All three share a large common articular cavity and an extensive synovial lining.

Muscle Groups and Additional Structures. Muscles traversing the elbow include the *biceps* and *brachioradialis* (flexion), the *triceps* (extension), the *pronator teres* (pronation), and the *supinator* (supination).

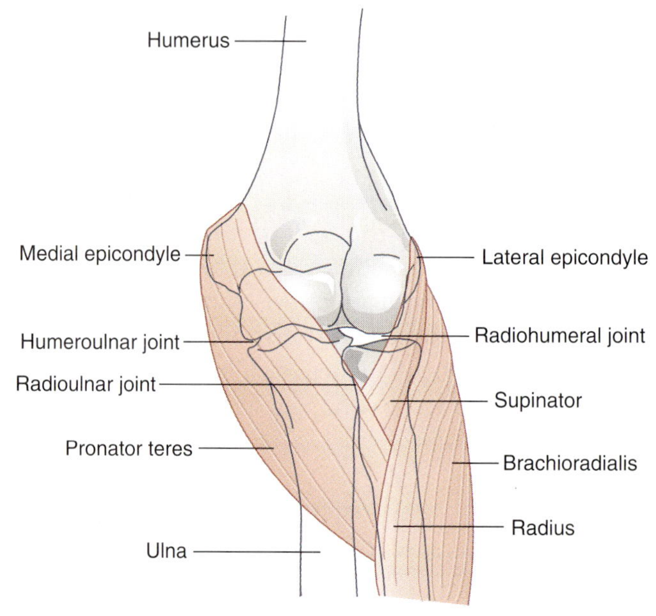

LEFT ELBOW—ANTERIOR VIEW

Note the location of the *olecranon bursa* between the olecranon process and the skin. The bursa is not normally palpable but swells and becomes tender when inflamed. The *ulnar nerve* runs posteriorly between the medial epicondyle and the olecranon process. On the ventral forearm, the *median nerve* is just medial to the brachial artery.

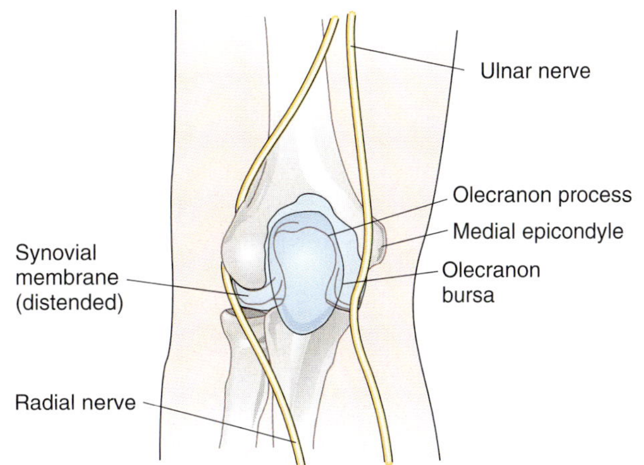

LEFT ELBOW—POSTERIOR VIEW

The Wrist and Hands

Overview. The wrist and hands form a complex unit of small, highly active joints used almost continuously during waking hours. There is little protection from overlying soft tissue, increasing vulnerability to trauma and disability.

Bony Structures. The wrist includes the distal radius and ulna and eight small carpal bones. At the wrist, identify the bony tips of the radius and the ulna.

The carpal bones lie distal to the wrist joint within each hand. Identify the carpal bones, each of the five metacarpals, and the proximal, middle, and distal phalanges. Note that the thumb lacks a middle phalanx.

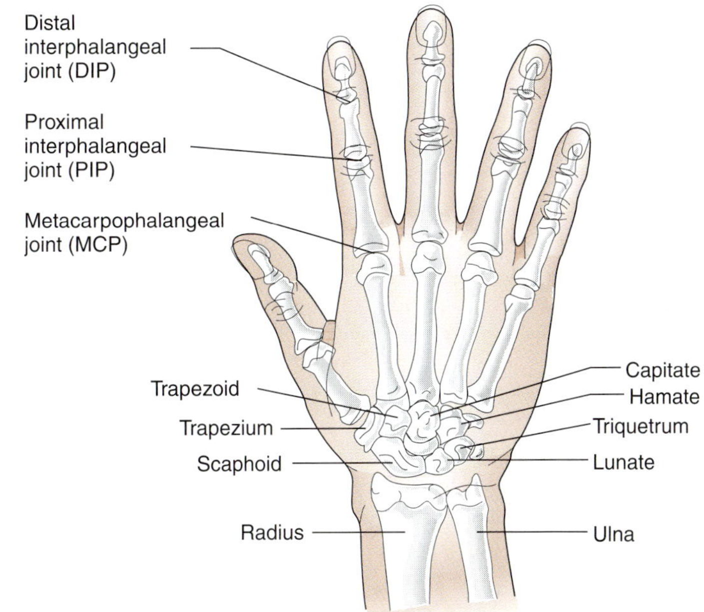

Joints. The numerous joints of the wrist and hand lend unusual dexterity to the hands.

- *Wrist joints.* The wrist joints include the *radiocarpal* or *wrist joint*, the *distal radioulnar joint*, and the *intercarpal joints.* The joint capsule, articular disc, and synovial membrane of the wrist join the radius to the ulna and to the proximal carpal bones. On the dorsum of the wrist, locate the groove of the radiocarpal joint.

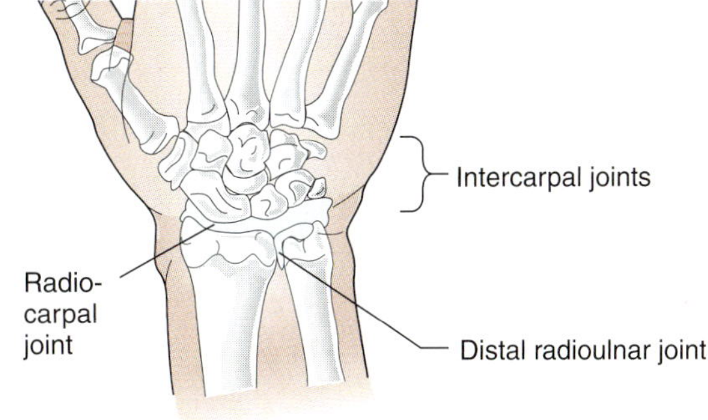

- *Hand joints.* The joints of the hand include the *metacarpophalangeal joints* (MCPs), the *proximal interphalangeal joints* (PIPs), and the *distal interphalangeal joints* (DIPs). Flex the hand and find the groove marking the MCP joint of each finger. It is distal to the knuckle and is best felt on either side of the extensor tendon.

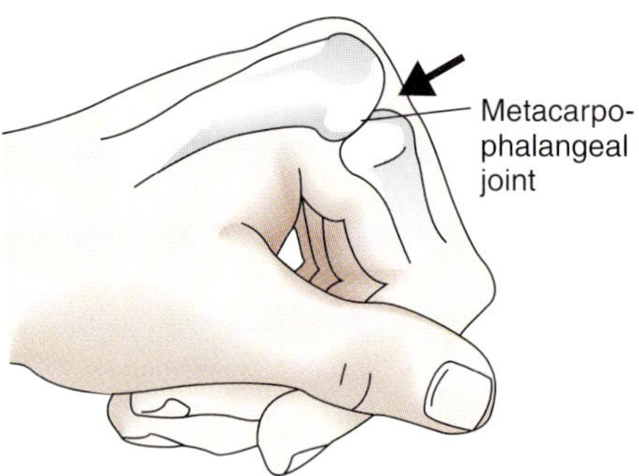

Muscle Groups. Wrist flexion arises from the two carpal muscles, located on the radial and ulnar surfaces. Two radial and one ulnar muscle provide wrist extension. Supination and pronation result from muscle contraction in the forearm.

The thumb is powered by three muscles that form the thenar eminence and provide flexion, abduction, and opposition. The muscles of extension are at the base of the thumb along the radial margin. Movement in the digits depends on action of the flexor and extensor tendons of muscles in the forearm and wrist.

The intrinsic muscles of the hand attaching to the metacarpal bones are involved in flexion (*lumbricals*), abduction (*dorsal interossei*), and adduction (*palmar interossei*) of the fingers.

Additional Structures. Soft-tissue structures, especially tendons and tendon sheaths, are extremely important in the wrist and hand. Six extensor tendons and two flexor tendons pass across the wrist and hand to insert on the fingers. Through much of their course these tendons travel in tunnel-like sheaths, generally palpable only when swollen or inflamed.

Be familiar with the structures in the *carpal tunnel,* a channel beneath the palmar surface of the wrist and proximal hand. The canal contains the sheath and flexor tendons of the forearm muscles and the *median nerve.*

Holding the tendons and tendon sheath in place is a transverse ligament, the *flexor retinaculum.* The median nerve lies between the flexor retinaculum and the tendon sheath. It provides sensation to the palm and the palmar surface of most of the thumb, the second and third digits, and half of the fourth digit. It also innervates the thumb muscles of flexion, abduction, and opposition.

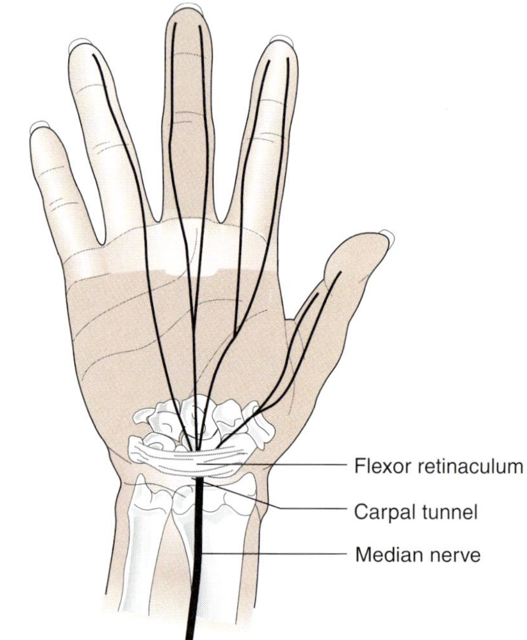

The Spine

Overview. The vertebral column, or spine, is the central supporting structure of the trunk and back. Note the *concave curves* of the cervical and lumbar spine and the *convex curves* of the thoracic and sacrococcygeal spine. These curves help distribute upper body weight to the pelvis and lower extremities and cushion the concussive impact of walking or running.

The complex mechanics of the back reflect the coordinated action of:

- The vertebrae and intervertebral discs
- An interconnecting system of ligaments between anterior vertebrae and posterior vertebrae, ligaments between the spinous processes, and ligaments between the lamina of two adjacent vertebrae
- Large superficial muscles, deeper intrinsic muscles, and muscles of the abdominal wall.

Viewing the patient from behind, identify the following landmarks:

1. Spinous processes, usually more prominent at C7 and T1 and more evident on forward flexion
2. Paravertebral muscles on either side of the midline
3. Scapulae
4. Iliac crests
5. Posterior superior iliac spines, usually marked by skin dimples.

A line drawn above the posterior iliac crests crosses the spinous process of L4.

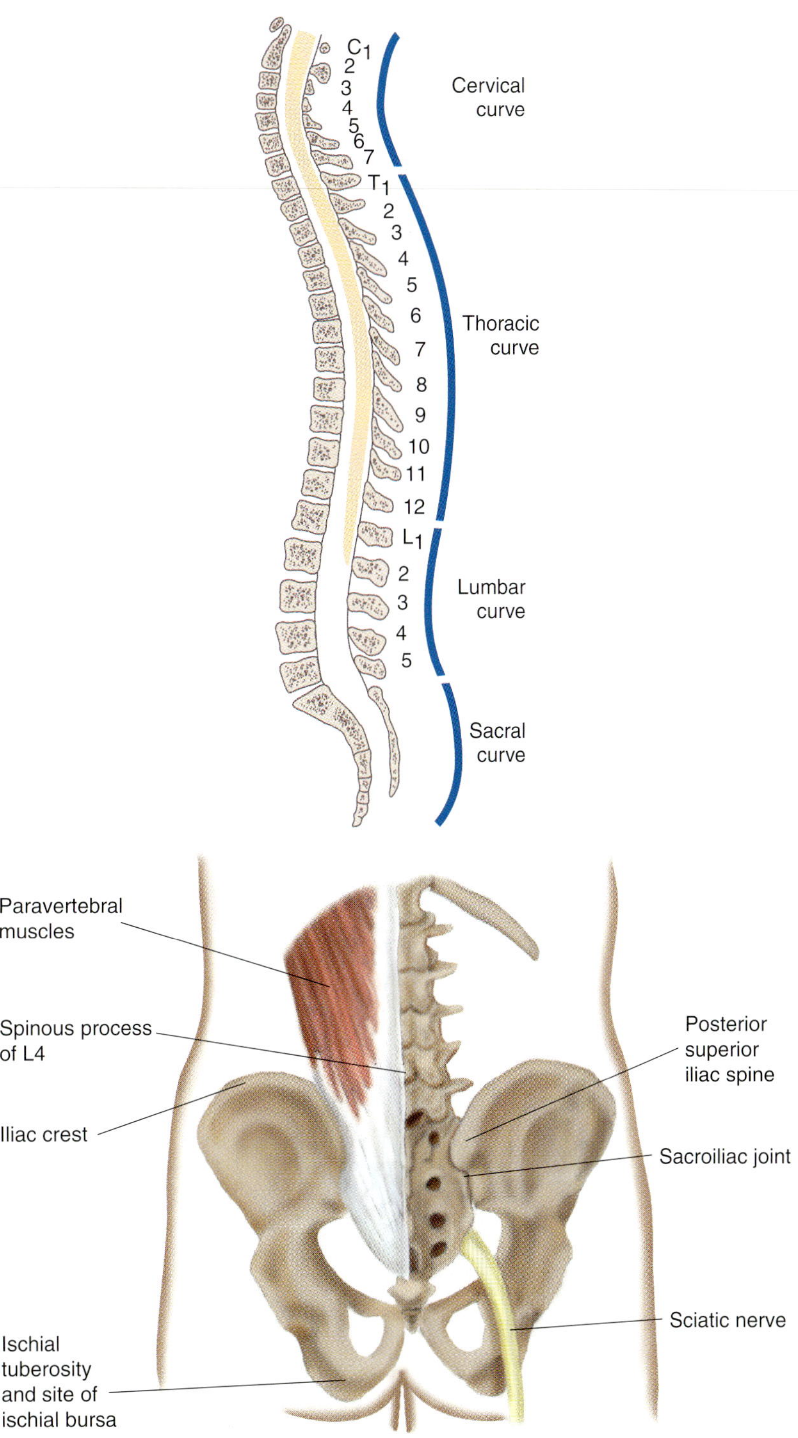

Bony Structures. The vertebral column contains 24 vertebrae stacked on the sacrum and coccyx. A typical vertebra contains sites for joint articulations, weight bearing, and muscle attachments, as well as foramina for the spinal nerve roots and peripheral nerves. Anteriorly, the *vertebral body* supports weight bearing. The posterior *vertebral arch* encloses the spinal cord. Review the location of the vertebral processes and foramina, with particular attention to:

- The *spinous process* projecting posteriorly in the midline and the two transverse processes at the junction of the *pedicle* and the *lamina*. Muscles attach at these processes.
- The *articular processes*—two on each side of the vertebra, one facing up and one facing down, at the junction of the pedicles and laminae, often called *articular facets*
- The *vertebral foramen,* which encloses the spinal cord, the *intervertebral foramen,* formed by the inferior and superior articulating process of adjacent vertebrae, creating a channel for the spinal nerve roots; and in the cervical vertebrae, the *transverse foramen* for the vertebral artery.

The proximity of the spinal cord and spinal nerve roots to their bony vertebral casing and the intervertebral discs makes them especially vulnerable to disc herniation, impingement from degenerative changes in the vertebrae, and trauma.

Joints. The spine has slightly movable cartilaginous joints between the vertebral bodies and between the articular facets. Between the vertebral bodies are the *intervertebral discs,* each consisting

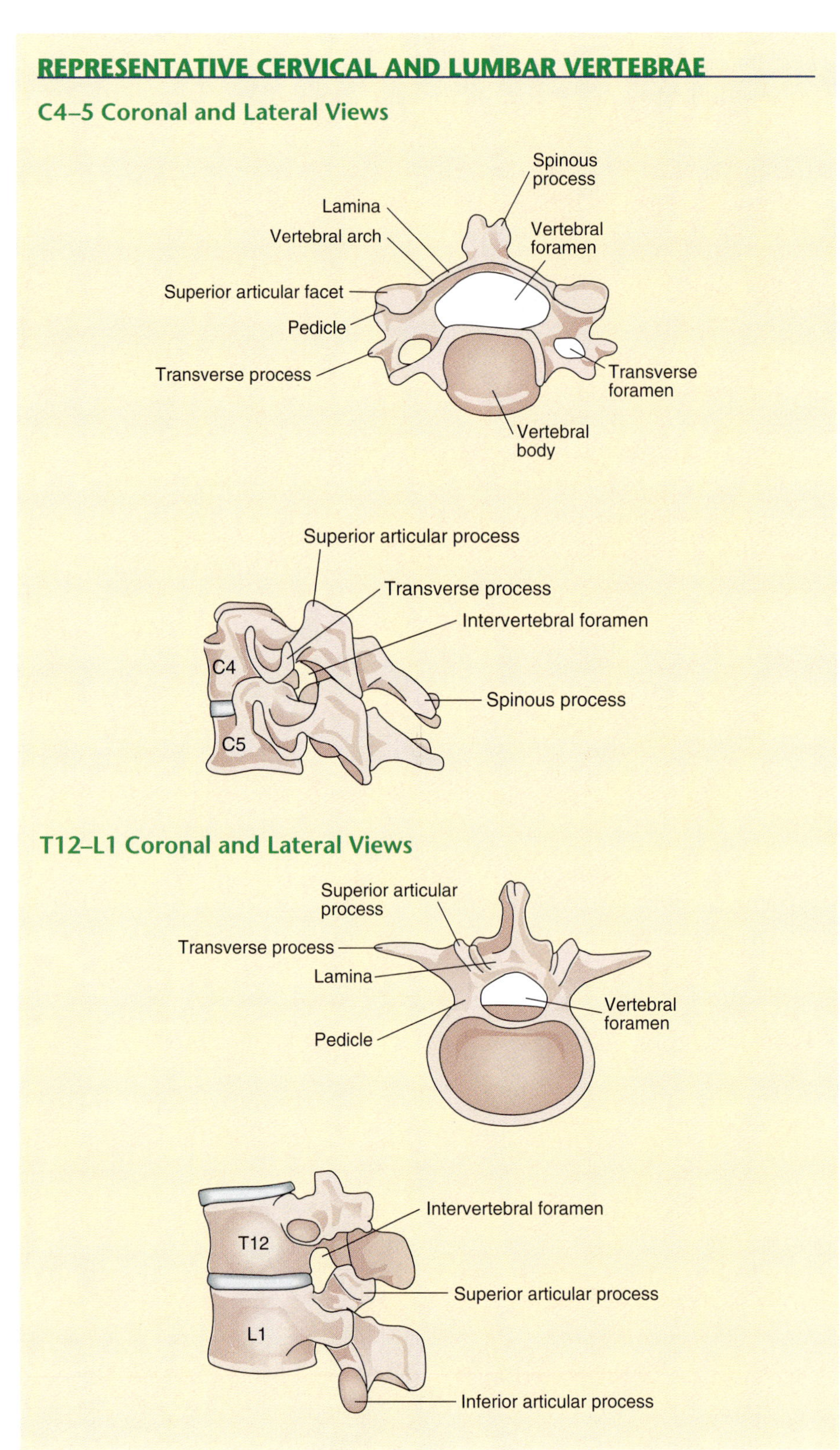

of a soft mucoid central core, the *nucleus pulposus*, rimmed by the tough fibrous tissue of the *annulus fibrosis.* The intervertebral discs cushion movement between vertebrae and allow the vertebral column to curve, flex, and bend. The flexibility of the spine is largely determined by the angle of the articular facet joints relative to the plane of the vertebral body, and varies at different levels of the spine. Note that the vertebral column angles sharply posterior at the *lumbosacral junction* and becomes immovable. The mechanical stress at this angulation contributes to the risk of disc herniation and subluxation, or slippage, of L5 on S1.

Muscle Groups. The *trapezius* and *latissimus dorsi* form the large outer layer of muscles attaching to each side of the spine. They overlie two deeper muscle layers—a layer attaching to the head, neck, and spinous processes (*splenius capitis, splenius cervicis,* and *sacrospinalis*) and a layer of smaller intrinsic muscles between vertebrae. Muscles attaching to the anterior surface of the vertebrae, including the *psoas* muscle and muscles of the abdominal wall, assist with flexion.

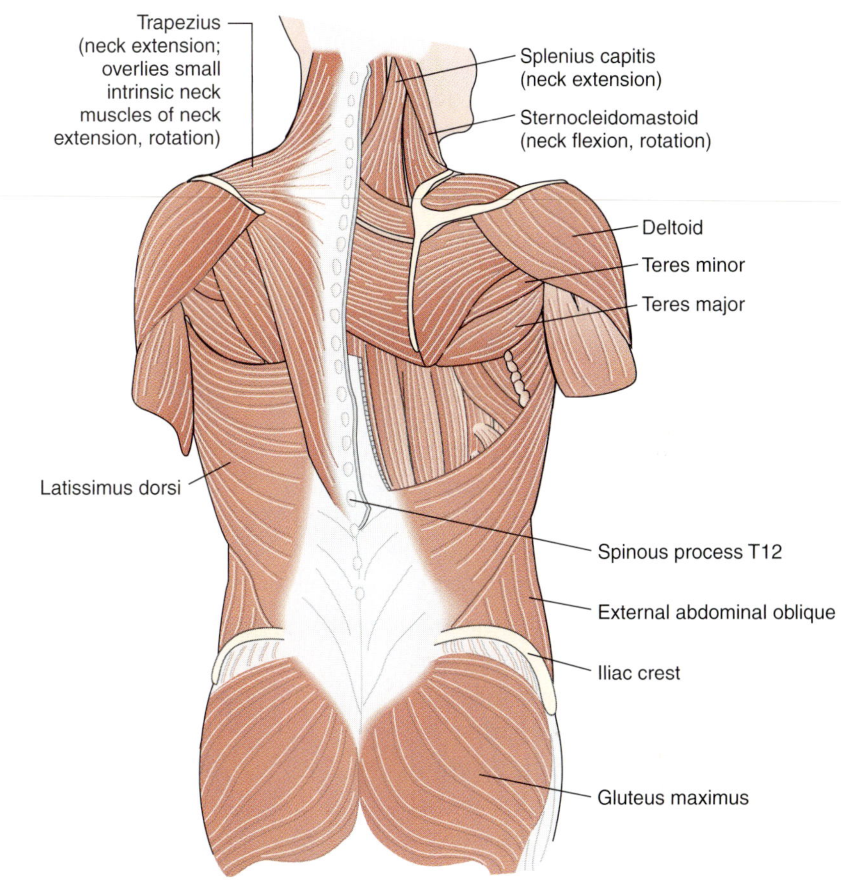

Muscles moving the neck and lower vertebral column are summarized below.

Movement	Principal Muscle Group
Cervical Spine (neck)	
Flexion	Sternocleidomastoid, scalene, and prevertebral muscles
Extension	Splenius, trapezius, small intrinsic neck muscles
Rotation	Sternocleidomastoid, small intrinsic neck muscles
Lateral bending	Scalene and small intrinsic neck muscles
Lumbar Spine	
Flexion	Psoas major, psoas minor, quadratus lumborum; abdominal muscles such as the internal and external obliques and rectus abdominis, attaching to the anterior vertebrae
Extension	Intrinsic muscles of the back, sacrospinalis
Rotation	Abdominal muscles, intrinsic muscles of the back
Lateral bending	Abdominal muscles, intrinsic muscles of the back

The Hip

Overview. The hip joint is deeply embedded in the pelvis, and is notable for its strength, stability, and wide range of motion. The stability of the hip joint, so essential for weight bearing, arises from the deep fit of the head of the femur into the *acetabulum*, its strong fibrous articular capsule, and the powerful muscles crossing the joint and inserting below the femoral head, providing leverage for movement of the femur.

Bony Structures and Joints. The hip joint lies below the middle third of the inguinal ligament but in a deeper plane. It is a ball-and-socket joint—note how the rounded head of the femur articulates with the cuplike cavity of the acetabulum. Because of its overlying muscles and depth, it is not readily palpable. Review the bones of the pelvis—the *acetabulum*, the *ilium*, and the *ischium*—and the connection inferiorly at the *symphysis pubis* and posteriorly with the sacroiliac bone.

On the *anterior aspect* of the hip, identify the *iliac crest* at the upper margin of the pelvis at the level of L4. Follow the downward anterior curve and locate the *iliac tubercle*, marking the widest point of the crest, and continue tracking downward to the *anterior superior iliac spine*. Place your thumbs on the anterior superior spines and move your fingers downward from the iliac tubercles to the *greater trochanter* of the femur. Then move your thumbs medially and obliquely to the *pubic symphysis*, which lies at the same level as the greater trochanter.

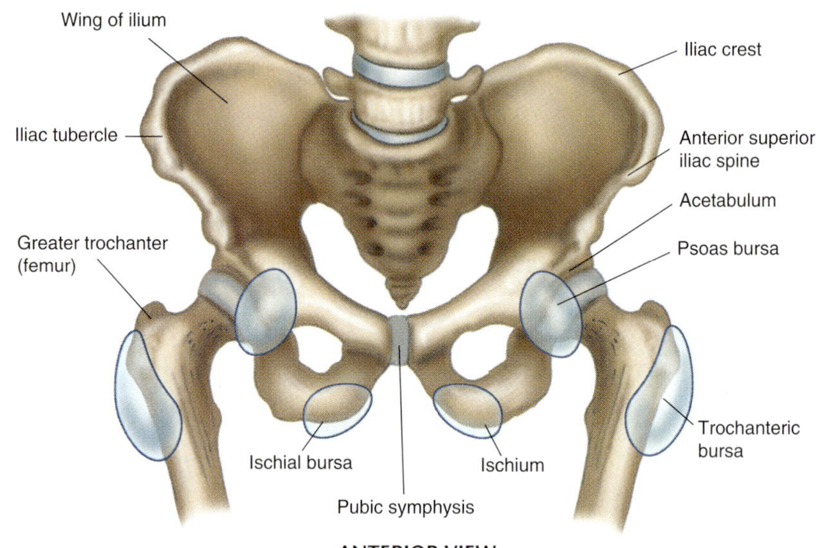

ANTERIOR VIEW

On the *posterior aspect* of the hip, locate the *posterior superior iliac spine* directly underneath the visible dimples just above the buttocks. Placing your left thumb and index finger over the posterior superior iliac spine, next locate the *greater trochanter* laterally with your fingers at the level of the gluteal fold and place your thumb medially on the *ischial tuberosity*. The *sacroiliac joint* is not palpable. Note that an imaginary line between the posterior superior iliac spines crosses the joint at S2.

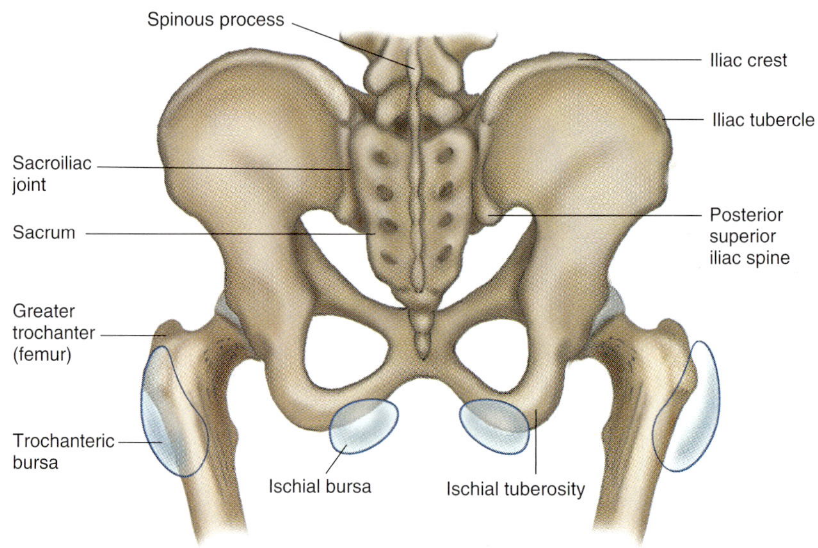

POSTERIOR VIEW

Muscle Groups. Four powerful muscle groups move the hip. To remember these groups, try to picture where muscles need to cross joints to move limbs such as the femur in a given direction. The *flexor group* lies anteriorly and flexes the thigh. The primary hip flexor is the *iliopsoas,* extending from above the iliac crest to the lesser trochanter. The *extensor group* lies posteriorly and extends the thigh. The *gluteus maximus* is the primary extensor of the hip. It forms a band crossing from its origin along the medial pelvis to its insertion below the trochanter.

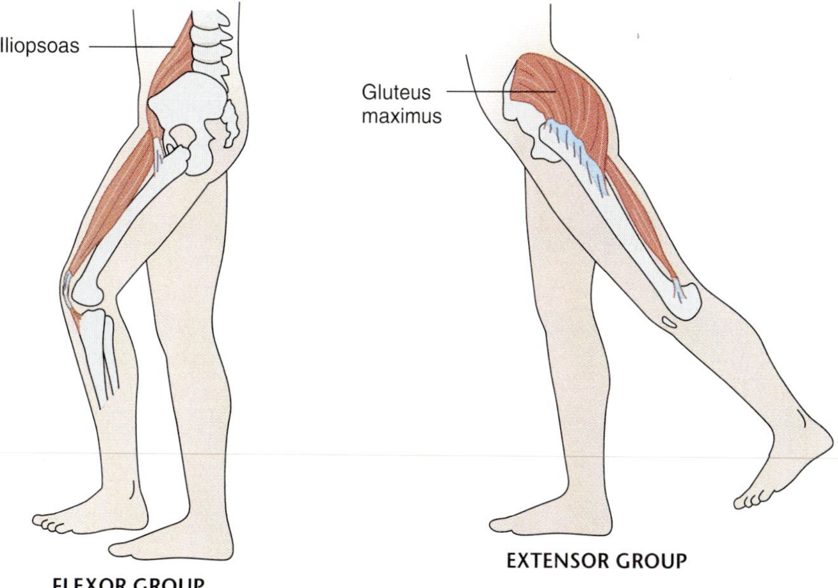

FLEXOR GROUP

EXTENSOR GROUP

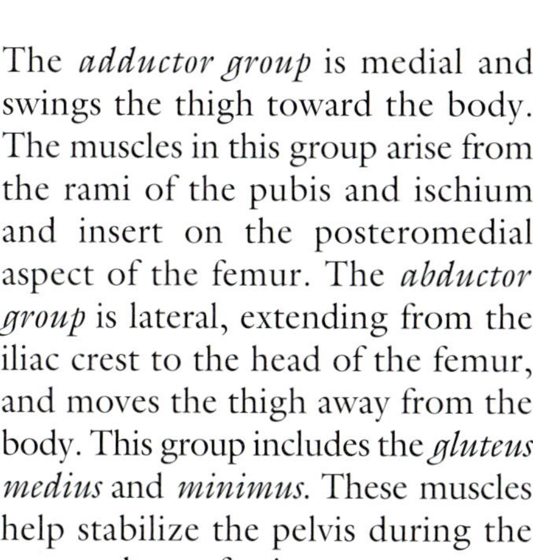

The *adductor group* is medial and swings the thigh toward the body. The muscles in this group arise from the rami of the pubis and ischium and insert on the posteromedial aspect of the femur. The *abductor group* is lateral, extending from the iliac crest to the head of the femur, and moves the thigh away from the body. This group includes the *gluteus medius* and *minimus.* These muscles help stabilize the pelvis during the stance phase of gait.

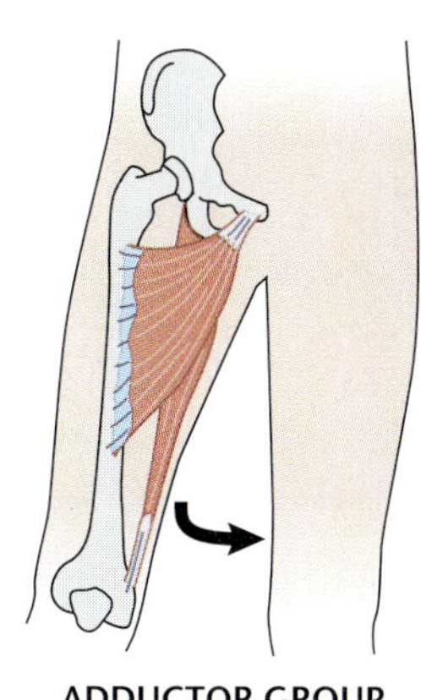

ADDUCTOR GROUP

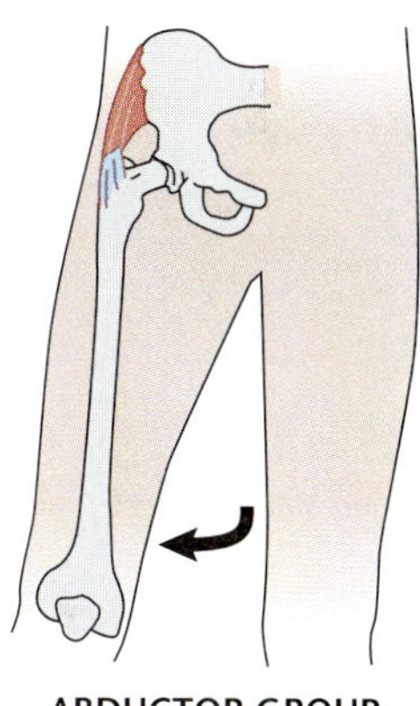

ABDUCTOR GROUP

Additional Structures. A strong dense articular capsule, extending from the acetabulum to the femoral neck, encases and strengthens the hip joint, reinforced by three overlying ligaments and lined with synovial membrane. There are three principal bursae at the hip. Anterior to the joint is the *iliopectineal* (or *iliopsoas*) *bursa,* overlying the articular capsule and the psoas muscle. Find the bony prominence lateral to the hip joint—the *greater trochanter* of the femur. The large multilocular *trochanteric bursa* lies on its posterior surface. The *ischiogluteal bursa*—not always present—lies under the *ischeal tuberosity,* on which a person sits. Note their proximity to the sciatic nerve, as shown on p. 475.

The Knee

Overview. The knee joint is the largest joint in the body. It involves three bones: the femur, the tibia, and the patella (or knee cap), with three articular surfaces, two between the femur and the tibia and one between the femur and the patella. Note how the two rounded condyles of the femur rest on the relatively flat tibial plateau. There is no inherent stability in the knee joint itself, making it dependent on ligaments to hold its articulating bones in place. This feature, in addition to the lever action of the femur on the tibia and lack of padding from fat or muscle, makes the knee highly vulnerable to injury.

Bony Structures. Landmarks in and around the knee will orient you to this complicated joint. Bring your fingertips firmly down the medial surface of the thigh along a line analogous to the inner seam of a pant leg. Your fingers will run up against an abrupt bony prominence, the *adductor tubercle.* Just below this is the *medial epicondyle.* The *lateral epicondyle* is comparably situated on the other side.

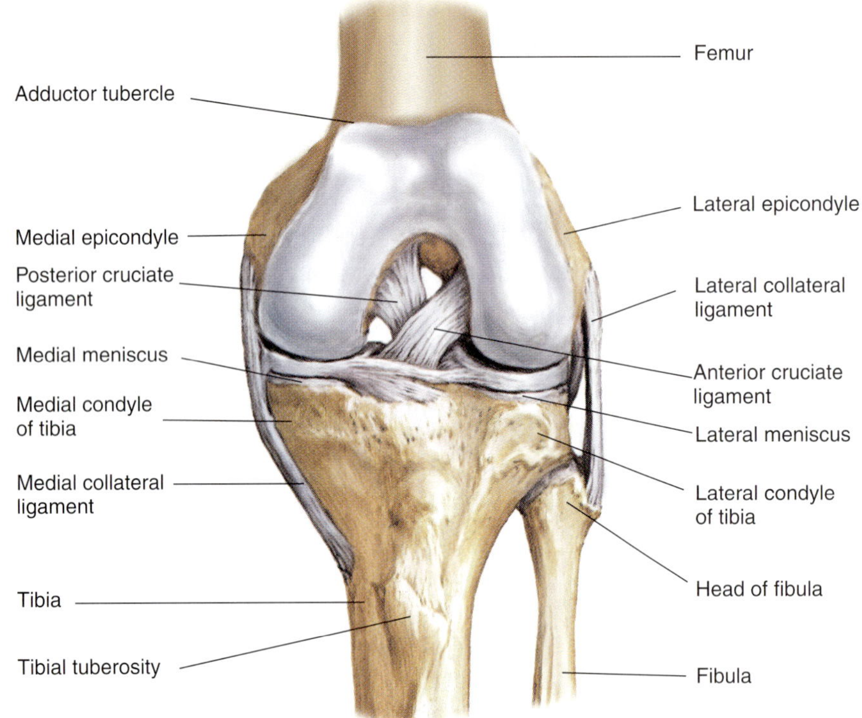

ANTERIOR ASPECT OF THE KNEE

Identify the flat medial surface of the tibia—the shin. Follow its anterior border upward to the *tibial tuberosity* (**A**). Mark this point with a dot of ink. Now follow the medial border of the tibia upward until it merges into a bony prominence—the *medial condyle* of the tibia (**B**). This is somewhat higher than the tibial tuberosity. In a comparable location on the other side of the knee, find a similar prominence—the *lateral condyle* (**C**). Mark both condyles with ink. These three points form an isosceles triangle. On the lateral surface of the knee, somewhat below the level of the lateral tibial condyle, find the head of the fibula.

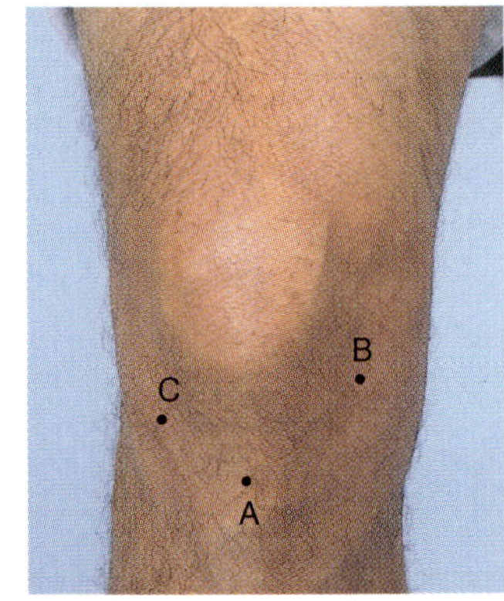

The *patella* rests on the anterior articulating surface of the femur, midway between the epicondyles, embedded in the tendon of the quadriceps muscle. This tendon continues below the knee joint as the *patellar tendon* and inserts on the tibial tuberosity.

Joints. Two condylar *tibiofemoral joints* are formed by the convex curves of the medial and lateral condyles of the femur as they articulate with the concave condyles of the tibia. The third articular surface is the *patellofemoral joint.* The patella slides in a groove on the anterior aspect of the distal femur, called the *trochlear groove,* during flexion and extension of the knee.

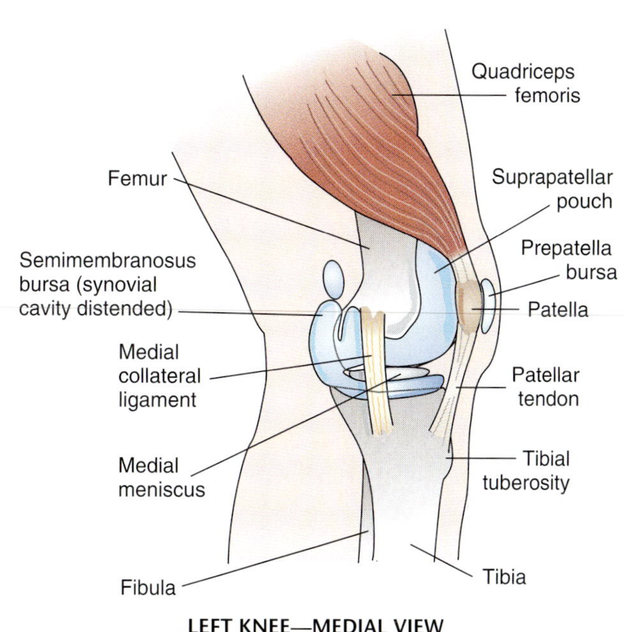

LEFT KNEE—MEDIAL VIEW

With the knee flexed about 90°, you can press your thumbs—one on each side of the patellar tendon—into the groove of the tibiofemoral joint. Note that the patella lies just above this joint line. As you press your thumbs downward, you can feel the edge of the tibial plateau, the upper surface of the tibia. Follow it medially, then laterally until you are stopped by the converging femur and tibia. By moving your thumbs upward toward the midline to the top of the patella, you can follow the articulating surface of the femur and identify the margins of the joint.

Muscle Groups. Powerful muscles move and support the knee. The *quadriceps femoris* extends the leg, covering the anterior, medial, and lateral aspects of the thigh. The *hamstring muscles* lie on the posterior aspect of the thigh and flex the knee.

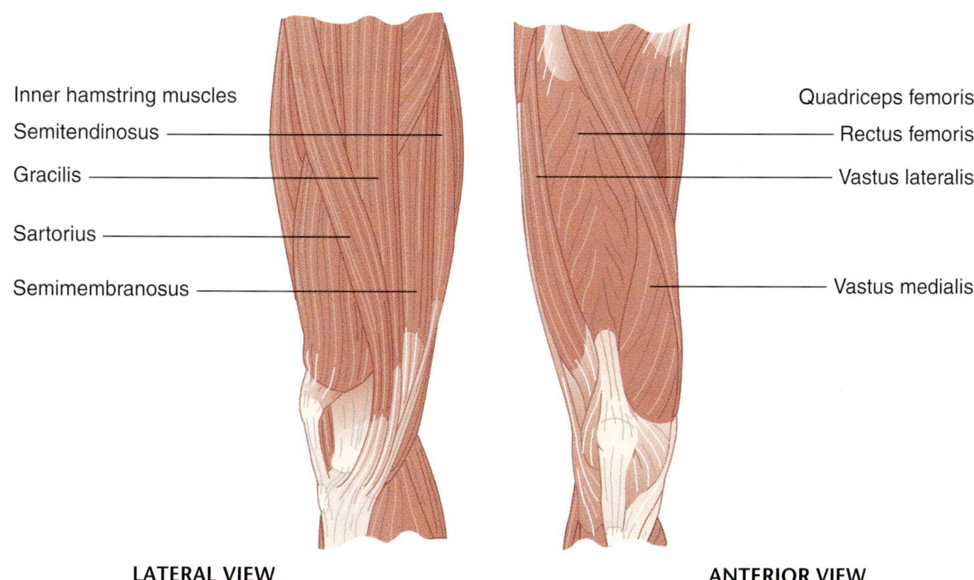

LATERAL VIEW

ANTERIOR VIEW

Additional Structures. Two important pairs of ligaments, the collateral ligaments and the cruciate ligaments, and the menisci provide stability to the knee (see drawing on pp. 480 and 481).

- The *medial collateral ligament* (MCL), not easily palpable, is a broad flat ligament connecting the medial condyles of the femur and the tibia. To locate the anatomic region of the MCL, move your fingers medially and posteriorly along the joint line, then palpate along the ligament from its origin to insertion.

- The *lateral collateral ligament* (LCL) connects the lateral femoral condyle and the head of the fibula. To feel the LCL, cross one leg so the ankle rests on the opposite knee and find the firm cord that runs from the lateral epicondyle of the femur to the head of the fibula. The MCL and LCL provide medial and lateral stability to the knee.

- The *anterior cruciate ligament* (ACL) crosses obliquely from the lateral femoral condyle to the medial tibia, preventing the tibia from sliding forward on the femur.

- The *posterior cruciate ligament* (PCL) crosses from the lateral tibia and lateral meniscus to the medial femoral condyle, preventing the tibia from slipping backward on the femur. Since these ligaments lie within the knee joint, they are not palpable. They are nonetheless crucial to the anteroposterior stability of the knee.

- The *medial and lateral menisci* cushion the action of the femur on the tibia. These crescent-shaped fibrocartilaginous discs add a cuplike surface to the otherwise flat tibial plateau. Palpate the *medial meniscus* by pressing on the medial soft-tissue depression along the upper edge of the tibial plateau. Place the knee in slight flexion and palpate the *lateral meniscus* along the lateral joint line.

Observe the concavities that are usually evident at each side of the patella and also above it. Occupying these areas is the synovial cavity of the knee, the largest joint cavity in the body. This cavity includes an extension 6 centimeters above the upper border of the patella, lying upward and deep to the quadriceps muscle—the *suprapatellar pouch.* The joint cavity covers the anterior, medial, and lateral surfaces of the knee, as well as the condyles of the femur and tibia posteriorly. Although the synovium is not normally detectable, these areas may become swollen and tender when the joint is inflamed.

Several bursae lie near the knee. The *prepatellar bursa* lies between the patella and the overlying skin. The *anserine bursa* lies 1 to 2 inches below the knee joint on the medial surface and cannot be palpated due to overlying tendons. Now identify the large *semimembranosus bursa* that communicates with the joint cavity, also on the posterior and medial surfaces of the knee.

The Ankle and Foot

Overview. The total weight of the body is transmitted through the ankle to the foot. The ankle and foot must balance the body and absorb the impact of the heel strike and gait. Despite thick padding along the toes, sole, and heel and stabilizing ligaments at the ankles, the ankle and foot are frequent sites of sprain and bony injury.

Bony Structures and Joints. The ankle is a hinge joint formed by the *tibia*, the *fibula*, and the *talus.* The tibia and fibula act as a mortise, stabilizing the joint while bracing the talus like an inverted cup.

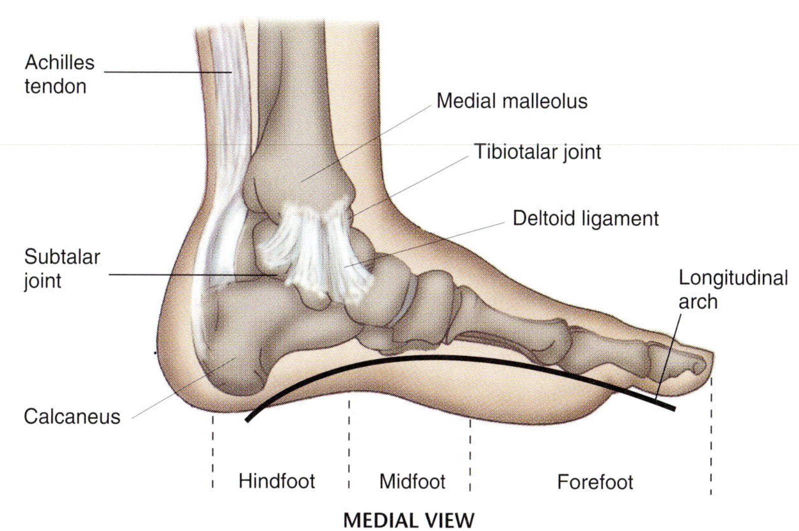

The principal joints of the ankle are the *tibiotalar joint*, between the tibia and the talus, and the *subtalar (talocalcaneal) joint.*

Note the principal landmarks of the ankle: the *medial malleolus*, the bony prominence at the distal end of the tibia, and the *lateral malleolus*, at the distal end of the fibula. Lodged under the talus and jutting posteriorly is the *calcaneus*, or heel.

An imaginary line, the *longitudinal arch*, spans the foot, extending from the calcaneus of the hind foot along the tarsal bones of the midfoot (see cuneiforms, navicular, and cuboid bones below) to the forefoot metatarsals and toes. The *heads of the metatarsals* are palpable in the ball of the foot. In the forefoot, identify the *metatarsophalangeal joints*, proximal to the webs of the toes, and the *proximal and distal interphalangeal joints* of the toes.

Muscle Groups and Additional Structures. Movement at the ankle joint is limited to dorsiflexion and plantar flexion. *Plantar flexion* is powered by the gastrocnemius, the posterior tibial muscle, and the toe flexors. Their tendons run behind the malleoli. The *dorsiflexors* include the anterior tibial muscle and the toe extensors. They lie prominently on the anterior surface, or dorsum, of the ankle, anterior to the malleoli.

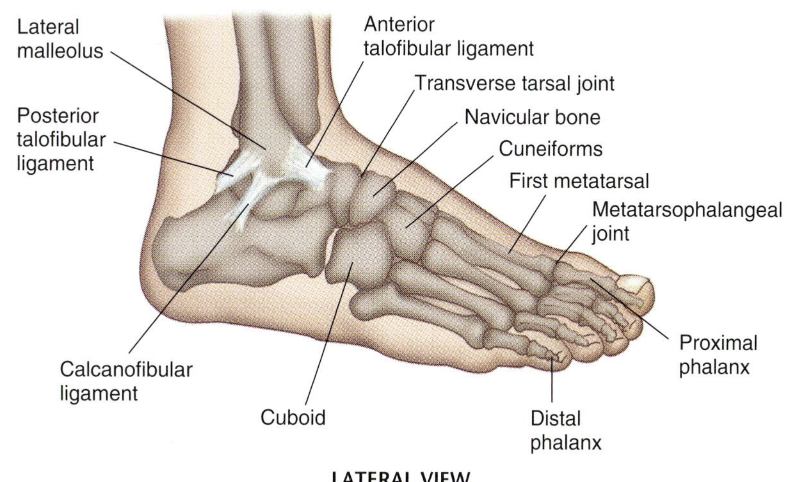

Ligaments extend from each malleolus onto the foot. Medially, the triangle-shaped *deltoid ligament* fans out from the inferior surface of the medial malleolus to the talus and proximal tarsal bones, protecting against stress from eversion (ankle bows inward). The three ligaments on the lateral side are less substantial, with higher risk of injury: the *anterior talofibular ligament*—most at risk in injury from inversion (ankle bows outward) injuries; the *calcaneofibular ligament*; and the *posterior talofibular ligament*. The strong Achilles tendon inserts on the heel posteriorly.

Changes With Aging

Musculoskeletal changes continue through the adult years. Soon after maturity adults begin to lose height subtly, and significant shortening becomes obvious in old age. Most loss of height occurs in the trunk as intervertebral discs become thinner and the vertebral bodies shorten or even collapse because of osteoporosis. Flexion at the knees and hips may contribute to shortened stature. The limbs of an elderly person thus tend to look long in proportion to the trunk.

The alterations in discs and vertebrae contribute too to the kyphosis of aging and increase the anteroposterior diameter of the chest, especially in women.

With aging, skeletal muscles decrease in bulk and power, and ligaments lose some of their tensile strength. Range of motion diminishes, partly because of osteoarthritis.

THE HEALTH HISTORY

Common or Concerning Symptoms

- Low back pain
- Neck pain
- Monoarticular or polyarticular joint pain
- Inflammatory or infectious joint pain
- Joint pain with systemic features such as fever, chills, rash, anorexia, weight loss, weakness
- Joint pain with symptoms from other organ systems

Joint pain is a common complaint of patients seeking health care. The health history is especially important in guiding you to the correct assessment.

You may wish to begin with "Any pains in your back?" since *backache* is the most common and widespread disorder of the musculoskeletal system. Using your usual interviewing style, get a clear picture of the problem, especially its

See Table 15-1, Low Back Pain, p. 522.

location. Establish whether the pain is on midline, in the area of the vertebrae, or off the midline. If the pain radiates into the legs, ask about any associated numbness, tingling, or weakness.

Causes of midline back pain include musculoskeletal strain, vertebral collapse, disc herniation, or spinal cord metastases. Pain off the midline may arise from sacroiliitis, trochanteric bursitis, sciatica, or arthritis in the hips.

Neck pain is also common, especially after trauma. Approach it in the same manner. For both neck and back pain, be especially alert for symptoms such as weakness, loss of sensation, or loss of bladder or bowel function.

See Table 15-2, Pains in the Neck, p. 523.

Motor or sensory deficits, loss of bladder or bowel function in spinal cord compression at S2–S4

To pursue other musculoskeletal disorders, ask "Do you have any pains in your joints?" If yes, you will need to determine whether the pain is *localized or widespread, acute or chronic, inflammatory or noninflammatory*.

Joint pain may be localized, diffuse, or systemic. Ask the patient to *point to the pain*. If the joint pain is localized and involves only one joint, it is *monoarticular*. Pain originating in the small joints of the hands and feet is more sharply localized than that from the larger joints. Pain from the hip joint is especially deceptive. Although it is typically felt in the groin or buttock, it is sometimes felt in the anterior thigh or partly or solely in the knee.

Pain in one joint suggests trauma, monoarticular arthritis, possible tendinitis, or bursitis. Hip pain near the greater trochanter suggests *trochanteric bursitis.*

More diffuse joint pain may be *polyarticular*, involving several joints. Ask whether the pain involves one joint or several joints. If polyarticular, what is the pattern of involvement . . . migrating from joint to joint or steadily spreading from one joint to multiple joint involvement? Is the involvement symmetric, affecting similar joints on both sides of the body?

Migratory pattern of spread in rheumatic fever or gonococcal arthritis; progressive additive pattern with symmetric involvement typically in rheumatoid arthritis

Note that joint pain may also be *nonarticular*, involving bones, muscles, and tissues around the joint such as the tendons, bursae, or even overlying skin. Generalized "aches and pains" are called *myalgias* if in muscles and *arthralgias* if there is pain but no evidence of arthritis.

Problems in tissues around joints include inflammation of bursae (*bursitis*), tendons (*tendinitis*), or tendon sheaths (*tenosynovitis*); also *sprains* from stretching or tearing of ligaments

Assess the timing, quality, and severity of the joint symptoms. *Timing* is especially important. Did the pain or discomfort develop rapidly over the course of a few hours or insidiously over weeks or even months? Has the pain progressed slowly or fluctuated, with periods of improvement and worsening? How long has the pain lasted? What is it like over the course of a day? . . . In the morning? . . . As the day wears on?

Severe pain of rapid onset in a swollen joint in the absence of trauma seen in acute septic arthritis or gout. In children consider osteomyelitis in bone contiguous to a joint.

If more rapid in onset, how did the pain arise? Was there an acute injury or overuse from repetitive motion of the same part of the body? If the pain comes from trauma, what was the *mechanism of injury* or the series of events that caused the joint pain? Further, what aggravates or relieves the pain? What are the effects of exercise, rest, and treatment?

See Table 15-3, Patterns of Pain In and Around the Joints, pp. 524–525.

Try to determine if the problem is *inflammatory* or *noninflammatory*. Is there *tenderness, warmth,* or *redness*? These features are best assessed on examination, but patients can sometimes guide you to points of tenderness. Ask about systemic symptoms such as fever or chills.

Fever, chills, warmth, redness in septic arthritis; also consider gout or possible rheumatic fever

Additional symptoms can help you decide if the pain is *articular* in origin, such as *swelling, stiffness,* or *decreased range of motion.* Localize any *swelling* as accurately as possible. If *stiffness* is present, it may be difficult to assess because people use the term differently. In the context of musculoskeletal problems, stiffness refers to a perceived tightness or resistance to movement, the opposite of feeling limber. It is often associated with discomfort or pain. If the patient does not report stiffness spontaneously, ask about it and try to calculate its duration. Find out when the patient gets up in the morning and when the joints feel the most limber. Healthy people experience stiffness and muscular soreness after unusually strenuous muscular exertion; such symptoms tend to peak around the second day after exertion.

Pain, swelling, loss of active and passive motion, "locking," deformity in *articular joint pain;* loss of active but not passive motion, tenderness outside the joint, absence of deformity often in *nonarticular pain*

Stiffness and limited motion after inactivity, sometimes called *gelling,* in degenerative joint disease but usually lasts only a few minutes; stiffness lasting ≥30 minutes in rheumatoid arthritis and other inflammatory arthritides Stiffness also with *fibromyalgia* and *polymyalgia rheumatica (PMR)*

To assess *limitations of motion,* ask about changes in level of activity because of problems with the involved joint. When relevant, inquire specifically about the patient's ability to walk, stand, lean over, sit, sit up, rise from a sitting position, climb, pinch, grasp, turn a page, open a door handle or jar, and care for bodily needs such as combing hair, brushing teeth, eating, dressing, and bathing.

Finally, some joint problems have *systemic* features such as fever, chills, rash, anorexia, weight loss, and weakness.

Generalized symptoms are common in rheumatoid arthritis, *systemic lupus erythematosus (SLE), PMR,* and other inflammatory arthritides. High fever and chills suggest an infectious cause.

Other joint disorders may be linked to *organ systems outside the musculoskeletal system.* Symptoms elsewhere in the body can give important clues to these conditions. Be alert to such symptoms as:

- *Skin conditions*

  A butterfly rash on the cheeks — Systemic lupus erythematosus

  The scaly rash and pitted nails of psoriasis — Psoriatic arthritis

  A few papules, pustules, or vesicles on reddened bases, located on the distal extremities — Gonococcal arthritis

  An expanding erythematous patch early in an illness — Lyme disease

  Hives — Serum sickness, drug reaction

  Erosions or scale on the penis and crusted scaling papules on the soles and palms — Reiter's syndrome, which also includes arthritis, urethritis, and ureitis

The maculopapular rash of rubella — Arthritis of rubella

Clubbing of the fingernails (see p. 110) — Hypertrophic osteoarthropathy

- Red, burning, and itchy eyes (*conjunctivitis*) — Reiter's syndrome, Behçet's syndrome
- Preceding *sore throat* — Acute rheumatic fever or gonococcal arthritis
- *Diarrhea, abdominal pain, cramping* — Arthritis with ulcerative colitis, regional enteritis, scleroderma
- Symptoms of *urethritis* — Reiter's syndrome or possibly gonococcal arthritis
- Mental status change, facial or other weakness, stiff neck. — Lyme disease with central nervous system involvement

HEALTH PROMOTION AND COUNSELING

Important Topics for Health Promotion and Counseling

- Balanced nutrition, exercise, appropriate weight
- Lifting and the biomechanics of the back
- Risk factor screening and prevention of falls
- Counseling about prevention and treatment of osteoporosis

Maintaining the integrity of the musculoskeletal system brings many features of daily life into play—balanced nutrition, regular exercise, appropriate weight. As shown in this chapter, each joint has its specific vulnerabilities to trauma and wear. Care with lifting, avoidance of falls, household safety measures, and, for selected postmenopausal women, hormone replacement therapy help to protect and preserve well-functioning muscles and joints.

The habits of a healthy lifestyle convey direct benefit to the skeleton. Good nutrition supplies calcium needed for bone mineralization and bone density. Exercise appears to maintain and possibly increase bone mass, in addition to improving outlook and management of stress. Weight appropriate to height and body frame reduces excess mechanical wear on weight-bearing joints such as hips and knees. (For further discussion of these topics, see pp. 59–62.)

One of the most vulnerable parts of the skeleton is the low back, especially L5–S1, where the sacral vertebrae make a sharp posterior angle. More than 80% of the population experiences low back pain at least once in a lifetime. Usually symptoms are short lived, but there is a pattern of recurrence in 30%

to 60% of individuals when onset is work related. Exercises to strengthen the low back, especially in flexion and extension, are often recommended (although studies have not consistently demonstrated a reduction in sick days from work). Alternatively, general fitness exercises appear equally effective. Education on lifting strategies, posture, and the biomechanics of injury is prudent for patients doing repetitive lifting such as nurses, heavy-machinery operators, and construction workers.

Among elderly persons in the United States, falls exact a heavy toil in morbidity and mortality. They are the leading cause of nonfatal injuries and account for a dramatic rise in death rates after age 65, increasing from ~5/100,000 in the general population to ~10/100,000 between the ages of 65 and 74 to ~147/100,000 after age 85.* Approximately 5% of falls result in fractures, usually of the wrist, hip, pelvis, or femur. Risk factors are both cognitive and physiological, including unstable gait, imbalanced posture, reduced strength, cognitive loss as in dementia, deficits in vision and proprioception, and osteoporosis. Poor lighting, stairs, chairs at awkward heights, slippery or irregular surfaces, and ill-fitting shoes are environmental dangers that can often be corrected. Clinicians should work with patients and families to help modify such risks whenever possible. Medications affecting balance, especially benzodiazepines, vasodilators, and diuretics, should be scrutinized. Home health assessments have proven useful in reducing environmental hazards, as have exercise programs to improve patient balance and strength.

Finally, it is important to counsel selected postmenopausal women about hormone replacement therapy and osteoporosis, defined as bone density >2.5 standard deviations below normal bone mass in young women.† Bone density reflects the interaction between bone mass (highest in the second decade), new bone formation, and bone resorption. A 10% drop in bone mineral density, equivalent to one standard deviation, is associated with a 20% increase in risk of fracture. Most fractures in patients over age 45 are attributable to postmenopausal osteoporosis. The decline in bone mass begins in the third decade and then accelerates in early menopause, especially in the trabecular bone of the vertebrae. At highest risk are women of Caucasian origin, slender build, or prior history of bilateral oophorectomy before menopause.

A number of agents inhibit bone resorption—calcium, vitamin D, calcitonin, bisphosphonates, and estrogen—but consensus on several clinical management decisions has yet to emerge. Criteria are unclear for identifying those women at menopause at greatest risk of bone loss and fractures one to two decades later. In addition, guidelines for tailoring dosage of medication to level of bone density have yet to be determined. Estrogen therapy appears to prevent vertebral trabecular bone resorption, and is most beneficial when started near menopause. Lifetime use is recommended because bone loss

---

* U.S. Preventive Services Task Force: "Counseling to Prevent Household and Recreational Injuries," In Guide to Clinical Preventive Services. Baltimore, Williams & Wilkins, pp. 659–685, 1996.

† U.S. Preventive Services Task Force: In Guide to Clinical Preventive Services. Baltimore, Williams & Wilkins, pp. 509–516, 1996.

resumes once therapy is discontinued. Although hormone replacement protects against osteoporosis and possibly cardiovascular disease, use of estrogen must be weighed carefully in each patient against risk of breast cancer, endometrial cancer (risk is decreased by progesterone), and thrombosis. Cognitive, environmental, and other physiologic risk factors for falls and fractures should also be addressed.

Preview: Recording the Examination—The Musculoskeletal System

The examples below contain phrases appropriate for most write-ups. Unfamiliar terms are explained in the next section, *Techniques of Examination.* Note that use of the anatomic terms specific to the structure and function of individual joint problems makes your write-up of musculoskeletal findings more meaningful and informative.

"Good range of motion in all joints. No evidence of swelling or deformity."

OR

"Good range of motion in all joints. Hand with degenerative changes of Heberden's nodes at the distal interphalangeal joints, Bouchard's nodes at proximal interphalangeal joints. Mild pain with flexion, extension, and rotation of both hips. Good range of motion in the knees, with moderate crepitus; no effusion but boggy synovium and osteophytes along the tibiofemoral joint line bilaterally. Both feet with hallux valgus at the first metatarsophalangeal joints."

Suggests osteoarthritis

OR

"Right knee with moderate effusion and tenderness over medial meniscus along the joint line. Moderate laxity of anterior cruciate ligament (ACL) on anterior drawer test; posterior cruciate ligament (PCL) and medial and lateral collateral ligaments (MCL, LCL) intact—no posterior drawer sign or tenderness with varus or valgus stress. Patellar tendon intact—patient able to extend lower extremity. All other joints with good range of motion, no other deformity or swelling."

Suggests partial tear of medial meniscus and ACL, possibly from sports injury or trauma

TECHNIQUES OF EXAMINATION

Important Areas of Examination for Each of the Major Joints

- Inspection for joint symmetry, alignment, bony deformities
- Inspection and palpation of surrounding tissues for skin changes, nodules, muscle atrophy, crepitus
- Range of motion and maneuvers to test joint function and stability, integrity of ligaments, tendons, bursae, especially if pain or trauma
- Assessment of inflammation or arthritis, especially swelling, warmth, tenderness, redness

As you examine the musculoskeletal system, direct your attention to function as well as structure. During the interview you have evaluated the patient's ability to carry out normal activities of daily living. Keep these abilities in mind during your physical examination.

In your initial survey of the patient you have assessed general appearance, body proportions, and ease of movement. Now, as you apply techniques of examination to the musculoskeletal system, visualize the underlying anatomy and recall the key elements of the history—for example, the mechanism of injury if there is trauma, or the time course of symptoms and limitations in function in arthritis.

Your examination should be systematic. It should include inspection, palpation of bony landmarks as well as related joint and soft-tissue structures, assessment of range of motion, and *special maneuvers* to test specific movements. These steps are described for each of the major joints. Recall that the anatomic shape of each joint determines its range of motion. This range is greatest in synovial or ball-and-socket joints.

Remember the following clues to guide your examination.

- During inspection, it is especially important to note *symmetry* of involvement. Is there a symmetric change in joints on both sides of the body, or is the change only in one or two joints?

  Acute involvement of only one joint suggests trauma, septic arthritis, gout. Rheumatoid arthritis typically involves several joints, symmetrically distributed.

  Also note any *joint deformities* or *malalignment of bones*.

  Dupuytren's contracture (p. 531), bowlegs or knock-knees (p. 779)

- Use inspection and palpation to assess the *surrounding tissues*, noting skin changes, subcutaneous nodules, and muscle atrophy. Note any *crepitus*, an audible and/or palpable crunching during movement of tendons or ligaments over bone. This may occur in normal joints but is more significant when associated with symptoms or signs.

  Subcutaneous nodules in rheumatoid arthritis or rheumatic fever; effusions in trauma; crepitus over inflamed joints, in osteoarthritis, or inflamed tendon sheaths

- Testing range of motion and maneuvers (described for each joint) may demonstrate *limitations in range of motion* or increased mobility and joint instability from excess mobility of joint ligaments, called *ligamentous laxity.*

Decreased range of motion in arthritis, inflammation of tissues around a joint, fibrosis in or around a joint, or bony fixation (*ankylosis*). Ligamentous laxity of the ACL in knee trauma

- Finally, testing *muscle strength* may aid in the assessment of joint function (for these techniques, see Chap. 16).

Muscle atrophy or weakness in rheumatoid arthritis

Be especially alert to *signs of inflammation and arthritis.*

- *Swelling.* Palpable swelling may involve: (1) the synovial membrane, which can feel boggy or doughy; (2) effusion from excess synovial fluid within the joint space; or (3) soft-tissue structures such as bursae, tendons, and tendon sheaths.

Palpable bogginess or doughiness of the synovial membrane indicates synovitis, which is often accompanied by effusion. Palpable joint fluid in effusion, tenderness over the tendon sheaths in tendinitis

- *Warmth.* Use the backs of your fingers to compare the involved joint with its unaffected contralateral joint, or with nearby tissues if both joints are involved.

Arthritis, tendinitis, bursitis, osteomyelitis

- *Tenderness.* Try to identify the specific anatomic structure that is tender. Trauma may also cause tenderness.

Tenderness and warmth over a thickened synovium may suggest arthritis or infection.

- *Redness.* Redness of the overlying skin is the *least* common sign of inflammation near the joints.

Redness over a tender joint suggests septic or gouty arthritis, or possibly rheumatoid arthritis.

If the person has painful joints, move the person gently. Patients may move more comfortably by themselves. Let them show you how they manage. If joint trauma is present, consider an x-ray before attempting movement.

The detail needed for examining the musculoskeletal system may vary widely. This section presents examination techniques for both comprehensive and targeted assessment of joint function. Patients with extensive or severe musculoskeletal problems will require more time. A briefer survey for those without musculoskeletal symptoms is outlined in Chapter 3 (see p. 69).

The Temporomandibular Joint (TMJ)

INSPECTION AND PALPATION

Inspect the joint for swelling or redness. Swelling may appear as a rounded bulge about 1 inch anterior to the external auditory meatus.

Swelling, tenderness, and decreased range of motion suggest an inflamed joint.

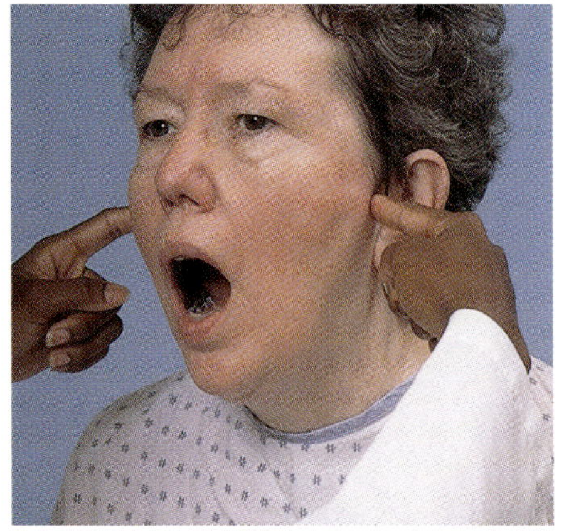

To locate and palpate the joint, place the tips of your index fingers just in front of the tragus of each ear and ask the patient to open his or her mouth. The fingertips should drop into the joint spaces as the mouth opens. Check for smooth range of motion; note any swelling or tenderness. Snapping or clicking may be felt or heard in normal people.

Dislocation of the TMJ may be seen in trauma.

Swelling, tenderness, and decreased range of motion suggest arthritis.

Palpable crepitus or clicking may occur in poor occlusion, meniscus injury, or synovial swelling from trauma.

RANGE OF MOTION AND MANEUVERS

The temporomandibular joint has glide and hinge motions in its upper and lower portions, respectively. Grinding or chewing consists primarily of gliding movements in the upper compartments.

Range of motion is three-fold: ask the patient to demonstrate opening and closing, protrusion and retraction (by jutting the jaw forward), and lateral, or side-to-side, motion. Normally as the mouth is opened wide, three fingers can be inserted between incisors. During normal protrusion of the jaw, the bottom teeth can be placed in front of the upper teeth.

The Shoulder

INSPECTION

Observe the shoulder and shoulder girdle anteriorly, and inspect the scapulae and related muscles posteriorly. Note any swelling, deformity, or muscle atrophy or fasciculations (fine tremors of the muscles).

Muscle atrophy points to lesions in the cervical nerves.

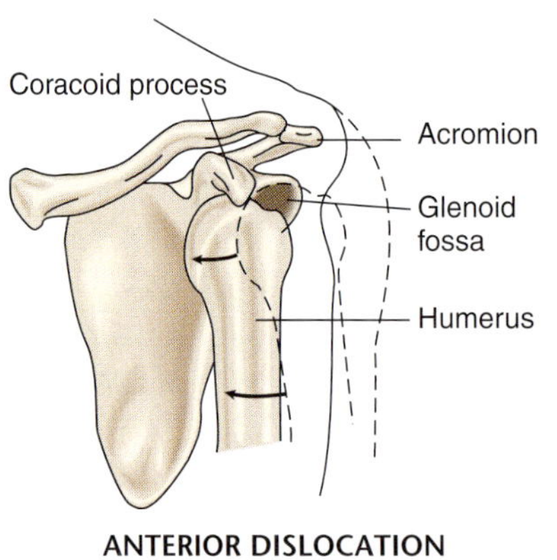

ANTERIOR DISLOCATION OF HUMERUS

Scoliosis may cause elevation of one shoulder. With anterior dislocation of the shoulder, the rounded lateral aspect of the shoulder appears flattened.

With posterior dislocation of the shoulder (relatively rare), the anterior aspect of the shoulder is flattened and the humeral head appears more prominent.

Look for swelling of the joint capsule anteriorly or a bulge in the subacromial bursa under the deltoid muscle. Survey the entire upper extremity for color change, skin alteration, or abnormal positioning.

A significant amount of synovial fluid is needed before the joint capsule appears distended.

PALPATION

If there is a history of shoulder pain, ask the patient to point to the painful area. The location of the pain may provide clues as to its origin:

See Table 15-4, Painful Shoulders (pp. 526–527).

- Top of the shoulder, radiating toward the neck—acromioclavicular joint
- Lateral aspect of the shoulder, radiating toward the deltoid insertion—rotator cuff
- Anterior shoulder—bicipital tendon

Now identify the bony landmarks of the shoulder and then palpate the area of pain. Locate the *acromion process* and press medially to locate the distal tip of the clavicle at the *acromioclavicular joint.* Palpate laterally and down a short step to the greater tubercle of the humerus, and then press medially to locate the *coracoid process* of the scapula. Next palpate the painful area and identify the structures involved.

RANGE OF MOTION AND MANEUVERS

The six motions of the shoulder girdle are flexion, extension, abduction, adduction, and internal and external rotation.

Inability to perform these movements may reflect weakness or soft-tissue changes from bursitis, capsulitis, rotator cuff tears or sprains, or tendinitis.

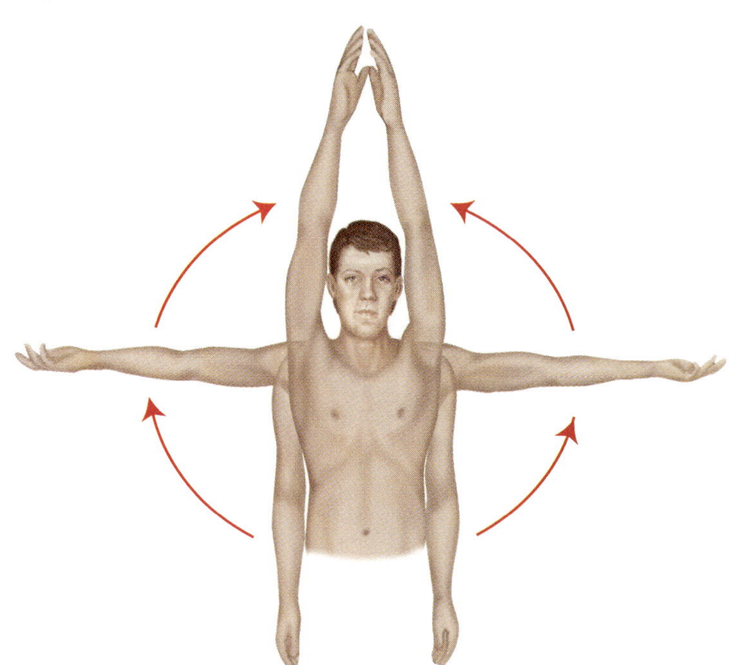

Watch for smooth, fluid movement as you stand in front of the patient and ask the patient to (1) raise (*abduct*) the arms to shoulder level (90°) with palms facing down (tests pure glenohumeral motion); (2) raise the arms to a vertical position above the head with the palms facing each other (tests scapulothoracic motion for 60°, and combined glenohumeral and scapulothoracic motion during adduction for the final 30°; (3) place both hands behind the neck, with elbows out to the side (tests *external rotation* and *abduction*); and (4) place both hands behind the small of the back (tests *internal rotation* and *adduction*). (Placing your hand on the shoulder during these movements allows you to detect any crepitus.)

The examination of the shoulder often requires selective evaluation of the acromioclavicular joint, the subacromial and subdeltoid bursae, the rotator cuff, the bicipital groove and tendon, and the articular capsule and synovial membrane of the glenohumeral joint. Techniques for examining these structures are described on following pages.

Structure	Techniques for Examining the Shoulder	Examples of Abnormalities
Acromioclavicular Joint	Palpate and compare both joints for swelling or tenderness. Adduct the patient's arm across the chest, sometimes called the *"crossover test."*	Localized tenderness or pain with adduction suggests inflammation or arthritis of the acromioclavicular joint. See Table 15-4, Painful Shoulders (pp. 526–527).
Subacromial and Subdeltoid Bursae	Passively extend the shoulder by lifting the elbow posteriorly. This exposes the bursae anterior to the acromion. Palpate carefully over the subacromial and subdeltoid bursae.	Localized tenderness arises from subacromial or subdeltoid bursitis, degenerative changes or calcific deposits in the rotator cuff. Swelling suggests a bursal tear with communication into the articular cavity.
Rotator Cuff	With the patient's arm hanging at the side, palpate the three "SITS" muscles that insert on the greater tuberosity of the humerus. (The fourth muscle, the subscapularis, inserts anteriorly and is not palpable.) ▪ **Supraspinatus**—directly under the acromion ▪ **Infraspinatus**—posterior to supraspinatus ▪ **Teres minor**—posterior and inferior to the supraspinatus Passively extend the shoulder by lifting the elbow posteriorly. This maneuver also moves the rotator cuff out from under the acromion. Palpate the rounded SITS muscle insertions near the greater tuberosity of the humerus.	Tenderness over the "SITS" muscle insertions and inability to lift the arm above shoulder level are seen in sprains, tears, and tendon rupture of the rotator cuff, most commonly the *supraspinatus*. See Table 15-4, Painful Shoulders (pp. 526–527).

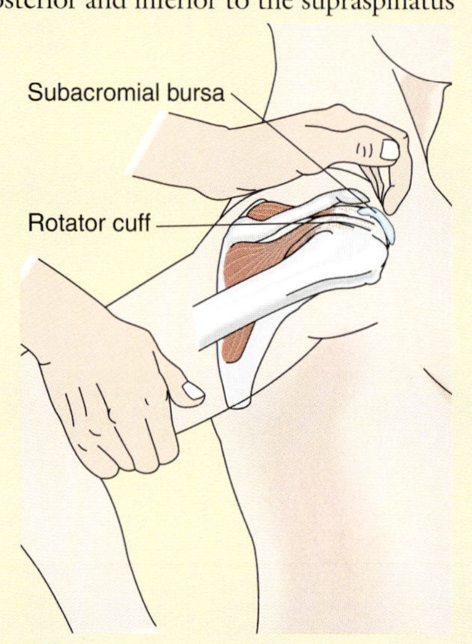

Structure	Techniques for Examining the Shoulder	Examples of Abnormalities
	Check the *"drop-arm" sign*. Ask the patient to fully abduct the arm to shoulder level (or up to 90°) and lower it slowly. (Note that abduction above shoulder level, from 90° to 120°, reflects action of the deltoid muscle.)	If the patient is unable to hold the arm fully abducted at shoulder level, the "drop arm" test is positive, indicating a tear in the rotator cuff.
Bicipital Groove and Tendon	Rotate the arm and forearm externally and locate the biceps muscle distally near the elbow. Track the muscle and its tendon proximally into the bicipital groove along the anterior aspect of the humerus. As you check for tendon tenderness, rolling the tendon under the fingertips may be helpful. **PALPATION OF THE BICIPITAL GROOVE AND TENDON**	See also Bicipital Tendinitis in Table 15-4 Painful Shoulders (pp. 526–527).
	Finally, hold the patient's elbow against the body with the forearm flexed at a right angle. Ask the patient to supinate the forearm against resistance.	Tenderness or pain against resistance occurs with tenosynovitis of the bicipital tendon sheath, tendinitis, or biceps tendon rupture.
Articular Capsule, Synovial Membrane, and Glenohumeral Joint	The fibrous articular capsule and the broad flat tendons of the rotator cuff are so closely associated that they must be examined simultaneously. Swelling in the capsule and synovial membrane is often best detected by looking down on the shoulder from above. Palpate the capsule and synovial membrane beneath the anterior and posterior acromion.	Tenderness and effusion suggest synovitis of the glenohumeral joint. If the margins of the capsule and synovial membrane are palpable, a moderate to large effusion is present. Minimal degrees of synovitis at the glenohumeral joint cannot be detected on palpation.

The following maneuvers test individual muscles of the shoulder girdle and help localize pain. Note that medial rotation against resistance also tests the pectoralis major, teres major, and latissimus dorsi. Additional evaluation of muscle strength, sensation over the neck, shoulder, and arm, and upper extremity reflexes is often warranted to complete your assessment (see pp. 573–575).

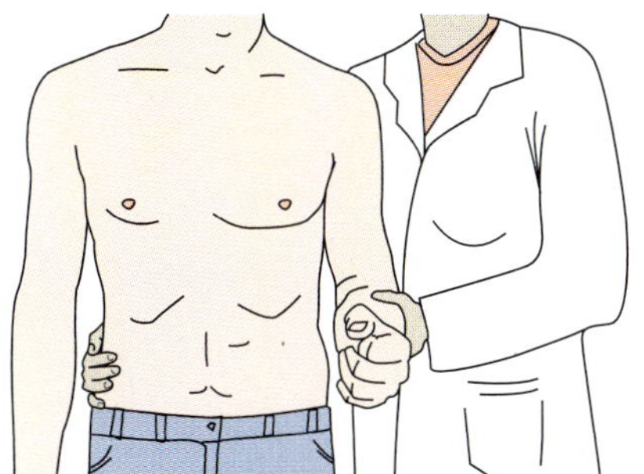

Supraspinatus: Patient abducts against resistance.

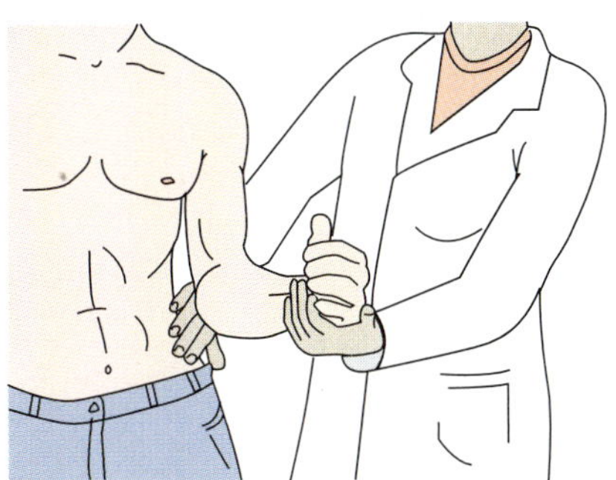

Subscapularis: Patient rotates forearm medially against resistance.

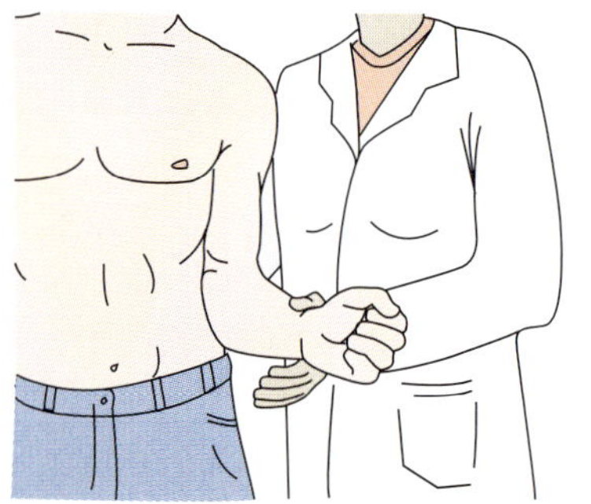

Infraspinatus, teres minor: Patient rotates forearm laterally against resistance.

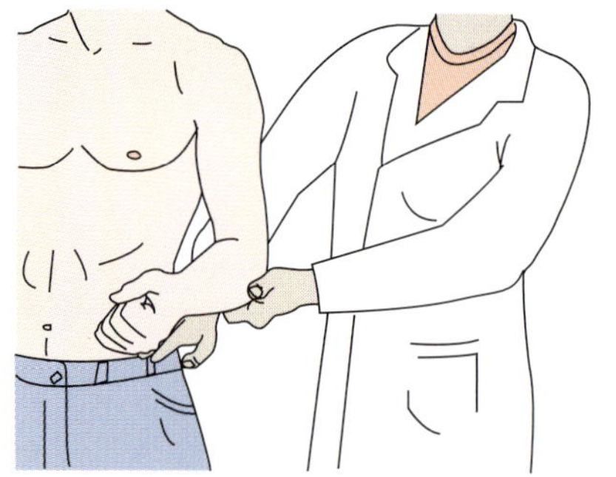

Thoracohumeral group: Patient adducts forearm against resistance.

The Elbow

INSPECTION AND PALPATION

Support the patient's forearm with your opposite hand so the elbow is flexed to about 70°. Identify the medial and lateral epicondyles and the olecranon process of the ulna. Inspect the contours of the elbow, including the extensor surface of the ulna and the olecranon process. Note any nodules or swelling.

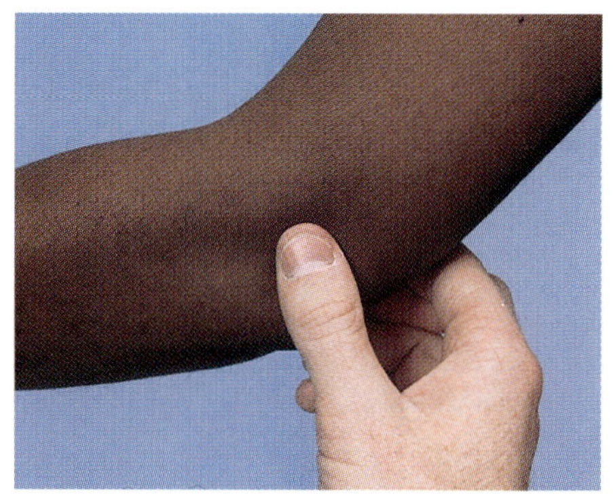

See Table 15-5, Swollen or Tender Elbows (p. 528).

Swelling over the olecranon process in olecranon bursitis; inflammation or synovial fluid in arthritis.

Palpate the olecranon process and press on the epicondyles for tenderness. Note any displacement of the olecranon.

Tenderness in *lateral epicondylitis* (tennis elbow) and in *medial epicondylitis* (pitcher's or golfer's elbow)

The olecranon is displaced posteriorly in *posterior dislocation of the elbow* and *supracondylar fracture.*

Palpate the grooves between the epicondyles and the olecranon, noting any tenderness, swelling, or thickening. The synovium is most accessible to examination between the olecranon and the epicondyles. (Normally neither synovium nor bursa is palpable.) The sensitive ulnar nerve can be felt posteriorly between the olecranon process and the medial epicondyle.

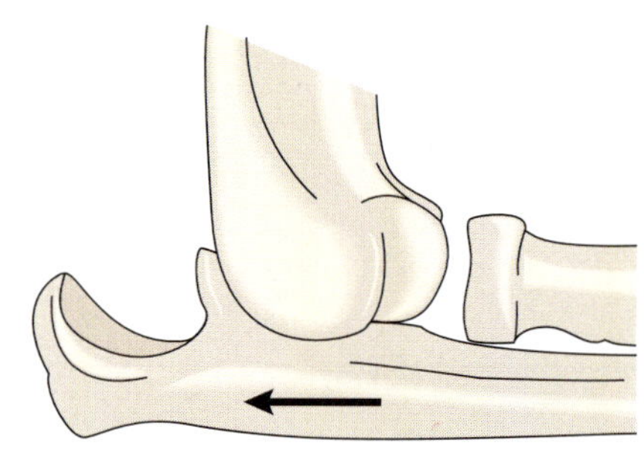

POSTERIOR DISLOCATION OF THE ELBOW

RANGE OF MOTION AND MANEUVERS

Range of motion includes *flexion* and *extension* at the elbow and *pronation* and *supination* of the forearm. To test flexion and extension, ask the patient to bend and straighten the elbow.

With the patient's arms at the sides and elbows flexed to minimize shoulder movement, ask the patient *supinate*, or turn up the palms, and to *pronate*, or turn down the palms.

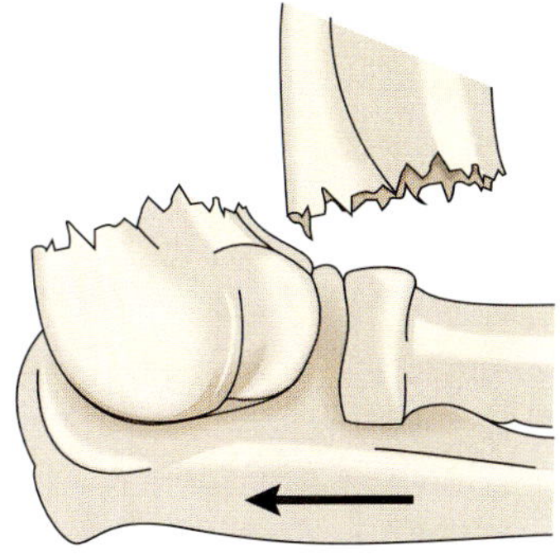

SUPRACONDYLAR FRACTURE OF THE ELBOW

The Wrist and Hand

INSPECTION

Observe the position of the hands in motion to see if movements are smooth and natural. At rest the fingers should be slightly flexed and aligned almost in parallel.

Guarded movement suggests injury. Poor finger alignment is seen in flexor tendon damage.

Inspect the palmar and dorsal surfaces of the wrist and hand carefully for swelling over the joints.

Diffuse swelling in arthritis or infection; localized swelling or ganglia from cystic enlargement. See Table 15-6, Swellings and Deformities of the Hands (pp. 529–531).

Note any deformities of the wrist, hand, or finger bones, as well as any angulation from radial or ulnar deviation.

In osteoarthritis, Heberden's nodes at the DIP joints, Bouchard's nodes at the PIP joints. In rheumatoid arthritis, symmetric deformity in the PIP, MCP, and wrist joints, with ulnar deviation

Observe the contours of the palm, namely the thenar and hypothenar eminences.

Thenar atrophy in median nerve compression from carpal tunnel syndrome; hypothenar atrophy in ulnar nerve compression.

Note any thickening of the flexor tendons or flexion contractures in the fingers.

Flexion contractures in the ring, 5th and 3rd fingers, or *Dupuytren's contractures*, arise from thickening of the palmar fascia (see p. 531).

PALPATION

At the wrist, palpate the distal radius and ulna on the lateral and medial surfaces. Palpate the groove of each wrist joint with your thumbs on the dorsum of the wrist, your fingers beneath it. Note any swelling, bogginess, or tenderness.

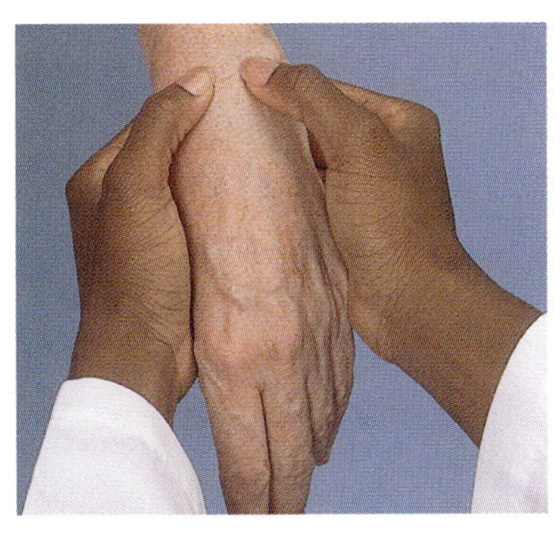

Tenderness over the distal radius in *Colles' fracture*. Any tenderness or bony step-offs are suspicious for fracture.

Swelling and/or tenderness suggests rheumatoid arthritis if bilateral and of several weeks' duration.

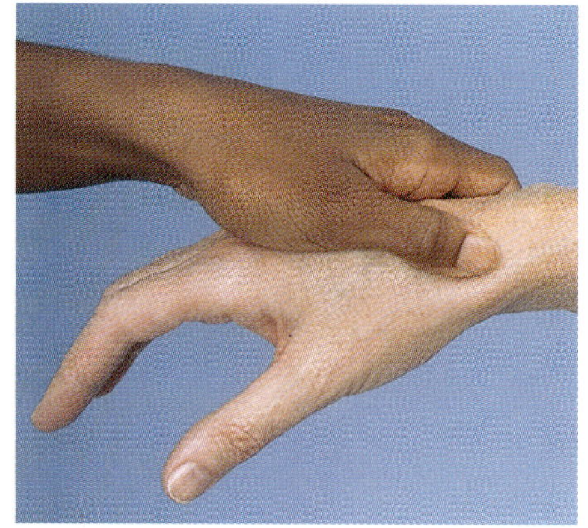

Palpate the *anatomic snuffbox,* a hollowed depression just distal to the radial styloid process formed by the abductor and extensor muscles of the thumb. The "snuffbox" becomes more visible with lateral extension of the thumb away from the hand.

Gonococcal infection may involve the wrist joint (arthritis) or the tendon sheaths at the wrist (gonococcal tenosynovitis).

Tenderness over the "snuffbox" suggests a scaphoid fracture.

Palpate the eight carpal bones lying distal to the wrist joint, and then each of the five metacarpals and the proximal, middle, and distal phalanges.

Palpate any other area where you suspect an abnormality.

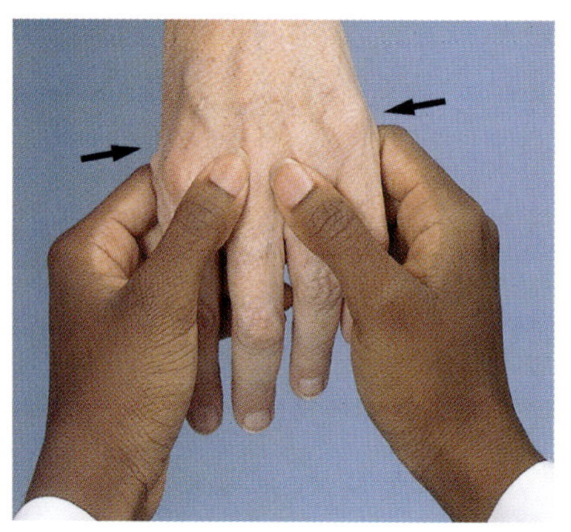

Compress the MCP joints by squeezing the hand from each side between the thumb and fingers. Alternatively, use your thumb to palpate each MCP joint just distal to and on each side of the knuckle as your index finger feels the head of the metacarpal in the palm. Note any swelling, bogginess, or tenderness.

Synovitis in the MCPs is painful with this pressure—a point to remember when shaking hands.

The MCPs are often boggy or tender in rheumatoid arthritis (but rarely involved in osteoarthritis).

Now examine the fingers. Palpate the medial and lateral aspects of each PIP joint between your thumb and index finger, again checking for swelling, bogginess, bony enlargement, or tenderness.

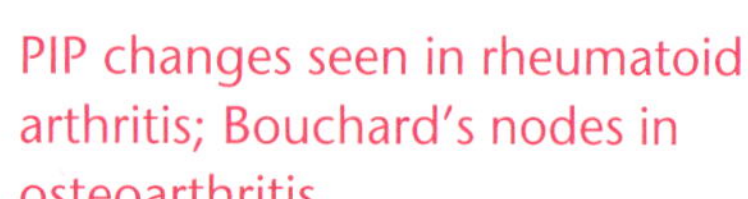

PIP changes seen in rheumatoid arthritis; Bouchard's nodes in osteoarthritis

Using the same techniques, examine the DIP joints.

Hard dorsolateral nodules on the DIP joints, or *Heberden's nodes,* common in osteoarthritis

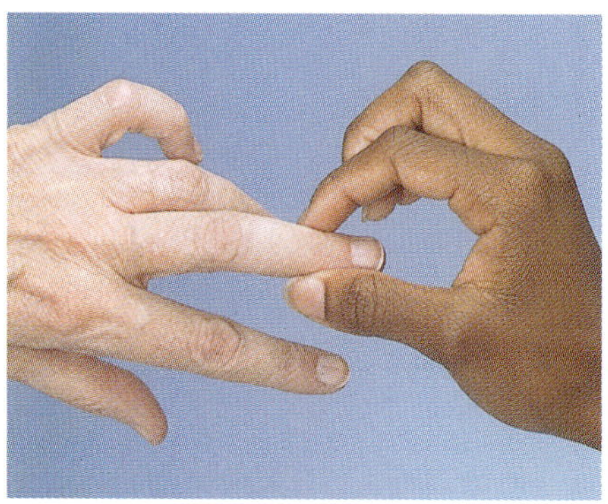

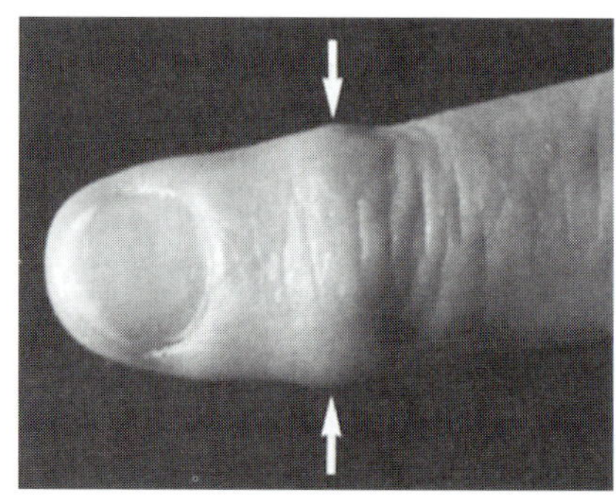

In any area of swelling or inflammation, palpate along the tendons inserting on the thumb and fingers.

Tenderness and swelling in *tenosynovitis,* or inflammation of the tendon sheaths. *De Quervain's tenosynovitis* over the extensor and abductor tendons of the thumb as they cross the radial styloid

RANGE OF MOTION AND MANEUVERS

Now assess range of motion for the wrists, fingers, and thumbs. At the *wrist,* test flexion, extension, and ulnar and radial deviation.

Conditions that impair range of motion include arthritis, tenosynovitis, Dupuytren's contracture. See Table 15-6, Swelling and Deformities of the Hands (pp. 529–531).

- *Flexion.* With the patient's forearm stabilized, place the wrist in extension and place your fingertips in the patient's palm. Ask the patient to flex the wrist against gravity, then against graded resistance.

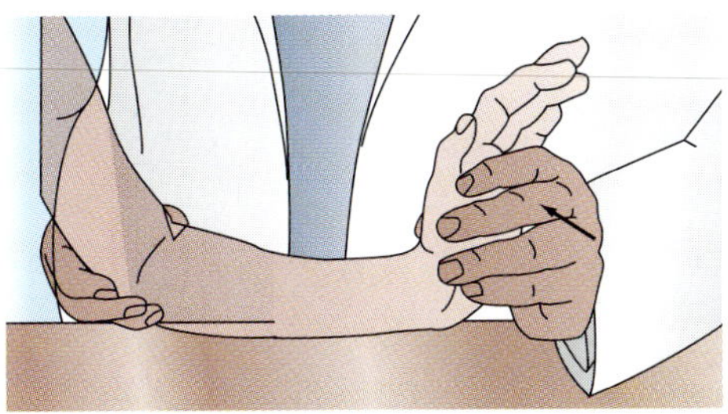

FLEXION

- *Extension.* With the patient's forearm stabilized, place the wrist in flexion and put your hand on the patient's dorsal metacarpals. Ask the patient to extend the wrist against gravity, then against graded resistance.

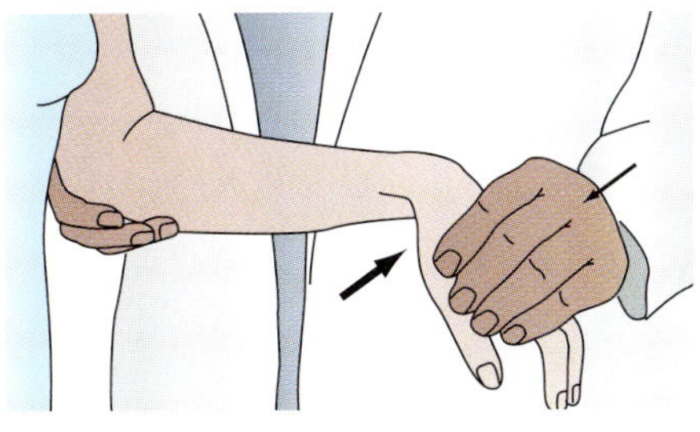

EXTENSION

- *Ulnar and radial deviation.* With palms down, ask the patient to move the wrists laterally and medially.

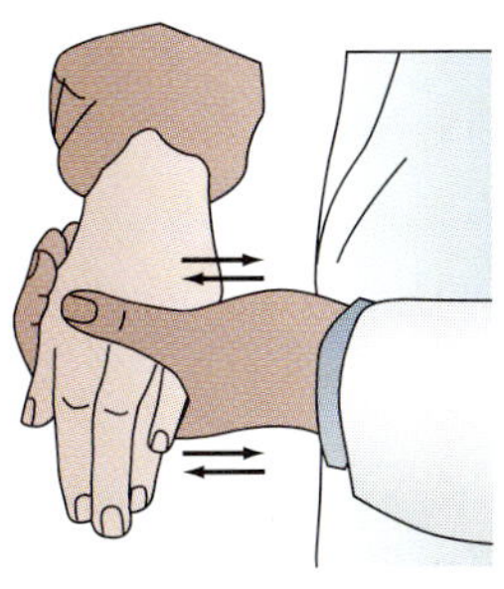

ULNAR AND RADIAL DEVIATION

Test flexion, extension, abduction, and adduction of the *fingers:*

- *Flexion and extension.* Ask the patient to make a tight fist with each hand, thumb across the knuckles, and then extend and spread the fingers. The fingers should close and open smoothly and easily. At the MCPs, the

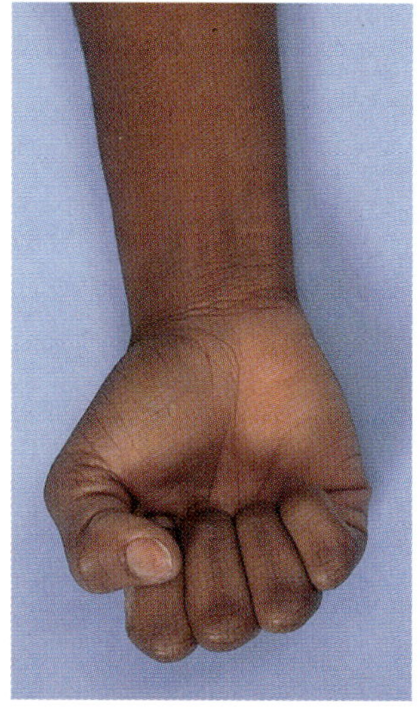

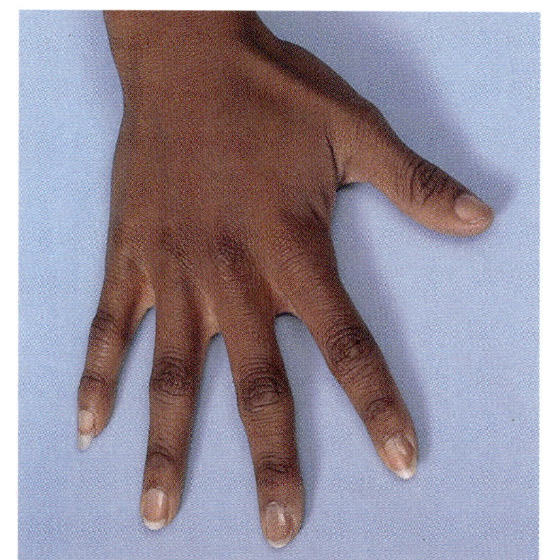

fingers may extend beyond the neutral position. Also test flexion and extension at the PIP and DIP joints.

- *Abduction and adduction.* Ask the patient to spread the fingers apart (abduction) and back together (adduction). Check for smooth, coordinated movement.

At the *thumb*, assess *flexion, extension, abduction, adduction,* and *opposition.* Ask the patient to move the thumb across the palm and touch the base of the 5th finger to test *flexion*, and then to move the thumb back across the palm and away from the fingers to test *extension.*

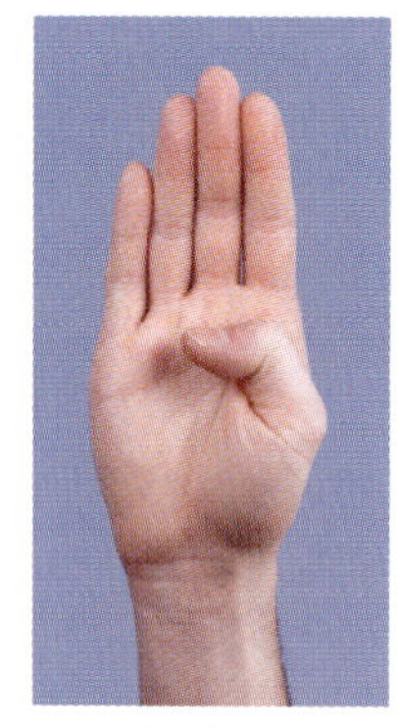

FLEXION

EXTENSION

Next, ask the patient to place the fingers and thumb in the neutral position with the palm up, then have the patient move the thumb anteriorly away from the palm to assess *abduction* and back down for *adduction.* To test *opposition,* or movements of the thumb across the palm, ask the patient to touch the thumb to each of the other fingertips.

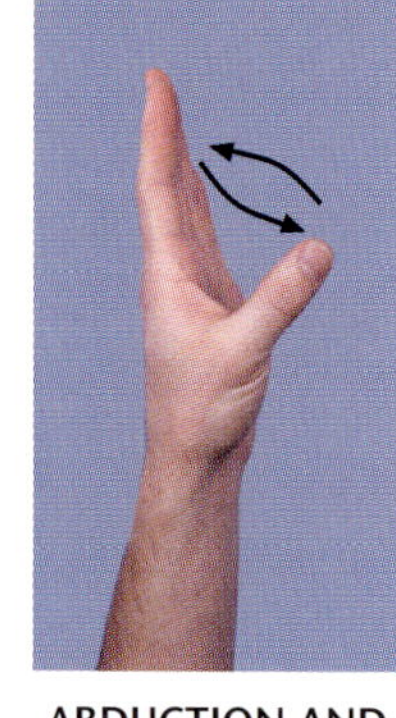

ABDUCTION AND ADDUCTION

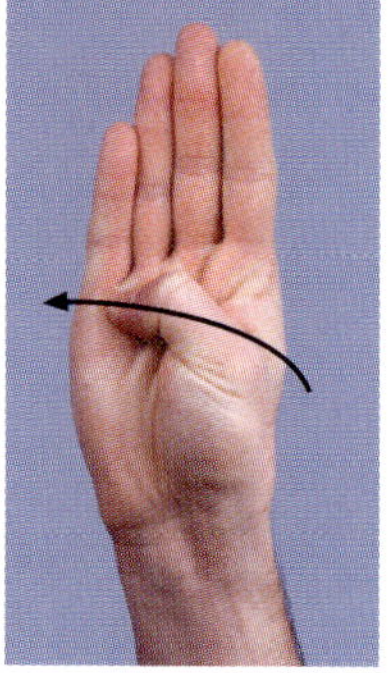

OPPOSITION

Test sensation in the fingers only along the lateral and medial surfaces to isolate any alterations in the digital nerves. Test median, ulnar, and radial nerve function by checking sensation as follows:

- Pulp of the index finger—median nerve
- Pulp of the 5th finger—ulnar nerve

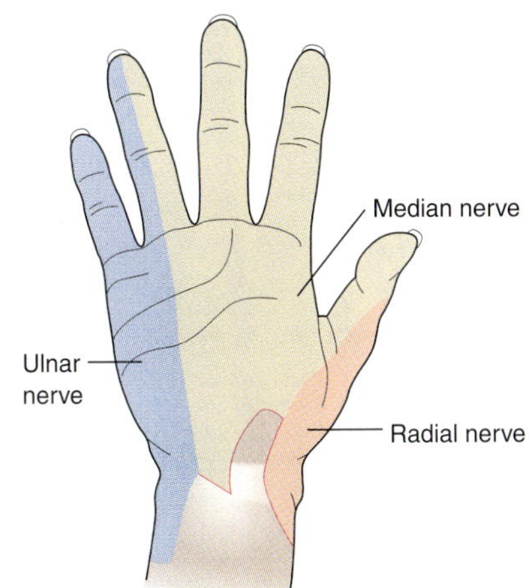

VOLAR SURFACE

- Dorsal web space of the thumb and index finger—radial nerve

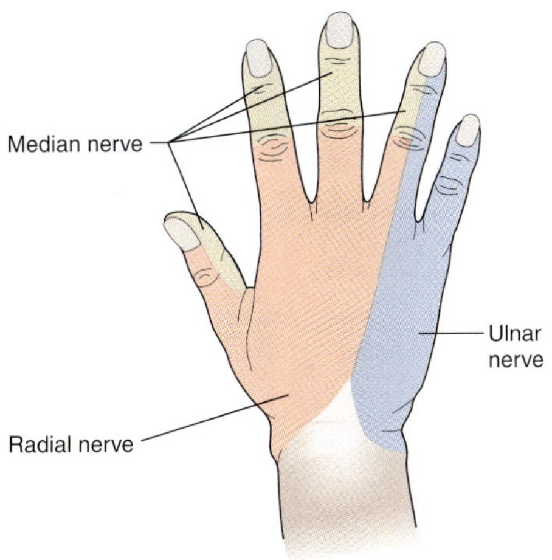

DORSAL SURFACE

The Spine

INSPECTION

Begin by observing the patient's posture, including the position of both neck and trunk, when entering the room.

Assess the patient for erect position of the head, smooth, coordinated neck movement, and ease of gait.

Neck stiffness signals arthritis, muscle strain, or other underlying pathology that should be pursued.

Drape or gown the patient to expose the entire back for complete inspection. If possible, the patient should be upright in the patient's natural standing position—with feet together and arms hanging at the sides. The head should be midline in the same plane as the sacrum, and the shoulders and pelvis should be level.

Lateral deviation and rotation of the head suggests *torticollis*, from contraction of the sternocleidomastoid muscle.

Inspect the patient from the side. Evaluate the spinal curvatures.

Inspection of the Spine

View of Patient	Focus of Inspection	Examples of Abnormalities
From the side	Cervical, thoracic, and lumbar curves.	Increased thoracic kyphosis occurs with aging. In children a correctable structural deformity should be pursued.
From behind	Upright spinal column (an imaginary line should fall from C7 through the gluteal cleft)	In *scoliosis,* there is lateral and rotatory curvature of the spine to bring the head back to midline. Scoliosis often becomes evident during adolescence, before symptoms appear.
	Alignment of the shoulders, the iliac crests, and the skin creases below the buttocks (gluteal folds)	*Unequal shoulder heights* seen in Sprengel's deformity of the scapula (from the attachment of an extra bone or band between the upper scapula and C7); in "winging" of the scapula (from loss of innervation of the serratus anterior muscle by the long thoracic nerve), and in contralateral weakness of the trapezius. *Unequal heights of the iliac crests,* or *pelvic tilt,* suggest unequal lengths of the legs and disappear when a block is placed under the short leg and foot. Scoliosis and hip abduction or adduction may also cause a pelvic tilt. "Listing" of the trunk to one side is seen with a herniated lumbar disc.
	Skin markings, tags, or masses	Birthmarks, port-wine stains, hairy patches, and lipomas often overlie bony defects such as *spina bifida.* Café-au-lait spots (discolored patches of skin), skin tags, and fibrous tumors in *neurofibromatosis*

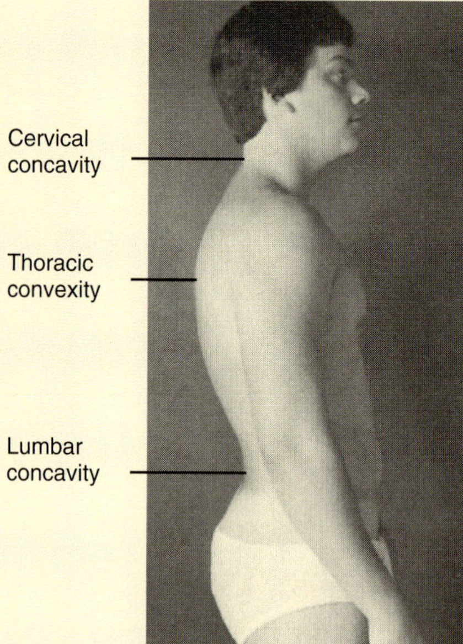

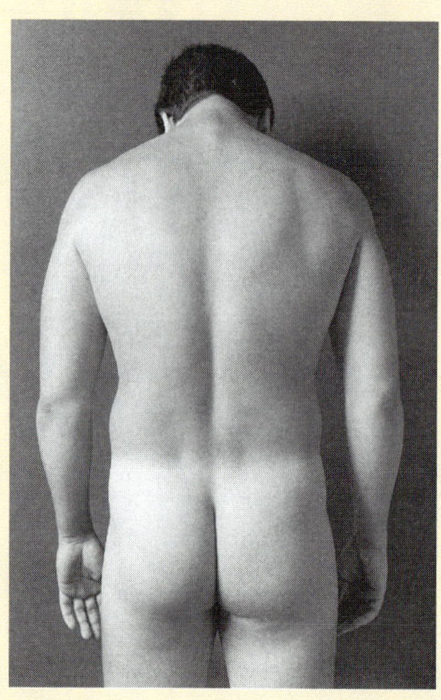

PALPATION

From a sitting or standing position, palpate the *spinous processes* of each vertebra with your thumb.

Tenderness suggests fracture or dislocation if preceded by trauma, underlying infection, or arthritis.

In the neck, also palpate the *facet joints* that lie between the cervical vertebrae about 1 inch lateral to the spinous processes of C2–C7. These joints lie deep to the trapezius muscle and may not be palpable unless the neck muscles are relaxed.

Tenderness occurs with arthritis, especially at the facet joints between C5 and C6.

In the lower lumbar area, check carefully for any vertebral "step-offs" to determine if one spinous process seems unusually prominent (or recessed) in relation to the one above it. Identify any tenderness.

Step-offs in *spondylolisthesis,* or forward slippage of one vertebra, which may compress the spinal cord. Vertebral tenderness is suspicious for fracture or infection.

Palpate over the sacroiliac joint, often identified by the dimple overlying the posterior superior iliac spine.

Tenderness over the sacroiliac joint pinpoints a common cause of low back pain. Ankylosing spondylitis may produce sacroiliac tenderness.

You may wish to percuss the spine for tenderness by thumping, but not too roughly, with the ulnar surface of your fist.

Pain on percussion may arise from osteoporosis, infection, or malignancy.

Inspect and palpate the paravertebral muscles for tenderness and spasm. Muscles in spasm feel firm and knotted and may be visible.

Spasm occurs in degenerative and inflammatory processes of muscles, prolonged contraction from abnormal posture, or anxiety.

With the hip flexed and the patient lying on the opposite side, palpate the sciatic nerve, the largest nerve in the body, consisting of nerve roots from L4, L5, S1, S2, and S3. The nerve lies midway between the greater trochanter and the ischial tuberosity as it leaves the pelvis through the sciatic notch.

Sciatic nerve tenderness suggests a herniated disc or mass lesion impinging on the contributing roots.

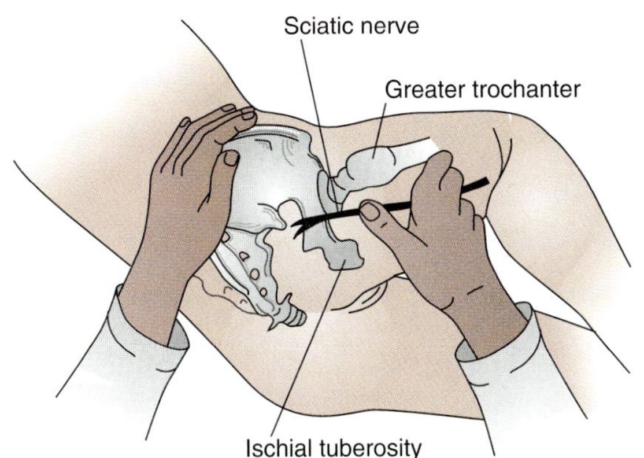

Palpate for tenderness in any other areas that are suggested by the patient's symptoms. Recall that low back pain warrants careful assessment for cord compression, the most serious cause of pain due to risk of paralysis of the affected limb.

Herniated intervertebral discs, most common between L5 and S1 or between L4 and L5, may produce tenderness of the spinous processes, the intervertebral joints, the paravertebral muscles, the sacrosciatic notch, and the sciatic nerve.

Rheumatoid arthritis may also cause tenderness of the intervertebral joints.

Remember that tenderness in the costovertebral angles may signify kidney infection rather than a musculoskeletal problem.

See Table 15-1, Low Back Pain (p. 522).

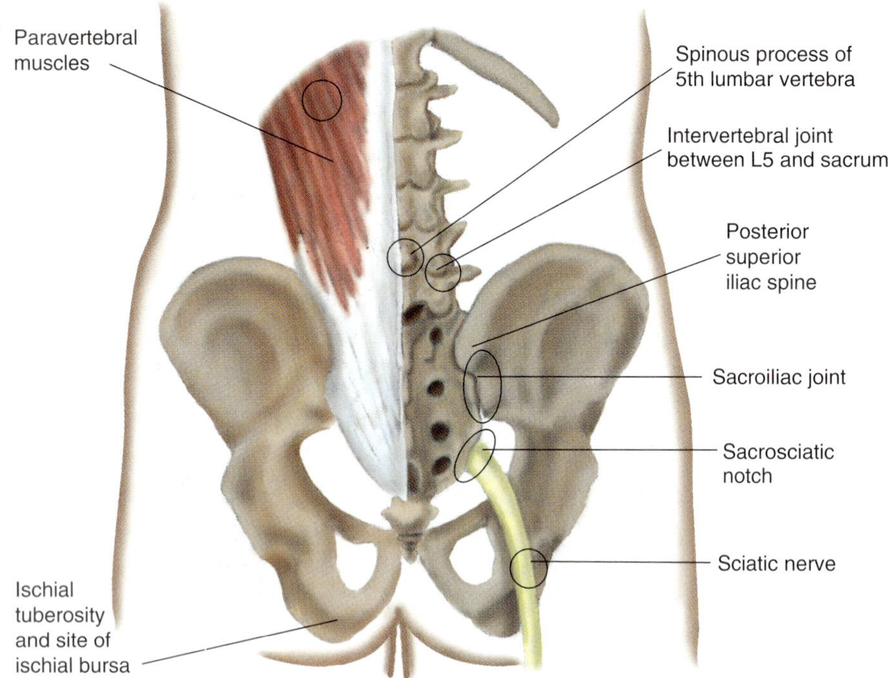

RANGE OF MOTION AND MANEUVERS

The neck is the most mobile portion of the spine, remarkable for its seven fragile vertebrae supporting the 10- to 15-pound ball of the head. Flexion and extension occur primarily between the skull and C1 (the atlas), rotation at C1–C2 (the axis), and lateral bending at C2–C7.

Limitations in range of motion may reflect stiffness from arthritis, pain from trauma, or muscle spasm such as *torticollis.*

Ask the patient to perform the following maneuvers, and check for smooth, coordinated motion:

- *Flexion.* Touch the chin to the chest.
- *Extension.* Look up at the ceiling.
- *Rotation.* Turn the head to each side, looking directly over the shoulder.
- *Lateral bending.* Tilt the head, touching each ear to the corresponding shoulder.

It is important to assess any complaints or findings of neck, shoulder, or arm pain or numbness for possible cervical cord or nerve root compression. See Table 15-2, Pains in the Neck (p. 523).

Tenderness, loss of sensation, or impaired movement warrants careful neurologic testing of the neck and upper extremities.

Now assess range of motion in the spinal column.

Tenderness at C1–C2 in rheumatoid arthritis suggests possible risk of subluxation and high cervical cord compression.

- *Flexion.* Ask the patient to bend forward to touch the toes (flexion). Note the smoothness and symmetry of movement, the range of motion, and the curve in the lumbar area. As flexion proceeds, the lumbar concavity should flatten out.

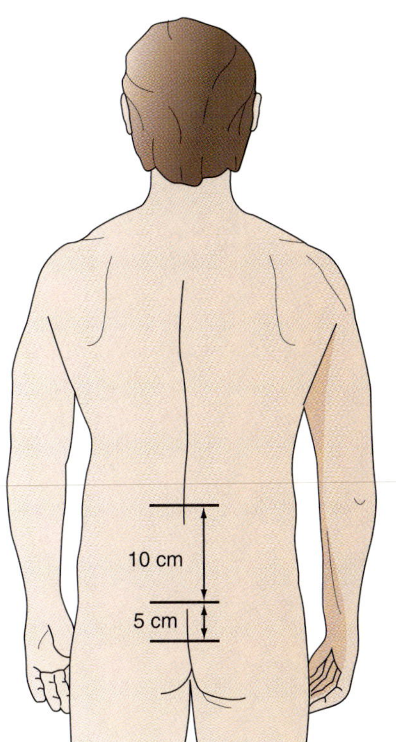

Deformity of the thorax on forward bending in scoliosis.

Persistence of lumbar lordosis suggests muscle spasm or ankylosing spondylitis.

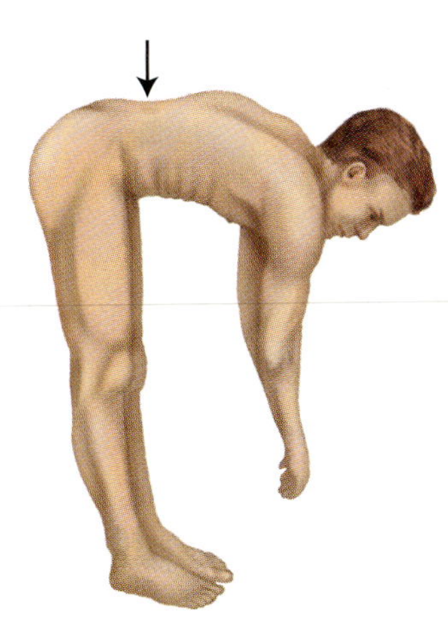

You may wish to measure the degree of flexion of the spine with the patient standing and bending forward. Mark the spine at the lumbosacral junction, then 10 cm above and 5 cm below this point. A 4-cm increase between the two upper marks is normally seen The distance between the lower two marks should be unchanged.

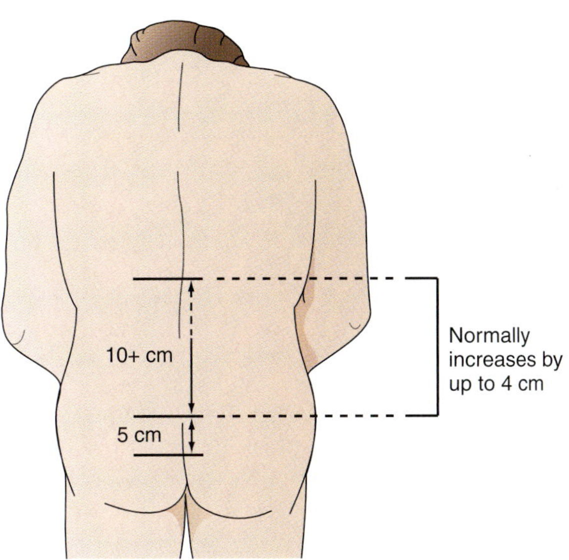

- *Extension.* Place your hand on the posterior superior iliac spine, with your fingers pointing toward the midline, and ask the patient to bend backward as far as possible.

Decreased spinal mobility in osteoarthritis and ankylosing spondylitis, among other conditions

- *Rotation.* Stabilize the pelvis by placing one hand on the patient's hip and the other on the opposite shoulder. Then rotate the trunk by pulling the shoulder and then the hip posteriorly. Repeat these maneuvers for the opposite side.

- *Lateral bending.* Again stabilize the pelvis by placing your hand on the patient's hip. Ask the patient to lean to both sides as far as possible.

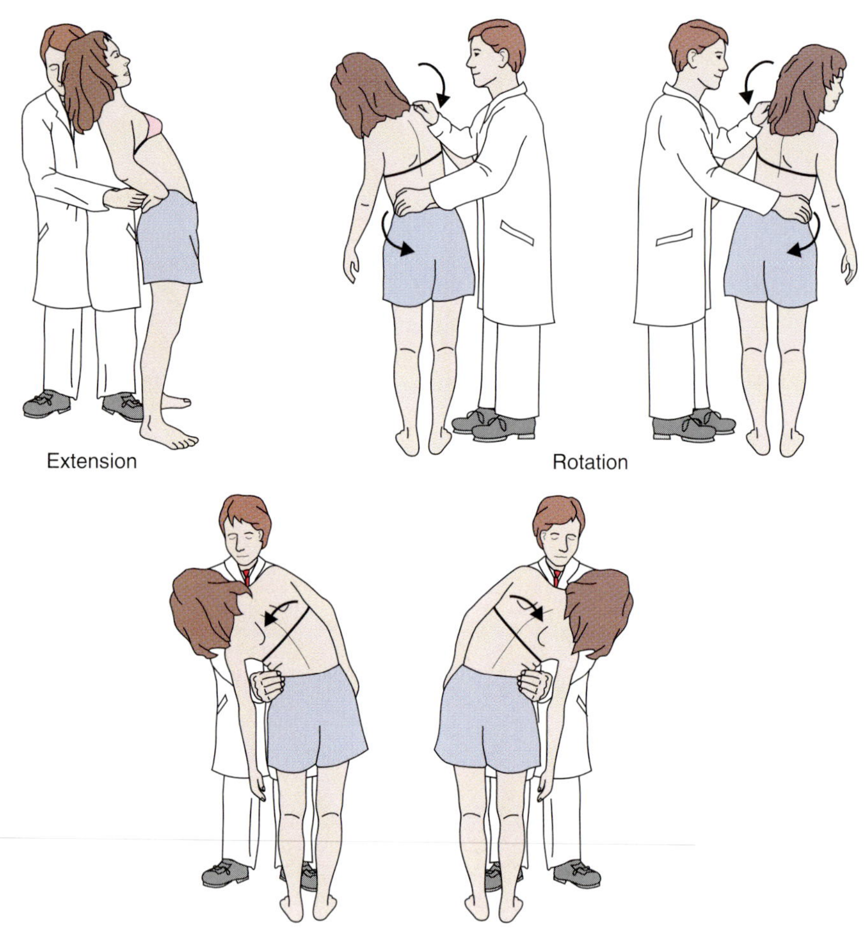

As with the neck, pain or tenderness with these maneuvers, particularly with radiation into the leg, warrants careful neurologic testing of the lower extremities.

Underlying cord or nerve root compression should be considered. Note that arthritis or infection in the hip, rectum, or pelvis may cause symptoms in the lumbar spine. See Table 15-1, Low Back Pain (p. 522).

The Hip

INSPECTION

Inspection of the hip begins with careful observation of the patient's gait on entering the room. Observe the two phases of gait:

- *Stance*—when the foot is on the ground and bears weight (60% of the walking cycle)

Most problems appear during the weight-bearing stance phase.

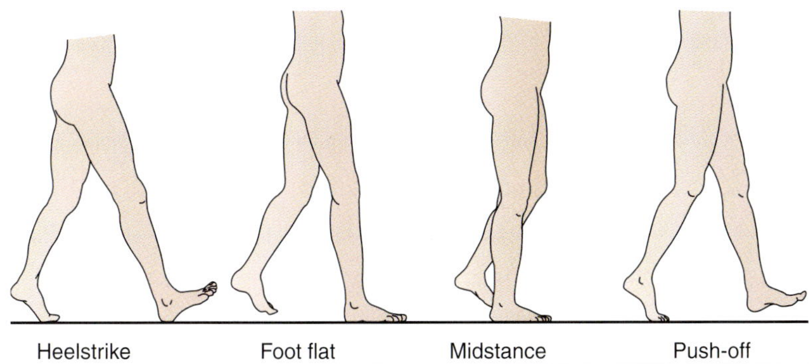

THE STANCE PHASE OF GAIT

- *Swing*—when the foot moves forward and does not bear weight (40% of the cycle)

Observe the gait for the width of the base, the shift of the pelvis, and flexion of the knee. The width of the base should be 2 to 4 inches from heel to heel. Normal gait has a smooth, continuous rhythm, achieved in part by contraction of the abductors of the weight-bearing limb. Abductor contraction stabilizes the pelvis and helps maintain balance, raising the opposite hip. The knee should be flexed throughout the stance phase, except when the heel strikes the ground to counteract motion at the ankle.

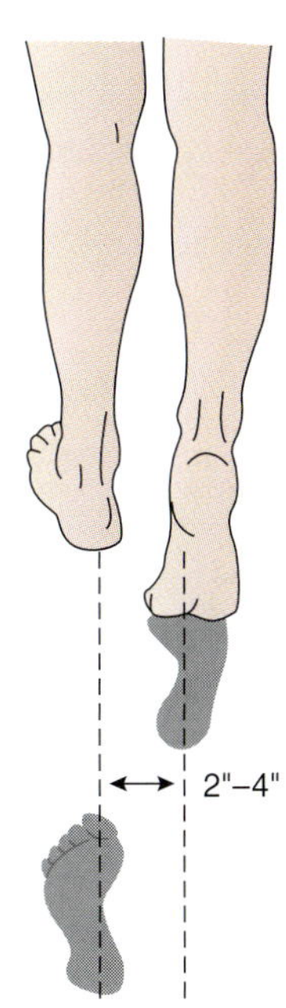

A wide base suggests cerebellar disease or foot problems.

Hip dislocation, arthritis, or abductor weakness can cause the pelvis to drop on the opposite side, producing a waddling gait.

Lack of knee flexion interrupts the smooth pattern of gait.

Observe the lumbar portion of the spine for slight lordosis and, with the patient supine, assess the length of the legs for symmetry. (To measure leg length, see Special Techniques, pp. 520–521).

Loss of lordosis may reflect paravertebral spasm; excess lordosis suggests a flexion deformity of the hip.

Changes in leg length are seen in abduction or adduction deformities and scoliosis. Leg shortening and external rotation suggest hip fracture.

Inspect the anterior and posterior surfaces of the hip for any areas of muscle atrophy or bruising.

PALPATION

Review the surface landmarks of the hip. On the *anterior surface* locate the *iliac crest*, the *iliac tubercle*, and the *anterior superior iliac spine*. On the *posterior surface* identify the *posterior superior iliac spine*, the *greater trochanter*, the *ischial tuberosity*, and the *sciatic nerve*.

With the patient supine, ask the patient to place the heel of the leg being examined on the opposite knee. Then palpate along the *inguinal ligament*, which extends from the anterior superior iliac spine to the pubic tubercle. The femoral nerve, artery, and vein bisect the overlying inguinal ligament; lymph nodes lie medially. The mnemonic **NAVEL** may help you remember the lateral-to-medial sequence of **N**erve—**A**rtery—**V**ein—**E**mpty space—**L**ymph node.

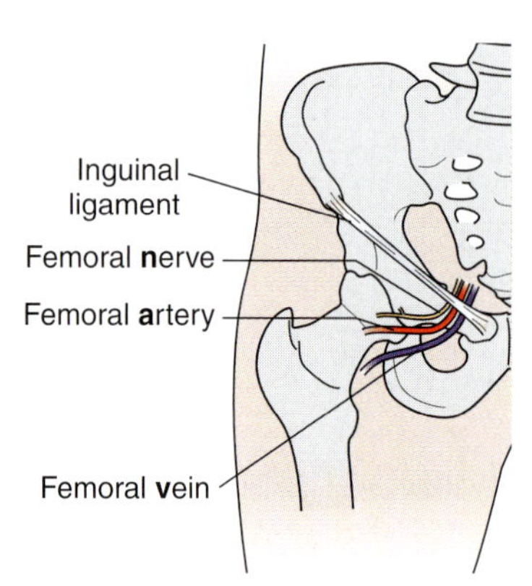

Bulges along the ligament may suggest an *inguinal hernia* or, on occasion, an *aneurysm.*

Enlarged lymph nodes suggest infection in the lower extremity or pelvis.

Tenderness may be due to synovitis of the hip joint, bursitis, or possibly psoas abscess.

If the hip is painful, palpate the *iliopectineal (iliopsoas) bursa,* below the inguinal ligament but on a deeper plane.

With the patient resting on one side and the hip flexed and internally rotated, palpate the *trochanteric bursa* lying over the greater trochanter. Normally, the *ischiogluteal bursa,* over the ischial tuberosity, is not palpable unless inflamed.

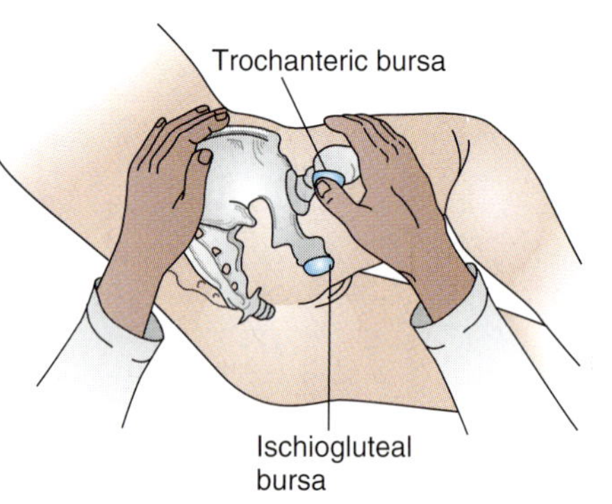

TROCHANTERIC BURSA

Swelling with tenderness suggests *trochanteric bursitis.* Tenderness without swelling on the posterolateral surface of the greater trochanter suggests localized tendinitis or muscle spasm from referred hip pain.

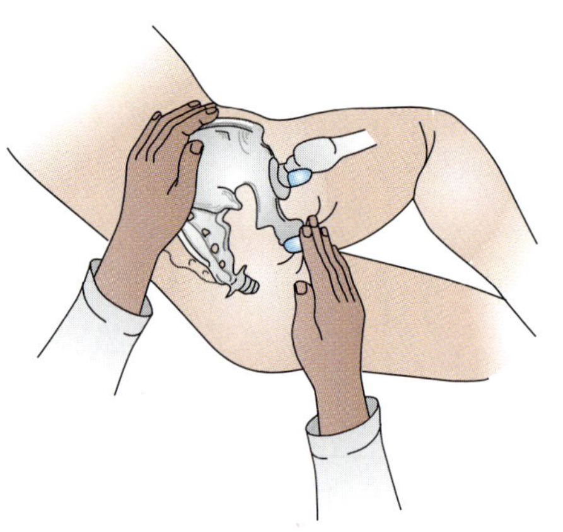

ISCHIOGLUTEAL BURSA

Tenderness and swelling in ischiogluteal bursitis or "weaver's bottom"—because of the adjacent sciatic nerve, this may mimic sciatica.

RANGE OF MOTION AND MANEUVERS

Motions at the hip include *flexion, extension, abduction, adduction*, and *rotation*. Note that the hip can flex farther when the knee is also flexed. Rotation at the hip while the knee is flexed may be confusing at first: when the lower leg swings laterally, the femur rotates internally. It is the motion of the femur at the hip joint that identifies these movements.

- *Flexion*. With the patient supine, place your hand under the patient's lumbar spine. Ask the patient to bend each knee in turn up to the chest and pull it firmly against the abdomen. Note when the back touches your hand, indicating normal flattening of the lumbar lordosis—further flexion must arise from the hip joint itself.

In flexion deformity of the hip, as the opposite hip is flexed (with the thigh against the chest), the affected hip does not allow full leg extension and the affected thigh appears flexed.

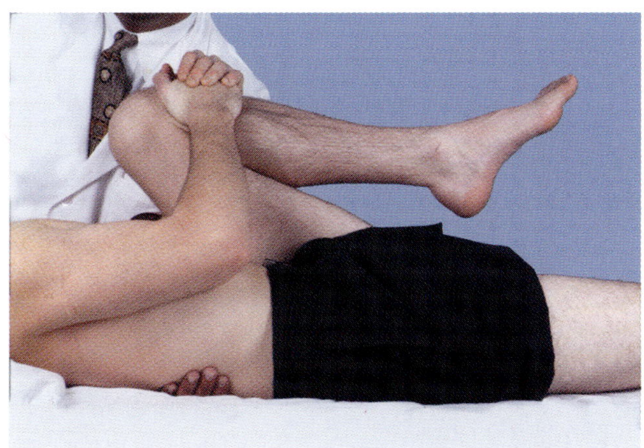

HIP FLEXION AND FLATTENING OF LUMBAR LORDOSIS

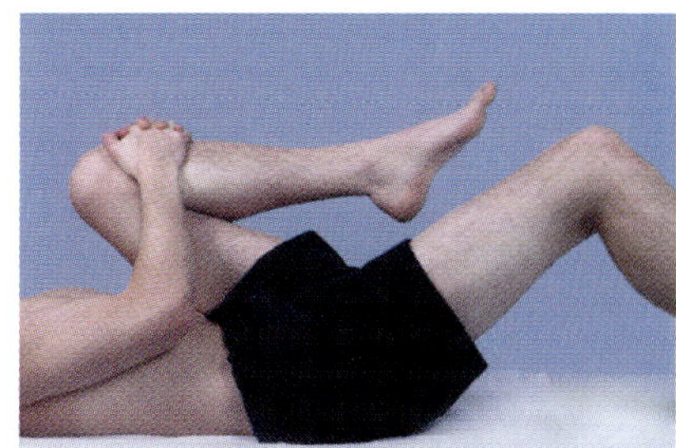

As the thigh is held against the abdomen, observe the degree of flexion at the hip and knee. Normally the anterior portion of the thigh can almost touch the chest wall. Note whether the opposite thigh remains fully extended, resting on the table.

Flexion deformity may be masked by an increase, rather than flattening, in lumbar lordosis and an anterior pelvic tilt.

- *Extension*. With the patient lying face down, extend the thigh toward you in a posterior direction.

- *Abduction*. Stabilize the pelvis by pressing down on the opposite anterior superior iliac spine with one hand. With the other hand, grasp the ankle and abduct the extended leg until you feel the iliac spine move. This movement marks the limit of hip abduction.

Restricted abduction is common in hip disease from osteoarthritis.

Alternatively, stand at the foot of the table, grasp both ankles, and spread them maximally, abducting both extended legs at the hips. This method

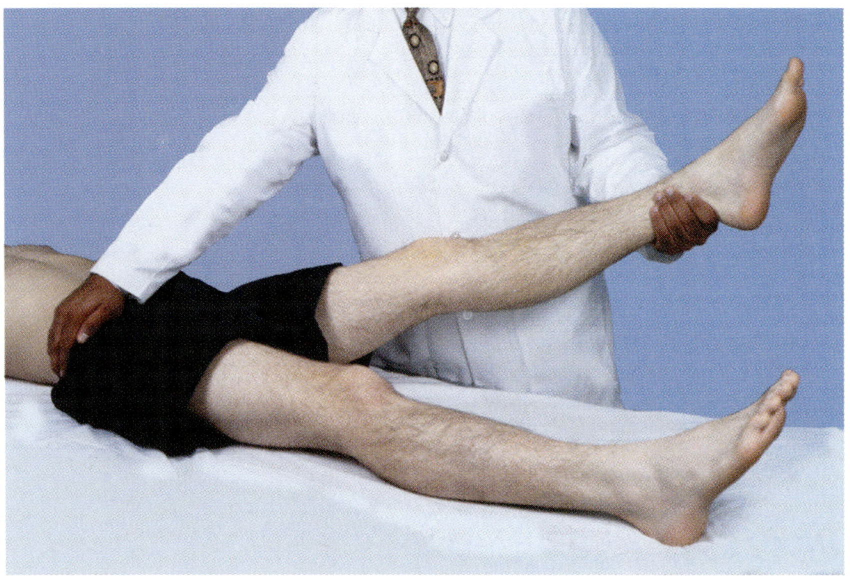

provides easy comparison of two sides when movements are restricted, but it is impractical when range of motion is full.

- *Adduction.* With the patient supine, stabilize the pelvis, hold one ankle, and move the leg medially across the body and over the opposite extremity.

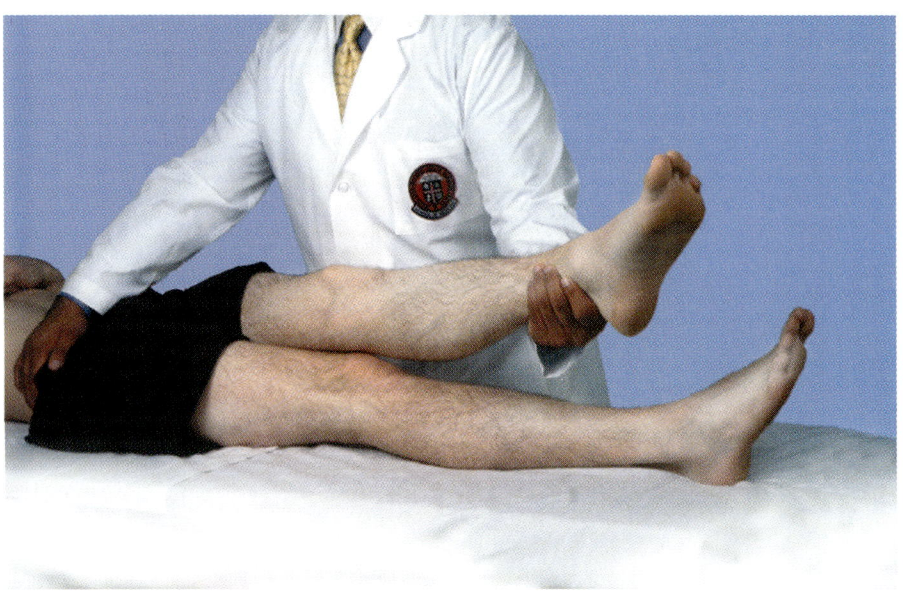

- *Rotation.* Flex the leg to 90° at hip and knee, stabilize the thigh with one hand, grasp the ankle with the other, and swing the lower leg—medially for external rotation at the hip and laterally for internal rotation.

Restriction of internal rotation is an especially sensitive indicator of hip disease such as arthritis. External rotation is also often restricted.

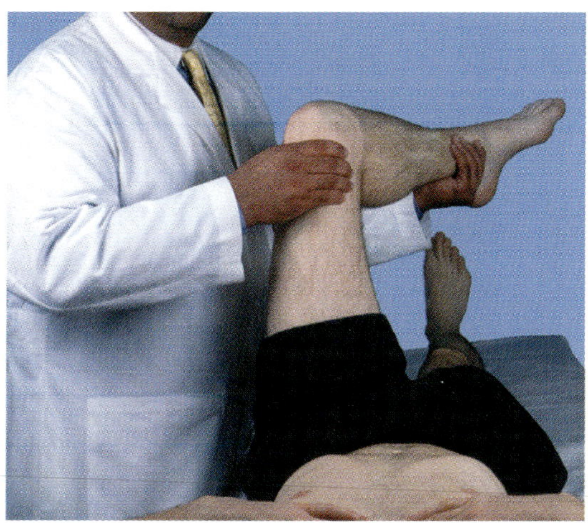

The Knee and Lower Leg

INSPECTION

Observe the gait for a smooth, rhythmic flow as the patient enters the room. The knee should be extended at heel strike and flexed at all other phases of swing and stance.

Stumbling or pushing the knee into extension with the hand during heel strike suggests quadriceps weakness.

Check the alignment and contours of the knees. Observe any atrophy of the quadriceps muscles.

Bowlegs (*genu varum*) and knock-knees (*genu valgum*) are common; flexion contracture (inability to extend fully) in limb paralysis

Look for loss of the normal hollows around the patella, a sign of swelling in the knee joint and suprapatellar pouch; note any other swelling in or around the knee.

Swelling over the patella suggests *prepatellar bursitis.* Swelling over the tibial tubercle suggests *infrapatellar* or, if more medial, *pes anserine bursitis.*

PALPATION

Ask the patient to sit on the edge of the examining table with the knees in flexion. In this position, bony landmarks are more visible and the muscles, tendons, and ligaments are more relaxed, making them easier to palpate.

First review the important bony landmarks of the knee. Facing the knee, place your thumbs in the soft-tissue depressions on either side of the *patellar tendon.* On the medial aspect, move your thumb upward and then downward and identify the *medial femoral condyle* and the upper margin of the *medial tibial plateau.* Trace the patellar tendon distally to the *tibial tubercle.* The *adductor tubercle* is posterior to the *medial femoral condyle.*

Lateral to the patellar tendon, identify the *lateral femoral condyle* and the *lateral tibial plateau*. The medial and lateral femoral *epicondyles* are lateral to the condyles with the knee in flexion. Locate the *patella*.

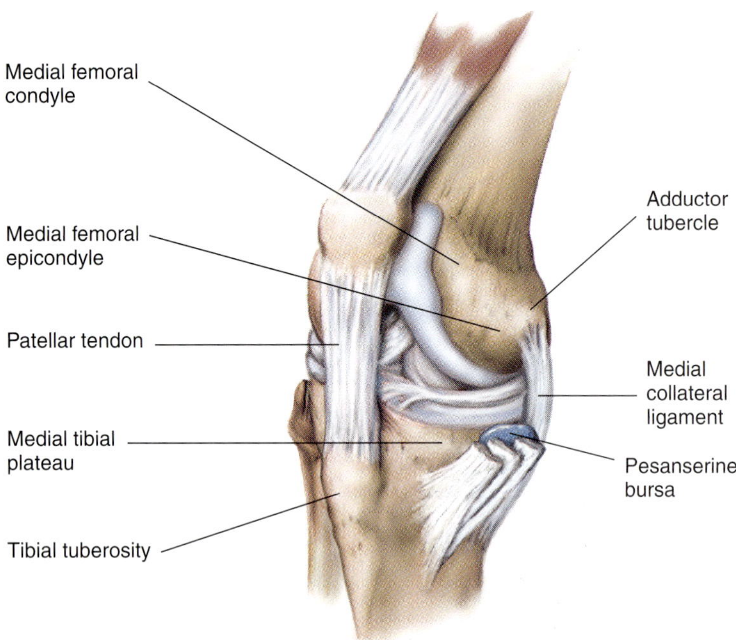

Palpate the ligaments, the borders of the menisci, and the bursae of the knee, paying special attention to any areas of tenderness. Pain is a common complaint in knee problems, and localizing the structure causing pain is important for accurate evaluation.

In the *patellofemoral compartment*, palpate the patellar tendon and ask the patient to extend the leg to make sure the tendon is intact.

Tenderness over the tendon or inability to extend the leg suggests a partial or complete tear of the patellar tendon.

With the patient supine and the knee extended, push the patella against the underlying femur. Ask the patient to tighten the quadriceps as the patella moves distally in the trochlear groove. Check for a smooth sliding motion (the *patellofemoral grinding test*).

Pain and crepitus suggest roughening of the patellar undersurface that articulates with the femur. Similar pain may occur with climbing stairs or getting up from a chair.

Pain with patellar movement during quadriceps contraction suggests *chondromalacia,* or degenerative patella.

Now assess the *medial and lateral compartments* of the *tibiofemoral joint*. Flex the patient's knee to about 90°. The patient's foot should rest on the examining table. Palpate the *medial collateral ligament* (MCL) between the medial femoral epicondyle and the femur; then palpate the cordlike *lateral*

MCL tenderness after injury is suspicious for an MCL tear. (The LCL is less subject to injury.)

collateral ligament (LCL) between the lateral femoral epicondyle and the fibular head.

Palpate the *medial and lateral menisci* along the medial and lateral joint lines. It is easier to palpate the medial meniscus if the tibia is internally rotated. Note any swelling or tenderness.

Tenderness from tears following injury are more common in the medial than in the lateral meniscus.

Note any irregular bony ridges along the joint margins.

Bony ridges along the joint margins may be felt in osteoarthritis.

Try to feel any thickening or swelling in the suprapatellar pouch and along the sides of the patella. Start 10 centimeters above the superior border of the patella (well above the pouch) and feel the soft tissues between your thumb and fingers. Move your hand distally in progressive steps, trying to identify the pouch. Continue your palpation along the sides of the patella. Note any tenderness or warmth greater than in the surrounding tissues.

Swelling above and adjacent to the patella suggests synovial thickening or effusion in the knee joint.

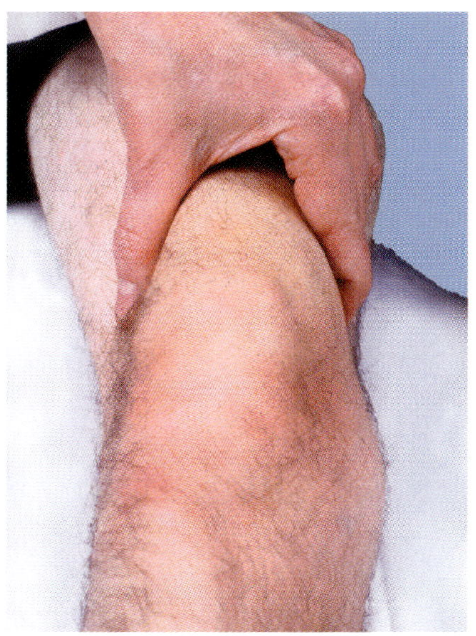

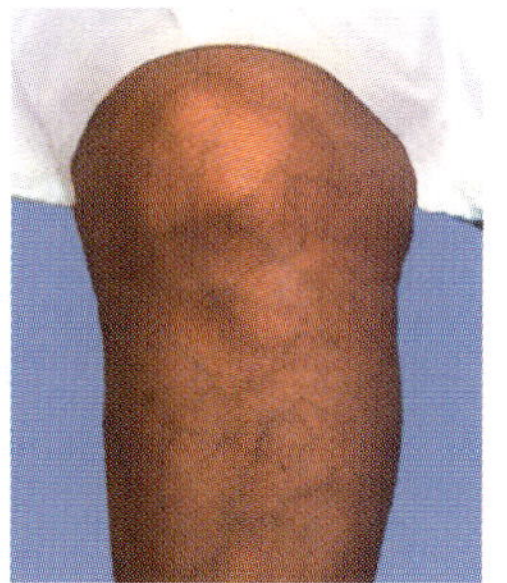

Thickening, bogginess, or warmth in these areas indicates synovitis or nontender effusions from osteoarthritis.

Check three other bursae for bogginess or swelling. Palpate the *prepatellar bursa,* and over the *anserine bursa* on the posteromedial side of the knee between the medial collateral ligament and the tendons inserting on the medial tibial and plateau. On the posterior surface, with the leg extended, check the medial aspect of the popliteal fossa.

Prepatellar bursitis ("housemaid's knee") from excessive kneeling. *Anserine bursitis* from running, valgus knee deformity, fibromyalgias, osteoarthritis. A *popliteal or "baker's" cyst* from distention of the gastrocnemius semimembranosus bursa

Three further tests will help you detect fluid in the knee joint.

- The *Bulge Sign* (*for minor effusions*). With the knee extended, place the left hand above the knee and apply pressure on the suprapatellar pouch, displacing or "milking" fluid downward. Stroke downward on the medial aspect of the knee and apply pressure to force fluid into the lateral area. Tap the knee just behind the lateral margin of the patella with the right hand.

A fluid wave or bulge on the medial side between the patella and the femur is considered a positive bulge sign consistent with an effusion.

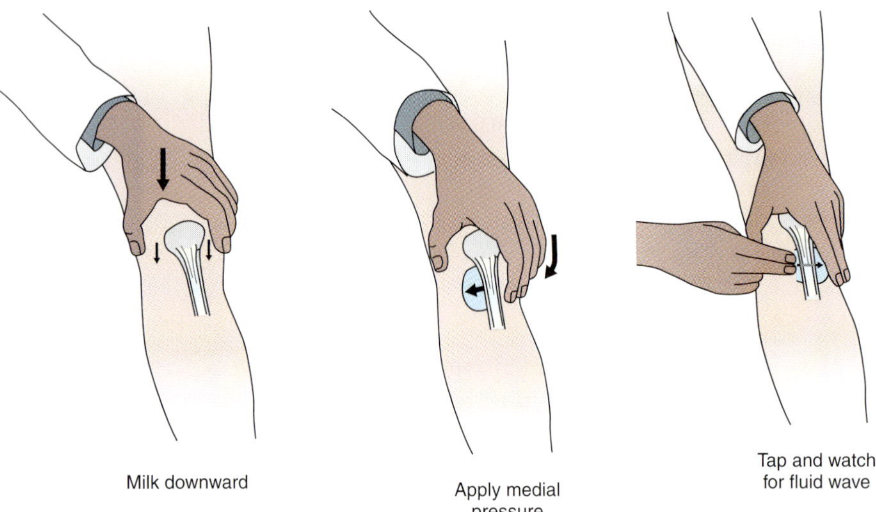

- The *Balloon Sign (for major effusions)*. Place the thumb and index finger of your right hand on each side of the patella; with the left hand, compress the suprapatellar pouch against the femur. Feel for fluid entering (or ballooning into) the spaces next to the patella under your right thumb and index finger.

When the knee joint contains a large effusion, suprapatellar compression ejects fluid into the spaces adjacent to the patella. A palpable fluid wave signifies a positive "balloon sign." A returning fluid wave into the suprapatellar pouch confirms an effusion.

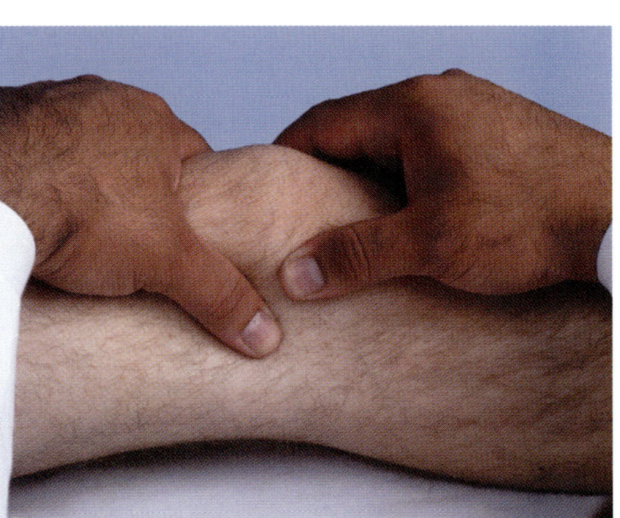

- *Ballotting the patella*. To assess large effusions, you can also compress the suprapatellar pouch and "ballotte" or push the patella sharply against the femur. Watch for fluid returning to the suprapatellar pouch.

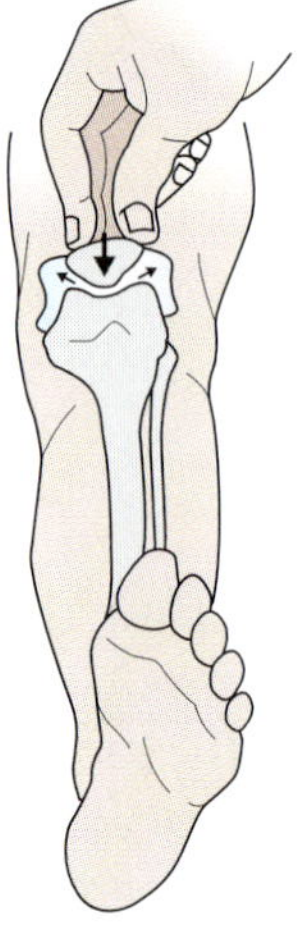

Palpable fluid returning into the pouch further confirms the presence of a large effusion.

A palpable patellar click with compression may also occur, but yields more false positives.

RANGE OF MOTION AND MANEUVERS

The principal movements of the knee are flexion, extension, and internal and external rotation. Ask the patient to flex and extend the knee while sitting. To check internal and external rotation, instruct the patient to rotate the foot medially and laterally. Knee flexion and extension can also be assessed by asking the patient to squat and stand up—provide support if needed to maintain balance.

You will often need to test ligamentous stability and integrity of the menisci, particularly when there is a history of trauma or palpable tenderness. Always examine both knees and compare findings.

Techniques for Examining the Knee

Structure	Maneuver	Examples of Abnormalities
Medial collateral ligament (MCL)	*Abduction Stress Test.* With the patient supine and the knee slightly flexed, move the thigh about 30° laterally to the side of the table. Place one hand against the lateral knee to stabilize the femur and the other hand around the medial ankle. Push medially against the knee and pull laterally at the ankle to open the knee joint on the medial side (*valgus stress*).	Pain or a gap in the medial joint line points to ligamentous laxity and a partial tear of the *medial collateral ligament.* Most injuries are on the medial side.
Lateral collateral ligament (LCL)	*Adduction Stress Test.* Now, with the thigh and knee in the same position, change your position so you can place one hand against the medial surface of the knee and the other around the lateral ankle. Push medially against the knee and pull laterally at the ankle to open the knee joint on the lateral side (*varus stress*).	Pain or a gap in the lateral joint line points to ligamentous laxity and a partial tear of the *lateral collateral ligament.*
Anterior cruciate ligament (ACL)	*Anterior Drawer Sign.* With the patient supine, hips flexed and knees flexed to 90° and feet flat on the table, cup your hands around the knee with the thumbs on the medial and lateral joint line and the fingers on the medial and lateral insertions of the hamstrings. Draw the tibia forward and observe if it slides forward (like a drawer) from under the femur. Compare the degree of forward movement with that of the opposite knee.	A few degrees of forward movement are normal if equally present on the opposite side. A forward jerk showing the contours of the upper tibia is a *positive anterior drawer sign* and suggests a tear of the *ACL.*

Techniques for Examining the Knee (Continued)

Structure	Maneuver	Examples of Abnormalities
	Lachman Test. Place the knee in 15° of flexion and external rotation. Grasp the distal femur with one hand and the upper tibia with the other. With the thumb of the tibial hand on the joint line, simultaneously move the tibia forward and the femur back. Estimate the degree of forward excursion.	Significant forward excursion indicates an ACL tear.
Posterior cruciate ligament (PCL)	*Posterior Drawer Sign.* Position the patient and place your hands in the positions described for the anterior drawer test. Push the tibia posteriorly and observe the degree of backward movement in the femur.	Isolated PCL tears are rare.
Medial meniscus and lateral meniscus	*McMurray Test.* If a click is felt or heard at the joint line during flexion and extension of the knee, or if tenderness is noted along the joint line, further assess the meniscus for a posterior tear.	
	With the patient supine, grasp the heel and flex the knee. Cup your other hand over the knee joint with fingers and thumb along the medial and lateral joint line. From the heel, rotate the lower leg internally and externally. Then push on the lateral side to apply a valgus stress on the medial side of the joint. At the same time, rotate the leg externally and slowly extend it.	A click or pop along the medial joint with valgus stress, external rotation, and leg extension suggests a probable tear of the posterior portion of the medial meniscus.

Palpate the *gastrocnemius* and *soleus muscles* on the posterior surface of the lower leg. Their common tendon, the Achilles, is palpable from about the lower third of the calf to its insertion on the calcaneus.

A defect in the muscles with tenderness and swelling in a *ruptured Achilles tendon;* tenderness and thickening of the tendon above the calcaneus, sometimes with a protuberant posterolateral bony process of the calcaneus in *Achilles tendinitis*

To test the integrity of the *Achilles tendon,* place the patient prone with the knee and ankle flexed at 90°, or alternatively, ask the patient to kneel on a chair. Squeeze the calf and watch for plantar flexion at the ankle.

Absence of plantar flexion is a positive test indicating rupture of the Achilles tendon. Sudden severe pain "like a gunshot wound," an ecchymosis from the calf into the heel, and a flat-footed gait with absence of "toe-off" may also be present.

The Ankle and Foot

INSPECTION

Observe all surfaces of the ankles and feet, noting any deformities, nodules, or swellings, and any calluses or corns.

See Table 15-7, Abnormalities of the Feet and Toes (pp. 532–533).

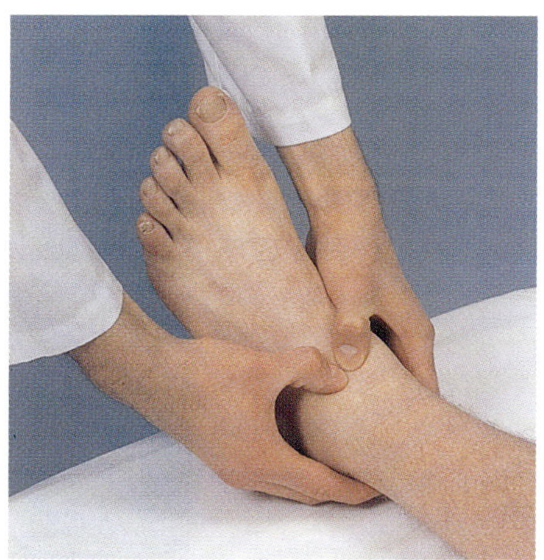

PALPATION

With your thumbs, palpate the anterior aspect of each *ankle joint,* noting any bogginess, swelling, or tenderness.

Localized tenderness in arthritis, ligamentous injury, or infection of the ankle

Feel along the *Achilles tendon* for nodules and tenderness.

Rheumatoid nodules; tenderness in Achilles tendinitis, bursitis, or partial tear from trauma

Palpate the heel, especially the posterior and inferior calcaneus, and the plantar fascia for tenderness.

Bone spurs may be present on the calcaneus; pain over the plantar fascia suggests *plantar fasciitis.*

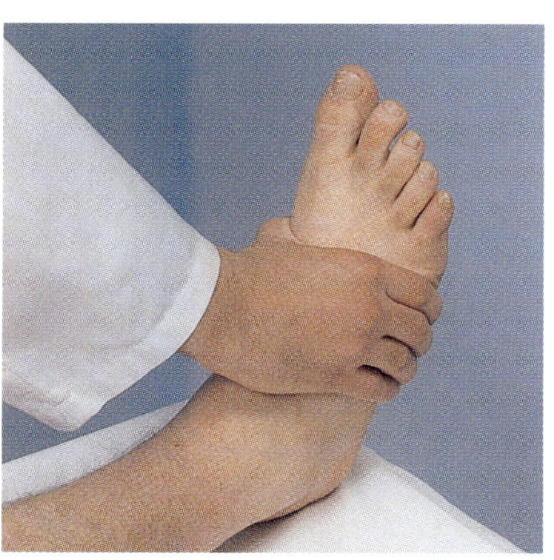

Palpate the *metatarsophalangeal joints* for tenderness. Compress the forefoot between the thumb and fingers. Exert pressure just proximal to the heads of the 1st and 5th metatarsals.

Tenderness on compression is an early sign of rheumatoid arthritis. Acute inflammation of the first metatarsophalangeal joint is associated with gout.

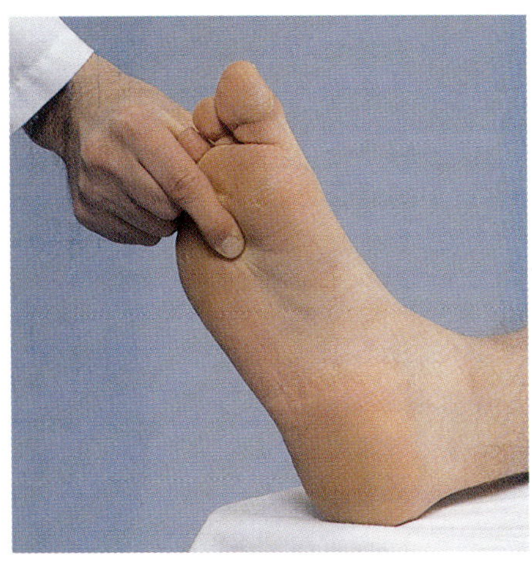

Palpate the heads of the five metatarsals and the grooves between them with your thumb and index finger. Place your thumb on the dorsum of the foot and your index finger on the plantar surface.

Pain and tenderness, called *metatarsalgia,* seen in trauma, arthritis, vascular compromise

RANGE OF MOTION AND MANEUVERS

Range of motion at the ankle includes *flexion* and *extension at the ankle (tibiotalar) joint* and, *in the foot, inversion* and *eversion* at the subtalar and transverse tarsal joints.

- *The Ankle (Tibiotalar) Joint.* Dorsiflex and plantar flex the foot at the ankle.

Pain during movements of the ankle and the foot helps to localize possible arthritis.

- *The Subtalar (Talocalcaneal) Joint.* Stabilize the ankle with one hand, grasp the heel with the other, and invert and evert the foot.

An arthritic joint is frequently painful when moved in any direction, while a ligamentous sprain produces maximal pain when the ligament is stretched. For example, in a common form of sprained ankle, inversion and plantar flexion of the foot cause pain, while eversion and plantar flexion are relatively pain free.

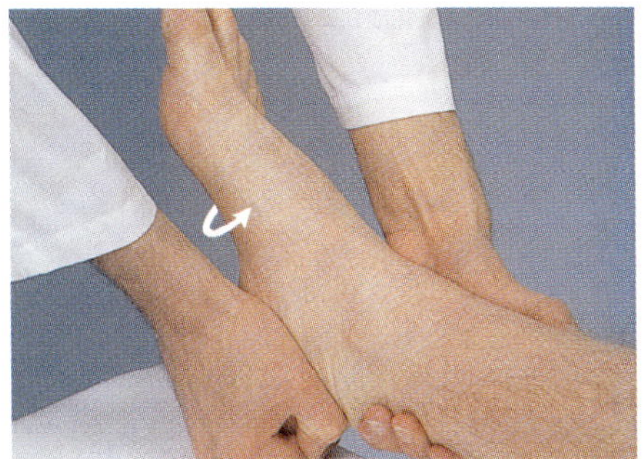

INVERSION

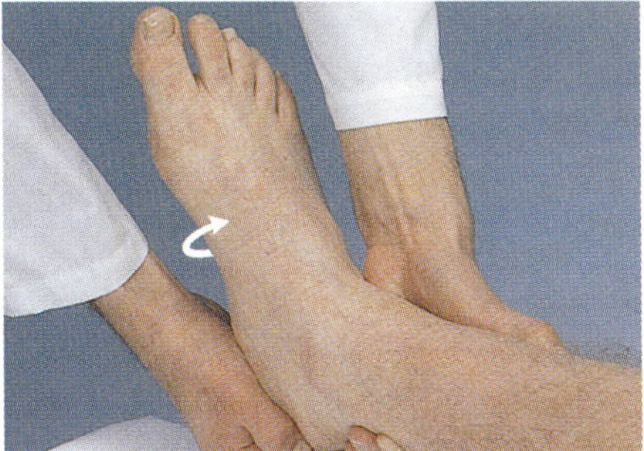

EVERSION

- *The Transverse Tarsal Joint.* Stabilize the heel and invert and evert the forefoot.

- *For the Metatarsophalangeal joints,* flex the toes in relation to the feet.

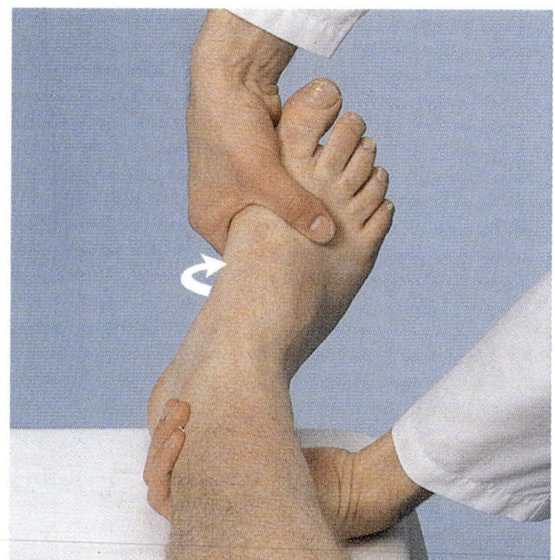
INVERSION

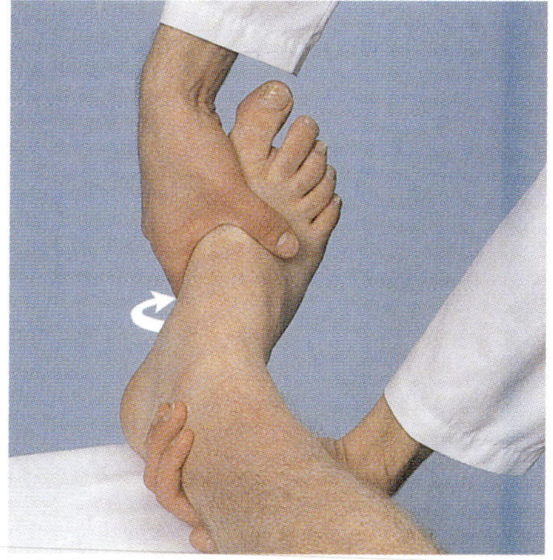
EVERSION

Special Techniques

For the Carpal Tunnel Syndrome. Pain and numbness on the ventral surface of the first three digits of the hand (but not in the palm), especially at night, suggest median nerve compression in the carpal tunnel, which lies between the carpal bones dorsally and a ventral band of more superficial fascia, the *flexor retinaculum*.

Onset often related to repetitive motion with wrists flexed (e.g., keyboard use, mail-sorting), pregnancy, rheumatoid arthritis, diabetes, hypothyroidism

Appropriate symptoms and objective loss of sensation on the ventral surface of the hand in the distribution of the median nerve (see p. 473 and p. 474), and *weak abduction of the thumb* on muscle strength testing are the most helpful for making the diagnosis. Two additional clinical tests are also used—when positive, Tinel's test appears more likely to be confirmed by further diagnostic testing.

Thenar atrophy may also be present.

Thumb Abduction. Ask the patient to raise the thumb perpendicular to the palm as you apply downward pressure on the distal phalanx. (This maneuver reliably tests the strength of the abductor pollicis brevis, which is innervated only by the median nerve.)

Tinel's Sign. With your finger, percuss lightly over the course of the median nerve in the carpal tunnel at the spot indicated by the arrow.

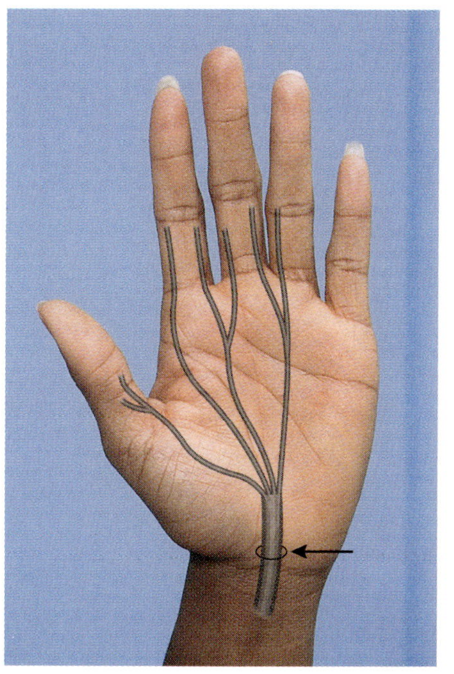

Tingling or electric sensations in the distribution of the median nerve constitute a positive test, suggesting carpal tunnel syndrome.

Phalen's Test. Hold the patient's wrists in acute flexion for 60 seconds. Alternatively, ask the patient to press the backs of both hands together to form right angles. These maneuvers compress the median nerve.

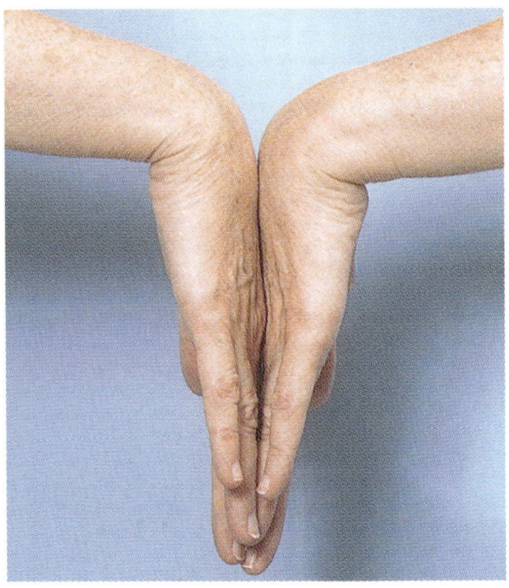

If numbness and tingling develop over the distribution of the median nerve (e.g., the palmar surface of the thumb, and the index, middle, and part of the ring fingers), the sign is positive, suggesting carpal tunnel syndrome.

For Low Back Pain With Radiation Into the Leg. If the patient has noted low back pain that radiates down the leg, check straight leg raising on each side in turn. The patient should be lying supine. Raise the patient's relaxed and straightened leg until pain occurs. Then dorsiflex the foot.

Record the degree of elevation at which pain occurs, the quality and distribution of the pain, and the effects of dorsiflexion. Tightness and mild discomfort in the hamstrings with these maneuvers are common and do not indicate radicular pain.

Sharp pain radiating from the back down the leg in an L5 or S1 distribution (*radicular pain*) suggests tension on or compression of the nerve root(s), often caused by a herniated lumbar disc. Dorsiflexion of the foot increases the pain. Increased pain in the affected leg when the opposite leg is raised strongly confirms radicular pain and constitutes a positive *crossed straight leg-raising sign.*

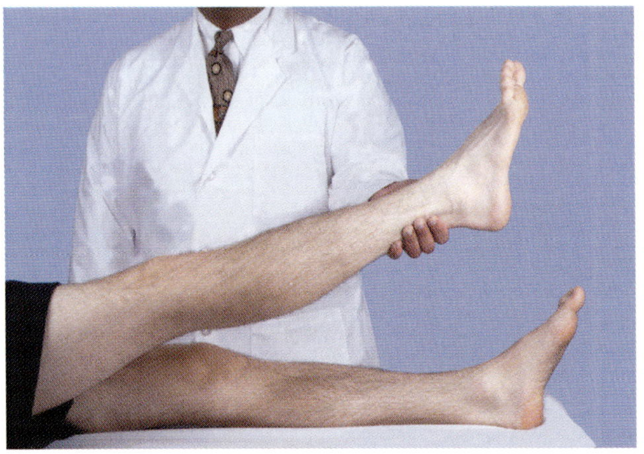

Examine the patient neurologically, focusing on the motor and sensory functions and the reflexes at the lumbosacral levels. These are outlined in the next chapter.

See Table 15-1 Low Back Pain (p. 522).

Measuring the Length of Legs. If you suspect that the patient's legs are unequal in length, measure them. Get the patient relaxed in the supine

Unequal leg length may explain a scoliosis.

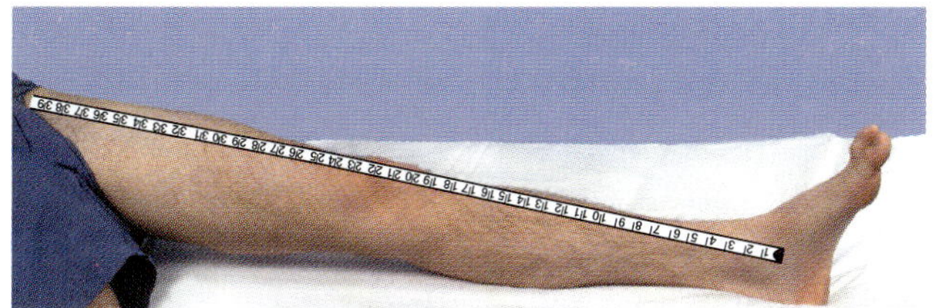

position and symmetrically aligned with legs extended. With a tape, measure the distance between the anterior superior iliac spine and the medial malleolus. The tape should cross the knee on its medial side.

Describing Limited Motion of a Joint. Although measurement of motion is seldom necessary, limitations can be described in degrees. Pocket goniometers are available for this purpose. In the two examples shown below, the red lines indicate the range of the patient's movement and the black lines suggest the normal range.

Observations may be described in several ways. The numbers in parentheses are suitably abbreviated recordings.

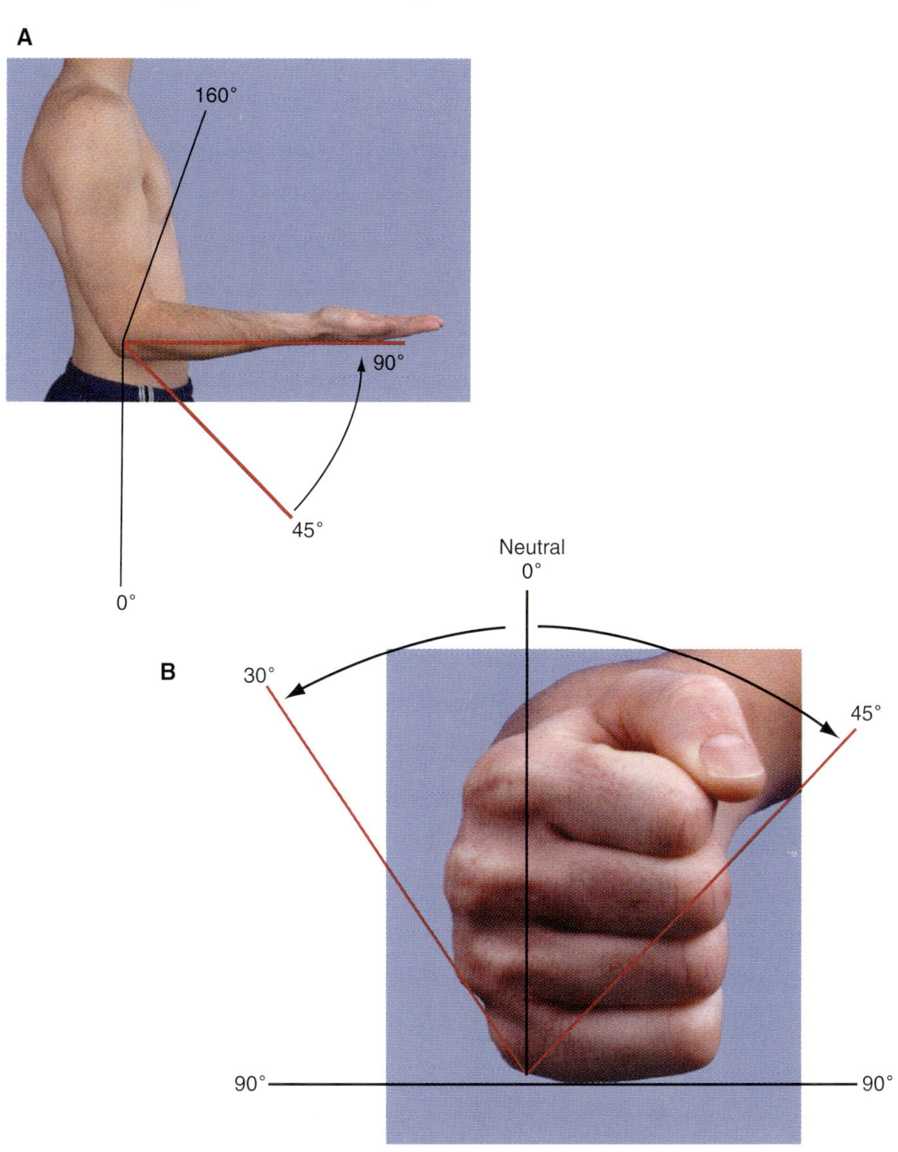

A. The elbow flexes from 45° to 90° (45° → 90°),
-or-
The elbow has a flexion deformity of 45° and can be flexed farther to 90° (45° → 90°).

B. Supination at elbow = 30° (0° → 30°)
Pronation at elbow = 45° (0° → 45°)

TABLE 15-1 ■ Low Back Pain

Patterns	Possible Causes	Possible Physical Signs
Mechanical Low Back Pain Acute, often recurrent, or possibly chronic aching pain in the lumbosacral area, possibly radiating into the posterior thighs but not below the knees. The pain is often precipitated or aggravated by moving, lifting, or twisting motions and is relieved by rest. Spinal movements are typically limited by pain. This is the back pain common from the teenage years through the 40s.	The exact cause cannot usually be proven. Intervertebral disc disease is probably involved in many cases. Congenital disorders of the spine, such as spondylolisthesis, may be present in a small percentage. In older women or in persons on long-term corticosteroid therapy, consider osteoporosis complicated by a collapsed vertebra.	Local tenderness, muscle spasm, pain on movement of the back, and loss of the normal lumbar lordosis, but no motor or sensory loss or reflex abnormalities. In osteoporosis there may be a thoracic kyphosis, percussion tenderness over a spinous process, or fractures elsewhere such as in the thoracic spine or in a hip.
Radicular Low Back Pain A radicular (nerve root) pain, usually superimposed on low back pain. The sciatic pain is shooting and radiates down one or both legs, usually to below the knee(s) in a dermatomal distribution, often with associated numbness and tingling and possibly local weakness. The pain is usually worsened by spinal movement such as bending and by sneezing, coughing, or straining.	A herniated intervertebral disc with compression or traction of nerve root(s) is the most common cause in persons under age 50. The nerve roots of L5 or S1 are most often affected. Spinal cord tumors or abscesses are much less common causes. Compared to a disc, they tend to affect more nerve roots and to produce more neurologic deficits.	Pain on straight leg raising (see p. 520), tenderness of the sciatic nerve, loss of sensation in a dermatomal distribution, local muscular weakness and atrophy, and decreased to absent reflex(es), especially affecting the ankle jerks. Dermatomal signs and reflex changes may be absent when only a single root is affected.
Back and Leg Pain From Lumbar Stenosis Pseudoclaudication is a pain in the back or legs that worsens with walking and improves with flexing of the spine, as by sitting or bending forward.	Lumbar stenosis, which is a combination of degenerative disc disease and osteoarthritis that narrows the spinal canal and impinges on the spinal nerves. It is a common cause of pain after age 60.	The posture may become flexed forward. Motor weakness and hyporeflexia in the lower extremities may be present.
Chronic Persistent Low Back Stiffness	Ankylosing spondylitis, a chronic inflammatory polyarthritis, most common in young men	Loss of the normal lumbar lordosis, muscle spasm, and limitation of anterior and lateral flexion
	Diffuse idiopathic skeletal hyperostosis (DISH), which affects middle-aged and older men	Flexion and immobility of the spine
Aching Nocturnal Back Pain, Unrelieved by Rest	Consider metastatic malignancy in the spine, as from cancer of the prostate, breast, lung, thyroid, and kidney, and multiple myeloma.	Variable with the source. Local bone tenderness may be present.
Back Pain Referred From the Abdomen or Pelvis Usually a deep, aching pain, the level of which varies with the source	Peptic ulcer, pancreatitis, pancreatic cancer, chronic prostatitis, endometriosis, dissecting aortic aneurysm, retroperitoneal tumor, and other causes	Spinal movements are not painful and range of motion is not affected. Look for signs of the primary disorder.

TABLE 15-2 ■ Pains in the Neck

Patterns	Possible Causes	Possible Physical Signs
"Simple Stiff Neck" Acute, episodic, localized pain in the neck, often appearing on awakening and lasting 1–4 days. No dermatomal radiation	The mechanisms are not understood.	Local muscular tenderness and pain on certain movements
Aching Neck A persistent dull aching in the back of the neck, often spreading to the occiput. This is common with postural strain, as with prolonged typing or studying, and may also accompany tension and depression.	Poorly understood; may be related to sustained muscle contraction	Local muscular tenderness. When areas of pain and tenderness are also present elsewhere in the body, consider the fibromyalgia syndrome (see Table 15-3, Patterns of Pain In and Around the Joints).
"Cervical Sprain" Acute and often recurrent neck pains that are often more severe and last longer than simple stiff neck. There may be a precipitating factor such as a whiplash injury, heavy lifting, or a sudden movement, but there is no dermatomal radiation.	Poorly understood	Local tenderness and pain on movement
Neck Pain With Dermatomal Radiation Neck pain as in cervical sprain, but with radiation of the pain to the shoulder, back, or arm in a dermatomal distribution. This radicular pain is typically sharp, burning, or tingling in quality.	Compression of one or more nerve roots caused by either a herniated cervical disc or degenerative disease of the intervertebral discs with bony spurring*	Muscle tenderness and spasm, a limited range of neck motion, increase in the pain on coughing or straining, and possible sensory loss, weakness, muscular atrophy, and decreased reflexes in the areas involved
Neck Pain From Possible Compression of the Cervical Spinal Cord Associated here is weakness or paralysis of the legs, often with a decrease in or loss of sensation. These symptoms may occur in addition to the radicular symptoms or by themselves. The neck pain may be mild or even absent.	Compression of the spinal cord in the neck caused by either a herniated cervical disc or degenerative disease of the intervertebral discs with bony spurring. Trauma may also be the cause.*	Limited range of motion in the neck, weakness or paralysis in the legs of the central nervous system type, Babinski responses, loss of position and vibration sense in the legs, and, less commonly, loss of pain and temperature sensation. Radicular signs in the arms may also be present.

* Tumors or abscesses of the cervical spinal cord, though less common, should also be considered.

TABLE 15-3 ■ Patterns of Pain In and Around the Joints

Problem	Process	Common Locations	Pattern of Spread	Onset	Progression and Duration
Rheumatoid Arthritis	Chronic inflammation of synovial membranes with secondary erosion of adjacent cartilage and bone, and damage to ligaments and tendons	Hands (proximal interphalangeal and metacarpophalangeal joints), feet (metatarsophalangeal joints), wrists, knees, elbows, ankles	Symmetrically additive: progresses to other joints while persisting in the initial ones	Usually insidious	Often chronic, with remissions and exacerbations
Osteoarthritis *(degenerative joint disease)*	Degeneration and progressive loss of cartilage within the joints, damage to underlying bone, and formation of new bone at the margins of the cartilage	Knees, hips, hands (distal, sometimes proximal interphalangeal joints), cervical and lumbar spine, and wrists (first carpometacarpal joint); also joints previously injured or diseased	Additive; however, only one joint may be involved.	Usually insidious	Slowly progressive, with temporary exacerbations after periods of overuse
Gouty Arthritis					
Acute Gout	An inflammatory reaction to microcrystals of sodium urate	Base of the big toe (the first metatarsophalangeal joint), the instep or dorsum of feet, the ankles, knees, and elbows	Early attacks are usually confined to one joint.	Sudden, often at night, often after injury, surgery, fasting, or excessive food or alcohol intake	Occasional isolated attacks lasting days up to 2 weeks; they may get more frequent and severe, with persisting symptoms.
Chronic Tophaceous Gout	Multiple local accumulations of sodium urate in the joints and other tissues (tophi), with or without inflammation	Feet, ankles, wrists, fingers, and elbows	Additive, not so symmetric as rheumatoid arthritis	Gradual development of chronicity with repeated attacks	Chronic symptoms with acute exacerbations
Polymyalgia Rheumatica	A disease of unclear nature seen in people over age 50, especially women; may be associated with giant cell arteritis	Muscles of the hip girdle and shoulder girdle; symmetric		Insidious or abrupt, even appearing overnight	Chronic but ultimately self-limiting
Fibromyalgia Syndrome	Widespread musculoskeletal pain and tender points. May accompany other diseases. Mechanisms unclear	"All over," but especially in the neck, shoulders, hands, low back, and knees	Shifts unpredictably or worsens in response to immobility, excessive use, or chilling	Variable	Chronic, with "ups and downs"

The vagueness of these characteristics is in itself a clue to the fibromyalgia syndrome.

Associated Symptoms				
Swelling	*Redness, Warmth, and Tenderness*	*Stiffness*	*Limitation of Motion*	*Generalized Symptoms*
Frequent swelling of synovial tissue in joints or tendon sheaths; also subcutaneous nodules	Tender, often warm, but seldom red	Prominent, often for an hour or more in the mornings, also after inactivity	Often develops	Weakness, fatigue, weight loss, and low fever are common.
Small effusions in the joints may be present, especially in the knees; also bony enlargement.	Possibly tender, seldom warm, and rarely red	Frequent but brief (usually 5–10 min), in the morning and after inactivity	Often develops	Usually absent
Present, within and around the involved joint	Exquisitely tender, hot, and red	Not evident	Motion is limited primarily by pain.	Fever may be present.
Present, as tophi, in joints, bursae, and subcutaneous tissues	Tenderness, warmth, and redness may be present during exacerbations.	Present	Present	Possibly fever; patient may also develop symptoms of renal failure and renal stones.
None	Muscles often tender, but not warm or red	Prominent, especially in the morning	Usually none	Malaise, a sense of depression, possibly anorexia, weight loss, and fever, but no true weakness
None	Multiple specific and symmetric tender "trigger points," often not recognized until the examination	Present, especially in the morning	Absent, though stiffness is greater at the extremes of movement	A disturbance of sleep, usually associated with morning fatigue

TABLE 15-4 ■ Painful Shoulders

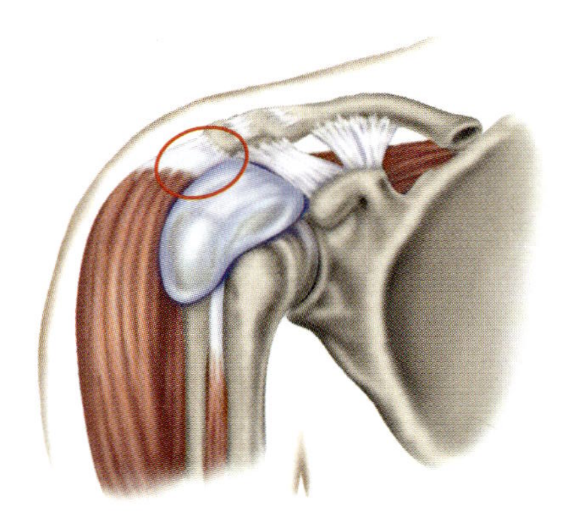

Rotator Cuff Tendinitis

Repeated shoulder motion, as in throwing or swimming, can cause edema and hemorrhage followed by inflammation, most commonly involving the supraspinatus tendon. Acute, recurrent, or chronic pain may result, often aggravated by activity. Patients may report sharp catches of pain, grating, and weakness when lifting the arm overhead. When the supraspinatus tendon is involved, tenderness is maximal just below the tip of the acromion. Patients are typically athletically active.

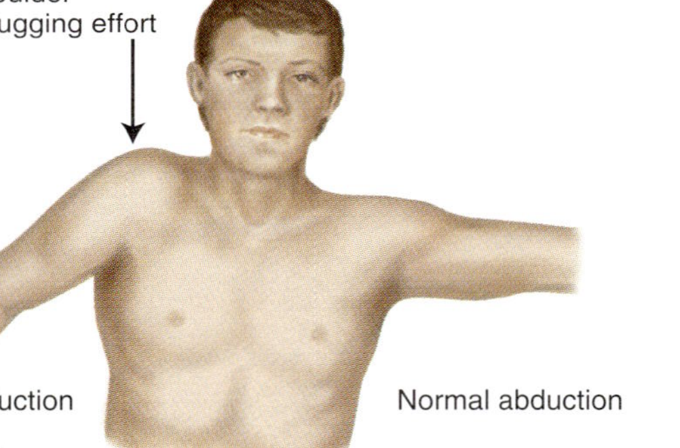

Rotator Cuff Tears

When the arm is raised in forward flexion, the rotator cuff may impinge against the undersurface of the acromion and the coracoacromial ligament. Injury from a fall or repeated impingement may weaken the rotator cuff, causing a partial or complete tear, usually after age 40. Weakness, atrophy of the supraspinatus and infraspinatus muscles, pain, and tenderness may ensue. In a complete tear of the supraspinatus tendon (illustrated), active abduction and forward flexion at the glenohumeral joint is severely impaired, producing a characteristic shrugging of the shoulder.

Calcific Tendinitis

Calcific tendinitis refers to a degenerative process in the tendon that is associated with the deposition of calcium salts. Like rotator cuff tendinitis, it usually involves the supraspinatus tendon. Acute, disabling attacks of shoulder pain may occur, usually in patients over 30 years of age and more often in women. The arm is held close to the side, and all motions are severely limited by pain. Tenderness is maximal below the tip of the acromion. The subacromial bursa, which overlies the supraspinatus tendon, may become involved in the inflammation. Chronic, less severe pain may also occur.

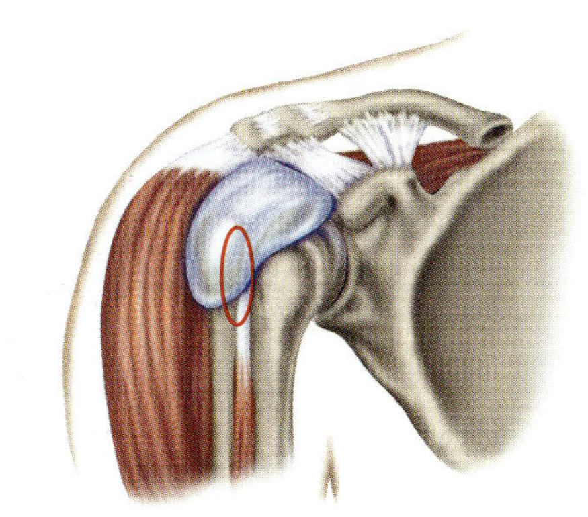
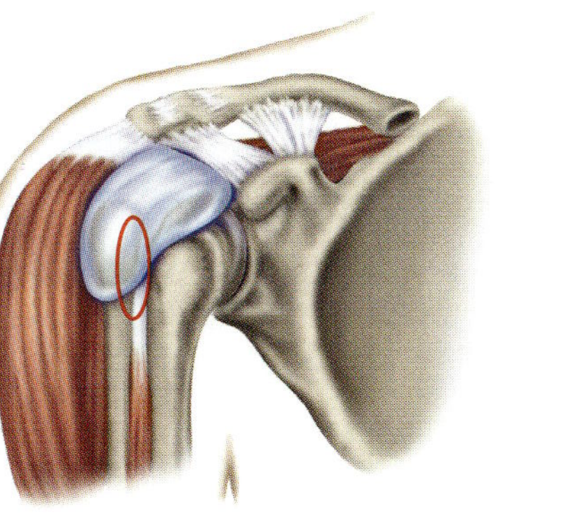

Bicipital Tendinitis

Inflammation of the long head of the biceps tendon and its sheath causes anterior shoulder pain that may resemble rotator cuff tendinitis and may coexist with it. Often this is a sign of shoulder instability. This tendon, like the cuff, may suffer impingement injury. Tenderness is maximal in the bicipital groove. By externally rotating and abducting the arm, you can more easily separate this area from the subacromial tenderness of supraspinatus tendinitis. With the patient's arm at the side, elbow flexed to 90°, ask the patient to supinate the forearm against your resistance. Increased pain in the bicipital groove confirms this condition.

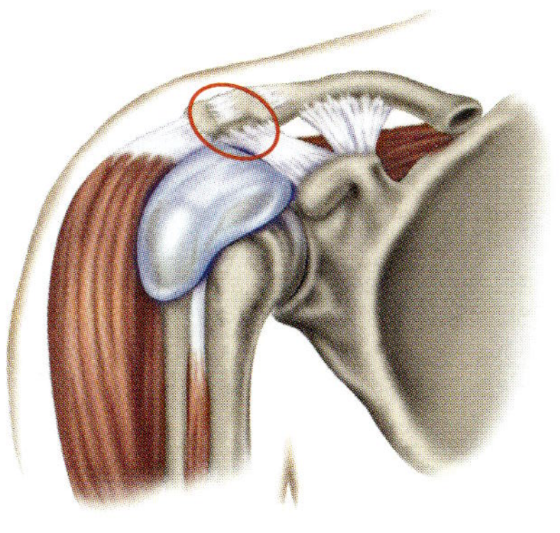

Acromioclavicular Arthritis

Acromioclavicular arthritis is not a common cause of shoulder pain. When present, it usually is the result of direct injury to the shoulder girdle with resulting degenerative changes. Tenderness is localized over the acromioclavicular joint. Although motion in the glenohumeral joint is not painful in acromioclavicular arthritis, as it is in many other painful conditions of the shoulder, movements of the scapula, such as shoulder shrugging, are.

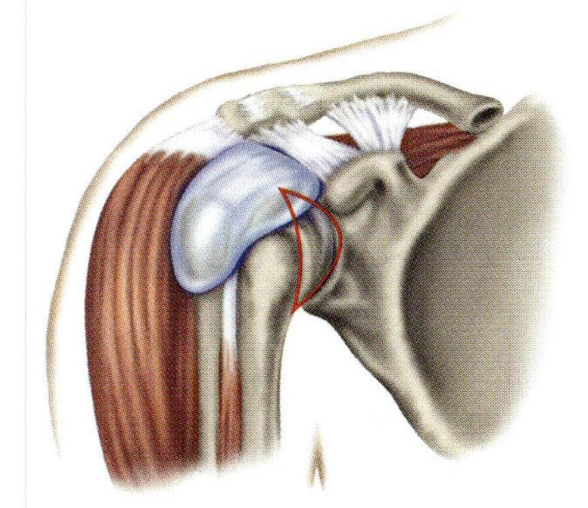

Adhesive Capsulitis (Frozen Shoulder)

Adhesive capsulitis refers to a mysterious fibrosis of the glenohumeral joint capsule, manifested by diffuse, dull, aching pain in the shoulder and progressive restriction of active and passive range of motion, but usually no localized tenderness. The condition is usually unilateral and occurs in persons aged 50 to 70. There is often an antecedent painful disorder of the shoulder or possibly another condition (such as myocardial infarction) that has decreased shoulder movements. The course is chronic, lasting months to years, but the disorder often resolves spontaneously, at least partially.

TABLE 15-5 ■ Swollen or Tender Elbows

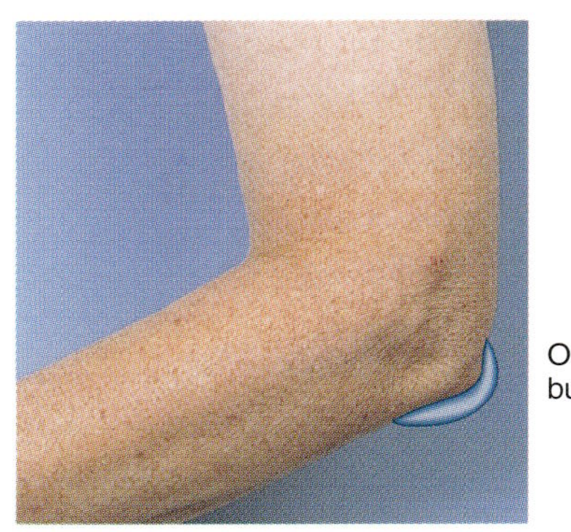

Olecranon Bursitis

Swelling and inflammation of the olecranon bursa may result from trauma or may be associated with rheumatoid or gouty arthritis. The swelling is superficial to the olecranon process.

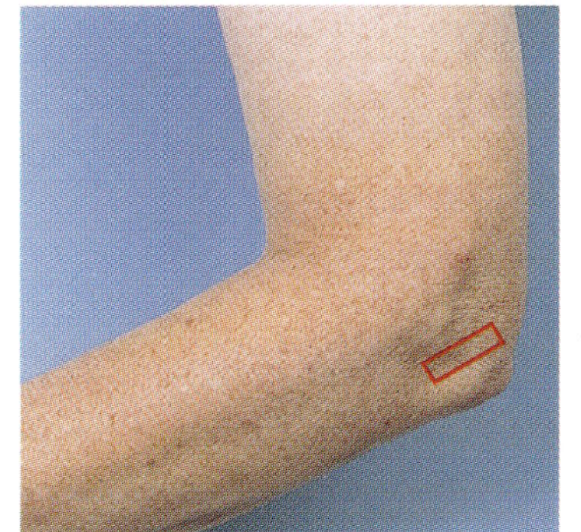

Arthritis of the Elbow

Synovial inflammation or fluid is felt best in the grooves between the olecranon process and the epicondyles on either side. Palpate for a boggy, soft, or fluctuant swelling and for tenderness.

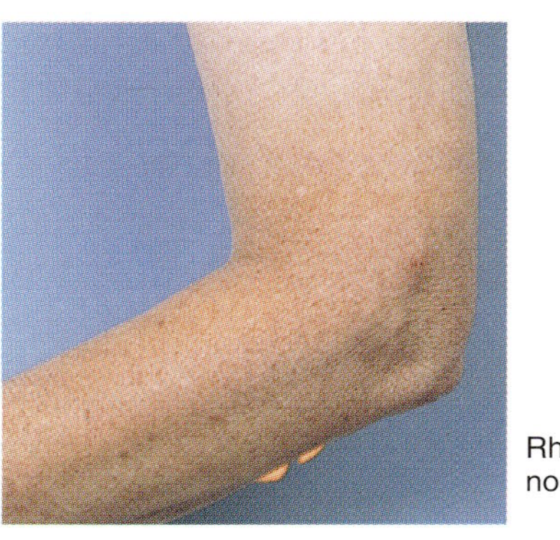

Rheumatoid Nodules

Subcutaneous nodules may develop at pressure points along the extensor surface of the ulna in patients with rheumatoid arthritis or acute rheumatic fever. They are firm and nontender, and are not attached to the overlying skin. They may or may not be attached to the underlying periosteum. Although they may develop in the area of the olecranon bursa, they often occur more distally.

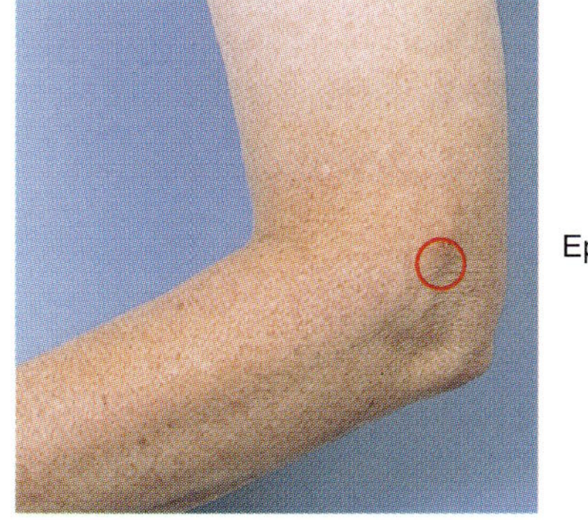

Epicondylitis

Lateral epicondylitis (tennis elbow) follows repetitive extension of the wrist or pronation–supination of the forearm. Pain and tenderness develop at the lateral epicondyle and possibly in the extensor muscles close to it. When the patient tries to extend the wrist against resistance, pain increases.
Medial epicondylitis (pitcher's, golfer's, or Little League elbow) follows repetitive wrist flexion, as in throwing. Tenderness is maximal at the medial epicondyle. Wrist flexion against resistance increases the pain.

TABLE 15-6 ■ Swellings and Deformities of the Hands

Osteoarthritis *(Degenerative Joint Disease)*

Radial deviation of distal phalanx
Heberden's node
Bouchard's node
Metacarpophalangeal joints uninvolved

Nodules on the dorsolateral aspects of the distal interphalangeal joints (*Heberden's nodes*) are due to the bony overgrowth of osteoarthritis. Usually hard and painless, they affect the middle-aged or elderly and often, although not always, are associated with arthritic changes in other joints. Flexion and deviation deformities may develop. Similar nodules on the proximal interphalangeal joints (*Bouchard's nodes*) are less common. The metacarpophalangeal joints are spared.

Acute Rheumatoid Arthritis

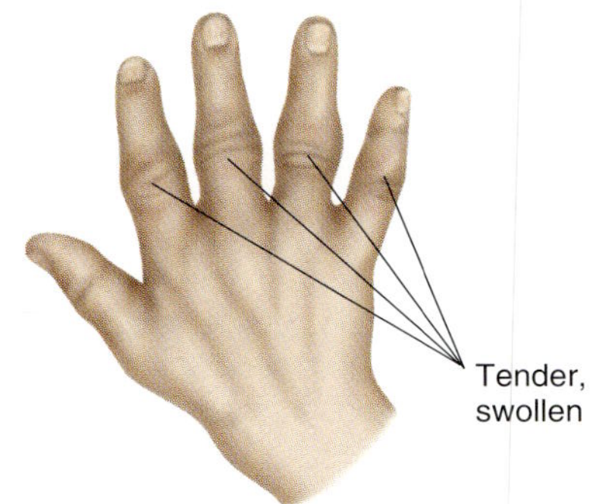

Tender, painful, stiff joints characterize rheumatoid arthritis. Symmetric involvement on both sides of the body is typical. The proximal interphalangeal, metacarpophalangeal, and wrist joints are frequently affected; the distal interphalangeal joints are rarely so. Patients with acute disease often have fusiform or spindle-shaped swelling of the proximal interphalangeal joints.

Chronic Rheumatoid Arthritis

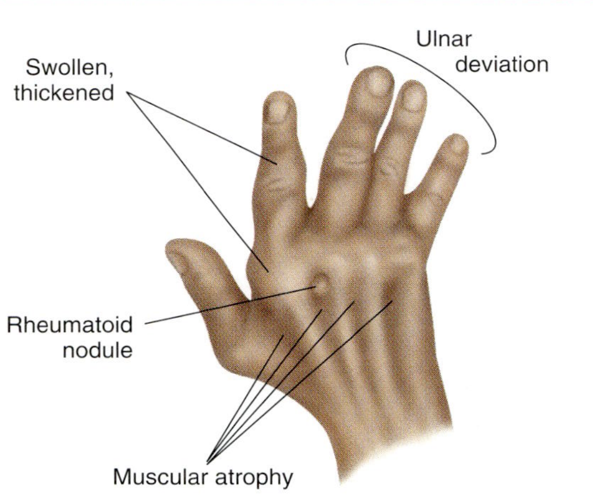

As the arthritic process continues and worsens, chronic swelling and thickening of the metacarpophalangeal and proximal interphalangeal joints appear. Range of motion becomes limited and the fingers may deviate toward the ulnar side. The interosseous muscles atrophy. The fingers may show *"swan neck" deformities* (i.e., hyperextension of the proximal interphalangeal joints with fixed flexion of the distal interphalangeal joints). Less common is a *boutonnière deformity* (i.e., persistent flexion of the proximal interphalangeal joint with hyperextension of the distal interphalangeal joint).

Rheumatoid nodules may accompany either the acute or the chronic stage.

Boutonnière deformity
Swan neck deformity

(table continues next page)

TABLE 15-6 ■ Swellings and Deformities of the Hands *(Continued)*

Chronic Tophaceous Gout

Swollen

Draining tophus

Knobby swelling

The deformities that develop in long-standing chronic tophaceous gout can sometimes mimic those of rheumatoid and osteoarthritis. Joint involvement is usually not so symmetric as in rheumatoid arthritis. Acute inflammation may be present. Knobby swellings around the joints sometimes ulcerate and discharge white chalklike urates.

Ganglion

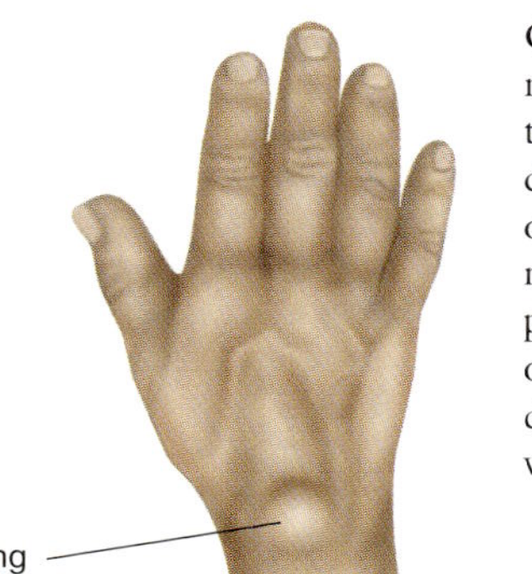

Ganglia are cystic, round, usually nontender swellings located along tendon sheaths or joint capsules. The dorsum of the wrist is a frequent site of involvement. Flexion of the wrist makes ganglia in this location more prominent; extension tends to obscure them. Ganglia may also develop elsewhere on the hands, wrists, ankles, and feet.

Tendon Sheath and Palmar Space Infections

Acute Tenosynovitis

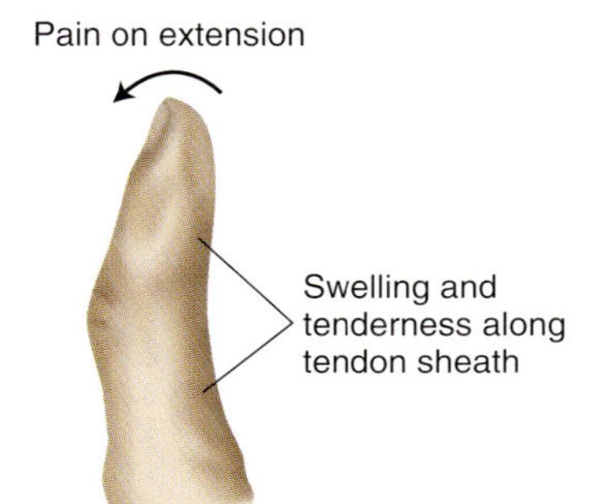

Infection of the flexor tendon sheaths (acute tenosynovitis) may follow local injury, even of apparently trivial nature. Unlike in arthritis, tenderness and swelling develop not in the joint but along the course of the tendon sheath, from the distal phalanx to the level of the metacarpophalangeal joint. The finger is held in slight flexion; attempts to extend it are very painful.

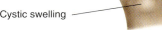

Acute Tenosynovitis and Thenar Space Involvement

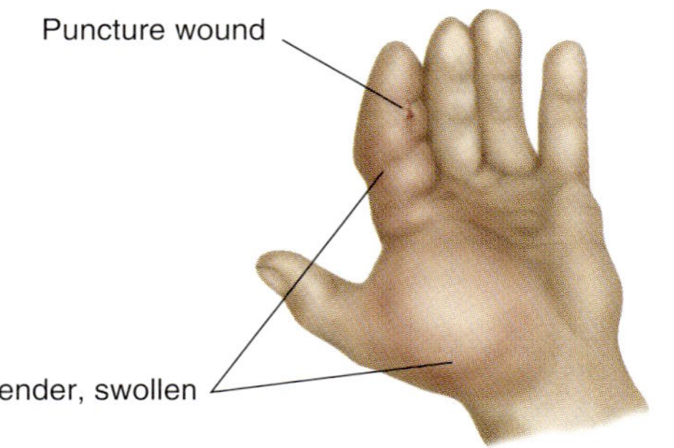

If the infection progresses, it may escape the bounds of the tendon sheath to involve one of the adjacent fascial spaces within the palm. Infections of the index finger and thenar space are illustrated.
Early diagnosis and treatment are important.

Felon

Puncture wound

Swollen, tender, dusky red

Injury to the fingertip may result in infection in the enclosed fascial spaces of the finger pad. Severe pain, localized tenderness, swelling, and dusky redness are characteristic. Early diagnosis and treatment are important.

Dupuytren's Contracture

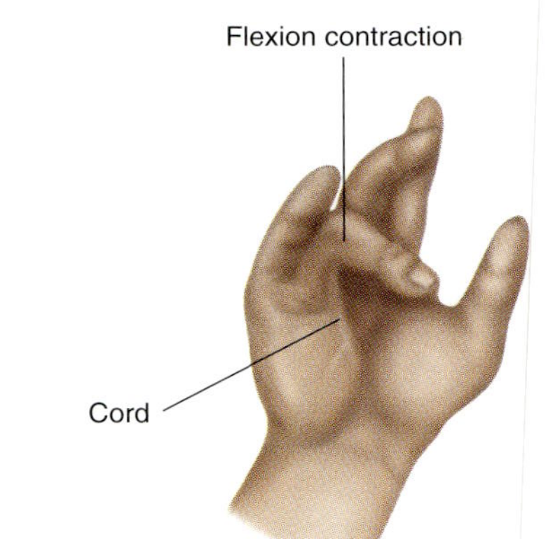

The first sign of a Dupuytren's contracture is a thickened plaque overlying the flexor tendon of the ring finger and possibly the little finger at the level of the distal palmar crease. Subsequently, the skin in this area puckers, and a thickened fibrotic cord develops between palm and finger. Flexion contracture of the fingers may gradually ensue.

Trigger Finger

A trigger finger is caused by a painless nodule in a flexor tendon in the palm, near the head of the metacarpal. The nodule is too big to enter easily into the tendon sheath when the person tries to extend the fingers from a flexed position. With extra effort or assistance, the finger extends with a palpable and audible snap as the nodule pops into the tendon sheath. This snap may also be evident during flexion. Watch and listen as the patient flexes and extends the fingers, and feel for both the nodule and the snap.

Thenar Atrophy

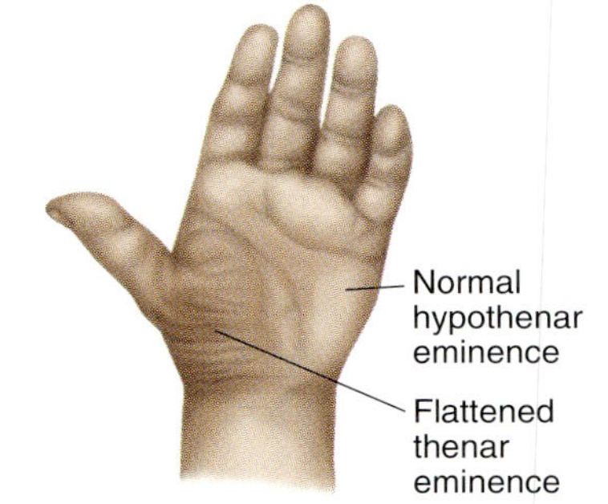
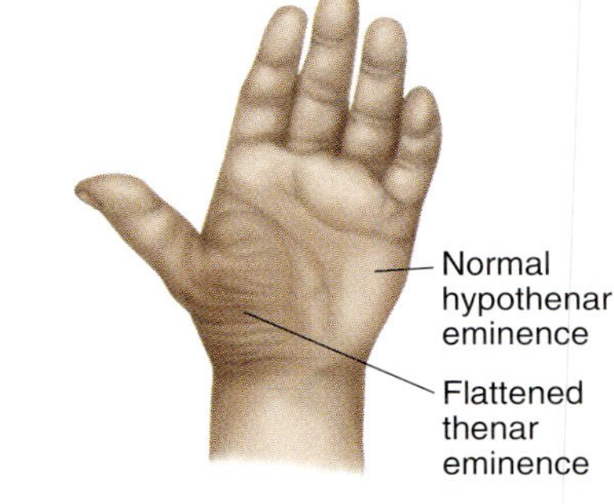

Muscular atrophy localized to the thenar eminence suggests a disorder of the median nerve or its components. Pressure on the nerve at the wrist is a common cause (*carpal tunnel syndrome*). Hypothenar atrophy suggests an ulnar nerve disorder.

TABLE 15-7 ■ Abnormalities of the Feet and Toes

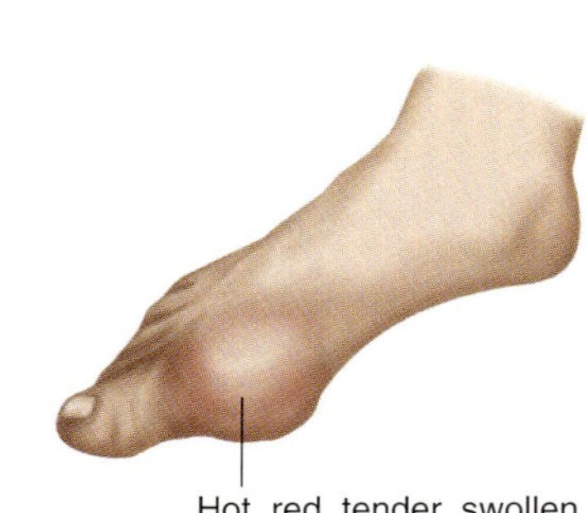

Acute Gouty Arthritis

The metatarsophalangeal joint of the great toe may be the first joint involved in acute gouty arthritis. It is characterized by a very painful and tender, hot, dusky red swelling that extends beyond the margin of the joint. It is easily mistaken for a cellulitis. Acute gout may also involve the dorsum of the foot.

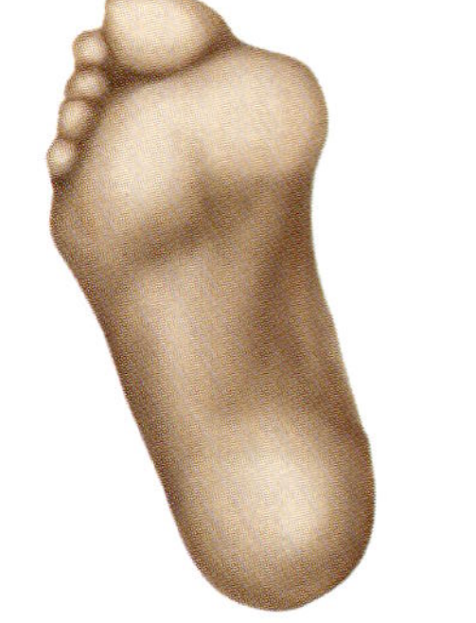

Hallux Valgus

In hallux valgus, the great toe is abnormally abducted in relationship to the first metatarsal, which itself is deviated medially. The head of the first metatarsal may enlarge on its medial side, and a bursa may form at the pressure point. This bursa may become inflamed.

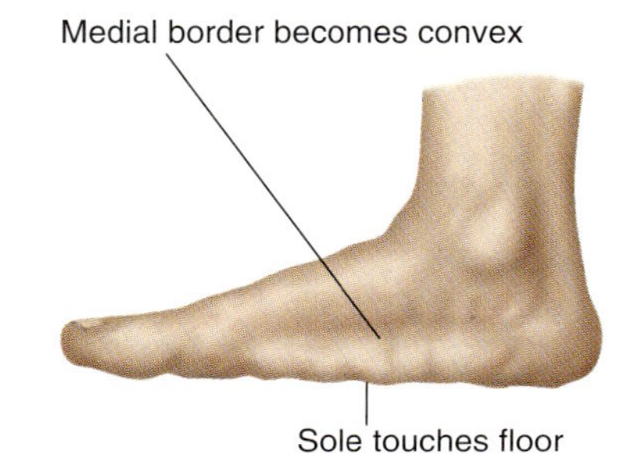

Flat Feet

Signs of flat feet may be apparent only when the patient stands, or they may become permanent. The longitudinal arch flattens so that the sole approaches or touches the floor. The normal concavity on the medial side of the foot becomes convex. Tenderness may be present from the medial malleolus down along the medial-plantar surface of the foot. Swelling may develop anterior to the malleoli. Inspect the shoes for excess wear on the inner side of the soles and heels.

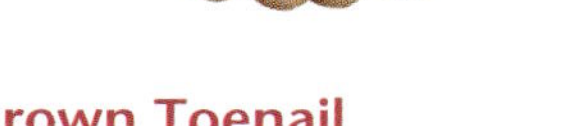

Ingrown Toenail

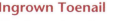

The sharp edge of a toenail may dig into and injure the lateral nail fold, resulting in inflammation and infection. A tender, reddened, overhanging nail fold, sometimes with granulation tissue and purulent discharge, results. The great toe is most often affected.

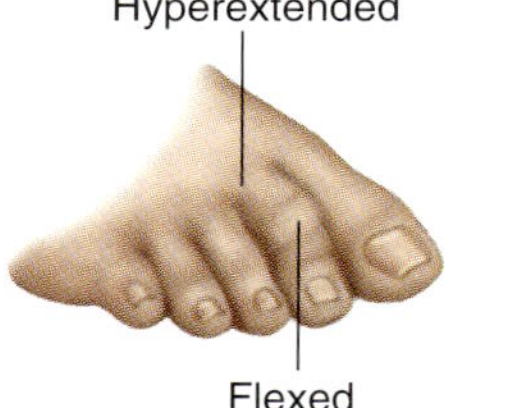

Hammer Toe

Most commonly involving the second toe, a hammer toe is characterized by hyperextension at the metatarsophalangeal joint with flexion at the proximal interphalangeal joint. A corn frequently develops at the pressure point over the proximal interphalangeal joint.

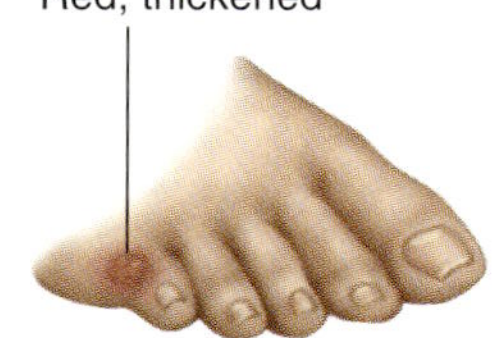

Corn

A corn is a painful conical thickening of skin that results from recurrent pressure on normally thin skin. The apex of the cone points inward and causes pain. Corns characteristically occur over bony prominences (e.g., the 5th toe). When located in moist areas (e.g., at pressure points between the 4th and 5th toes), they are called soft corns.

TABLE 15-7 ■ Abnormalities of the Feet and Toes

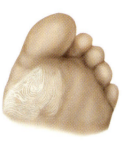

Callus

Like a corn, a callus is an area of greatly thickened skin that develops in a region of recurrent pressure. Unlike a corn, however, a callus involves skin that is normally thick, such as the sole, and is usually painless. If a callus is painful, suspect an underlying plantar wart.

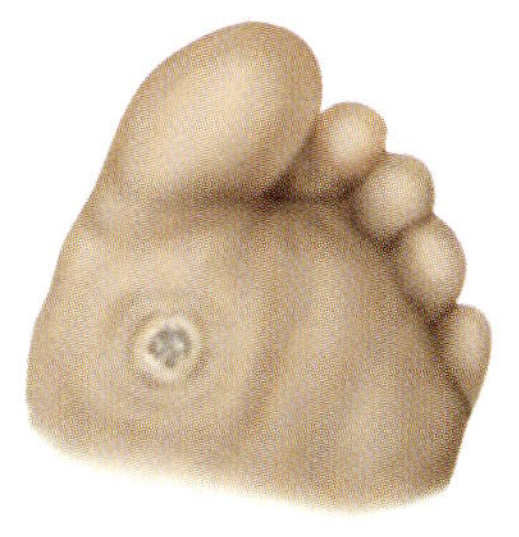

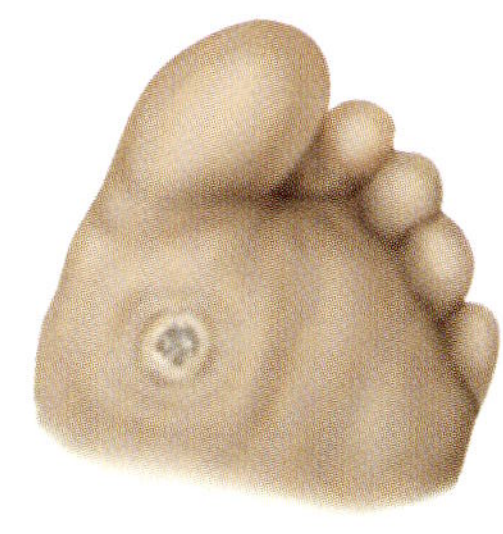

Plantar Wart

A plantar wart is a common wart (verruca vulgaris) located in the thickened skin of the sole. It may look somewhat like a callus or even be covered by one. Look for the characteristic small dark spots that give a stippled appearance to a wart. Normal skin lines stop at the wart's edge.

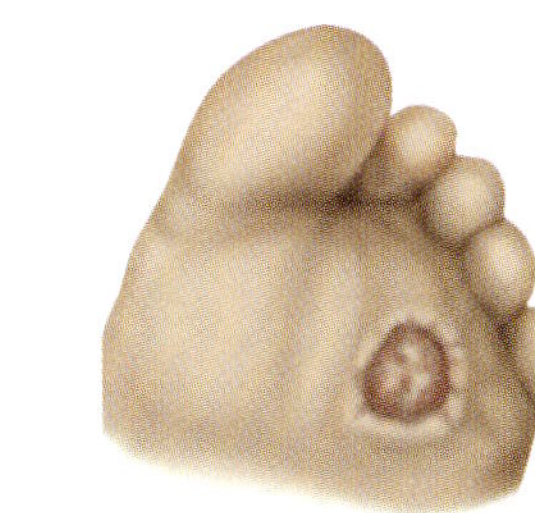

Neuropathic Ulcer

When pain sensation is diminished or absent (as in diabetic neuropathy, for example), neuropathic ulcers may develop at pressure points on the feet. Although often deep, infected, and indolent, they are painless. Callus formation about the ulcer is diagnostically helpful. Like the ulcer itself, it results from chronic pressure.

CHAPTER

16

The Nervous System

ANATOMY AND PHYSIOLOGY

This section deals briefly with structures, functions, and concepts that relate directly to the neurologic examination. After a short description of the brain, spinal cord, cranial and peripheral nerves, and reflexes, it summarizes important motor and sensory pathways. Common or concerning symptoms, health promotion and counseling, and a preview of the pertinent write-up then follow. Next comes *Techniques of Examination* for the nervous system, including mental status, the cranial nerves, the motor and sensory systems, and reflexes.

As you review this material, note that the *central nervous system* consists of the brain and the spinal cord. The *peripheral nervous system* consists of the 12 pairs of cranial nerves and the spinal and peripheral nerves. Most of the peripheral nerves contain both motor and sensory fibers.

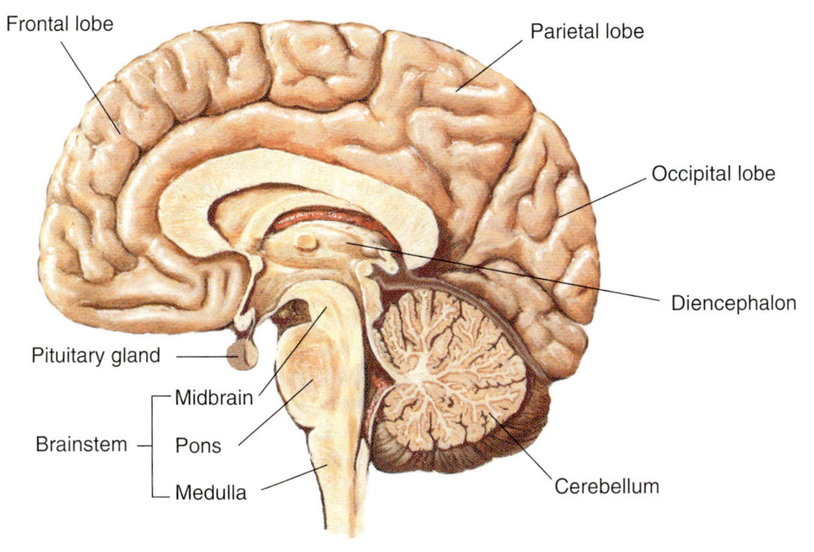

RIGHT HALF OF THE BRAIN, MEDIAL VIEW

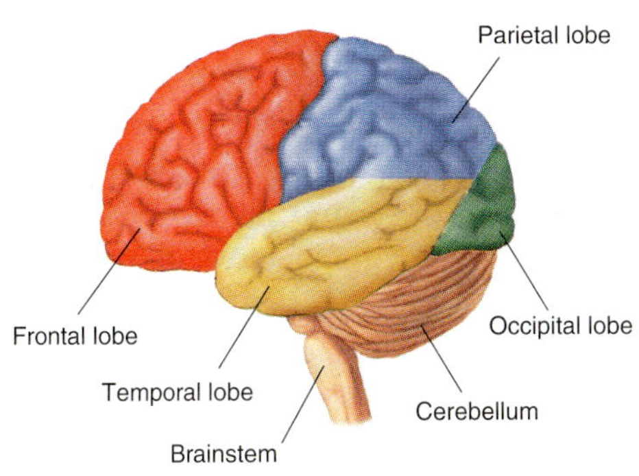

LEFT LATERAL VIEW OF THE BRAIN

Central Nervous System

THE BRAIN

The brain has four regions: the cerebrum, the diencephalon, the brainstem, and the cerebellum. The cerebral hemispheres contain the greatest mass of brain tissue. Each hemisphere is subdivided into frontal, parietal, temporal, and occipital lobes.

The brain is a vast network of interconnecting *neurons* (nerve cells). These consist of cell bodies and their *axons*—single long fibers that conduct impulses to other parts of the nervous system.

Brain tissue may be gray or white. *Gray matter* consists of aggregations of neuronal cell bodies. It rims the surfaces of the cerebral hemispheres, forming the cerebral cortex. *White matter* consists of neuronal axons that are coated with myelin. The myelin sheaths, which create the white color, allow nerve impulses to travel more rapidly.

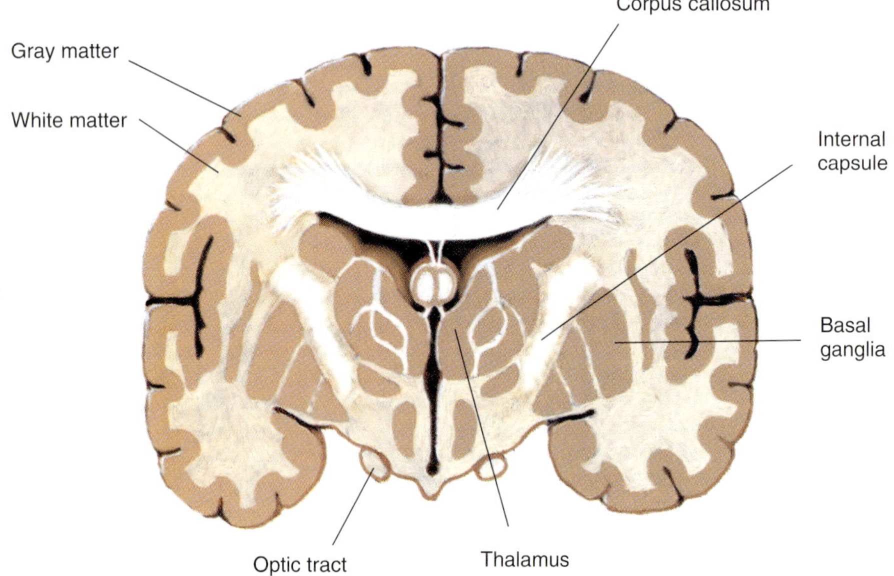

CORONAL SECTION OF THE BRAIN

Deep in the brain lie additional clusters of gray matter. These include the *basal ganglia,* which affect movement, and the thalamus and the hypothalamus (structures in the diencephalon). The *thalamus* processes sensory impulses and relays them to the cerebral cortex. The *hypothalamus* maintains homeostasis and regulates temperature, heart rate, and blood pressure. The hypothalamus affects the endocrine system and governs emotional behaviors such as anger and sexual drive. Hormones secreted in the hypothalamus act directly on the pituitary gland.

In contrast, note the *internal capsule,* a white matter structure where myelinated fibers converge from all parts of the cerebral cortex and descend into the brainstem. The *brainstem,* which connects the upper part of the brain with the spinal cord, has three sections: the midbrain, the pons, and the medulla.

Consciousness depends on the interaction between intact cerebral hemispheres and an important structure in the diencephalon and upper brainstem, the *reticular activating (arousal) system.*

The *cerebellum,* which lies at the base of the brain, coordinates all movement and helps maintain the body upright in space.

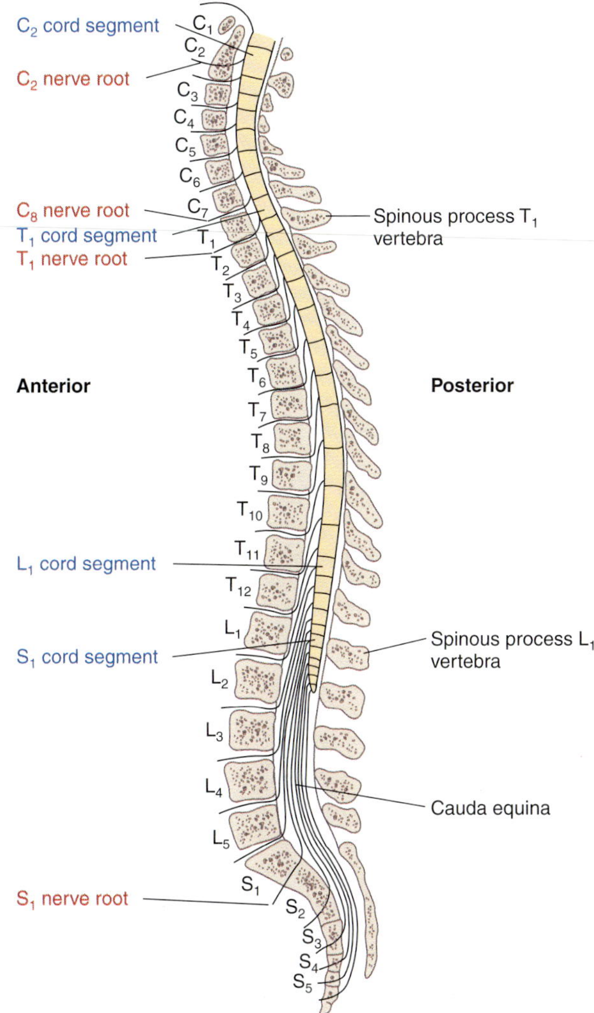

THE SPINAL CORD, LATERAL VIEW

THE SPINAL CORD

The *spinal cord* is a cylindrical mass of nerve tissue encased within the bony vertebral column, extending from the medulla to the first or second lumbar vertebra. It contains important motor and sensory nerve pathways that exit and enter the cord via anterior and posterior nerve roots and spinal and peripheral nerves. The spinal cord also mediates reflex activity of the deep tendon (or spinal nerve) reflexes. Motor and sensory tracts and the deep tendon reflexes are further discussed on pp. 541–546).

The spinal cord is divided into five segments: cervical (C1–8), thoracic (T1–12), lumbar (L1–5), sacral (S1–5), and coccygeal.

Note that the spinal cord is not as long as the vertebral canal. The level of the nerve roots exiting the cord differs from the adjacent vertebral level. The lumbar and sacral roots travel the longest intraspinal distance. These roots fan out like a horse's tail at L1–2, giving rise to the term *cauda equina*. (To avoid injury to the cord, most lumbar punctures are performed at the L3–4 vertebral interspace.)

Peripheral Nervous System

THE CRANIAL NERVES

Twelve pairs of special nerves called *cranial nerves* emerge from within the skull or *cranium*. Cranial Nerves II through XII arise from the diencephalon and the brainstem, as illustrated below. (Cranial Nerves I and II are actually fiber tracts emerging from the brain.) Some cranial nerves are limited to general motor or sensory functions, whereas others are specialized, producing smell, vision, or hearing (I, II, VIII).

Functions of the cranial nerves (CN) most relevant to physical examination are summarized on the next page.

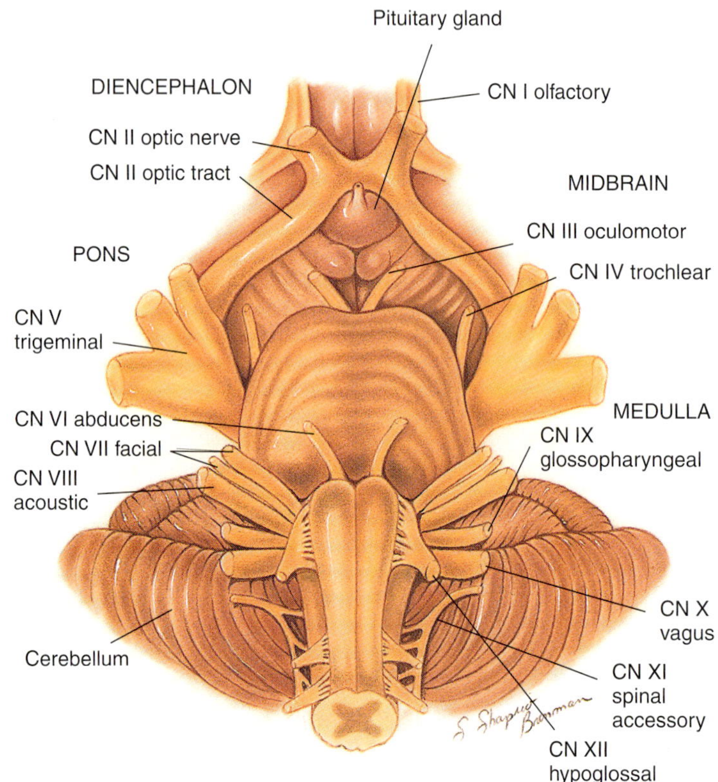

INFERIOR SURFACE OF THE BRAIN

THE PERIPHERAL NERVES

In addition to cranial nerves, the peripheral nervous system also includes spinal and peripheral nerves that carry impulses to and from the cord. Thirty-one pairs of nerves attach to the spinal cord: 8 cervical, 12 thoracic, 5 lumbar,

No.	Cranial Nerve	Function
I	**Olfactory**	Sense of smell
II	**Optic**	Vision
III	**Oculomotor**	Pupillary constriction, opening the eye, and most extraocular movements
IV	**Trochlear**	Downward, inward movement of the eye
VI	**Abducens**	Lateral deviation of the eye
V	**Trigeminal**	*Motor*—temporal and masseter muscles (jaw clenching), also lateral movement of the jaw *Sensory*—facial. The nerve has three divisions: (1) ophthalmic, (2) maxillary, and (3) mandibular.
VII	**Facial**	*Motor*—facial movements, including those of facial expression, closing the eye, and closing the mouth *Sensory*—taste for salty, sweet, sour, and bitter substances on the anterior two thirds of the tongue
VIII	**Acoustic**	Hearing (cochlear division) and balance (vestibular division)
IX	**Glossopharyngeal**	*Motor*—pharynx *Sensory*—posterior portions of the eardrum and ear canal, the pharynx, and the posterior tongue, including taste (salty, sweet, sour, bitter)
X	**Vagus**	*Motor*—palate, pharynx, and larynx *Sensory*—pharynx and larynx
XI	**Spinal accessory**	*Motor*—the sternomastoid and upper portion of the trapezius
XII	**Hypoglossal**	*Motor*—tongue

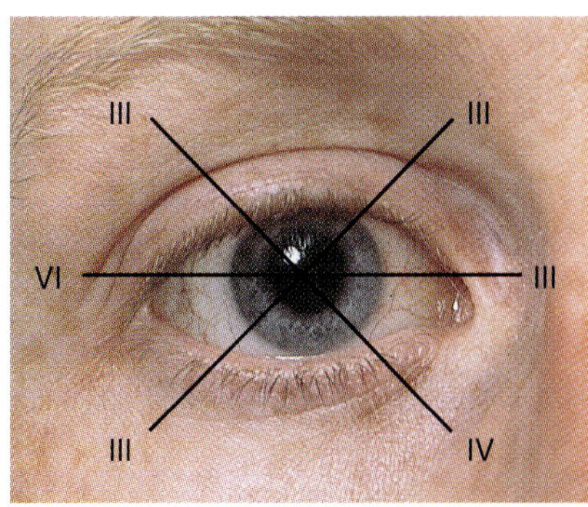

RIGHT EYE (CN III, IV, VI)

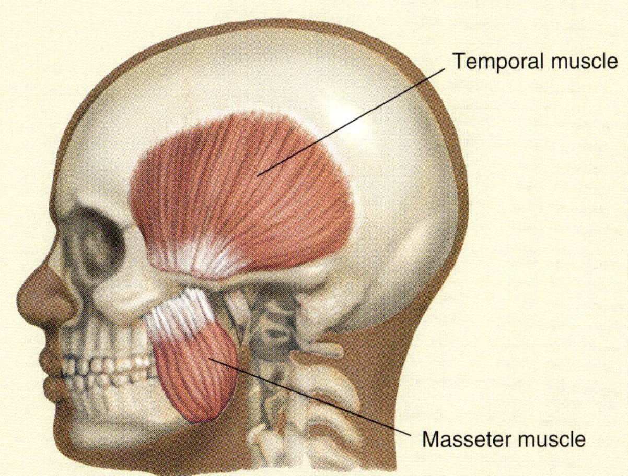

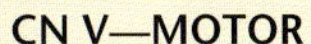
CN V—MOTOR

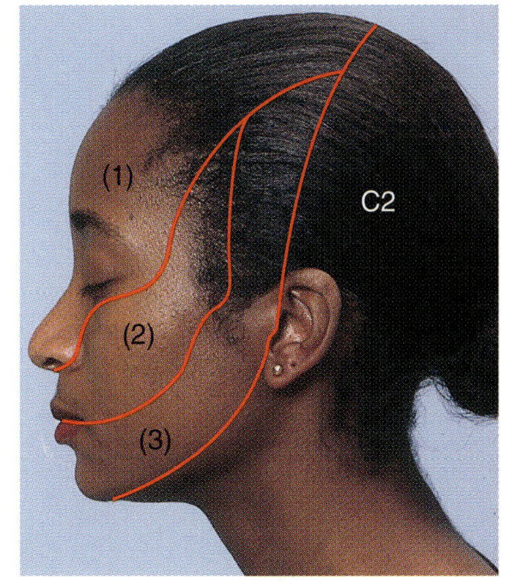

CN V—SENSORY

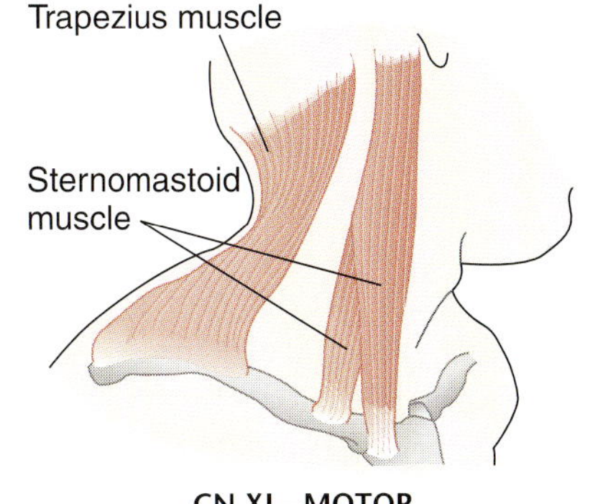

CN XI—MOTOR

5 sacral, and 1 coccygeal. Each nerve has an anterior (ventral) root containing motor fibers, and a posterior (dorsal) root containing sensory fibers. The anterior and posterior roots merge to form a short (<5 mm) *spinal nerve.* Spinal nerve fibers commingle with similar fibers from other levels to form *peripheral nerves.* Most peripheral nerves contain both *sensory* (afferent) and *motor* (efferent) fibers.

Like the brain, the spinal cord contains both gray matter and white matter. Nuclei of gray matter, which are aggregations of nerve cell bodies, are surrounded by white tracts of nerve fibers connecting the brain to the peripheral nervous system. Note the butterfly appearance of the gray matter nuclei, with anterior and posterior horns.

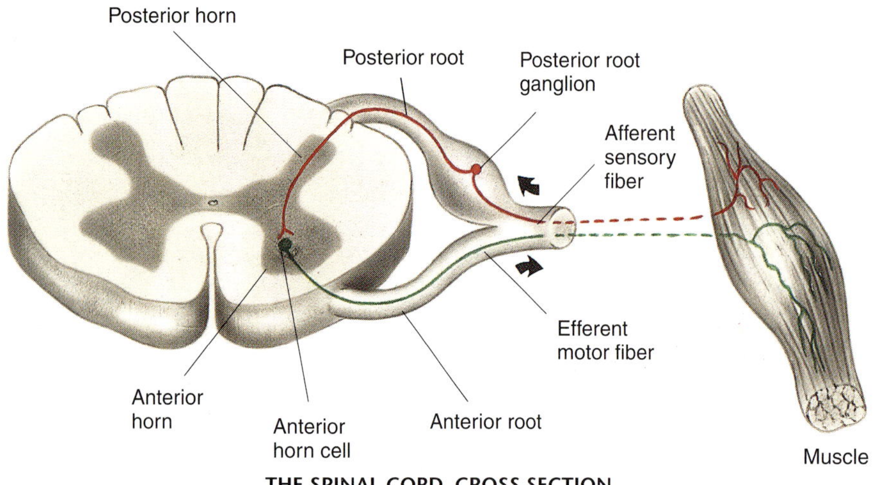

THE SPINAL CORD, CROSS SECTION

Spinal Reflexes: The Deep Tendon Response

The deep tendon or muscle stretch reflexes are relayed over structures of both the central and peripheral nervous systems. Recall that a *reflex* is an involuntary stereotypical response that may involve as few as two neurons, one afferent (sensory) and one efferent (motor), across a single synapse. The deep tendon reflexes in the arms and legs are such monosynaptic reflexes. They illustrate the simplest unit of sensory and motor function. (Other reflexes are polysynaptic, involving interneurons interposed between sensory and motor neurons.)

To elicit a deep tendon reflex, briskly tap the tendon of a partially stretched muscle. For the reflex to fire, all components of the reflex arc must be intact: sensory nerve fibers, spinal cord synapse, motor nerve fibers, neuromuscular junction, and muscle fibers. Tapping the tendon activates special sensory fibers in the partially stretched muscle, triggering a sensory impulse that travels to the spinal cord via a peripheral nerve. The stimulated sensory fiber synapses directly with the anterior horn cell innervating the same muscle. When the impulse crosses the neuromuscular junction, the muscle suddenly contracts, completing the reflex arc.

Because each deep tendon reflex involves specific spinal segments, together with their sensory and motor fibers, an abnormal reflex can help you to locate a pathologic lesion. You should know the segmental levels of the deep tendon reflexes. You can remember them easily by their numerical sequence in ascending order from ankle to triceps: S1—L2, 3, 4,—C5, 6, 7.

Ankle reflex	Sacral 1 primarily
Knee reflex	Lumbar 2, 3, 4
Supinator (brachioradialis) reflex	Cervical 5, 6
Biceps reflex	Cervical 5, 6
Triceps reflex	Cervical 6, 7

Reflexes may be initiated by stimulating skin as well as muscle. Stroking the skin of the abdomen, for example, produces a localized muscular twitch. These superficial (cutaneous) reflexes and their corresponding spinal segments include:

Abdominal reflexes—upper	Thoracic 8, 9, 10
—lower	Thoracic 10, 11, 12
Plantar responses	Lumbar 5, Sacral 1

Motor Pathways

Motor pathways contain upper motor neurons, synapses in the brainstem or spinal cord, and lower motor neurons. Nerve cell bodies or *upper motor neurons* lie in the motor strip of the cerebral cortex and in several brainstem nuclei; their axons synapse with motor nuclei in the brainstem (for cranial nerves) and in the spinal cord (for peripheral nerves). *Lower motor neurons* have cell bodies in the spinal cord, termed anterior horn cells; their axons transmit impulses through the anterior roots and spinal nerves into peripheral nerves, terminating at the neuromuscular junction.

Three kinds of motor pathways impinge on the anterior horn cells: the corticospinal tract, the basal ganglia system, and the cerebellar system. There are additional pathways originating in the brainstem that mediate flexor and extensor tone in limb movement and posture; most notable in coma (see Table 16-16, p. 622).

All of these higher motor pathways affect movement only through the lower motor neurons—sometimes called the "final common pathway." Any movement, whether initiated voluntarily in the cortex, "automatically" in the

THE PRINCIPAL MOTOR PATHWAYS

- The ***corticospinal (pyramidal) tract***. The corticospinal tracts mediate voluntary movement and integrate skilled, complicated, or delicate movements by stimulating selected muscular actions and inhibiting others. They also carry impulses that inhibit *muscle tone,* the slight tension maintained by normal muscle even when it is relaxed. The corticospinal tracts originate in the motor cortex of the brain. Motor fibers travel down into the lower medulla, where they form an anatomical structure resembling a pyramid. There most of these fibers cross to the opposite or *contralateral* side of the medulla, continue downward, and synapse with anterior horn cells or with intermediate neurons. Tracts synapsing in the brainstem with motor nuclei of the cranial nerves are termed *corticobulbar.*
- The ***basal ganglia system***. This exceedingly complex system includes motor pathways between the cerebral cortex, basal ganglia, brainstem, and spinal cord. It helps to maintain muscle tone and to control body movements, especially gross automatic movements such as walking.
- The ***cerebellar system***. The cerebellum receives both sensory and motor input and coordinates motor activity, maintains equilibrium, and helps to control posture.

basal ganglia, or reflexly in the sensory receptors, must ultimately be translated into action via the anterior horn cells. A lesion in any of these areas will affect movement or reflex activity.

When the corticospinal tract is damaged or destroyed, its functions are reduced or lost below the level of injury. *When upper motor neurons are damaged above the crossover of its tracts in the medulla, motor impairment develops on the opposite or contralateral side. In damage below the crossover, motor impairment occurs on the same or ipsilateral side of the body.* The affected limb becomes weak or paralyzed, and skilled, complicated, or delicate movements are performed especially poorly when compared to gross movements. Muscle tone is increased and deep tendon reflexes are exaggerated.

Damage to the lower motor neurons causes ipsilateral weakness and paralysis, but in this case muscle tone and reflexes are decreased or absent.

Disease of the basal ganglia system or cerebellar system does not cause paralysis, but can be disabling. Damage to the basal ganglia system produces changes in muscle tone (most often an increase), disturbances in posture and gait, a slowness or lack of spontaneous and automatic movements termed *bradykinesia*, and a variety of involuntary movements. Cerebellar damage impairs coordination, gait, and equilibrium, and decreases muscle tone.

Sensory Pathways

Sensory impulses not only participate in reflex activity, as previously described, but also give rise to conscious sensation, calibrate body position in space, and help regulate internal autonomic functions like blood pressure, heart rate, and respiration.

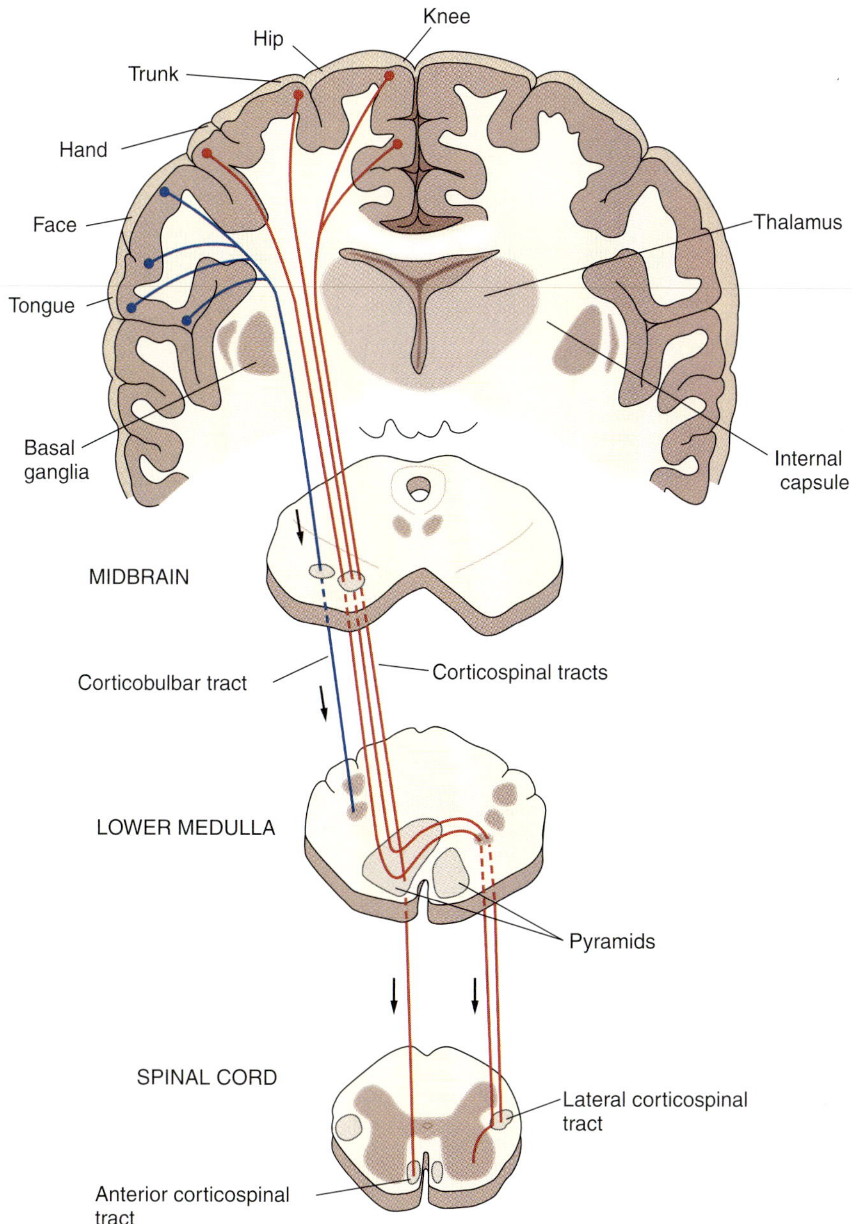

MOTOR PATHWAYS: CORTICOSPINAL AND CORTICOBULBAR TRACTS

A complex system of sensory receptors relays impulses from skin, mucous membranes, muscles, tendons, and viscera. Sensory fibers registering sensations such as pain, temperature, position, and touch, pass through the peripheral nerves and posterior roots and enter the spinal cord. Once inside the cord, sensory impulses reach the sensory cortex of the brain via one of the two pathways: the spinothalamic tracts or the posterior columns.

Within one or two spinal segments from their entry into the cord, fibers conducting the sensations of *pain* and *temperature* pass into the posterior horn of the spinal cord and synapse with secondary sensory neurons. Fibers conducting *crude touch*—a sensation perceived as light touch but without accurate localization—also pass into the posterior horn and synapse with secondary neurons. The secondary neurons then cross to the opposite side and pass upward in the *spinothalamic tract* into the thalamus.

Fibers conducting the sensations of *position* and *vibration* pass directly into the *posterior columns* of the cord and travel upward to the medulla, together with fibers transmitting *fine touch*—touch that is accurately localized and finely discriminating. These fibers synapse in the medulla with secondary sensory neurons. Fibers projecting from secondary neurons cross to the opposite side at the medullary level and continue on to the thalamus.

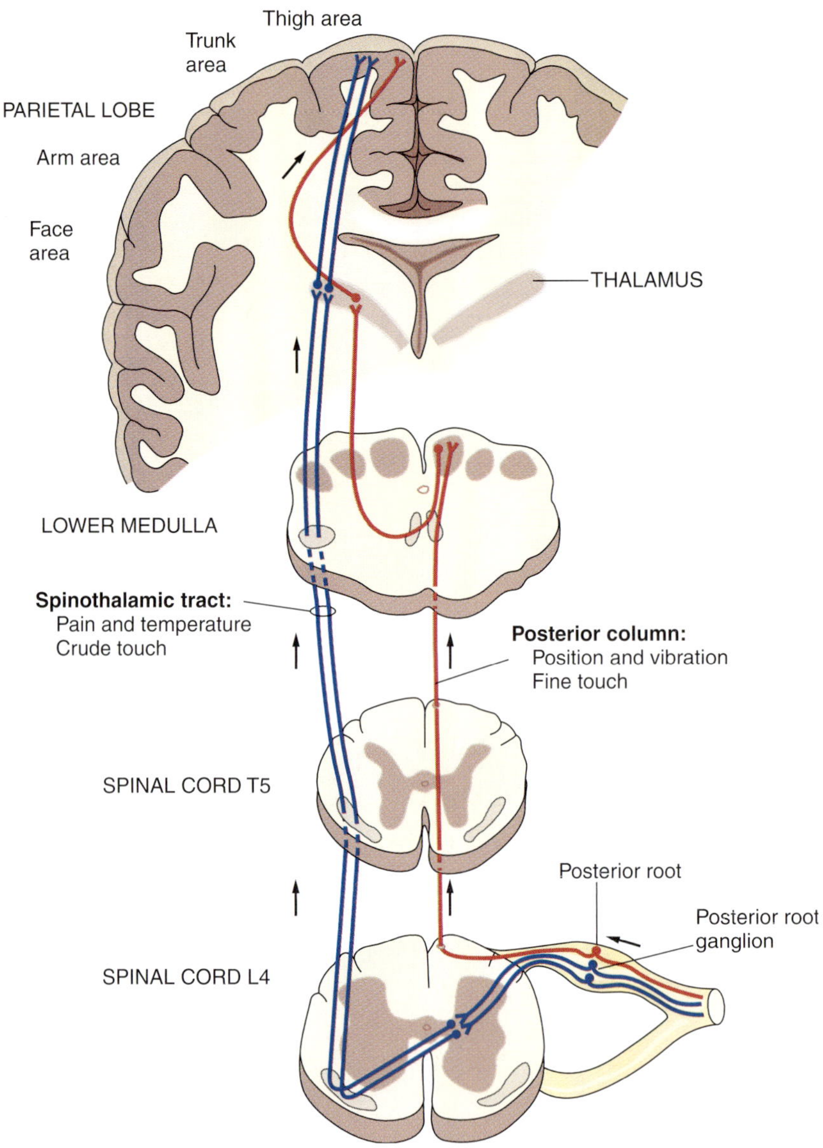

SENSORY PATHWAYS: SPINOTHALAMIC TRACT AND POSTERIOR COLUMNS

At the *thalamic level,* the general quality of sensation is perceived (e.g., pain, cold, pleasant and unpleasant), but fine distinctions are not made. For full perception, a third group of sensory neurons sends impulses from the thalamus to the *sensory cortex* of the brain. Here stimuli are localized and discriminations made among them.

Lesions at different points in the sensory pathways produce different kinds of sensory loss. Patterns of sensory loss, together with their associated motor findings, help you to identify where the causative lesions might be. A lesion in the sensory cortex may not impair the perception of pain, touch, and position, for example, but does impair finer discrimination. A person so affected cannot appreciate the size, shape, or texture of an object by feeling it and therefore cannot identify it. Loss of position and vibration sense with preservation of other sensations points to disease of the posterior columns, while loss of all sensations from the waist down, together with paralysis and hyperactive reflexes in the legs, indicates transection of the spinal cord (see Table 16-5, p. 603). Crude and light touch are often preserved despite partial damage to the cord because impulses originating on one side of the body travel up both sides of the cord.

A knowledge of *dermatomes* also aids in localizing neurologic lesions. *A dermatome is the band of skin innervated by the sensory root of a single spinal nerve.* Dermatome patterns are mapped in the next two figures. Their lev-

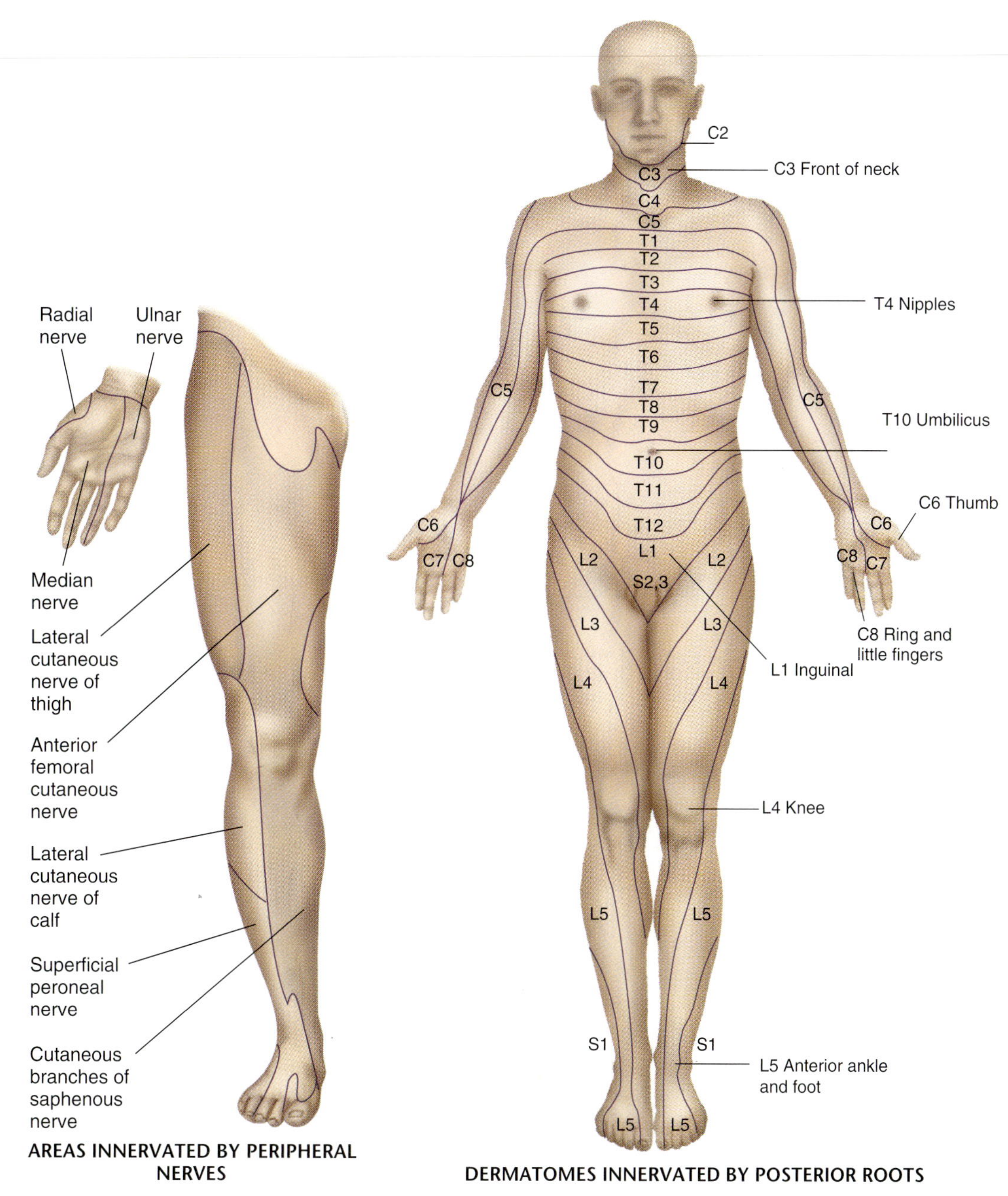

AREAS INNERVATED BY PERIPHERAL NERVES

DERMATOMES INNERVATED BY POSTERIOR ROOTS

els are considerably more variable than the diagrams suggest, and dermatomes overlap each other. The sensory nerves from each side of the body overlap slightly across the midline. The distribution of a few key peripheral nerves is shown in the inserts on the left.

Do not try to memorize all the dermatomes. It is useful, however, to remember the locations of some, such as those shaded in yellow on the right side of the diagrams.

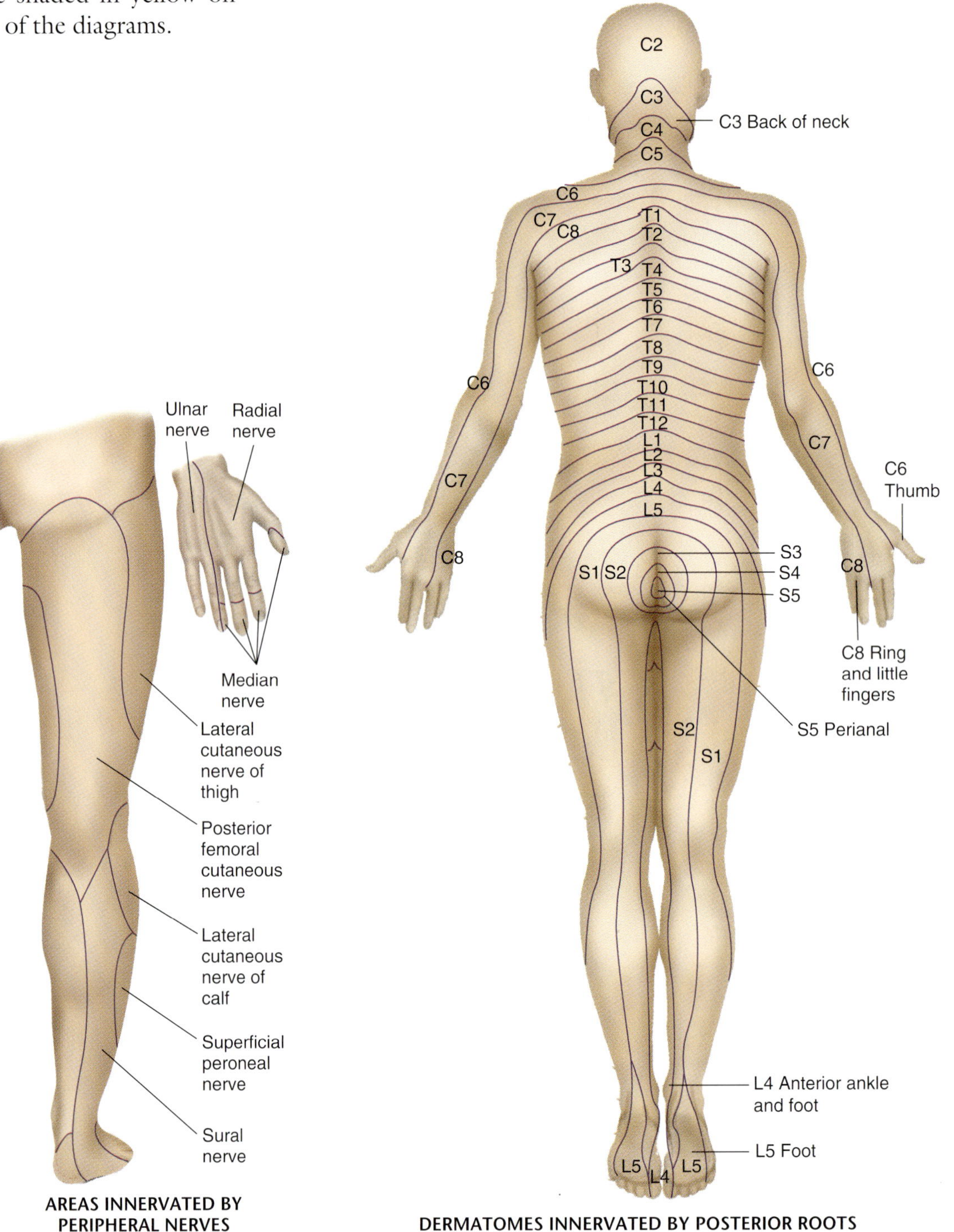

AREAS INNERVATED BY PERIPHERAL NERVES

DERMATOMES INNERVATED BY POSTERIOR ROOTS

Changes With Aging

Aging may affect all aspects of the nervous system, from mental status to motor and sensory function and reflexes. Age-related losses may take their toll on the mental function of an elderly person. These include the deaths of loved ones and friends, retirement from valued employment, diminution in income, decreased physical capacities including impairments in vision and hearing, and perhaps decreased stimulation or growing isolation. In addition, biologic changes affect the aging brain. Brain volume and the number of cortical brain cells decrease, and both microanatomic and biochemical changes have been identified. Nevertheless, most men and women adapt well to getting older. They maintain their self-esteem, they alter their activities in ways that are appropriate to their changing capacities and circumstances, and eventually they ready themselves for death.

In assessing the nervous system of an older person, it is sometimes difficult to distinguish the changes of normal aging from those of age-related or other diseases. Some findings that you would consider abnormal in younger people, however, occur often enough in the elderly that you may attribute them to aging alone. Alterations in hearing, vision, extraocular movements, and pupillary size, shape, and reactivity have been described in Chapter 5 (see pp. 134–136).

Changes in the motor system are common. Older persons move and react with less speed and agility than younger ones, and skeletal muscles decrease in bulk. The hands of an aged person often look thin and bony because their small muscles have atrophied. Look for such muscular wasting in the backs of the hands, where atrophy of the dorsal interosseous muscles may leave concavities or grooves. As illustrated on page 572, this change is often most evident between the thumb and the hand (1st and 2nd metacarpals) but may also be seen between the other metacarpals. Atrophy of small muscles may also flatten the thenar and hypothenar eminences of the palms. Muscle strength, though diminished, is relatively well maintained. Arm and leg muscles may also show atrophy. This sometimes exaggerates the apparent size of adjacent joints.

Occasionally, an older person develops a benign essential tremor in the head, jaw, lips, or hands that may be confused with parkinsonism (p. 608). Unlike parkinsonian tremors, however, benign tremors are slightly faster and disappear at rest, and there is no associated muscle rigidity.

Vibration sense is frequently decreased or lost in the feet and ankles (but not in the fingers or over the shins). Less commonly, position sense may diminish or disappear.

Aging may also alter some of the reflexes. The gag reflex may be diminished or absent. Ankle reflexes may be symmetrically decreased or absent, even when reinforced. Less commonly, knee reflexes are similarly affected. Abdominal reflexes may diminish or disappear and, partly because of musculoskeletal changes in the feet, the plantar responses become less obvious and more difficult to interpret.

If changes such as those described are accompanied by other neurologic abnormalities, or if atrophy and reflex changes are asymmetric, you should search for an explanation other than age alone.

Most elderly people do well on a mental status examination, but functional impairments may become evident, especially at advanced ages. Many older people complain about their memories. "Benign forgetfulness" is the usual explanation and may occur at any age. This term refers to a difficulty in recalling the names of people or objects or certain details of specific events. Naming this common phenomenon, when appropriate, may help to reassure a person who is worried that it signifies Alzheimer's disease. In addition to this circumscribed forgetfulness, elderly people retrieve and process data more slowly, and they take more time to learn new material. Their motor responses may slow, and their ability to perform complex tasks may become impaired.

The clinician must often try to distinguish these age-related changes from the manifestations of specific mental disorders, some of which are more prevalent with aging, such as depression and dementia. Sorting out these ailments from medical complaints may be difficult, particularly since both mood disturbances and cognitive changes may impair the patient's ability to recognize or report symptoms. Older patients are also more susceptible to delirium, a temporary confusional state that may be the first clue to infection or problems with medications. The clinician must learn to recognize these conditions promptly and to protect the patient from harm. (Information on detection of these conditions can be found on pp. 549–551, the Health History, on pp. 551–553, Health Promotion and Counseling, and in Table 16-1, Disorders of Mood, p. 599, and Table 16-5, Delirium and Dementia, p. 603.)

THE HEALTH HISTORY

Common or Concerning Symptoms

- Changes in mood, attention, or speech
- Changes in orientation, memory, insight, or judgment
- Delirium or dementia
- Headache
- Dizziness or vertigo
- Generalized, proximal, or distal weakness
- Numbness, abnormal or loss of sensations
- Loss of consciousness, syncope, or near-syncope
- Seizures
- Tremors or involuntary movements

Much of the information about the patient's *mental status* becomes evident during the interview. As you talk to the patient and listen to the patient's story, you should assess *level of consciousness*, general *appearance and mood*, and *ability to pay attention*, *remember*, *understand*, and *speak*. By placing the patient's vocabulary and general fund of information in the context of the patient's cultural and educational background, you can often make a rough estimate of intelligence. Likewise, the patient's responses to illness and life circumstances often tell you about his or her degree of *insight and judgment*. If the patient has unusual thoughts, preoccupations, beliefs, or perceptions, you should explore them as they arise during the interview. If you suspect a problem in *orientation and memory*, you can ask, "Let's see, your last clinic appointment was when . . . ?" . . . "And the date today?" The more you can integrate your exploration of mental status into a sensitive patient history, the less it will seem like an interrogation.

See Table 16-1, Disorders of Mood, p. 599, and Table 16-2, Disorders of Speech, p. 600.

See Table 16-3, Anxiety Disorders, p. 601, and Table 16-4, Psychotic Disorders, p. 602.

For some patients, you will need to supplement your interview with questions in specific areas. You may determine the need to go further and pursue a formal mental status examination. The components of the mental status examination are described in the section on Techniques of Examination, pp. 556–557.

All patients with documented or suspected brain lesions, psychiatric symptoms, or reports of vague or changed behavioral symptoms by family members need further systematic assessment. Patients may have subtle behavioral changes, difficulty taking medications properly, problems attending to household chores or paying bills, or loss of interest in their usual activities. Other patients may behave strangely after surgery or during an acute illness. Each problem should be identified as expeditiously as possible. Mental function influences the ability to hold a job and is often important in evaluating disability.

Possible signs of depression or dementia

See Table 16-5, Delirium and Dementia, p. 603.

Two of the most common symptoms in neurologic disorders are *headache* and *dizziness*. Turn to p. 136 and p. 139 to review the health history pertinent to these symptoms.

For *headache*, be sure to ask about location, severity, how long it lasts, and any associated symptoms, such as visual changes, weakness, or loss of sensation. Ask if the headache is affected by coughing, sneezing, or sudden movements of the head.

See Table 5-1, Headaches, pp. 170–173.

Subarachnoid hemorrhage may evoke "the worst headache of my life." Dull headache affected by such maneuvers, especially on awakening and recurring in the same location, is seen with mass lesions such as a brain tumor.

The complaint of *dizziness* can have many meanings. You will need to elicit exactly what the patient has experienced. Is the patient light-headed or feeling faint? Or is there *vertigo*, a perception that the room is spinning or rotating?

Light-headedness in palpitations, near syncope from vasovagal stimulation, low blood pressure, febrile illness, and others. Vertigo in middle-ear conditions, brainstem tumor. See Table 5-2, p. 174.

Especially in older patients, are any medications contributing to the dizziness? Are there any associated symptoms such as double vision, or *diplopia*, difficulty forming words, or *dysarthria*, or difficulty with gait or balance, or *ataxia*?

Diplopia, dysarthria, ataxia in posterior circulation transient ischemic attack (TIA) or stroke

What about any associated *weakness*, either generalized or in the face or a part of the body? Weakness is another common symptom and requires careful attention to detail. Probe for exactly what it means to the patient. Explore whether there is any *paralysis*, or inability to move a part or side of the body. Did the weakness start slowly or suddenly? Has it progressed? How? What areas of the body are involved? Does the weakness affect one or both sides? What movements are affected?

Weakness or paralysis in transient ischemic attack or stroke

Focal weakness may arise from ischemic, vascular, or mass lesions in the central nervous system; also from peripheral nervous system disorders, neuromuscular disorders, or the muscles themselves.

For weakness without light-headedness, try to distinguish between *proximal* and *distal weakness*. For proximal weakness, ask about combing hair, trying to reach something on a high shelf, or difficulty getting up out of a chair or taking a high step up. Does the weakness increase with repeated effort and improve after rest? Are there associated sensory or other symptoms? For distal weakness in the arms, inquire about hand movements such as opening a jar or can, or using hand tools such as scissors, pliers, or a screwdriver. For distal weakness in the legs, ask about frequent tripping.

Bilateral proximal weakness in myopathy. Bilateral, predominantly distal weakness in polyneuropathy. Weakness made worse with repeated effort and improved with rest suggests myasthenia gravis.

Find out if the patient has had any *loss of sensation*. Ask if there has been any *numbness*, but clarify its meaning and location. Has there been loss of sensation, difficulty moving a limb, or altered sensations such as tingling or pins and needles? There may be peculiar sensations without an obvious stimulus, called *paresthesias*. These occur commonly when an arm or leg "goes to sleep" following compression of a nerve, and may be described as tingling, prickling, or feelings of warmth, coldness, or pressure. *Dysesthesias* are distorted sensations in response to a stimulus and may last longer than the stimulus itself. For example, a person may perceive a light touch or pinprick as a burning or tingling sensation that is irritating or unpleasant. *Pain* may arise from neurologic causes but is usually reported with symptoms of other body systems, such as the head and neck or the musculoskeletal system.

Loss of sensation, paresthesias, and dysesthesias in central lesions in the brain and spinal cord, as well as disorders of peripheral sensory roots and nerves; paresthesias in the hands and around the mouth in hyperventilation.

See Table 5-1, Headaches, pp. 170–173, Table 15-2, Pains in the Neck, p. 523, and Table 15-1, Low Back Pain, p. 522.

"Have you ever fainted or passed out?" leads the discussion to any *loss of consciousness*. It is important to begin by exploring what the patient means by loss of consciousness. Did the patient black out completely, or could voices be heard throughout the episode, indicating some consciousness? Be sure to use descriptive terms carefully and precisely. *Syncope* is the sudden but temporary loss of consciousness that occurs with decreased blood flow to the brain, commonly described as *fainting*. Symptoms of feeling faint, lightheaded, or weak, but without actual loss of consciousness, are called *near syncope* or *presyncope*.

See Table 16-6, Syncope and Similar Disorders, pp. 604–605.

Get as complete and unbiased a description of the event as you can. What brought on the episode? Were there any warning symptoms? Was the patient standing, sitting, or lying down when the episode began? How long did it last? Could voices be heard while passing out and coming to? How rapidly did the patient recover? In retrospect, were onset and offset slow or fast?

Young people with emotional stress and warning symptoms of flushing, warmth, or nausea may have *vasodepressor (or vasovagal) syncope* of slow onset, slow offset. *Cardiac syncope* from arrhythmias, more common in older patients, often with sudden onset, sudden offset.

Also ask if anyone observed the episode. If so, what did the patient look like before losing consciousness, during the episode, and afterward? Was there any seizure-like movement of the arms or legs? Any incontinence of the bladder or bowel? Any drowsiness or impaired memory after the episode ended?

Tonic-clonic motor activity, bladder or bowel incontinence, and *postictal state* suggest a generalized *seizure.* Unlike syncope, injury such as tongue biting or bruising of limbs may occur.

A *seizure* is a paroxysmal disorder caused by sudden excessive electrical discharge in the cerebral cortex or its underlying structures. Seizures can be of several types. Depending on the type, there may or may not be loss of consciousness. With some types of seizures, there may be abnormal feelings, thought processes, and sensations, including smells, as well as abnormal movements. Asking "Have you ever had any seizures or 'spells'?" . . . "Any fits or convulsions?" can open the discussion. As with syncope, aim for a full and complete description, including precipitating circumstances, warnings, and behavior and feelings both during the attack and afterward. Ask about age at onset, frequency, any change in frequency or symptom pattern, and use of medications. Is there any history of prior head injury or other conditions that may be causally related?

See Table 16-7, Seizure Disorders, pp. 606–607.

Tremors and other *involuntary movements* occur with or without additional neurologic manifestations. Ask about any trembling, shakiness, or body movements that the patient seems unable to control.

See Table 16-8, Involuntary Movements, pp. 608–609.

Distinct from these symptoms is an almost indescribable *restlessness of the legs* that typically develops at rest and is accompanied by an urge to move about. Walking gives relief.

The common but often overlooked restless legs syndrome, usually benign

HEALTH PROMOTION AND COUNSELING

Important Topics for Health Promotion and Counseling

- Screening for depression and suicidality
- Screening for dementia
- Prevention of TIAs or stroke

Up to a third of all primary care visits involve mental health—depressed mood, anxiety, somatic concerns, and more serious disorders of mood and mental function. The burden of suffering imposed by these disorders is great. For the general population, focus health promotion and counseling on depression, suicidality, and dementia, three important conditions often overlooked. You should also screen for use of drugs or alcohol (see pp. 43–45).

The lifetime prevalence of major depression meeting formal diagnostic criteria is 5% to 10% in men and 10% to 20% in women. Primary-care providers fail to diagnose major depression in up to 50% of affected patients, often missing early clues such as low self-esteem, anhedonia (failure to find pleasure in daily activities), sleep disorders, and difficulty in concentrating or making decisions. Routine general screening has not been shown to improve outcomes; rather, target diagnosis and treatment to patients who are symptomatic. Watch carefully for depressive symptoms, especially in patients who are young, female, single, divorced, separated, seriously or chronically ill, or bereaved. Patients with a prior history of depression or positive family history are also at risk. Failure to diagnose depression can have consequences that are fatal—suicide rates in patients with major depression are eight times higher than in the general population.*

Clinicians must be adept at eliciting suicidal ideation or intent (see Chap 2, p. 47). Suicide rates are highest among men over age 65, but have been increasing in teenagers and young adults. Risk factors include any history of psychiatric illness (especially if linked to a hospital admission), substance abuse, personality disorder, prior suicide attempt, or family history of suicide. Clinicians should ask about domestic firearms and screen for alcohol dependence: guns are present in the home of more than half of all suicide victims, and alcohol intoxication is associated with nearly 25% of suicide deaths. Any evidence of suicidal ideation must be further assessed. Has a weapon been obtained? Is there a plan or a note? Such patients should be promptly referred for mental health and psychiatric care and for treatment of any related problems of alcohol or drug abuse.

Dementia, a "global impairment of cognitive function that interferes with normal activities,"† affects 16% of Americans over 65. Prominent features include short- and long-term memory deficits and impaired judgment. Thought processes are impoverished and speech may be hesitant due to difficulty in finding words. Loss of orientation to place may make navigating by foot or car problematic or even dangerous. Most dementias represent Alzheimer's disease (~50%–85%) or vascular multi-infarct dementia (~10%–20%). Be watchful for Alzheimer's disease in individuals with a pos-

*U.S. Preventive Services Task Force: Ch. 49: "Screening for Depression." In *Guide to Clinical Preventive Services.* Baltimore, Williams and Wilkins, pp. 541–546, 1996.

†U.S. Preventive Services Task Force: Ch. 48: "Screening for Dementia." In *Guide to Clinical Preventive Services.* Baltimore, Williams and Wilkins, pp. 531–541, 1996.

itive family history, since their risk is three times higher than in the general population.

Dementia often has a slow, insidious onset and may escape detection by both families and clinicians, especially in its initial stages. Currently there are no reliable screening tests to help you detect dementia early in its course. Clinicians should be alert to evidence of change in cognitive function or activities of daily living, and to family complaints about new or unusual patient behaviors. Use of the Mini-Mental State Examination is helpful for assessing cognitive impairment (although scores may be affected by level of education and cultural variables such as language). Once cognitive change is identified, be sure to address the possible role of medications, depression, or metabolic abnormalities. Couple cognitive and behavioral assessment with a careful neurologic examination during your evaluation of the patient. Be sure to look for other medical and psychiatric conditions that could be contributing to changes in behavior or level of daily activity. For demented patients and affected families, counseling about the potential for disruptive behavior, accidents and falls, and termination of driving privileges is warranted. Clinicians can foster discussion of legal matters such as power of attorney and advanced directives while the patient is still able to contribute to decision-making.

Finally, direct clinical attention to averting cerebrovascular accidents (CVAs). Strokes, or CVAs, are the third leading cause of death in the United States and contribute to extensive disability in the workforce and general population. The incidence of stroke increases with age and is 60% higher in African Americans compared to Caucasians. The clinician's first task in stroke prevention is to control hypertension. Hypertension accelerates atherosclerotic changes in the carotid, vertebral, and cerebral arteries and disturbs autoregulation of cerebral blood pressure. It is the leading risk factor for both ischemic and hemorrhagic stroke, which account for approximately 85% and approximately 10% of all CVAs, respectively. In addition, clinicians should counsel patients to modify conditions contributing to atherosclerosis: smoking, hyperlipidemia, and diabetes. Drug users should be warned of the link between stroke and cocaine.

Clinicians should be alert to symptoms of transient ischemic attacks (TIAs), generally defined as neurologic events that resolve within 24 hours. TIAs can be viewed as CVA warning signals, the anginal equivalent of the brain. In the first year after a TIA, risk of CVA is 6%–7%, and the CVA usually occurs in the same vascular distribution as the TIA. Common symptoms of TIAs include visual loss (especially transient monocular blindness from emboli), aphasia, dysarthria, and changes in facial movement or sensation. For TIAs affecting motor or sensory pathways, watch for clumsiness, weakness, paralysis, or tingling or paresthesias of the arm, leg, or hemibody.

Preview: Recording the Examination—The Nervous System

Note that initially you may use sentences to describe your findings; later you will use phrases. The style below contains phrases appropriate for most write-ups. Unfamiliar terms are explained in the next section, Techniques of Examination. Note that there are five components to the examination and write-up of the nervous system.

"*Mental Status:* Alert, relaxed, and cooperative. Thought process coherent. Oriented to person, place, and time. Detailed cognitive testing deferred. *Cranial Nerves:* I—not tested; II through XII intact. *Motor:* Good muscle bulk and tone. Strength 5/5 throughout. Cerebellar: Rapid alternating movements (RAMs), finger-to-nose (F→N), heel-to-shin (H→S) intact. Gait with normal base. Romberg—maintains balance with eyes closed. No pronator drift. *Sensory:* Pinprick, light touch, position, and vibration intact. *Reflexes:* 2+ and symmetric with plantar reflexes downgoing."

OR

"*Mental Status:* The patient is alert and tries to answer questions but has difficulty finding words. *Cranial Nerves:* I—not tested; II—visual acuity intact; visual fields full; III, IV, VI—extraocular movements intact; V motor—temporal and masseter strength intact, sensory corneal reflexes present; VII motor—prominent right facial droop and flattening of right nasolabial fold, left facial movements intact, sensory—taste not tested; VIII—hearing intact bilaterally to whispered voice; IX, X—gag intact; XI—strength of sternomastoid and trapezius muscles 5/5; XII—tongue midline. *Motor:* strength in right biceps, triceps, iliopsoas, gluteals, quadriceps, hamstring, and ankle flexor and extensor muscles 3/5 with good bulk but increased tone and spasticity; strength in comparable muscle groups on the left 5/5 with good bulk and tone. Gait—unable to test. Cerebellar—unable to test on right due to right arm and leg weakness; RAMs, F→N, H→S intact on left. Romberg—unable to test due to right leg weakness. Right pronator drift present. *Sensory:* decreased sensation to pinprick over right face, arm, and leg; intact on the left. Stereognosis and two-point discrimination not tested. *Reflexes* (can record in two ways):

Suggests left hemispheric CVA in distribution of the left middle cerebral artery, with right-sided hemiparesis

	Biceps	Triceps	Brach	Knee	Ankle	Pl
RT	4+	4+	4+	4+	4+	↑
LT	2+	2+	2+	2+	1+	↓

OR

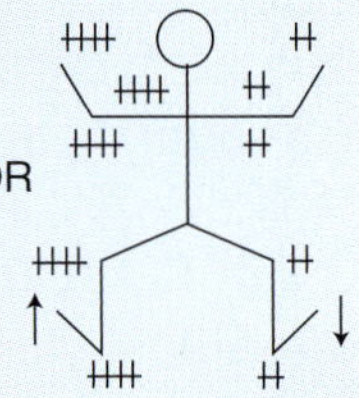

TECHNIQUES OF EXAMINATION

Important Areas of Examination

- Mental status: appearance and behavior, speech and language, mood, thoughts and perceptions, cognition
- Cranial Nerves I through XII
- Motor system: muscle bulk, tone, and strength; coordination, gait, and stance
- Sensory system: pain and temperature, position and vibration, light touch, discrimination
- Deep tendon, abdominal, and plantar reflexes

Three important questions govern the neurologic examination:

- Is the mental status intact?
- Are right-sided and left-sided findings symmetric?
- And, if the findings are asymmetric or otherwise abnormal, does the causative lesion lie in the central nervous system or the peripheral nervous system?

In this section, you will learn the techniques for a practical and reasonably comprehensive examination of the nervous system. It is important to master the techniques for a thorough examination. At first these techniques may seem difficult, but with practice, dedication, and supervision you will come to feel comfortable evaluating neurologic symptoms and disease. You should be active in your learning and ask your instructors or even neurologists to review your skills.

The detail of an appropriate neurologic examination varies widely. As you gain experience, you will find that in healthy persons your examination will come to be relatively brief. When you detect abnormal findings, your examination will become more comprehensive. Be aware that neurologists may use many other techniques in specific situations.

For efficiency, you should integrate certain portions of the neurologic assessment with other parts of your examination. Survey the patient's mental status and speech during the interview, for example, even though you may wish to do further testing during your neurologic evaluation. Assess some of the cranial nerves as you examine the head and neck, and inspect the arms and legs for neurologic abnormalities while you also observe the peripheral vascular and musculoskeletal systems. Chapter 3 provides an outline for this kind of integrated approach. Think about and describe your findings, however, in terms of the nervous system as a unit.

Organize your thinking into five categories: (1) mental status, speech and language, (2) cranial nerves, (3) the motor system, (4) the sensory system, and (5) reflexes. If your findings are abnormal, begin to group them into patterns of central or peripheral disorders.

Mental Status

Your assessment of mental status, such as the General Survey, begins with the first words of the interview. As you gather the health history, you will quickly discern the patient's level of *alertness* and *orientation, mood, attention,* and *memory.* As the history unfolds, you will learn about the patient's *insight* and *judgment,* as well as any *recurring or unusual thoughts or perceptions.* For some, you will need to supplement your interview with specific questions and a more formal evaluation of mental status. Just as symptoms, blood pressure, and valvular murmurs help you to distinguish, for example, health from disease in the cardiovascular system, specific components of mental function illuminate the workings of the mind. Although these components do not encompass all the aspects of human thought and feeling, they serve as useful and continually important clinical tools.

Components of the mental status examination include:

- Appearance and behavior
- Speech and language
- Mood
- Thoughts and perceptions
- Cognitive function, including memory, attention, information and vocabulary, calculations, and abstract thinking and constructional ability.

Many of these terms are familiar to you from social conversation. Take the time to learn their special meaning in the context of a formal mental status evaluation.

COMPONENTS OF THE MENTAL STATUS EXAMINATION

Level of consciousness	Alertness or state of awareness of the environment
Attention	The ability to focus or concentrate over time on one task or activity—an inattentive or distractible person with impaired consciousness has difficulty giving a history or responding to questions.
Memory	The process of registering or recording information, tested by asking for immediate repetition of material, followed by storage or retention of information. *Recent or short-term memory* covers minutes, hours, or days; *remote or long-term memory* refers to intervals of years.

Orientation	Awareness of personal identity, place, and time; requires both memory and attention
Perceptions	Sensory awareness of objects in the environment and their interrelationships (external stimuli); also refers to internal stimuli such as dreams or hallucinations
Thought processes	The logic, coherence, and relevance of the patient's thought as it leads to selected goals, or *how* people think
Thought content	*What* the patient thinks about, including level of insight and judgment
Insight	Awareness that symptoms or disturbed behaviors are normal or abnormal; for example, distinguishing between daydreams and hallucinations that seem real
Judgment	Process of comparing and evaluating alternatives when deciding on a course of action; reflects values that may or may not be based on reality and social conventions or norms
Affect	An observable, usually episodic, feeling tone expressed through voice, facial expression, and demeanor
Mood	A more sustained emotion that may color a person's view of the world (mood is to affect as climate is to weather)
Language	A complex symbolic system for expressing, receiving, and comprehending words; as with consciousness, attention, and memory, language is essential for assessing other mental functions
Higher cognitive functions	Assessed by vocabulary, fund of information, abstract thinking, calculations, construction of objects that have two or three dimensions

Distinguishing the interplay of body and mind in relation to these attributes is very important but not always easy. Mental disorders such as anxiety or depression may take the form of somatic complaints. Likewise, physical illness can cause mental and emotional responses and in older patients, can impair mental function without causing typical symptoms or signs such as fever or pain. Always look carefully for physical or pharmacologic causes as you try to understand the context and emotional meaning of changes in mental status. Some mental status evaluations are complicated by personality factors, psychodynamics, or the patient's personal experiences, areas that can be explored during the interview (but not covered in this chapter). By integrating and correlating all the relevant data, the clinician tries to understand the person as a whole.

As a student, you may feel reluctant to perform mental status examinations, wondering if they will upset patients, invade their privacy, or result in labeling their thoughts or behavior as pathologic. Such concerns are understandable and appropriate. An insensitive examination of mental status may alarm a patient, and even a skillful examination may bring to conscious awareness an embarrassing or upsetting deficit that the patient was trying to ignore. You may wish to discuss some of these concerns with your instructor or other experienced clinicians. As with other realms of interviewing and assessment, your skills and confidence will improve with practice and rewards will follow. Remember that many patients will appreciate an understanding listener, and some will owe their health, their safety, or even their lives to your attention.

The format that follows should help to organize your observations, but it is not intended as a step-by-step guide. When a full examination is indicated, you should be flexible in your approach but thorough in what you cover. In some situations, however, sequence is important. If during your initial interview the patient's consciousness, attention, comprehension of words, or ability to speak seems impaired, assess this attribute promptly. Such a patient cannot give a reliable history and you will not be able to test most of the other mental functions.

APPEARANCE AND BEHAVIOR

Use here all the relevant observations made throughout the course of your history and examination. Include these areas:

Level of Consciousness. Is the patient awake and alert? Does the patient seem to understand your questions and respond appropriately and reasonably quickly, or is there a tendency to lose track of the topic and fall silent or even asleep?

See the table on Level of Consciousness (Arousal), p. 595.

If the patient does not respond to your questions, escalate the stimulus in steps:

- Speak to the patient by name and in a loud voice.

Lethargic patients are drowsy but open their eyes and look at you, respond to questions, and then fall asleep.

- Shake the patient gently, as if awakening a sleeper.

Obtunded patients open their eyes and look at you, but respond slowly and are somewhat confused.

If there is no response to these stimuli, promptly assess the patient for stupor or coma—severe reductions in the level of consciousness (see p. 595).

Posture and Motor Behavior. Does the patient lie in bed, or prefer to walk about? Note body posture and the patient's ability to relax. Observe the pace, range, and character of movements. Do they seem to be under voluntary control? Are certain parts immobile? Do posture and motor activity change with topics under discussion or with activities or people around the patient?

Tense posture, restlessness, and fidgetiness of anxiety; crying, pacing, and handwringing of agitated depression; hopeless, slumped posture and slowed movements of depression; singing, dancing, and expansive movements of a manic episode.

Dress, Grooming, and Personal Hygiene. How is the patient dressed? Is clothing clean, pressed, and properly fastened? How does it compare with clothing worn by people of comparable age and social group? Note the patient's hair, nails, teeth, skin, and, if present, beard. How are they groomed? How do the person's grooming and hygiene compare with those of other people of comparable age, lifestyle, and socioeconomic group? Compare one side of the body with the other.

Grooming and personal hygiene may deteriorate in depression, schizophrenia, and dementia. Excessive fastidiousness may be seen in an obsessive–compulsive disorder. One-sided neglect may result from a lesion in the opposite parietal cortex, usually the non-dominant side.

Facial Expression. Observe the face, both at rest and when the patient is interacting with others. Watch for variations in expression with topics under discussion. Are they appropriate? Or is the face relatively immobile throughout?

Expressions of anxiety, depression, apathy, anger, elation. Facial immobility of parkinsonism

Manner, Affect, and Relationship to Persons and Things. Using your observations of facial expressions, voice, and body movements, assess the patient's affect. Does it vary appropriately with topics under discussion, or is the affect labile, blunted, or flat? Does it seem inappropriate or extreme at certain points? If so, how? Note the patient's openness, approachability, and reactions to others and to the surroundings. Does the patient seem to hear or see things that you do not or seem to be conversing with someone who is not there?

Anger, hostility, suspiciousness, or evasiveness of paranoid patients. Elation and euphoria of the manic syndrome. Flat affect and remoteness of schizophrenia. Apathy (dulled affect with detachment and indifference) in dementia. Anxiety, depression

SPEECH AND LANGUAGE

Throughout the interview, note the characteristics of the patient's speech, including the following:

Quantity. Is the patient talkative or relatively silent? Are comments spontaneous or only responsive to direct questions?

Rate. Is speech fast or slow?

Slow speech of depression; accelerated rapid, loud speech in mania

Loudness. Is speech loud or soft?

Articulation of Words. Are the words spoken clearly and distinctly? Is there a nasal quality to the speech?

Dysarthria refers to defective articulation. *Aphasia* refers to a disorder of language. See Table 16-2, Disorders of Speech, p. 600.

Fluency. This involves the rate, flow, and melody of speech and the content and use of words. Be alert for abnormalities of spontaneous speech such as these:

- Hesitancies and gaps in the flow and rhythm of words
- Disturbed inflections, such as a monotone
- Circumlocutions, in which phrases or sentences are substituted for a word the person cannot think of, such as "what you write with" for "pen"

These abnormalities suggest aphasia. The patient may have so much difficulty in talking or in understanding others that you may not be able to obtain a history. You may also falsely suspect a psychotic disorder.

- Paraphasias, in which words are malformed ("I write with a den"), wrong ("I write with a bar"), or invented ("I write with a dar").

If the patient's speech lacks meaning or fluency, proceed with further testing as outlined in the following table.

Testing for Aphasia

Word Comprehension	Ask the patient to follow a one-stage command, such as "Point to your nose." Try a two-stage command: "Point to your mouth, then your knee."
Repetition	Ask the patient to repeat a phrase of one-syllable words (the most difficult repetition task): "No ifs, ands, or buts."
Naming	Ask the patient to name the parts of a watch.
Reading Comprehension	Ask the patient to read a paragraph aloud.
Writing	Ask the patient to write a sentence.

These tests help you to decide what kind of aphasia the patient may have. Remember that deficiencies in vision, hearing, intelligence, and education may also affect performance. Two common kinds of aphasia—Wernicke's and Broca's—are compared in Table 16-2, Disorders of Speech, p. 600.

A person who can write a correct sentence does not have aphasia.

MOOD

Assess mood during the interview by exploring the patient's own perceptions of it. Find out about the patient's usual mood level and how it has varied with life events. "How did you feel about that?", for example, or, more generally, "How are your spirits?" The reports of relatives and friends may be of great value.

Moods include sadness and deep melancholy; contentment, joy, euphoria, and elation; anger and rage; anxiety and worry; and detachment and indifference.

What has the patient's mood been like? How intense has it been? Has it been labile or fairly unchanging? How long has it lasted? Is it appropriate to the patient's circumstances? In case of depression, have there also been episodes of an elevated mood, suggesting a bipolar disorder?

For depressive and bipolar disorders, see Table 16-1, Disorders of Mood, p. 599.

If you suspect depression, assess its depth and any associated risk of suicide. A series of questions such as the following is useful, proceeding as far as the patient's positive answers warrant.

> Do you get pretty discouraged (or depressed or blue)?
> How low do you feel?
> What do you see for yourself in the future?
> Do you ever feel that life isn't worth living? Or that you would just as soon be dead?
> Have you ever thought of doing away with yourself?
> How did (do) you think you would do it?
> What would happen after you were dead?

Asking about suicidal thoughts does not implant the idea in the patient's mind, and it may be the only way to get the information. Although many student clinicians feel uneasy about exploring this topic, most patients can discuss their thoughts and feelings about it freely with you, sometimes with considerable relief. By such discussion, you demonstrate your interest and concern for what may well be the patient's most serious and threatening problem. By avoiding the issue, you may miss the most important feature of the patient's illness.

THOUGHT AND PERCEPTIONS

Thought Processes. Assess the logic, relevance, organization, and coherence of the patient's thought processes as they are revealed in words and speech throughout the interview. Does speech progress in a logical manner toward a goal? Here you are using the patient's speech as a window into the patient's mind. Listen for patterns of speech that suggest disorders of thought processes, as outlined in the table below.

Variations and Abnormalities in Thought Processes

Circumstantiality	Speech characterized by indirection and delay in reaching the point because of unnecessary detail, although the components of the description have a meaningful connection. Many people without mental disorders speak circumstantially.	Observed in obsessional persons
Derailment (Loosening of Associations)	Speech in which a person shifts from one subject to others that are unrelated or only obliquely related without realizing that the subjects are not meaningfully connected. Ideas slip off the track between clauses, not within them.	Observed in schizophrenia, manic episodes, and other psychotic disorders
Flight of Ideas	An almost continuous flow of accelerated speech in which a person changes abruptly from topic to topic. Changes are usually based on understandable associations, plays on words, or distracting stimuli, but the ideas do not progress to sensible conversation.	Most frequently noted in manic episodes
Neologisms	Invented or distorted words, or words with new and highly idiosyncratic meanings	Observed in schizophrenia, other psychotic disorders, and aphasia
Incoherence	Speech that is largely incomprehensible because of illogic, lack of meaningful connections, abrupt changes in topic, or disordered grammar or word use. Shifts in meaning occur within clauses. Flight of ideas, when severe, may produce incoherence.	Observed in severely disturbed psychotic persons (usually schizophrenic)
Blocking	Sudden interruption of speech in midsentence or before completion of an idea. The person attributes this to losing the thought. Blocking occurs in normal people.	Blocking may be striking in schizophrenia.
Confabulation	Fabrication of facts or events in response to questions, to fill in the gaps in an impaired memory	Common with amnesia
Perseveration	Persistent repetition of words or ideas	Occurs in schizophrenia and other psychotic disorders
Echolalia	Repetition of the words and phrases of others	Occurs in manic episodes and schizophrenia
Clanging	Speech in which a person chooses a word on the basis of sound rather than meaning, as in rhyming and punning speech. For example, "Look at my eyes and nose, wise eyes and rosy nose. Two to one, the ayes have it!"	Occurs in schizophrenia and manic episodes

Thought Content. You should ascertain most of the information relevant to thought content during the interview. Follow appropriate leads as they occur rather than using stereotyped lists of specific questions. For example, "You mentioned a few minutes ago that a neighbor was responsible for your entire illness. Can you tell me more about that?" Or, in another situation, "What do you think about at times like these?"

You may need to make more specific inquiries. If so, couch them in tactful and accepting terms. "When people are upset like this, they sometimes can't keep certain thoughts out of their minds," or ". . . things seem unreal. Have you experienced anything like this?"

In these ways find out about any of the patterns shown in the following table.

Abnormalities of Thought Content

Compulsions	Repetitive behaviors or mental acts that a person feels driven to perform in order to produce or prevent some future state of affairs, although expectation of such an effect is unrealistic	Compulsions, obsessions, phobias, and anxieties are often associated with neurotic disorders. See Table 16-3, Anxiety Disorders (p. 601).
Obsessions	Recurrent, uncontrollable thoughts, images, or impulses that a person considers unacceptable and alien	
Phobias	Persistent, irrational fears, accompanied by a compelling desire to avoid the stimulus	
Anxieties	Apprehensions, fears, tensions, or uneasiness that may be focused (phobia) or free floating (a general sense of ill-defined dread or impending doom)	
Feelings of Unreality	A sense that things in the environment are strange, unreal, or remote	
Feelings of Depersonalization	A sense that one's self is different, changed, or unreal, or has lost identity or become detached from one's mind or body	Delusions and feelings of unreality or depersonalization are more often associated with psychotic disorders. See Table 16-4, Psychotic Disorders (p. 602). Delusions may also occur in delirium, severe mood disorders, and dementia.
Delusions	False, fixed, personal beliefs that are not shared by other members of the person's culture or subculture. Examples include: ▪ *Delusions of persecution* ▪ *Grandiose delusions* ▪ *Delusional jealousy* ▪ *Delusions of reference,* in which a person believes that external events, objects, or people have a particular and unusual personal significance (e.g., that the radio or television might be commenting on or giving instructions to the person) ▪ *Delusions of being controlled* by an outside force ▪ *Somatic delusions* of having a disease, disorder, or physical defect ▪ *Systematized delusions,* a single delusion with many elaborations or a cluster of related delusions around a single theme, all systematized into a complex network	

Perceptions. Inquire about false perceptions in a manner similar to that used for thought content. For example, "When you heard the voice speaking to you, what did it say? How did it make you feel?" Or, "After you've been drinking a lot, do you ever see things that aren't really there?" Or, "Sometimes after major surgery like this, people hear peculiar or frightening things. Have you experienced anything like that?" In these ways find out about the following abnormal perceptions.

Abnormalities of Perception		
Illusions	Misinterpretations of real external stimuli	Illusions may occur in grief reactions, delirium, acute and posttraumatic stress disorders, and schizophrenia.
Hallucinations	Subjective sensory perceptions in the absence of relevant external stimuli. The person may or may not recognize the experiences as false. Hallucinations may be auditory, visual, olfactory, gustatory, tactile, or somatic. (False perceptions associated with dreaming, falling asleep, and awakening are not classified as hallucinations.)	Hallucinations may occur in delirium, dementia (less commonly), post-traumatic stress disorder, schizophrenia, and alcoholism.

Insight and Judgment. These attributes are usually best assessed during the interview.

Insight. Some of your very first questions to the patient often yield important information about insight: "What brings you to the hospital?" "What seems to be the trouble?" "What do you think is wrong?" More specifically, note whether or not the patient is aware that a particular mood, thought, or perception is abnormal or part of an illness.

Patients with psychotic disorders often lack insight into their illness. Denial of impairment may accompany some neurologic disorders.

Judgment. You can usually assess judgment by noting the patient's responses to family situations, jobs, use of money, and interpersonal conflicts. "How do you plan to get the help you'll need after leaving the hospital?" "How are you going to manage if you lose your job?" "If your husband starts to abuse you again, what will you do?" "Who will attend to your financial affairs while you are in the nursing home?"

Judgment may be poor in delirium, dementia, mental retardation, and psychotic states. Judgment is affected also by anxiety, mood disorders, intelligence, education, socioeconomic options, and cultural values.

Note whether decisions and actions are based on reality or, for example, on impulse, wish fulfillment, or disordered thought content. What values seem to underlie the patient's decisions and behavior? Allowing for cultural variations, how do these compare with mature adult standards? Because judgment is part of the maturational response, it may be variable and unpredictable during adolescence.

COGNITIVE FUNCTIONS

Orientation. By skillful questioning you can often determine the patient's orientation in the context of the interview. For example, you can ask quite naturally for specific dates and times, the patient's address and

Disorientation occurs especially when memory or attention is impaired, as in delirium.

telephone number, the names of family members, or the route taken to the hospital. At times—when rechecking the status of a delirious patient, for example—simple, direct questions may be indicated.

"Can you tell me what time it is now . . . and what day is it?" In either of these ways, determine the patient's orientation for the following:

- *Time* (e.g., the time of day, day of the week, month, season, date and year, duration of hospitalization)
- *Place* (e.g., the patient's residence, the names of the hospital, city, and state)
- *Person* (e.g., the patient's own name, and the names of relatives and professional personnel)

Attention. These tests of attention are commonly used:

Digit Span. Explain that you would like to test the patient's ability to concentrate, perhaps adding that people tend to have trouble with that when they are in pain, or ill, or feverish. Recite a series of digits, starting with two at a time and speaking each number clearly at a rate of about one per second. Ask the patient to repeat the numbers back to you. If this repetition is accurate, try a series of three numbers, then four, and so on as long as the patient responds correctly. Jotting down the numbers as you say them helps to ensure your own accuracy. If the patient makes a mistake, try once more with another series of the same length. Stop after a second failure in a single series.

Causes of poor performance include delirium, dementia, mental retardation, and performance anxiety.

In choosing digits you may use street numbers, zip codes, telephone numbers, and other numerical sequences that are familiar to you, but avoid consecutive numbers, easily recognized dates, and sequences that possibly are familiar to the patient.

Now, starting again with a series of two, ask the patient to repeat the numbers to you backward.

Normally, a person should be able to repeat correctly at least five digits forward and four backward.

Serial 7s. Instruct the patient, "Starting from a hundred, subtract 7, and keep subtracting 7. . . ." Note the effort required and the speed and accuracy of the responses. (Writing down the answers helps you keep up with the arithmetic.) Normally, a person can complete serial 7s in 1½ minutes, with fewer than four errors. If the patient cannot do serial 7s, try 3s or counting backward.

Poor performance may be due to delirium, the late stage of dementia, mental retardation, loss of calculating ability, anxiety, or depression. Also consider the possibility of limited education.

Spelling Backward. This can substitute for serial 7s. Say a five-letter word, spell it, e.g., W-O-R-L-D, and ask the patient to spell it backward.

Remote Memory. Inquire about birthdays, anniversaries, social security number, names of schools attended, jobs held, or past historical events such as wars relevant to the patient's past.

Remote memory may be impaired in the late stage of dementia.

Recent Memory (e.g., the events of the day). Ask questions with answers that you can check against other sources so that you will know whether or not the patient is confabulating (making up facts to compensate for a defective memory). These might include the day's weather, today's appointment time, and medications or laboratory tests taken during the day. (Asking what the patient had for breakfast may be a waste of time unless you can check the accuracy of the answer.)

Recent memory is impaired in dementia and delirium. See Table 16-5, Delirium and Dementia, p. 603. *Amnestic disorders* impair memory or new learning ability significantly and reduce a person's social or occupational functioning, but they do not have the global features of delirium or dementia. Anxiety, depression, and mental retardation may also impair recent memory.

New Learning Ability. Give the patient three or four words such as "83 Water Street and blue," or "table, flower, green, and hamburger." Ask the patient to repeat them so that you know that the information has been heard and registered. This step, like digit span, tests registration and immediate recall. Then proceed to other parts of the examination. After about 3 to 5 minutes, ask the patient to repeat the words. Note the accuracy of the response, awareness of whether or not it is correct, and any tendency to confabulate. Normally, a person should be able to remember the words.

HIGHER COGNITIVE FUNCTIONS

Information and Vocabulary. Information and vocabulary, when observed clinically, provide a rough estimate of a person's intelligence. Assess them during the interview. Ask a student, for example, about favorite courses, or inquire about a person's work, hobbies, reading, favorite television programs, or current events. Explore such topics first with simple questions, then with more difficult ones. Note the person's grasp of information, the complexity of the ideas expressed, and the vocabulary used.

If considered in the context of cultural and educational background, information and vocabulary are fairly good indicators of intelligence. They are relatively unaffected by any but the most severe psychiatric disorders, and may be helpful for distinguishing mentally retarded adults (whose information and vocabulary are limited) from those with mild or moderate dementia (whose information and vocabulary are fairly well preserved).

More directly, you can ask about specific facts, such as these:

The name of the president, vice president, or governor
The names of the last four or five presidents
The names of five large cities in the country

Calculating Ability. Test the patient's ability to do arithmetical calculations, starting at the rote level with simple addition ("What is 4 + 3? . . . 8 + 7?") and multiplication ("What is 5 × 6? . . . 9 × 7?"). The task can be made more difficult by using two-digit numbers ("15 + 12" or "25 × 6") or longer, written examples.

Poor performance may be a useful sign of dementia or may accompany aphasia, but it must be assessed in terms of the patient's intelligence and education.

Alternatively, pose practical and functionally important questions, such as "If something costs 78 cents and you give the clerk one dollar, how much should you get back?"

Abstract Thinking. The capacity to think abstractly can be tested in two ways.

Concrete responses are often given by persons with mental retardation, delirium, or dementia, but may also be simply a function of limited education. Schizophrenics may respond concretely or with personal, bizarre interpretations.

Proverbs. Ask the patient what people mean when they use some of the following proverbs:

A stitch in time saves nine.
Don't count your chickens before they're hatched.
The proof of the pudding is in the eating.
A rolling stone gathers no moss.
The squeaking wheel gets the grease.

Note the relevance of the answers and their degree of concreteness or abstractness. For example, "You should sew a rip before it gets bigger" is concrete, while "Prompt attention to a problem prevents trouble" is abstract. Average patients should give abstract or semiabstract responses.

Similarities. Ask the patient to tell you how the following are alike:

An orange and an apple	A church and a theater
A cat and a mouse	A piano and a violin
A child and a dwarf	Wood and coal

Note the accuracy and relevance of the answers and their degree of concreteness or abstractness. For example, "A cat and a mouse are both animals" is abstract, "They both have tails" is concrete, and "A cat chases a mouse" is not relevant.

Constructional Ability. The task here is to copy figures of increasing complexity onto a piece of blank unlined paper. Show each figure one at a time and ask the patient to copy it as well as possible.

The three diamonds below are rated poor, fair, and good (but not excellent).

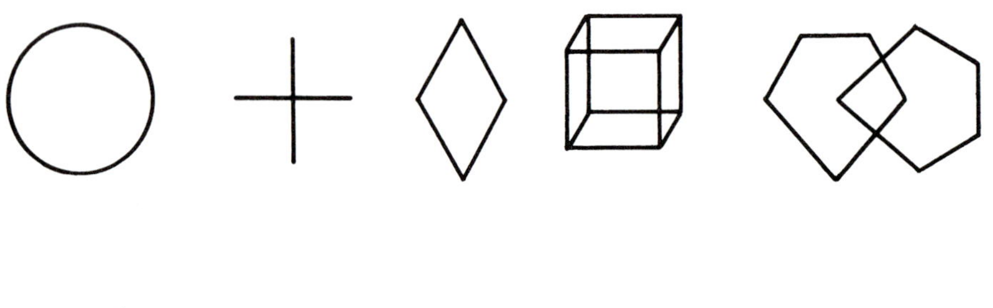

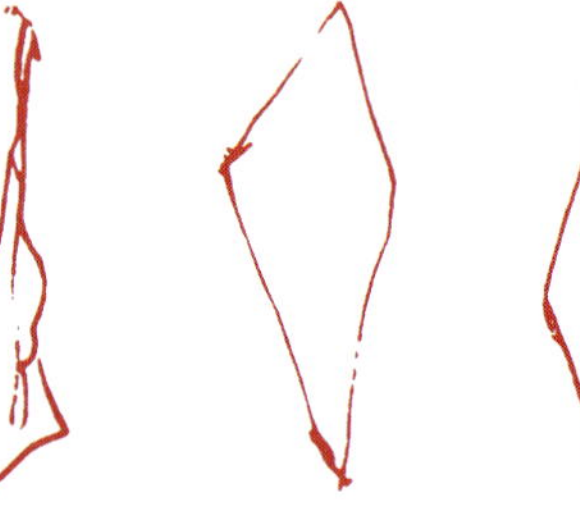

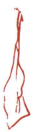

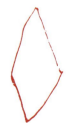

(Strub RL, Black FW: The Mental Status Examination in Neurology, 2nd ed. Philadelphia, FA Davis, 1985)

In another approach, ask the patient to draw a clock face complete with numbers and hands. The example below is rated excellent.

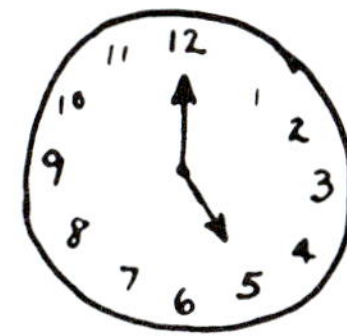

(Strub RL, Black FW: The Mental Status Examination in Neurology, 2nd ed. Philadelphia, FA Davis, 1985)

These three clocks are poor, fair, and good.

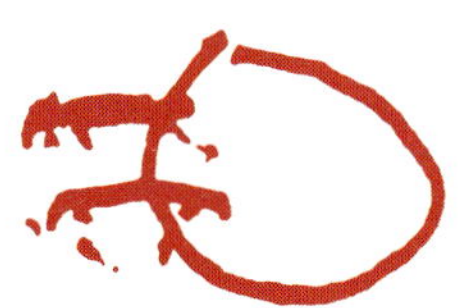

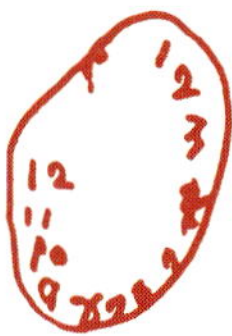

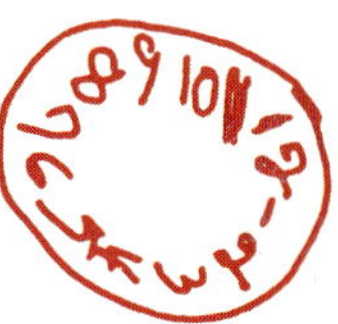

If vision and motor ability are intact, poor constructional ability suggests dementia or parietal lobe damage. Mental retardation may also impair performance.

The Cranial Nerves

Overview. The examination of the cranial nerves (often abbreviated as CN) can be summarized as follows:

I	Smell
II	Visual acuity, visual fields, and ocular fundi
II, III	Pupillary reactions
III, IV, VI	Extraocular movements
V	Corneal reflexes, facial sensation, and jaw movements
VII	Facial movements
VIII	Hearing
IX, X	Swallowing and rise of the palate, gag reflex
V, VII, X, XII	Voice and speech
XI	Shoulder and neck movements
XII	Tongue symmetry and position

Cranial Nerve I—Olfactory. Test the *sense of smell* by presenting the patient with familiar and nonirritating odors. First be sure that each nasal passage is open by compressing one side of the nose and asking the patient to sniff through the other. The patient should then close both eyes. Occlude one nostril and test smell in the other with such substances as cloves, coffee, soap, or vanilla. Ask if the patient smells anything and, if so, what. Test the other side. A person should normally perceive odor on each side, and can often identify it.

Loss of smell has many causes, including nasal disease, head trauma, smoking, aging, and the use of cocaine. It may be congenital.

Cranial Nerve II—Optic. Test *visual acuity* (see pp. 144–145).

Inspect the *optic fundi* with your ophthalmoscope, paying special attention to the optic discs (see pp. 151–155).

Optic atrophy, papilledema

Screen the visual fields by confrontation (see pp. 145–146). Occasionally—in a stroke patient, for example—screening indicates a visual field defect, such as a homonymous hemianopsia, that you cannot confirm by testing one eye at a time. This screening observation, nevertheless, is significant.

These findings suggest visual *extinction,* a subtle impairment detectable only when testing both eyes simultaneously. It suggests a lesion in the parietal cortex.

Cranial Nerves II and III—Optic and Oculomotor. Inspect the size and shape of the pupils, and compare one side with the other. Test the *pupillary reactions to light*; if these are abnormal, examine the *near response* also (see p. 149).

See Table 5-9, Pupillary Abnormalities (p. 181).

Cranial Nerves III, IV, and VI—Oculomotor, Trochlear, and Abducens. Test the *extraocular movements* in the six cardinal directions of gaze, and look for loss of conjugate movements in any of the six directions. Check convergence of the eyes. Identify any nystagmus, noting the direction of gaze in which it appears, the plane in which movements occur (horizontal, vertical, rotary, or mixed), and the direction of the quick and slow components (see pp. 149–151).

See Table 5-10, Deviations of the Eyes (p. 182).

See Table 16-9, Nystagmus (pp. 610–611).

Look for *ptosis* (drooping of the upper eyelids). A slight difference in the width of the palpebral fissures may be noted in about one third of all normal people.

Ptosis in 3rd nerve palsy, Horner's syndrome (ptosis, meiosis, anhidrosis), myasthenia gravis

Cranial Nerve V—Trigeminal

Motor. While palpating the temporal and masseter muscles in turn, ask the patient to clench his or her teeth. Note the strength of muscle contraction.

Weak or absent contraction of the temporal and masseter muscles on one side suggests a lesion of CN V. Bilateral weakness may result from peripheral or central involvement. When the patient has no teeth, this test may be difficult to interpret.

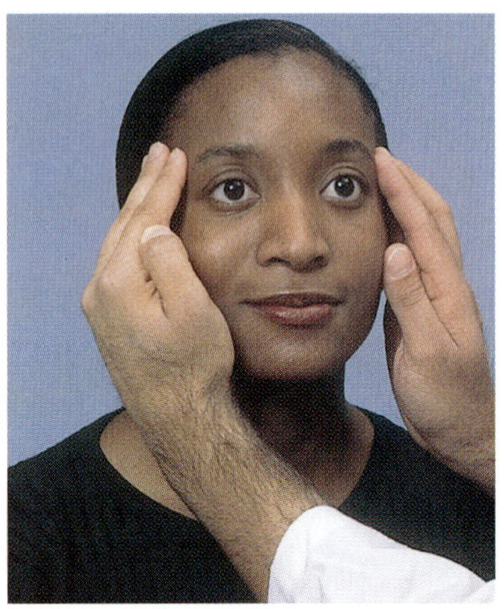

PALPATING TEMPORAL MUSCLES

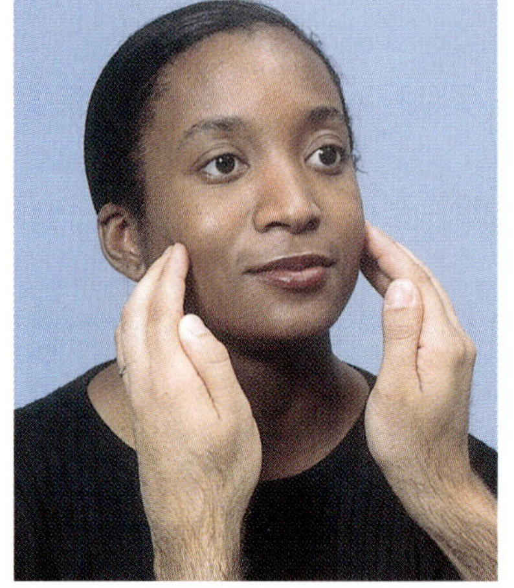

PALPATING MASSETER MUSCLES

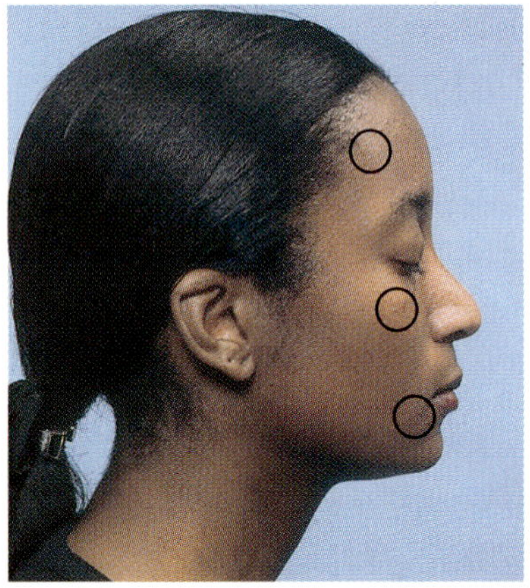

Sensory. After explaining what you plan to do, test the forehead, cheeks, and jaw on each side for *pain sensation*. Suggested areas are indicated by the circles. The patient's eyes should be closed. Use a safety pin or other suitable sharp object,* occasionally substituting the blunt end for the point as a stimulus. Ask the patient to report whether it is "sharp" or "dull" and to compare sides.

Unilateral decrease in or loss of facial sensation suggests a lesion of CN V or of interconnecting higher sensory pathways. Such a sensory loss may also be associated with a conversion reaction.

*To avoid transmitting infection, use a new object with each patient. You can create a sharp wood splinter by breaking or twisting a cotton swab. The cotton end of the swab can also be used as a dull stimulus.

If you find an abnormality, confirm it by testing *temperature sensation*. Two test tubes, filled with hot and ice-cold water, are the traditional stimuli. A tuning fork may also be used. It usually feels cool. If you are near running water, the fork is easily made colder or warm. Dry it before use. Touch the skin and ask the patient to identify "hot" or "cold."

Then test for *light touch*, using a fine wisp of cotton. Ask the patient to respond whenever you touch the skin.

Test *the corneal reflex*. Ask the patient to look up and away from you. Approaching from the other side, out of the patient's line of vision, and avoiding the eyelashes, touch the cornea (not just the conjunctiva) lightly with a fine wisp of cotton. If the patient is apprehensive, however, first touching the conjunctiva may allay fear.

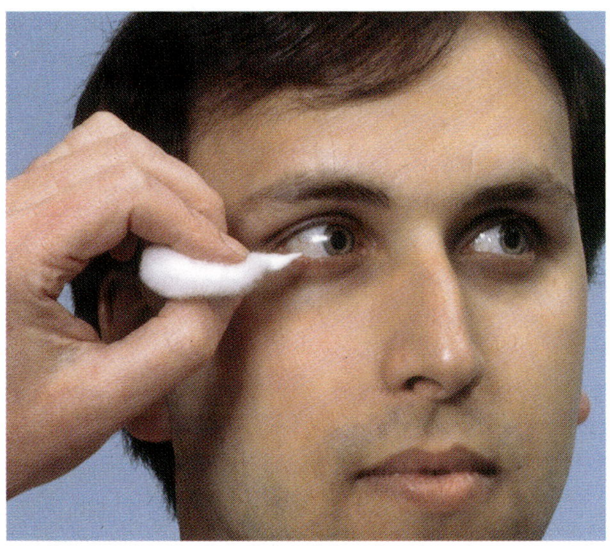

Look for blinking of the eyes, the normal reaction to this stimulus. (The sensory limb of this reflex is carried in CN V, the motor response in CN VII.) Use of contact lenses frequently diminishes or abolishes this reflex.

Absence of blinking suggests a lesion of CN V. A lesion of CN VII (the nerve to the muscles that close the eyes) may also impair this reflex.

Cranial Nerve VII—Facial. Inspect the face, both at rest and during conversation with the patient. Note any asymmetry (e.g., of the nasolabial folds), and observe any tics or other abnormal movements.

Flattening of the nasolabial fold and drooping of the lower eyelid suggest facial weakness.

Ask the patient to:

1. Raise both eyebrows.

2. Frown.

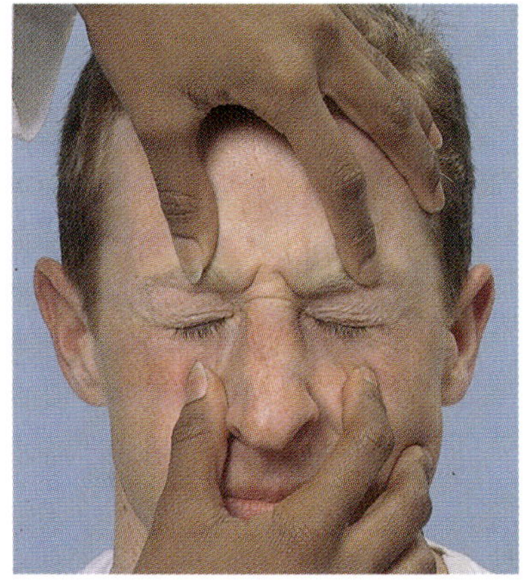

A peripheral injury to CN VII, as in Bell's palsy, affects both the upper and the lower face; a central lesion affects mainly the lower face. See Table 16-10, Types of Facial Paralysis (pp. 612–613).

3. Close both eyes tightly so that you cannot open them. Test muscular strength by trying to open them, as illustrated.
4. Show both upper and lower teeth.
5. Smile.
6. Puff out both cheeks.

In unilateral facial paralysis, the mouth droops on the paralyzed side when the patient smiles or grimaces.

Note any weakness or asymmetry.

Cranial Nerve VIII—Acoustic. Assess *hearing*. If hearing loss is present, (1) test for *lateralization,* and (2) compare *air and bone conduction* (see pp. 156–158).

See Table 5-19, Patterns of Hearing Loss (pp. 196–197).

Specific tests of *vestibular function* are seldom included in the usual neurologic examination. Consult textbooks of neurology or otolaryngology as the need arises.

Nystagmus may indicate vestibular dysfunction. See Table 16-9, Nystagmus (pp. 610–611).

Cranial Nerves IX and X—Glossopharyngeal and Vagus. Listen to the patient's *voice*. Is it hoarse or does it have a nasal quality?

Hoarseness in vocal cord paralysis; a nasal voice in paralysis of the palate

Is there difficulty in swallowing?

Pharyngeal or palatal weakness

Ask the patient to say "ah" or to yawn as you watch the *movements of the soft palate and the pharynx*. The soft palate normally rises symmetrically, the uvula remains in the midline, and each side of the posterior pharynx moves medially, like a curtain. The slightly curved uvula seen occasionally in a normal person should not be mistaken for a uvula deviated by a 10th nerve lesion.

The palate fails to rise with a bilateral lesion of the vagus nerve. In unilateral paralysis, one side of the palate fails to rise and, together with the uvula, is pulled toward the normal side (see p. 162).

Warn the patient that you are going to test the *gag reflex*. Stimulate the back of the throat lightly on each side in turn and note the gag reflex. It may be symmetrically diminished or absent in some normal people.

Unilateral absence of this reflex suggests a lesion of CN IX, perhaps CN X.

Cranial Nerve XI—Spinal Accessory. From behind, look for atrophy or fasciculations in the trapezius muscles, and compare one side with the

Weakness with atrophy and fasciculations indicates a peripheral nerve disorder. When the trapezius is paralyzed, the shoulder droops and the scapula is displaced downward and laterally.

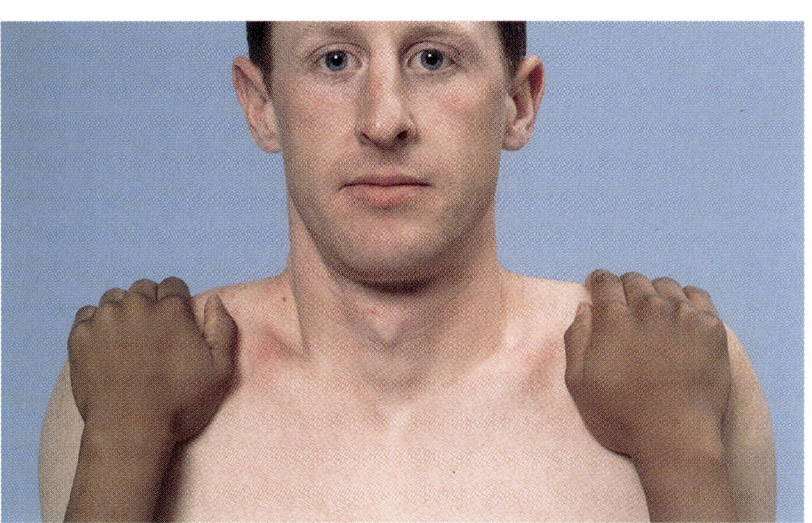

other. Ask the patient to shrug both shoulders upward against your hands. Note the strength and contraction of the trapezii.

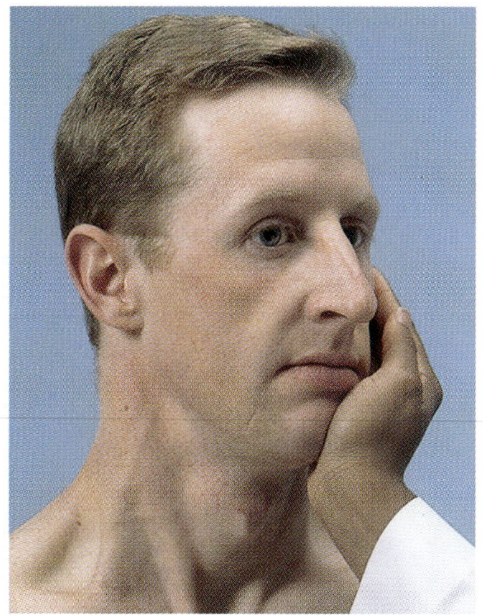

Ask the patient to turn his or her head to each side against your hand. Observe the contraction of the opposite sternomastoid and note the force of the movement against your hand.

A supine patient with bilateral weakness of the sternomastoids has difficulty raising the head off the pillow.

Cranial Nerve XII—Hypoglossal. Listen to the articulation of the patient's words. This depends on Cranial Nerves V, VII, and X as well as XII. Inspect the patient's tongue as it lies on the floor of the mouth. Look for any atrophy or *fasciculations* (fine, flickering, irregular movements in small groups of muscle fibers). Some coarser restless movements are often seen in a normal tongue. Then, with the patient's tongue protruded, look for asymmetry, atrophy, or deviation from the midline. Ask the patient to move the tongue from side to side, and note the symmetry of the movement. In ambiguous cases, ask the patient to push the tongue against the inside of each cheek in turn as you palpate externally for strength.

For poor articulation, or *dysarthria*, see Table 16-2, Disorders of Speech (p. 600). Atrophy and fasciculations in amyotrophic lateral sclerosis, polio

In a unilateral cortical lesion, the protruded tongue deviates transiently in a direction away from the side of the cortical lesion.

The Motor System

As you assess the motor system, focus on body position, involuntary movements, characteristics of the muscles (bulk, tone, and strength), and coordination. These components are described below in sequence. You may either use this sequence or check each component in the arms, legs, and trunk in turn. If you see an abnormality, identify the muscle(s) involved. Think about whether the abnormality is central or peripheral in origin, and begin to learn which nerves innervate the affected muscles.

Body Position. Observe the patient's body position during movement and at rest.

Abnormal positions alert you to neurologic deficits such as paralysis.

Involuntary Movements. Watch for involuntary movements such as tremors, tics, or fasciculations. Note their location, quality, rate, rhythm, and amplitude, and their relation to posture, activity, fatigue, emotion, and other factors.

See Table 16-8, Involuntary Movements (pp. 608–609).

Muscle Bulk. Compare the size and contours of muscles. Do the muscles look flat or concave, suggesting atrophy? If so, is the process unilateral or bilateral? Is it proximal or distal?

When looking for atrophy, pay particular attention to the hands, shoulders, and thighs. The thenar and hypothenar eminences should be full and convex, and the spaces between the metacarpals, where the dorsal interosseous muscles lie, should be full or only slightly depressed. Atrophy of hand muscles may occur with normal aging, however, as shown on the right below.

Muscular *atrophy* refers to a loss of muscle bulk (wasting). It results from diseases of the peripheral nervous system such as diabetic neuropathy, as well as diseases of the muscles themselves. *Hypertrophy* refers to an increase in bulk with proportionate strength, while increased bulk with diminished strength is called *pseudohypertrophy* (seen in the Duchenne form of muscular dystrophy).

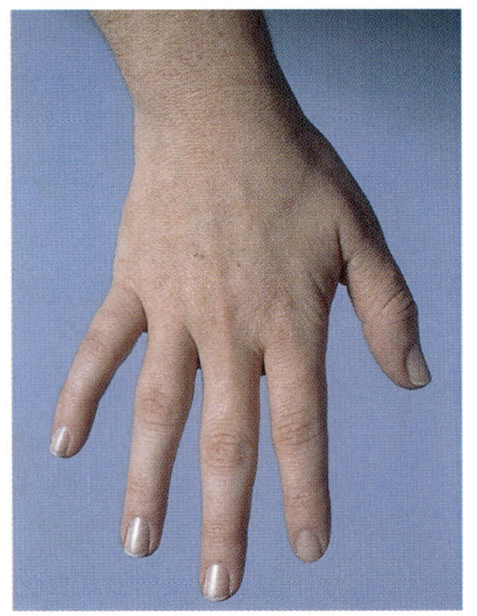

Hand of a 44-year-old woman

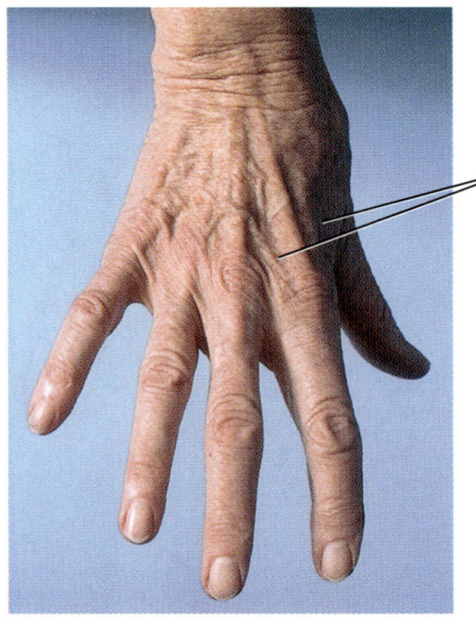

Hand of an 84-year-old woman

Flattening of the thenar and hypothenar eminences and furrowing between the metacarpals suggest atrophy. Localized atrophy of the thenar and hypothenar eminences suggests damage to the median and ulnar nerves, respectively.

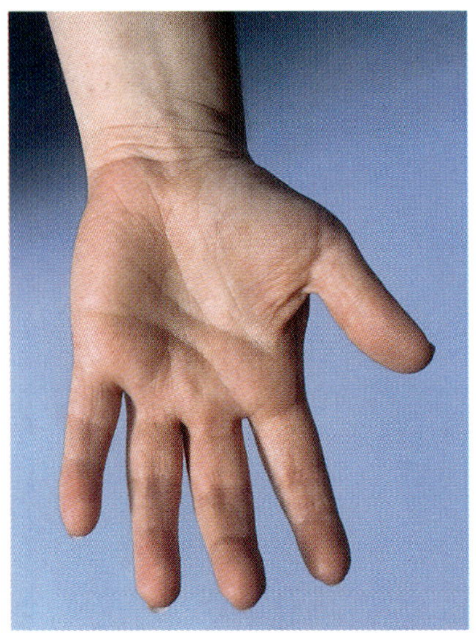

Hand of a 44-year-old woman

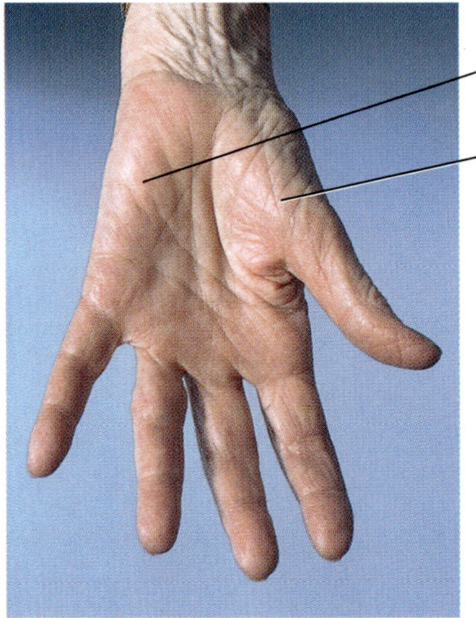

Hand of an 84-year-old woman

Other causes of muscular atrophy include motor neuron diseases, disuse of the muscles, rheumatoid arthritis, and protein-calorie malnutrition.

Be alert for fasciculations in atrophic muscles. If you see none, a tap on the muscle with a reflex hammer may stimulate them.

Fasciculations suggest lower motor neuron disease as a cause of atrophy.

Muscle Tone. When a normal muscle with an intact nerve supply is relaxed voluntarily, it maintains a slight residual tension known as muscle tone. This can be assessed best by feeling the muscle's resistance to passive stretch. Persuade the patient to relax. Take one hand with yours and, while supporting the elbow, flex and extend the patient's fingers, wrist, and elbow, and put the shoulder through a moderate range of motion. With practice, these actions can be combined into a single smooth movement. On each side, note muscle tone—the resistance offered to your movements. Tense patients may show increased resistance. You will learn the feel of normal resistance only with repeated practice.

Decreased resistance suggests disease of the peripheral nervous system, cerebellar disease, or the acute stages of spinal cord injury. See Table 16-11, Disorders of Muscle Tone (p. 614).

If you suspect decreased resistance, hold the forearm and shake the hand loosely back and forth. Normally the hand moves back and forth freely but is not completely floppy.

Marked floppiness indicates *hypotonic* or flaccid muscles.

If resistance is increased, determine whether it varies as you move the limb or whether it persists throughout the range of movement and in both directions, for example, during both flexion and extension. Feel for any jerkiness in the resistance.

Increased resistance that varies, commonly worse at the extremes of the range, is called *spasticity.* Resistance that persists throughout the range and in both directions is called *lead-pipe rigidity.*

To assess muscle tone in the legs, support the patient's thigh with one hand, grasp the foot with the other, and flex and extend the patient's knee and ankle on each side. Note the resistance to your movements.

Muscle Strength. Normal individuals vary widely in their strength, and your standard of normal, while admittedly rough, should allow for such variables as age, sex, and muscular training. A person's dominant side is usually slightly stronger than the other side. Keep this difference in mind when you compare sides.

Test muscle strength by asking the patient to move actively against your resistance or to resist your movement. Remember that a muscle is strongest when shortest, and weakest when longest.

If the muscles are too weak to overcome resistance, test them against gravity alone or with gravity eliminated. When the forearm rests in a pronated position, for example, dorsiflexion at the wrist can be tested against gravity alone. When the forearm is midway between pronation and supination, extension at the wrist can be tested with gravity eliminated. Finally, if the patient fails to move the body part, watch or feel for weak muscular contraction.

Impaired strength is called weakness (*paresis*). Absence of strength is called paralysis (*plegia*). *Hemiparesis* refers to weakness of one half of the body; *hemiplegia* to paralysis of one half of the body. *Paraplegia* means paralysis of the legs; *quadriplegia,* paralysis of all four limbs.

See Table 16-12, Disorders of the Central and Peripheral Nervous Systems (pp. 615–617).

Muscle strength is graded on a 0 to 5 scale:

0—No muscular contraction detected
1—A barely detectable flicker or trace of contraction
2—Active movement of the body part with gravity eliminated
3—Active movement against gravity
4—Active movement against gravity and some resistance
5—Active movement against full resistance without evident fatigue. This is normal muscle strength.

More experienced clinicians make further distinctions by using plus or minus signs toward the stronger end of this scale. Thus 4+ indicates good but not full strength, while 5− means a trace of weakness.

Methods for testing the major muscle groups are described below. The spinal root innervations and the muscles affected are shown in parentheses. To localize lesions in the spinal cord or the peripheral nervous system more precisely, additional testing may be necessary. For these specialized methods, refer to detailed texts of neurology.

Test flexion (C5, C6—biceps) *and extension* (C6, C7, C8—triceps) *at the elbow* by having the patient pull and push against your hand.

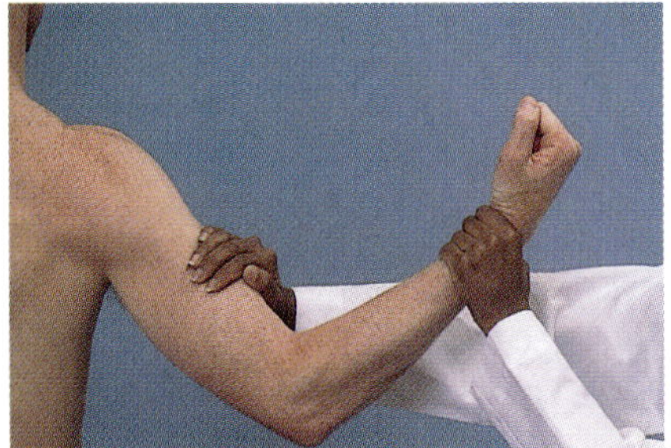

FLEXION

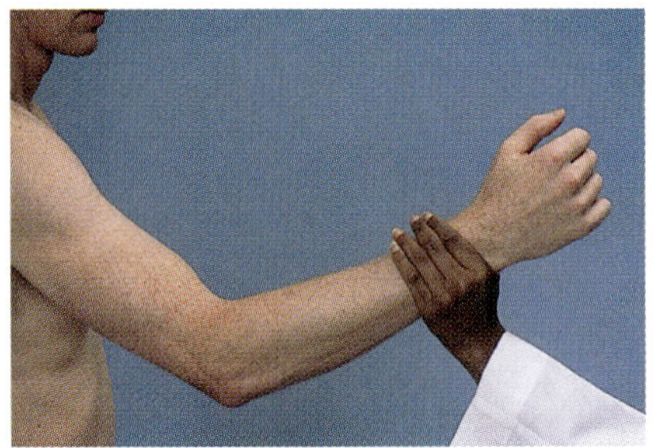

EXTENSION

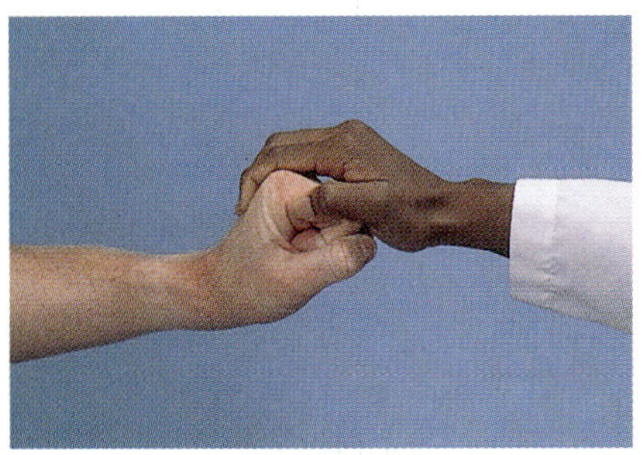

EXTENSION AT WRIST

Test extension at the wrist (C6, C7, C8, radial nerve) by asking the patient to make a fist and resist your pulling it down.

Weakness of extension is seen in peripheral nerve disease (e.g., radial nerve damage) and in central nervous system disease producing hemiplegia (e.g., stroke or multiple sclerosis).

Test the grip (C7, C8, T1). Ask the patient to squeeze two of your fingers as hard as possible and not let them go. (To avoid getting hurt by hard squeezes, place your own middle finger on top of your index finger.) You should normally have difficulty removing your fingers from the patient's grip. Testing both grips simultaneously with arms extended or in the lap facilitates comparison.

A weak grip may be due to either central or peripheral nervous system disease. It may also result from painful disorders of the hands.

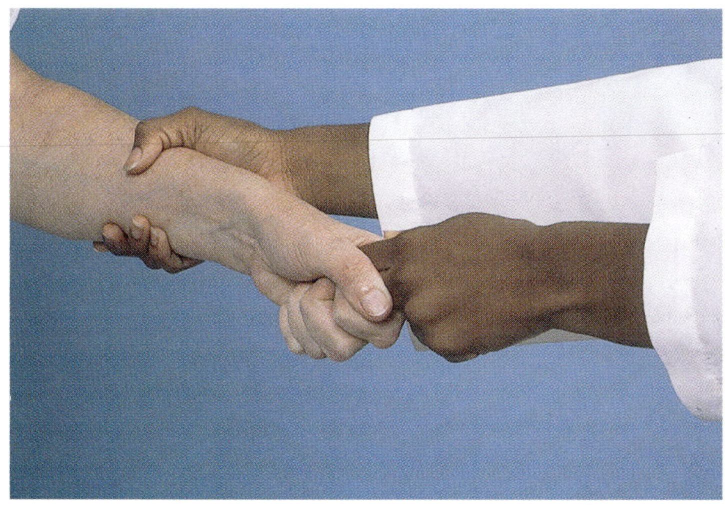

Test finger abduction (C8, T1, ulnar nerve). Position the patient's hand with palm down and fingers spread. Instructing the patient not to let you move the fingers, try to force them together.

Weak finger abduction in ulnar nerve disorders

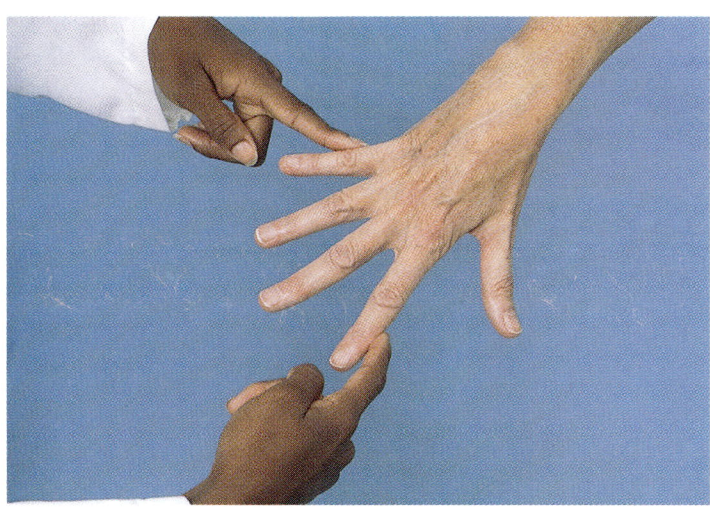

Test opposition of the thumb (C8, T1, median nerve). The patient should try to touch the tip of the little finger with the thumb, against your resistance.

Weak opposition of the thumb in median nerve disorders such as carpal tunnel syndrome

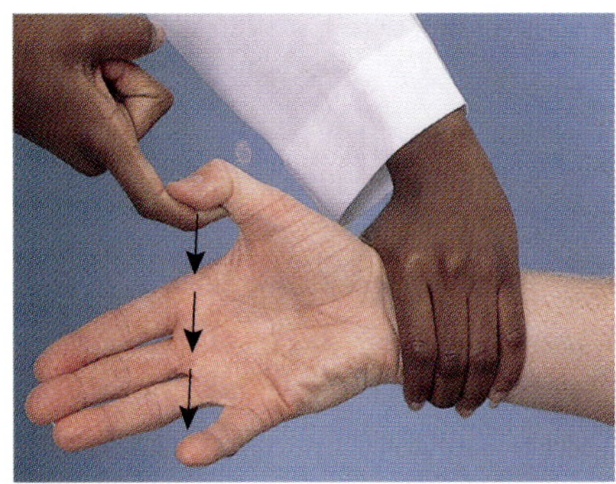

Assessment of *muscle strength of the trunk* may already have been made in other segments of the examination. It includes:

- Flexion, extension, and lateral bending of the spine, and
- Thoracic expansion and diaphragmatic excursion during respiration

Test flexion at the hip (L2, L3, L4—iliopsoas) by placing your hand on the patient's thigh and asking the patient to raise the leg against your hand.

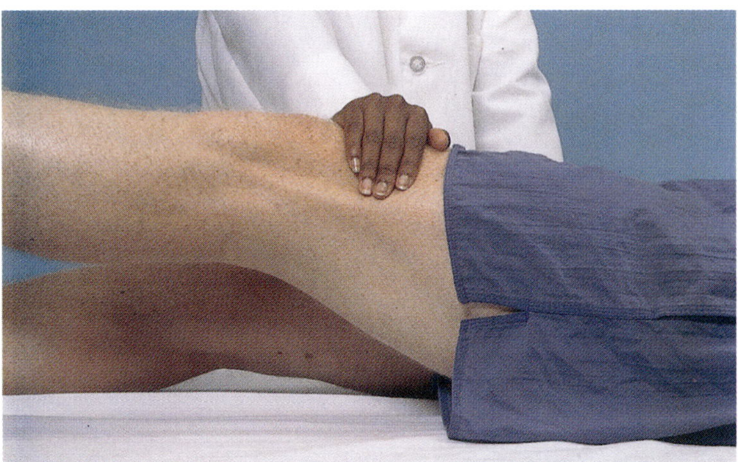

Test adduction at the hips (L2, L3, L4—adductors). Place your hands firmly on the bed between the patient's knees. Ask the patient to bring both legs together.

Symmetric weakness of the proximal muscles suggests a *myopathy* or muscle disorder; symmetric weakness of distal muscles suggests a *polyneuropathy,* or disorder of peripheral nerves.

Test abduction at the hips (L4, L5, S1—gluteus medius and minimus). Place your hands firmly on the bed outside the patient's knees. Ask the patient to spread both legs against your hands.

Test extension at the hips (S1—gluteus maximus). Have the patient push the posterior thigh down against your hand.

Test extension at the knee (L2, L3, L4—quadriceps). Support the knee in flexion and ask the patient to straighten the leg against your hand. The quadriceps is the strongest muscle in the body, so expect a forceful response.

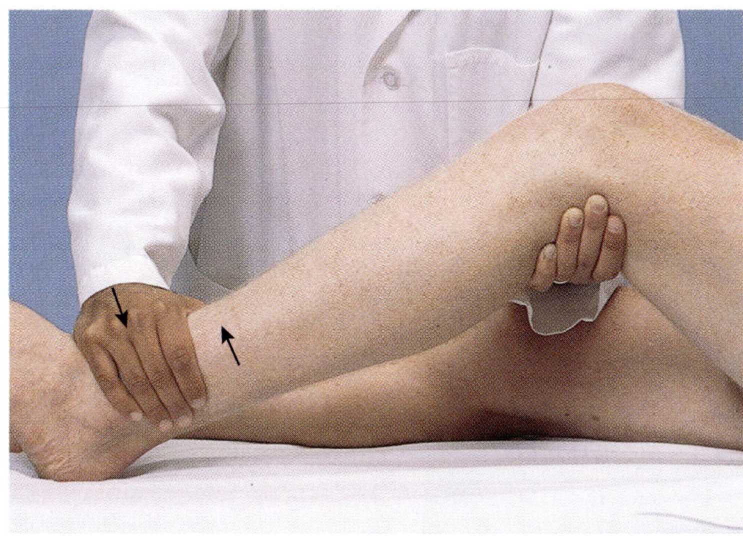

EXTENSION AT THE KNEE

Test flexion at the knee (L4, L5, S1, S2—hamstrings) as shown below. Place the patient's leg so that the knee is flexed with the foot resting on the bed. Tell the patient to keep the foot down as you try to straighten the leg.

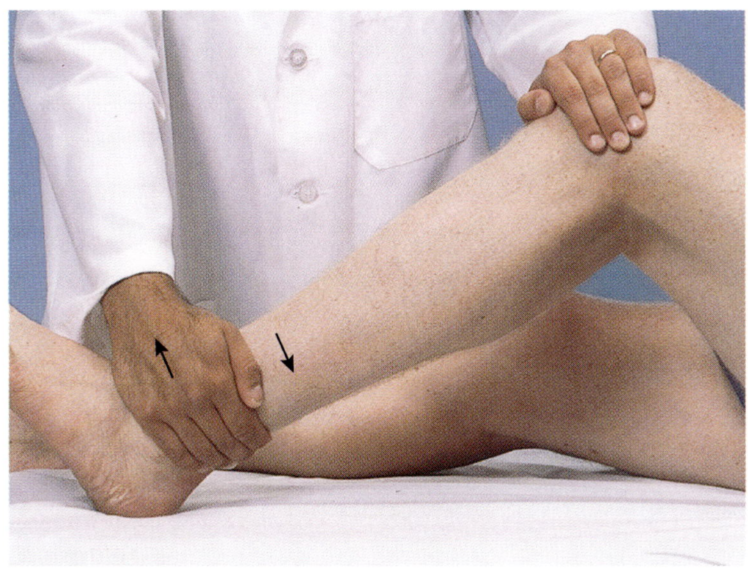

FLEXION AT THE KNEE

Test dorsiflexion (mainly L4, L5) and *plantar flexion* (mainly S1) at the ankle by asking the patient to pull up and push down against your hand.

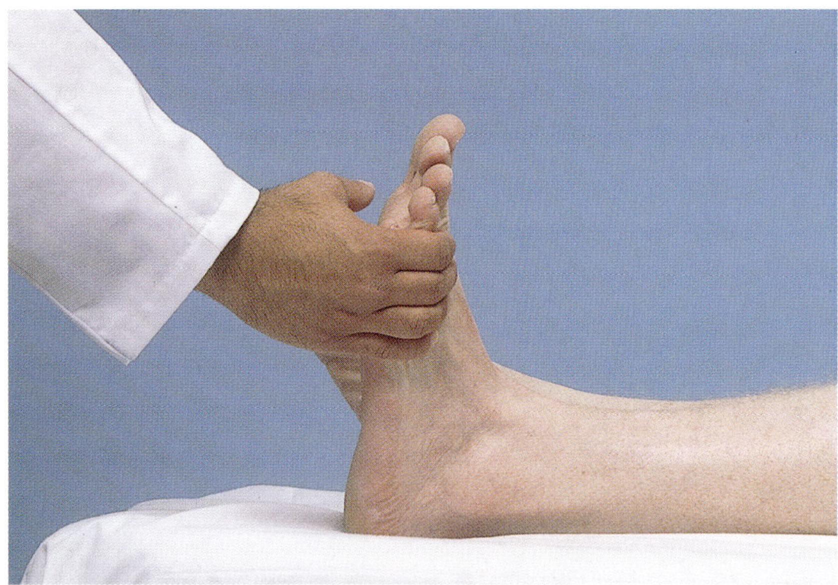

DORSIFLEXION

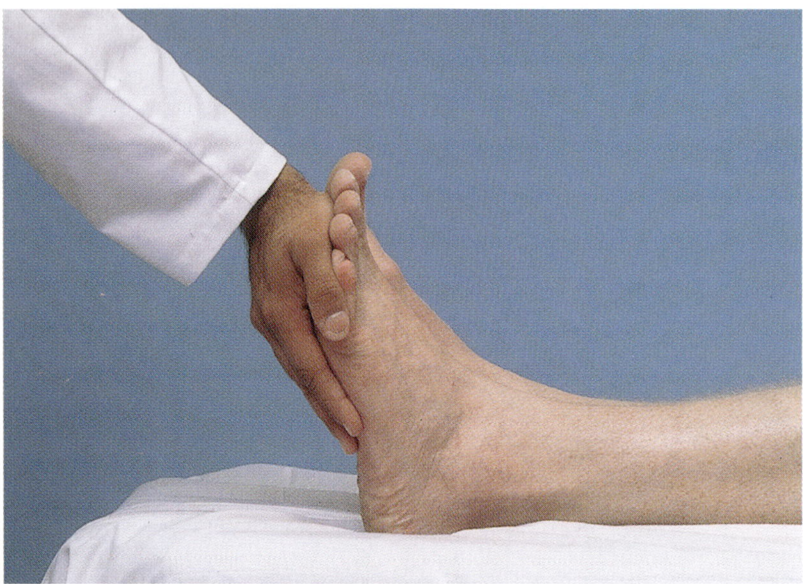

PLANTAR FLEXION

Coordination. Coordination of muscle movement requires that four areas of the nervous system function in an integrated way:

- The motor system, for muscle strength
- The cerebellar system (also part of the motor system), for rhythmic movement and steady posture

- The vestibular system, for balance and for coordinating eye, head, and body movements
- The sensory system, for position sense.

To assess coordination, observe the patient's performance in:

- Rapid alternating movements
- Point-to-point movements
- Gait and other related body movements
- Standing in specified ways.

Rapid Alternating Movements

ARMS. Show the patient how to strike one hand on the thigh, raise the hand, turn it over, and then strike the back of the hand down on the same place. Urge the patient to repeat these alternating movements as rapidly as possible.

Observe the speed, rhythm, and smoothness of the movements. Repeat with the other hand. The nondominant hand often performs somewhat less well.

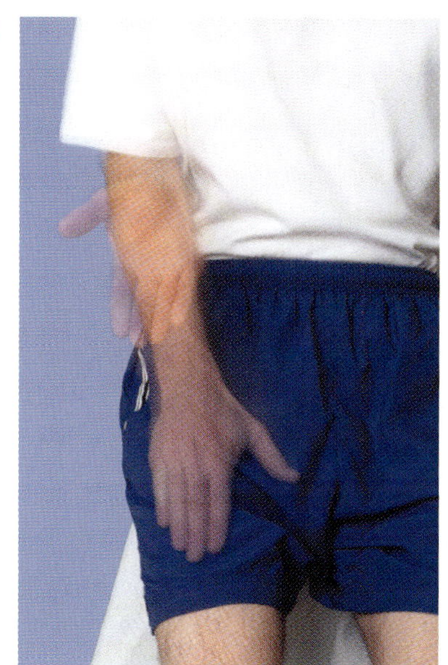

In cerebellar disease, one movement cannot be followed quickly by its opposite and movements are slow, irregular, and clumsy. This abnormality is called *dysdiadochokinesis.* Upper motor neuron weakness and basal ganglia disease may also impair rapid alternating movements, but not in the same manner.

Show the patient how to tap the distal joint of the thumb with the tip of the index finger, again as rapidly as possible. Again, observe the speed, rhythm, and smoothness of the movements. The nondominant side often performs less well.

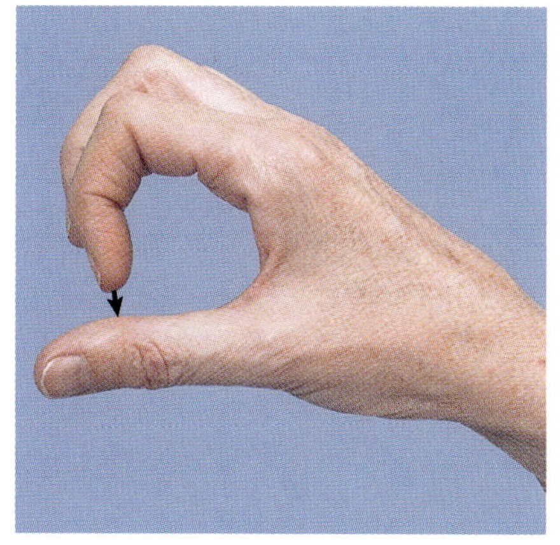

LEGS. Ask the patient to tap your hand as quickly as possible with the ball of each foot in turn. Note any slowness or awkwardness. The feet normally perform less well than the hands.

Dysdiadochokinesis in cerebellar disease

Point-To-Point Movements

ARMS. Ask the patient to touch your index finger and then his or her nose alternately several times. Move your finger about so that the patient has to alter directions and extend the arm fully to reach it. Observe the accuracy and smoothness of movements and watch for any tremor. Normally the patient's movements are smooth and accurate.

In cerebellar disease, movements are clumsy, unsteady, and inappropriately varying in their speed, force, and direction. The finger may initially overshoot its mark, but finally reaches it fairly well. Such movements are termed *dysmetria.* An intention tremor may appear toward the end of the movement (see p. 608).

Now hold your finger in one place so that the patient can touch it with one arm and finger outstretched. Ask the patient to raise the arm overhead and lower it again to touch your finger. After several repeats, ask the patient to close both eyes and try several more times. Repeat on the other side. Normally a person can touch the examiner's finger successfully with eyes open or closed. These maneuvers test position sense and the functions of both the labyrinth and the cerebellum.

Cerebellar disease causes incoordination that may get worse with eyes closed. Inaccuracy that appears with eyes closed suggests loss of position sense. Repetitive and consistent deviation to one side (referred to as *past pointing*), worse with the eyes closed, suggests cerebellar or vestibular disease.

LEGS. Ask the patient to place one heel on the opposite knee, and then run it down the shin to the big toe. Note the smoothness and accuracy of the movements. Repetition with the patient's eyes closed tests for position sense. Repeat on the other side.

In cerebellar disease, the heel may overshoot the knee and then oscillate from side to side down the shin. When position sense is lost, the heel is lifted too high and the patient tries to look. With eyes closed, performance is poor.

Gait. Ask the patient to:

Abnormalities of gait increase risk of falls.

- *Walk across the room* or down the hall, then turn, and come back. Observe posture, balance, swinging of the arms, and movements of the legs. Normally balance is easy, the arms swing at the sides, and turns are accomplished smoothly.

A gait that lacks coordination, with reeling and instability, is called *ataxic.* Ataxia may be due to cerebellar disease, loss of position sense, or intoxication. See Table 16-13, Abnormalities of Gait and Posture (pp. 618–619).

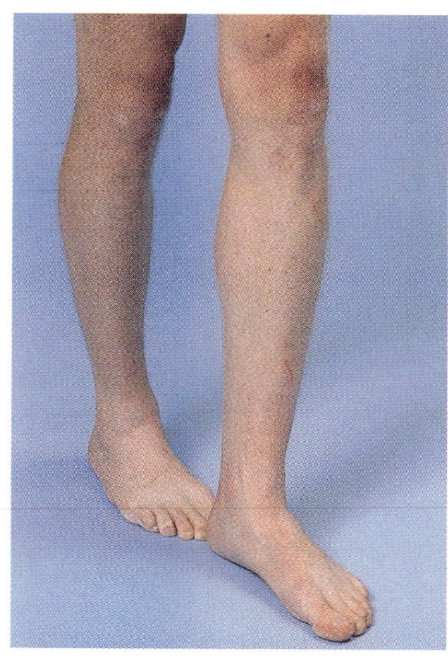

- *Walk heel-to-toe* in a straight line—a pattern called *tandem walking.*

Tandem walking may reveal an ataxia not previously obvious.

- *Walk on the toes,* then *on the heels*—sensitive tests respectively for plantar flexion and dorsiflexion of the ankles, as well as for balance.

Walking on toes and heels may reveal distal muscular weakness in the legs. Inability to heel-walk is a sensitive test for corticospinal tract weakness.

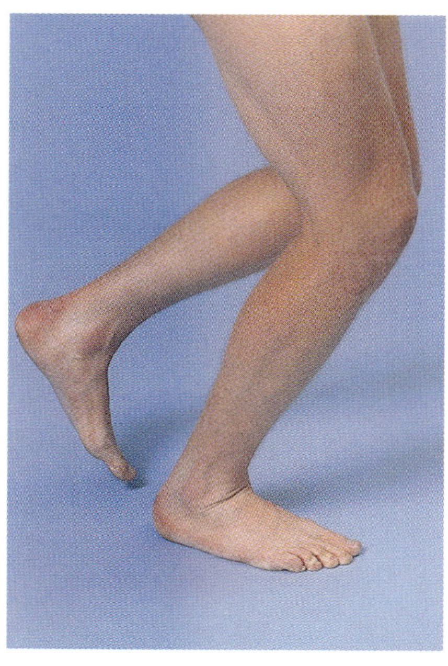

- *Hop in place* on each foot in turn (if the patient is not too ill). Hopping involves the proximal muscles of the legs as well as the distal ones and requires both good position sense and normal cerebellar function.

Difficulty with hopping may be due to weakness, lack of position sense, or cerebellar dysfunction.

- *Do a shallow knee bend,* first on one leg, then on the other. Support the patient's elbow if you think the patient is in danger of falling.

Difficulty here suggests proximal weakness (extensors of the hip), weakness of the quadriceps (the extensor of the knee), or both.

- *Rising from a sitting position* without arm support and *stepping up* on a sturdy stool are more suitable tests than hopping or knee bends when patients are old or less robust.

People with proximal muscle weakness involving the pelvic girdle and legs have difficulty with both of these activities.

Stance. The following two tests can often be performed concurrently. They differ only in the patient's arm position and in what you are looking for. In each case, stand close enough to the patient to prevent a fall.

THE ROMBERG TEST. This is mainly a test of position sense. The patient should first stand with feet together and eyes open and then close both eyes for 20 to 30 seconds without support. Note the patient's ability to maintain an upright posture. Normally only minimal swaying occurs.

In ataxia due to loss of position sense, vision compensates for the sensory loss. The patient stands fairly well with eyes open but loses balance when they are closed, a *positive Romberg sign.* In cerebellar ataxia, the patient has difficulty standing with feet together whether the eyes are open or closed.

TEST FOR PRONATOR DRIFT. The patient should stand for 20 to 30 seconds with both arms straight forward, palms up, and with eyes closed. A person who cannot stand may be tested for a pronator drift in the sitting position. In either case, a normal person can hold this arm position well.

The pronation of one forearm suggests a contralateral lesion in the corticospinal tract; downward drift of the arm with flexion of fingers and elbow may also occur. These movements are called a *pronator drift,* shown below.

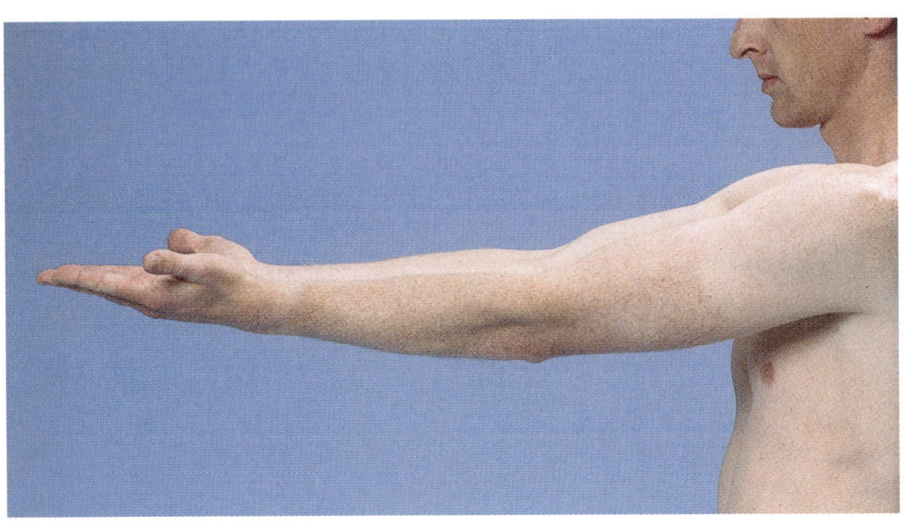

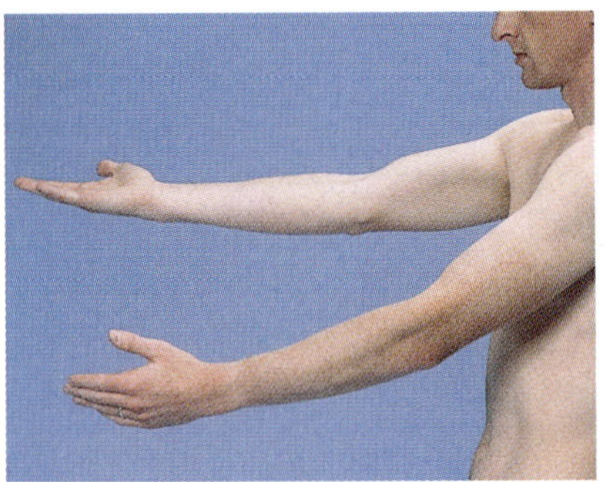

A sideward or upward drift, sometimes with searching, writhing movements of the hands, suggests loss of position sense.

Now, instructing the patient to keep the arms up and eyes shut, as shown above, *tap the arms briskly downward.* The arms normally return smoothly to the horizontal position. This response requires muscular strength, coordination, and a good sense of position.

A weak arm is easily displaced and often remains so. A patient lacking position sense may not recognize the displacement and, if told to correct it, does so poorly. In cerebellar incoordination, the arm returns to its original position but overshoots and bounces.

The Sensory System

To evaluate the sensory system, you will test several kinds of sensation:

- Pain and temperature (spinothalamic tracts)
- Position and vibration (posterior columns)
- Light touch (both of these pathways)
- Discriminative sensations, which depend on some of the above sensations but also involve the cortex

Familiarize yourself with each kind of test so that you can use it as indicated. When you detect abnormal findings, correlate them with motor and reflex activity. Is the underlying lesion central or peripheral?

See Table 16-12, Disorders of the Central and Peripheral Nervous Systems (pp. 615–617).

Patterns of Testing. Because sensory testing quickly fatigues many patients and then produces unreliable results, conduct the examination as efficiently as possible. Pay special attention to those areas (1) where there are symptoms such as numbness or pain, (2) where there are motor or reflex abnormalities that suggest a lesion of the spinal cord or peripheral nervous system, and (3) where there are trophic changes, such as absent or excessive sweating, atrophic skin, or cutaneous ulceration). Repeated testing at another time is often required to confirm abnormalities.

Meticulous sensory mapping helps to establish the level of a spinal cord lesion and to determine if a more peripheral lesion is in a nerve root, a major peripheral nerve, or one of its branches.

The following patterns of testing help you to identify sensory deficits accurately and efficiently.

- *Compare symmetric areas* on the two sides of the body, including the arms, legs, and trunk.

Hemisensory loss due to a lesion in the spinal cord or higher pathways

- When testing pain, temperature, and touch sensation, also *compare the distal with the proximal areas* of the extremities. Further, scatter the stimuli so as to sample most of the dermatomes and major peripheral nerves (see pp. 542–546). One suggested pattern includes both shoulders (C4), the inner and outer aspects of the forearms (C6 and T1), the thumbs and little fingers (C6 and C8), the fronts of both thighs (L2), the medial and lateral aspects of both calves (L4 and L5), the little toes (S1), and the medial aspect of each buttock (S3).

Symmetric distal sensory loss suggests a polyneuropathy, as described in the example on the next page. You may miss this finding unless you compare distal and proximal areas.

- When testing vibration and position sensation, first test the fingers and toes. If these are normal, you may safely assume that more proximal areas will also be normal.
- *Vary the pace of your testing.* This is important so that the patient does not merely respond to your repetitive rhythm.

- When you detect an area of sensory loss or hypersensitivity, *map out* its *boundaries* in detail. Stimulate first at a point of reduced sensation, and move by progressive steps until the patient detects the change. An example is shown at right.

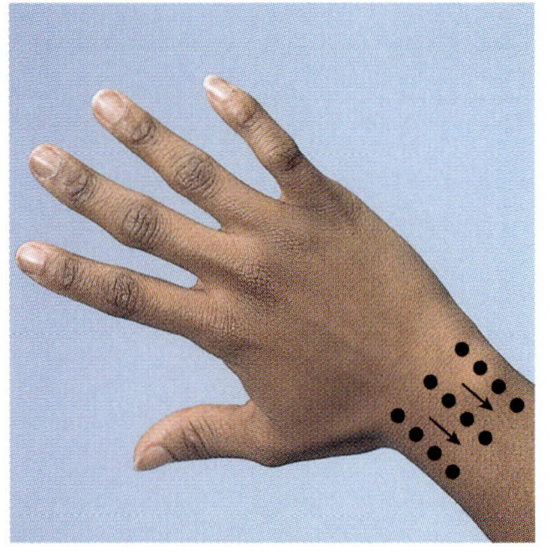

Here all sensation in the hand is lost. Repetitive testing in a proximal direction reveals a gradual change to normal sensation at the wrist. This pattern fits neither a peripheral nerve nor a dermatome (see pp. 542–546). If bilateral, it suggests the "glove and stocking" sensory loss of a polyneuropathy, often seen in alcoholism and diabetes.

By identifying the distribution of sensory abnormalities and the kinds of sensations affected, you can infer where the causative lesion might be. Any motor deficit or reflex abnormality also helps in this localizing process.

Before each test below, show the patient what you plan to do and what responses you want. Unless otherwise specified, the patient's eyes should be closed during actual testing.

Pain. Use a sharp safety pin or other suitable tool. Occasionally, substitute the blunt end for the point. Ask the patient, "Is this sharp or dull?" or, when making comparisons, "Does this feel the same as this?" Apply the lightest pressure needed for the stimulus to feel sharp, and try not to draw blood.

Analgesia refers to absence of pain sensation, *hypalgesia* to decreased sensitivity to pain, and *hyperalgesia* to increased sensitivity.

To prevent transmitting a blood-borne infection, discard the pin or other device safely. Do not reuse it on another person.

Temperature. (This is often omitted if pain sensation is normal, but include it if there is any question.) Use two test tubes, filled with hot and cold water, or a tuning fork heated or cooled by water. Touch the skin and ask the patient to identify "hot" or "cold."

Light Touch. With a fine wisp of cotton, touch the skin lightly, avoiding pressure. Ask the patient to respond whenever a touch is felt, and to compare one area with another. Calloused skin is normally relatively insensitive and should be avoided.

Anesthesia is absence of touch sensation, *hypesthesia* is decreased sensitivity, and *hyperesthesia* is increased sensitivity.

Vibration. Use a relatively low-pitched tuning fork of 128 Hz . Tap it on the heel of your hand and place it firmly over a distal interphalangeal joint of the patient's finger, then over the interphalangeal joint of the big toe. Ask what the patient feels. If you are uncertain whether it is pressure or vibration, ask the patient to tell you when the vibration stops, and then touch the fork to stop it. If

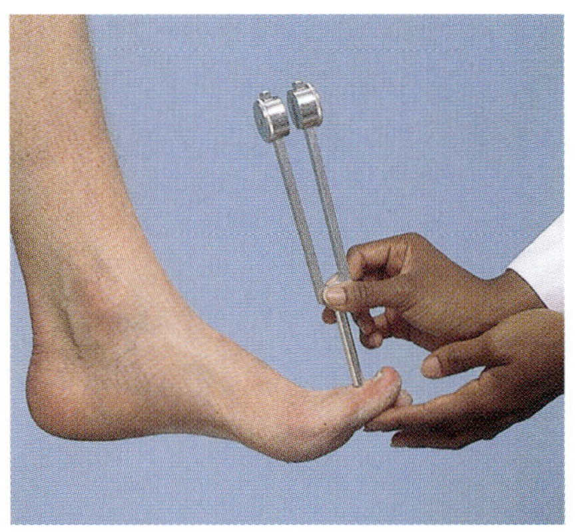

Vibration sense is often the first sensation to be lost in a peripheral neuropathy. Common causes include diabetes and alcoholism. Vibration sense is also lost in posterior column disease, as in tertiary syphilis or vitamin B_{12} deficiency.

Testing vibration sense in the trunk may be useful in estimating the level of a cord lesion.

vibration sense is impaired, proceed to more proximal bony prominences (e.g., wrist, elbow, medial malleolus, patella, anterior superior iliac spine, spinous processes, and clavicles).

Position. Grasp the patient's big toe, holding it by its sides between your thumb and index finger, and then pull it away from the other toes so as to avoid friction. (These precautions prevent extraneous tactile stimuli from revealing position changes that might not otherwise be detected.) Demonstrate "up" and "down" as you move the patient's toe clearly upward and downward. Then, with the patient's eyes closed, ask for a response of "up" or "down" when moving the toe in a small arc.

Loss of position sense, like loss of vibration sense, suggests either posterior column disease or a lesion of the peripheral nerve or root.

Repeat several times on each side, avoiding simple alternation of the stimuli. If position sense is impaired, move proximally to test it at the ankle joint. In a similar fashion, test position in the fingers, moving proximally if indicated to the metacarpophalangeal joints, wrist, and elbow.

Discriminative Sensations. Several additional techniques test the ability of the sensory cortex to correlate, analyze, and interpret sensations. Because discriminative sensations are dependent on touch and position sense, they are useful only when these sensations are either intact or only slightly impaired.

When touch and position sense are normal or only slightly impaired, a disproportionate decrease in or loss of discriminative sensations suggests disease of the sensory cortex. Stereognosis, number identification, and two-point discrimination are also impaired by posterior column disease.

Screen a patient with *stereognosis,* and proceed to other methods if indicated. The patient's eyes should be closed during all these tests.

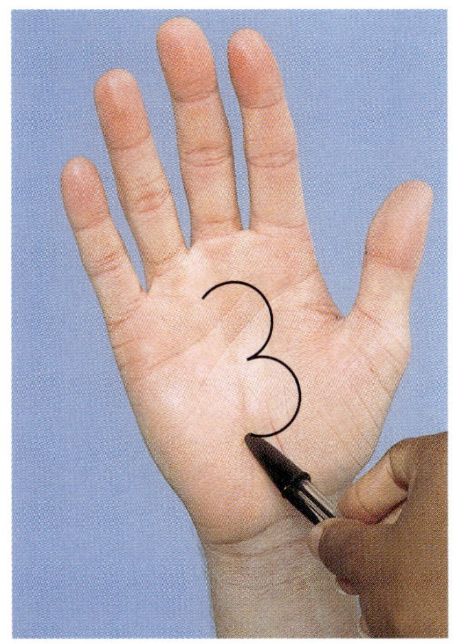

- *Stereognosis.* Stereognosis refers to the ability to identify an object by feeling it. Place in the patient's hand a familiar object such as a coin, paper clip, key, pencil, or cotton ball, and ask the patient to tell you what it is. Normally a patient will manipulate it skillfully and identify it correctly. Asking the patient to distinguish "heads" from "tails" on a coin is a sensitive test of stereognosis.

Astereognosis refers to the inability to recognize objects placed in the hand.

- *Number identification (graphesthesia).* When motor impairment, arthritis, or other conditions pre-

The inability to recognize numbers, like astereognosis, suggests a lesion in the sensory cortex.

vent the patient from manipulating an object well enough to identify it, test the ability to identify numbers. With the blunt end of a pen or pencil, draw a large number in the patient's palm. A normal person can identify most such numbers.

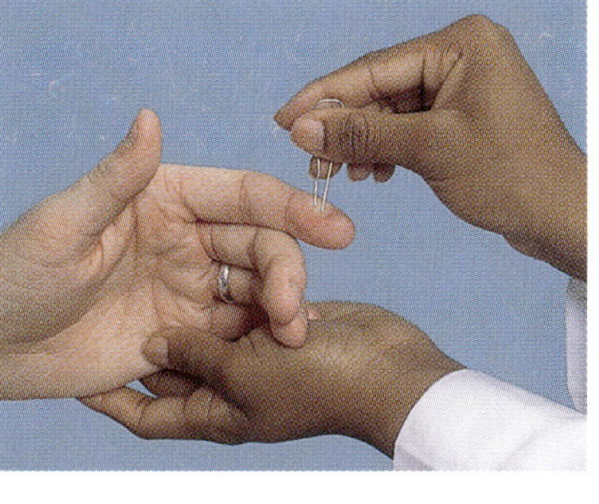

- *Two-point discrimination.* Using the two ends of an opened paper clip, or the sides of two pins, touch a finger pad in two places simultaneously. Alternate the double stimulus irregularly with a one-point touch. Be careful not to cause pain.

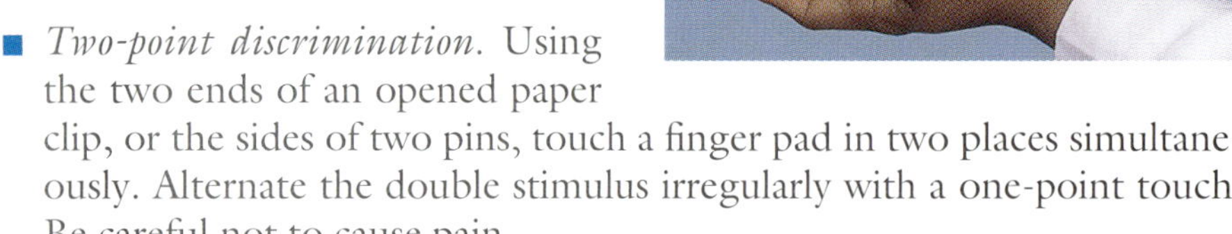

Find the minimal distance at which the patient can discriminate one from two points (normally less than 5 mm on the finger pads). This test may be used on other parts of the body, but normal distances vary widely from one body region to another.

Lesions of the sensory cortex increase the distance between two recognizable points.

- *Point localization.* Briefly touch a point on the patient's skin. Then ask the patient to open both eyes and point to the place touched. Normally a person can do so accurately. This test, together with the test for extinction, is especially useful on the trunk and the legs.

Lesions of the sensory cortex impair the ability to localize points accurately.

- *Extinction.* Simultaneously stimulate corresponding areas on both sides of the body. Ask where the patient feels your touch. Normally both stimuli are felt.

With lesions of the sensory cortex, only one stimulus may be recognized. The stimulus on the side opposite the damaged cortex is extinguished.

Deep Tendon Reflexes

To elicit a *deep tendon reflex,* persuade the patient to relax, position the limbs properly and symmetrically, and strike the tendon briskly, using a rapid wrist movement. Your strike should be quick and direct, not glancing. You may use either the pointed or the flat end of the hammer. A properly weighted hammer is important. The pointed end is useful in striking small areas, such as your finger as it overlies the biceps tendon, while the flat end gives the patient less discomfort over the brachioradialis. Hold the reflex hammer between your thumb and index

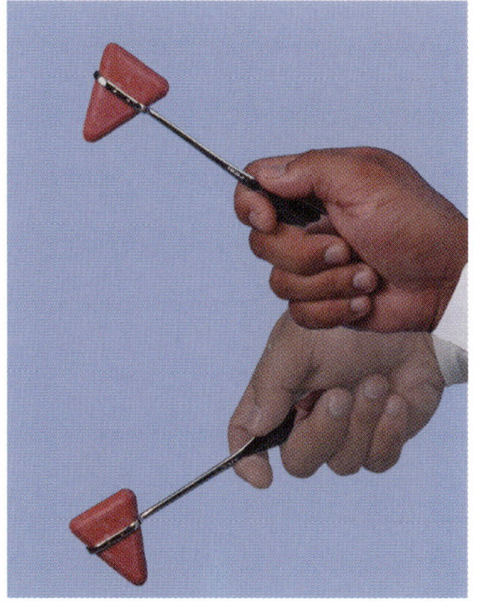

finger so that it swings freely within the limits set by your palm and other fingers. Note the speed, force, and amplitude of the reflex response. Always compare one side with the other.

Reflexes are usually graded on a 0 to 4+ scale:

4+	Very brisk, hyperactive, with *clonus* (rhythmic oscillations between flexion and extension)
3+	Brisker than average; possibly but not necessarily indicative of disease
2+	Average; normal
1+	Somewhat diminished; low normal
0	No response

Hyperactive reflexes suggest central nervous system disease. Sustained clonus confirms it. Reflexes may be diminished or absent when sensation is lost, when the relevant spinal segments are damaged, or when the peripheral nerves are damaged. Diseases of muscles and neuromuscular junctions may also decrease reflexes.

Reflex response depends partly on the force of your stimulus. Use no more force than you need to provoke a definite response. Differences between sides are usually easier to assess than symmetric changes. Symmetrically diminished or even absent reflexes may be found in normal people.

If the patient's reflexes are symmetrically diminished or absent, use *reinforcement*, a technique involving isometric contraction of other muscles that may increase reflex activity. In testing arm reflexes, for example, ask the patient to clench his or her teeth or to squeeze one thigh with the opposite hand. If leg reflexes are diminished or absent, reinforce them by asking the patient to lock fingers and pull one hand against the other. Tell the patient to pull just before you strike the tendon.

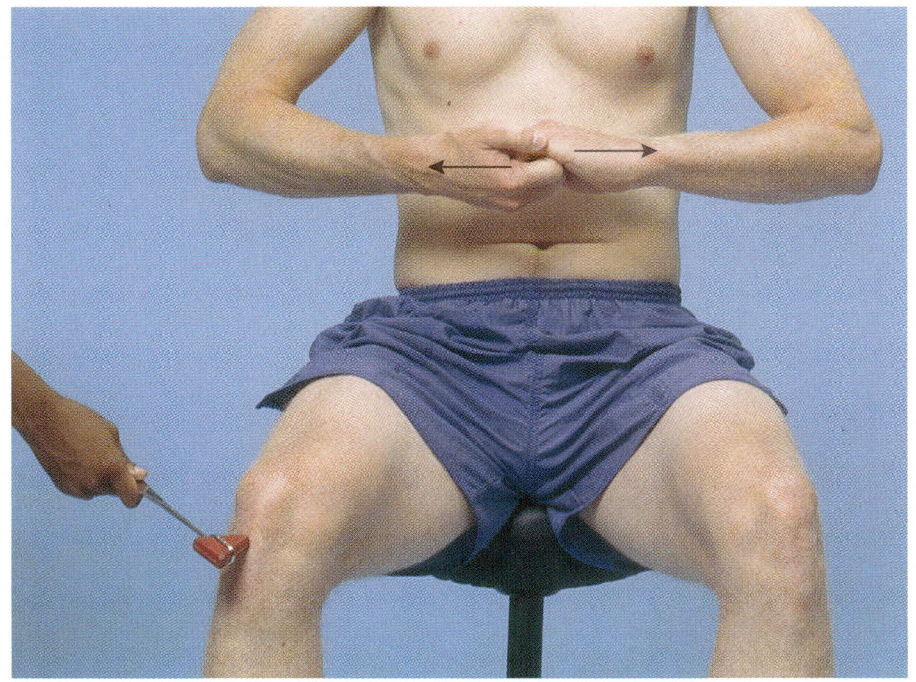

REINFORCEMENT OF KNEE REFLEX

The Biceps Reflex (C5, C6). The patient's arm should be partially flexed at the elbow with palm down. Place your thumb or finger firmly on the biceps tendon. Strike with the reflex hammer so that the blow is aimed directly through your digit toward the biceps tendon.

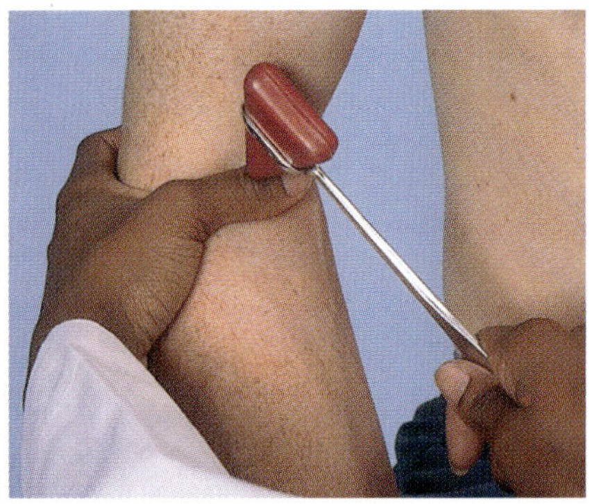

PATIENT SITTING

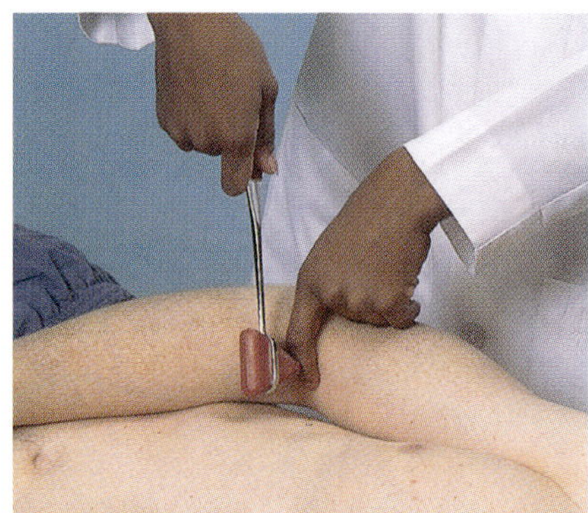

PATIENT LYING DOWN

Observe flexion at the elbow, and watch for and feel the contraction of the biceps muscle.

The Triceps Reflex (C6, C7). Flex the patient's arm at the elbow, with palm toward the body, and pull it slightly across the chest. Strike the triceps tendon above the elbow. Use a direct blow from directly behind it. Watch for contraction of the triceps muscle and extension at the elbow.

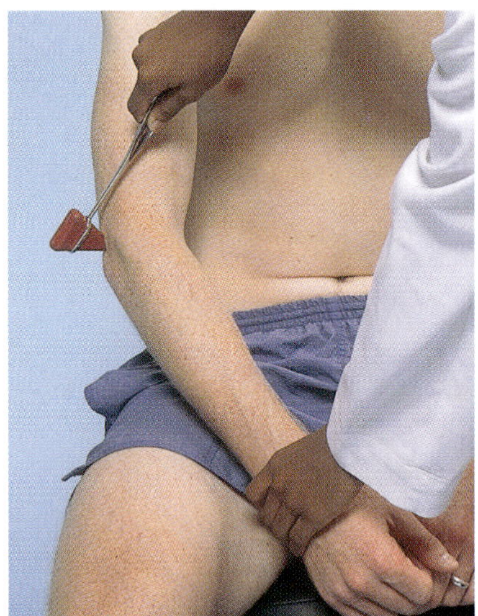

PATIENT SITTING

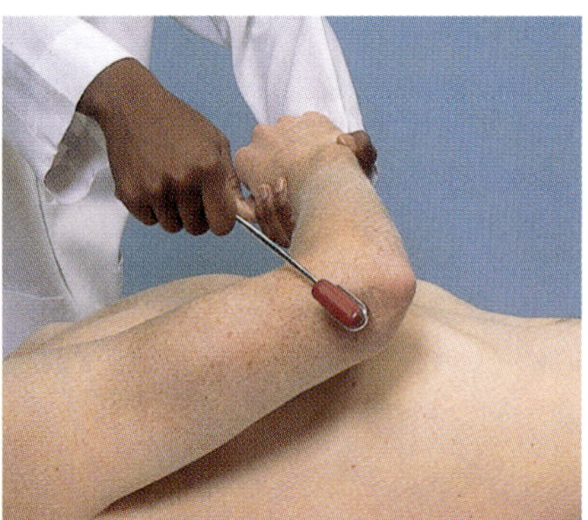

PATIENT LYING DOWN

If you have difficulty getting the patient to relax, try supporting the upper arm as illustrated on the right. Ask the patient to let the arm go limp, as if it were "hung up to dry." Then strike the triceps tendon.

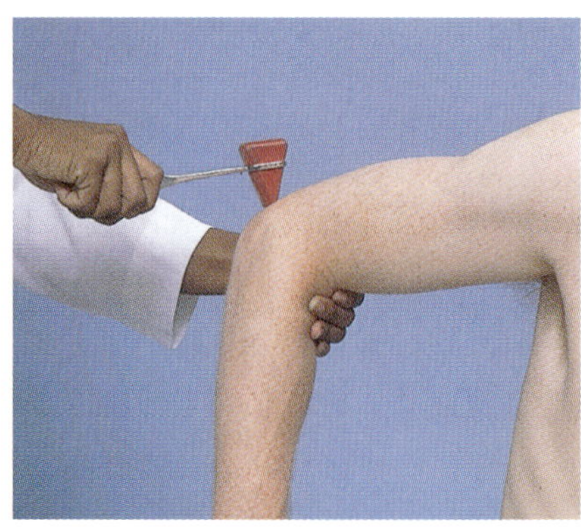

The Supinator or Brachioradialis Reflex (C5, C6). The patient's hand should rest on the abdomen or the lap, with the forearm partly pronated. Strike the radius about 1 to 2 inches above the wrist. Watch for flexion and supination of the forearm.

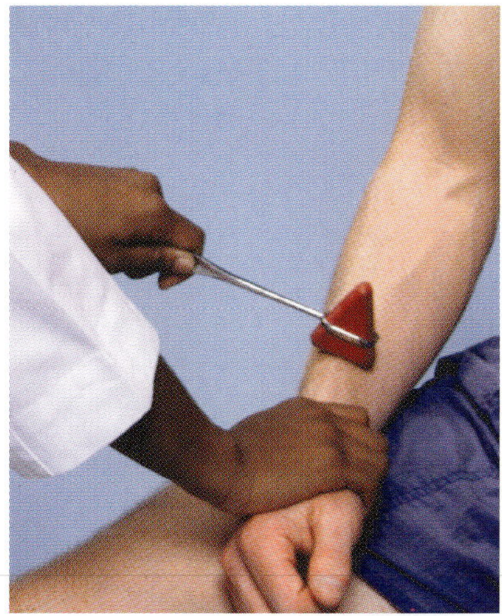

The Abdominal Reflexes. Test the abdominal reflexes by lightly but briskly stroking each side of the abdomen, above (T8, T9, T10) and below (T10, T11, T12) the umbilicus, in the directions illustrated. Use a key, the wooden end of a cotton-tipped applicator, or a tongue blade twisted and split longitudinally. Note the contraction of the abdominal muscles and deviation of the umbilicus toward the stimulus. Obesity may mask an abdominal reflex. In this situation, use your finger to retract the patient's umbilicus away from the side to be stimulated. Feel with your retracting finger for the muscular contraction.

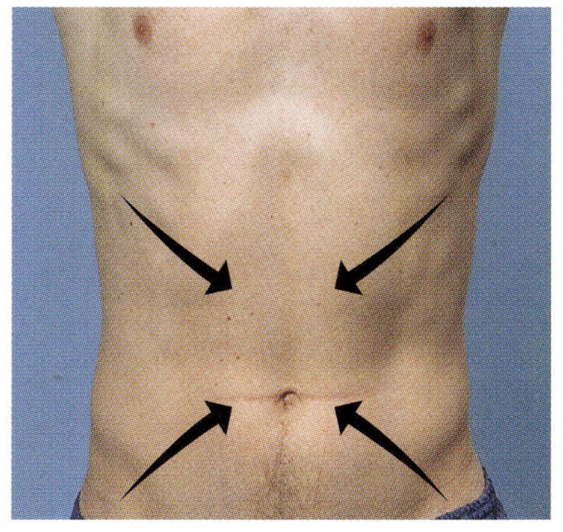

Abdominal reflexes may be absent in both central and peripheral nervous system disorders.

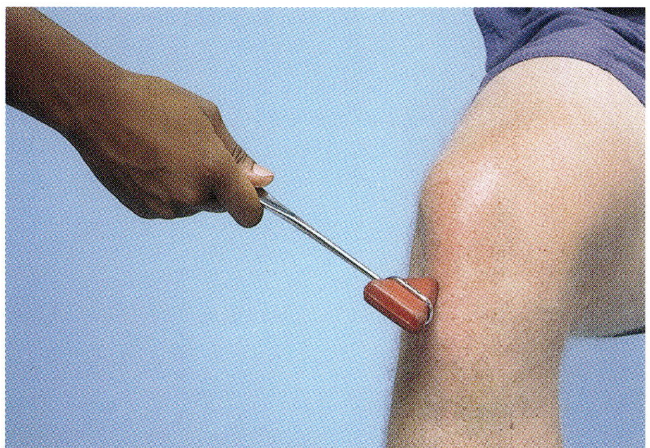

PATIENT SITTING

The Knee Reflex (L2, L3, L4). The patient may be either sitting or lying down as long as the knee is flexed. Briskly tap the patellar tendon just below the patella. Note contraction of the quadriceps with extension at the knee. A hand on the patient's anterior thigh lets you feel this reflex.

Two methods are useful when examining the supine patient. Supporting both knees at once, as shown below on the left, allows you to assess small differences between knee reflexes by repeatedly testing one reflex and then the other. Sometimes, however, supporting both legs is uncomfortable for both the examiner and the patient. You may wish to rest your supporting arm under the patient's leg, as shown below on the right. Some patients find it easier to relax with this method.

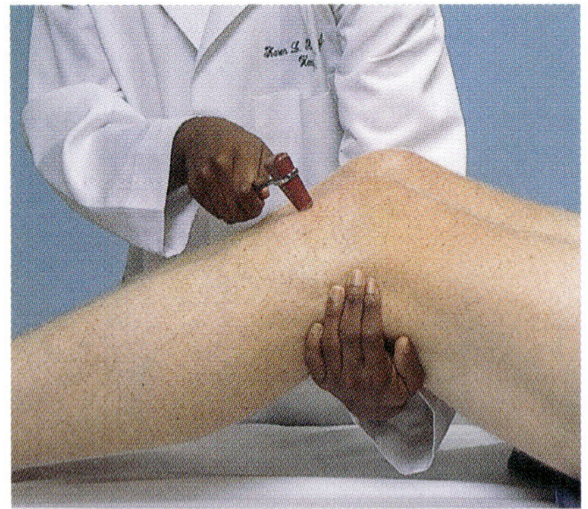

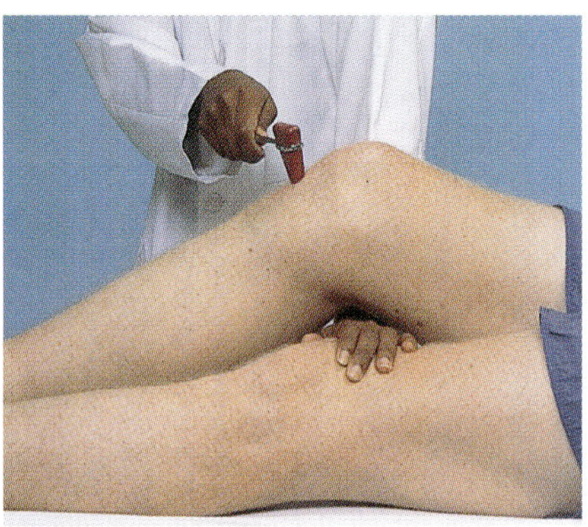

The Ankle Reflex (primarily S1). If the patient is sitting, dorsiflex the foot at the ankle. Persuade the patient to relax. Strike the Achilles tendon. Watch and feel for plantar flexion at the ankle. Note also the speed of relaxation after muscular contraction.

The slowed relaxation phase of reflexes in hypothyroidism is often easily seen and felt in the ankle reflex.

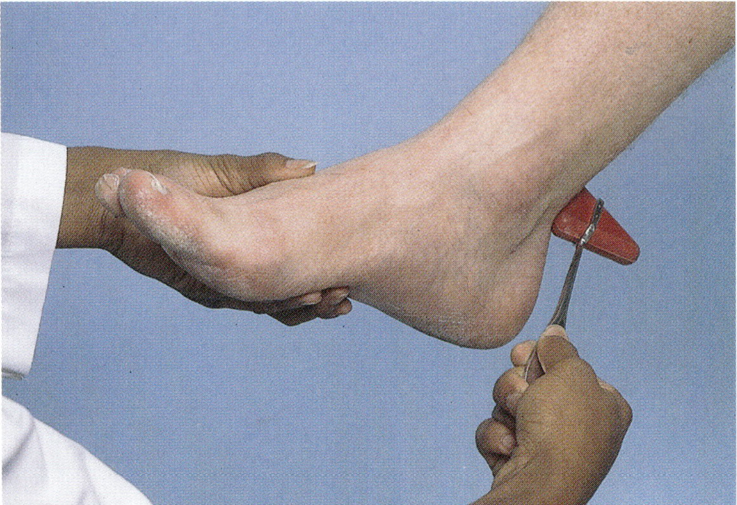

PATIENT SITTING

When the patient is lying down, flex one leg at both hip and knee and rotate it externally so that the lower leg rests across the opposite shin. Then dorsiflex the foot at the ankle and strike the Achilles tendon.

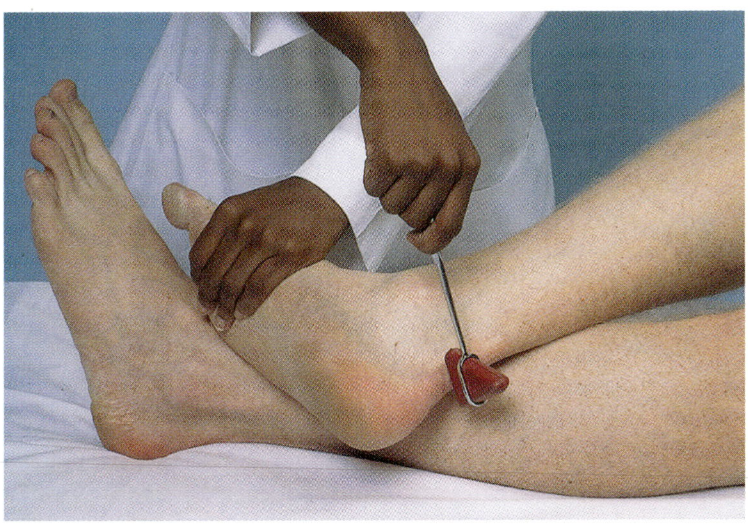

PATIENT LYING DOWN

The Plantar Response (L5, S1). With an object such as a key or the wooden end of an applicator stick, stroke the lateral aspect of the sole from the heel to the ball of the foot, curving medially across the ball. Use the lightest stimulus that will provoke a response, but be increasingly firm if necessary. Note movement of the toes, normally flexion.

Dorsiflexion of the big toe, often accompanied by fanning of the other toes, constitutes a Babinski response. It often indicates a central nervous system lesion in the corticospinal tract.

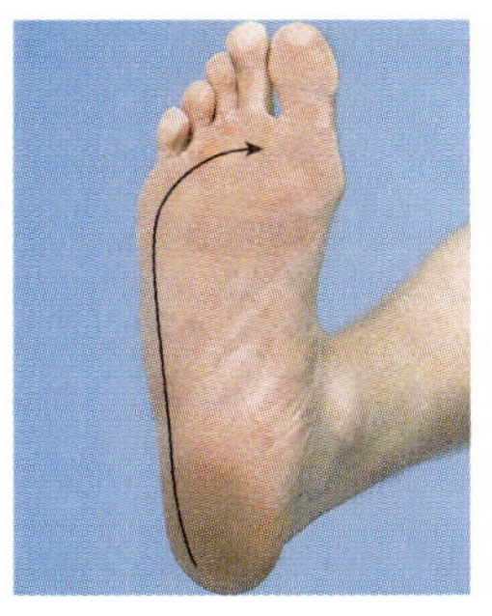

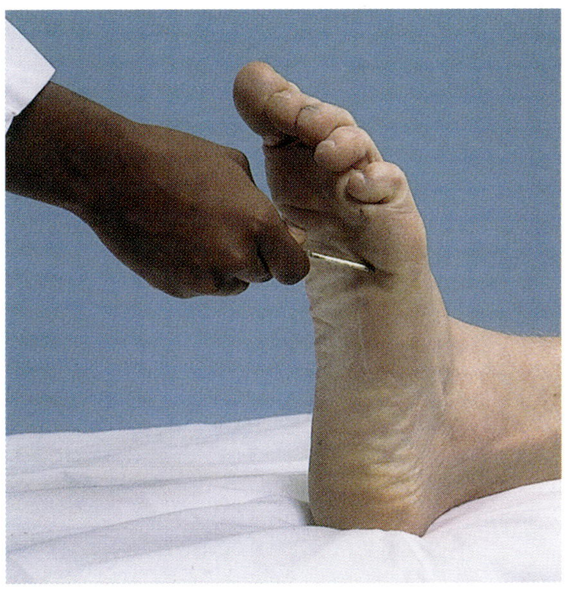

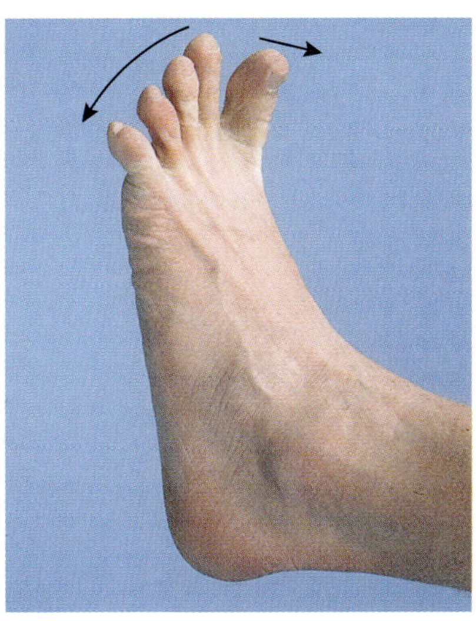

A Babinski response may also be seen in unconscious states due to drug or alcohol intoxication or in the postictal period following a seizure.

Some patients withdraw from this stimulus by flexing the hip and the knee. Hold the ankle, if necessary, to complete your observation. It is sometimes difficult to distinguish withdrawal from a Babinski response.

A marked Babinski response is occasionally accompanied by reflex flexion at hip and knee.

Clonus. If the reflexes seem hyperactive, test for *ankle clonus.* Support the knee in a partly flexed position. With your other hand, dorsiflex and plantar flex the foot a few times while encouraging the patient to relax, and then sharply dorsiflex the foot and maintain it in dorsiflexion. Look and feel for rhythmic oscillations between dorsiflexion and plantar flexion. In most normal people, the ankle does not react to this stimulus. A few clonic beats may be seen and felt, especially when the patient is tense or has exercised.

Sustained clonus indicates central nervous system disease. The ankle plantar flexes and dorsiflexes repetitively and rhythmically.

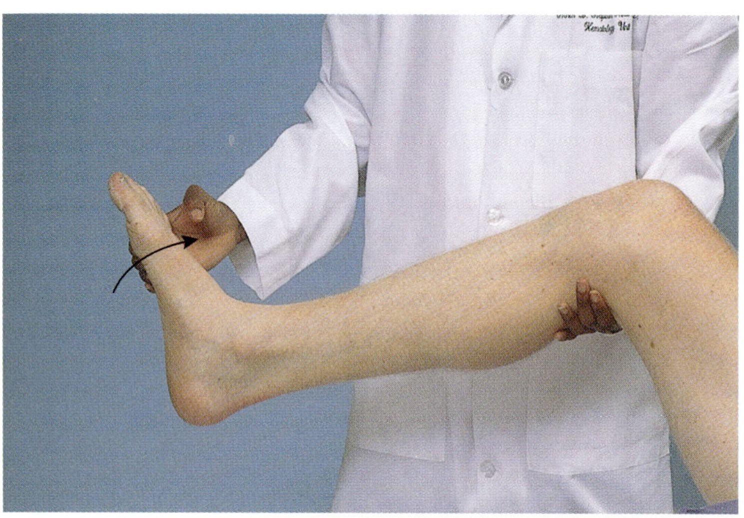

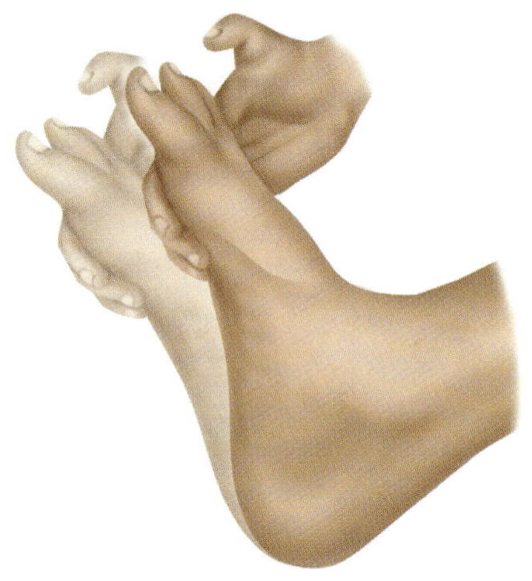

Clonus may also be elicited at other joints. A sharp downward displacement of the patella, for example, may elicit patellar clonus in the extended knee.

Special Techniques

Mini-Mental State Examination (MMSE). This brief test is useful in screening for cognitive dysfunction or dementia and following their course over time. For more detailed information regarding the MMSE, contact the Publisher, Psychological Assessment Resources, Inc., 16204 North Florida Avenue, Lutz, Florida 33549.

Asterixis. Asterixis helps identify a metabolic encephalopathy in patients whose mental functions are impaired. Ask the patient to "stop traffic" by extending both arms, with hands cocked up and fingers spread. Watch for 1 to 2 minutes, coaxing the patient as necessary to maintain this position.

Sudden, brief, nonrhythmic flexion of the hands and fingers indicates asterixis.

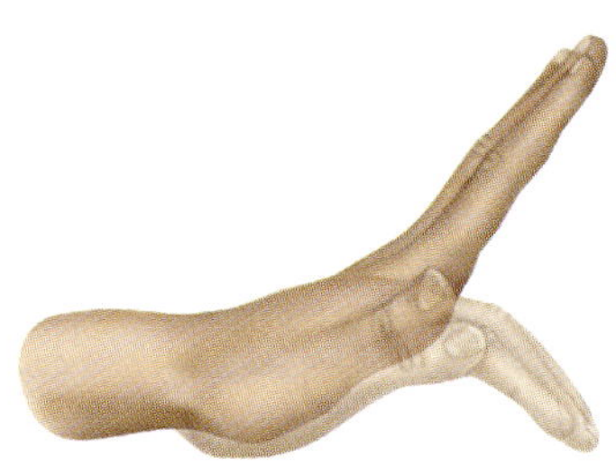

Winging of the Scapula. When the shoulder muscles seem weak or atrophic, look for winging. Ask the patient to extend both arms and push against your hand or against a wall. Observe the scapulae. Normally they lie close to the thorax.

In winging, shown below, the medial border of the scapula juts backward. It suggests weakness of the serratus anterior muscle, as in muscular dystrophy or injury to the long thoracic nerve.

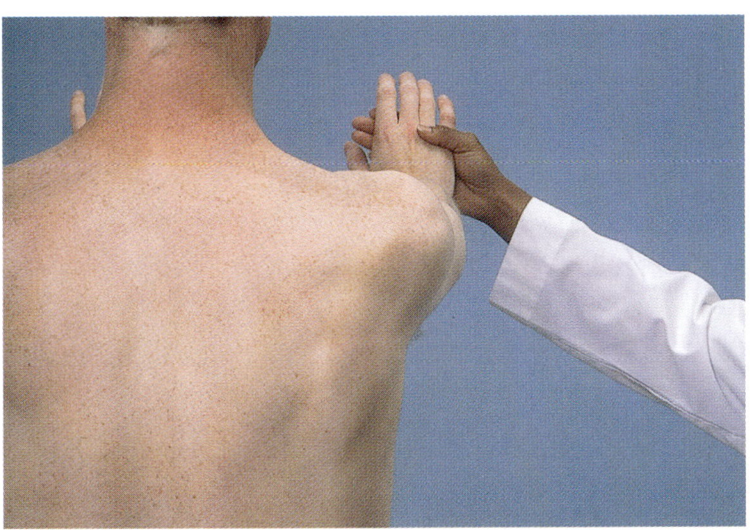

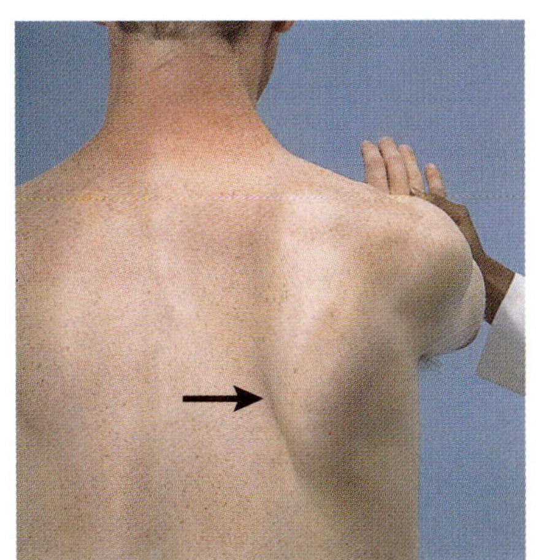

In very thin but normal people, the scapulae may appear "winged" even when the musculature is intact.

Meningeal Signs. Testing for these signs is important if you suspect meningeal inflammation from infection or subarachnoid hemorrhage.

Neck Mobility. First make sure there is no injury to the cervical vertebrae or cervical cord. (In settings of trauma, this may require evaluation by x-ray.) Then, with the patient supine, place your hands behind the patient's head and flex the neck forward, until the chin touches the chest if possible. Normally the neck is supple and the patient can easily bend the head and neck forward.

Pain in the neck and resistance to flexion can arise from meningeal inflammation, arthritis, or neck injury.

Brudzinski's Sign. As you flex the neck, watch the hips and knees in reaction to your maneuver. Normally they should remain relaxed and motionless.

Flexion of the hips and knees is a *positive Brudzinski's sign* and suggests meningeal inflammation.

Kernig's Sign. Flex the patient's leg at both the hip and the knee, and then straighten the knee. Discomfort behind the knee during full extension occurs in many normal people, but this maneuver should not produce pain.

Pain and increased resistance to extending the knee are a *positive Kernig's sign.* When bilateral, it suggests meningeal irritation.

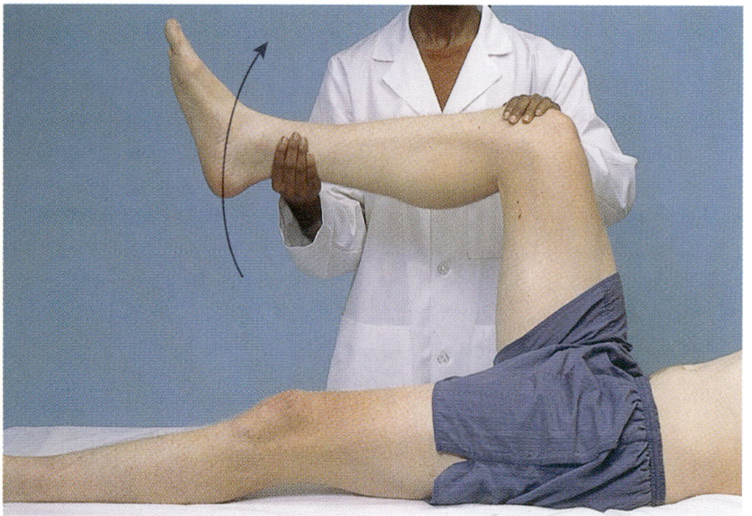

Compression of a lumbosacral nerve root may also cause resistance, together with pain in the low back and the posterior thigh. Only one leg is usually involved.

Anal Reflex. Using a dull object, such as a cotton swab, stroke outward in the four quadrants from the anus. Watch for reflex contraction of the anal musculature.

Loss of the anal reflex suggests a lesion in the S2–3–4 reflex arc, as in a cauda equina lesion.

The Stuporous or Comatose Patient. Coma signals a potentially life-threatening event affecting the two hemispheres, the brainstem, or both. The usual sequence of history, physical examination, and laboratory evaluation does not apply. Instead, you must:

- First assess the ABCs (airway, breathing, and circulation)
- Establish the patient's level of consciousness
- Examine the patient neurologically. Look for focal or asymmetric findings, and determine whether impaired consciousness arises from a metabolic or a structural cause.

See Table 16-14, Metabolic and Structural Coma (p. 620).

Interview relatives, friends, or witnesses to establish the speed of onset and duration of unconsciousness, any warning symptoms, precipitating factors, or previous episodes, and the prior appearance and behavior of the patient. Any history of past medical and psychiatric illnesses is also useful.

As you proceed to the examination, remember two cardinal DON'T s:

1. *Don't* dilate the pupils, the single most important clue to the underlying cause of coma (structural vs. metabolic), and
2. *Don't* flex the neck if there is any question of trauma to the head or neck. Immobilize the cervical spine and get an x-ray first to rule out fractures of the cervical vertebrae that could compress and damage the spinal cord.

Airway, Breathing, and Circulation. Quickly check the patient's color and pattern of breathing. Inspect the posterior pharynx and listen over the trachea for stridor to make sure the airway is clear. If respirations are slowed or shallow, or if the airway is obstructed by secretions, consider intubating the patient as soon as possible while stabilizing the cervical spine.

Assess the remaining vital signs: pulse, blood pressure, and *rectal* temperature. If hypotension or hemorrhage is present, establish intravenous access and begin intravenous fluids. (Further emergency management and laboratory studies are beyond the scope of this text.)

Level of Consciousness. Level of consciousness primarily reflects the patient's capacity for arousal, or wakefulness. It is determined by the level of activity that the patient can be aroused to perform in response to escalating stimuli from the examiner.

Five clinical levels of consciousness are described in the table below, together with the techniques that may be used to elicit their characteristics. Increase your stimuli in a stepwise manner, depending on the patient's response.

When you examine patients with an altered level of consciousness, describe and record exactly what you see and hear. Summary terms such as lethargy, obtundation, stupor, or coma may have different meanings for other examiners.

Level of Consciousness (Arousal): Techniques and Patient Response

Level	Technique	Abnormal Response
Alertness	Speak to the patient in a normal tone of voice. An alert patient opens the eyes, looks at you, and responds fully and appropriately to stimuli (arousal intact).	
Lethargy	Speak to the patient in a loud voice. For example, call the patient's name or ask "How are you?"	A lethargic patient appears drowsy but opens the eyes and looks at you, responds to questions, and then falls asleep.
Obtundation	Shake the patient gently as if awakening a sleeper.	An obtunded patient opens the eyes and looks at you, but responds slowly and is somewhat confused. Alertness and interest in the environment are decreased.
Stupor	Apply a painful stimulus. For example, pinch a tendon, rub the sternum, or roll a pencil across a nail bed. (No stronger stimuli needed!)	A stuporous patient arouses from sleep only after painful stimuli. Verbal responses are slow or even absent. The patient lapses into an unresponsive state when the stimulus ceases. There is minimal awareness of self or the environment.
Coma	Apply repeated painful stimuli.	A comatose patient remains unarousable with eyes closed. There is no evident response to inner need or external stimuli.

Neurologic Evaluation

RESPIRATIONS. Observe the rate, rhythm, and pattern of respirations. Because neural structures that govern breathing in the cortex and brainstem overlap those that govern consciousness, abnormalities of respiration often occur in coma.

See Table 16-14, Metabolic and Structural Coma (p. 620), and Table 3-12, Abnormalities in Rate and Rhythm of Breathing (p. 93).

PUPILS. Observe the size and equality of the pupils and test their reaction to light. The presence or absence of the light reaction is one of the most important signs distinguishing structural from metabolic causes of coma. The light reaction often remains intact in metabolic coma.

See Table 16-15, Pupils in Comatose Patients (p. 621).

Structural lesions such as stroke may lead to asymmetrical pupils and loss of light reaction.

OCULAR MOVEMENT. Observe the position of the eyes and eyelids at rest. Check for horizontal deviation of the eyes to one side (*gaze preference*). When the oculomotor pathways are intact, the eyes look straight ahead.

In structural hemispheric lesions, the eyes "look at the lesion" in the affected hemisphere.

In irritative lesions due to epilepsy or early cerebral hemorrhage, the eyes "look away" from the affected hemisphere.

OCULOCEPHALIC REFLEX (DOLL'S EYE MOVEMENTS). This reflex helps to assess brainstem function in a comatose patient. Holding open the upper eyelids so that you can see the eyes, turn the head quickly, first to one side and then to the other. (Make sure the patient has no neck injury before performing this test.)

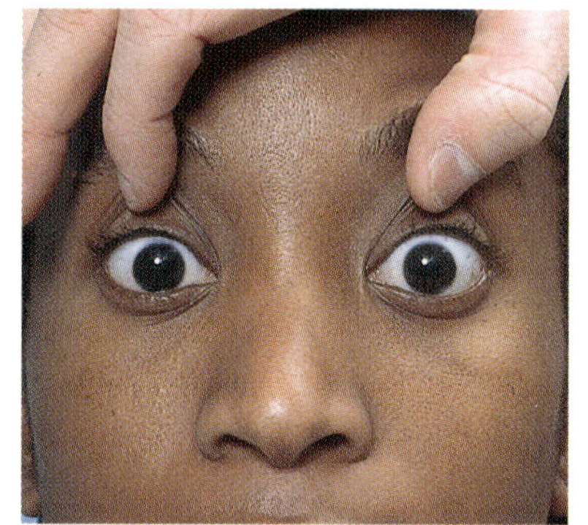

In a comatose patient with absence of doll's eye movements, shown below, the ability to move both eyes to one side is lost, suggesting a lesion of midbrain or pons.

In a comatose patient with an intact brainstem, as the head is turned the eyes move toward the opposite side (the doll's eye movements). In the adjacent photo, for example, the patient's head has been turned to the right; her eyes have moved to the left. Her eyes still seem to gaze at the camera. The doll's eye movements are intact.

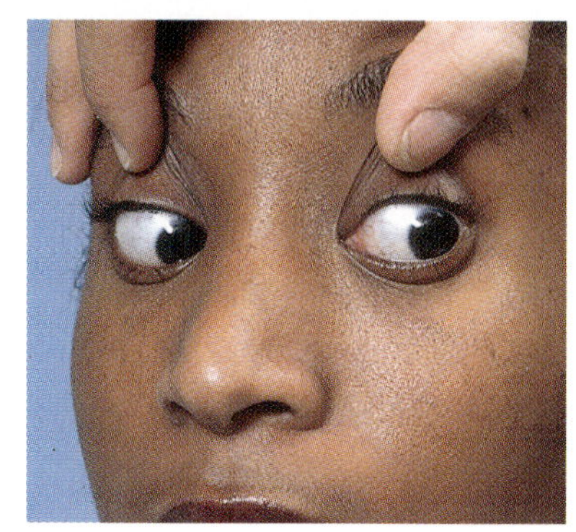

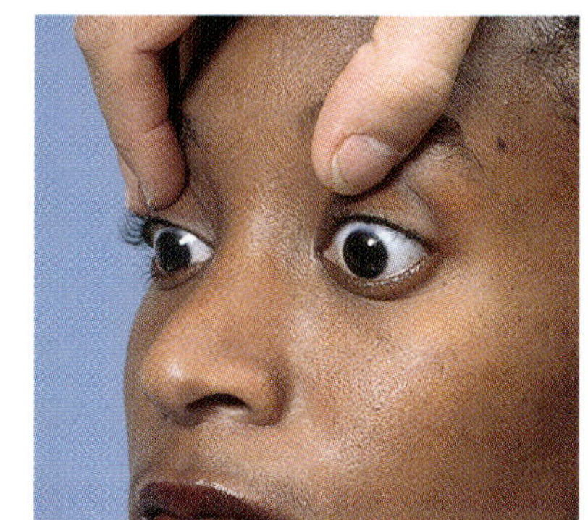

OCULOVESTIBULAR REFLEX (WITH CALORIC STIMULATION). If the oculocephalic reflex is absent and you seek further assessment of brainstem function, test the oculovestibular reflex. Note that this test is almost never performed in an awake patient.

Make sure the eardrums are intact and the canals clear. You must elevate the patient's head to 30° to perform the test accurately. Place a kidney basin under the ear to catch any overflowing water. With a large syringe, inject ice water through a small catheter that is lying in (but not plugging) the ear canal. Watch for deviation of the eyes in the horizontal plane. You may need to use up to 120 ml of ice water to elicit a response. In the comatose patient with an intact brainstem, the eyes drift *toward* the irrigated ear. Repeat on the opposite side, waiting 3 to 5 minutes if necessary for the first response to disappear.

No response to stimulation suggests brainstem injury.

POSTURE AND MUSCLE TONE. Observe the patient's posture. If there is no spontaneous movement, you may need to apply a painful stimulus (see p. 595). Classify the resulting pattern of movement as:

See Table 16-16, Abnormal Postures in the Comatose Patient (p. 622).

- *Normal–avoidant*—the patient pushes the stimulus away or withdraws.
- *Stereotypic*—the stimulus evokes abnormal postural responses of the trunk and extremities.

Two stereotypic responses predominate: *decorticate rigidity* and *decerebrate rigidity* (see Table 16-16, Abnormal Postures in the Comatose Patient, p. 622).

- *Flaccid paralysis or no response*

No response on one side suggests a corticospinal tract lesion.

Test muscle tone by grasping each forearm near the wrist and raising it to a vertical position. Note the position of the hand, usually only slightly flexed at the wrist.

The hemiplegia of sudden cerebral accidents is usually flaccid at first. The limp hand drops to form a right angle with the wrist.

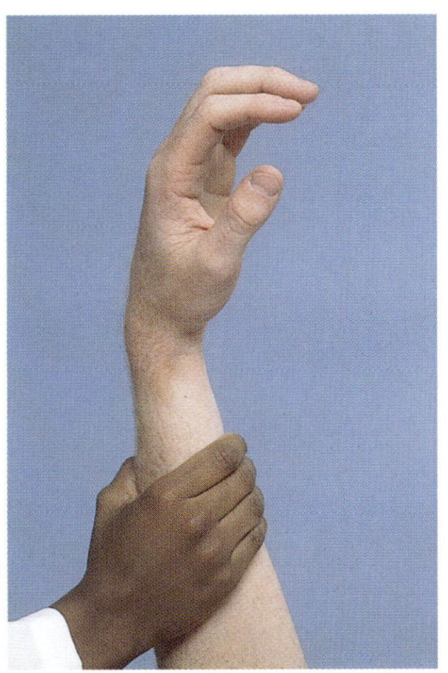

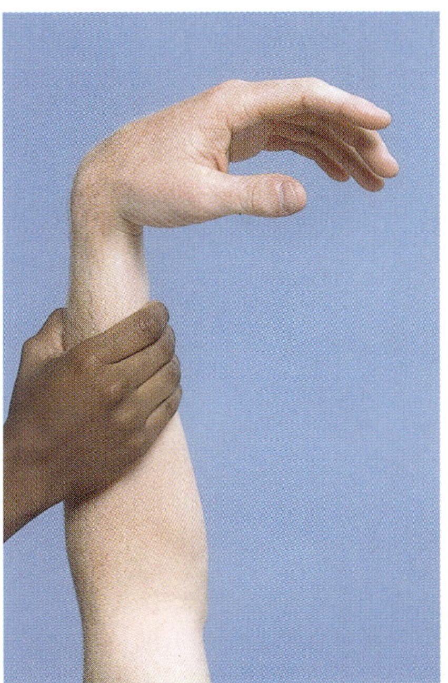

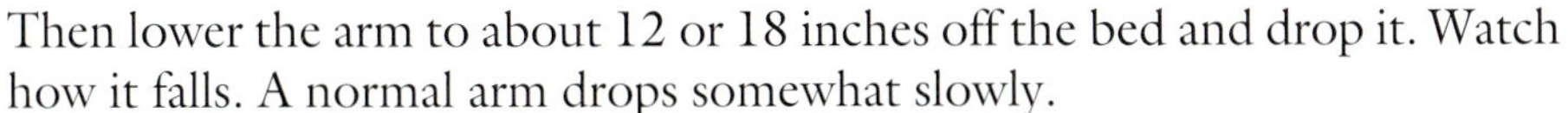

Then lower the arm to about 12 or 18 inches off the bed and drop it. Watch how it falls. A normal arm drops somewhat slowly.

A flaccid arm drops rapidly, like a flail.

Support the patient's flexed knees. Then extend one leg at a time at the knee and let it fall (see next page). Compare the speed with which each leg falls.

In acute hemiplegia, the flaccid leg falls more rapidly

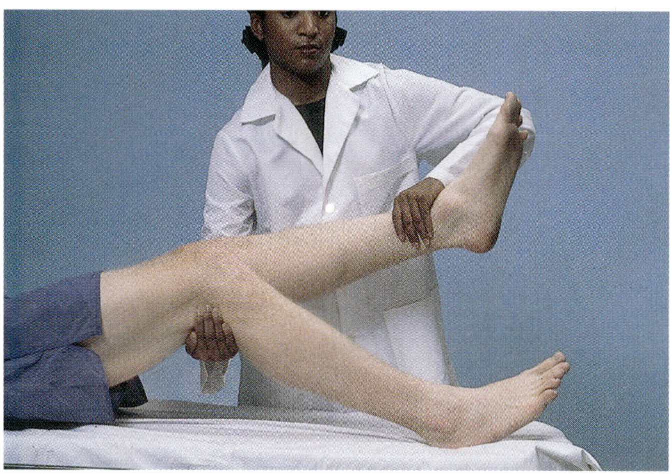

Flex both legs so that the heels rest on the bed and then release them. The normal leg returns slowly to its original extended position.

In acute hemiplegia, the flaccid leg falls rapidly into extension, with external rotation at the hip.

Further Examination

As you complete the neurologic examination, check for facial asymmetry and asymmetries in motor, sensory, and reflex function. Test for meningeal signs if indicated.

Meningitis, subarachnoid hemorrhage.

As you proceed to the general physical examination, check for unusual odors.

Alcohol, liver failure, uremia

Look for abnormalities of the skin, including color, moisture, evidence of bleeding disorders, needle marks, and other lesions.

Jaundice, cyanosis, cherry red color of carbon monoxide poisoning

Examine the scalp and skull for signs of trauma.

Bruises, lacerations, swelling

Examine the fundi carefully.

Papilledema, hypertensive retinopathy

Check to make sure the corneal reflexes are intact. (Remember that use of contact lenses may abolish these reflexes.)

Reflex loss in coma and lesions affecting CN V or CN VII

Inspect the ears and nose, and examine the mouth and throat.

Blood or cerebrospinal fluid in the nose or the ears suggests a skull fracture; otitis media suggests a possible brain abscess.

Tongue injury suggests a seizure.

Be sure to evaluate the heart, lungs, and abdomen.

Tables 16-1 through 16-7 summarize the manifestations of selected disorders. They show how the data collected can be used diagnostically, and will help you to recognize and think about certain patterns of illness.

Tables 16-1, 16-3, and 16-4 are based, with permission, on the *Diagnostic and Statistical Manual of Mental Disorders,* Fourth Edition, Text Revision (DSM IV-TR) Washington, D.C., American Psychiatric Association, 2000. For further details and criteria, the reader should consult this manual, its successor, or comprehensive textbooks of psychiatry.

TABLE 16-1 ■ Disorders of Mood

Mood disorders may be either depressive or bipolar. A bipolar disorder includes manic or hypomanic features as well as depressive ones. Four types of *episodes,* described below, are combined in different ways in diagnosis of *mood disorders.* A major depressive disorder includes only one or more major depressive episodes. A *bipolar I disorder* includes one or more manic or mixed episodes, usually accompanied by major depressive episodes. A *bipolar II disorder* includes one or more major depressive episodes accompanied by at least one hypomanic episode.

Dysthymic and *cyclothymic disorders* are chronic and less severe conditions that do not meet the criteria of the other disorders. *Mood disorders due to general medical conditions or substance abuse* are classified separately.

Major Depressive Episode

At least five of the symptoms listed below (including one of the first two) must be present during the same 2-week period. They must also represent a change from the person's previous state.

- Depressed mood (may be an irritable mood in children and adolescents) most of the day, nearly every day
- Markedly diminished interest or pleasure in almost all activities most of the day, nearly every day
- Significant weight gain or loss (not dieting) or increased or decreased appetite nearly every day
- Insomnia or hypersomnia nearly every day
- Psychomotor agitation or retardation nearly every day
- Fatigue or loss of energy nearly every day
- Feelings of worthlessness or inappropriate guilt nearly every day
- Inability to think or concentrate or indecisiveness nearly every day
- Recurrent thoughts of death or suicide, or a specific plan for or attempt at suicide

The symptoms cause significant distress or impair social, occupational, or other important functions. In severe cases, hallucinations and delusions may occur.

Mixed Episode

A mixed episode, which must last at least 1 week, meets the criteria for both manic and major depressive episodes.

Dysthymic Disorder

A depressed mood and symptoms for most of the day, for more days than not, over at least 2 years (1 year in children and adolescents). Freedom from symptoms lasts no more than 2 months at a time.

Manic Episode

A distinct period of abnormally and persistently elevated, expansive, or irritable mood must be present for at least a week (any duration if hospitalization is necessary). During this time, at least three of the symptoms listed below have been persistent and significant. (Four of the these symptoms are required if the mood is only irritable).

- Inflated self-esteem or grandiosity
- Decreased need for sleep (feels rested after sleeping 3 hours)
- More talkative than usual or pressure to keep talking
- Flight of ideas or racing thoughts
- Distractibility
- Increased goal-directed activity (either socially at work or school, or sexually) or psychomotor agitation
- Excessive involvement in pleasurable high-risk activities (buying sprees, foolish business ventures, sexual indiscretions)

The disturbance is severe enough to impair social or occupational functions or relationships. It may necessitate hospitalization for the protection of self or others. In severe cases, hallucinations and delusions may occur.

Hypomanic Episode

The mood and symptoms resemble those in a manic episode but are less impairing, do not require hospitalization, do not include hallucinations or delusions, and have a shorter minimum duration—4 days.

Cyclothymic Episode

Numerous periods of hypomanic and depressive symptoms that last for at least 2 years (1 year in children and adolescents). Freedom from symptoms lasts no more than 2 months at a time.

TABLE 16-2 ■ Disorders of Speech

Disorders of speech fall into three groups: those affecting (1) the voice, (2) the articulation of words, and (3) the production and comprehension of language.

Aphonia refers to a loss of voice that accompanies disease affecting the larynx or its nerve supply. *Dysphonia* refers to less severe impairment in the volume, quality, or pitch of the voice. For example, a person may be hoarse or only able to speak in a whisper. Causes include laryngitis, laryngeal tumors, and a unilateral vocal cord paralysis (Cranial Nerve X).

Dysarthria refers to a defect in the muscular control of the speech apparatus (lips, tongue, palate, or pharynx). Words may be nasal, slurred, or indistinct, but the central symbolic aspect of language remains intact. Causes include motor lesions of the central or peripheral nervous system, parkinsonism, and cerebellar disease.

Aphasia refers to a disorder in producing or understanding language. It is often caused by lesions in the dominant cerebral hemisphere (usually the left).

Compared below are two common types of aphasia: (1) Wernicke's, a fluent (receptive) aphasia, and (2) Broca's, a nonfluent (or expressive) aphasia. There are other less common kinds of aphasia, which may be distinguished from each other by differing responses on the specific tests listed. Neurologic consultation is usually indicated.

	Wernicke's Aphasia	Broca's Aphasia
Qualities of Spontaneous Speech	Fluent; often rapid, voluble, and effortless. Inflection and articulation are good, but sentences lack meaning and words are malformed (paraphasias) or invented (neologisms). Speech may be totally incomprehensible.	Nonfluent; slow, with few words and laborious effort. Inflection and articulation are impaired but words are meaningful, with nouns, transitive verbs, and important adjectives. Small grammatical words are often dropped.
Word Comprehension	Impaired	Fair to good
Repetition	Impaired	Impaired
Naming	Impaired	Impaired, though the patient recognizes objects
Reading Comprehension	Impaired	Fair to good
Writing	Impaired	Impaired
Location of Lesion	Posterior superior temporal lobe	Posterior inferior frontal lobe

While it is important to recognize aphasia early in your encounter with a patient, its full diagnostic meaning does not become clear until you integrate this information with your neurologic examination.

TABLE 16-3 ■ Anxiety Disorders

Anxiety disorders cause great distress and impair function, but those affected are not psychotic. The disorders are distinguished by the symptoms, the entities feared, or the stressors.

Panic Disorder	A panic disorder is defined by recurrent, unexpected panic attacks, at least one of which has been followed by a month or more of persistent concern about further attacks, worry over their implications or consequences, or a significant change in behavior in relation to the attacks. A *panic attack* is a discrete period of intense fear or discomfort that develops abruptly and peaks within 10 minutes. It involves at least four of the following symptoms: (1) palpitations, pounding heart, or accelerated heart rate, (2) sweating, (3) trembling or shaking, (4) shortness of breath or a sense of smothering, (5) a feeling of choking, (6) chest pain or discomfort, (7) nausea or abdominal distress, (8) feeling dizzy, unsteady, lightheaded, or faint, (9) feelings of unreality or depersonalization, (10) fear of losing control or going crazy, (11) fear of dying, (12) paresthesias (numbness or tingling), (13) chills or hot flushes. Panic disorder may occur with or without agoraphobia.
Agoraphobia	Agoraphobia is an anxiety about being in places or situations where escape may be difficult or embarrassing or help for sudden symptoms unavailable. Such situations are avoided, require a companion, or cause marked anxiety.
Specific Phobia	A specific phobia is a marked, persistent, and excessive or unreasonable fear that is cued by the presence or anticipation of a specific object or situation, such as dogs, injections, or flying. The person recognizes the fear as excessive or unreasonable, but exposure to the cue provokes immediate anxiety. Avoidance or fear impairs the person's normal routine, occupational or academic functioning, or social activities or relationships.
Social Phobia	A social phobia is a marked, persistent fear of one or more social or performance situations that involve exposure to unfamiliar people or to scrutiny by others. Those afflicted fear that they will act in embarrassing or humiliating ways, as by showing their anxiety. Exposure creates anxiety and possibly a panic attack, and the person avoids precipitating situations. He or she recognizes the fear as excessive or unreasonable. Normal routines, occupational or academic functioning, or social activities or relationships are impaired.
Obsessive–Compulsive Disorder	This disorder involves obsessions or compulsions that cause marked anxiety or distress. While they are recognized at some point as excessive or unreasonable, they are very time consuming and interfere with the person's normal routine, occupational functioning, or social activities or relationships.
Acute Stress Disorder	The person has been exposed to a traumatic event that involved actual or threatened death or serious injury to self or others and responded with intense fear, helplessness, or horror. During or immediately after this event, the person has at least three of these dissociative symptoms: (1) a subjective sense of numbing, detachment, or absence of emotional responsiveness; (2) a reduced awareness of surroundings, as in a daze; (3) feelings of unreality; (4) feelings of depersonalization; and (5) amnesia for an important part of the event. The event is persistently reexperienced, as in thoughts, images, dreams, illusions, and flashbacks, or distress from reminders of the event. The person is very anxious or shows increased arousal and tries to avoid stimuli that evoke memories of the event. The disturbance causes marked distress or impairs social, occupational, or other important functions. The symptoms occur within 4 weeks of the event and last from 2 days to 4 weeks.
Posttraumatic Stress Disorder	The event, the fearful response, and the persistent reexperiencing of the traumatic event resemble those in acute stress disorder. Hallucinations may occur. The person has increased arousal, tries to avoid stimuli related to the trauma, and has numbing of general responsiveness. The disturbance causes marked distress, impairs social, occupational, or other important functions, and lasts for more than a month.
Generalized Anxiety Disorder	This disorder lacks a specific traumatic event or focus for concern. Excessive anxiety and worry, which the person finds hard to control, are about a number of events or activities. At least three of the following symptoms are associated: (1) feeling restless, keyed up, or on edge, (2) being easily fatigued, (3) difficulty in concentrating or mind going blank, (4) irritability, (5) muscle tension, (6) difficulty in falling or staying asleep, or restless, unsatisfying sleep. The disturbance causes significant distress or impairs social, occupational, or other important functions.

TABLE 16-4 ■ Psychotic Disorders

Psychotic disorders involve grossly impaired reality testing. Specific diagnoses depend on the nature and duration of the symptoms and on a cause when it can be identified. Seven disorders are outlined below.

Schizophrenia	Schizophrenia impairs major functioning, as at work or school or in interpersonal relations or self care. For this diagnosis, performance of one or more of these functions must have decreased for a significant time to a level markedly below prior achievement. In addition, the person must manifest at least two of the following for a significant part of 1 month: (1) delusions, (2) hallucinations, (3) disorganized speech, (4) grossly disorganized or catatonic behavior,* and (5) negative symptoms such as a flat affect, alogia (lack of content in speech), or avolition (lack of interest, drive, and ability to set and pursue goals). Continuous signs of the disturbance must persist for at least 6 months. Subtypes of this disorder include paranoid, disorganized, and catatonic schizophrenia.
Schizophreniform Disorder	A schizophreniform disorder has symptoms similar to those of schizophrenia but they last less than 6 months, and the functional impairment seen in schizophrenia need not be present.
Schizoaffective Disorder	A schizoaffective disorder has features of both a major mood disturbance and schizophrenia. The mood disturbance (depressive, manic, or mixed) is present during most of the illness and must, for a time, be concurrent with symptoms of schizophrenia (listed above). During the same period of time, there must also be delusions or hallucinations for at least 2 weeks without prominent mood symptoms.
Delusional Disorder	A delusional disorder is characterized by nonbizarre delusions that involve situations in real life, such as having a disease or being deceived by a lover. The delusion has persisted for at least a month, but the person's functioning is not markedly impaired and behavior is not obviously odd or bizarre. The symptoms of schizophrenia except for tactile and olfactory hallucinations related to the delusion have not been present.
Brief Psychotic Disorder	In this disorder, at least one of the following psychotic symptoms must be present: delusions, hallucinations, disordered speech such as frequent derailment or incoherence, or grossly disorganized or catatonic behavior. The disturbance lasts at least 1 day but less than 1 month, and the person returns to his or her prior functional level.
Psychotic Disorder Due to a General Medical Condition	Prominent hallucinations or delusions may be experienced during a medical illness. For this diagnosis, they should not occur exclusively during the course of delirium. The medical condition should be documented and judged to be causally related to the symptoms.
Substance-Induced Psychotic Disorder	Prominent hallucinations or delusions may be induced by intoxication or withdrawal from a substance such as alcohol, cocaine, or opioids. For this diagnosis, these symptoms should not occur exclusively during the course of delirium. The substance should be judged to be causally related to the symptoms.

*Catatonic behaviors are psychomotor abnormalities that include stupor, mutism, negativistic resistance to instructions or attempts to move the person, rigid or bizarre postures, and excited, apparently purposeless activity.

TABLE 16-5 ■ Delirium and Dementia

Delirium and dementia are common and very important disorders that affect multiple aspects of mental status. Both have many possible causes. Some clinical features of these two conditions and their effects on mental status are compared below. A delirium may be superimposed on dementia.

	Delirium	Dementia
Clinical Features		
Onset	Acute	Insidious
Course	Fluctuating, with lucid intervals; worse at night	Slowly progressive
Duration	Hours to weeks	Months to years
Sleep/Wake Cycle	Always disrupted	Sleep fragmented
General Medical Illness or Drug Toxicity	Either or both present	Often absent, especially in Alzheimer's disease
Mental Status		
Level of Consciousness	Disturbed. Person less clearly aware of the environment and less able to focus, sustain, or shift attention	Usually normal until late in the course of the illness
Behavior	Activity often abnormally decreased (somnolence) or increased (agitation, hypervigilance)	Normal to slow; may become inappropriate
Speech	May be hesitant, slow or rapid, incoherent	Difficulty in finding words, aphasia
Mood	Fluctuating, labile, from fearful or irritable to normal or depressed	Often flat, depressed
Thought Processes	Disorganized, may be incoherent	Impoverished. Speech gives little information.
Thought Content	Delusions common, often transient	Delusions may occur.
Perceptions	Illusions, hallucinations, most often visual	Hallucinations may occur.
Judgment	Impaired, often to a varying degree	Increasingly impaired over the course of the illness
Orientation	Usually disoriented, especially for time. A known place may seem unfamiliar.	Fairly well maintained, but becomes impaired in the later stages of illness
Attention	Fluctuates. Person easily distracted, unable to concentrate on selected tasks	Usually unaffected until late in the illness
Memory	Immediate and recent memory impaired	Recent memory and new learning especially impaired
Examples of Cause	Delirium tremens (due to withdrawal from alcohol) Uremia Acute hepatic failure Acute cerebral vasculitis Atropine poisoning	*Reversible:* Vitamin B_{12} deficiency, thyroid disorders *Irreversible:* Alzheimer's disease, vascular dementia (from multiple infarcts), dementia due to head trauma

TABLE 16-6 ■ Syncope and Similar Disorders

Problem	Mechanism	Precipitating Factors
Vasodepressor Syncope *(the common faint)*	Sudden peripheral vasodilatation, especially in the skeletal muscles, without a compensatory rise in cardiac output. Blood pressure falls.	A strong emotion such as fear or pain
Postural *(orthostatic)* **Hypotension**	▪ *Inadequate vasoconstrictor reflexes* in both arterioles and veins, with resultant venous pooling, decreased cardiac output, and low blood pressure	▪ Standing up
	▪ *Hypovolemia,* a diminished blood volume insufficient to maintain cardiac output and blood pressure, especially in the upright position	▪ Standing up after hemorrhage or dehydration
Cough Syncope	Several possible mechanisms associated with increased intrathoracic pressure	Severe paroxysm of coughing
Micturition Syncope	Unclear	Emptying the bladder after getting out of bed to void
Cardiovascular Disorders		
Arrhythmias	Decreased cardiac output secondary to rhythms that are too fast (usually more than 180) or too slow (less than 35–40)	A sudden change in rhythm
Aortic Stenosis and Hypertrophic Cardiomyopathy	Vascular resistance falls with exercise, but cardiac output cannot rise.	Exercise
Myocardial Infarction	Sudden arrhythmia or decreased cardiac output	Variable
Massive Pulmonary Embolism	Sudden hypoxia or decreased cardiac output	Variable
Disorders Resembling Syncope		
Hypocapnia (decreased carbon dioxide) Due to Hyperventilation	Constriction of cerebral blood vessels secondary to hypocapnia that is induced by hyperventilation	Possibly a stressful situation
Hypoglycemia	Insufficient glucose to maintain cerebral metabolism; secretion of epinephrine contributes to symptoms.	Variable, including fasting
*Hysterical Fainting Due to a Conversion Reaction**	The symbolic expression of an unacceptable idea through body language	Stressful situation

* Important diagnostic observations in hysterical fainting include normal skin color and normal vital signs, sometimes bizarre and purposive movements, and occurrence in the presence of other people.

Predisposing Factors	Prodromal Manifestations	Postural Associations	Recovery
Fatigue, hunger, a hot, humid environment	Restlessness, weakness, pallor, nausea, salivation, sweating, yawning	Usually occurs when standing, possibly when sitting	Prompt return of consciousness when lying down, but pallor, weakness, nausea, and slight confusion may persist for a time.
■ Peripheral neuropathies and disorders affecting the autonomic nervous system; drugs such as antihypertensives and vasodilators; prolonged bed rest	■ Often none	■ Occurs soon after the person stands up	■ Prompt return to normal when lying down
■ Bleeding from the GI tract or trauma, potent diuretics, vomiting, diarrhea, polyuria	■ Lightheadedness and palpitations (tachycardia) on standing up	■ Usually occurs soon after the person stands up	■ Improvement on lying down
Chronic bronchitis in a muscular man	Often none except for cough	May occur in any position	Prompt return to normal
Nocturia, usually in elderly or adult men	Often none	Standing to void	Prompt return to normal
Organic heart disease and old age decrease the tolerance to abnormal rhythms.	Often none	May occur in any position	Prompt return to normal unless brain damage has resulted
Cardiac disorders	Often none. Onset is sudden.	Occurs with or after exercise	Usually a prompt return to normal
Coronary artery disease	Often none	May occur in any position	Variable
Deep venous thrombosis	Often none	May occur in any position	Variable
A predisposition to anxiety attacks and hyperventilation	Dyspnea, palpitations, chest discomfort, numbness and tingling of the hands and around the mouth lasting for several minutes. Consciousness is often maintained.	May occur in any position	Slow improvement as hyperventilation ceases
Insulin therapy and a variety of metabolic disorders	Sweating, tremor, palpitations, hunger; headache, confusion, abnormal behavior, coma. True syncope is uncommon.	May occur in any position	Variable, depending on severity and treatment
Hysterical personality traits	Variable	A slump to the floor, often from a standing position without injury	Variable, may be prolonged, often with fluctuating responsiveness

TABLE 16-7 ■ Seizure Disorders

Partial seizures are those that start with focal manifestations. They are further divided into *simple partial seizures,* which do not impair consciousness, and *complex partial seizures,* which do. Each of these two types may remain localized or progress into a third type, *partial seizures that become generalized*. Partial seizures of all kinds usually indicate a structural lesion in the cerebral cortex, such as a scar, tumor, or infarction. The quality of such seizures helps the clinician to localize the causative lesion in the brain.

Problem	Clinical Manifestations	Postictal *(Postseizure)* State
Partial Seizures		
Simple Partial Seizures		
■ With motor symptoms		
Jacksonian	Tonic and then clonic movements that start unilaterally in the hand, foot, or face and spread to other body parts on the same side	Normal consciousness
Other motor	Turning of the head and eyes to one side, or tonic and clonic movements of an arm or leg without the Jacksonian spread	Normal consciousness
■ With sensory symptoms	Numbness, tingling; simple visual, auditory, or olfactory hallucinations such as flashing lights, buzzing, or odors	Normal consciousness
■ With autonomic symptoms	A "funny feeling" in the epigastrium, nausea, pallor, flushing, lightheadedness	Normal consciousness
■ With psychiatric symptoms	Anxiety or fear; feelings of familiarity (déjà vu) or unreality; dreamy states; fear or rage; flashback experiences; more complex hallucinations	Normal consciousness
Complex Partial Seizures May start with simple partial seizures or with impaired consciousness. Automatisms may develop.	The seizure may or may not start with the autonomic or psychic symptoms that are outlined above. Consciousness is impaired and the person appears confused. Automatisms include automatic motor behaviors such as chewing, smacking the lips, walking about, and unbuttoning clothes; also more complicated and skilled behaviors such as driving a car.	The patient may remember initial autonomic or psychic symptoms (which are then termed an *aura*), but is amnesic for the rest of the seizure. Temporary confusion and headache may occur.
Partial Seizures That Become Generalized	Partial seizures that become generalized resemble tonic–clonic seizures (see next page). Unfortunately, the patient may not recall the focal onset and observers may overlook it.	As in a tonic–clonic seizure, described on the next page. *Two attributes indicate a partial seizure that has become generalized: (1) the recollection of an aura, and (2) a unilateral neurologic deficit during the postictal period.*

TABLE 16-7 ■ Seizure Disorders *(Continued)*

Generalized seizures, in contrast to partial ones, begin with either bilateral bodily movements or impairment of consciousness, or both. They suggest a widespread, bilateral cortical disturbance that may be either hereditary or acquired. When generalized seizures of the tonic–clonic (grand mal) variety start in childhood or young adulthood, they are often hereditary. When tonic–clonic seizures begin after the age of 30, suspect either a partial seizure that has become generalized or a general seizure caused by a toxic or metabolic problem. Toxic and metabolic causes include withdrawal from alcohol or other sedative drugs, uremia, hypoglycemia, hyperglycemia, hyponatremia and water intoxication, and bacterial meningitis.

Problem	Clinical Manifestations	Postictal *(Postseizure)* State
Generalized Seizures		
*Tonic–Clonic Convulsion (grand mal)**	The person loses consciousness suddenly, sometimes with a cry, and the body stiffens into tonic extensor rigidity. Breathing stops and the person becomes cyanotic. A clonic phase of rhythmic muscular contraction follows. Breathing resumes and is often noisy, with excessive salivation. Injury, tongue biting, and urinary incontinence may occur.	Confusion, drowsiness, fatigue, headache, muscular aching, and sometimes the temporary persistence of bilateral neurologic deficits such as hyperactive reflexes and Babinski responses. The person has amnesia for the seizure and recalls no aura.
Absence	A sudden brief lapse of consciousness, with momentary blinking, staring, or movements of the lips and hands but no falling. Two subtypes are recognized. *Petit mal absences* last less than 10 sec and stop abruptly. *Atypical absences* may last more than 10 sec.	No aura recalled. In petit mal absences, a prompt return to normal; in atypical absences, some postictal confusion
Atonic Seizure, or Drop Attack	Sudden loss of consciousness with falling but no movements. Injury may occur.	Either a prompt return to normal or a brief period of confusion
Myoclonus	Sudden, brief, rapid jerks, involving the trunk or limbs. Associated with a variety of disorders	Variable
Pseudoseizures		
May mimic seizures but are due to a conversion reaction (a psychological disorder).	The movements may have personally symbolic significance and often do not follow a neuroanatomic pattern. Injury is uncommon.	Variable

* *Febrile convulsions* that resemble brief tonic–clonic seizures may occur in infants and young children. They are usually benign but occasionally may be the first manifestation of a seizure disorder.

TABLE 16-8 ■ Involuntary Movements

Tremors

Tremors are relatively rhythmic oscillatory movements, which may be roughly subdivided into three groups: resting (or static) tremors, intention tremors, and postural tremors.

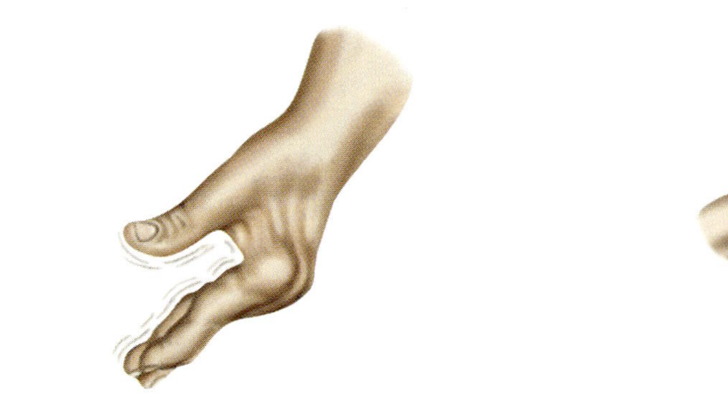

Resting (Static) Tremors

These tremors are most prominent at rest, and may decrease or disappear with voluntary movement. Illustrated is the common, relatively slow, fine, pill-rolling tremor of parkinsonism, about 5 per second.

Postural Tremors

These tremors appear when the affected part is actively maintaining a posture. Examples include the fine, rapid tremor of hyperthyroidism, the tremors of anxiety and fatigue, and benign essential (and sometimes familial) tremor. Tremor may worsen somewhat with intention.

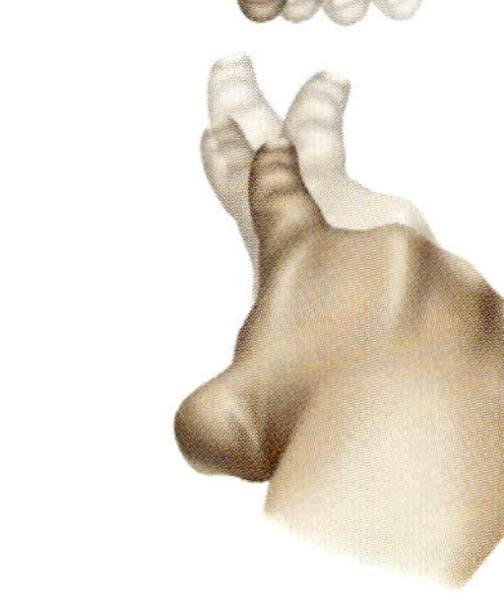

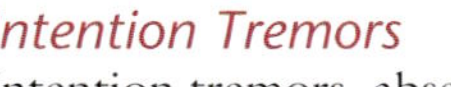

Intention Tremors

Intention tremors, absent at rest, appear with activity and often get worse as the target is neared. Causes include disorders of cerebellar pathways, as in multiple sclerosis.

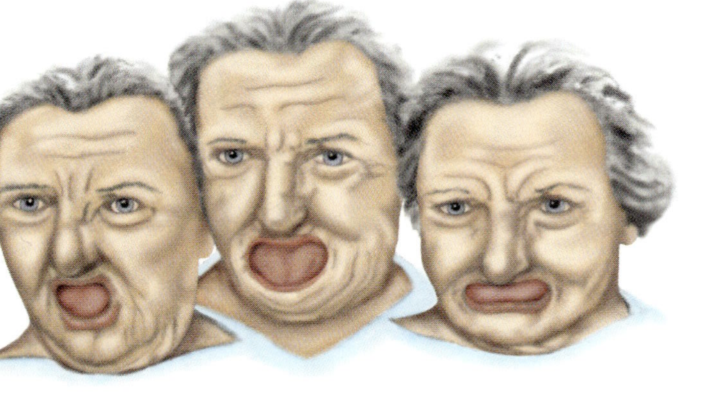

Oral–Facial Dyskinesias

Oral–facial dyskinesias are rhythmic, repetitive, bizarre movements that chiefly involve the face, mouth, jaw, and tongue: grimacing, pursing of the lips, protrusions of the tongue, opening and closing of the mouth, and deviations of the jaw. The limbs and trunk are involved less often. These movements may be a late complication of psychotropic drugs such as phenothiazines, and have then been termed *tardive* (late) dyskinesias. They also occur in long-standing psychoses, in some elderly individuals, and in some edentulous persons.

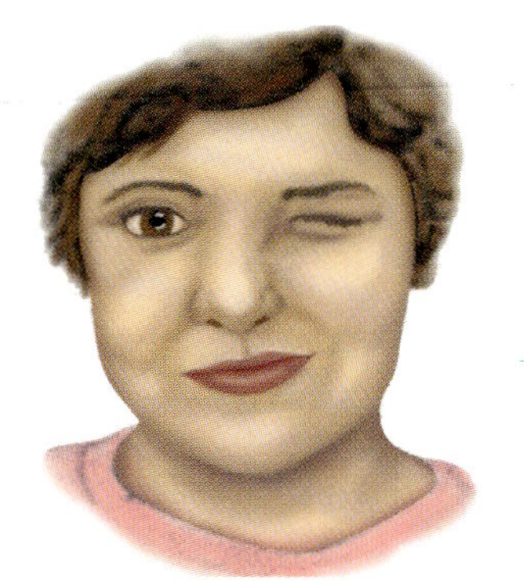

Tics

Tics are brief, repetitive, stereotyped, coordinated movements occurring at irregular intervals. Examples include repetitive winking, grimacing, and shoulder shrugging. Causes include Tourette's syndrome and drugs such as phenothiazines and amphetamines.

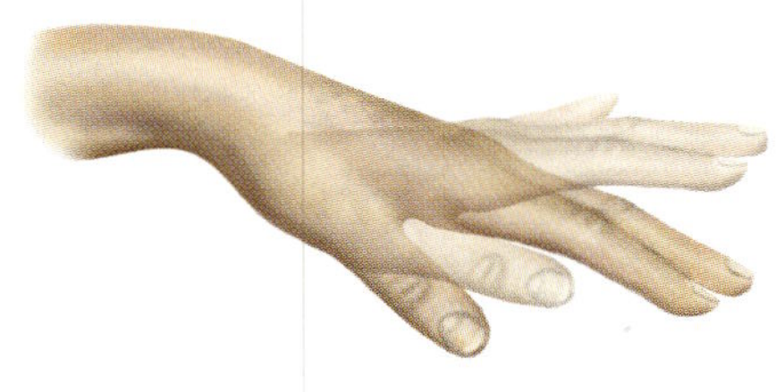

Chorea

Choreiform movements are brief, rapid, jerky, irregular, and unpredictable. They occur at rest or interrupt normal coordinated movements. Unlike tics, they seldom repeat themselves. The face, head, lower arms, and hands are often involved. Causes include Sydenham's chorea (with rheumatic fever) and Huntington's disease.

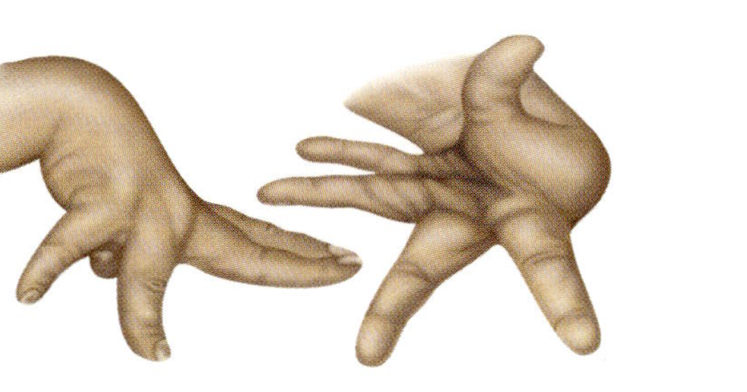

Athetosis

Athetoid movements are slower and more twisting and writhing than choreiform movements, and have a larger amplitude. They most commonly involve the face and the distal extremities. Athetosis is often associated with spasticity. Causes include cerebral palsy.

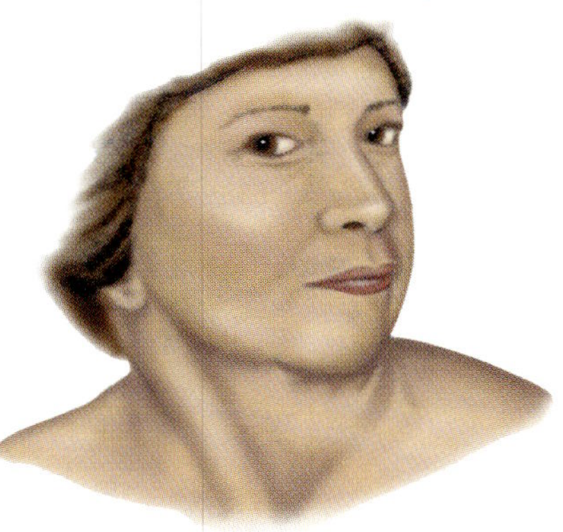

Dystonia

Dystonic movements are somewhat similar to athetoid movements, but often involve larger portions of the body, including the trunk. Grotesque, twisted postures may result. Causes include drugs such as phenothiazines, primary torsion dystonia and, as illustrated, spasmodic torticollis.

TABLE 16-9 ■ Nystagmus

Nystagmus is a rhythmic oscillation of the eyes, analogous to a tremor in other parts of the body. Its causes are multiple, including impairment of vision in early life, disorders of the labyrinth and the cerebellar system, and drug toxicity. Nystagmus occurs normally when a person watches a rapidly moving object (e.g., a passing train). Observe the three characteristics of nystagmus listed below and on the following page. Then refer to textbooks of neurology for differential diagnosis.

Direction of the Quick and Slow Components

Example: Nystagmus to the Left—A Slow Drift to the Right, Then a Quick Jerk to the Left in Each Eye

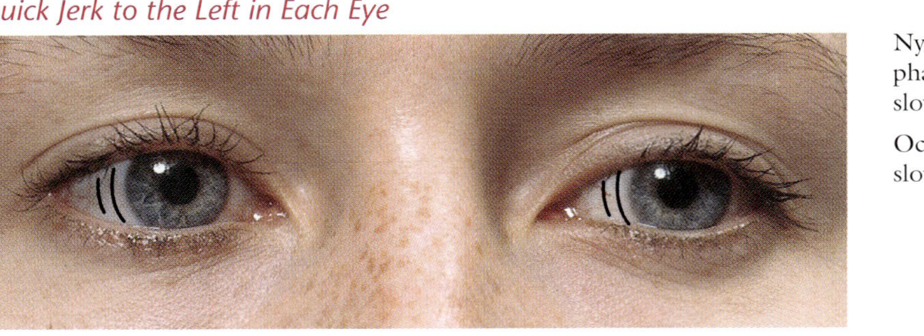

Nystagmus usually has both fast and slow movements, but is defined by its fast phase. For example, if the eyes jerk quickly to the patient's left and drift back slowly to the right, the patient is said to have nystagmus to the left.

Occasionally, nystagmus consists only of coarse oscillations without quick and slow components. It is then said to be *pendular*.

Plane of the Movements

Horizontal Nystagmus

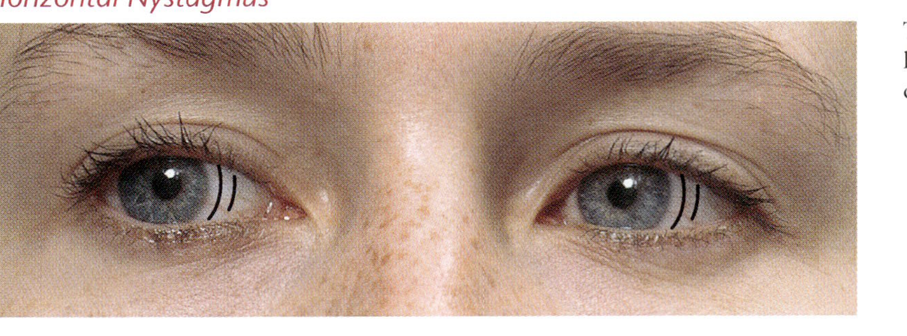

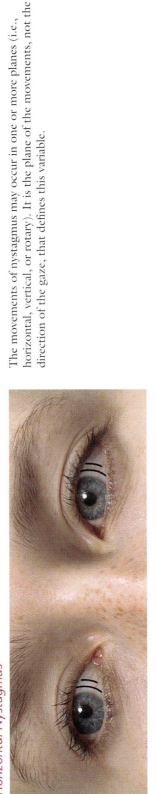

The movements of nystagmus may occur in one or more planes (i.e., horizontal, vertical, or rotary). It is the plane of the movements, not the direction of the gaze, that defines this variable.

Vertical Nystagmus

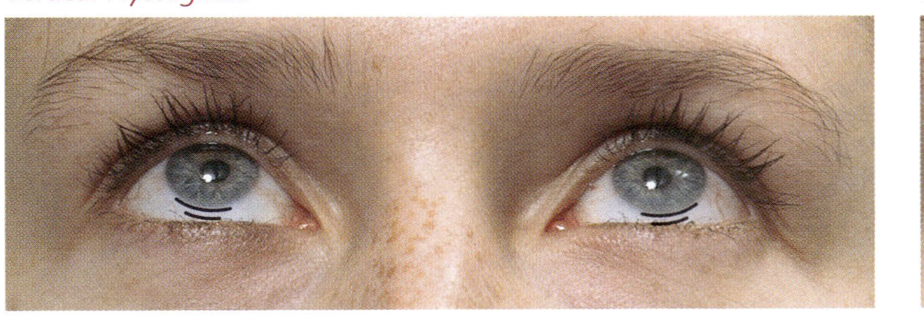

Rotary Nystagmus

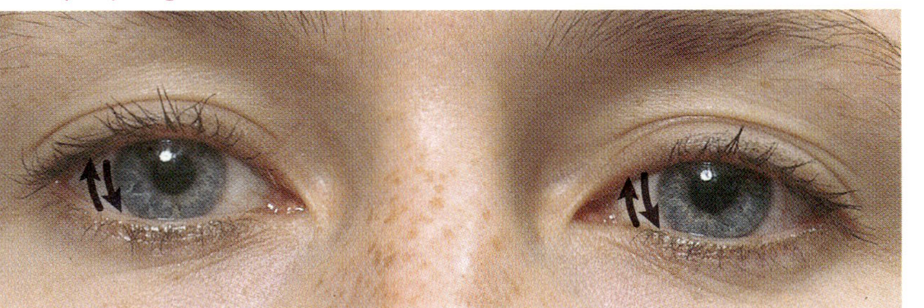

Direction of Gaze in Which Nystagmus Appears

Example: Nystagmus on Right Lateral Gaze

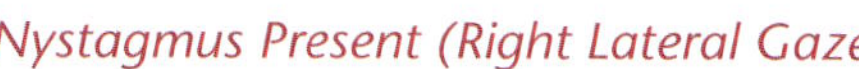

Nystagmus Present (Right Lateral Gaze)

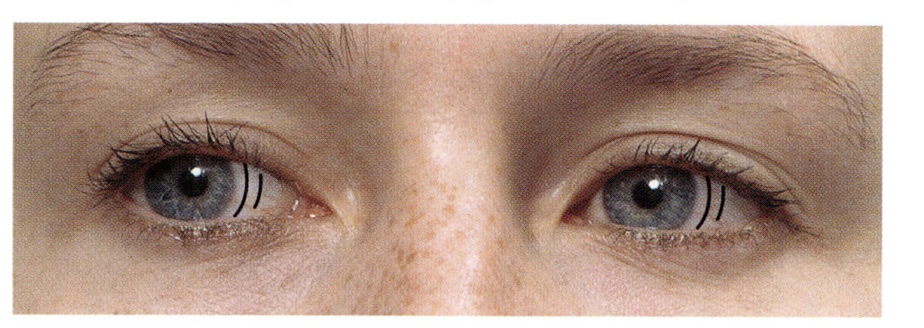

Nystagmus Not Present (Left Lateral Gaze)

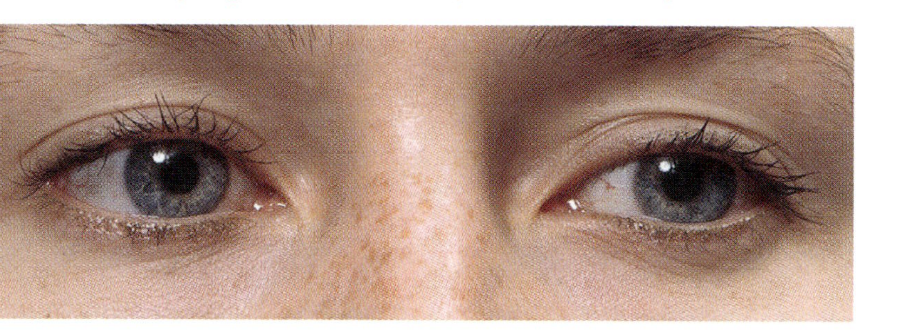

Although nystagmus may be present in all directions of gaze, it may appear or become accentuated only on deviation of the eyes (e.g., to the side or upward). On extreme lateral gaze, the normal person may show a few beats resembling nystagmus. Avoid making assessments in such extreme positions, and observe for nystagmus only within the field of full binocular vision.

TABLE 16-10 ■ Types of Facial Paralysis

Facial weakness or paralysis may result either (1) from a peripheral lesion of CN VII, the facial nerve, anywhere from its origin in the pons to its periphery in the face, or (2) from a central lesion involving the upper motor neurons between the cortex and the pons. A peripheral lesion of CN VII, exemplified here by a Bell's palsy, is compared with a central lesion, exemplified by a left hemispheric cerebrovascular accident. Note their different effects on the upper part of the face, by which they can be distinguished.

CN VII—Peripheral Lesion

Peripheral nerve damage to CN VII paralyzes the entire right side of the face, including the forehead.

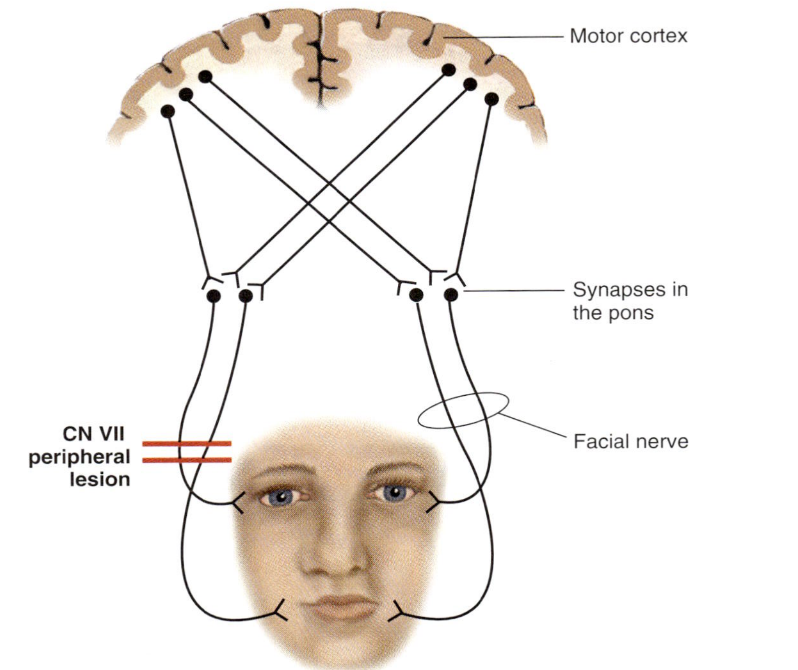

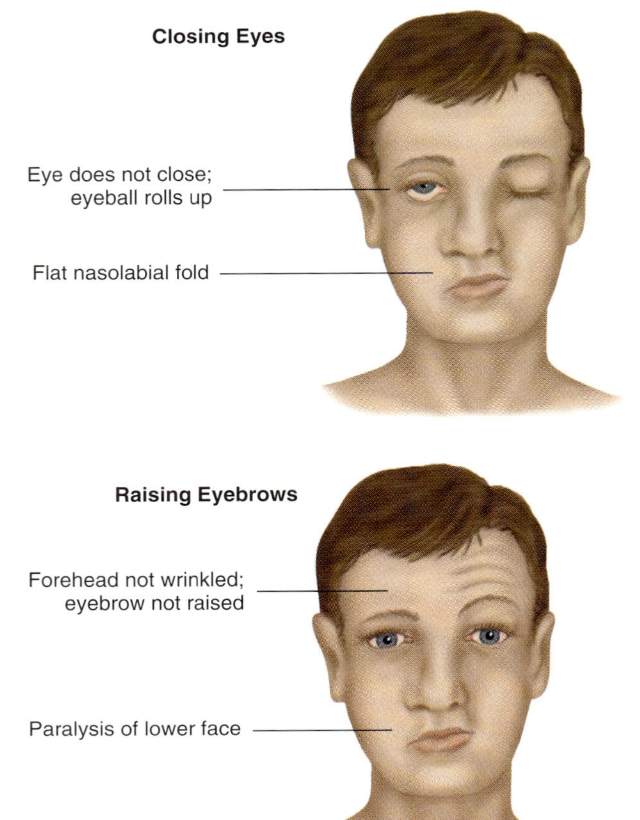

CN VII—Central Lesion

The lower part of the face normally is controlled by upper motor neurons located on only one side of the cortex—the opposite side. *Left-sided damage to these pathways, as in a stroke, paralyzes the right lower face.* The upper face, however, is controlled by pathways from both sides of the cortex. Even though the upper motor neurons on the left are destroyed, others on the right remain and the right upper face continues to function fairly well.

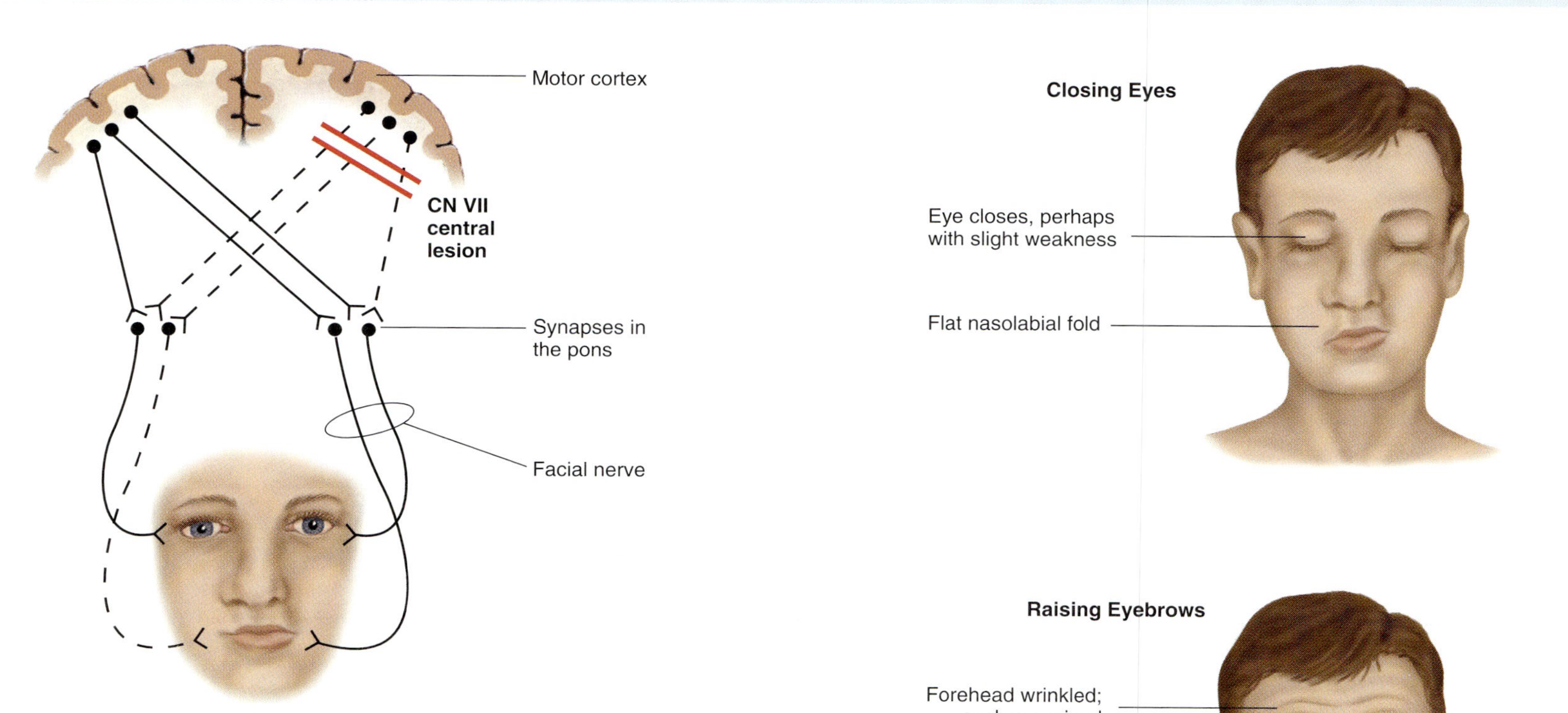

TABLE 16-11 ■ Disorders of Muscle Tone

	Spasticity	Rigidity	Flaccidity	Paratonia
Location of Lesion	Upper motor neuron of the corticospinal tract at any point from the cortex to the spinal cord	Basal ganglia system	Lower motor neuron at any point from the anterior horn cell to the peripheral nerves	Both hemispheres, usually in the frontal lobes
Description	Increased muscle tone (*hypertonia*) that is rate-dependent. Tone is greater when passive movement is rapid, and less when passive movement is slow. Tone is also greater at the extremes of the movement arc. During rapid passive movement, initial hypertonia may give way suddenly as the limb relaxes. This spastic "catch" and relaxation is known as "clasp-knife" resistance.	Increased resistance that persists throughout the movement arc, independent of rate of movement, is called *lead-pipe rigidity*. With flexion and extension of the wrist or forearm, a superimposed rachetlike jerkiness is called *cogwheel rigidity*.	Loss of muscle tone (*hypotonia*), causing the limb to be loose or floppy. The affected limbs may be hyperextensible or even flail-like.	Sudden changes in tone with passive range of motion. Sudden loss of tone that increases the ease of motion is called *mitgehen* (moving with). Sudden increase in tone making motion more difficult is called *gegenhalten* (holding against).
Common Cause	Stroke, especially late or chronic stage	Parkinsonism	Guillain–Barré syndrome; also initial phase of spinal cord injury (spinal shock) or stroke	Dementia

TABLE 16-12 ■ Disorders of the Central and Peripheral Nervous Systems

Central Nervous System Disorders

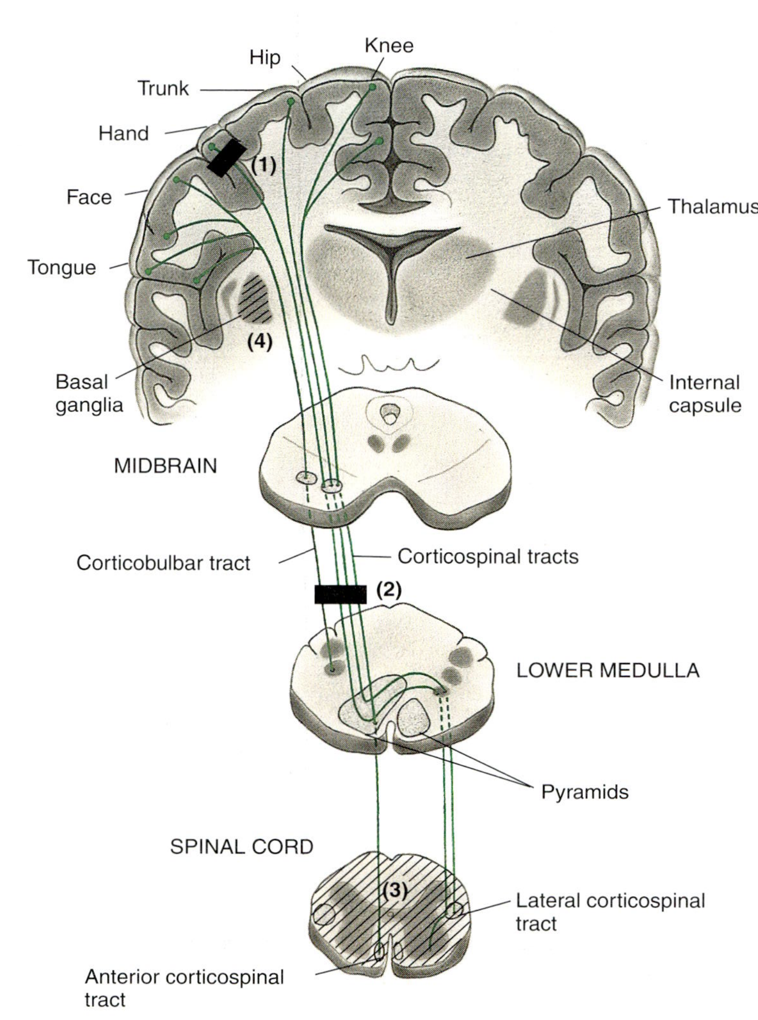

(table continues next page)

TABLE 16-12 ■ Disorders of the Central and Peripheral Nervous Systems *(Continued)*

Central Nervous System Disorders

Location of Lesion	Typical Findings: *Motor*	Typical Findings: *Sensory*	Typical Findings: *Deep Tendon Reflexes*	Examples of Cause
Cerebral Cortex (1)	Chronic contralateral upper motor neuron weakness and spasticity. Flexion is stronger than extension in the arm, plantar flexion is stronger than dorsiflexion in the foot, and the leg is externally rotated at the hip.	Contralateral sensory loss on the limbs and trunk on the same side as the motor deficits	↑	Cortical stroke
Brainstem (2)	Weakness and spasticity as above, plus cranial nerve deficits such as diplopia (from weakness of the extraocular muscles) and dysarthria	Variable. No typical sensory findings	↑	Brainstem stroke, acoustic neuroma
Spinal Cord (3)	Weakness and spasticity, as above, but often affecting both sides (when cord damage is bilateral), causing paraplegia or quadriplegia depending on the level of injury	Dermatomal sensory deficit on the trunk bilaterally at the level of the lesion, and sensory loss from tract damage below the level of the lesion	↑	Trauma, causing cord compression
Subcortical Gray Matter: Basal Ganglia (4)	Slowness of movement (bradykinesia), rigidity, and tremor	Sensation not affected	Normal or ↓	Parkinsonism
Cerebellar (not illustrated)	Hypotonia, ataxia, and other abnormal movements, including nystagmus, dysdiadochokinesis, and dysmetria	Sensation not affected	Normal or ↓	Cerebellar stroke, brain tumor

Peripheral Nervous System Disorders

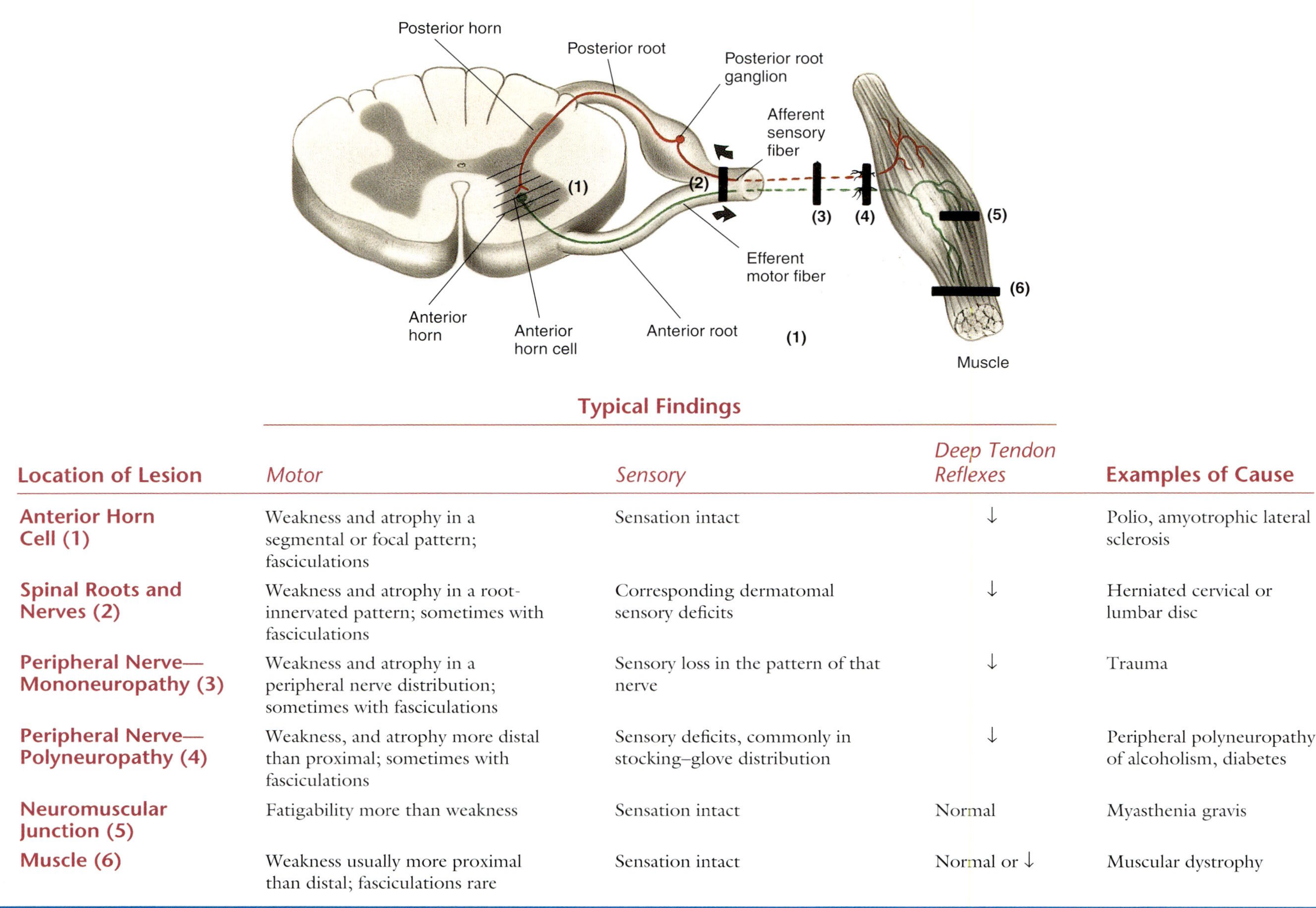

Location of Lesion	Typical Findings: *Motor*	*Sensory*	*Deep Tendon Reflexes*	Examples of Cause
Anterior Horn Cell (1)	Weakness and atrophy in a segmental or focal pattern; fasciculations	Sensation intact	↓	Polio, amyotrophic lateral sclerosis
Spinal Roots and Nerves (2)	Weakness and atrophy in a root-innervated pattern; sometimes with fasciculations	Corresponding dermatomal sensory deficits	↓	Herniated cervical or lumbar disc
Peripheral Nerve—Mononeuropathy (3)	Weakness and atrophy in a peripheral nerve distribution; sometimes with fasciculations	Sensory loss in the pattern of that nerve	↓	Trauma
Peripheral Nerve—Polyneuropathy (4)	Weakness, and atrophy more distal than proximal; sometimes with fasciculations	Sensory deficits, commonly in stocking–glove distribution	↓	Peripheral polyneuropathy of alcoholism, diabetes
Neuromuscular Junction (5)	Fatigability more than weakness	Sensation intact	Normal	Myasthenia gravis
Muscle (6)	Weakness usually more proximal than distal; fasciculations rare	Sensation intact	Normal or ↓	Muscular dystrophy

TABLE 16-13 ■ Abnormalities of Gait and Posture

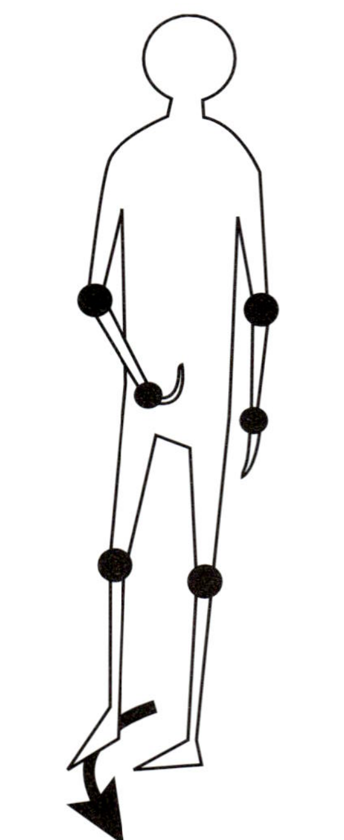

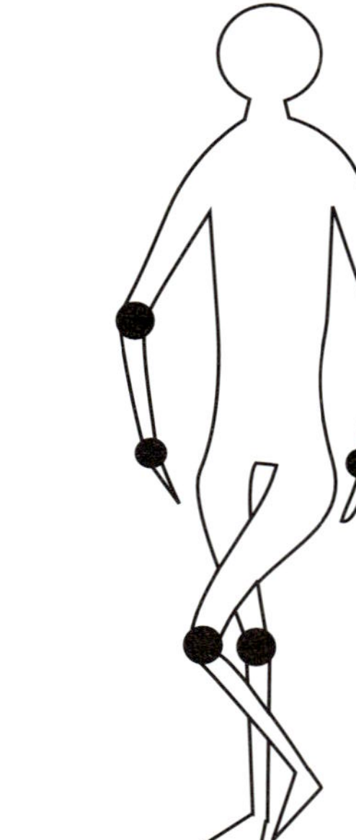

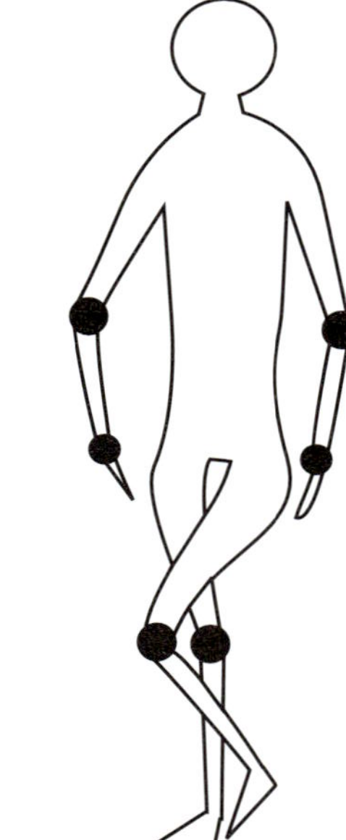

	Spastic Hemiparesis	Scissors Gait	Steppage Gait
Underlying Defect	Associated with lesion in corticospinal tract, as with stroke	Associated with bilateral spastic paresis of the legs	Associated with foot drop, usually secondary to lower motor neuron disease
Description	One arm is held immobile and close to the side, with elbow, wrist, and interphalangeal joints flexed. The leg is extended, with plantar flexion of the foot. On walking, the patient either drags the foot, often scraping the toe, or circles it stiffly outward and forward (*circumduction*).	The gait is stiff. Each leg is advanced slowly, and the thighs tend to cross forward on each other at each step. The steps are short. The patient appears to be walking through water.	These patients either drag their feet or lift them high, with knees flexed, and bring them down with a slap onto the floor, thus appearing to be walking up stairs. They are unable to walk on their heels. The steppage gait may involve one or both sides.

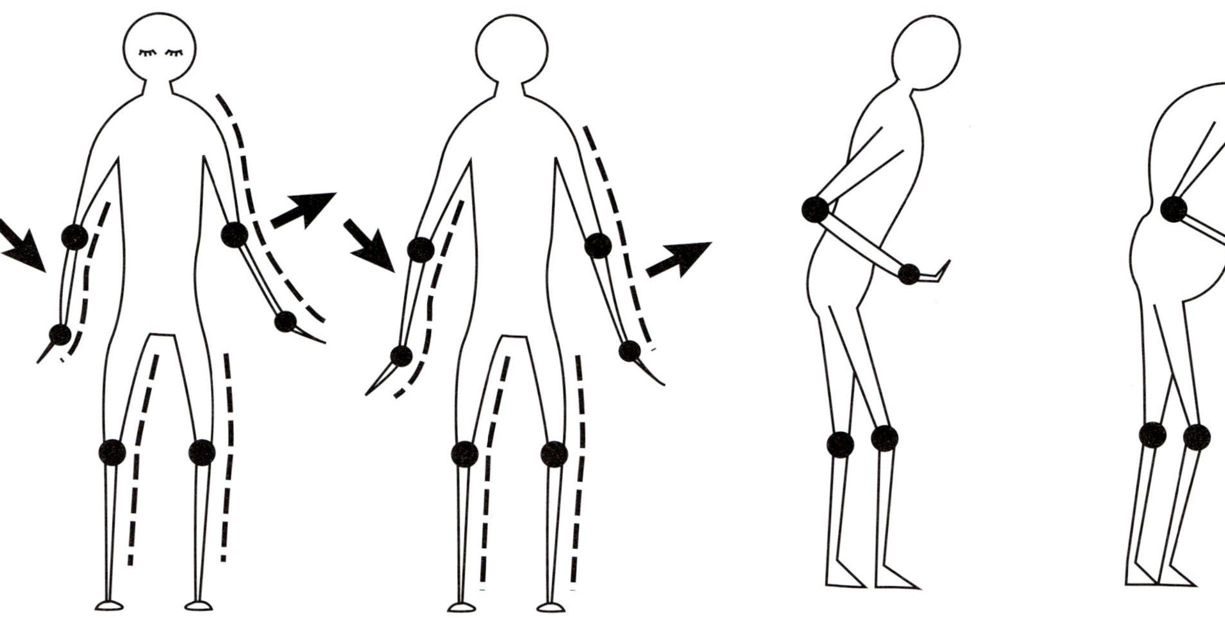

	Sensory Ataxia	Cerebellar Ataxia	Parkinsonian Gait	Gait of Older Age
Underlying Defect	Associated with loss of position sense in the legs, as from polyneuropathy or posterior column damage	Associated with disease of the cerebellum or associated tracts	Associated with the basal ganglia defects of Parkinson's disease	The aging process
Description	The gait is unsteady and wide based (with feet wide apart). These patients throw their feet forward and outward and bring them down, first on the heels and then on the toes, with a double tapping sound. They watch the ground for guidance while walking. With eyes closed, they cannot stand steadily with feet together (a positive Romberg sign) and the staggering gait worsens.	The gait is staggering, unsteady, and wide based, with exaggerated difficulty on the turns. These patients cannot stand steadily with feet together, whether their eyes are open or closed.	The posture is stooped, with head and neck forward and hips and knees slightly flexed. Arms are flexed at elbows and wrists. The patient is slow in getting started. Steps are short and often shuffling. Arm swings are decreased and the patient turns around stiffly—"all in one piece."	Speed, balance, and agility decrease with aging. Steps become short, uncertain, and even shuffling. The legs may be flexed at hips and knees. A cane may bolster lost confidence.

TABLE 16-14 ■ Metabolic and Structural Coma

Although there are many causes of coma, most can be classified as either structural or metabolic. Findings vary widely in individual patients; the features listed are general guidelines rather than strict diagnostic criteria. Remember that psychiatric disorders may mimic coma.

	Toxic–Metabolic	Structural
Pathophysiology	Arousal centers poisoned or critical substrates depleted	Lesion destroys or compresses brainstem arousal areas, either directly or secondary to more distant expanding mass lesions.
Clinical Features		
■ Respiratory pattern	If regular, may be normal or hyperventilation. If irregular, usually Cheyne–Stokes	Irregular, especially Cheyne–Stokes or ataxic breathing
■ Pupillary size and reaction	Equal, reactive to light. If *pinpoint* from opiates or cholinergics, you may need a magnifying glass to see the reaction. May be unreactive if *fixed and dilated* from anticholinergics or hypothermia	Unequal or unreactive to light (fixed) *Midposition, fixed*—suggests midbrain compression *Dilated, fixed*—suggests compression of CN III from herniation
■ Level of consciousness	Changes after pupils change	Changes before pupils change
Examples of Cause	Uremia, hyperglycemia	Epidural, subdural, or intracerebral hemorrhage
	Alcohol, drugs, liver failure	Cerebral infarct or embolus
	Hypothyroidism, hypoglycemia	Tumor, abscess
	Anoxia, ischemia	Brainstem infarct, tumor, or hemorrhage
	Meningitis, encephalitis	Cerebellar infarct, hemorrhage, tumor, or abscess
	Hyperthermia, hypothermia	

TABLE 16-15 ■ Pupils in Comatose Patients

Pupillary size, equality, and light reactions help in assessing the cause of coma and in determining the region of the brain that is impaired. Remember that unrelated pupillary abnormalities, including miotic drops for glaucoma or mydriatic drops for a better view of the ocular fundi, may have preceded the coma.

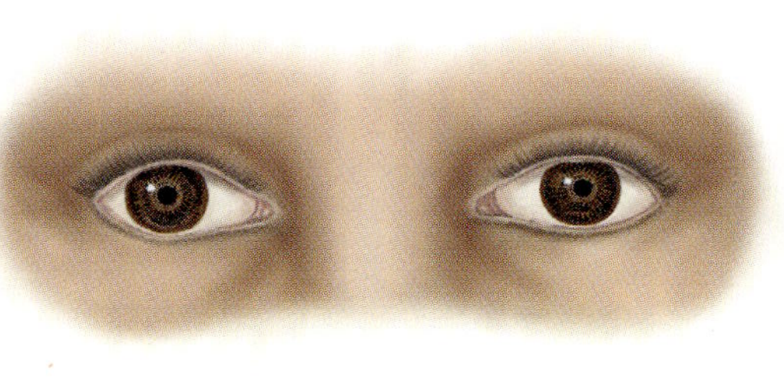

Small or Pinpoint Pupils

Bilaterally small pupils (1–2.5 mm) suggest (1) damage to the sympathetic pathways in the hypothalamus, or (2) metabolic encephalopathy (a diffuse failure of cerebral function that has many causes, including drugs). Light reactions are usually normal.

Pinpoint pupils (< 1 mm) suggest (1) a hemorrhage in the pons, or (2) the effects of morphine, heroin, or other narcotics. The light reactions may be seen with a magnifying glass.

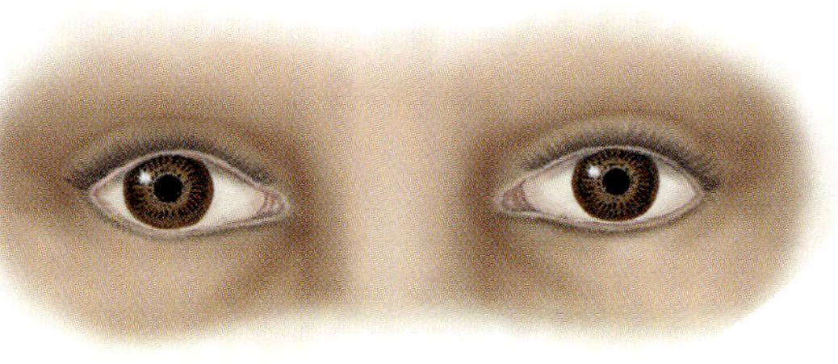

Midposition Fixed Pupils

Pupils that are in the *midposition* or *slightly dilated* (4–6 mm) and are *fixed to light* suggest structural damage in the midbrain.

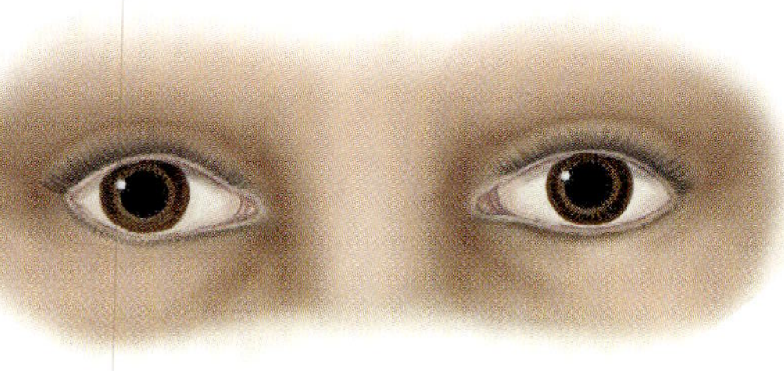

Large Pupils

Bilaterally fixed and dilated pupils may be due to severe anoxia and its sympathomimetic effects, as seen after cardiac arrest. They may also result from atropinelike agents, phenothiazines, or tricyclic antidepressants.

Bilaterally large reactive pupils may be due to cocaine, amphetamine, LSD, or other sympathetic nervous system agonists.

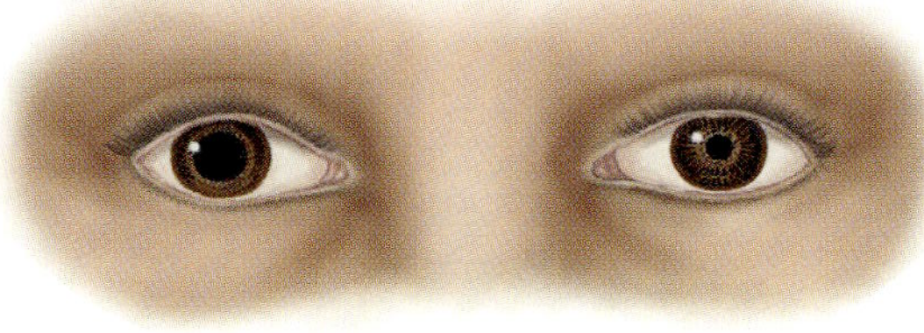

One Large Pupil

A pupil that is *fixed and dilated* warns of herniation of the temporal lobe, causing compression of the oculomotor nerve and midbrain.

TABLE 16-16 ■ Abnormal Postures in Comatose Patients

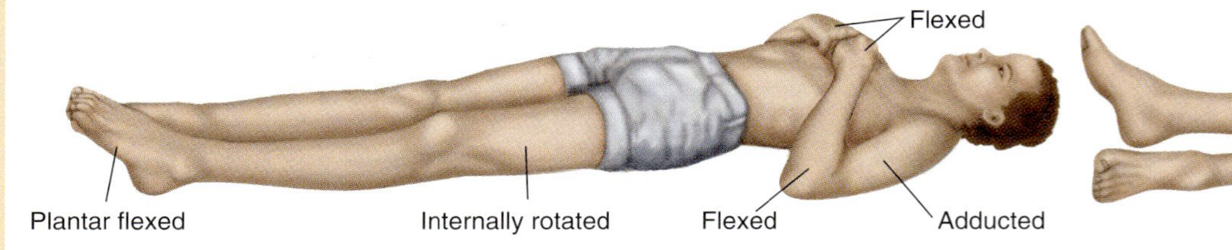

Decorticate Rigidity (Abnormal Flexor Response)

In decorticate rigidity, the upper arms are held tight to the sides with elbows, wrists, and fingers flexed. The legs are extended and internally rotated. The feet are plantar flexed. This posture implies a destructive lesion of the corticospinal tracts within or very near the cerebral hemispheres. When unilateral, this is the posture of chronic spastic hemiplegia.

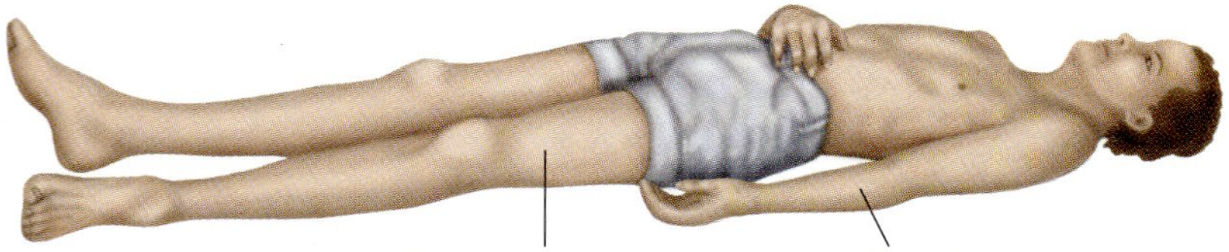

Externally rotated

Flaccid

Hemiplegia (Early)

Sudden unilateral brain damage involving the corticospinal tract may produce a hemiplegia (one-sided paralysis), which early in its course is flaccid. Spasticity will develop later. The paralyzed arm and leg are slack. They fall loosely and without tone when raised and dropped to the bed. Spontaneous movements or responses to noxious stimuli are limited to the opposite side. The leg may lie externally rotated. One side of the lower face may be paralyzed, and that cheek puffs out on expiration. Both eyes may be turned away from the paralyzed side.

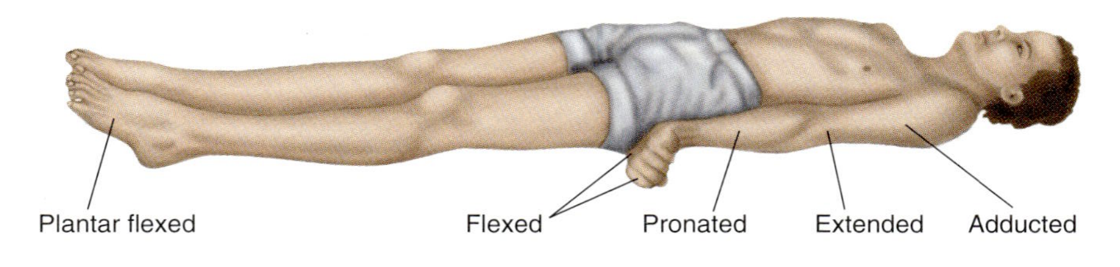

Decerebrate Rigidity (Abnormal Extensor Response)

In decerebrate rigidity, the jaws are clenched and the neck is extended. The arms are adducted and stiffly extended at the elbows, with forearms pronated, wrists and fingers flexed. The legs are stiffly extended at the knees, with the feet plantar flexed. This posture may occur spontaneously or only in response to external stimuli such as light, noise, or pain. It is caused by a lesion in the diencephalon, midbrain, or pons, although severe metabolic disorders such as hypoxia or hypoglycemia may also produce it.

CHAPTER

17

Assessing Children: Infancy Through Adolescence

Peter G. Szilagyi, MD, MPH

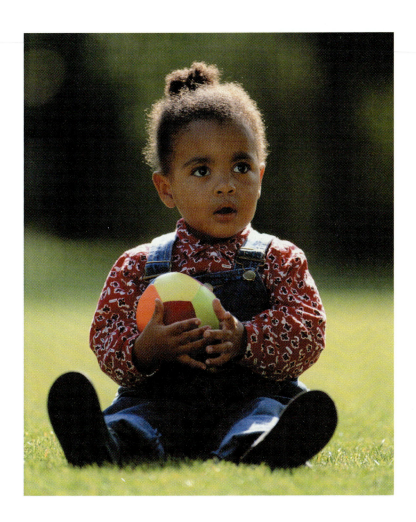

Before you can effectively talk to and examine a child, you need to understand children and their development. Children are anatomically and physiologically different from adults, and many techniques for assessment, physical findings, and abnormalities in young patients differ as well. Children display tremendous variations in physical, cognitive, and social development compared with adults. This chapter opens with the section on Child Development to help you assess children at all ages and to distinguish normal from abnormal symptoms and signs.

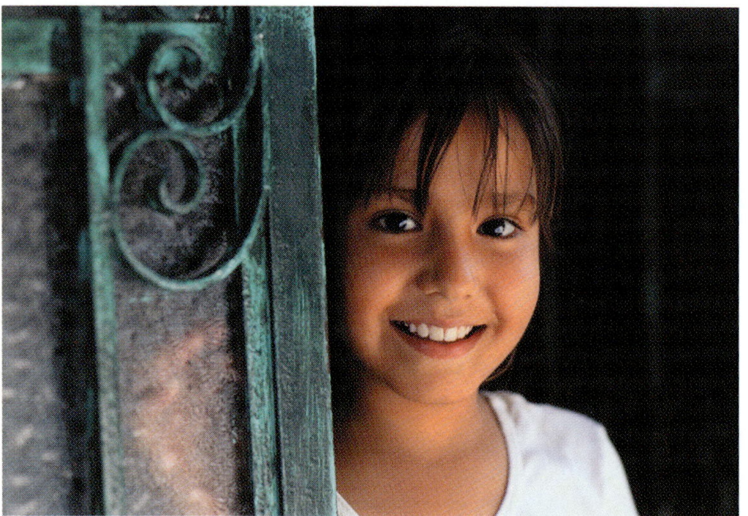

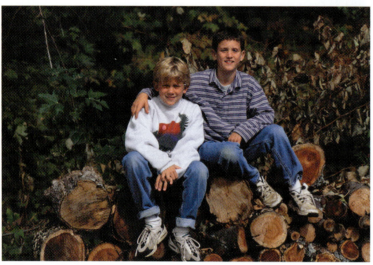

Health promotion and counseling are central to children's health care and should almost always be addressed whenever health care providers are examining children. The section on Health Promotion and Counseling outlines some critical areas to consider.

Children change rapidly, and it is important to understand the milestones for normal development for children at any age. Normal for a 2-year-old may be abnormal for a 10-year-old. Table 17-4, Growth Charts, (pp. 742–749) has key parameters of children's growth and development.

The major section of this chapter, Techniques of Examination, details the physical examination of regional systems as in the rest of the book and follows a head-to-toe sequence. The section on Approach to the Examination of Children at Different Ages provides particular strategies useful for each age group. The section is divided by age group: *infancy* (the first year), *early childhood* (years 1 through 4), and *middle childhood* (years 5 through 10). The physical examination of *adolescents* (years 11 through

20) is similar to that of adults, although cognitively and emotionally they are far from alike!

The Tables of Abnormalities (pp. 780–782) follow the order of the chapter and highlight major pediatric abnormalities.

CHILD DEVELOPMENT

When I approach a child, he inspires in me two sentiments: tenderness for what he is, and respect for what he may become.
—Louis Pasteur

Key Principles

Childhood is a period of remarkable growth and change, by far the greatest in a person's lifetime. During a few short years, a child will physically increase in size 20-fold, mature into an adult, acquire sophisticated language and reasoning, and develop complex psychosocial interactions. What a journey!

The first principle of *child development* is that it *proceeds along a predictable pathway* governed by the maturing brain. You can measure age-specific milestones and characterize a child's development as normal or abnormal according to established criteria. Once a milestone is achieved, the child proceeds to the next. Loss of milestones is concerning. Because your physical examination takes place at one point in time, you need to learn where the child fits within a developmental trajectory.

The second principle is that the *range of normal development is wide*. It is critical to recognize that children mature at different rates.

The third principle recognizes that *a variety of physical, disease-related, social, and environmental factors affect child development and health*. For example, chronic diseases and social problems such as child abuse and poverty can result not only in detectable physical abnormalities but in alterations in the rate and course of developmental advancement. Children with physical or cognitive disabilities may not follow the expected age-specific developmental trajectory outlined here. Tailor the physical examination to the child's developmental level.

A fourth principle, specific to the pediatric examination, is that *the child's developmental level affects the nature of the medical history and physical examination*. For example, interviewing a 5-year-old is fundamentally different from interviewing an adolescent—the physical examination of a rambunctious toddler who is dismantling the examination room has little in common with that of a shy teenager. Both order and style are quite different from the traditional examination of an adult. You will be faced simultaneously with adjusting your physical examination to the developmental level of the child while attempting to ascertain that developmental level. An understanding of normal child development helps you achieve these tasks.

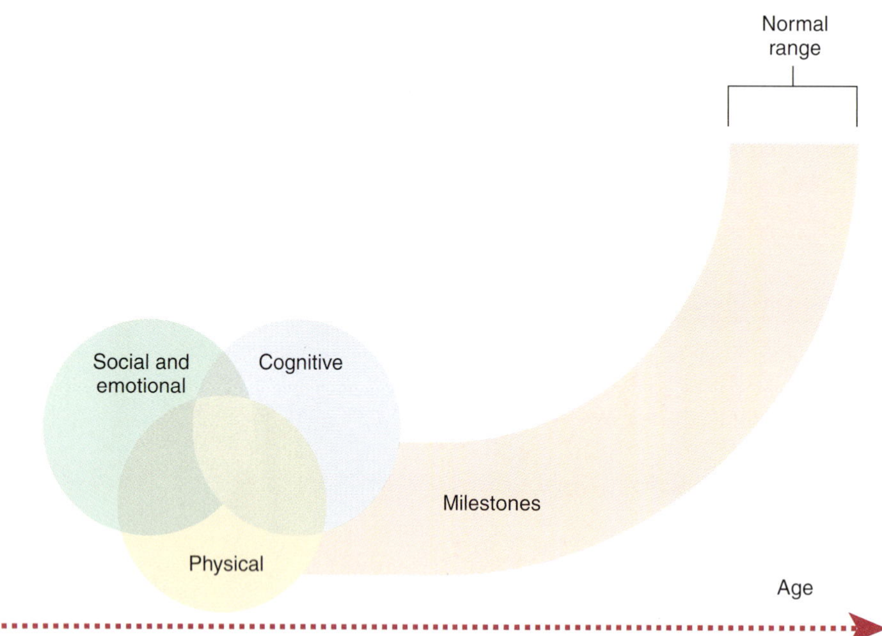

Every age has its pleasures, its style of wit, and its own ways.
—Nicholas Boileau-Despreaux

Infancy: The First Year of Life

Physical Development. The rate of physical growth during the first year of life is the most rapid of any age. By 1 year of age, the child should triple the birth weight and increase in height by 50%. Body proportions change, and the head becomes smaller relative to the body.

The figure on p. 628 shows the amazing developmental progression from birth to 1 year of age. Even a newborn has cognitive abilities that may surprise you. For example, a newborn can fix upon and follow a human face and respond to voices. Neurologic development progresses in a central to peripheral direction. Thus, a newborn learns head control before trunk control and use of arms and legs before use of hands and fingers.

Every child is born a genius.
—R. Buckminster Fuller

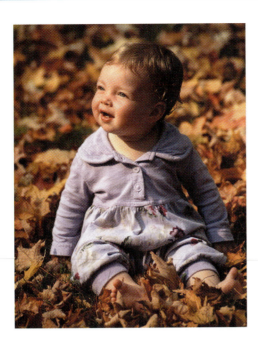

By 3 months, the normal infant will lift up his head and clasp his hands. By 6 months, the infant will roll over, reach for objects, turn to voices, and may sit with support. Learning occurs through activity, exploration, and manipulation of the environment. As peripheral coordination increases, the infant learns to reach for objects, to transfer from hand to hand, to crawl, to stand by holding on, and to play with objects by banging and grabbing. A 1-year-old may be standing, exploring the environment, and putting everything in her mouth.

Cognitive and Language Development. With this exploration comes an increased understanding of the infant's self and environment. The infant learns about cause and effect (such as shaking a rattle to produce a sound), the permanence of objects, and the use of tools to explore the environment. By 9 months of age, the child may recognize you as a stranger deserving wary cooperation, seek comfort from parents during the examination, and actively manipulate objects within reach (such as your clothes). Language development proceeds from cooing at 2 months, to babbling at 6 months, to 1 to 3 words by 1 year.

Social and Emotional Development. An infant's understanding of self and family also matures. Social tasks include bonding, attachment to caregivers, and trust that loved ones will meet needs. This may result in a reluctance to play with a strange examiner. Temperaments vary greatly. Some infants are predictable, adaptable, and respond positively to new stimuli; others are less adaptable and respond intensely or negatively to new stimuli. Because social development is affected by the environment, observe the child's interactions with caretakers.

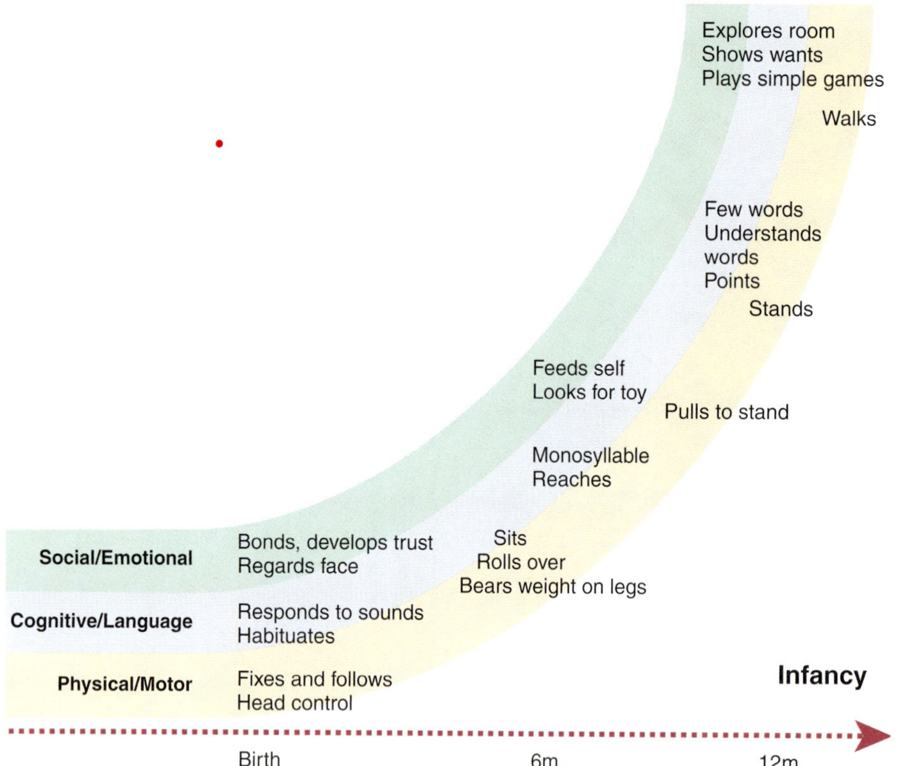

Early Childhood: 1 Through 4 Years

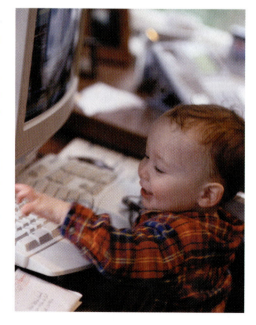

Physical Development. After 1 year of age, the rate of physical growth slows to half that of infancy. After age 2 years, toddlers gain about 2 to 3 kg and grow 5 cm per year. Growth can proceed in spurts. Physical changes are impressive, and during a few short years, children are transformed from chubby, clumsy toddlers into leaner, more muscular preschoolers. Even more significant are the changes in motor and cognitive development.

Gross motor skills develop quickly during this period. Most children walk by 15 months, run well by 2 years, and pedal a tricycle and jump around by 3 years. These new skills make the world a dangerous place for toddlers and pose inherent challenges during your examination. Fine motor skills develop through neurologic maturation and experience with manipulation of the environment. The 18-month-old who scribbles fleetingly, develops into a 2-year-old who imitates lines, and a 4-year-old who draws and copies circles.

Children are the keys of paradise.
—Richard Stoddard

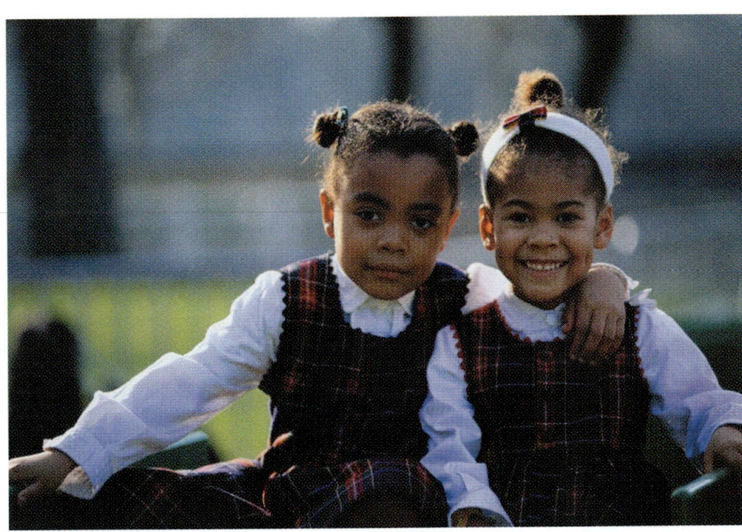

Cognitive and Language Development. Intellectually, a toddler makes the transition from learning about the environment through touching and looking (sensorimotor learning), to symbolic thinking, simple problem-solving, remembering songs, and imitating through play. Take advantage of these changes by making your examination seem like you are playing.

Language develops at extraordinary speed. An 18-month-old with 10 to 20 words emerges as a 2-year-old with two- to three-word sentences, and then a 3-year-old who converses well, asks "why" repeatedly, and entertains you with songs and often uproariously illogical symbolic stories. By 4 years of age, preschoolers form complex sentences. Recall that these ambitious and creative youngsters are still preoperational in thinking and lack sustained logical thought processes.

Social and Emotional Development. The toddler's march to new intellectual pursuits is only surpassed by a new drive for independence. Expect a struggle during parts of your examination. Because toddlers are impulsive, temper tantrums are common. Don't get into a battle of wills with a 2-year-old! Also, don't ask a toddler "May I listen to your chest?" After all, what will you do when the toddler emphatically says "No!"? Just tell the toddler gently what you will do. Note interactions between toddlers and caregivers, assessing both strengths and areas of concern.

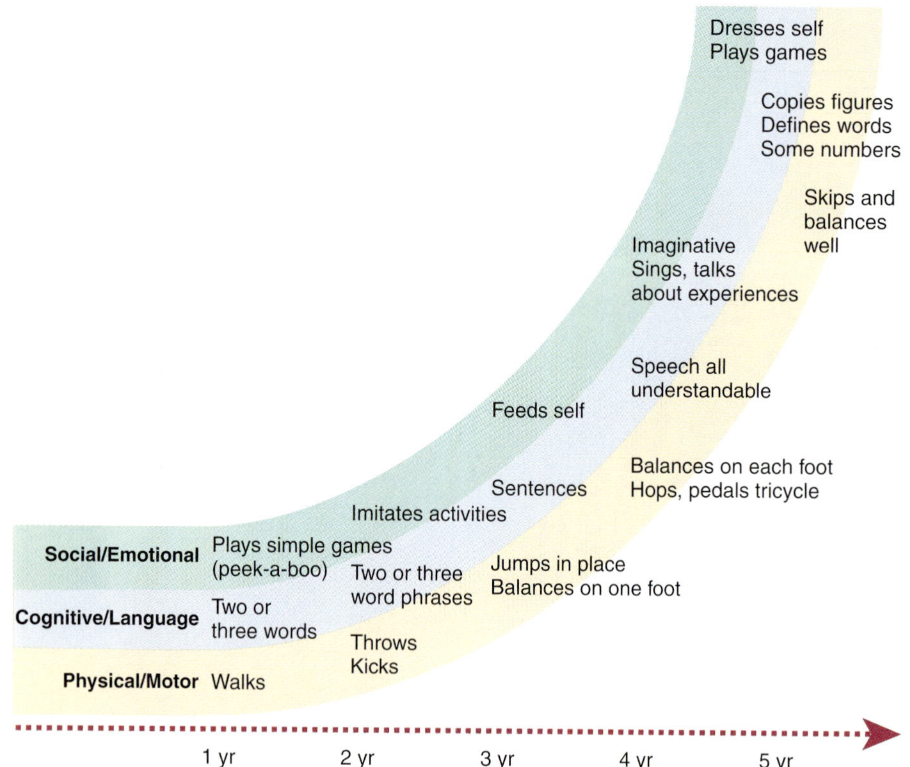

Middle Childhood: 5 Through 10 Years

Despite Freud's viewpoint, the middle childhood years are certainly not latent. Rather, this period is marked by goal-directed exploration of the world, increasing physical and cognitive abilities and achievements, and trials and errors. The physical examination is more straightforward in this age group, but keep in mind the developmental stages and tasks facing these school-age children.

Physical Development. Physically, children in this age group grow steadily but at a slower rate than during the preschool and adolescent periods. Nevertheless, you will see major improvements in strength and coordination, leading to increasing participation in activities. This is also a time when children with physical disabilities or chronic illnesses begin to face their limitations.

Cognitive and Language Development. Children become "concrete operational"—capable of limited logical thinking and increasingly complicated learning, yet still rooted in the present, with little ability to understand consequences or abstract issues. A tremendous amount of learning from school and family takes place, and this is greatly influenced by environmental factors. A major developmental task is the achievement of self-efficacy, or the knowledge and ability to thrive in different situations. Moral development remains simple, with a clear sense of "right

and wrong." Language becomes increasingly complex during this age period.

You know children are growing up when they start asking questions that have answers.
—*John Plomp*

Social and Emotional Development. School-age children become progressively more independent, initiating their own activities and enjoying their own accomplishments. This is a period of achievements and a critical time for developing self-esteem and an appropriate "fit" within the child's major social structures—the family, the school, and peer activity groups. Guilt and poor self-esteem can also appear. The child's family and environment are crucial to the achievement of a positive self-image. Moral and value systems mature, though they remain relatively simple and concrete.

Middle Childhood

Developmental Task	Characteristic	Health Care Needs
Physical	Enhanced strength and coordination Competence on a variety of tasks and activities	Screening for strengths, assessing problems Involvement of parents in competence Support for disabilities or problems Anticipatory guidance about safety
Cognitive	"Concrete operational": focus on the present Achievement of knowledge and skills, self-efficacy	Emphasis on short-term consequences Support; screening about skills
Social	Achieving good "fit" with family, friends, school Sustained self-esteem Reconciling individuality with conformity Evolving self-identity	Assessment, support, advice about interactions Support Confidentiality, understanding, advice Understanding, support

Adolescence: 11 Through 20 Years

Adolescence can be divided into three stages: early, middle, and late, as shown in the table on p. 633. You need to understand the physical, cognitive, and social/emotional stage of each adolescent, because your interview and examination techniques will vary widely depending on the adolescent's level of development.

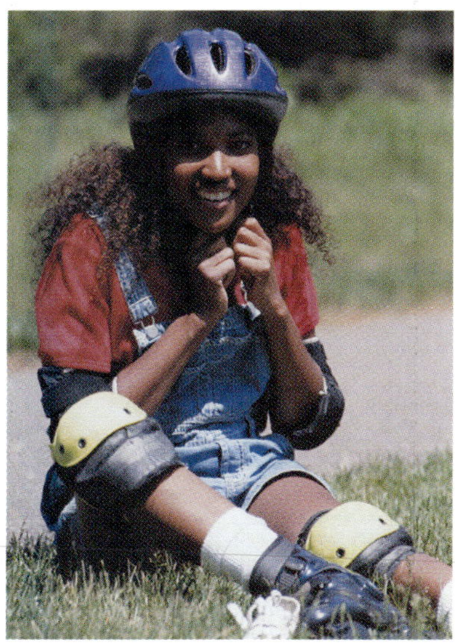

Physical Development. Adolescence is the period of transition from childhood to adulthood. The physical transformation generally occurs over a period of years, beginning at an average age of 10 in girls and 11 in boys. On average, girls end pubertal development with a growth spurt by age 14 and boys by age 16. The age of onset and duration of puberty varies widely, although the stages are predictable. Early adolescents are preoccupied with these physical changes.

A boy becomes an adult three years before his parents think he does, and about two years after he thinks he does.
—Lewis B. Hershey

Cognitive Development. Although not as obvious, cognitive changes during adolescence are as dramatic as changes in physique. Most adolescents progress from concrete to formal operational thinking, acquiring an ability to reason logically and abstractly and to consider future implications of current actions. Although the interview and examination resemble those of adults, keep in mind the wide variability in cognitive development of adolescents and their often erratic and still limited ability to see beyond simple solutions. Moral thinking becomes sophisticated, with lots of time spent debating issues.

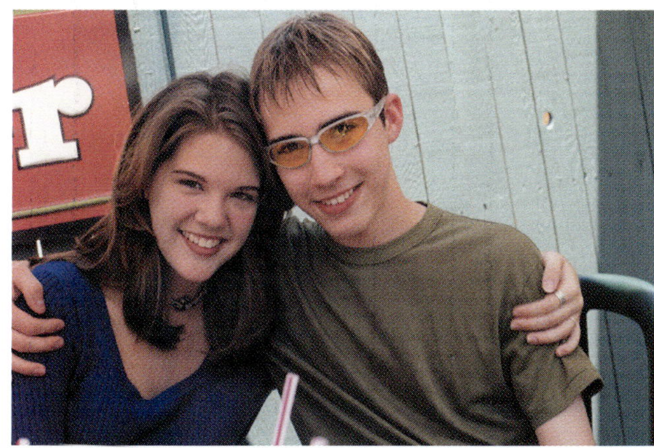

Social and Emotional Development. Adolescence is a tumultuous time, marked by the transition from family-dominated influences to increasing autonomy and peer influence. The struggle for identity, independence, and eventually intimacy leads to much stress, many health-related problems, and, often, high-risk behaviors. This struggle also provides you with an important opportunity for health promotion.

Adolescence

Developmental Task	Characteristic	Health Care Needs
Early Adolescence (10–14-year-olds)		
Physical	Puberty (F: 10–14; M: 11–16) variable	Confidentiality; privacy
Cognitive	"Concrete operational": focus on the present	Emphasis on immediate consequences
Social		
Identity	Am I normal? Peers increasingly important	Reassurance and positive attitude
Independence	Ambivalence (family, self, peers)	Support for growing autonomy
Middle Adolescence (15–16-year-olds)		
Physical	Females more comfortable, males awkward	Support if patient varies from "normal"
Cognitive	Transition to formal operational; many ideas	Problem-solving; decision-making; teaching
Social		
Identity	Who am I? Much introspection; global issues	Nonjudgmental acceptance
Independence	Limit testing; "experimental" behaviors; dating	Consistency; limit-setting
Late Adolescence (17–20-year-olds)		
Physical	Adult appearance; slow changes	Minimal needs, except if chronic illness
Cognitive	"Formal operational"; thinking about future	Approach as an adult
Social		
Identity	Role with respect to others; sexuality; future	Encouragement of identity to allow growth
Independence	Separation from family; toward real independence	Support

HEALTH PROMOTION AND COUNSELING

An ounce of prevention is worth a pound of cure.
—Benjamin Franklin

The heart of pediatrics is health promotion. Pediatric health care clinicians dedicate substantial time to health supervision visits and health promotion activities. The sage saying above is particularly true for children and adolescents because prevention at a young age can result in improved health outcomes for many decades.

Several national and international organizations have identified guidelines for health promotion for children. Current concepts of health promotion include not only the detection and prevention of disease, but active promotion of the well-being of children and their families, spanning physical, cognitive, emotional, and social health.

Every interaction with a child and family is an opportunity for health promotion! From your interview questions to your detailed physical examination, think about your interactions as having two opportunities: the traditional detection of normality and medical problems, and the ability to promote health. What a priceless gift!

Key components of pediatric health promotion are shown below. Not every issue is relevant for each visit or age. Tailor your health promotion to the relevant developmental phase of your patient.

KEY COMPONENTS OF HEALTH PROMOTION FOR CHILDREN AND ADOLESCENTS

1. Age-appropriate developmental achievement of the child
   - Physical (maturation, growth, puberty)
   - Motor (gross and fine motor skills)
   - Cognitive (achievement of milestones, language, school performance)
   - Emotional (self-efficacy and mastery, self-esteem, independence, morality)
   - Social (social competence, self-responsibility, integration with family and community)
2. Health supervision visits
   - Periodic assessment of medical and oral health, per health supervision schedules (see p. 637)
   - Adjustment of frequency for children or families with special needs
3. Integration of physical examination findings (assure normality, relate findings to healthy lifestyle)
4. Immunizations
5. Screening procedures
6. Anticipatory guidance
   - Healthy habits
   - Nutrition and healthy eating
   - Emotional and mental health
   - Oral health

(continued)

KEY COMPONENTS OF HEALTH PROMOTION FOR CHILDREN AND ADOLESCENTS (Continued)

- Safety and prevention of injury
- Sexual development and sexuality
- Self-responsibility and efficacy
- Family relationships (interactions, strengths, supports)
- Community interactions (childcare, school)
- Prevention or recognition of illness
- Prevention of risky behaviors and addictions
- School and vocational achievement
- Peer relationships

7. Partnership between health care provider and child, adolescent, and family

Promotion of development should be age-appropriate. Health promotion is developmental and most effective if encouraged over multiple visits. Promotion regarding development includes suggestions about stimulation (reading, conversing, music, optimizing opportunities for gross and fine motor development). Advise parents about upcoming developmental stages and needs of children to help them promote their child's development. Remember, parents are the major agent of health promotion in children, and your advice is implemented through them.

EXAMPLES OF ANTICIPATORY GUIDANCE DURING HEALTH SUPERVISION VISITS

1-Year-Old	*16-Year-Old*
Development	Development
Walking, language, social games	School, social, self, physical
Nutrition	Nutrition
Nutritious snacks	Healthy meals, dieting, prevention of obesity
Choking	
Oral health	Oral health
Brushing	Brushing, dentist
No bottle in bed	Braces
Safety and prevention of injury	Safety and prevention of injury
Safety in home, car, childcare	Seat belts, driving, and alcohol
Exposures: smoke, drugs	Violence, abuse prevention
Ipecac for poisoning	Protective gear for activities
Self-efficacy, behavior	Self-efficacy
Praising good behavior	Competence, self worth, future
Setting limits	Managing stress
Discipline	Mental health, depression
Family relationships	Family relationships
Siblings, spending individual time	Communication
Sharing meals and activities	Separation
	Sexuality
	Advice, information, puberty
	Saying no, safer sex, HIV and STDs
Community and peer interactions	Community and peer interactions
Assessing child care	Peers, significant others
Community resources and services	Positive activities, financial, culture

The American Academy of Pediatrics (AAP) publishes guidelines for *health supervision visits* and key age-appropriate components of these visits (p. 637). Remember that children and adolescents who have a chronic illness or are from high-risk family or environmental circumstances will probably require more frequent visits and more intensive health promotion.

Integrate explanations of your physical findings with health promotion. For example, provide advice about expected maturational changes or how health behaviors can impact physical findings (e.g., exercise may reduce blood pressure and obesity). It is particularly powerful to demonstrate the relationship between healthy lifestyles and physical health.

Childhood immunizations are a mainstay for health promotion and have been recognized as the most significant medical achievement of public health worldwide. The childhood immunization schedule changes yearly and updates are widely disseminated.

Screening procedures are performed at certain ages. For all children, these include growth parameters and developmental screening at all ages, blood pressure after infancy, and vision and hearing screening at certain key ages. Screening procedures that are particularly recommended for high-risk patients include tests for lead poisoning, tuberculosis exposure, anemia, cholesterol, urinary tract infections, and sexually transmitted diseases. There is variation worldwide in recommendations for screening tests; the AAP recommendations are provided on the next page.

Anticipatory guidance is a major component of the pediatric visit. Key areas are shown in the Recommendations for Preventive Pediatric Health Care and cover a broad range of topics, from purely "medical" to social and emotional health. The examples of anticipatory guidance (p. 635) for a 1-year-old and a 16-year-old highlight key components for two different age groups. The health of children is affected by all of these factors. If we are to achieve a healthier world, we *must* emphasize comprehensive and broadly defined health promotion during childhood. Our children's future depends on it!

APPROACH TO THE EXAMINATION OF CHILDREN AT DIFFERENT AGES

Each child is an adventure into a better life—an opportunity to change the old pattern and make it new.

—Hubert H. Humphrey

Often, neophyte (and some veteran) examiners are intimidated when approaching a tiny baby or a screaming child, especially under the critical eyes of anxious parents. Although it takes a bit of courage, you will come to accept the challenge easily and to enjoy almost all such encounters. This section provides guidelines for a reassuring yet thorough approach to children in the various age groups.

Recommendations for Preventive Pediatric Health Care

Each child and family is unique; therefore, these Recommendations are designed for the care of children who are receiving competent parenting, have no manifestations of any important health problems, and are growing and developing in satisfactory fashion. Additional visits may become necessary if circumstances suggest variations from normal.

	INFANCY								EARLY CHILDHOOD					MIDDLE CHILDHOOD				ADOLESCENCE									
AGE	2-4 days[1]	By 1 mo	2 mo	4 mo	6 mo	8 mo	10 mo	12 mo	15 mo	18 mo	24 mo	3 y	4 y	5 y	6 y	8 y	10 y	11 y	12 y	13 y	14 y	15 y	16 y	17 y	18 y	19 y	20 y+
HISTORY																											
Initial / Interval	•	•	•	•	•	•	•	•	•	•	•	•	•	•	•	•	•	•	•	•	•	•	•	•	•	•	•
MEASUREMENTS																											
Height and Weight	•	•	•	•	•	•	•	•	•	•	•	•	•	•	•	•	•	•	•	•	•	•	•	•	•	•	•
Head Circumference	•	•	•	•	•	•	•	•	•	•	•																
Blood Pressure												•	•	•	•	•	•	•	•	•	•	•	•	•	•	•	•
SENSORY SCREENING																											
Vision	S	S	S	S	S	S	S	S	S	S	S	O	O	O	O	O	O	S	O	S	S	O	S	S	O	S	S
Hearing	S	S	S	S	S	S	S	S	S	S	S	S	O	O	O	O	O	S	O	S	S	O	S	S	O	S	S
DEVELOPMENTAL/ BEHAVIORAL ASSESSMENT[2]	•	•	•	•	•	•	•	•	•	•	•	•	•	•	•	•	•	•	•	•	•	•	•	•	•	•	•
PHYSICAL EXAMINATION[3]	•	•	•	•	•	•	•	•	•	•	•	•	•	•	•	•	•	•	•	•	•	•	•	•	•	•	•

1. For newborns discharged in less than 48 hours after delivery
2. By history and appropriate physical examination: if suspicious, by specific objective development testing
3. At each visit, a complete physical examination is essential, with infant totally unclothed, older child undressed and suitably draped

Key: • = to be performed S = subjective, by history
O = objective, by a standard testing method

Adapted from Recommendations For Preventive Pediatric Health Care promulgated by the American Academy of Pediatrics Committee on Practice and Ambulatory Medicine. Pediatrics 96:373, 1995. Additional recommendations made by the Committee regarding screening for metabolic disorders, tuberculosis, anemia, and urinary tract diseases, administration of immunizations, provision of anticipatory guidance, and initial dental referral are not included in the above summation.

An important and unique aspect of examining younger children is that parents are usually watching and taking part in the interaction, providing you the opportunity to observe the parent–child interaction. Note whether the child displays age-appropriate behaviors. Assess the "goodness of fit" between parents and child. While some abnormal interactions may be due to the unnatural setting of the examination room, others may be due to interactional problems. Careful *observation* of the child's interactions with parents and the child's unstructured play in the examination room can reveal *abnormalities in physical, cognitive, and social development.*

Normal toddlers are occasionally terrified, more commonly angry at the examiner, and often completely uncooperative. Most eventually warm up. If this behavior continues and is not developmentally appropriate (e.g., stranger anxiety of the infant or shyness of the early adolescent), there may be an *underlying behavioral* or *developmental abnormality.*

SOME TIPS FOR EXAMINING YOUNG CHILDREN (1–4-YEAR-OLDS)

Useful Strategies for Examination	*Useful Toys and Aids*
Examine a child sitting on parent's lap. Try to be at the child's eye level.	"Blow out" the otoscope light.
First examine the child's toy or teddy bear, then the child.	"Beep" the stethoscope on your nose.
Let the child do some of the exam (e.g., move the stethoscope). Then go back and "get the places we missed."	Make tongue-depressor puppets.
Ask the toddler who keeps pushing you away to "hold your hand." Then have the toddler "help you" with the exam.	Use the child's own toys for play.
Some toddlers believe that if they can't see you, then you aren't there. Perform the exam while the child stands on the parent's lap, facing the parent.	Jingle your keys to test for hearing.
If 2-year-olds are holding something in each hand (such as tongue depressors), they can't fight or resist!	Shine the otoscope through the tip of your finger, "lighting it up," and then examine the child's ears with it.

Sequence of the Examination. Begin by reviewing Chapter 3, Beginning the Physical Examination: General Survey and Vital Signs, for the methods and sequence of examining adults. When examining infants and children, the sequence should vary according to the child's age and comfort level. *Perform nondisturbing maneuvers early on and potentially distressing maneuvers near the end of the examination.* For example, palpate the head and neck and auscultate the heart and lungs early, and examine the ears and mouth and palpate the abdomen near the end. If the child reports pain in one area, examine that part last.

The format of the pediatric medical record is the same as that of the adult record, so although the sequence of the physical examination may vary, you should then convert your written findings back into the traditional format.

Assessing the Newborn

The first year of life, infancy, is divided into the neonatal period (the first 28 days) and the postneonatal period (29 days to 1 year). Often, the first pediatric examination outside the delivery room is performed in the hospital within 24 hours of birth.

If possible, do the physical examination in front of the parents so that they can interact with you and ask questions. Often parents have specific questions about their baby's physical appearance, so stating normal findings as you go can be quite reassuring. This is also an excellent time to observe parental bonding with the newborn, and to observe how well the breast-feeding baby latches and sucks. To detect problems early, try to observe breast-feeding firsthand. Breast-feeding is physiologically and psychologically optimal, but many mothers will need help and support. Early detection of difficulties and anticipatory guidance can promote and sustain healthy breast-feeding.

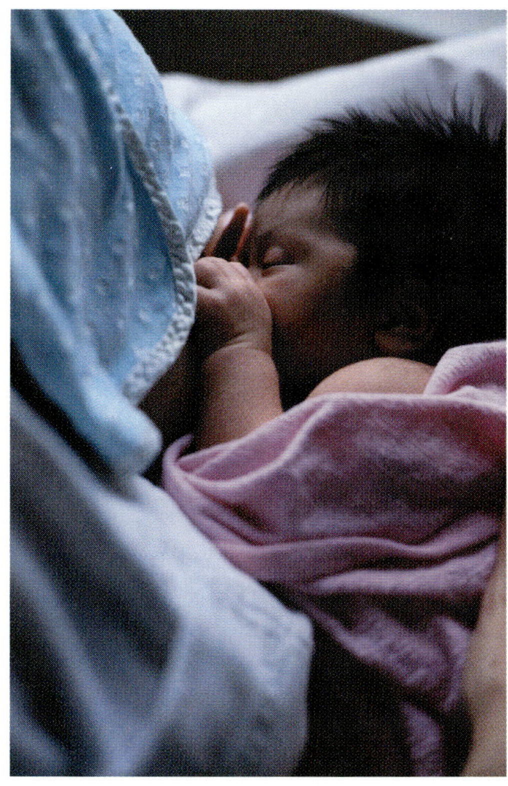

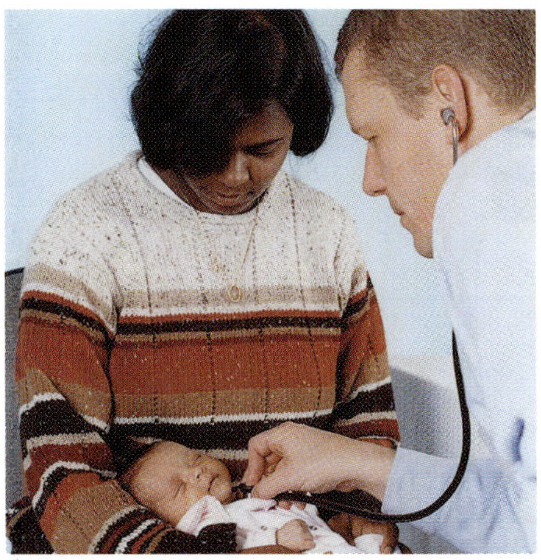

Newborns are most responsive 1 to 2 hours after a feeding, when they are neither too satiated (becoming less responsive) nor too hungry (and often agitated). It is helpful to start with the newborn swaddled and comfortable. Then undress the newborn as the examination proceeds, for gradual stimulation and arousal. If the newborn becomes agitated, use a pacifier or a bottle of formula (if not breast-feeding), or allow the baby to suck on your gloved finger or the baby's own hand. You can also try reswaddling to silence the baby long enough to complete the parts of the examination that require a quiet baby.

A child is fed with milk and praise.
—*Mary Lamb*

TIPS FOR EXAMINING NEWBORNS

- Examine the newborn in the presence of the parents.
- Swaddle and then undress the newborn as the examination proceeds.
- Dim the lights and rock the baby back and forth to encourage the baby's eyes to open.
- Observe feeding if possible (particularly breast-feeding).
- Demonstrate calming maneuvers to parents (swaddling, holding techniques, use of pacifier).
- Observe transitions as baby arouses, and teach parents about these transitions.
- A typical sequence for the newborn examination (for minimal disruption of the baby):
  - Careful observation
  - Head, neck, heart, lungs, abdomen, genitourinary system
  - Lower extremities, back
  - Ears, mouth
  - Eyes, whenever they are spontaneously open
  - Skin, as you go along
  - Neurologic system
  - Hips

ASSESSMENT OF NEWBORNS

A number of techniques help you assess the developmental level of newborns. These techniques are often part of a limited-screening pediatric physical examination performed immediately after birth.

Immediate Assessment at Birth: Adaptation to Extrauterine Life. Examining newborns immediately after birth is important for determining the general condition, developmental status, abnormalities in gestational development, and presence of congenital abnormalities. The examination may reveal diseases of cardiac, respiratory, or neurologic origin. Listen to the anterior thorax with your stethoscope, palpate the abdomen, and inspect the head, face, oral cavity, extremities, genitalia, and perineum.

Apgar Score. The Apgar score is the key initial assessment of the baby immediately after birth. It contains five components for classifying the newborn's neurologic recovery from the birth process and immediate adaptation to extrauterine life. Score each newborn according to the following table, at 1 and 5 minutes after birth. Scoring is based on a 3-point scale (0, 1, or 2) for each component. Total scores may range from 0 to 10. Scoring may continue at 5-minute intervals until the score is greater than 7. If the 5-minute Apgar score is 8 or more, proceed to a more complete examination.

The Apgar Scoring System

Assigned Score			
Clinical Sign	*0*	*1*	*2*
Heart rate	Absent	<100	>100
Respiratory effort	Absent	Slow and irregular	Good; strong
Muscle tone	Flaccid	Some flexion of the arms and legs	Active movement
Reflex irritability*	No responses	Grimace	Crying vigorously, sneeze, or cough
Color	Blue, pale	Pink body, blue extremities	Pink all over

*Reaction to suction of nares with bulb syringe

1-Minute Apgar Score		5-Minute Apgar Score	
0–4	Severe depression, requiring immediate resuscitation	0–7	High risk for subsequent central nervous system and other organ system dysfunction
5–7	Some nervous system depression	8–10	Normal
8–10	Normal		

Gestational Age and Birthweight. Once newborns have successfully adapted to their new environment, it is important to classify them by birth weight and gestational age (maturity). These classifications help predict medical problems and morbidity.

CLASSIFICATION BY BIRTH WEIGHT AND GESTATIONAL AGE

Birth Weight

Classification	*Weight*
■ Extremely low birth weight	<1000 grams
■ Very low birth weight	<1500 grams
■ Low birth weight	<2500 grams
■ Normal birth weight	≥ 2500 grams

Gestational Age

Classification	*Gestational Age*
■ Preterm	< 37 wks (<259th day)
■ Term	37–42 wks
■ Postterm	> 42 wks (>294th day)

Gestational age is based on specific neuromuscular signs and physical characteristics that change with gestational maturity. Several scores have been developed to estimate gestational age using these characteristics.

The *Ballard scoring system* estimates gestational age to within 2 weeks, even in extremely premature infants. Table 17-1 (p. 737) includes a complete Ballard scoring system, with instructions for assessing neuromuscular and physical maturity.

A useful classification includes both birth weight and gestational age components, and is based on the birth weight of the newborn on the intrauterine growth curve.

Category	Abbreviation	Percentile
Small for gestational age	SGA	<10th
Appropriate for gestational age	AGA	10–90th
Large for gestational age	LGA	>90th

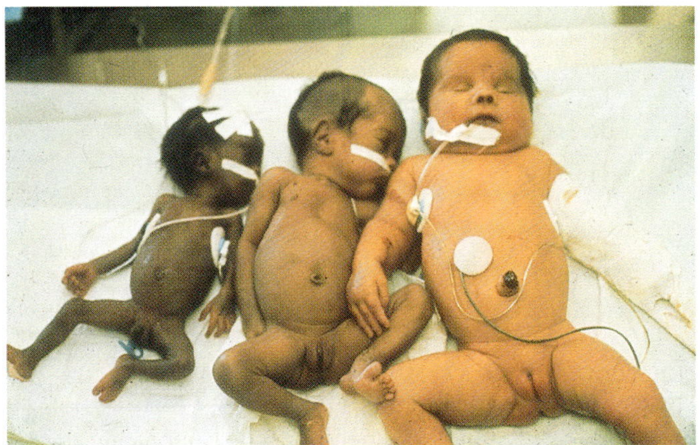

(Reprinted with permission from Korones SB: High-Risk Newborn Infants: The Basis for Intensive Nursing Care, 4th ed. St. Louis, CV Mosby, 1986.)

The figure below shows the intrauterine growth curves for the 10th and 90th percentiles, and depicts the different categories of maturity for newborn infants based on birth weight and gestational age. The three babies shown on the previous page were all born at 32 weeks' gestational age, and weighed 600 g (SGA), 1400 g (AGA), and 2750 g (LGA).

Each of these categories has a different mortality rate, highest for preterm SGA and AGA infants, and lowest for term AGA infants.

Preterm AGA infants are more prone to respiratory distress syndrome, apnea, patent ductus arteriosus with left-to-right shunt, and infection. *Preterm SGA infants* are more likely to experience asphyxia, hypoglycemia, and hypocalcemia.

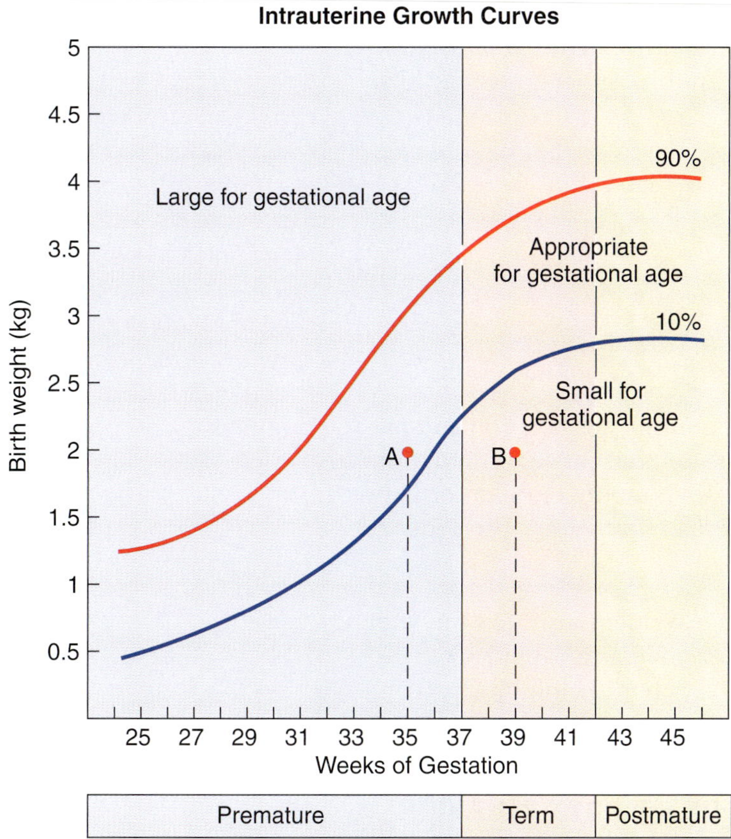

Level of intrauterine growth based on birth weight and gestational age of liveborn, single, white infants. Point A represents a premature infant, while point B indicates an infant of similar birth weight who is mature but small for gestational age; the growth curves are representative of the 10th and 90th percentiles for all of the newborns in the sampling. (Adapted from Sweet YA: Classification of the low-birth-weight infant. In Klaus MH, Fanaroff AA: Care of the High-Risk Neonate, 3rd ed. Philadelphia, WB Saunders, 1986. Reproduced with permission.)

Examination Several Hours After Birth. During the first day of life, and optimally within 8 hours of birth, newborns should have a comprehensive examination. Wait until 1 or 2 hours after a feeding, when the baby is most responsive, and ask the parents to remain in the room.

Observe the baby, first when lying undisturbed and then almost completely undressed if the baby is quiet. Observe the baby's color, size, body proportions, nutritional status, and posture, as well as respirations and movements of the head and extremities.

Most normal, full-term newborns lie in a symmetric position, with the limbs semiflexed and the legs partially abducted at the hip.

In *breech babies*, the legs and head are extended; the legs of a *frank breech baby* are abducted and externally rotated.

Normally there is spontaneous motor activity, with flexion and extension alternating between the arms and legs. The fingers are usually flexed in a tight fist, but may extend in slow, athetoid posturing movements. Brief tremors of the arms, legs, and body are commonly seen for a short time after birth during vigorous crying, and even at rest.

By 4 days after birth, tremors occurring at rest signal central nervous system disease from a variety of possible causes, ranging from *asphyxia* to *drug withdrawal.* Asymmetric movements of the arms or legs at any time suggest the possibility of *central or peripheral neurologic deficits, birth injury* (such as a fractured clavicle or brachial plexus injury), or *congenital anomalies.*

Throughout the examination, and particularly during auscultation and palpation, it is important to have the baby quiet to optimize your examination. Place the tip of your gloved finger in a crying baby's mouth to quiet the baby long enough to complete these portions of the examination. The order of the examination is unimportant.

Studies by Dr. T. Berry Brazelton and others have demonstrated the wide range of abilities in newborns. Demonstrating some of the abilities of newborns during your comprehensive examination is both helpful for you and wonderful for the parents. Here are some of these newborn abilities:

WHAT A NEWBORN CAN DO: ABILITY FOR COMPLEX BEHAVIOR*

Core Elements

- Newborns can use all five of their senses.
  For example, they prefer to look at a human face and will turn to a parent's voice.
- Newborns are unique individuals, with wide variations in their abilities to interact with their environment.
  Marked differences exist in temperaments, personality, behavior, learning, and interactions.
- Newborns interact dynamically with their caregivers.
  It is a two-way street! Newborns affect caregivers as much as caregivers influence newborns.

(continued)

WHAT A NEWBORN CAN DO: ABILITY FOR COMPLEX BEHAVIOR* (Continued)

Examples of Complex Newborn Behavior

Habituation	Ability of newborn to selectively and progressively shut out negative stimuli (such as a repetitive sound)
Attachment	A reciprocal, dynamic process of interacting and bonding with the caregiver
State Regulation	A newborn's ability to modulate the level of arousal under different degrees of stimulation (e.g., ability to console self and calm down)
Perception	Newborn's ability to regard faces, turn to voices, quiet in presence of singing, track colorful objects, respond to touch, and recognize familiar scents

*Points from T. Berry Brazelton, MD.

The potential possibilities of any child are the most intriguing and stimulating in all creation.
—*Ray L. Wilbur*

Assessing the Infant

The key to a successful examination of the infant is using developmentally appropriate methods such as distraction and play. Because infants usually pay attention to only one thing at a time, it is relatively easy to bring the baby's attention to something other than the examination being performed. Distract the infant with a moving object, a flashing light, a game of peek-a-boo, tickling, or any sort of noise.

If you cannot distract the infant or make the awake infant attend to an object, your face, or a sound, consider a possible *visual or hearing deficit.*

Start the examination with the infant sitting or lying in the parent's lap. If the infant is tired, hungry, or ill, you might ask the parent to hold him against the chest. Make sure there are appropriate toys, a blanket, or other familiar objects nearby. A hungry infant may need to be fed before you can proceed with a complete examination.

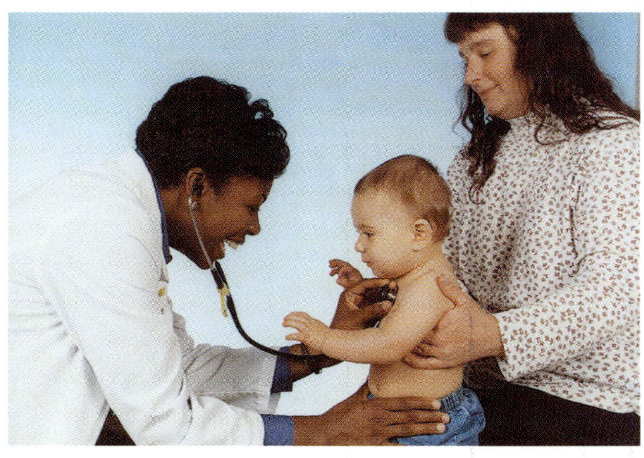

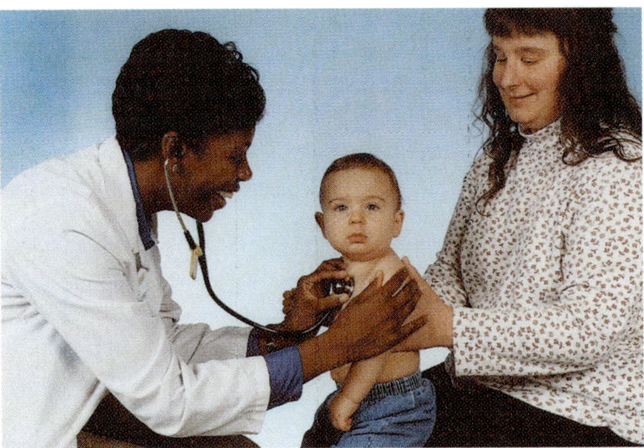

Observe parent–infant interactions. Watch the parent's affect when talking about the infant. Note the parent's manner of holding, moving, and dressing the baby, and response to situations that produce any discomfort for the infant.

Observation of the infant's communication with the parent can reveal abnormalities such as *developmental delay, language delay, hearing deficits*, or *inadequate parental attachment*. Likewise, observations of the parent–infant interaction may identify maladaptive nurturing patterns that may stem from *maternal depression* or *inadequate social support.*

Infants usually do not object to removal of their clothing. Indeed, most seem to prefer being nude, perhaps because of greater tactile stimulation. To keep yourself and your surroundings dry, it is wise to leave the diaper in place throughout the examination; remove it only to examine the genitals, rectum, lower spine, and hips.

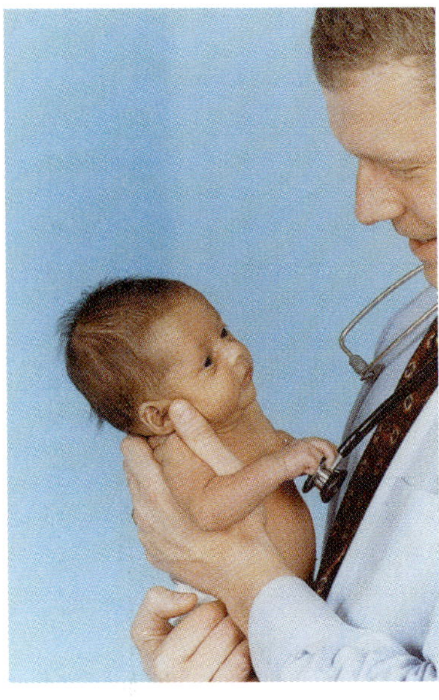

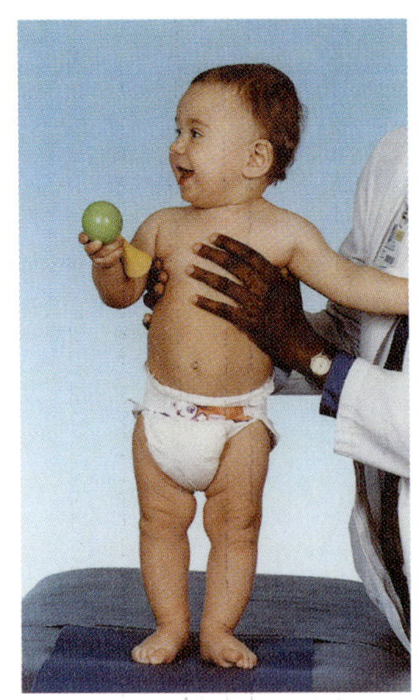

TIPS FOR EXAMINING INFANTS

- Approach the older infant gradually, using a toy or object to distract the infant.
- Do as much of the examination as possible with the infant in the parent's lap.
- Speak softly to the infant or mimic the infant's sounds to attract attention and to keep the infant occupied.
- Ask a parent about the infant's strengths to elicit useful developmental and parenting information.
- If the infant is cranky, make sure he or she is well fed before proceeding with the examination.

TESTING FOR DEVELOPMENTAL MILESTONES

Because you'll want to measure the infant's best performance, checking milestones is best achieved at the end of the interview, just before the examination. This "fun and games" interlude also enhances cooperation during the examination. Experienced clinicians can weave the developmental examination into the other parts of the examination. The graph at the bottom of p. 628 shows some key physical/motor, cognitive/language, and social/emotional milestones during the first year of life. The standard for measuring developmental milestones throughout infancy and childhood is the Denver Developmental Screening Test (DDST). The DDST is designed to detect developmental delays in personal–social, fine motor–adaptive, language, and gross motor dimensions from birth through 6 years of age.

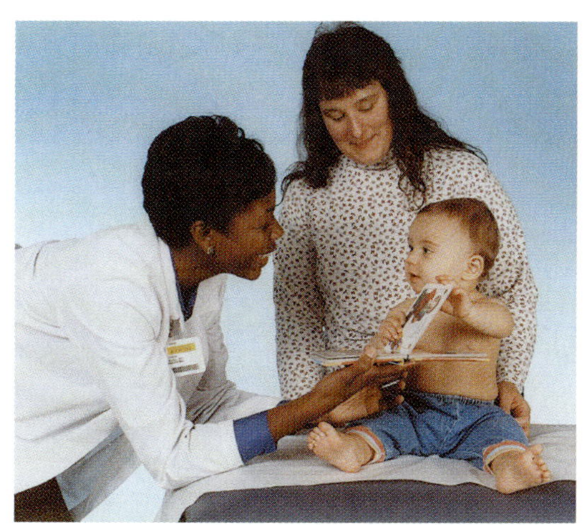

The DDST form is shown on p. 738 in Table 17-2 and includes instructions for recording specific observations. Each test item is represented on the form under the age by a bar, which indicates when 25%, 50%, 75%, and 90% of children attain the milestones depicted. It must be emphasized that the DDST is only a measure of developmental attainment in the categories indicated and not a measure of intelligence.

COMMON CAUSES OF DEVELOPMENTAL DELAY IN INFANTS*

In the largest group of children with developmental delay, the causes are unknown. The following are some *known causes:*

Abnormality in Embryonic Development
- Prenatal insult (e.g., intrauterine, drug)
- Chromosomal (e.g., Down syndrome)

Hereditary and Genetic Disorders
- Inborn errors of metabolism
- Preconceptual genetic abnormalities

Environmental and Social Problems
- Parental psychological/social problems with insufficient stimulation of child
- Childhood mental health disease

Other Pregnancy or Perinatal Problems
- Fetal (e.g., placental insufficiency)
- Perinatal (e.g., prematurity)

Childhood Diseases
- Infection (e.g., meningitis)
- Trauma
- Severe chronic disease

*Many disorders cause delays in more than one milestone.

The DDST is a highly specific screening test, so most normal children score as normal, but it is not very sensitive. Many children with mild developmental delay also score as normal. In particular, the language section of the DDST is sparse; it will miss children with mild language delay. While the DDST is a useful screening test, other more sophisticated tests are available for specialists to use to assess motor, language, and social development. You should use the DDST as an adjunct to a comprehensive de-

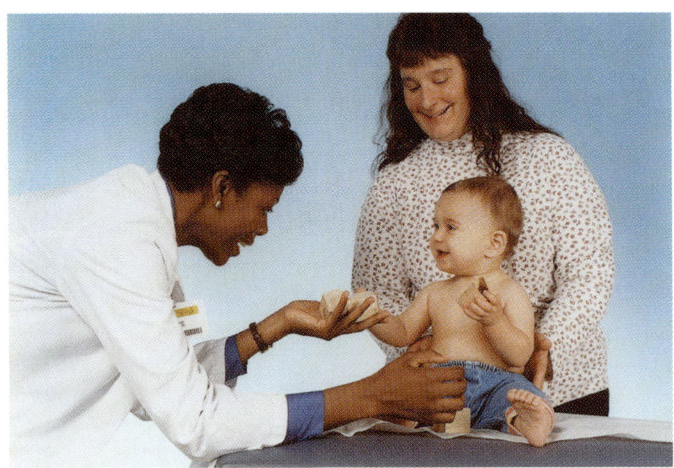

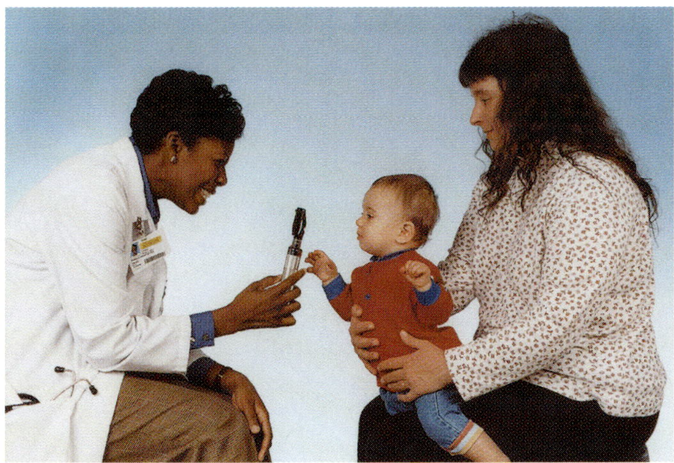

velopmental examination. When delays are suspected from the general examination or DDST, further evaluation is warranted.

For babies born prematurely, adjust the expected developmental milestones for the gestational age up to about 12 months of age.

> ***All kids are gifted; some just open their packages earlier than others.***
> —*Michael Carr*

Assessing Early Childhood

One of the most difficult challenges facing the clinician examining children in this age group is avoiding a physical struggle, a crying child, or a distraught parent. Accomplishing this successfully is satisfying to all and is one aspect of the "art of medicine" in the practice of pediatrics.

Gaining the child's confidence and allaying the child's fears begin at the start of the encounter. The approach varies with the circumstances of the visit. A health supervision visit for a well child allows greater rapport than a visit when the child is acutely ill.

Letting the child remain dressed during the interview makes her less apprehensive. It also allows you to interact more naturally and observe the child playing, interacting with her parents, and undressing and dressing.

Toddlers who are 9 to 15 months may have *stranger anxiety,* a fear of strangers that is developmentally normal. It signals the infant's growing awareness that the stranger is "new." You should not approach these infants

THE "POWER OF OBSERVATION": ABNORMALITIES THAT CAN BE DETECTED WHILE OBSERVING PLAY

*Behavioral Problems**
- Poor parent–child interactions
- Sibling rivalry
- Inappropriate parental discipline
- "Difficult temperament"

Developmental Delay (see DDST)
- Gross motor delay
- Fine motor delay
- Language delay (expressive, receptive)
- Delay in social or emotional tasks

Social or Environmental Problems
- Parental problem, e.g., stress, depression
- Risk for abuse or neglect

Neurologic Problems
- Weakness
- Abnormal posture
- Spasticity
- Clumsiness
- Attentional problems and hyperactivity
- Autistic features

Specific Systems

The initial paragraphs of each section in this chapter describe components of the examination that can be accomplished by observation alone.

*Note: The child's behavior during the visit may not represent typical behavior, but your observations may serve as a springboard for discussion with parents.

quickly. Make sure they remain solidly in their parent's lap throughout much of the examination.

Engage children in conversation appropriate to their ages, and then ask simple questions about themselves, their illness, or their toys. It is helpful to compliment them about their appearance or behavior, tell a story, or play a simple game or trick to "break the ice." If a child is shy and reticent, turn your attention to the parent to allow the child to warm up to you gradually.

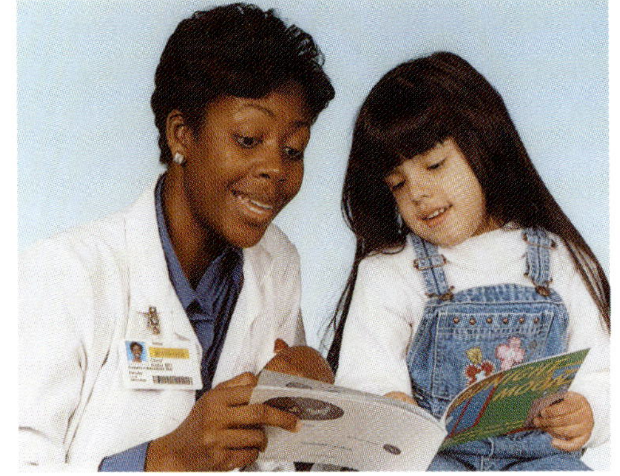

You can observe a lot just by watching.
—Yogi Berra

The physical examination, with certain exceptions, does not need to take place on the examining table; it can occur on the floor or with the child sitting on the parent's lap. The key is to engage the child's cooperation. For the few young children who resist undressing, expose only the part of the body being examined. When examining two or more siblings, it is wise to begin with the older one, who is more likely to cooperate and set a good example.

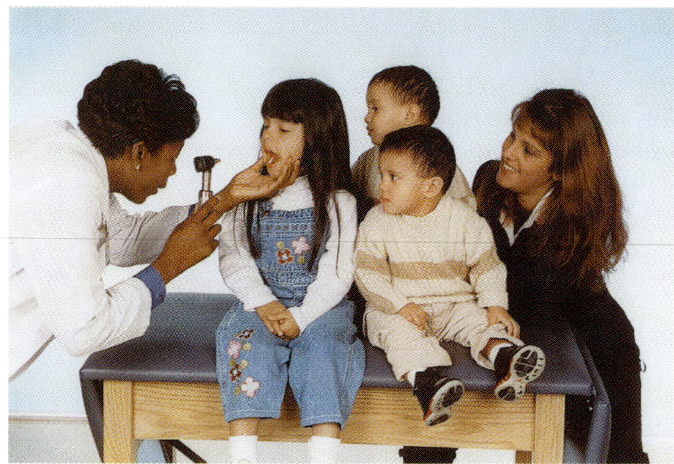

Your approach to the child should be pleasant. Explain each step of the examination as you are performing it. Keep up a running conversation with the parent or the child during the examination to provide distraction.

Plan the order of the examination so that you do the least distressing procedures first and the most distressing (which tend to involve the throat and ears) last. Start with the parts that can be accomplished while the child is sitting—for example, examination of the eyes, palpation of the neck, percussion, and auscultation.

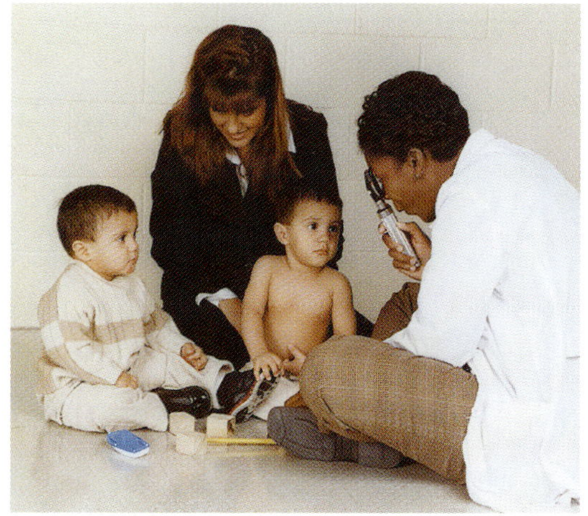

Lying down may make the child feel more vulnerable and more likely to resist further examination, so make this change with care. Once the child is supine, examine the abdomen first, saving either the throat and ears or genitalia for last.

Remember that the physical examination is designed to gather essential information, and an incomplete examination is frustrating for both you and the parents. Thus, patience, distraction, play, flexibility in the order of the examination, and a caring but firm and gentle approach are all keys to successfully examining the young child.

Usually, resistance to the examination is developmentally appropriate. Many toddlers will strive to stay upright and seek the comfort of their parents. In these cases, avoid conveying frustration and reassure the parents that this behavior is normal. Some parents become embarrassed and scold the child, compounding the problem. Involve the parent in the examination (by removing diapers or palpating the abdomen) and play with the child. If needed, pause to allow the child to recover. Learn which techniques work best for you and which approach you find most comfortable. It is not unusual to require a parent's help to restrain the child for examination of the ears or throat. However, use of formal restraints is not appropriate.

SOME MORE TIPS FOR EXAMINING THE YOUNG CHILD

- Let the child see and touch the tools you will be using during the examination.
- Use a reassuring voice throughout the examination.
- Avoid asking permission to examine a body part because you will do the examination anyway. Instead, ask the child which ear or which part of the body he or she would like you to examine "first."
- Examine an apprehensive child in the parent's lap, and let the parent undress the child.
- If unable to console the child, complete the examination expediently or give the child a short break.
- Make a game out of the examination! For example, "Let's see how big your tongue is!" or "Is Barney in your ear? Let's see!"

Assessing Middle Childhood

Usually you will find little difficulty in examining children after they reach school age. While some may have unpleasant memories of previous clinical encounters, most children will respond well when the examiner is attuned to their level of development.

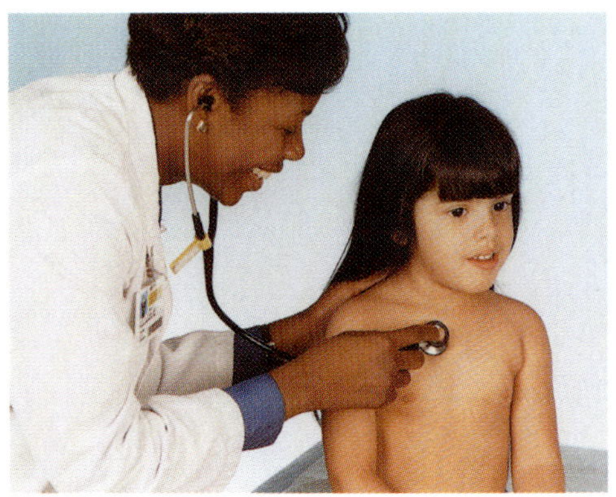

Many children at this age are modest. It is wise to provide gowns and to leave underwear in place until removal is required. It is also helpful to have children disrobe behind a curtain. Consider leaving the room when the children change with parents' help. Some children may prefer that siblings of the opposite sex depart, but most prefer to have a parent of either sex remain in the room, and parents of children under 11 years should remain with them. The order of the examination now begins to follow that used for adults. As at any age, examine painful areas last, and forewarn children about areas you are going to examine. If a child resists part of the examination, you can return to it at the end.

Assessing the Adolescent

The key to successfully examining adolescents is a comfortable, confidential environment. This makes the examination more relaxed and informative. Consider the cognitive and social development of the adolescent when deciding issues of privacy, parental involvement, and confidentiality.

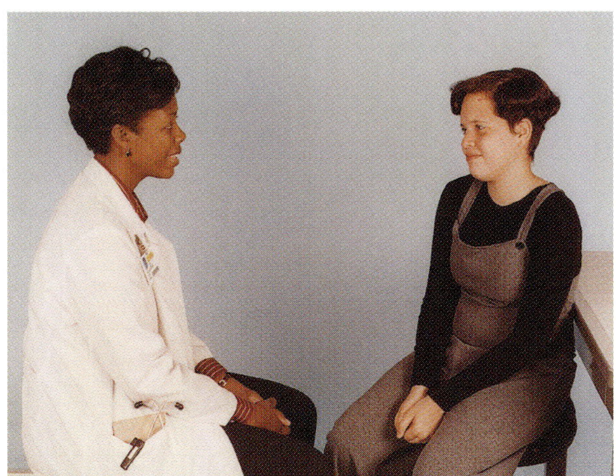

As in middle childhood, modesty is important. The patient should remain dressed until the examination begins, and you should leave the room while the patient gowns. Most adolescents older than age 13 prefer to be examined without a parent in the room, but this depends on the patient's developmental level, familiarity with the examiner, relationship with the parent, and medical issues. For younger adolescents, ask the adolescent and parent their preferences. While the examination of the adolescent can be anxiety-provoking for the novice clinician, with practice, these interactions can be very rewarding for both the adolescent and the clinician.

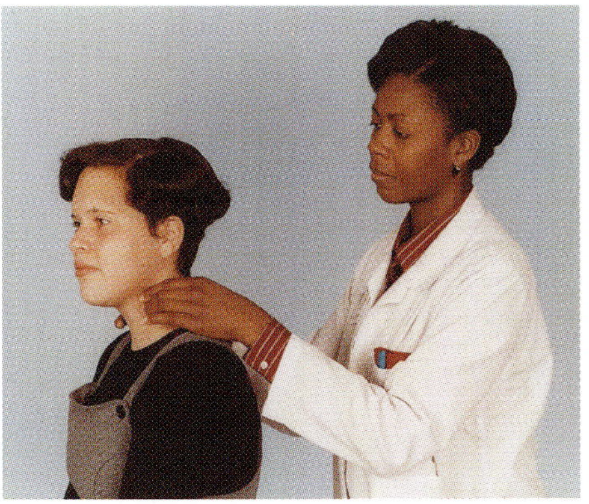

The sequence and content of the physical examination are similar to that of the adult. However, pay particular attention to issues unique to adolescents, such as puberty, growth, development, family and peer relationships, sexuality, decision-making, and risk behaviors.

It is important to have a chaperone (parent or nurse) present during the genital examination of adolescent females.

Now that you have formed your approach to the child before you, you are ready to begin the physical examination.

Children need models rather than critics.
—Joseph Joubert

TECHNIQUES OF EXAMINATION

Important components of the physical examination of children include measurement of body size (height, weight, and head circumference) and vital signs (blood pressure, pulse, respiratory rate, and temperature). Table 17-3, Blood Pressure, and Table 17-4, Growth Charts, (pp. 740–749) show norms for blood pressure, height, weight, body mass index (BMI), and head circumference. Deviations from normal may be the first and only indicators of disease (see Table 17-5, Abnormal Growth Patterns in Infancy and Childhood, pp. 750–759). Except for body temperature, it is important to compare the child's vital signs or body proportions to age-specific norms, because they change dramatically as children grow older. Recently, an increasing number of pediatric practitioners are also assessing pain on a regular basis, using standardized pain scales.

General Survey

SOMATIC GROWTH: HEIGHT, WEIGHT, AND HEAD CIRCUMFERENCE

Measurement of growth is one of the most important indicators of the health of children, and deviations from normal may provide an early indication of an underlying problem. To assess growth, it is important to compare a child's growth parameters with respect to

Table 17-5, pp. 750–759, shows several common *abnormal growth patterns.*

- Normal values according to age and sex
- Prior readings on the same child to assess trends

Failure to thrive is inadequate weight gain for age. Common scenarios are:

- Growth <5th percentile for age
- Growth drop >2 percentiles in 6 months
- Weight for height <5th percentile

Causes include *environmental* or *psychosocial,* and a variety of *gastrointestinal, neurologic, cardiac, endocrine, renal,* and other diseases.

To be clinically meaningful, growth parameters should be measured carefully, using a consistent technique and, optimally, the same scales to measure height and weight.

The most important tools for assessing somatic growth are growth charts, which recently have been modified and published by the National Center for Health Statistics. These charts include height, weight, and head circumference for age, with one set for children up to 36 months and a second set for children ages 2 to 18 years. Charts plotting weight by length are also available. These growth charts have percentile lines indicating the percentage of normal children above and below the child's measurement by chronologic age. Table 17-4, Growth Charts, pp. 742–749, displays these growth charts.

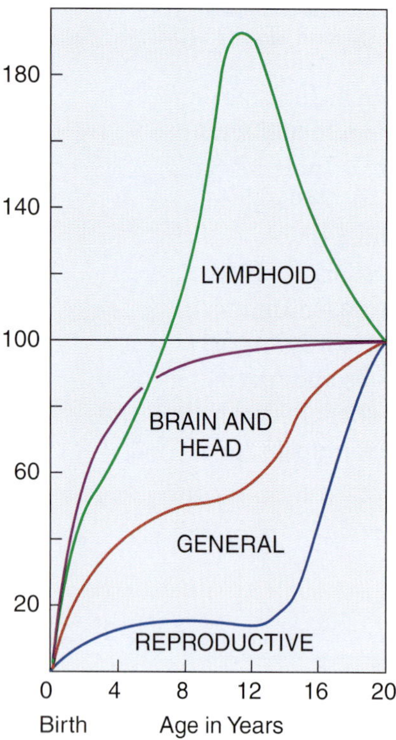

Height. For children older than age 2 years, measure standing height, optimally using wall-mounted stadiometers. Have the child stand with heels, back, and head against a wall or the back of the stadiometer. If using a wall with a marked ruler, make sure to place a flat board or surface against the top of the child's head and at right angles to the ruler. Stand-up weight scales with a height attachment are not very accurate.

Reduced growth in height may indicate *endocrine disease,* other causes of *short stature,* or, if weight is also low, other *chronic diseases.*

Rule of thumb on height: After age 2 years, children should grow at least 5 centimeters per year.

Short stature, defined as subnormal height for age, can be a normal variant or due to endocrine or other diseases. Normal variants include *familial short stature* and *constitutional delay.* Chronic diseases include *growth hormone deficiency,* other endocrine diseases, *gastrointestinal disease* (e.g., inflammatory bowel disease or celiac disease), *renal* or *metabolic disease,* and *genetic syndromes.*

For children under the age of 2 years, measure body length by placing the child supine on a measuring board or in a measuring tray, as shown on the following page. Direct measurement of the infant using a tape measure is inaccurate unless an assistant holds the child still with hips and knees extended. Velocity growth curves, such as the one on the next page, are helpful in older children, especially those who are suspected of having endocrine disorders.

Weight. Weigh infants directly with an infant scale; this is more accurate than an indirect method based on weighing the parent and child together and subtracting the weight of the parent from the total weight. Infants should be clothed only in a diaper or weighed naked.

Children who can stand should be weighed in their underpants on a stand-up scale. While initially nervous, most young children can be coaxed onto such scales. School-age children and adolescents can wear gowns. This is particu-

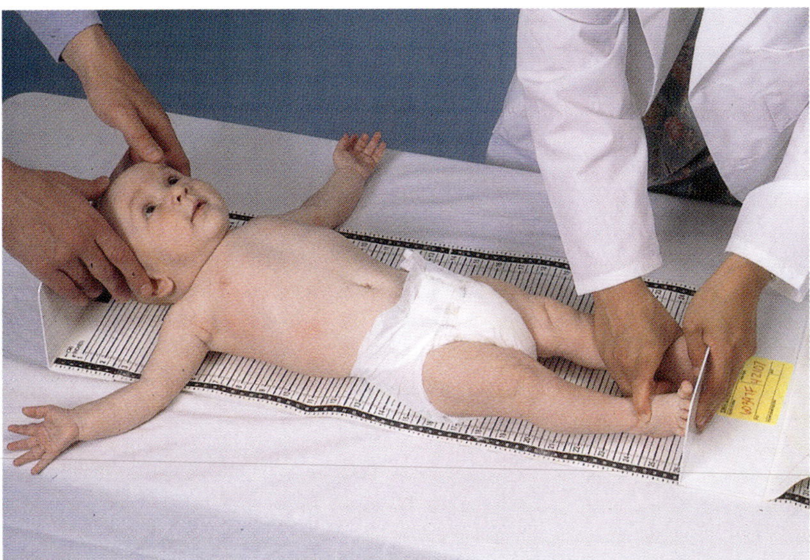

larly important for adolescent girls being evaluated for underweight problems. Ideally, serial weights (and heights) should use the same scales.

Head Circumference. The head circumference of infants should be measured during the first 2 years of life, but measurement can be useful at any age to assess growth of the head. The head circumference in infants reflects the rate of growth of the cranium and the brain. In older children, head

A small head size may be due to *premature closure of the sutures* or to *microcephaly.* Microcephaly may be familial or due to a variety of *chromosomal abnormalities, congenital infections, maternal metabolic disorders,* and *neurologic insults.*

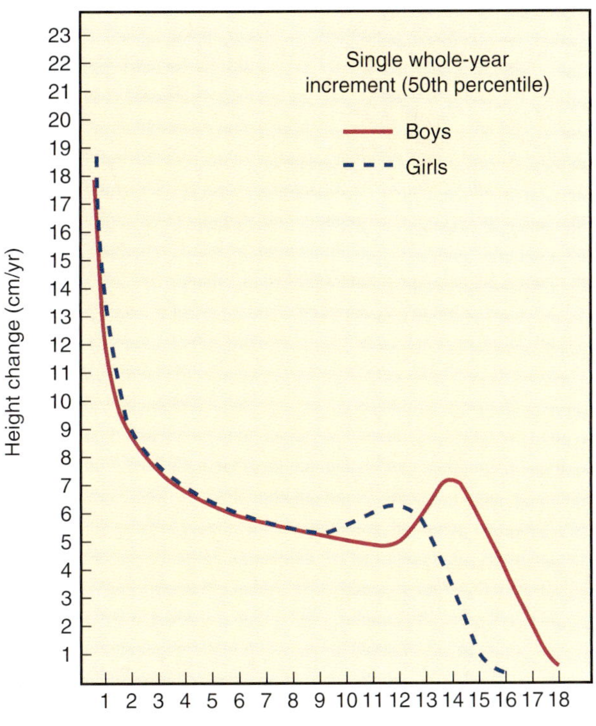

Velocity curves for length and height for boys and girls based on intervals of 1 year. (From Lowrey GH: Growth and development of children, *ed 8, Chicago, 1986, Mosby.)*

size is affected by genetic factors, and it may be useful to measure the head circumference of parents when children have abnormal head sizes.

To measure head circumference, place the measuring tape over the occipital, parietal, and frontal prominences to obtain the maximum circumference. During infancy this is done best with the patient supine. You may need to make several measurements and use the largest one. Measurements of chest and abdominal circumference are not clinically useful.

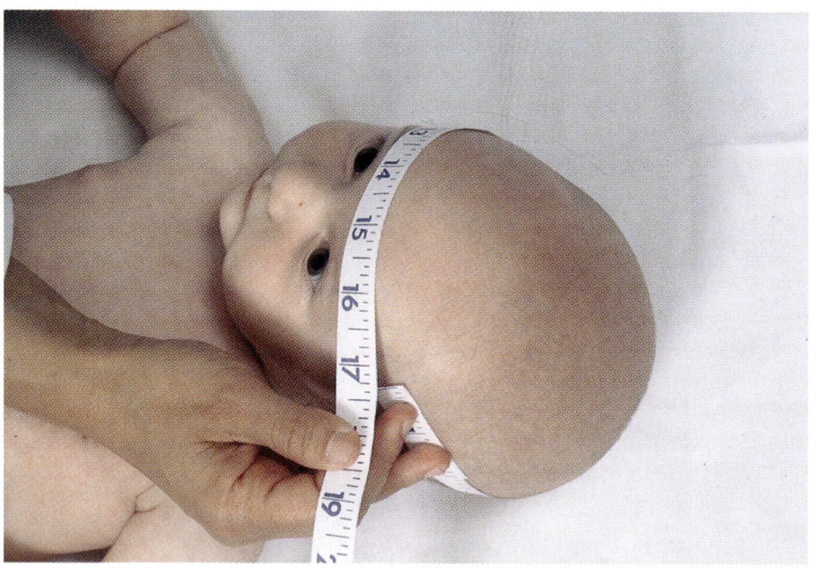

An abnormally large head size (>97th percentile or 2 standard deviations above the mean) is *macrocephaly,* which may be due to *hydrocephalus, subdural hematoma,* or rare causes like *brain tumor or inherited syndromes. Familial megaloencephaly* (large head) is a benign familial condition with normal brain growth.

BODY MASS INDEX-FOR-AGE

Age- and sex-specific charts are now available to assess body mass index (BMI) in children (see the following table). BMI in children is associated with body fat, related to health risks of obesity, and measurements are helpful for children over the age of 2 years.

Interpreting BMI in Children

Group	BMI-for-Age
Underweight	<5th percentile
At risk of overweight	≥85th percentile
Overweight	≥95th percentile

Vital Signs

BLOOD PRESSURE

Although there are special challenges to obtaining accurate blood pressure readings in young infants, this measurement, nevertheless, is important and should be part of the physical examination of every child older than 2 years of age, and of any younger child whose history or physical examination suggests that the blood pressure may be abnormal. *Hypertension during childhood is more common than previously thought, and it is important to recognize, confirm, and appropriately manage it.*

Children have elevated blood pressure during exercise, crying, and anxiety. Although young children may be anxious at first, when the procedure is explained and demonstrated beforehand, most children are cooperative. If the blood pressure is initially elevated, you can perform blood pressure readings again at the end of the examination; one trick is to leave the cuff on the arm (deflated) and repeat the reading later. Elevated readings must always be confirmed by subsequent measurements.

The most frequent "cause" of an elevated blood pressure in children is probably an *improperly performed examination,* often due to an incorrect cuff size.

Select the blood pressure cuff as you would in adults. It should be wide enough to cover two thirds of the upper arm or leg. A narrower cuff falsely elevates the blood pressure reading, while a wider cuff lowers it and may interfere with proper placement of the stethoscope diaphragm over the artery. *Thus, a proper cuff size is essential for accurate determinations of blood pressure in children.*

In children, as in adults, blood pressure readings from the thigh are approximately 10 mm Hg higher than those from the upper arm. If they are the same or lower, *coarctation of the aorta* should be suspected.

With children, as with adults, the point at which the Korotkoff sounds disappear constitutes the diastolic pressure. At times, especially among chubby young children, the Korotkoff sounds are not easily heard. In such instances, you can use palpation to determine the systolic blood pressure (see pp. 76–77), remembering that the systolic pressure is approximately 10 mm Hg lower by palpation than by auscultation.

A relatively inaccurate means is to use "inspection." Watch for the needle to bounce about 10 mm Hg higher than it does in auscultation. While this technique is suboptimal, in squirming children sometimes it is all you can get.

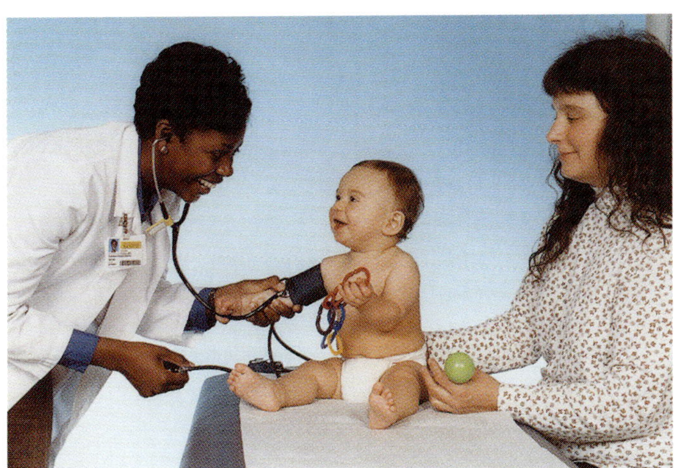

The most easily used measure of the systolic blood pressure of infants and young children is obtained with the *Doppler method,* which detects arterial blood flow vibrations, converts them to systolic blood pressure levels, and transmits them to a digital read-out device. However, Doppler instruments are expensive, and readings tend to be higher than by auscultation.

The systolic blood pressure gradually increases throughout infancy and childhood. For example, normal systolic pressure in males is about 70 mm Hg

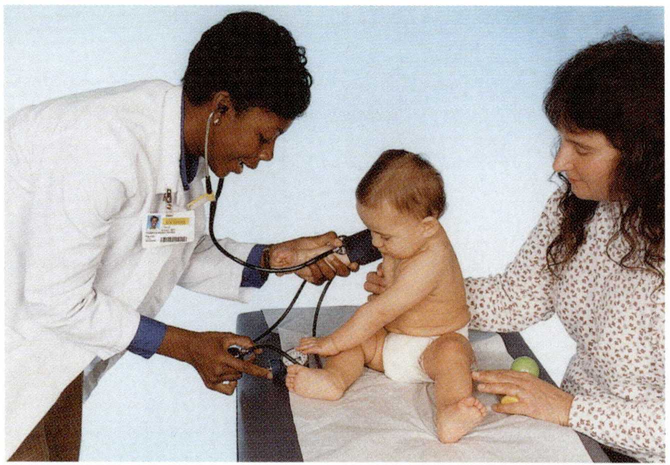

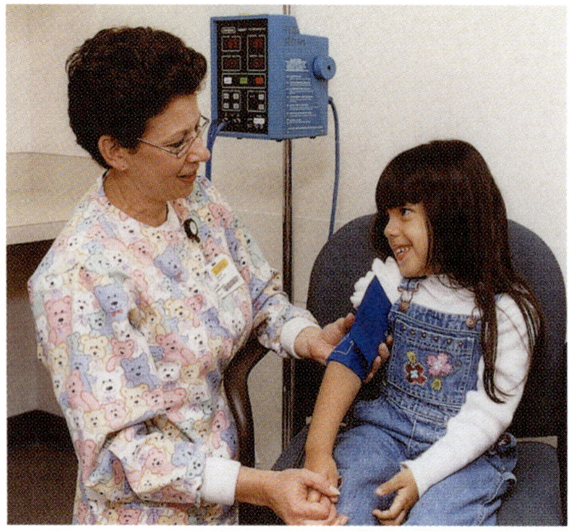

at birth, 85 mm Hg at 1 month, and 90 mm Hg at 6 months. Turn to Table 17-3, pp. 740–741, for normal blood pressure levels by year of life for boys and girls, including percentiles specific to age and height.

In 1995, the National Heart, Lung, and Blood Institute's National High Blood Pressure Working Group on Hypertension Control in Children and Adolescents defined normal, high-normal, and high blood pressure as follows, with measurements on at least three separate occasions:

Although most adults with hypertension have normal blood pressure as children, *essential hypertension* often is detectable in adolescents.

Blood Pressure Category	Average Systolic and/or Diastolic Blood Pressure for Age, Sex, and Height
Normal	<90th percentile
High Normal	90th–95th percentile
High	≥95th percentile

Children who have hypertension should be evaluated extensively to determine the cause. For infants and young children, a specific cause can usually be found. In older children and adolescents, however, an increasing proportion

It is also important not to *falsely label* a child or adolescent as having hypertension, because of

has essential or primary hypertension. In all cases, it is important to repeat measurements to reduce the possibility that the elevation reflects anxiety. Sometimes repeating measurements in school is a way to obtain readings in a more relaxed environment.

the stigmata of labeling, potential limitations to activities, and possible side effects of treatment.

Causes of Sustained Hypertension in Children

Newborn	Middle Childhood
Renal artery disease (stenosis, thrombosis) Congenital renal malformations Coarctation of the aorta	Renal parenchymal or arterial disease Primary hypertension Coarctation of the aorta
Infancy and Early Childhood	**Adolescence**
Renal parenchymal or artery disease Coarctation of the aorta	Primary hypertension Renal parenchymal disease Drug induced

PULSE

The heart rate of infants and children is quite variable. It is more sensitive to the effects of illness, exercise, and emotion than that of adults. Average heart rates are shown in the table below:

A pulse rate that is too rapid to count (usually >180–200/min) usually indicates *paroxysmal supraventricular tachycardia.*

Average Heart Rate of Infants and Children at Rest

Age	Average Rate	Range (Two Standard Deviations)
Birth	140	90–190
1st 6 months	130	80–180
6–12 months	115	75–155
1–2 years	110	70–150
2–6 years	103	68–138
6–10 years	95	65–125
10–14 years	85	55–115

You may have trouble obtaining an accurate pulse rate in a squirming infant or child. The best strategy is to palpate the femoral arteries in the inguinal area or the brachial arteries in the antecubital fossa, or to auscultate the heart. In older children who are cooperative, palpate the radial artery at the wrist.

Bradycardia in infants or young children may be due to *drug ingestion, hypoxia, intracranial* or *neurologic conditions,* or, rarely, *cardiac arrhythmia* such as *heart block.*

To measure the man, measure his heart.
—*Malcolm Stevenson Forbes*

Bradycardia in a thin adolescent female may be due to *anorexia nervosa.*

RESPIRATORY RATE

As with heart rate, compared to that of adults, the respiratory rate in infants and children has a greater range and is more responsive to illness, exercise, and emotion. The rate of respirations per minute ranges between 30 and 60

Extremely rapid and shallow respiratory rates are seen in newborns with *cyanotic cardiac disease* who

in the newborn, 20 and 40 during early childhood, and 15 and 25 during late childhood, reaching adult levels at age 15 years.

have normal lungs but right-to-left shunting, and in conditions of *metabolic acidosis.*

The respiratory rate may vary considerably from moment to moment in newborn infants, with alternating periods of rapid and slow breathing. The sleeping respiratory rate is most reliable. However, respiratory rates during active sleep compared to quiet sleep may be up to 10 breaths per minute faster. The respiratory pattern should be observed for at least 60 seconds. In infancy and early childhood, diaphragmatic breathing is predominant; thoracic excursion is minimal.

Children with respiratory diseases such as *bronchiolitis* or *pneumonia* have rapid respirations (up to 80–90/min), but *also* increased work of breathing such as grunting, nasal flaring, or use of accessory muscles.

For young children, observe the movements of the chest wall for two 30-second intervals or over 1 minute, preferably prior to stimulating them. Direct auscultation of the chest or placing the stethoscope in front of the mouth is also useful for counting respirations, but the measurement may be falsely elevated if the child becomes agitated. For older children, use the same technique as used for adults.

Commonly accepted cutoffs for defining *tachypnea* are:

Infants 0–2 months	>60/min
Infants 2–12 months	>50/min
Children >12 months	>40/min

The best single physical finding for ruling out *pneumonia* is an absence of tachypnea.

Fever can raise respiratory rates in infants. In the absence of pneumonia, an infant's respiratory rate can increase by up to 10 respirations per minute for each degree centigrade of fever.

TEMPERATURE

Because fever is so common in children, obtaining an accurate body temperature is helpful whenever you suspect infection, collagen vascular disease, or malignancy. The techniques for obtaining rectal, oral, and auditory canal temperatures in adults are described on pp. 81–82. Axillary and thermal-tape (temporal artery) skin temperature recordings in children are inaccurate.

Fever (>38.0°C or >100.0°F) in infants <2–3 months may be a sign of *serious infection* or disease. These infants should be evaluated promptly.

In children and adolescents, auditory canal temperature recordings are preferable because they can be obtained quickly with essentially no discomfort. For infants under 2 months of age, rectal temperatures are preferred because clinical guidelines for evaluating serious bacterial infections use rectal temperature levels as a major criterion.

The technique for obtaining the *rectal temperature* is relatively simple. One method is illustrated on the next page. Place the infant or child prone on the examining table, on the parent's lap, or on your own lap. While you separate the buttocks with the thumb and forefinger on one hand, with the other hand gently insert a well-lubricated rectal thermometer, inclined approximately 20° from the table or lap, through the anal sphincter to a depth of approximately 2 to 3 centimeters. Keep the thermometer in place for at least 2 minutes.

Body temperature in infants and children is less constant than in adults. The average rectal temperature is higher in infancy and early childhood, usually not falling below 99.0°F (37.2°C) until after age 3 years. Body temperature may fluctuate as much as 3°F during a single day, approaching 101°F (38.3°C) in normal children, particularly in late afternoon and after vigorous activity.

During early childhood, extremely high fever (up to 104°F or 40°C) is common, even with minor infections.

Anxiety may elevate the body temperature of children. *Excessive bundling* of infants may elevate the skin but not the core temperature.

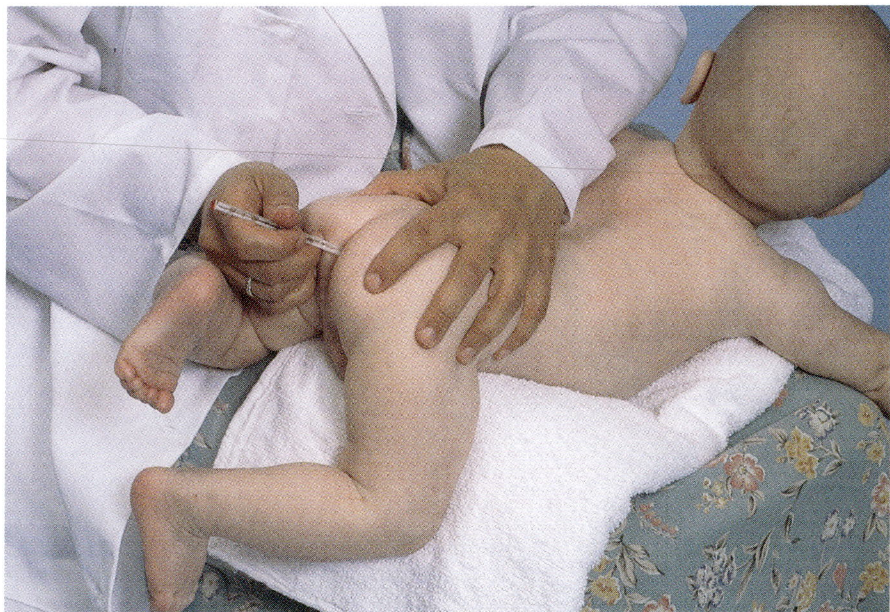

The Skin

NEWBORN AND EARLY INFANCY

The newborn infant's skin has a unique characteristic *texture and appearance*. The texture is soft and smooth because it is thinner than the skin of older children. Within the first 10 minutes after birth, a normal newborn progresses from generalized cyanosis to pinkness. In lighter-skinned infants, an erythematous flush, giving the skin the appearance of a "boiled lobster," is common during the first 8 to 24 hours, then the normal pale pink coloring predominates.

Cutis marmorata is prominent in *premature infants,* and in infants with *congenital hypothyroidism* and *Down syndrome.*

Vasomotor changes in the dermis and subcutaneous tissue—a response to cooling or chronic exposure to radiant heat—can produce a latticelike, bluish mottled appearance (*cutis marmorata*), particularly on the trunk, arms, and legs. This response to cold may last for months in normal infants. *Acrocyanosis,* a blue cast to the hands and feet when exposed to cold (see the photo on the next page), is very common in newborns for the first few days, and may recur throughout early infancy. Occasionally in newborns, a striking color change (*harlequin dyschromia*) appears with transient cyanosis of one half of the body or one extremity, presumably due to temporary vascular instability.

If acrocyanosis does not disappear within 8 hours or with warming, *cyanotic congenital heart disease* should be considered.

The amount of melanin in the skin of newborns varies, affecting *pigmentation.* Black newborns may have a lighter skin color initially than later on, except in the nail beds and genitalia, which are dark at birth. A dark or bluish pigmentation over the buttocks and lower lumbar regions is common in newborns of African, Asian, and Mediterranean descent. These areas, formerly called Mongolian spots, are due to the presence of pigmented cells in the deep layers of the skin; they become less noticeable with age and usually disappear during childhood. It is important to document these pigmented areas to avoid later concern about bruising.

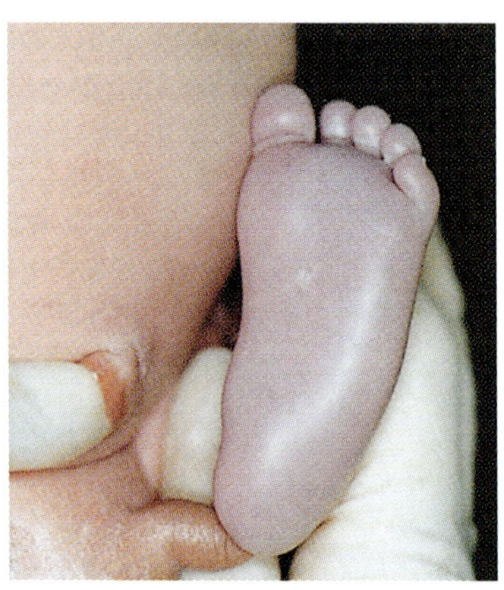

Acrocyanosis in the first half hour of life in a 32-week infant. (From Fletcher M: Physical Diagnosis in Neonatology, Philadelphia, Lippincott-Raven Publishers, 1998.)

Central cyanosis in a baby or child of any age should raise suspicion of *congenital heart disease.* The best area to look for central cyanosis is the tongue and oral mucosa, not the nail beds or the extremities.

At birth there is a fine, downy growth of hair called *lanugo* over the entire body, but especially the shoulders and back. This hair is shed within the first few weeks. Lanugo is prominent in premature infants. Hair thickness on the head varies considerably among newborns, and fortunately is not predictive of later hair growth. All of the original hair is shed within months, replaced with a new crop, sometimes of a different color.

Pigmented light-brown lesions (<1–2 cm at birth) are *café-au-lait spots.* Isolated lesions have no significance, but multiple lesions with smooth borders may suggest *neurofibromatosis* (see Table 17-6, p. 761).

Inspect the newborn closely for a series of common skin conditions. At birth, a cheesy white material called *vernix caseosa,* composed of sebum and desquamated epithelial cells, covers the body. Some newborns have *edema* over their hands, feet, lower legs, pubis, and sacrum; this disappears within a few days. Superficial desquamation of the skin is often noticeable 24 to 36 hours after birth.

Skin desquamation at birth occurs in some normal babies, and frequently in *post-term babies* (>40 wks gestation). Rarely, it is a sign of placental circulatory insufficiency or *congenital ichthyosis.*

You should be able to identify four common dermatologic conditions in newborns. None is clinically significant. *Milia,* pinhead-sized smooth, white raised areas without surrounding erythema on the nose, chin, and forehead, are caused by retention of sebum in the openings of the sebaceous glands. While occasionally present at birth, milia usually appear within the first few weeks and disappear over several weeks. *Miliaria rubra* consists of scattered vesicles on an erythematous base, usually on the face and trunk, caused by sweat gland duct obstruction; it also disappears spontaneously within weeks. *Erythema toxicum,* which usually appears on the 2nd or 3rd day of life, consists of erythematous macules with central pinpoint vesicles scattered diffusely over the entire body, appearing much like flea bites. These lesions are of unknown etiology, but disappear within a week after birth. *Pustular melanosis,* seen more commonly in black infants, is present at birth as small vesiculopustules over a brown macular base and can last for several months.

Midline hair tufts over the lumbosacral spine region suggest a *spinal cord defect.*

Both erythema toxicum and pustular melanosis may appear similar to the pathologic vesicular rash of *herpes simplex* or *staphylococcus aureus skin infection,* which are serious infections requiring rapid treatment.

Note any signs of trauma from the birth process and the use of forceps or suction; these signs disappear but should prompt a careful neurologic examination.

Normal "physiologic" *jaundice,* which occurs in half of all newborns, appears on the 2nd or 3rd day, peaks at about the 5th day, and usually disappears within a week. Jaundice can best be appreciated in natural daylight rather than artificial light. Newborn jaundice seems to progress from head to toe, with more intense jaundice on the upper body and less intense yellow color in the lower extremities. To detect jaundice, apply pressure to the skin as shown below to press the normal pink or brown color out. Look for the presence of a yellowish "blanching," which indicates jaundice. Another technique is to press a glass slide against the skin to empty the capillary bed and observe for color contrast. Also see Table 17-7, p. 762.

Jaundice that appears within the first 24 hours of birth is likely to be pathologic jaundice due to *hemolytic disease of the newborn.*

Jaundice that persists beyond 2–3 weeks should raise suspicions of *biliary obstruction* or *liver disease.*

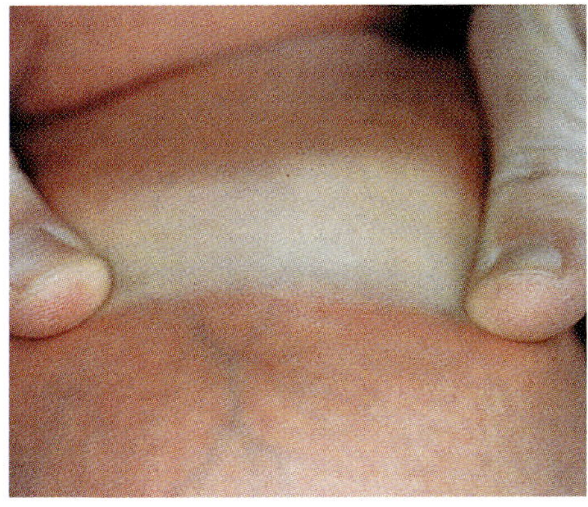

Pressing the red color from the skin allows better recognition of the yellow of jaundice. Infant with no appreciable jaundice at chest level. (From Fletcher M: Physical Diagnosis in Neonatology, Philadelphia, Lippincott-Raven Publishers, 1998.)

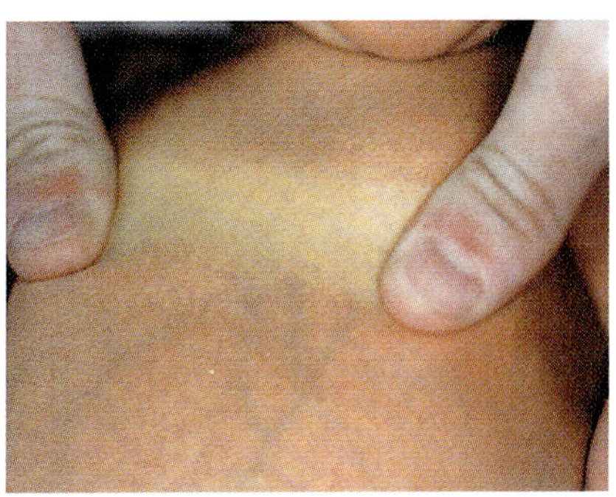

Infant with bilirubin level of 13 mg/d (222 µmol/L). (From Fletcher M: Physical Diagnosis in Neonatology, Philadelphia, Lippincott-Raven Publishers, 1998.)

A common *vascular marking,* found in 40% of newborns, is the "salmon patch" (also known as *nevus simplex,* telangiectatic nevus, or capillary hemangioma). These flat, irregular, light pink patches are most often seen on the nape of the neck ("stork bite"), upper eyelids, forehead, or upper lip ("angel kisses"). They are not true nevi, but are due to distended dermal capillaries; they almost all disappear by 1 year of age. Darker, purplish lesions on the face or extremities are "port wine stains" and do not fade.

Nuchal salmon patch at hairline. (From Fletcher M: Physical Diagnosis in Neonatology, Philadelphia, Lippincott-Raven Publishers, 1998.)

A unilateral port wine stain over the distribution of the ophthalmic branch of the trigeminal nerve may be a sign of *Sturge-Weber syndrome,* which is associated with seizures, hemiparesis, glaucoma, and mental retardation.

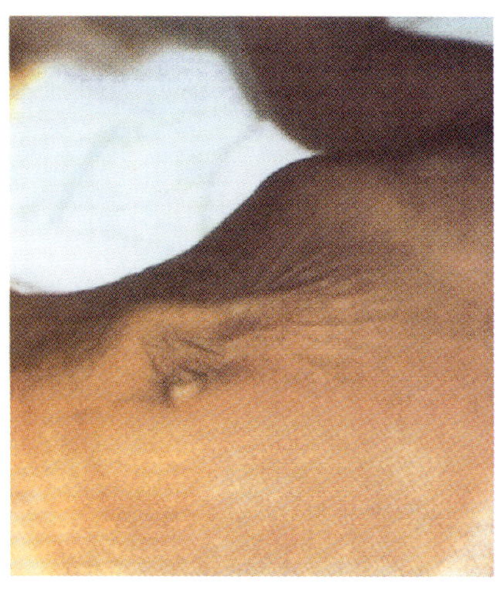

From Zitelli BJ and Davis HW: Atlas of Pediatric Diagnosis, ed. 3, St. Louis, 1997, Mosby-Year Book.

The examination of the skin should include palpation to assess the degree of hydration or *turgor*. Roll a fold of loosely adherent skin on the abdominal wall between your thumb and forefinger to determine its consistency. The skin in well-hydrated infants and children returns to its normal position immediately upon release.

Significant edema of the hands and feet of a newborn girl may be suggestive of *Turner's syndrome.*

Delay in return to normal skin position as shown on the left, a phenomenon called "tenting," usually occurs in children with significant *dehydration.*

EARLY AND LATE CHILDHOOD

After a child's first year of life, the techniques of examination are the same as those for the adult (see Chap. 4, The Skin).

The Head

In examining the head and neck, tailor your examination to the child's stage of growth and development.

Even before touching the child, carefully observe the shape of the head, its symmetry, and the presence of abnormal facies. Next, measure the head circumference in children under 2 years (described on p. 657). At birth, a baby's head may seem relatively large to you. A newborn's head accounts for one fourth of the body length and one third of the body weight; these proportions change, so that by adulthood the head accounts for one eighth of the body length and about one tenth of the body weight.

INFANCY

Examine the *sutures* and *fontanelles* carefully (see the figure on the next page). The bones of the skull are separated from one another by membranous tissue spaces called *sutures.* The areas where the major sutures intersect in the anterior and posterior portions of the skull are known as *fontanelles.*

An enlarged posterior fontanelle may be present in *congenital hypothyroidism.*

On palpation, the sutures feel like ridges and the fontanelles like soft concavities. The *anterior fontanelle* at birth measures 4 cm to 6 cm in diameter and usually closes between 4 and 26 months of age (90% between 7–19 mos). The *posterior fontanelle* measures 1 cm to 2 cm at birth and usually closes by 2 months.

A bulging, tense fontanelle is observed in infants with *increased intracranial pressure,* which may be due to *central nervous system infections, neoplastic disease,* or *hydrocephalus* (obstruction of the circulation of cerebrospinal fluid within the ventricles of the brain).

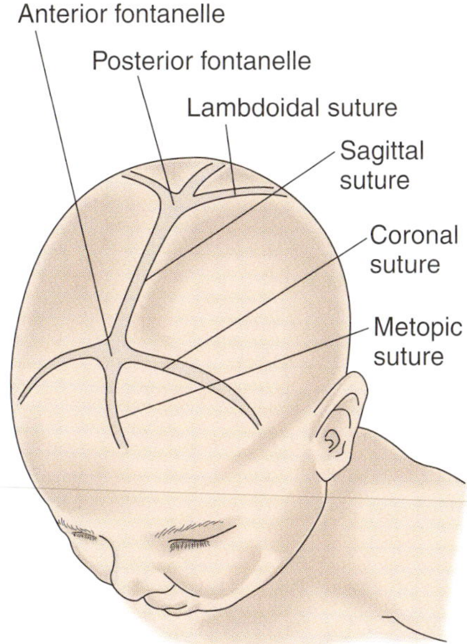

Careful examination of the fontanelle is important because the fullness of the fontanelle reflects *intracranial pressure.* It is best to palpate the fontanelle while the baby is sitting quietly or being held upright. Experienced pediatric health care providers often have the habit of palpating the fontanelles at the beginning of the examination. In normal infants, the anterior fontanelle is soft and flat. Increased intracranial pressure produces a bulging, full anterior fontanelle and is seen when a baby cries, vomits, or has underlying pathology. Pulsations of the fontanelle reflect the peripheral pulse.

A depressed anterior fontanelle may be a sign of *dehydration.*

Overlap of the cranial bones at the sutures at birth, called *molding,* results from passage of the head through the birth canal; it disappears within 2 days.

Inspect the scalp veins carefully to assess for dilatation.

Dilated scalp veins are indicative of long-standing *increased intracranial pressure.*

Assess the *symmetry of the skull.* A number of conditions can cause asymmetry of the skull in newborns and infants; some are normal or benign, while others reflect underlying pathology.

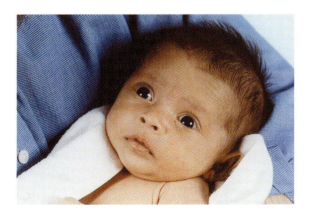

A newborn's scalp is often swollen from localized subcutaneous edema over the occipitoparietal region, called *caput succedaneum,* caused by distension of capillaries and extravasation of blood and fluid resulting from the vacuum

Another type of localized swelling of the scalp is a *cephalohematoma,* due to subperiosteal hemorrhage

effect of rupture of the amniotic sac. This swelling often crosses over suture lines and resolves in 1 to 2 days.

from the trauma of birth. This swelling does not cross over suture lines and resolves within 3 weeks. As the hemorrhage resolves and calcifies, there may be a palpable bony rim with a soft center.

The premature infant's head at birth is relatively long in the occipitofrontal diameter and narrow in the bitemporal diameter (*dolichocephaly*). Usually the skull shape normalizes within 1 to 2 years.

Asymmetry of the cranial vault (*plagiocephaly*) occurs when an infant lies mostly on one side, resulting in a flattening of the parieto-occipital region on the dependent side and a prominence of the frontal region on the opposite side. It disappears as the baby becomes more active and spends less time in one position, and symmetry is almost always restored. Interestingly, the current trend to have newborns sleep on their backs to reduce the risk for sudden infant death syndrome has resulted in more cases of plagiocephaly.

While *plagiocephaly* may be due to positioning, it may also reflect pathology such as *torticollis* from injury to the sternocleidomastoid muscle at birth, or *lack of stimulation* of the infant.

Premature closure of one or more cranial sutures causes *craniosynostosis,* with an abnormally shaped skull. *Sagittal suture synostosis* causes a narrow head due to lack of growth of the parietal bones. Palpation may reveal a raised bony ridge at the suture line.

Measure the head circumference (p. 658) to detect abnormally large head size (*macrocephaly*) or small head (*microcephaly*), which may be due to an underlying disorder affecting the brain.

Examine the *skull.* You can perform the following maneuvers with care:

- On palpation of the infant's skull, you may note that the cranial bones appear "soft" or pliable; they will become firmer with increasing gestational age. An exception occurs in a condition known as *craniotabes,* which is found in some normal infants but also in some with diseases. In this condition, the cranial bones feel pliable and springy, much as a ping-pong ball springs back upon pressure.

Craniotabes can be due to increased intracranial pressure as in *hydrocephaly,* metabolic disturbances such as *rickets,* and infection (e.g., *congenital syphilis*).

- Percuss the parietal bone on each side of the skull using your index or middle finger. This will produce a "cracked pot" sound (*Macewen's sign*) in normal infants prior to closure of the cranial sutures.

Macewen's sign is noted in older infants with high intracranial pressure that causes closed cranial sutures to separate (e.g., due to *lead encephalopathy, brain tumor,* or *hydrocephalus*).

Auscultation of the skull is not useful in young children because a systolic or continuous bruit may be heard over the temporal areas in many normal children. Older children with significant anemia may have a cranial bruit.

An *arteriovenous fistula* in the brain can produce a loud bruit.

Transillumination of the skull may be helpful in the evaluation of an infant with possible central nervous system disease. In a completely darkened room, place a bright flashlight fitted with a soft rubber collar flush against the skull at various points. In normal infants, a 2-cm halo of light is present around the circumference of the flashlight placed over the frontoparietal area, and a 1-cm halo when placed over the occipital area.

If the entire head "lights up," *hydranencephaly* or *reduced size of the cerebral cortex* is suspected. Localized bright spots may be seen with *subdural effusions* and *porencephalic cysts.*

Check the *face* of infants for symmetry. In utero positioning may result in transient facial asymmetries. If the head is flexed on the sternum, a shortened chin (*micrognathia*) may result. Pressure of the shoulder on the jaw may create a temporary lateral displacement of the mandible.

Micrognathia may also be part of a syndrome, such as the *Pierre Robin syndrome.*

Examine the face for an overall impression of the *facies;* it is helpful to compare to the face of the parents. There are diagnostic facies in childhood (Table 17-12, pp. 768–769, shows several) that reflect chromosomal abnormalities, endocrine defects, chronic illness, and other disorders. While it is often difficult to distinguish abnormal facies from normal variants, here are some "pearls."

"PEARLS" TO EVALUATE A CHILD WITH POTENTIALLY ABNORMAL FACIES

Carefully review the history, especially:

- Family history
- Pregnancy
- Perinatal history

Note abnormalities on other parts of the physical examination, especially:

- Growth
- Development
- Other dysmorphic somatic features

Perform measurements (and plot percentiles), especially

- Head circumference
- Height
- Weight

Consider the three mechanisms of facial dysmorphogenesis.

- Deformations due to intrauterine constraint
- Disruptions due to amniotic bands or disruption from fetal tissue
- Malformations due to an intrinsic abnormality in either the face/head or the brain

Examine the parents and siblings.

- Similarity to a parent may be reassuring (e.g., large head) or may represent a familial disorder.

Try to determine whether the facial features fit a recognizable syndrome, comparing to:

- References (including measurements) and pictures of syndromes
- Tables/databases of combinations of features.

A child with abnormal shape or length of palpebral fissures:
 Upslanting (Down syndrome)
 Down-slanting (Noonan's syndrome)
 Short (fetal alcohol effects)

Percussion of the cheek is useful to check for *Chvostek's sign,* which is present in some metabolic disturbances and occasionally in normal infants. Percuss at the top of the cheek just below the zygomatic bone in front of the ear, using the tip of your index or middle finger.

A positive Chvostek's sign produces facial grimacing caused by repeated contractions of the facial muscles. A Chvostek sign is noted in cases of *hypocalcemic tetany, tetanus and tetany due to hyperventilation.*

EARLY AND LATE CHILDHOOD

The examination of the head in later childhood is the same as that for adults. Abnormal facies may not be apparent until later in childhood; therefore, carefully examine the face as well as the head of all children.

The Neck

Beyond infancy, the techniques for examining the neck are the same as for adults. Several important and somewhat unique aspects of the pediatric examination of the neck are described below.

Lymphadenopathy is usually due to viral or bacterial infections (see Table 17-13, Abnormalities of the Neck, p. 770).

Palpate the *lymph nodes of the neck* and assess the presence of any additional masses such as *congenital cysts*. Because the necks of infants are short, it is best to palpate the neck while infants are lying supine, whereas older children are best examined while sitting. Check the position of the thyroid cartilage and trachea.

Malignancy is more likely if the node is greater than 2 cm, is hard or fixed to the skin or underlying tissues (i.e., not mobile), is accompanied by serious systemic signs such as weight loss, and, in the case of cervical lymph nodes, if the chest x-ray findings are abnormal.

Lymphadenopathy is unusual during infancy but very common during childhood. As shown on p. 656, the child's lymphatic system reaches its zenith of growth at 12 years, and cervical or tonsillar lymph nodes reach their peak size between 8 and 16 years. The vast majority of enlarged lymph nodes in children are due to infections (mostly viral but frequently bacterial) and not to malignant disease, even though the latter is a concern for many parents. It is important to differentiate normal lymph nodes from abnormal ones or from congenital cysts of the neck.

In young children with small necks, it may be difficult to differentiate low posterior cervical lymph nodes from *supraclavicular lymph nodes* (which are always abnormal and raise suspicion for malignancy).

The following figure illustrates the typical location of congenital cysts, including thyroglossal duct cysts, branchial cleft cysts, cystic hygromas, epidermal (dermoid) cysts, and preauricular cysts or sinuses.

Branchial cleft cysts appear as small dimples or openings anterior to the midportion of the sternocleidomastoid muscle. They may be associated with a sinus tract.

Preauricular cysts and sinuses are common, pinhole-size pits, usually located anterior to the helix of the ear. They are often bilateral and may occasionally be associated with *hearing deficits.*

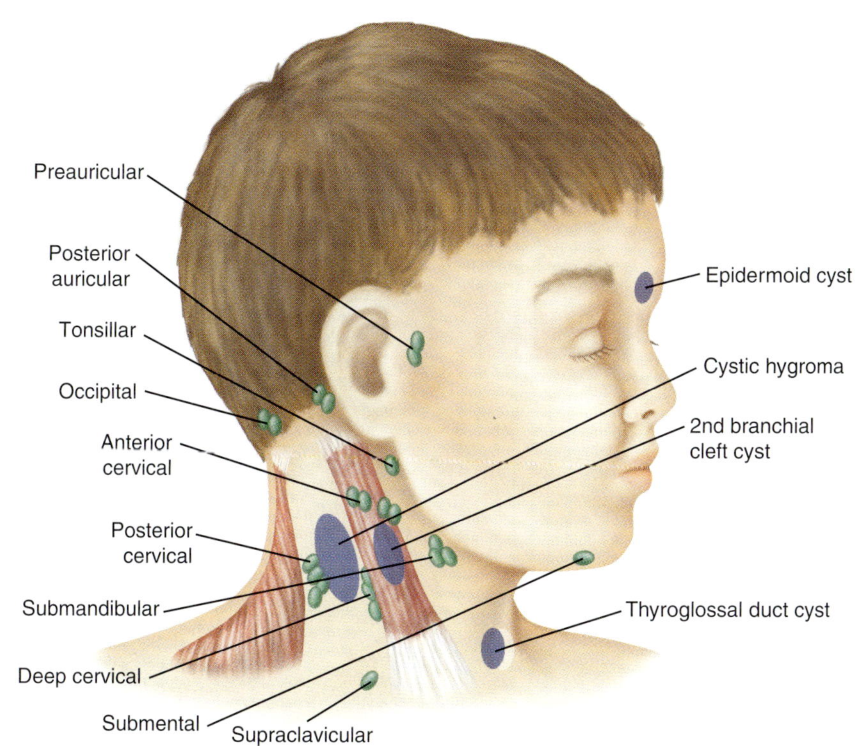

Thyroglossal duct cysts are located at the midline of the neck, just above the thyroid cartilage. These small, firm, mobile masses move upward with tongue protrusion or with swallowing. They are usually detected after 2 years.

Check for *neck mobility*. It is important to ensure that the neck of all infants and children is supple and easily mobile in all directions. This is particularly important when the patient is holding the head in an asymmetric manner, and when central nervous system disease such as meningitis is suspected.

Congenital torticollis, or a "wry neck," is due to bleeding into the sternocleidomastoid muscle during the stretching process of birth. A firm fibrous mass is felt within the muscle 2–3 weeks after birth and generally disappears over months.

In infants and children, the presence of nuchal rigidity is a more reliable indicator of meningeal irritation than *Brudzinski's sign* or *Kernig's sign*. To detect nuchal rigidity in older children, ask the child to sit with legs extended on the examining table. Normally, children should be able to sit upright and touch their chins to their chests. Younger children can be persuaded to flex their necks by having them follow a small toy or light beam. You also can test for nuchal rigidity with the child lying on the examining table, as shown on the next page. Nearly all children with nuchal rigidity will be extremely sick, irritable, and difficult to examine.

Nuchal rigidity is marked resistance to movement of the head in any direction. It suggests meningeal irritation due to *meningitis, bleeding, tumor,* or *other causes.* These children are extremely irritable and difficult to console and may have "paradoxical irritability"—increased irritability when being held.

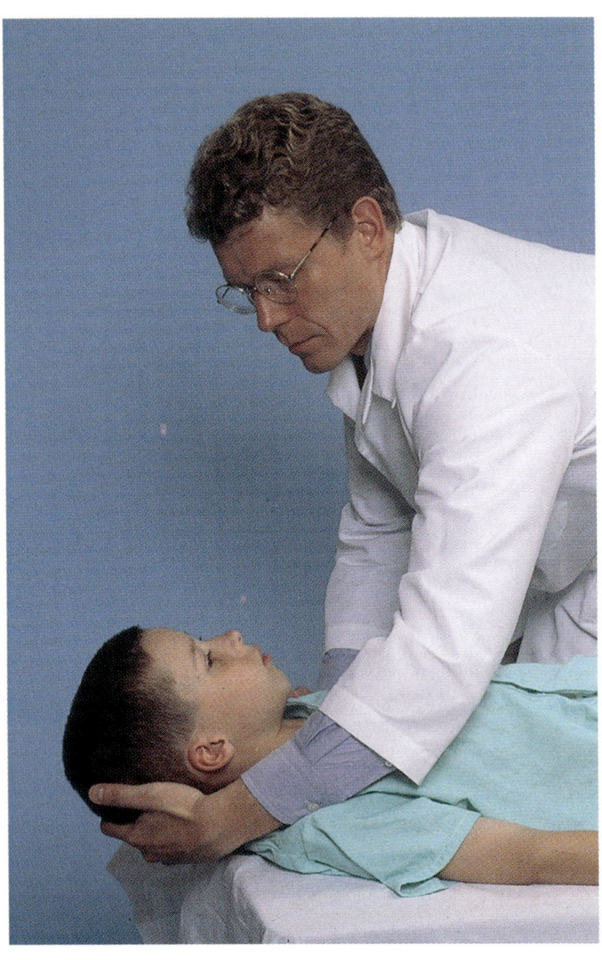

When meningeal irritation is present, the child assumes the *tripod position* and is unable to assume a full upright position to perform the chin-to-chest maneuver.

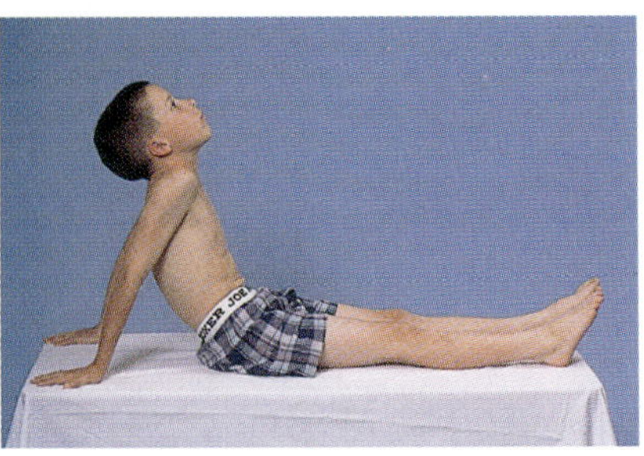

In newborns, palpate the *clavicles* and look for evidence of a fracture. If present, you may feel a break in the contour of the bone, tenderness, crepitus at the fracture site, and limited movement of the arm on the affected side.

A *fracture of the clavicle* may occur during delivery, particularly during difficult arm or shoulder extractions.

The Eye

We must teach our children to dream with their eyes open.
—Harry Edwards

You will have to be clever to examine the eyes of infants and young children and use some tricks to get them to cooperate. Small colorful toys are useful as fixation devices in examining the eyes.

INFANCY

Newborns keep their eyes closed except during brief awake periods. If you attempt to separate their eyelids, they will tighten them even more. Bright light causes infants to blink, so use subdued lighting. If you awaken the baby gently, turn down the lights, and support the baby in a sitting position, you will often find that the eyes open. The eyes of many newborns are edematous from the birth process.

Newborns may look at your face and follow a bright light if you catch them during an alert period. You can even get some newborns to follow your face and turn their heads 90° to each side, much to the delight of new parents.

If a newborn fails to gaze at you and follow your face during alert periods, pay particular attention to the rest of the ocular examination. This may still be a normal child, but may indicate *visual impairment.*

The photo below shows one way to examine young infants for *eye movements.* Hold the baby upright, supporting the head. Rotate yourself with the baby slowly in one direction. This usually causes the baby's eyes to open, allowing you to examine the sclerae, pupils, irides, and extraocular movements. The baby's eyes gaze in the direction you are turning. When the rotation stops, the eyes look in the opposite direction, after a few nystagmoid movements.

Nystagmus (wandering or shaking eye movements) persisting after a few days or persisting after the maneuver described on the left may indicate *poor vision* or *central nervous system disease.*

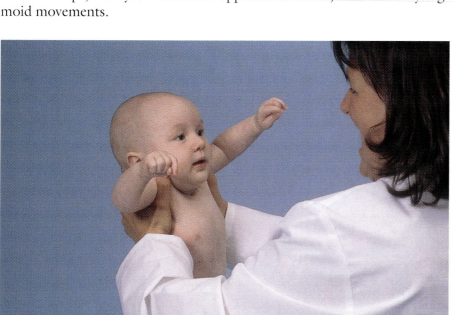

During the first 10 days of life, the eyes may be fixed, staring in one direction if just the head is turned without moving the body (*doll's eye reflex*). During the first few months of life, some infants have intermittent crossed eyes (*intermittent alternating convergent strabismus,* or *esotropia*) or intermittent laterally deviated eyes (*intermittent alternating divergent strabismus,* or *exotropia*).

Alternating convergent or divergent *strabismus* persisting beyond 3 months, or persistent strabismus of any type, may indicate *ocular motor weakness* or another abnormality in the visual system.

Look for abnormalities or congenital problems in the *sclerae* and *pupils.* Subconjunctival hemorrhages are common in newborns.

Colobomas (p. 188) may be seen with the naked eye, and represent defects in the iris.

Pupillary reactions can be observed either by response to light or by covering each eye with your hand and then uncovering it. Although there may be some initial asymmetry in the size of the pupils, over time they should be equal in size and reaction to light.

Inspect the irides carefully for abnormalities.

Brushfield spots are a ring of white specks in the iris (see Table 17-14, p. 771). While sometimes present in normal children, these strongly suggest *Down syndrome.*

Examine the *conjunctiva* for swelling or redness. Chemical conjunctivitis is common following application of silver nitrate at birth as prophylaxis against gonorrheal conjunctivitis (ophthalmia neonatorum). Most newborn nurseries have switched to using erythromycin ointment because it produces less irritation.

You will not be able to measure the *visual acuity* of newborns or infants. You can use visual reflexes to indirectly assess vision: direct and consensual pupillary constriction in response to light, blinking in response to bright light (*optic blink reflex*), and blinking in response to quick movement of an object toward the eyes. During the first year of life, visual acuity sharpens as the ability to focus improves. Infants achieve the following visual milestones:

Persistent ocular discharge and tearing since birth may be due to *dacryocystitis* or *nasolacrimal duct obstruction.*

Birth	Blinks, may regard face
1 month	Fixes on objects
1½–2 months	Coordinated eye movements
3 months	Eyes converge, baby reaches
12 months	Acuity around 20/50

Failure to progress along these visual developmental milestones may indicate *delayed visual maturation.*

For the *ophthalmoscopic examination,* with the newborn awake and eyes open, examine the red retinal (fundus) reflex by setting the ophthalmoscope at 0 diopters and viewing the pupil from about 10 inches. Normally, a red or orange color is reflected from the fundus through the pupil.

Cloudiness of the cornea may be caused by congenital glaucoma. A dark light reflex can be caused by *cataracts, retinopathy of prematurity,* or other disorders. A white retinal reflex (*leukokoria*) is abnormal and *cataract, retinal detachment, chorioretinitis, or retinoblastoma* should be suspected.

A thorough ophthalmoscopic examination is difficult in young infants, but may be needed if ocular or neurologic abnormalities are noted. Occasionally, a mydriatic solution may be required to examine the fundus successfully (e.g., using one drop of 2.5% phenylephrine with 0.5% cyclopentolate in each eye); this is usually done with the help of a neurologist or ophthalmologist. The cornea can ordinarily be seen at +20 diopters, the lens at +15 diopters, and the fundus at 0 diopters.

Examine the optic disc area as you would for an adult. In infants, the optic disk is lighter in color. There may be less macular pigmentation, and the foveal light reflection may not be visible. Look carefully for retinal hemorrhages. Papilledema is rare in infants because the fontanelles and open sutures accommodate any increased intracranial pressure, sparing the optic discs.

Small retinal hemorrhages may occur in normal newborns. Extensive hemorrhages may suggest severe *anoxia, subdural hematoma, subarachnoid hemorrhage,* or *severe trauma.*

Pigment changes in the retina can occur in newborns with *congenital toxoplasmosis, cytomegalovirus,* or *rubella.*

EARLY CHILDHOOD

The two most important aspects of the eye examination for young children are to test visual acuity in each eye and to determine whether the gaze is conjugate or symmetric.

Strabismus (see Table 17-14, p. 771) in children requires treatment by an ophthalmologist.

Use the methods described in Chapter 7 for adults to assess *conjugate gaze*, or the *position and alignment of the eyes*, and the function of the extraocular muscles. The corneal light reflex test and the cover–uncover test are particularly useful in young children.

Both *ocular strabismus* and *anisometropia* (eyes with significantly different refractive errors) can result in *amblyopia*, or reduced vision in an otherwise normal eye. *Amblyopia* can lead to a "lazy eye," with permanently reduced visual acuity if not corrected early (generally by 6 years).

You can perform the cover–uncover test as a game by having the young child watch your nose or tell you if you are smiling or not while you cover one of the child's eyes.

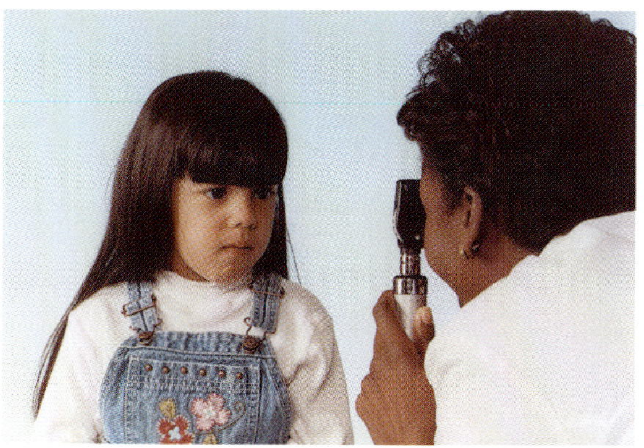

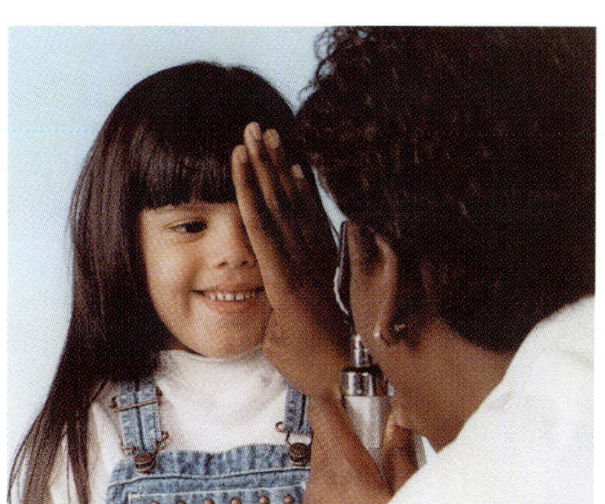

It may not be possible to measure the *visual acuity* of children under 3 years of age who cannot identify pictures on an eye chart. For these children, the simplest examination is to assess for fixation preference by alternately covering one eye; the child with normal vision will not object, but a child with poor vision in one eye will object to having the good eye covered. In all tests of visual acuity, it is important that both eyes show the same result.

3 months	Eyes converge, baby reaches
12 months	~20/200
Less than 4 years	20/40
4 years and older	20/30

Any difference in visual acuity between the eyes (e.g., 20/20 on the left and 20/30 on the right) is abnormal, and the patient should be referred to an ophthalmologist.

As shown on the next page, visual acuity in children 3 years and older can usually be formally tested using an eye chart with one of a variety of optotypes (characters or symbols). A child who does not know letters or numbers reliably can be tested using pictures, symbols, or the "E" chart. Using the "E" chart, most children will cooperate by telling you in which direction the "E" is pointing.

The *visual fields* can be examined in infants and young children with the child sitting on the parent's lap. One eye should be tested at a time with the other eye covered. Hold the child's head in the midline while bringing an object such as a toy into the field of vision from behind the child. The overall method is the same as that for adults, except that you will have to make this into a game for your patient.

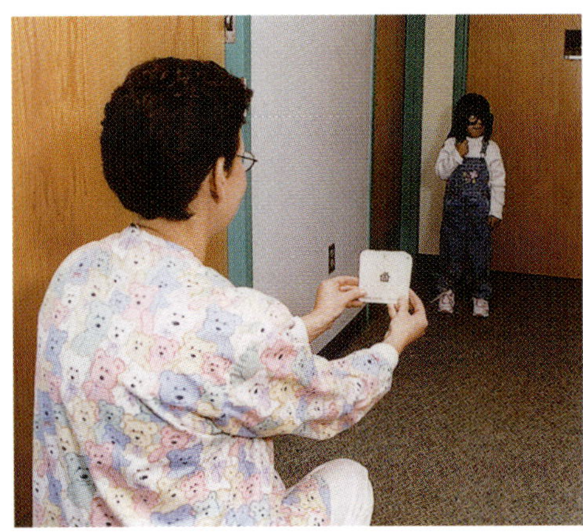

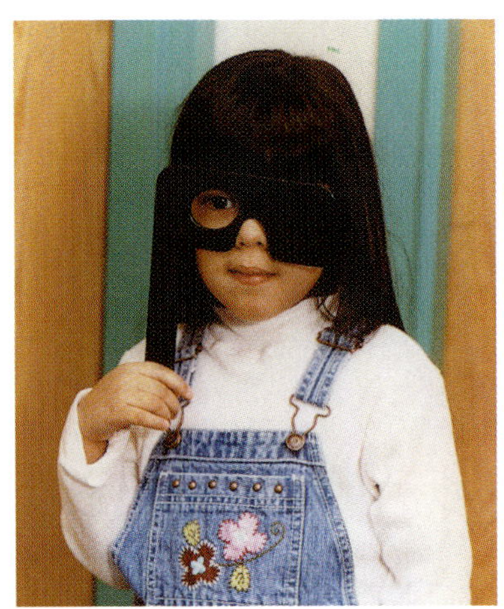

LATE CHILDHOOD AND ADOLESCENCE

The methods used to examine the eye, including testing for visual acuity, are the same as those for adults. Refractive errors become common, and it is important to test visual acuity monocularly at regular intervals, such as during the annual health supervision visit.

The Ear

The physical examination of the ear of infants and children is important because many abnormalities can be detected, including structural abnormalities of the ear, otitis media, and hearing loss. This means that you must hone your skills with the otoscope!

INFANCY

The major goals are to determine if the *position, shape, and features of the ear* are normal and to detect abnormalities. Note the position of the ears in relation to the eyes. An imaginary line drawn across the inner and outer canthi of the eyes should cross the pinna or auricle; if the pinna is below this line then the infant has low-set ears.

Small, deformed, or low-set auricles may indicate associated *congenital defects,* especially renal disease.

Examination of the newborn's ear with an otoscope can only detect patency of the *ear canal* because the tympanic membrane is obscured by accumulated vernix caseosa for the first few days of life. In infancy, the ear canal is directed downward from the outside; therefore, you may want to pull the auricle gently downward rather than upward for the best view of the ear drum. Once the tympanic membrane becomes visible, you may note that the light reflex is diffuse and does not become cone-shaped for several months.

A small skin tab, cleft, or pit found just forward of the tragus represents a remnant of the *first branchial cleft* and usually has no significance.

The *acoustic blink reflex* is a blinking of the infant's eyes in response to a sudden sharp sound; you can produce this by snapping your fingers or using a bell, beeper, or other noisemaking device about a foot from the infant's ear. Be sure that you are not producing an airstream that may cause the infant to

Perinatal problems raising the risk for *hearing defects* include birth weight <1500 grams, anoxia, treatment with potentially ototoxic

blink. The reflex may be difficult to elicit during the first 2 to 3 days of life. After it is elicited several times, the reflex will disappear, a phenomenon known as *habituation*. This is a crude test of hearing, and certainly does not determine normal hearing. Currently, there is an increased movement toward universal hearing screening of all newborns in addition to those at high risk for hearing problems.

medications, congenital infections, severe hyperbilirubinemia, and meningitis.

Many children with *hearing deficits* are not diagnosed until as old as 2 years. Clues to hearing deficits include parental concern about hearing, delayed speech, and lack of developmental indicators of hearing.

Age	Signs That an Infant Can Hear
0–2 months	Startle response and blink to a sudden noise Calming down with soothing voice or music
2–3 months	Change in body movements in response to sound Change in facial expression to familiar sounds
3–4 months	Turning eyes and head to sound
6–7 months	Turning to listen to voices and conversation

EARLY CHILDHOOD

You may feel as if you need 10 hands and a bag of tricks to examine the ear of toddlers and young children, who are sensitive to *examining the ear canal and drum* and fearful because they cannot observe the procedure. With a little practice you can master this technique. Unfortunately, many young children will need to be briefly restrained during this part of the examination, which is why you may want to leave it for the end.

If the child is not too fearful, you may be able to do the examination while the child is sitting on his parent's lap. It is helpful to make a game out of the otoscopic examination, such as finding an imaginary object in the child's ear, or talking playfully throughout the examination to allay any fears. It is sometimes helpful to place the otoscopic speculum gently into the external auditory canal of one ear and then withdraw it to have the child get used to the procedure, before performing the actual examination. Ask the parent for a preference regarding the positioning of the child for the examination.

There are two common positions—the child lying down and restrained, and the child sitting in the parent's lap. If the child is being held supine, have the parent hold the arms either extended or close to the sides to limit motions. You can hold the head and retract the tragus with one hand while you hold the otoscope with your other hand. If the child is on the parent's lap, the child's legs should be between the parent's legs. The parent could help with gentle restraint by placing one arm around the child's body and a second arm to steady the head.

Many students have difficulty even visualizing a child's tympanic membrane. In young children, the external auditory canal is directed upward and backward from the outside, and the auricle must be pulled upward, outward, and backward to afford the best view. Hold the child's head with one hand (your left hand if you are right-handed), and with that same hand pull up on the auricle. With your other hand, position the otoscope.

TIPS FOR CONDUCTING THE OTOSCOPIC EXAMINATION

Use the best angle of the otoscope.
Use the largest possible speculum.
 A larger speculum will allow you to visualize the tympanic membrane better.
 A small speculum may not provide a seal for pneumatic otoscopy.
Don't apply too much pressure.
 Too much pressure will cause the child to cry and may cause false–positives on pneumatic otoscopy.
Insert the speculum ¼ to ½ inch into the canal.
First find the landmarks.
 Sometimes the ear canal resembles the tympanic membrane—don't be fooled!
Note whether the tympanic membrane is abnormal.
Remove cerumen if it is blocking your view, using
 Special plastic curettes
 A moistened microtipped cotton swab
 Flushing of ears for older children
 Special instruments that can also be purchased.

Not only are there two positions for the child lying down or sitting, there are two ways to hold the otoscope, as illustrated by the following photos. The first is the method generally used in adults, with the otoscope handle pointing upward while you pull up on the auricle. Hold the lateral aspect of your hand that has the otoscope against the child's head to provide a buffer against sudden movements by the patient.

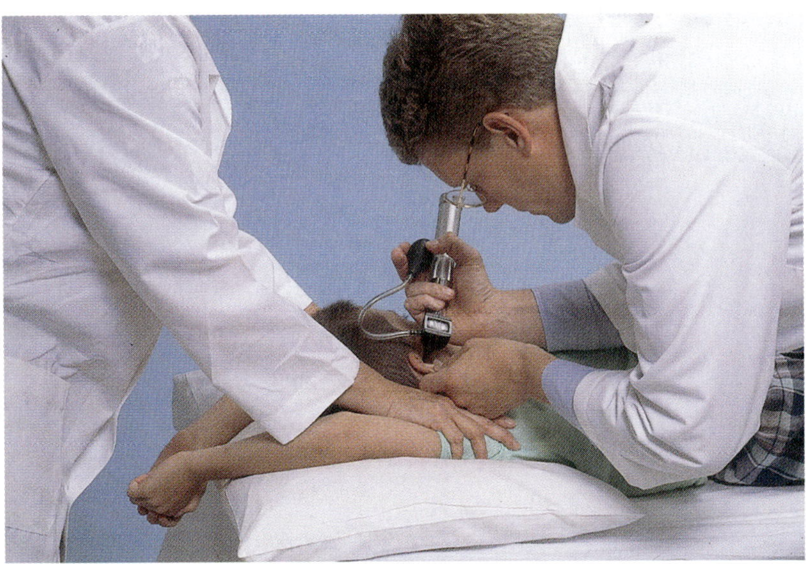

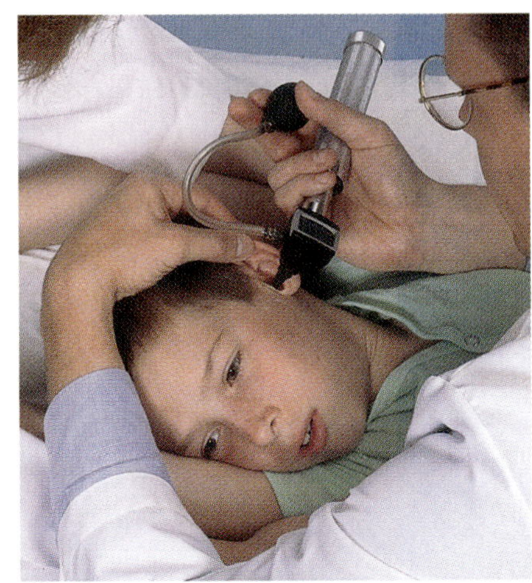

The second technique (see p. 679) is used by many pediatricians because of the different angle of the auditory canal in children. This involves holding the otoscope with the handle pointing down toward the child's feet while you pull up on the auricle. Hold the head and pull up on the auricle with one hand, while you hold the otoscope with the other hand.

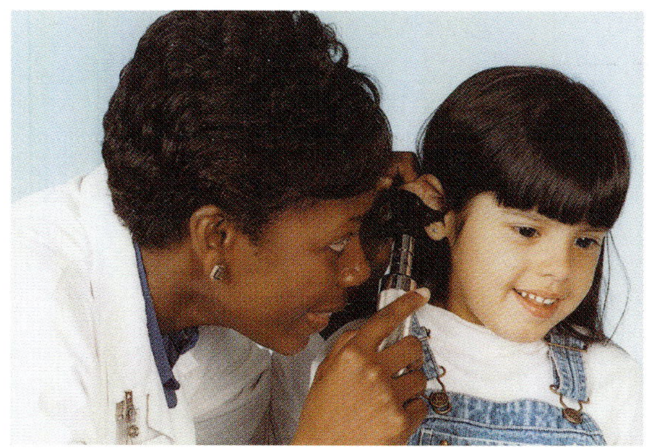

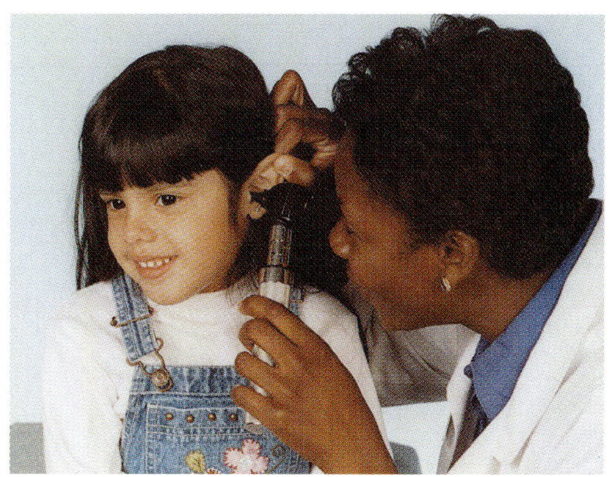

Learn to use a *pneumatic otoscope* to improve your accuracy of diagnosis of otitis media in children. This allows you to assess the mobility of the tympanic membrane as you increase or decrease the pressure in the external auditory canal by squeezing the rubber bulb of the pneumatic otoscope.

Acute otitis media is a common condition of childhood. A symptomatic child has a red, bulging tympanic membrane, with a dull or absent light reflex and diminished movement on pneumatic otoscopy. Purulent material may also be seen behind the tympanic membrane. See Table 17-14, Abnormalities of the Eyes and Ears, p. 771.

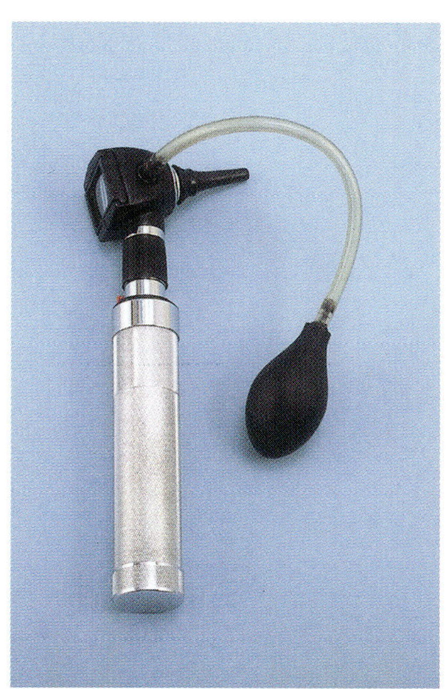

First, check the pneumatic otoscope for leaks by placing your finger over the tip of the speculum and squeezing the bulb. Note the pressure on the bulb. Then insert the speculum, obtaining a proper seal; this is critical because failure to obtain a seal can produce a false–positive finding (lack of movement of the tympanic membrane).

When air is introduced into the normal ear canal, the tympanic membrane and its light reflex move inward. When air is removed, the tympanic membrane moves outward, toward you. This to-and-fro movement of the tympanic membrane has been likened to the luffing of a sail. If the tympanic membrane fails to move perceptibly as you introduce positive or negative pressure, then the child is likely to have a middle ear effusion. A child with acute otitis media may flinch because of pain due to the air pressure.

This movement of the tympanic membrane is absent in middle ear effusion (*otitis media with effusion*).

Significant, temporary hearing loss for several months can accompany otitis media with effusion.

Gently move and pull on the *pinna* before or during your otoscopic examination. Carefully inspect the area behind the pinna, over the mastoid bone.

With *otitis externa* (but not otitis media), movement of the pinna elicits pain.

With acute *mastoiditis,* the auricle may protrude forward,

and the area over the mastoid bone will be red, swollen, and tender.

Although formal hearing testing is necessary for accurate detection of hearing deficits in young children, you can grossly *test for hearing* by whispering at a distance of 8 feet, asking the child questions or giving simple commands. All children above age 4 years should have a full-scale acoustic screening test.

Younger children who fail these screening maneuvers or who have speech delay should have audiometric testing.

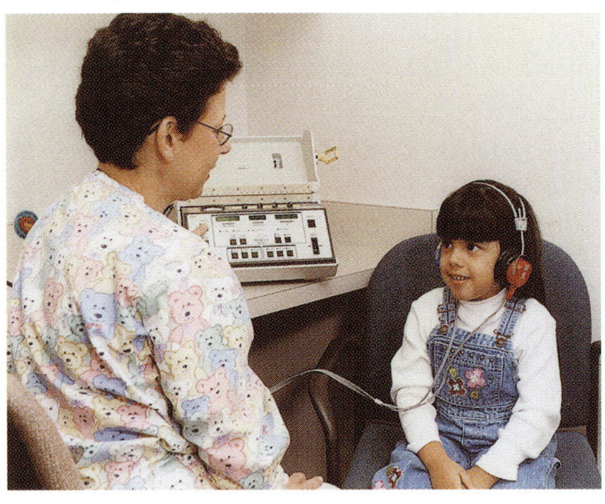

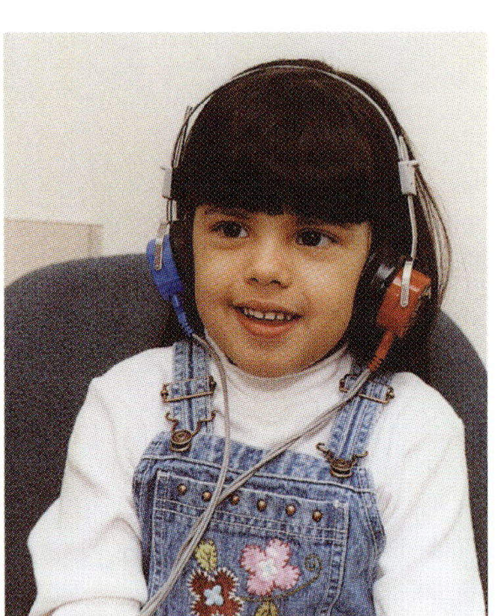

LATE CHILDHOOD AND ADOLESCENCE

As the child grows, the ease and techniques of examining the ears and testing the hearing approach the methods used for adults. There are no ear abnormalities or variations of normal unique to this age group. Of course, parents of older children routinely refer to the normal condition of "selective deafness," defined as choosing to hear what the child wishes to hear.

The Nose and Paranasal Sinuses

INFANCY

The most important component of the examination of the nose of newborns is to test for patency of the nasal passages. You can do this by gently occluding each nostril alternately while holding the infant's mouth closed. This will not cause stress in a normal baby, because most newborns are nasal breathers. Indeed, some infants are *obligate nasal breathers* and have difficulty breathing through their mouths. Do not occlude both nares simultaneously—this will cause considerable distress!

The nasal passages in newborns may be obstructed in *choanal atresia.* In severe cases, nasal obstruction can be assessed by attempting to pass a No. 8 feeding tube through each nostril into the posterior pharynx.

Inspect the nose to ensure that the nasal septum is midline. You can gently insert a wide nasal speculum of the otoscope into the nose.

At birth, only the ethmoid sinuses are developed. Palpation of the sinuses of newborns is not helpful.

EARLY AND LATE CHILDHOOD

You can inspect the anterior portion of the nose by using a large speculum on your otoscope. Inspect the nasal mucous membranes, noting their color and condition. Look for nasal septal deviation and the presence of polyps.

Pale, boggy nasal mucous membranes are found in children with *chronic (perennial) allergic rhinitis.*

Purulent rhinitis is common in viral infections, but may be part of the constellation of symptoms of *sinusitis.*

Foul-smelling purulent, unilateral discharge from the nose may be due to a *foreign body* in the nose.

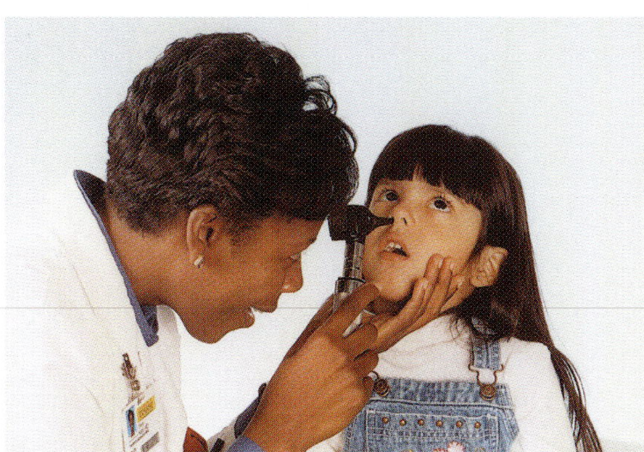

Maxillary sinuses are noted on x-rays by age 4 years, sphenoid sinuses by age 6, and frontal sinuses by age 6 to 7. The sinuses of older children can be palpated like adult sinuses, looking for tenderness. Traditionally, transillumination of the paranasal sinuses of younger children has been taught; however, this technique has poor sensitivity and specificity for diagnosing sinusitis or fluid in the sinuses.

The Mouth and Pharynx

The face of a child can say it all, especially the mouth part of the face.
—*Jack Handley*

INFANCY

Use both inspection (with a tongue blade and flashlight) and palpation to inspect the mouth and pharynx of newborns. The newborn's mouth is edentulous, and the alveolar mucosa is smooth, with finely serrated borders. Occasionally, pearl-like retention cysts are seen along the alveolar ridges and are easily mistaken for teeth—they disappear within a month or two. Petechiae are commonly found on the soft palate after birth. Palpate the upper hard palate to make sure it is intact.

Rarely, *supernumerary teeth* are noted. These are usually dysmorphic and are shed within days but are removed to prevent aspiration.

Epstein's pearls, tiny white or yellow rounded mucous retention cysts, are located along the posterior midline of the hard palate. They disappear within months.

Infants produce little saliva during the first 3 months, but you will note that older infants produce lots of saliva and drool frequently.

Inspect the tongue. The frenulum of the tongue varies, sometimes extending almost to the tip and other times being thick and short, limiting protrusion of the tongue (*ankyloglossia,* or *tongue tie*); these variations rarely interfere with speech or function.

Although unusual, a prominent, protruding tongue may signal *congenital hypothyroidism* or *Down syndrome.*

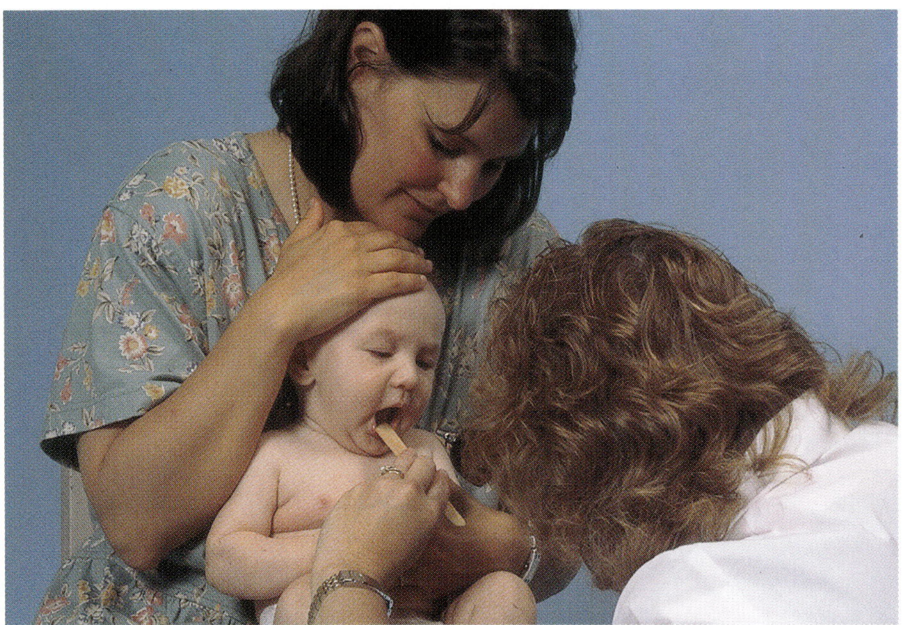

You will often see a whitish covering on the tongue. If this coating is due to milk, it can be easily removed by scraping or wiping it away.

Oral candidiasis (thrush) is common in infants. The lesions are difficult to wipe away and have an erythematous raw base (see Table 17-15, Abnormalities of the Mouth and Teeth, p. 772).

The pharynx of the infant is best seen while the baby is crying. You will likely have difficulty using a tongue blade because it produces a strong gag reflex. Do not expect to be able to visualize the tonsils.

Listen to the quality of the *infant's cry.* Normal infants have a lusty, strong cry. The following box lists some unusual types of infant cries.

INFANT CRIES

Type	*Possible Related Condition*
Shrill or high-pitched	Increased intracranial pressure. Such cries also occur in newborn infants born to narcotic-addicted mothers.
Hoarse	Hypocalcemic tetany or congenital hypothyroidism
Continuous inspiratory and expiratory stridor	Caused by upper airway obstruction due to a variety of lesions (e.g., a polyp or hemangioma), a relatively small larynx (*infantile laryngeal stridor*), or a delay in the development of the cartilage in the tracheal rings (*tracheomalacia*)
Absence of cry	Suggests severe illness, vocal cord paralysis, or profound brain damage

EARLY AND LATE CHILDHOOD

For anxious or young children, you may want to leave this part of the examination toward the end, because it may require parental restraint. The young, cooperative child may be more comfortable sitting in the parent's lap, as shown below.

The following figure demonstrates some tricks to getting children to open their mouths. The child who can say "ahhh" will usually offer a sufficient (albeit brief) view of the posterior pharynx so that a tongue blade is unnecessary. Healthy children are more likely to cooperate with this examination than sick children, especially if the sick child sees the tongue blade or has had previous experience with throat cultures.

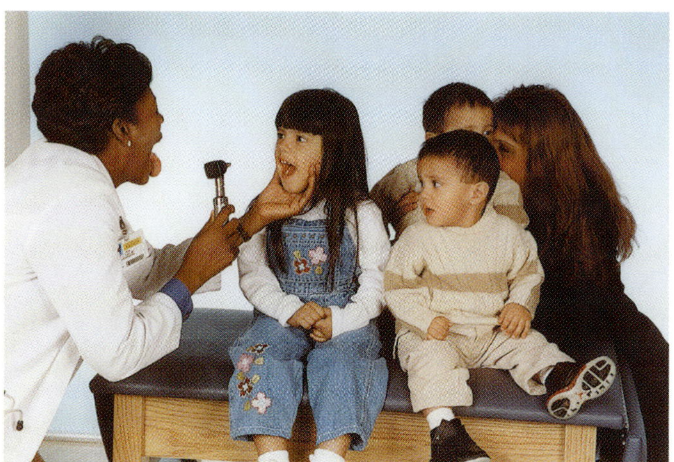

HOW TO GET CHILDREN TO OPEN THEIR MOUTHS (AKA, "WOULD YOU *PLEASE* SAY 'AHHH'?")

- Turn it into a game.
  - "Now let's see what's in your mouth."
  - "Can you stick out your *whole tongue*?"
  - "I bet you can't open your mouth *really wide*!"
  - "Let me see the inside of your teeth."
  - "Is Barney stuck in there?"
- Don't show a tongue blade unless really necessary.
- Demonstrate first on an older sibling (or even the parent).
- Offer enthusiastic praise for opening their mouths a little and encourage them to open even wider!

If you need to use the tongue blade, the best technique is to push down and pull slightly forward toward yourself while the child says "ahhh," being careful not to place the blade too far posteriorly, eliciting a gag reflex. Sometimes young and anxious children will need to be restrained and will clamp their teeth and purse their lips. In these cases, you will need to carefully slip the tongue depressor between the teeth and onto the tongue. This will either allow you to push down on the tongue or elicit a gag reflex, which should permit a brief look at the posterior pharynx and tonsils. Remember, an unplanned, direct frontal assault on the front teeth will only meet with failure and a splintered tongue blade; careful planning and parental help are needed.

Examine the *teeth* for the timing and sequence of eruption, number, character, condition, and position. Abnormalities of the enamel may reflect local or general disease.

Carefully inspect the inside of the upper teeth, as shown in the figure below. This is a common location for *nursing bottle caries.*

Dental caries are caused by bacterial activity. Caries are more likely among young children who have prolonged bottle-feeding ("nursing-bottle caries"). See Table 17-15, Abnormalities of the Mouth and Teeth, p. 772, for different stages of caries.

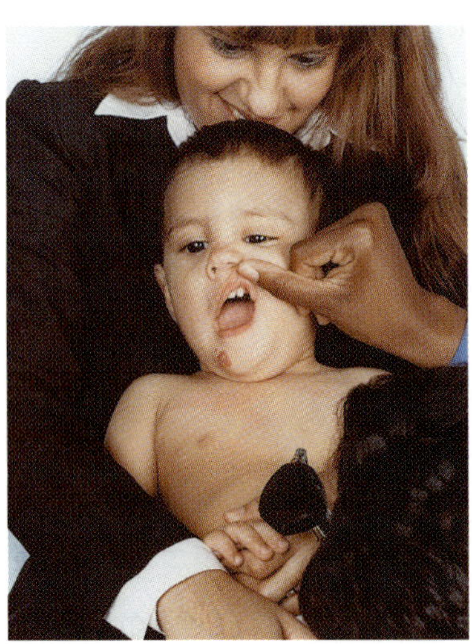

As in most developmental changes of childhood, there is a predictable progression of tooth eruption and also a wide variation in the age of eruption. A rule of thumb is that the infant will have one tooth for each month of age between 6 and 26 months, up to the full complement of 20 primary teeth. The table below displays a common pattern of teeth eruption. In general, lower teeth erupt a bit earlier than upper teeth.

Staining of the teeth may be intrinsic or extrinsic. Intrinsic stains may be due to tetracycline use prior to 8 years (yellow, gray, or brown stain). Iron preparation (black stain) is an example of extrinsic stain. Extrinsic stains can be polished off; intrinsic stains cannot (see Table 17-15, Abnormalities of the Mouth and Teeth, p. 772).

Tooth Types and Age of Eruption

	Approximate Age of Eruption	
Tooth Type	*Primary (mos)*	*Permanent (yrs)*
Central incisor	5–8	6–8
Lateral incisor	5–11	7–9
Cuspids	24–30	11–12
First bicuspids	—	10–12
Second bicuspids	—	10–12
First molars	16–20	6–7
Second molars	24–30	11–13
Third molars	—	17–22

Look for abnormalities of the position of the teeth. These include malocclusion, maxillary protrusion (*overbite*), and mandibular protrusion (*underbite*). You can demonstrate the latter two by asking the child to bite down hard and part the lips. Observe the true bite. In normal children, the lower teeth are contained within the arch formed by the upper teeth.

Malocclusion and misalignment of teeth is often due to excessive thumb sucking and is reversible if the habit is arrested by 6 or 7 years. Malocclusion can also be a hereditary condition, or due to premature loss of primary teeth.

Carefully inspect the *tongue*, including the underside. Most children will happily stick their tongue out at you, move it from side to side, and demonstrate its color (the blue tongue below is from eating candy!)

Common abnormalities include *coated tongue* in viral infections, *congenital geographic tongue*, and *strawberry tongue* found in scarlet fever.

Streptococcal pharyngitis typically produces a strawberry tongue, white exudates on the tonsils, beefy-red uvula, and palatal petechiae.

Note the size, position, symmetry, and appearance of the *tonsils*. The peak growth of tonsillar tissue is between 8 and 16 years (see figure on p. 656). The size of the tonsils varies considerably in children and is often categorized on a scale of 1+ to 4+, with 1+ being easy visibility of the gap between the tonsils, and 4+ being tonsils that touch in the midline with the mouth wide open. The tonsils in children often appear more obstructive than they really are.

A *peritonsillar abscess* is suggested by asymmetric enlargement of the tonsils and lateral displacement of the uvula.

Tonsils in children usually have deep crypts on their surfaces, which often have white concretions or food particles protruding from their depths. This does not indicate disease.

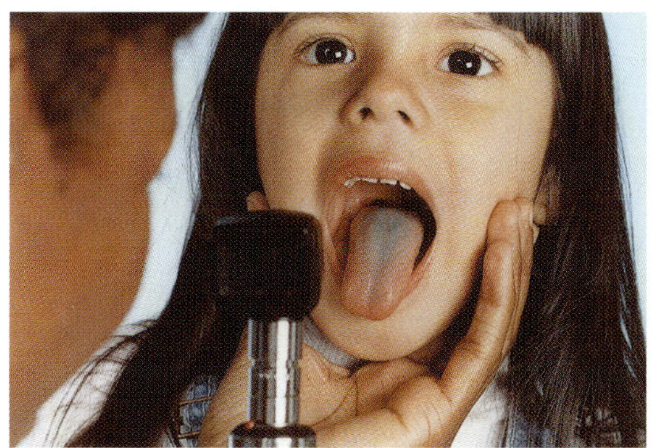

Look for clues of a submucosal cleft palate, such as notching of the posterior margin of the hard palate or a bifid *uvula*. Because the mucosa is intact, the underlying defect is easily missed.

There is one condition—*acute epiglottitis*—now thankfully rare in the United States due to immunization against *Hemophilus influenzae* type B, which is a contraindication to examination of the throat because of potential gagging and laryngeal obstruction.

Note the quality of the child's voice. Certain abnormalities can change the pitch and quality.

Voice Changes—Clues to Underlying Abnormalities

Voice Change	Possible Abnormality
Hypernasal speech	Submucosal cleft palate
Nasal voice plus snoring	Adenoidal hypertrophy
Hoarse voice plus cough	Viral infection (croup)
"Rocks in mouth"	Tonsillitis

You may note an abnormal breath odor, which may help lead to a diagnosis.

The Thorax and Lungs

INFANCY

The infant's *thorax* is more rounded than that of older children and adults. Also, the chest wall in infancy is thin, with little musculature, and therefore lung and heart sounds are transmitted quite clearly. The bony and cartilaginous rib cage is very soft and pliant. The tip of the xiphoid process is often seen protruding anteriorly immediately beneath the skin at the apex of the costal angle.

Two types of chest wall abnormalities noted in childhood include *pectus excavatum,* or "funnel chest," and *pectus carinatum,* or "chicken breast deformity" (see p. 239).

Carefully *assess respirations* and the pattern of breathing. Newborn infants, especially those born prematurely, exhibit irregular breathing characterized by periods of breathing at normal rates (30 to 40 per minute) alternating with "periodic breathing," during which the respiratory rate slows markedly and may even cease for 5 to 10 seconds.

Apnea is defined as cessation of breathing for more than 20 seconds. Apnea is often accompanied by bradycardia and may indicate the presence of a *respiratory disease, central nervous system disease,* or, rarely, a *cardiopulmonary condition.* Apnea is a high-risk factor for *sudden infant death syndrome (SIDS).*

An important tip for the examination of the respiratory status of infants and young children is *not* to rush to the stethoscope, but to observe the patient carefully as demonstrated in the photograph and the table on the next page. Visual inspection is best done when infants are not crying; thus work with the parents to settle the child. By observing infants for a significant time (perhaps 1 minute), you can note the general appearance, respiratory rate, color, nasal component of breathing, audible breath sounds, and work of breathing, as described on p. 662.

Because infants are obligate nasal breathers, observe their nose as they breathe, looking for *nasal flaring.* Observe the breathing with the infant's mouth closed or with the infant nursing or sucking on a bottle to assess for nasal patency.

In newborns and young infants, nasal flaring may be due simply to *upper respiratory infections* with subsequent obstruction of their small nares.

Listen to the sounds of the infant's breathing and note any *grunting, audible wheezing, or lack of breath sounds (obstruction).*

It is important to evaluate, by observation, two aspects of the infant: *audible breath sounds* and the *work of breathing.* These are particularly relevant in as-

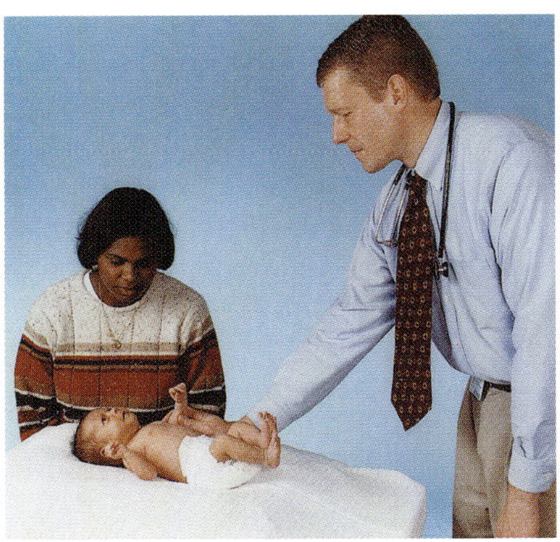

sessing both upper and lower respiratory illness. Studies in countries that have poor access to chest radiographs have found that these signs are at least as useful as auscultation in assessing both the upper and lower respiratory tract.

Examination of the Lungs in Infants—Before You Touch the Child!

Type of Assessment	Specific Observable Pathology
General appearance	Inability to feed or smile Lack of consolability
Respiratory rate	Tachypnea (see p. 662)
Color	Pallor or cyanosis
Nasal component of breathing	Nasal flaring (enlargement of both nasal openings during inspiration)
Audible breath sounds	Grunting (repetitive, short expiratory sound) Wheezing (musical expiratory sound) Stridor (high-pitched, inspiratory noise) Obstruction (lack of breath sounds)
Work of breathing	Nasal flaring (see above) Grunting (see above) Retractions (or chest indrawing): Supraclavicular (soft tissue above clavicles) Intercostal (indrawing of the skin between ribs) Subcostal (just below the costal margin)

Any of the abnormalities listed at the left should raise concern about underlying respiratory pathology.

Lower respiratory infections, defined as infections below the vocal cords, are common in infants, and include *bronchiolitis* and *pneumonia.*

Acute stridor is a potentially serious condition; causes include *laryngo-tracheo-bronchitis (croup), epiglottitis, bacterial tracheitis, foreign body,* or *a vascular ring.*

In infants, abnormal work of breathing, combined with abnormal findings on auscultation, is the best finding for ruling in *pneumonia.* The best single sign for ruling *out* pneumonia is the absence of tachypnea.

In healthy infants, the ribs do not move much during quiet breathing. If the ribs do move, outward movement is produced by descent of the diaphragm. Descent of the diaphragm compresses the abdominal contents, which in turn shifts the lower ribs outward.

Pulmonary disease causes an increase in abdominal breathing in infants, and can result in *retractions* (*chest indrawing*), a sign commonly used by the World Health Organization as an indicator of pulmonary disease in infants younger than 2 years of age. Chest indrawing is the inward movement of the ribs (or more precisely, the skin between the ribs) during inspiration. Breath-

Asymmetric chest movement may be a clue to a space-occupying lesion, such as *pleural effusion, hemothorax,* or *intrathoracic mass.*

ing is predominantly affected by movement of the diaphragm, with little assistance from the thoracic muscles. As mentioned in the table on the previous page, three types of retractions can be noted in infants: supraclavicular, intercostal, and subcostal.

Obstructive respiratory disease in infants can result in *Hoover's sign,* or paradoxical (seesaw) breathing, in which the abdomen moves outward while the chest moves inward during inspiration. *Thoracoabdominal paradox,* inward movement of the chest and outward movement of the abdomen during inspiration, is a normal finding in preterm and newborn infants. It continues to persist during active, or REM, sleep even when it is no longer seen during wakefulness or quiet sleep because of the decreased muscle tone of active sleep. As muscle strength increases and chest wall compliance decreases with age and growth, paradox is no longer discernable as a normal finding.

Children with *muscle weakness* may be noted to have thoracoabdominal paradox at several years of age.

Tactile fremitus can be assessed by *palpation.* Place your hand on the chest when the infant cries or makes noise. Place your hand or fingertips over each side of the infant's chest and feel for symmetry in the transmitted vibrations. Percussion is not helpful in infants except in extreme instances. The infant's chest is hyperresonant throughout, and it is difficult to detect abnormalities on percussion.

Because of the excellent transmission of sounds throughout the chest, any abnormalities of tactile fremitus or on percussion suggest severe pathology, such as a large *pneumonic consolidation.*

After performing these maneuvers, you are ready for *auscultation.* Breath sounds are louder and harsher than those in adults because the stethoscope is closer to the origin of the sounds. Also, it is often difficult to distinguish transmitted upper airway sounds from sounds originating in the chest. The table below has some useful hints. Upper airway sounds tend to be loud, transmitted symmetrically throughout the chest, and loudest as you move your stethoscope upward. They are usually inspiratory, coarse sounds. Lower airway sounds are loudest over the site of pathology, are often asymmetric, and often have an expiratory phase.

Biphasic sounds imply *severe obstruction from intrathoracic airway narrowing* or *severe obstruction from extrathoracic airway narrowing.*

Distinguishing Upper Airway From Lower Airway Sounds

Technique	Upper Airway	Lower Airway
Compare sounds from nose/stethoscope	Same sounds	Often different sounds
Listen to harshness of sounds	Often harsh and loud	Variable
Note symmetry (left/right)	Symmetric	Often asymmetric
Compare sounds at different locations (higher or lower)	Sounds get louder as stethoscope is moved up on the chest	Sounds often louder lower in chest
Inspiratory vs. expiratory	Almost always inspiratory	Often has expiratory phase

If you hear expiratory sounds, you can be relatively sure that they arise from an intrathoracic source. On the other hand, inspiratory sounds typically arise from an extrathoracic airway such as the trachea. During expiration, the diameter of the intrathoracic airways decreases because radial forces from the surrounding lung do not "tether" the airways open as occurs during inspiration. Higher flow rates during inspiration produce turbulent flow, resulting in appreciable sounds.

The characteristics of the breath sounds, such as vesicular and bronchovesicular, and of the adventitious lung sounds, such as crackles, wheezes, and rhonchi, are the same as those for adults, except that they may be more difficult to distinguish in infants and often occur together. Wheezes and rhonchi are common in infants. Wheezes, often audible without the stethoscope, occur more frequently in infants because of the smaller size of the tracheobronchial tree. Wheezes usually reflect narrowing of smaller airways, or bronchioles. Rhonchi reflect obstruction of larger airways, or bronchi. Crackles (rales) are discontinuous sounds (see p. 228), near the end of inspiration; they are usually due to lung disorders and are far less likely to represent cardiac failure in infants than in adults.

Wheezes in infants occur commonly from *asthma* or *bronchiolitis.*

Crackles (rales) can be heard with *pneumonia* and *bronchiolitis.*

EARLY AND LATE CHILDHOOD

As children become older, the examination of the lungs begins to approach that used in adults. Again, it is critical for children to cooperate with this examination. Auscultation is often best accomplished when the child is barely aware of the examination (as when he is in his parent's lap). If a toddler seems fearful of your stethoscope, you might let the child play with it before touching the chest.

If you ask young children to "take deep breaths," they will often hold their breath, making it even more difficult for you to auscultate the lungs. Thus it is easier, for preschool children, to let them breathe normally. For older children, you can demonstrate how to take nice, quiet, deep breaths, and make a game out of it. A forced expiratory maneuver can be accomplished by asking the child to blow out the candles on an imaginary birthday cake.

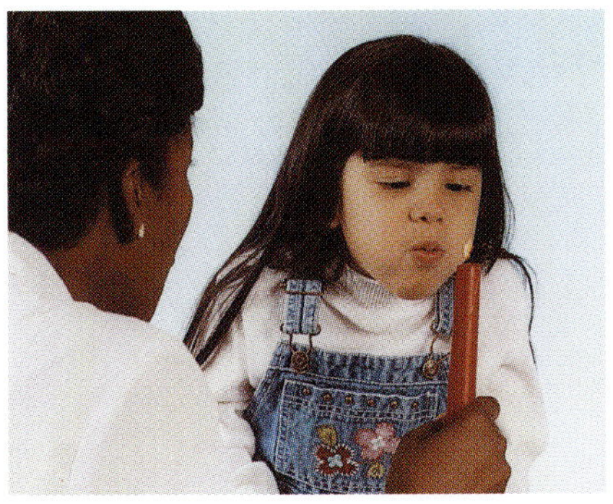

In examining children, assess the relative proportion of time spent on inspiration versus expiration. Normally, this ratio is about 1:1.

In the presence of upper airway obstruction such as croup, inspiration is prolonged and accompanied by other signs such as stridor, cough, or rhonchi. In the presence of lower airway obstruction such as asthma, expiration is prolonged

Older children will be cooperative for the respiratory examination and can even go through the maneuvers of assessing fremitus or listening to "E to A" changes (see p. 229). As children grow, the evaluation by observation discussed on the previous page, such as assessing the work of breathing, nasal flaring, and grunting, becomes less helpful in evaluating for respiratory pathology, and palpation, percussion, and auscultation achieve greater importance in a careful examination of the thorax and lungs.

and often accompanied by audible wheezing.

Childhood asthma is an extremely common condition throughout the world. Children with acute asthma present with varying severity and often have increased work of breathing. Expiratory wheezing and a prolonged expiratory phase, caused by reversible bronchospasm, can be heard without the stethoscope and are apparent on auscultation.

The Heart

The heart is the chief feature of a functioning mind.
—Frank Lloyd Wright

The examination of the heart and vascular systems in infants and children is similar to that in adults, but recognition of their fear, their inability to cooperate, and in many instances, their desire to play, will make the exam easier and more productive. Use your knowledge of the developmental stage of each child, recognizing that a 2-year-old may be easiest to examine while standing or sitting on the mother's lap, facing her shoulder, as shown below. Give young children something to hold in each hand. They cannot figure out how to drop the object and therefore have no hand free to push you away. Endless chatter to small children will hold their attention and they will forget you are examining them. Let children move the stethoscope themselves, going back to listen properly. Use your imagination to make the examination work!

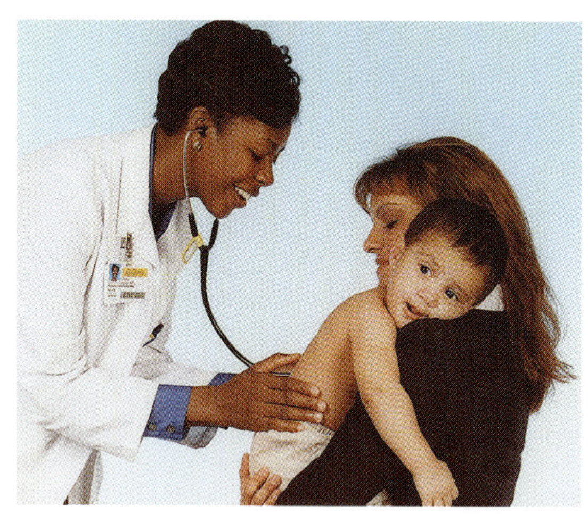

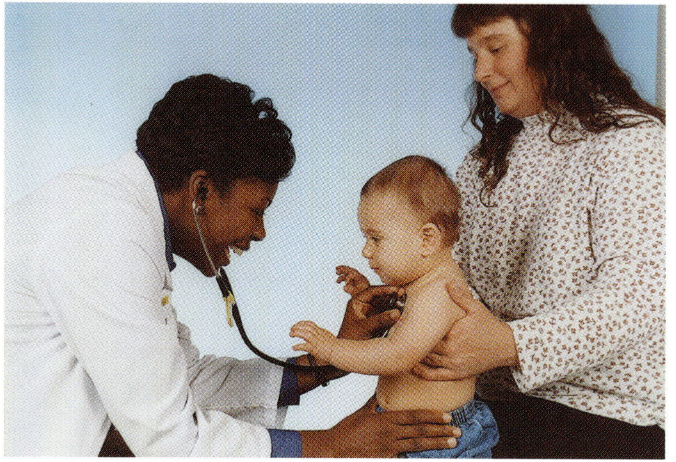

Inspection. Before examining the heart itself, *observe* the infant carefully for the presence or absence of cyanosis. Acrocyanosis in the newborn is discussed on p. 663. It is important to detect *central cyanosis* (Table 17-10, Cyanosis in Children, p. 766) because it is always abnormal and many congenital cardiac abnormalities, as well as respiratory diseases, present with cyanosis (see Table 17-16, Pathologic Findings: Heart Murmurs, pp. 773–775).

Cardiac Causes of Central Cyanosis in Children

Age of Onset	Potential Cardiac Cause
Immediately at birth	Transposition of the great arteries Pulmonary valve atresia Severe pulmonary valve stenosis Possibly Ebstein's malformation
Within a few days after birth	All of the above plus: Total anomalous pulmonary venous return Hypoplastic left heart syndrome Truncus arteriosus (sometimes) Single ventricle variants
Weeks, months, or years of life	All of the above plus: Pulmonary vascular disease with atrial, ventricular, or great vessel shunting

The recognition of minimal degrees of cyanosis requires care. Look where the inside of the body can be seen without having to peer through skin (i.e., the inside of the mouth, the tongue, the conjunctivae, and, to a lesser degree, the nail beds). A true pink is normal, while any hint of raspberry red suggests desaturation. The distribution of the cyanosis should be evaluated. An oxymetry reading will confirm desaturation.

Observe the infant for *general signs of health.* The infant's nutritional status, responsiveness, happiness, and irritability are all clues that may be useful in evaluating cardiac disease. Note that noncardiac findings can be present in infants with cardiac disease.

COMMON NONCARDIAC FINDINGS IN INFANTS WITH CARDIAC DISEASE

Poor feeding	Tachypnea
Failure to thrive	Hepatomegaly
Irritability	Clubbing

Observation of the respiratory rate and pattern is helpful in distinguishing the degree of illness and cardiac versus pulmonary diseases. An increase in respiratory effort is expected from pulmonary diseases, whereas in cardiac disease there may be tachypnea, but not increased work of breathing until congestive heart failure becomes significant.

A diffuse bulge outward of the left side of the chest suggests longstanding *cardiomegaly.*

While observing the respiratory pattern, note any abnormalities of the sternum as discussed on p. 686.

Palpation. The major branches of the aorta can be assessed by evaluation of the *peripheral pulses.* All neonates should have an evaluation of all pulses at the time of their newborn examination. In neonates and infants, the brachial artery pulse in the antecubital fossa is easier to feel than the radial artery pulse at the wrist. Both temporal arteries should be felt just in front of the ear. It is important to feel the femoral pulses. They lie in the midline just below the inguinal crease, between the iliac crest and the symphysis pubis. Take your time and search for femoral pulses; they are difficult to detect in chubby, squirming infants. If you first flex the infant's thighs on the abdomen, this may overcome the reflex flexion that occurs when you then extend the legs. The dorsalis pedis and posterior tibial pulses in neonates and infants (see photo below) may be difficult to feel unless there is an abnormality involving aortic run-off. Normal pulses should have a sharp rise, be firm, and well localized.

The absence or diminution of femoral pulses is indicative of *coarctation of the aorta.* If you can't detect femoral pulses, measure blood pressures of the lower and upper extremities. If they are equal or lower in the legs, coarctation is likely to be present.

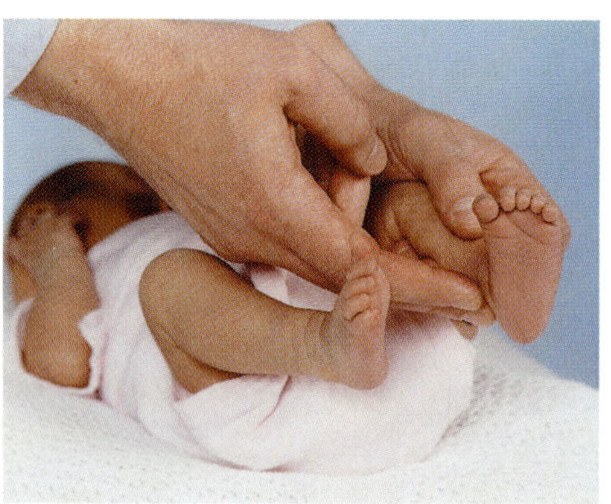

A weak or thready, difficult-to-feel, pulse may reflect *myocardial dysfunction* and *congestive heart failure,* particularly if associated with an unusual degree of tachycardia.

Although the pulses in the feet of neonates and infants are often faint, several conditions can cause full pulses, such as *patent ductus arteriosus* or *truncus arteriosus.*

As discussed on p. 658, carefully measure the *blood pressure* of infants and children as part of the cardiac examination. It may be helpful to measure the blood pressure in both arms and one leg at one time around age 3 to 4 years to check for possible *coarctation of the aorta.* Thereafter, only the right arm blood pressure needs to be measured.

The *point of maximal impulse,* or *PMI,* is not always palpable in infants and is affected by respiratory patterns, a full stomach, and the infant's positioning. It is usually an interspace higher than in adults during the first few years of life because the heart lies more horizontally within the chest.

Palpation of the chest wall will allow you to assess volume changes within the heart. For example, a hyperdynamic precordium reflects a big volume change.

A *"rolling" heave* at the left sternal border suggests an *increase in right ventricular work,* while the same kind of motion closer to the apex suggests the same thing for the left ventricle.

Thrills are palpable when there is enough turbulence within the heart or great vessels to be transmitted to the surface. Knowledge of the structures beneath the precordium will allow you to determine the origin of the thrill. Thrills are easiest to feel with your palm or the base of your fingers, not your fingertips. Thrills have a somewhat rough, vibrating quality. The figure that follows shows locations of thrills from various cardiac abnormalities that occur in infants and children.

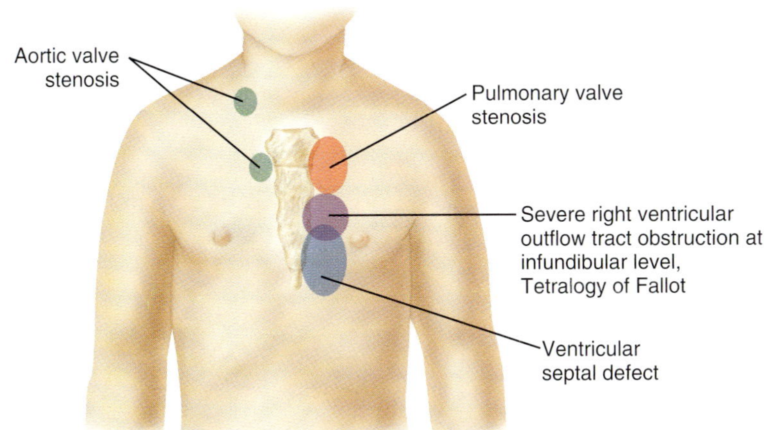

Auscultation. The *heart rhythm* is more easily evaluated in infants by listening to the heart than by feeling the peripheral pulses, but in older children can be done either way. Children commonly have a normal sinus dysrhythmia, with the heart rate increasing on inspiration and decreasing on expiration, sometimes quite abruptly. This is a normal finding and can be identified by its repetitive nature, its correlation with respiration, and by its involvement of several beats rather than a single beat.

The most common dysrhythmia in children is *paroxysmal supraventricular tachycardia, or paroxysmal atrial tachycardia (PSVT, or PAT).* It can occur at any age, including in utero. It is remarkably well tolerated by some children and is found on examination when the child looks perfectly healthy, may be mildly pale or has tachypnea, but has a rapid, sustained, completely regular heart rate of 240 beats per minute or more. Other children, particularly neonates, appear very ill with this condition. In older children, this dysrhythmia is more likely to be truly paroxysmal, with episodes of varying duration and varying frequency (see Table 17-5, p. 758).

Many children, particularly neonates, have premature atrial or ventricular beats that are often appreciated as "skipped" beats. They can usually be eradicated by increasing the intrinsic sinus rate by exercise, such as crying in an infant or jumping in an older child, although they may be more frequent in the postexercise period. In a completely healthy child, they are usually benign and rarely persist.

Pathologic arrhythmias in children can be due to *structural cardiac lesions,* but also to other causes such as *drug ingestion, metabolic abnormalities, endocrine disorders, serious infections, and postinfectious states,* or they may be related to conduction disturbances without structural heart disease.

The S_1 and S_2 *heart sounds* should be evaluated carefully. They are normally crisp. The second sounds (S_2) at the base are usually heard separately but should fuse into a single sound in deep expiration. In the neonate, it should be possible to detect a split second sound if the infant is examined when completely quiet or asleep; detecting this split eliminates many, but not all, of the more serious congenital cardiac defects.

Distant heart tones suggest *pericardial effusion;* mushy, less distinct heart sounds suggest *myocardial dysfunction.*

Characteristics of Normal Variants of Heart Rhythms in Children

Characteristics	Normal Sinus Arrhythmias	Atrial Premature Contractions (APCs) or Ventricular Premature Contractions (VPCs)
Most common age	After infancy Throughout childhood (less common in adults)	Neonates (but may occur at any time)
Correlation with respiration	Yes: Increases on inspiration Decreases on expiration	No
Effect of exercise on tachycardia	Disappears	Eradicated by exercise May be more frequent postexercise
Characteristic of rhythm	Gradually faster with inspiration Often suddenly slower on expiration	Skipped or missed beat Irregularly occurring
Number of beats	Several beats, usually in repetitive cycles	Usually single abnormal beats
Severity	Benign (by definition)	Usually benign

In addition to trying to detect splitting of the second heart sound, listen for the intensity of A_2 and P_2. The aortic, or first component of the second sound at the base, is normally louder than the pulmonic, or second component.

A louder-than-normal pulmonic component, particularly when louder than the aortic sound, suggests *pulmonary hypertension.*

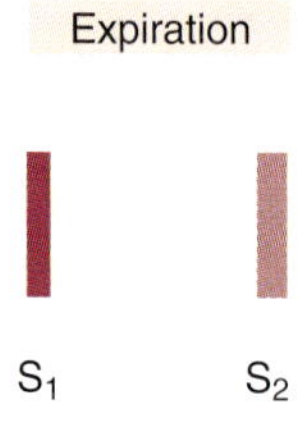

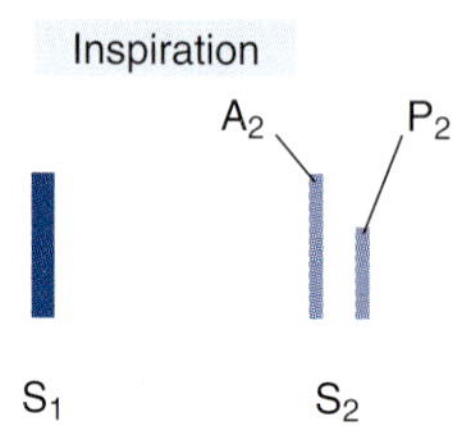

Persistent splitting of S_2 may indicate a right ventricular volume load such as *atrial septal defect, anomalies of pulmonary venous return,* or *chronic anemia.*

Third heart sounds, which are low-pitched, early diastolic sounds best heard at the lower left sternal border, or apex, are frequently heard in children and are normal. They reflect rapid ventricular filling.

Fourth heart sounds, which are not often heard in children, are low-frequency, late diastolic sounds, occurring just before the first heart sound.

Fourth heart sounds represent decreased ventricular compliance and are associated with *congestive heart failure.*

An *apparent gallop,* in the presence of a normal heart rate and rhythm, is a frequent finding in normal children and does not represent pathology.

A *gallop rhythm*—tachycardia plus a loud third and/or fourth heart sound—is pathologic and indicates *congestive heart failure* and *poor ventricular function.*

One of the most challenging aspects to the cardiac examination in children is the evaluation of *heart murmurs.* In addition to the task of trying to listen to a squirming, perhaps uncooperative child, a major challenge is to distinguish common benign murmurs from unusual or pathologic ones. Heart murmurs in children must be characterized by specific location (e.g., left upper sternal border, not just left sternal border), timing, intensity, and quality. If each murmur is delineated that completely, the diagnosis is usually made, and all that is needed is confirmation and amplification with laboratory tools such as ECG, chest x-ray, and echocardiography.

An important rule of thumb is that, by definition, *benign murmurs in children have no associated abnormal findings.* Many (but not all) children with serious cardiac malformations have signs and symptoms other than a heart murmur obtainable on careful history or examination. Many will also have other, noncardiac signs and symptoms as well, including evidence of genetic defects that may offer helpful diagnostic clues.

The presence of any of the *noncardiac findings* that frequently accompany cardiac disease in children markedly raises the possibility that a murmur that appears benign is really pathologic.

Most children (indeed, some say nearly all) will have one or more *functional, or benign, heart murmur* before reaching adulthood. It is important to identify functional murmurs by their specific qualities rather than by their softness. The common functional murmurs of infancy and childhood should be easily recognized by the practitioner and under most circumstances do not require evaluation.

Many *pathologic murmurs of congenital heart disease* are present at birth. Others are not apparent until later, depending on their severity, drop in pulmonary vascular resistance following birth, or changes associated with growth of the child. Table 17-16 on pp. 773–775 shows examples of pathologic murmurs of childhood.

The figure on the next page characterizes *benign* heart murmurs of children according to their location, key characteristics, and typical ages of presentation. These benign murmurs may be noted as children age:

Neonates	Closing ductus murmur
	Peripheral pulmonary flow murmur
Preschool or school-age	Still's murmur
	Venous hum
Preschool or later	Carotid bruit
Adolescence	Pulmonary flow murmur

Location and Characteristics of Benign Heart Murmurs in Children

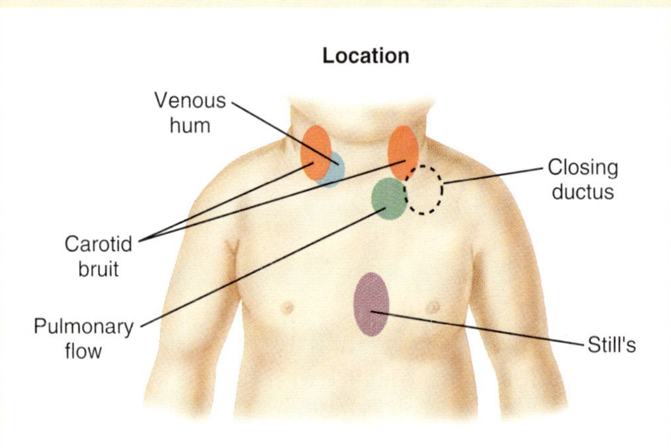

Typical Age	Name	Characteristics	Description and Location
Newborn	*Closing ductus*		Transient, soft, ejection Upper left sternal border
Newborn to 1 year	*Peripheral pulmonary flow murmur*		Soft, slightly ejectile, systolic To left of upper left sternal border and in lung fields and axillae
Preschool or early school age	*Still's murmur*		Grade I–II/VI, musical, vibratory Multiple overtones Early and midsystolic Mid/lower left sternal border Frequently also a carotid bruit
Preschool or early school age	*Venous hum*		Soft, hollow, continuous Louder in diastole Under clavicle Can be eliminated by maneuvers
Preschool and later	*Carotid bruit*		Early and midsystolic Usually louder on left Eliminated by carotid compression
Adolescence and later	*Pulmonary flow murmur*		Grade I–II/VI soft, nonharsh Ejection in timing Upper left sternal border Normal P_2

The neonate may have a transient, soft, ejection murmur at the upper left sternal border and to the left, as flow continues through a *closing ductus arteriosus.* This murmur usually disappears within a day or two after birth.

A pathologic *patent ductus arteriosus* transmits a continuous murmur at the upper left sternal border of neonates, and is frequently accompanied by a loud P_2, bounding pulses, and developing congestive heart failure.

Some neonates and infants will have a soft, somewhat ejectile murmur heard, not over the precordium, but over the lung fields, particularly in the axillae. This represents peripheral pulmonary artery flow and is partly the result of inadequate pulmonary artery growth in utero (when there is little pulmonary blood flow) and the sharp angle at which the pulmonary artery curves backward. In the absence of any physical findings to suggest additional underlying diseases, this *peripheral pulmonary flow murmur* can be considered benign and usually disappears by the age of 1 year.

A pulmonary flow murmur in the newborn who has signs of other disease is more likely to be pathologic. Diseases may include *Williams syndrome, congenital rubella syndrome, and Alagille syndrome.*

Preschool and school-aged children often have benign murmurs. The most common (*Still's murmur*) is a grade I–II/VI, musical, vibratory, early and midsystolic murmur with multiple overtones, located over the mid or lower left sternal border, but also frequently heard over the carotid arteries. Carotid artery compression will usually cause the precordial murmur to disappear. This murmur may be extremely variable and may be accentuated when cardiac output is increased, as occurs with fever or exercise.

The murmur heard in the carotid area or just above the clavicles is known as a *carotid bruit.* It is early and midsystolic, with a slightly harsh quality. It is usually louder on the left and may be heard alone or in combination with the Still's murmur, as noted above. It may be completely eradicated by carotid artery compression.

PHYSIOLOGIC BASIS FOR SOME PATHOLOGIC HEART MURMURS

Change in Pulmonary Vascular Resistance

Heart murmurs that are dependent on a postnatal drop in pulmonary vascular resistance, allowing turbulent flow from the high-pressured systemic circuit to the lower-pressured pulmonary circuit, are not audible until such a drop has occurred. Therefore, except in premature infants, murmurs of a *ventricular septal defect* or *patent ductus arteriosus* are not expected in the first few days of life and usually become audible after a week or 10 days.

Obstructive Lesions

Obstructive lesions, such as *pulmonary and aortic stenosis,* are caused by normal blood flow through two small valves, and, therefore, are not dependent on a drop in pulmonary vascular resistance and are audible at birth.

Pressure Gradient Differences

Murmurs of *atrioventricular valve regurgitation* are audible at birth because of the high pressure gradient between the ventricle and its atrium.

Changes Associated With Growth of Children

Some murmurs do not follow the rules above, but are audible due to alterations in normal blood flow and occur or change with growth. For example, even though it is an obstructive defect, *aortic stenosis* may not be audible until considerable growth has occurred, and, indeed, is frequently not heard until adulthood, although a congenitally abnormal valve is responsible. Similarly, the pulmonary flow murmur of an *atrial septal defect* may not be heard for a year or more, as right ventricular compliance gradually increases and the shunt becomes larger, eventually producing a murmur caused by too much blood flow across a normal pulmonary valve.

Also in preschool or school-aged children, you may detect a *venous hum*. This is a soft, hollow, continuous sound, louder in diastole, heard just below the right clavicle. It can be completely eliminated by maneuvers that affect venous return, such as lying supine, changing head position, or jugular venous compression. It has the same quality as breath sounds and therefore is frequently overlooked.

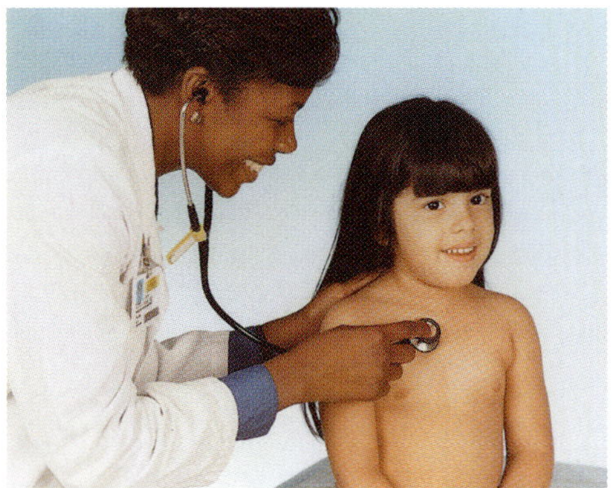

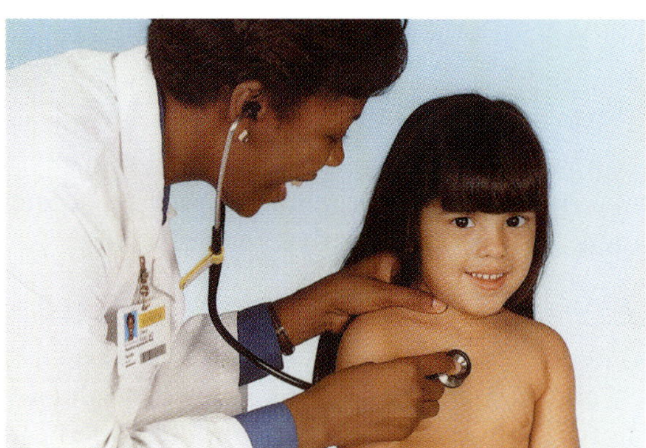

In adolescence, a *pulmonary flow murmur* may be heard. It is a grade I–II/VI soft, nonharsh murmur with the timing characteristics of an ejection murmur, beginning after the first sound and ending before the second sound but without the marked crescendo–decrescendo quality of an organic ejection murmur. If you hear this murmur, make sure to evaluate whether the pulmonary closure sound is of normal intensity and whether splitting of the second heart sound is eliminated during expiration. An adolescent with a benign pulmonary ejection murmur will have normal intensity and normally split second heart sounds.

A pulmonary flow murmur accompanied by a fixed split-second heart sound, suggests right-heart volume load such as an *atrial septal defect.*

This pulmonary flow murmur may also be heard in the presence of volume overload from any reason, such as chronic anemia, pregnancy, and following exercise. It may persist into adulthood.

Review the figures on p. 696 and learn to identify the locations of benign heart murmurs in children, and to understand the ages of presentation, characteristics, and qualities of these common murmurs.

When you detect any murmur in children, note all of the qualities as described in Chapter 7, The Cardiovascular System, to help you distinguish *pathologic murmurs* from the benign murmurs just described. Heart murmurs that reflect underlying structural heart disease are easier to evaluate if you have a good knowledge of intrathoracic anatomy and the functional cardiac changes following birth and if you understand the physiologic basis for heart murmurs. Understanding these physiologic changes can help you to distinguish pathologic murmurs from benign heart murmurs in children.

Characteristics of specific pathologic heart murmurs in children are described in Table 17-16 on pp. 773–775.

The Breasts

INFANCY

The breasts of the newborn in both males and females are often enlarged. This is due to maternal estrogen effect and may last several months. The breasts may also be engorged with a white liquid, sometimes colloquially called "witch's milk," which may last a week or two.

In *premature thelarche,* breast development occurs, most often between 6 months and 2 years of age. Other signs of puberty or hormonal abnormalities are not present.

OLDER CHILDREN AND ADOLESCENTS

The most important issues related to the examination of the breasts in older children involve assessment of normal maturational development. For years the established normal age range for onset of breast development was 8 to 13 years of age (average age of 11 years), with breast development occurring before 8 years being abnormal. Some recent studies suggest that the lower age cutoff should be 7 years for Caucasian females and 6 years for African-American (and probably Hispanic) females, though there remains some controversy about the exact age.

Supernumerary nipples occasionally are found on the thorax or the abdomen along a vertical line below the true nipple(s), as shown on p. 714. They appear as small, round, flat or slightly raised, pigmented lesions, and are not clinically significant.

Physical changes in a young girl's breasts are one of the first signs of puberty. As in most developmental changes, there is a systematic progression of maturational changes. Generally, over a 4-year period, the breasts progress through five stages, called Tanner stages or Tanner sex maturity rating (SMR) stages, as shown on the next page. These progress from a preadolescent stage, to the appearance of breast buds, to subsequent enlargement and change in the contour of the breasts and areola. These stages are accompanied by the development of pubic hair and other secondary sexual characteristics as shown on p. 713. Menarche usually occurs when a girl is in breast stage 3 or 4, and by then she has passed her peak growth spurt (see the figure on p. 700). These sequential changes in breast development are important to understand in relation to overall pubertal changes, and are helpful in counseling girls about their physical maturation.

Masses or nodules in the breasts of adolescent girls should be examined carefully. They are usually *benign fibroadenomas* or *cysts;* less likely etiologies include *abscesses* or *lipomas.* Breast carcinoma is extremely rare in adolescence, and nearly always occurs in families with a strong family history of the disease.

In about 10% of girls, the breasts develop at different rates and considerable asymmetry may result in either size or Tanner stage. This generally resolves, and reassurance to the patient is most helpful.

In older adolescent girls, a comprehensive breast examination should be accompanied by instructions for breast self-examination (p. 313).

In boys, the breasts consist of a small nipple and areola. During puberty, about one third of boys develop a firm button of breast tissue 2 cm or more in diameter, and these are often noted in one breast only. Obese boys can develop substantial breast tissue.

A substantial number of adolescent boys develop *gynecomastia,* or breast enlargement, on one or both sides. While usually slight, the enlargement can be substantial and quite embarrassing. It generally resolves within a few years.

SEX MATURITY RATINGS IN GIRLS: BREASTS

Stage 1

Preadolescent. Elevation of nipple only

Stage 2

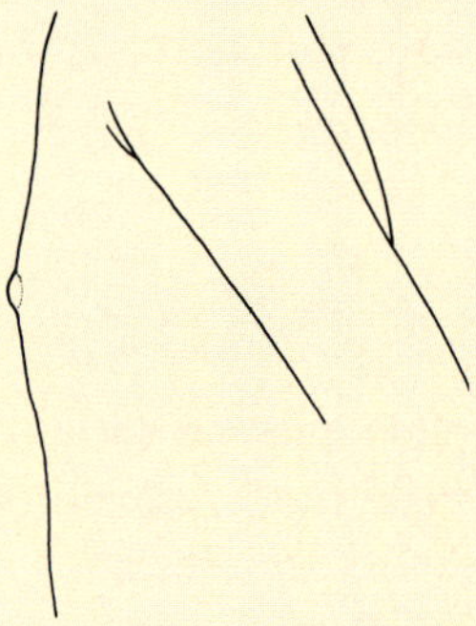

Breast bud stage. Elevation of breast and nipple as a small mound; enlargement of areolar diameter

Stage 3

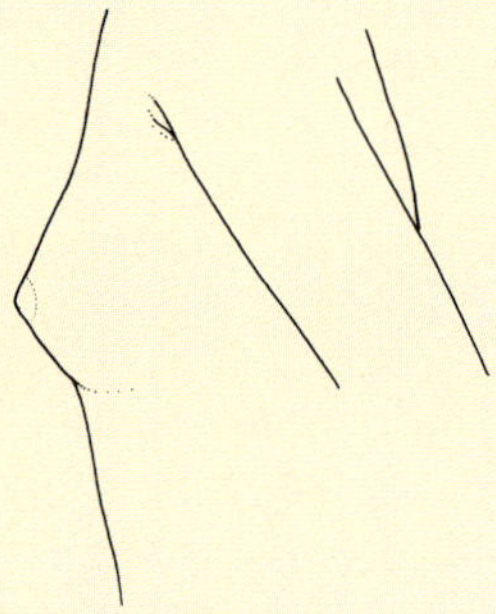

Further enlargement of elevation of breast and areola, with no separation of their contours

Stage 4

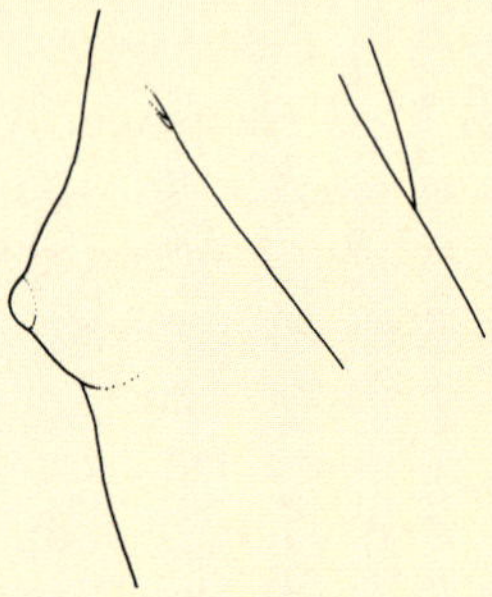

Projection of areola and nipple to form a secondary mound above the level of breast

Stage 5

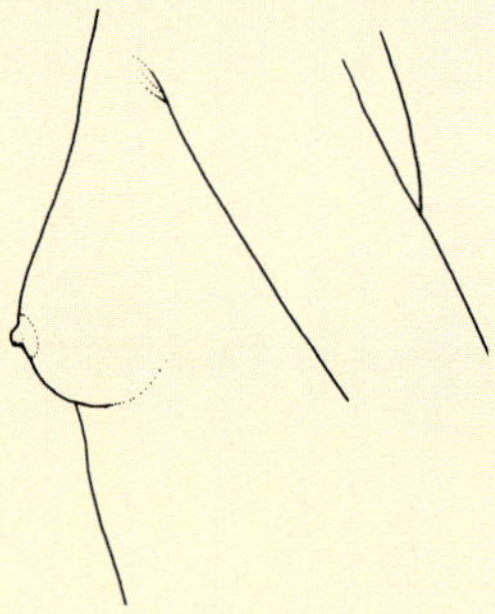

Mature stage; projection of nipple only. Areola has receded to general contour of the breast (although in some normal individuals the areola continues to form a secondary mound).

(Illustrations through the courtesy of W. A. Daniel, Jr., Professor Emeritus, Division of Adolescent Medicine, University of Alabama, Birmingham.)

The Abdomen

NEWBORN PERIOD AND INFANCY

Inspect the abdomen with the infant lying supine, optimally while asleep. The abdomen is protuberant due to poorly developed abdominal musculature. You will easily notice abdominal wall blood vessels and intestinal peristalsis.

Inspect the newborn's *umbilical cord* to detect abnormalities. Normally, there are two thick-walled umbilical arteries and one larger but thin-walled umbilical vein, which is usually located at the 12 o'clock position.

A *single umbilical artery* may be associated with congenital anomalies, but also occurs in normal infants as an isolated anomaly.

The umbilicus in the newborn may have a long cutaneous portion (*umbilicus cutis*), which is covered with skin, or an amniotic portion (*umbilicus amnioticus*), which is covered by a firm gelatinous substance. The amniotic portion dries up and falls off within 2 weeks, while the cutaneous portion retracts to be flush with the abdominal wall.

An *umbilical granuloma* at the base of the navel is the development of pink granulation tissue formed during the healing process.

Inspect the area around the umbilicus for redness or swelling. *Umbilical hernias* are detectable at a few weeks of age.

Umbilical hernias in infants are due to a defect in the abdominal wall, and can be up to 6 cm in diameter and quite protuberant when intra-abdominal pressure is increased. Most disappear by 1 year, nearly all by 5 years.

A *diastasis recti* may be noted in normal infants. This involves separation of the two rectus abdominis muscles, causing a midline ridge, most apparent on contraction of the abdominal muscles. A benign condition in most cases, it resolves during early childhood. Chronic abdominal distention may also predispose to this condition.

Auscultation of a quiet infant's abdomen is easy. Don't be surprised if you hear an orchestra of musical tinkling bowel sounds every 10 to 30 seconds.

An increase in pitch or frequency of bowel sounds is heard with *gastroenteritis* or, rarely, with *intestinal obstruction.*

You can *percuss* an infant's abdomen as you would for an adult, but be prepared to note greater tympanitic sounds due to the infant's propensity to swallow air. Percussion is useful for determining the size of organs and abdominal masses.

A silent, tympanic, distended abdomen suggests *peritonitis.*

You will find it easy to *palpate* an infant's abdomen because he likes being touched. A useful technique to relax the infant, shown here, is to hold the legs flexed at the knees and hips with one hand and palpate the abdomen with the other. You may also want to use a pacifier or bottle to quiet the infant in this position.

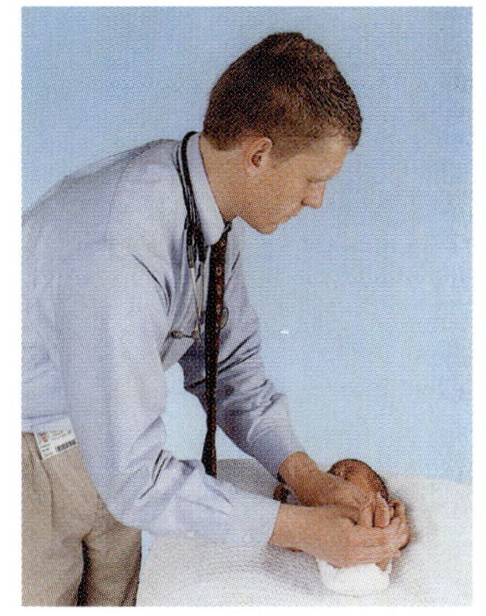

Start gently palpating the liver of infants low in the abdomen, moving upwards with your fingers. This technique helps you avoid missing an extremely enlarged liver that extends down into the pelvis. With a careful examination, you can feel the liver edge in most infants, 1 to 2 cm below the right costal margin.

An enlarged, tender liver may be due to *congestive heart failure* or to *storage diseases.*

Similarly, you can usually palpate the spleen tip. In fact, you may be able to palpate the kidneys of infants by carefully placing the fingers of one hand in front of and those of the other behind each kidney. The descending colon is a sausagelike mass in the left lower quadrant.

Once you have identified the normal structures in the infant's abdomen, use palpation to identify abnormal masses.

Abnormal abdominal masses in infants can be associated with the kidney (e.g., *hydronephrosis*), bladder (e.g., *urethral obstruction*), bowel (e.g., *Hirschsprung's disease,* or *intussusception*), and tumors.

In *pyloric stenosis,* deep palpation in the right upper quadrant or midline can reveal an "olive," or a 2-cm firm pyloric mass. While feeding, some infants with this condition will have visible peristaltic waves pass across their abdomen, followed by projectile vomiting.

EARLY AND LATE CHILDHOOD, AND ADOLESCENCE

Toddlers and young children commonly have protuberant abdomens, most apparent when they are upright. The examination can follow the same order as for adults, except that you may need to open your bag of tricks to distract the child during the examination.

An exaggerated "pot-belly appearance" may indicate malabsorption due to *celiac disease, cystic fibrosis,* or *constipation* or *aerophagia.*

Most children are ticklish when you first place your hand on their abdomens for *palpation*. This reaction tends to disappear, particularly if you distract the child with conversation and place your whole hand flush on the abdominal surface for a few moments without probing. For children who are particularly sensitive and who tighten their abdominal muscles, you can start by placing the child's hand under yours as shown in the following photo. Eventually you will be able to remove the child's hand and palpate the abdomen freely.

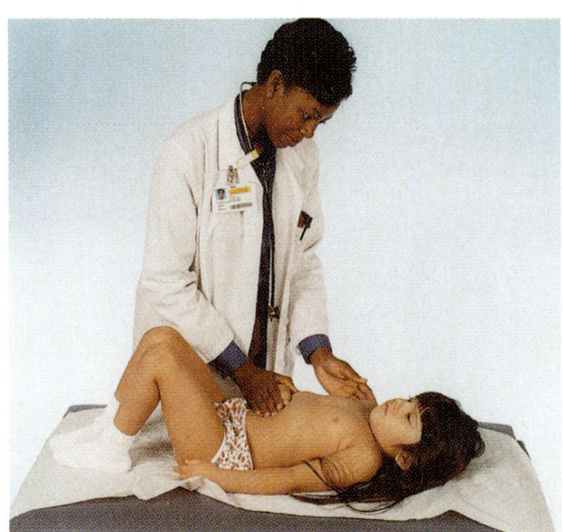

You can also try flexing the knees and hips to relax the child's abdominal wall. Palpate lightly in all areas, then deeply, leaving a site of potential pathology to the end.

To detect abdominal tenderness, have the young child tell you which specific area is tender, and note a change in his facial expression or cry.

The *liver* is easily palpated in most children. The edge of the liver is normally felt 1 cm to 2 cm below the right costal margin. It is sharp and soft and moves easily when pushed from below upward during deep inspiration. As in infants, you should start feeling for the liver edge in the right lower quadrant and work upwards, because a greatly enlarged liver can be missed in children.

Young children with respiratory illness and *lung hyperinflation* may appear to have an enlarged liver and abdomen based on the liver edge being several cm below the right costal margin. Percussion will determine accurate liver size.

The size of the liver is determined better by percussion than by palpation. The table below shows the expected liver span noted by percussion in the right midclavicular line.

A pathologically enlarged liver in children is usually palpable more than 2 cm below the costal margin, has a round, firm edge, and is often tender. Causes in older children include *neoplasms, infectious or inflammatory disease, metabolic or genetic diseases,* and *congestive heart failure.*

Expected Liver Span of Infants, Children, and Adolescents by Percussion

	Mean Estimated Liver Span (cm)			Mean Estimated Liver Span (cm)	
Age in Years	*Males*	*Females*	**Age in Years**	*Males*	*Females*
0.5 (6 mo)	2.4	2.8	8	5.6	5.1
1	2.8	3.1	10	6.1	5.4
2	3.5	3.6	12	6.5	5.6
3	4.0	4.0	14	6.8	5.8
4	4.4	4.3	16	7.1	6.0
5	4.8	4.5	18	7.4	6.1
6	5.1	4.8	20	7.7	6.3

One method to determine the lower border of the liver involves the *scratch test,* shown in the figure below. Place the diaphragm of your stethoscope just above the right costal margin at the midclavicular line. With your fingernail, lightly scratch the skin of the abdomen along the midclavicular line, moving from below the umbilicus toward the costal margin. When your scratching finger reaches the liver's edge, you will hear a change in the scratching sound as it passes through the liver to your stethoscope.

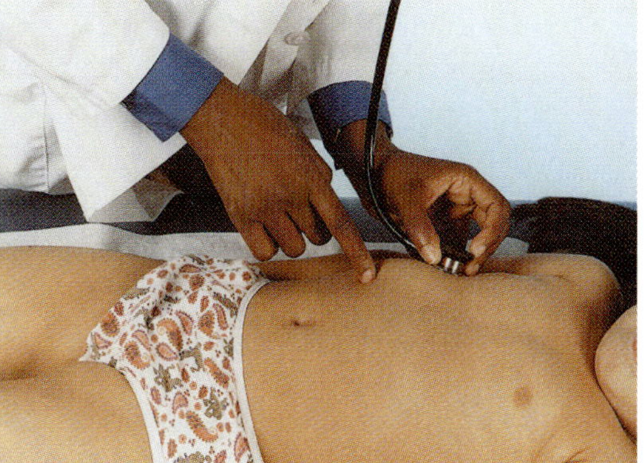

The *spleen,* like the liver, is felt easily in most children. It too is soft with a sharp edge, and it projects downward like a tongue from under the left costal margin. The spleen is moveable and rarely extends more than 1 cm to 2 cm below the costal margin.

Splenomegaly can be caused by a variety of diseases, including *infections, hematologic disorders* such as *hemolytic anemias, infiltrative disorders,* and *inflammatory* or *autoimmune diseases,* as well as congestion from *portal hypertension.*

Palpate the *other abdominal structures.* You will commonly note pulsations in the epigastrium caused by the aorta. This is felt most easily to the left of the midline, on deep palpation.

Palpating for abdominal tenderness in an older child is the same as for the adult; however, the causes of abdominal pain are often different, encompassing a wide spectrum of acute and chronic diseases. Localization of tenderness may help you pinpoint the abdominal structures most likely to be causing the abdominal pain.

In a child with an acute abdomen, as in *acute appendicitis,* special techniques are helpful, such as checking for involuntary rigidity, rebound tenderness, a Rovsing's sign, or a positive psoas or obturator sign (see p. 347–348).

Male Genitalia

NEWBORN PERIOD AND INFANCY

Inspect the male genitalia with the infant in the supine position, noting the appearance of the penis, testes, and scrotum. The *foreskin* completely covers the glans penis. It is nonretractable at birth, though you may be able to retract it enough to visualize the external urethral meatus. Retraction of the foreskin in the uncircumcised male occurs months to years later. The rate of circumcision has declined recently in North America and varies worldwide, depending on cultural practices.

A *hypospadias* is present when the urethral orifice appears at some point along the ventral surface of the glans or shaft of the penis (see Table 17-17, The Male Genitourinary System, p. 776). The foreskin is incompletely formed ventrally.

Inspect the shaft of the penis, noting any abnormalities on the ventral surface. Make sure the penis appears straight.

A fixed, downward bowing of the penis is a *chordee;* this may accompany a hypospadias.

Scrotal edema may be present for several days following delivery due to the effect of maternal estrogens.

Inspect the scrotum, noting rugae, which should be present by 40 weeks' gestation. Palpate the testes in the scrotal sacs, proceeding downward from the external inguinal ring to the scrotum. If you feel a testis up in the inguinal canal, gently milk it downward into the scrotum. The newborn's testes should be about 10 mm in width and 15 mm in length and should lie in the scrotal sacs most of the time.

In newborns with an *undescended testicle* (*cryptorchidism*), the scrotum often appears underdeveloped and tight, and palpation reveals an absence of scrotal contents (see Table 17-17, The Male Genitourinary System, p. 776).

In 3% of neonates, one or both testes cannot be felt in the scrotum or inguinal canal. This raises concern of *cryptorchidism.* In two thirds of these cases, both testes are descended by 1 year of age.

Examine the testes for swelling within the scrotal sac and over the inguinal ring. If you detect swelling in the scrotal sac, try to differentiate it from the testis. Note whether the size changes when the infant increases abdominal

Two common scrotal masses in newborns are *hydroceles* and *inguinal hernias;* frequently both

pressure by crying. See if your fingers can get above the mass, trapping it in the scrotal sac. Apply gentle pressure to try to reduce the size of the mass and note any tenderness. Note whether it transilluminates.

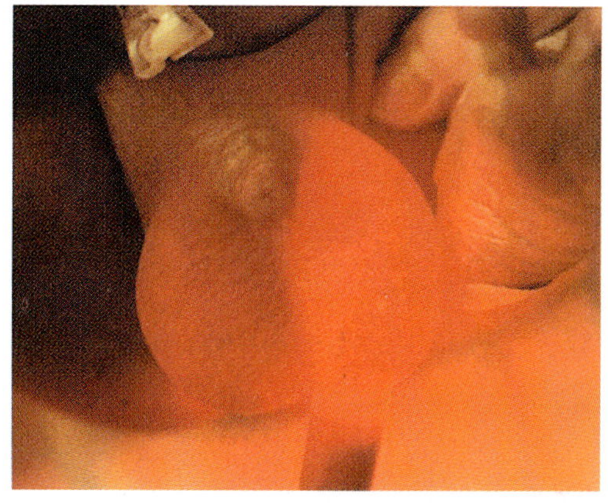

Fletcher M: Physical Diagnosis in Neonatology, Philadelphia, Lippincott-Raven Publishers, 1998.

coexist, and both are more common on the right side. Hydroceles overlie the testes and the spermatic cord, are not reducible, and can be transilluminated (see photo at left). Most resolve by 18 months. Hernias are separate from the testes, are usually reducible, and often do not transilluminate. They do not resolve. Sometimes a thickened spermatic cord is noted (called the *silk sign*).

EARLY AND LATE CHILDHOOD

Inspect the penis. The size in prepubertal children has little significance unless it is abnormally large. In obese boys, the fat pad over the symphysis pubis may obscure the penis.

In *precocious puberty,* the penis and testes are enlarged, with signs of pubertal changes. This is caused by a variety of conditions associated with excess androgens, including *adrenal or pituitary tumors.* Other pubertal changes also occur.

There is an art to *palpation* of the young boy's scrotum and testes because many have an extremely active cremasteric reflex that may cause the testis to retract upwards into the inguinal canal and thereby appear to be undescended. Examine the child when he is relaxed, because anxiety stimulates the cremasteric reflex. With warm hands, palpate the lower abdomen, working your way downward toward the scrotum along the inguinal canal. This will minimize retraction of the testes into the canal.

A useful technique is to have the boy sit cross-legged on the examining table, as shown here. You can also give him a balloon to inflate or an object to lift to increase intra-abdominal pressure. If you can detect the testis in the scrotum, it is descended even if it spends much time in the inguinal canal.

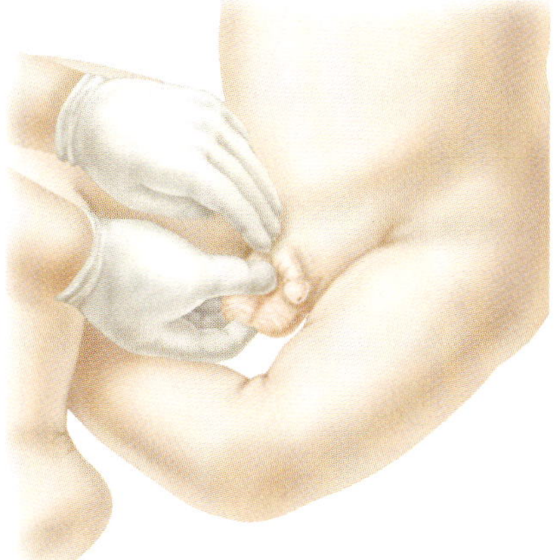

The cremasteric reflex can be tested by scratching the medial aspect of the thigh. The testes will move upward.

Cryptorchidism may be noted at this age. It requires surgical correction. It should be differentiated from a retractible testis.

A painful testicle requires rapid treatment; common causes include infection such as *epididymitis* or *orchitis, torsion of the testicle,* or *torsion of the appendix testis.*

Examine the inguinal canal as you would for adults, noting any swelling that may reflect an *inguinal hernia.*

Inguinal hernias in older boys present as they do in adult men, with swelling in the inguinal canal, particularly following a Valsalva maneuver.

ADOLESCENCE

The genital examination of the adolescent boy proceeds like the examination of the adult male. Be particularly aware of the embarrassment of many boys regarding this aspect of the examination.

Important anatomic changes in the male genitalia accompany puberty and help to define its progress. The first reliable sign of puberty, starting between ages 9 and 13.5 years, is an increase in the size of the testes. Next, pubic hair appears, along with progressive enlargement of the penis. The complete change from preadolescent to adult anatomy requires about 3 years, with a range of 1.8 to 5 years.

Delayed puberty is suspected in boys who have no signs of pubertal development by 14 years of age.

An important goal when examining the adolescent male is to assign a sexual maturity rating. The five stages of sexual development, first described by Tanner, are outlined and illustrated on the next page. These involve changes in the penis, testes, and scrotum. In addition, in about 80% of men, pubic hair spreads farther up the abdomen in a triangular pattern pointing toward the umbilicus; this phase is not completed until the 20s.

The most common cause of delayed puberty in males is *constitutional delay,* a frequently familial condition involving delayed bone and physical maturation but normal hormonal levels.

An important developmental principle is that physical pubertal changes progress along a well-established sequence, as diagrammed below. Although there are wide age ranges for the start and completion, the sequence for each boy is nevertheless the same. This is helpful in counseling an anxious adolescent regarding his current and future maturation, and regarding the normality of pubertal changes along a wide age range. It is also helpful for detecting abnormal physical changes.

While nocturnal or daytime ejaculation tends to begin around Sexual Maturity Rating 3, a finding on either history or physical examination of penile discharge may indicate a *sexually transmitted disease.*

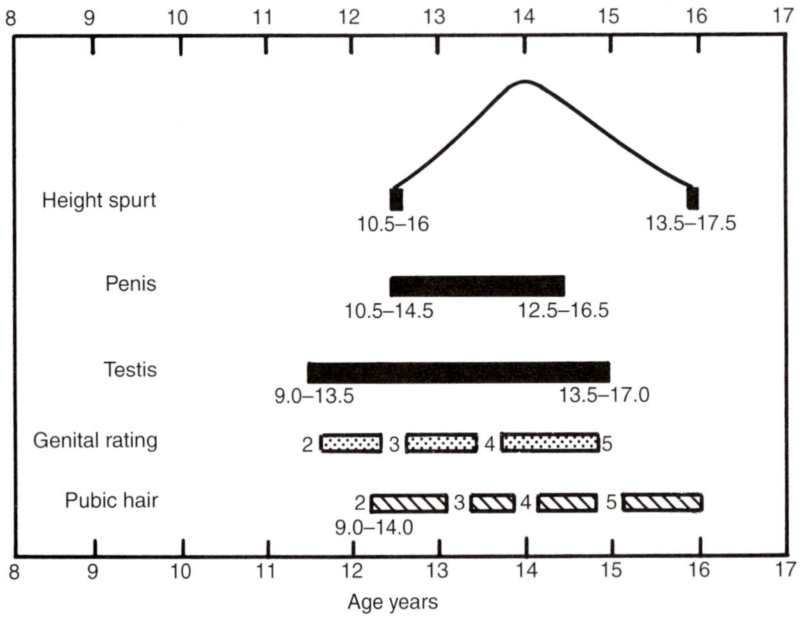

Numbers below the bars indicate the ranges in age within which certain changes occur. (Redrawn from Marshall WA, Tanner JM: Variations in the patterns of pubertal changes in boys. Arch Dis Child 45:22, 1970)

Sex Maturity Ratings in Boys

In assigning SMRs in boys, observe each of the three characteristics separately because they may develop at different rates. Record two separate ratings: pubic hair and genital. If the penis and testes differ in their stages, average the two into a single figure for the genital rating.

		Genital	
	Pubic Hair	*Penis*	*Testes and Scrotum*
Stage 1	Preadolescent—no pubic hair except for the fine body hair (vellus hair) similar to that on the abdomen	Preadolescent—same size and proportions as in childhood	Preadolescent—same size and proportions as in childhood
Stage 2	Sparse growth of long, slightly pigmented, downy hair, straight or only slightly curled, chiefly at the base of the penis	Slight or no enlargement	Testes larger; scrotum larger, somewhat reddened, and altered in texture
Stage 3	Darker, coarser, curlier hair spreading sparsely over the pubic symphysis	Larger, especially in length	Further enlarged
Stage 4	Coarse and curly hair, as in the adult; area covered greater than in stage 3 but not as great as in the adult and not yet including the thighs	Further enlarged in length and breadth, with development of the glans	Further enlarged; scrotal skin darkened
Stage 5	Hair adult in quantity and quality, spread to the medial surfaces of the thighs but not up over the abdomen	Adult in size and shape	Adult in size and shape

(Illustrations through the courtesy of W. A. Daniel, Jr., Professor Emeritus, Division of Adolescent Medicine, University of Alabama, Birmingham.)

Female Genitalia

Every health care provider should be familiar with the anatomy of a normal female. It is difficult to identify an abnormality unless you know what normal is. The genital examination can be anxiety-provoking for the older child and adolescent (especially if you are of the opposite sex), for parents, and for you; however, if not performed, a significant finding may be missed. Depending on the child's developmental stage, explain what parts of the body you will check, and that this is part of the routine examination.

NEWBORN PERIOD AND INFANCY

In the newborn female, the genitalia will be prominent due to the effects of maternal estrogen. The labia majora and minora have a dull pink color in light-skinned infants and may be hyperpigmented in dark-skinned infants. During the first few weeks of life, there is often a milky white discharge that may be blood-tinged. This estrogenized appearance of the genitalia decreases during the first year of life.

Ambiguous genitalia, involving masculinization of the female external genitalia, is a rare condition caused by endocrine disorders such as *congenital adrenal hyperplasia* (see Table 17-18, Abnormalities of the Female Genitourinary System, p. 777).

Examine the female genitalia with the infant in the supine position. One of the challenges is to determine the actual anatomy of the female infant's genitalia, which is shown below.

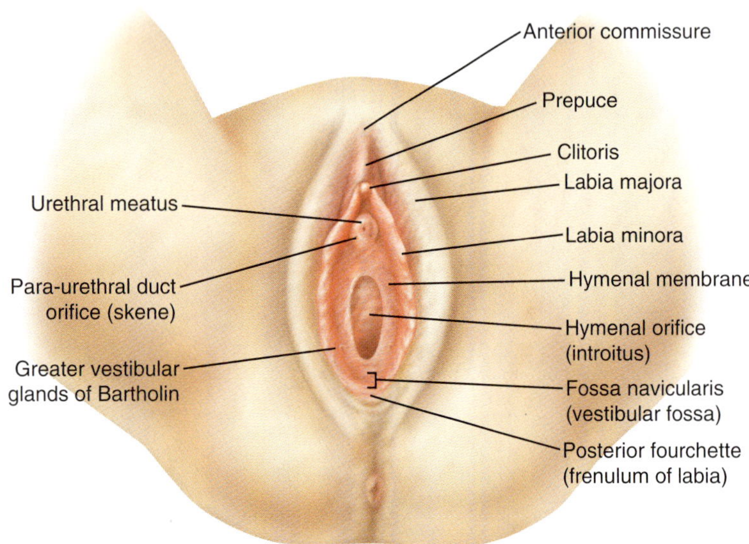

Examine the different structures systematically, including the size of the clitoris, the color and size of the labia majora, and the presence of rashes, bruises, or external lesions. Next, separate the labia majora at their midpoint with the thumb of each hand for young infants, or as shown in the diagrams on p. 710 for early and late childhood. Infants will not mind the examination as they are used to having their diapers changed and their bodies washed.

Inspect the urethral orifice and the labia minora. Assess the hymen, which in newborns and young infants is a thickened, avascular structure with a central orifice, covering the vaginal opening. You should be able to note a vaginal opening, although the hymen will be thickened and redundant. Note any discharge.

EARLY AND LATE CHILDHOOD

After infancy, the labia majora and minora flatten out, and the hymenal membrane becomes thin, translucent, and vascular, with the edges easily identified.

The appearance of pubic hair before the age of 7 years should be considered *precocious puberty* and requires evaluation to determine the cause.

The genital examination is the same for all ages of children, from late infancy until adolescence. Use a calm, gentle approach, including a developmentally appropriate explanation as you do the examination. A bright light source is essential. Most children can be examined in the supine, frog-leg position.

If the child seems reluctant, it may be helpful to have the parent sit on the examination table with the child; alternatively, the exam may be performed while the child sits in the parent's lap. Do not use stirrups as these may frighten the child. The following diagram demonstrates a 5-year-old child sitting on her parent's lap with the parent holding her knees outstretched.

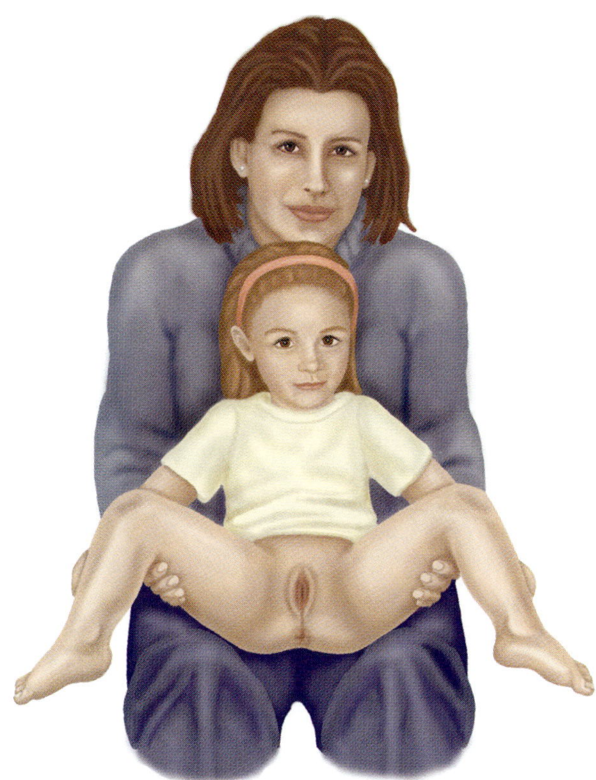

Examine the genitalia in an efficient and systematic manner. Inspect the external genitalia for the presence of pubic hair, the size of the clitoris, the color and size of the labia majora, and the presence of rashes, bruises, or other lesions.

Next, visualize the structures by separating the labia with your fingers as shown at the left on the following page. You can also apply gentle traction by grasping the labia between your thumb and index finger of each hand,

A *vaginal discharge* in early childhood can be due to *perineal irritation* (e.g., bubble baths or soaps),

and separating the labia majora laterally and posteriorly to examine the inner structures, as shown below. *Labial adhesions,* or fusion of the labia minora, may be noted in prepubertal children and can obscure the vaginal and urethral orifices. They may be a normal variant.

foreign body, vaginitis, or a *sexually transmitted disease* from sexual abuse.

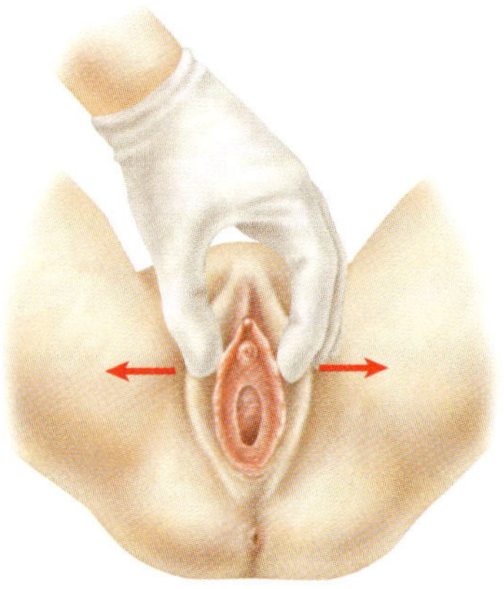

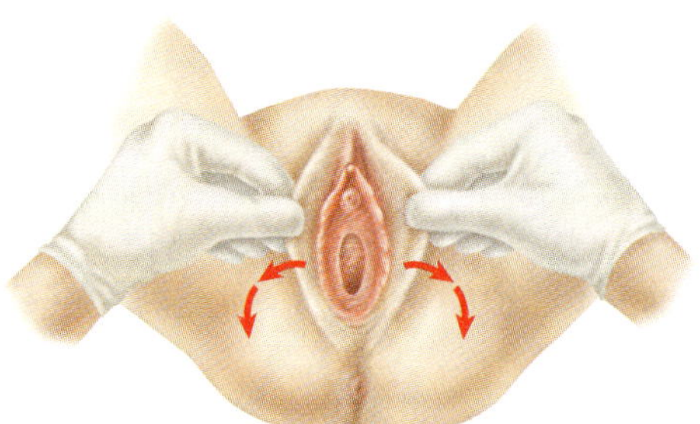

Vaginal bleeding is always concerning. Etiologies include *vaginal infection, accidental trauma, sexual abuse, foreign body,* and *tumors. Precocious puberty* from many causes can induce menses in a young girl.

Note the condition of the labia minora, urethra, hymen, and proximal vagina. If you are unable to visualize the edges of the hymen, ask the child to take a deep breath to relax the abdominal muscles. Another useful technique is to position her in the knee-chest position as shown on the right. These maneuvers will often open the hymen. You can also use saline drops to make the edges of the hymen less sticky.

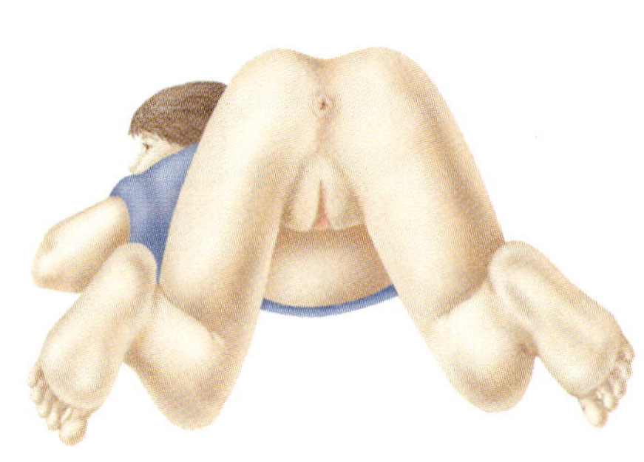

Purulent, profuse, malodorous, or blood-tinged discharge should be evaluated for the presence of *infection, foreign body,* or *trauma.*

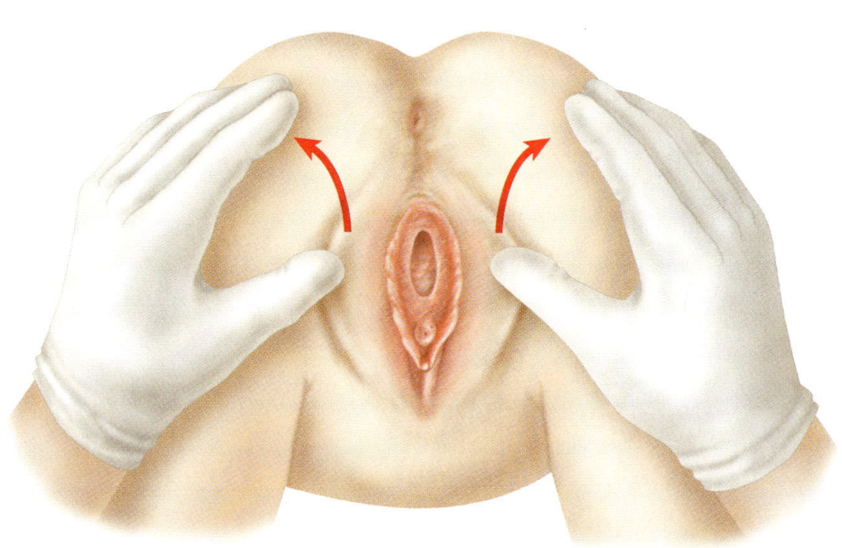

Avoid touching the hymenal edges as the hymen is exquisitely tender without the protective effects of hormones. Examine for discharge, labial adhesions, lesions, estrogenization (indicating onset of puberty), hymenal variations (such as imperforate or septate hymen, which is rare), and hygiene. A thin, white discharge (leukorrhea) is often present. A speculum examination of the vagina and cervix is not necessary in a prepubertal child unless there is suspicion of severe trauma or foreign body.

Abrasions or signs of trauma of the external genitalia can be due to benign causes such as masturbation, irritants, or accidental trauma, but should also raise the possibility of *sexual abuse.*

The normal hymen in infants and young children can have a variety of configurations, as shown in the following figures.

The physical examination may reveal signs that suggest *sexual abuse,* and the exam is particularly important if there are suspicious clues in the history. Bear in mind, that even with known abuse, the great majority of examinations will be unremarkable. Mounds, notches, and tags on the hymen may all be normal variants. The size of the orifice can vary with age and the examination technique. If the hymenal edges are smooth and without interruption in the inferior half, then the hymen is probably normal. Certain physical findings, however, suggest the possibility of sexual abuse and require more complete evaluation by an expert in the field.

PHYSICAL SIGNS THAT MAY INDICATE SEXUAL ABUSE IN CHILDREN*

1. Marked and immediate dilatation of the anus in knee–chest position, with no constipation, stool in the vault, or neurologic disorders
2. Hymenal notch or cleft that extends greater than 50% of the inferior hymenal rim (confirmed in knee–chest position)
3. Condyloma acuminata in a child over 3 years
4. Bruising, abrasions, lacerations, or bite marks of labia or perihymenal tissue
5. Herpes of the anogenital area beyond the neonatal period
6. Purulent or malodorous vaginal discharge in a young girl (all discharges should be cultured and viewed under a microscope for evidence of a sexually transmitted disease)

PHYSICAL SIGNS THAT STRONGLY SUGGEST SEXUAL ABUSE IN CHILDREN*

1. Lacerations, ecchymoses, and newly healed scars of the hymen or the posterior fourchette
2. Absence of hymenal tissue from 3 to 9 o'clock (confirmed in various positions)
3. Healed hymenal transections, especially between 3 and 9 o'clock (complete cleft)
4. Perianal lacerations extending to external sphincter

A child with concerning physical signs must be evaluated by a sexual abuse expert for a complete history and sexual abuse examination.

*Any physical sign must be evaluated in light of the entire history, other parts of the physical examination, and laboratory data.

NORMAL CONFIGURATIONS OF THE HYMEN IN PREPUBERTAL AND ADOLESCENT FEMALES

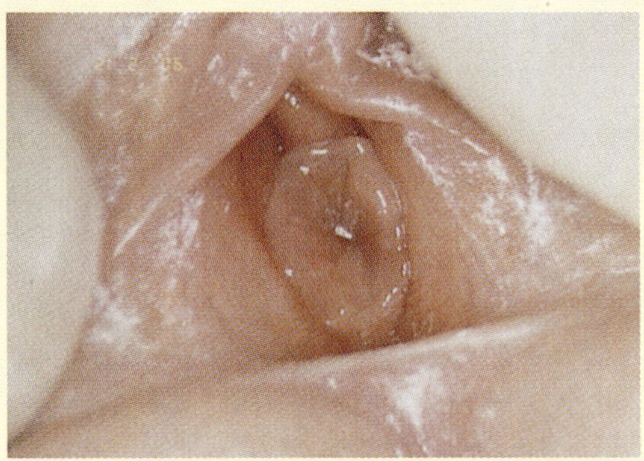

15-month-old infant with annular hymenal orifice

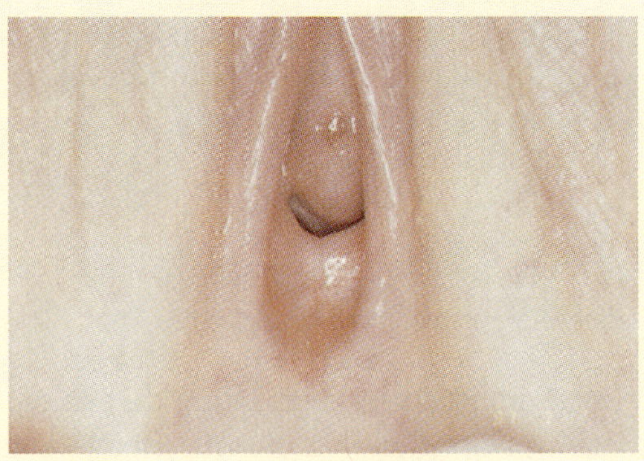

7-year-old girl with a crescent-shaped hymenal orifice

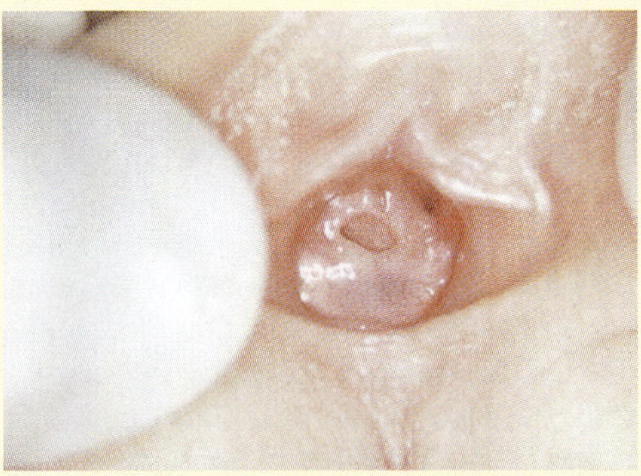

2-year-old with an annular orifice, located off-center, visible with labial traction

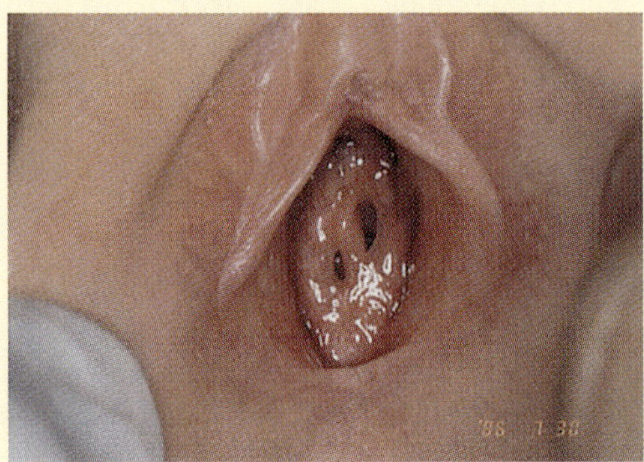

6-year-old with a septate hymen causing two orifices. Traction is needed to visualize the two openings.

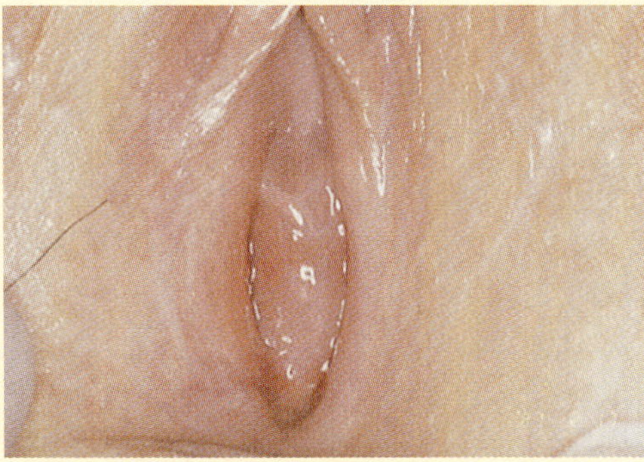

9-year-old girl with redundant labial tissue. Greater traction or a knee–chest position would reveal a normal orifice.

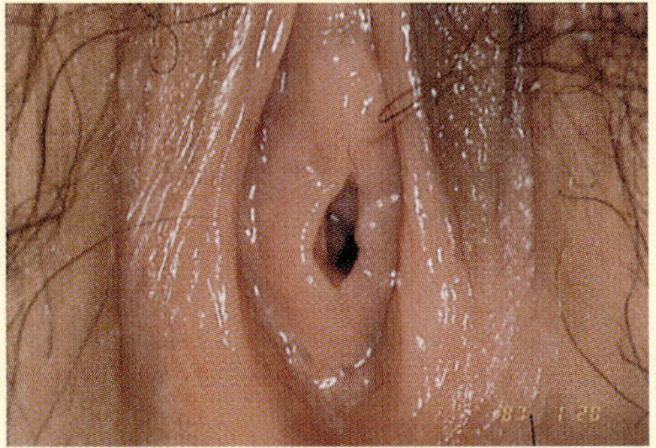

12-year-old girl with annular-shaped orifice and hormonal influence of puberty, causing thickened, pink tissue

(Source of photos: Reece R, Ludwig S (eds): Child Abuse: Medical Diagnosis and Management, 2nd ed., Philadelphia, Lippincott Williams & Wilkins, 2001.)

ADOLESCENCE

The external examination of adolescent female genitalia proceeds in the same manner as for the school-aged child. If it is necessary to complete a full pelvic exam on an adolescent, the actual technique is the same as that used for an adult. A full explanation of the steps of the examination, demonstration of the instruments, and a gentle, reassuring approach is necessary because the adolescent is usually quite anxious. An adolescent's first pelvic examination should be performed by an experienced health care provider.

The presence of a *vaginal discharge* in a young adolescent should be treated as in the adult. Causes include *physiologic* leukorrhea, *sexually transmitted diseases* from consensual sexual activity or *sexual abuse, bacterial vaginosis, foreign body,* and *external irritants.*

You should assign a sexual maturity rating to every female, irrespective of chronologic age. The assessment of sexual maturity in girls is based on both growth of pubic hair and the development of breasts. The assessment (Tanner staging) of pubic hair growth is shown in the figure illustrating the five Tanner stages of sexual maturity, below. See p. 700 for breast development assessment.

Although there is a wide variation in the age of onset and completion of puberty, remember that the stages occur in a predictable sequence, as shown here.

It is helpful to counsel girls about this sequence and their current maturational stage. A girl's initial signs of puberty are hymenal changes secondary to estrogen, widening of the hips, and beginning of a height spurt, although these changes are difficult to detect. The first easily detectable sign of pu-

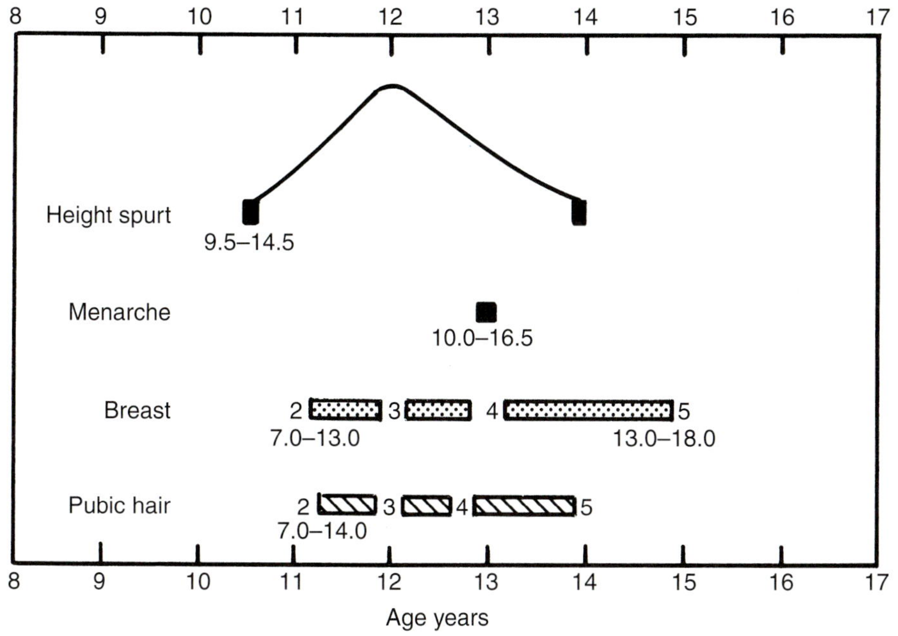

Numbers below the bars indicate the ranges in age within which certain changes occur. (Redrawn from Marshall WA, Tanner JM: Variations in the pattern of pubertal changes in girls. Arch Dis Child 45:22, 1970)

SEX MATURITY RATINGS IN GIRLS: PUBIC HAIR

Stage 1

Preadolescent—no pubic hair except for the fine body hair (vellus hair) similar to that on the abdomen

Stage 2

Sparse growth of long, slightly pigmented, downy hair, straight or only slightly curled, chiefly along the labia

Stage 3

Darker, coarser, curlier hair, spreading sparsely over the pubic symphysis

Stage 4

Coarse and curly hair as in adults; area covered greater than in stage 3 but not as great as in the adult and not yet including the thighs

Stage 5

Hair adult in quantity and quality, spread on the medial surfaces of the thighs but not up over the abdomen

(Illustration through the courtesy of W. A. Daniel, Jr., Professor Emeritus, Division of Adolescent Medicine, University of Alabama, Birmingham.)

berty is usually the appearance of breast buds, although pubic hair sometimes appears earlier. The average age of the appearance of pubic hair has decreased in recent years, and current consensus is that the appearance of pubic hair as early as 7 years can be normal, particularly in dark-skinned girls who develop secondary sexual characteristics at an earlier age.

The Rectal Examination

The rectal examination is not part of the routine pediatric examination, but should be done whenever intra-abdominal, pelvic, or perirectal disease is suspected.

The rectal examination of the young child can be performed with the child either in the side-lying or lithotomy position. For many young children, the lithotomy position is less threatening and easier to perform. Have the child lie on the back with the knees and hips flexed and the legs abducted. Drape the child from the waist down. Provide frequent reassurance during the examination, and ask the child to breathe in and out through the mouth to relax. Spread the buttocks and observe the anus. You can use your lubricated gloved index finger, even in small children. Palpate the abdomen with your other hand, both to distract the child and to note the abdominal structures between your hands. The prostate gland is not palpable in young boys.

Anal skin tags are present in *inflammatory bowel disease,* but are more often an incidental finding.

Tenderness noted on rectal examination of a child usually indicates an infectious or inflammatory cause, such as an *abscess,* or *appendicitis.*

In young girls, a rectal examination is useful for detecting tenderness or masses. The rectal examination for older girls who are undergoing a pelvic examination should proceed as it does for the adult patient.

The Musculoskeletal System

NEWBORN PERIOD AND INFANCY

Enormous changes in the musculoskeletal system occur during infancy. Much of the newborn musculoskeletal exam focuses on detection of congenital abnormalities, particularly in the hands, spine, hips, legs, and feet. With a little practice, you will be able to combine the musculoskeletal examination with the neurologic and developmental examination.

The *newborn's hands* are clenched. Because of the palmar grasp reflex (see the discussion on the nervous system), you will need to help the infant extend the fingers. Inspect the fingers carefully, noting any defects.

Skin tags, remnants of digits, polydactyly (extra fingers), or *syndactyly* (webbed fingers) are congenital defects noted at birth.

Palpate along the *clavicle* of the newborn, noting any lumps, tenderness, or crepitus; these may indicate a fracture.

A *fracture of the clavicle* can occur during a difficult delivery.

Inspect the *spine* carefully. While major defects of the spine such as *meningomyelocele* are obvious and often detected by ultrasound prior to birth, subtle abnormalities may include pigmented spots, hairy patches, or deep pits. These abnormalities, if present within 1 cm or so of the midline, may overlie external openings of sinus tracts that extend to the spinal canal. Do not probe sinus tracts because of the potential risk of infection. Palpate the spine, particularly in the lumbosacral region, noting any deformities of the vertebrae.

Spina bifida occulta (a defect of the vertebral bodies) may be associated with defects of the spinal cord, which can cause severe neurologic dysfunction.

Examine the newborn and infant's *hips* carefully at each examination for signs of dislocation. The following photos demonstrate the two major techniques, one to test for the presence of a posteriorly dislocated hip (*Ortolani test*), and the second to test for the ability to sublux or dislocate an intact but unstable hip (*Barlow test*).

A soft audible "click" heard with these maneuvers does not prove a dislocated hip, but should prompt a careful examination.

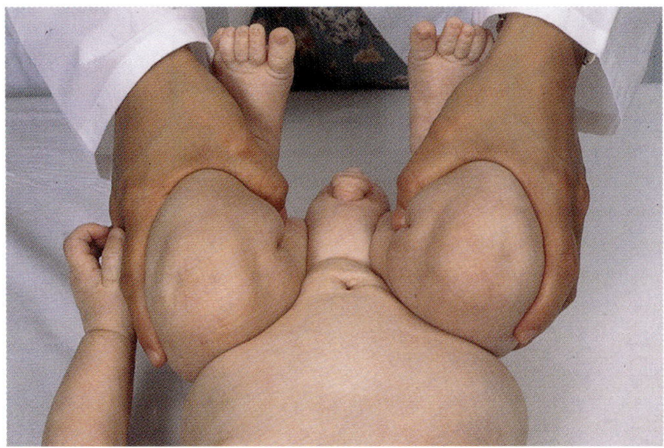

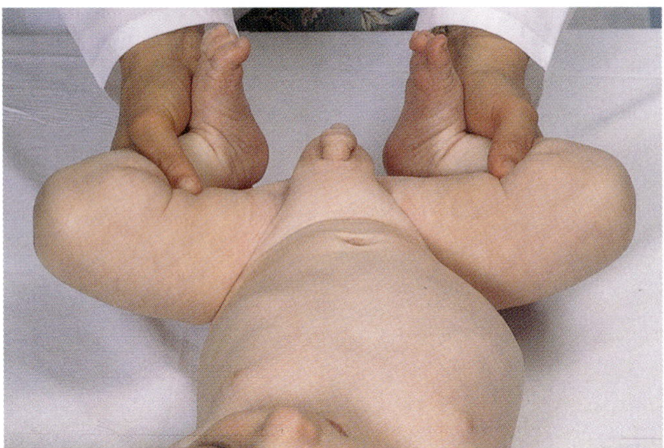

Make sure the baby is relaxed for the next two techniques, using a bottle or pacifier if appropriate. For the *Ortolani test*, place the baby supine with the legs pointing toward you. Flex the legs to form right angles at the hips and knees, placing your index fingers over the greater trochanter of each femur and your thumbs over the lesser trochanters. Abduct both hips simultaneously until the lateral aspect of each knee touches the examining table. A palpable movement of the femoral head back into place constitutes a *positive Ortolani sign*.

With a *hip dysplasia*, you feel a "clunk" as the femoral head, which lies posterior to the acetabulum, enters the acetabulum.

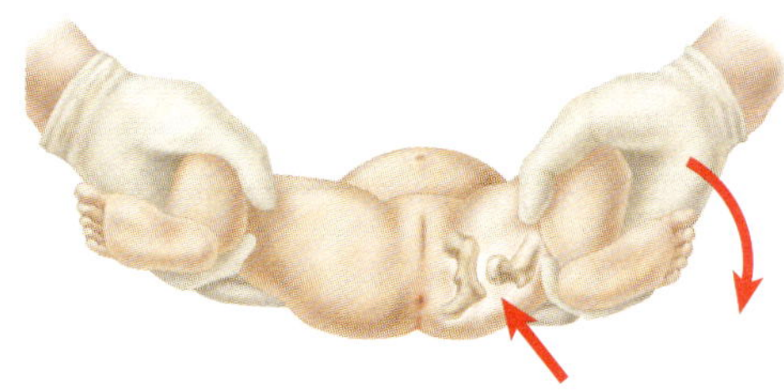

For the *Barlow test,* place your hands in the same position as for the Ortolani test. This time, press in the opposite direction with your thumbs moving down toward the table and outward. Feel for any movement of the head of the femur laterally. Normally there is no movement and the hip feels "stable." If you feel the head of the femur slipping out onto the posterior lip of the acetabulum, this constitutes a *positive Barlow's sign*. If you do feel this dislocation movement, abduct the hip by pressing with your index and middle fingers back inward and feel for the movement of the femoral head as it returns to the hip socket.

A positive Barlow's sign is not diagnostic of a *dysplastic hip,* but it indicates laxity and a dislocatable hip progressively, and the baby needs to be reexamined in the future.

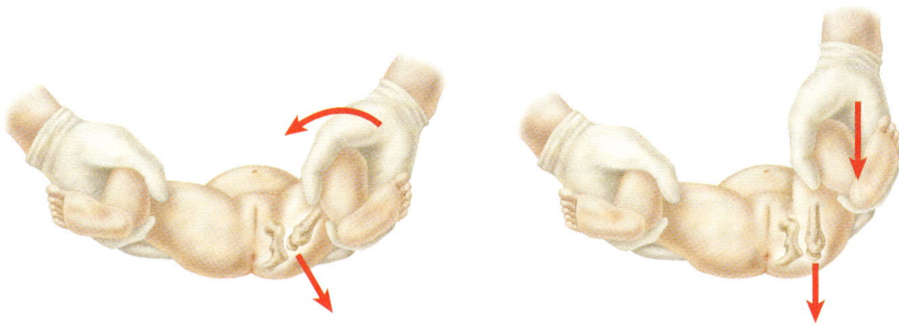

Children older than 3 months may have a negative Ortolani or Barlow sign and still have a *dislocated hip* due to tightening of the hip muscles and ligaments.

In addition to examining the hips, it is important to examine a newborn or infant's *legs and feet* to detect developmental abnormalities. Assess symmetry, bowing, and torsion of the legs. There should be no discrepancy in leg length. It is common for normal infants to have asymmetric thigh skinfolds, but if you do detect asymmetry, make sure you perform the instability tests because dislocated hips are commonly associated with this finding.

Most newborns are *bowlegged,* reflecting their curled up intrauterine position. During early infancy, there is a common and normal progression of increased bowlegged growth (as shown below, left), which begins to disappear at about 18 months of age, often followed by transition toward knock-knees. The *knock-knee pattern* (as shown below, right), is usually maximal by age 3 to 4 years, and gradually corrects by age 9 or 10 years.

Severe bowing of the legs (genu varum) may still be physiologic bowing and will spontaneously resolve. Extreme bowing or unilateral bowing may be due to pathologic causes such as *rickets* or *tibia vara (Blount's disease)*.

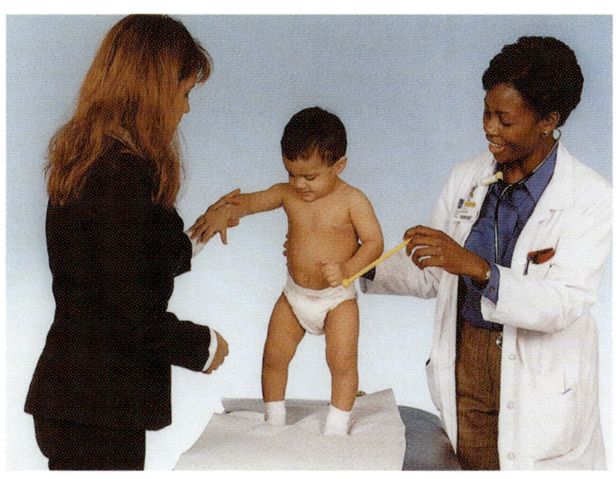

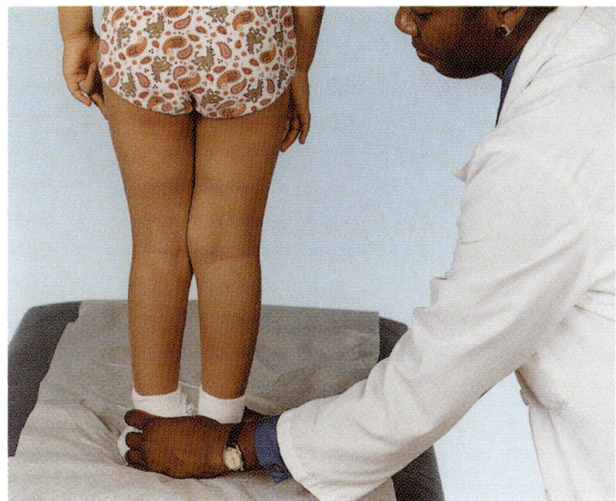

Another finding after 3 months of age is apparent femoral shortening (*positive Galeazzi* or *Alice test*). The picture below demonstrates this technique. Place the feet together and note any difference in knee heights.

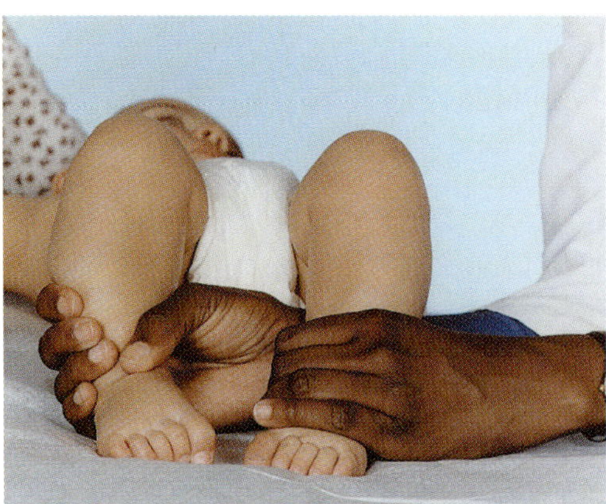

Some normal infants exhibit twisting or *torsion of the tibia* inwardly or outwardly on its longitudinal axis. Parents may be concerned about a toeing in or toeing out of the foot and an awkward gait, all of which are usually normal. Tibial torsion corrects itself during the second year of life after months of weight bearing.

Pathologic tibial torsion occurs only in association with *deformities of the feet or hips.*

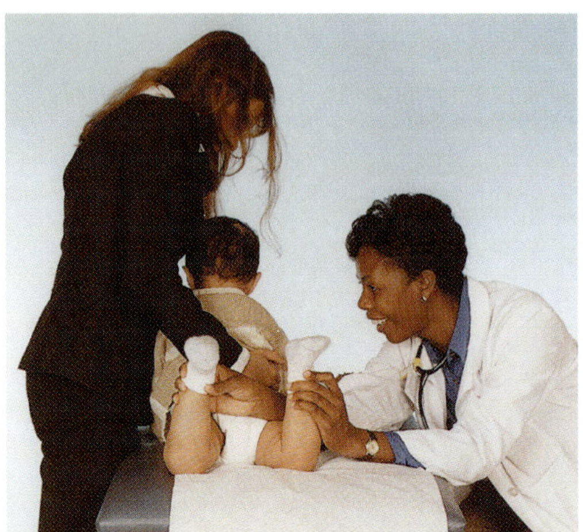

The presence of tibial torsion can be assessed in several ways; one method is shown above. Have the toddler lie prone on the examination table, with the knees flexed to 90°, as shown. Note the thigh–foot axis. Usually there is ±10° of internal or external rotation.

Children may *toe in* when they begin to walk. This may increase up to 4 years and then gradually disappear by around 10 years of age.

Now examine the feet of newborns and infants. At birth, the feet may appear deformed from retaining their intrauterine positioning, often turned inward as shown on the following page. Manipulate the affected foot—a

True *deformities of the feet* do not return to the neutral position even with manipulation.

normal foot should be easy to correct to the neutral and even to an overcorrected position. Also, you can scratch or stroke along the outer edge to see if the foot assumes a normal position.

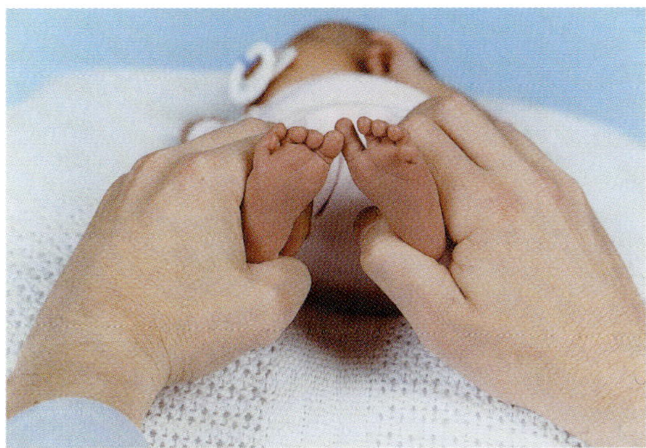

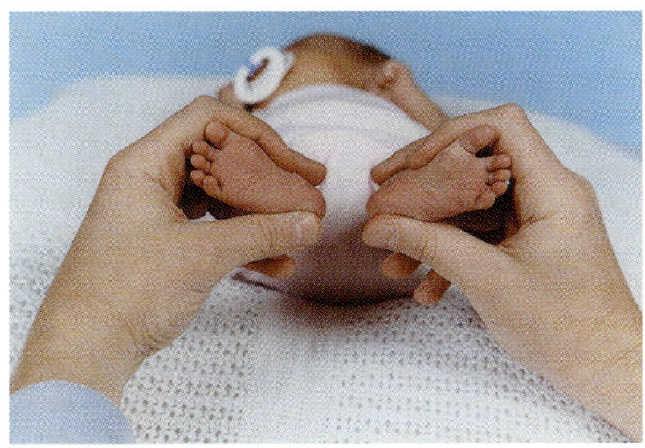

The normal newborn's foot has several features that may initially concern you. These features, shown on the next page, are benign. The newborn's foot appears flat because of a plantar fat pad. There is often inversion of the foot, elevating the medial margin. Other babies will have adduction of the forefoot without inversion, called *metatarsus adductus.* Still others will have adduction of the entire foot. Finally, most toddlers have some pronation during early stages of weight bearing, with eversion of the foot. In all of these normal variants, the abnormal position can be easily overcorrected past midline. They all tend to resolve within a year or two. The series of illustrations on the next page shows examples of pathologic foot deformities of newborns and infants.

EARLY AND LATE CHILDHOOD

In older children, abnormalities of the upper extremities are rare in the absence of injury.

Toddlers may acquire *nursemaid's elbow* or subluxation of the radial head due to a tugging injury.

The normal young child has increased lumbar concavity and decreased thoracic convexity compared with the adult, and often a protuberant abdomen.

Observe the child standing and walking barefoot. You can also ask the child to touch the toes, rise from a sitting position, run a short distance, and pick up objects. You will detect most abnormalities by watching carefully from

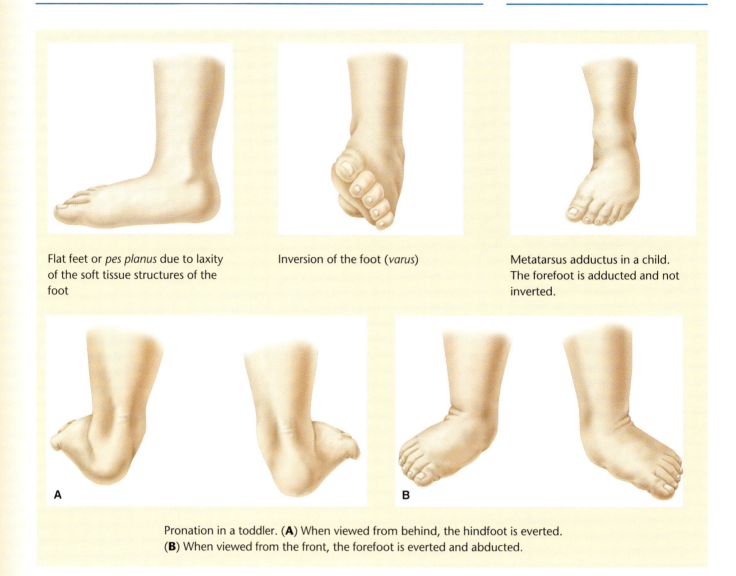

Flat feet or *pes planus* due to laxity of the soft tissue structures of the foot

Inversion of the foot (*varus*)

Metatarsus adductus in a child. The forefoot is adducted and not inverted.

A

B

Pronation in a toddler. (**A**) When viewed from behind, the hindfoot is everted. (**B**) When viewed from the front, the forefoot is everted and abducted.

both front and behind. To indirectly assess the gait pattern of the child, you can also note the soles of the shoes to see which side of the soles is worn down.

Inspect any child who can stand for *scoliosis* using techniques described below. Make sure to have the child bend forward with the knees straight (*Adams bend test*). Evaluate any asymmetry in positioning or gait. Scoliosis in a young child is unusual and abnormal; mild scoliosis in an older child is not uncommon.

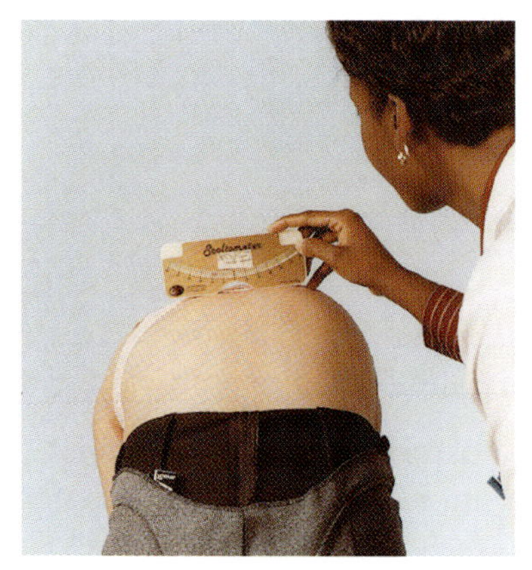

If you detect scoliosis, you can use a *scoliometer* to test for the degree of scoliosis. With the child standing, look for asymmetry of the shoulder blades or gluteal folds. Have the child bend forward as described.

Several types of *scoliosis* may present during childhood. Idiopathic scoliosis (75% of cases), seen mostly in girls, is usually detected in early adolescence.

Look for prominence of the posterior ribs. Place the scoliometer over the spine at a point of maximum prominence, making sure that the spine is parallel to the floor at that point, as shown on the previous page. Have the child bend fully forward to assess lumbar scoliosis, and less so to assess thoracic scoliosis.

You can also use a *plumb line,* a string with a weight attached, to assess symmetry of the back. Place the top of the plumb line at C-7 and have the child stand straight. The plumb line should extend to the gluteal crease (not shown here).

Test for severe hip disease, with its associated weakness of the gluteus medius muscle—observe the child from behind as the child shifts weight from one leg to the other. The pelvis should remain level when the weight is borne on the unaffected side, called a *negative Trendelenburg's sign.*

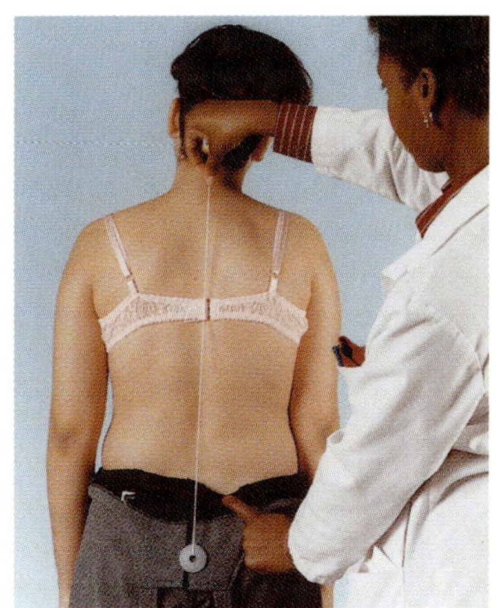

In *severe hip disease,* the pelvis tilts toward the unaffected hip when weight is borne on the affected side (an abnormal *positive Trendelenburg's sign*).

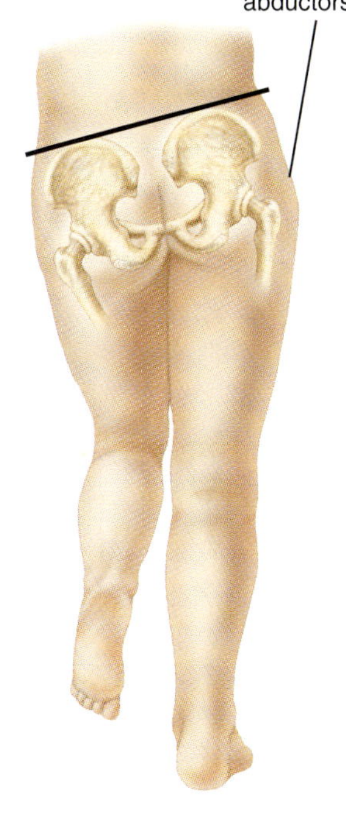

Determine any *leg shortening* that may accompany hip disease by comparing the distance from the anterior superior spine of the ilium to the medial malleolus on each side. First, straighten out the child by gently pulling on the legs and then compare the levels of the medial malleoli to each other. You can also put a small ink dot over the prominent malleoli and touch them together to give you a contact point to measure.

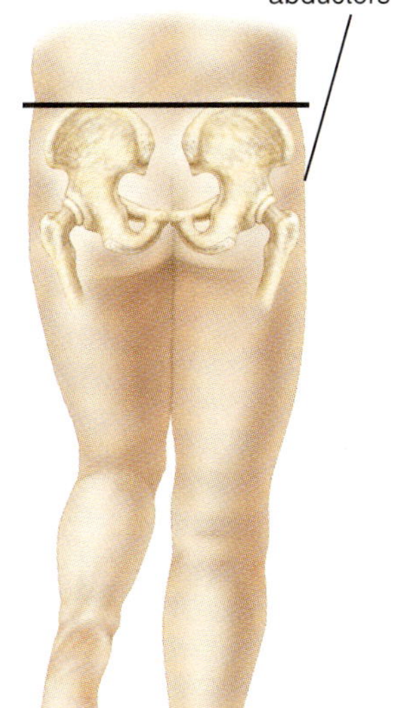

Also, have the child stand straight and place your hands horizontally over the iliac crests from behind, as shown in the photo on the next page. Small discrepancies in leg length can be appreciated. If such a discrepancy is noted, a clever trick is to place a book under the shorter leg; this should eliminate the discrepancy.

The musculoskeletal examination of the adolescent is similar to that of the adult. Pay particular attention to the possibility of scoliosis.

More than 25 million children and adolescents in the United States and a large number in other countries participate in organized sports and often

Important risk factors for sudden cardiovascular death during sports include episodes of *dizziness or palpitations, prior syncope* (particularly if associated with exercise), or family history of *sudden death* in young or middle-aged relatives.

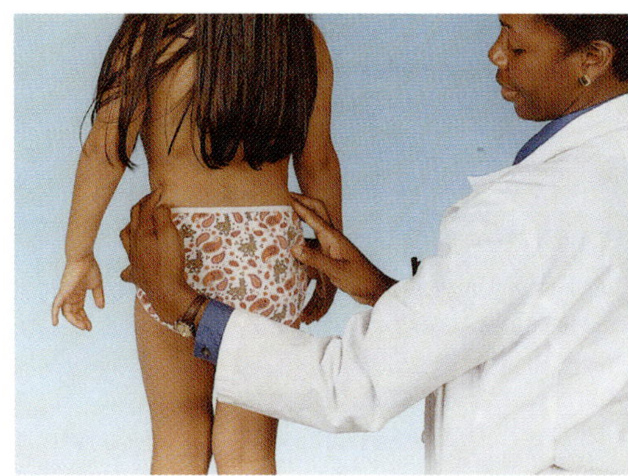

require "medical clearance." Start the exam with a thorough medical history, focusing on cardiovascular risk factors, prior surgeries, prior injuries, other medical problems, and a family history. The preparticipation physical exam is often the only time a healthy adolescent will see a medical professional, so it is important to include some screening questions and anticipatory guidance (see the discussion on Health Promotion and Counseling). Finally, perform a general physical, with special attention to the cardiac and lung exams and a vision and hearing screen. The preparticipation exam should then include a focused, thorough musculoskeletal exam, looking for weakness, limited range of motion, and evidence of previous injury.

During the preparticipation sports physical, assess carefully for cardiac *murmurs* and *wheezing* in the lungs.

A 2-minute preparticipation screening musculoskeletal examination has been recommended.

Screening Musculoskeletal Examination for Children Participating in Sports

Specific Components of the Musculoskeletal Examination		
Positioning	*Instructions to Patients*	**Common Abnormalities Due to Prior Injury**
	1. Stand straight, facing you.	Asymmetry, swelling of joints

(continued)

Screening Musculoskeletal Examination for Children Participating in Sports (Continued)

Specific Components of the Musculoskeletal Examination		
Positioning	*Instructions to Patients*	**Common Abnormalities Due to Prior Injury**
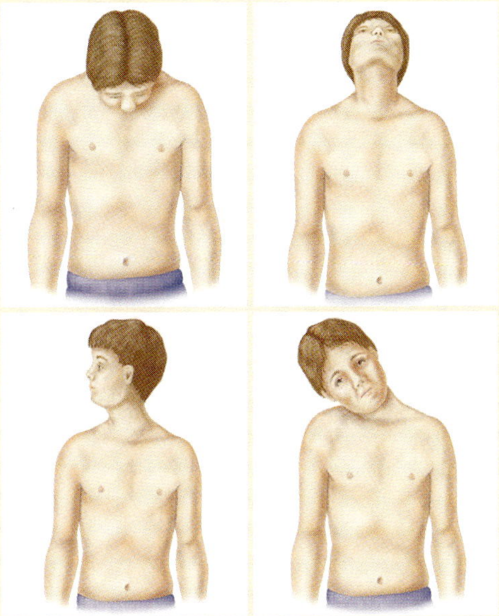	2. Move neck in all directions—look at the ceiling and floor, touch ears to shoulders.	Loss of range of motion
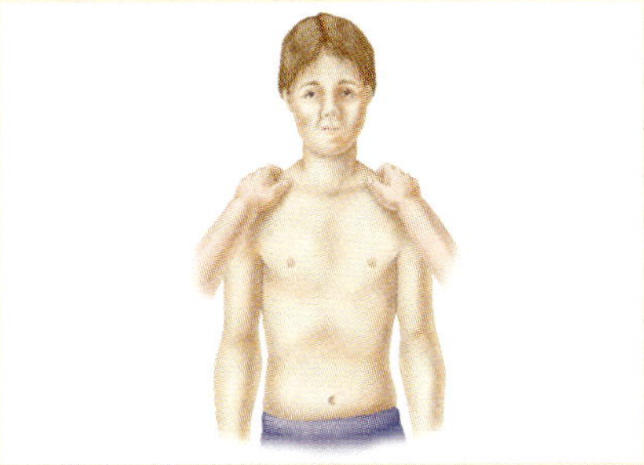	3. Shrug shoulders while you hold them down.	Weakness of shoulder, neck, or trapezius muscles
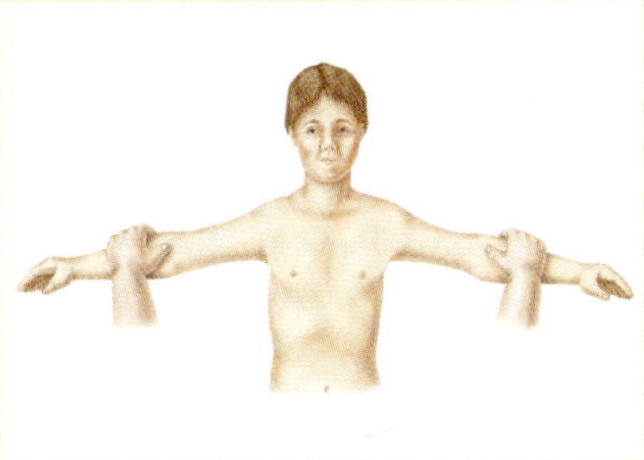	4. Hold arms out to side and lift arms while you press down.	Loss of strength of deltoid muscle

(continued)

Screening Musculoskeletal Examination for Children Participating in Sports *(Continued)*

Specific Components of the Musculoskeletal Examination		
Positioning	*Instructions to Patients*	**Common Abnormalities Due to Prior Injury**
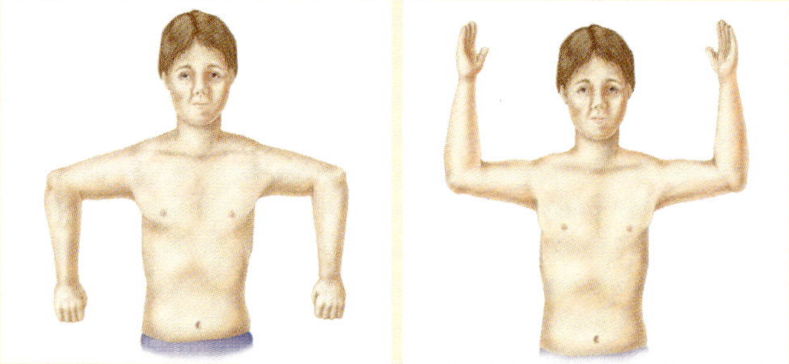	5. Hold arms out to side with elbows bent 90°, raise and lower arms.	Loss of external rotation and injury to glenohumeral joint
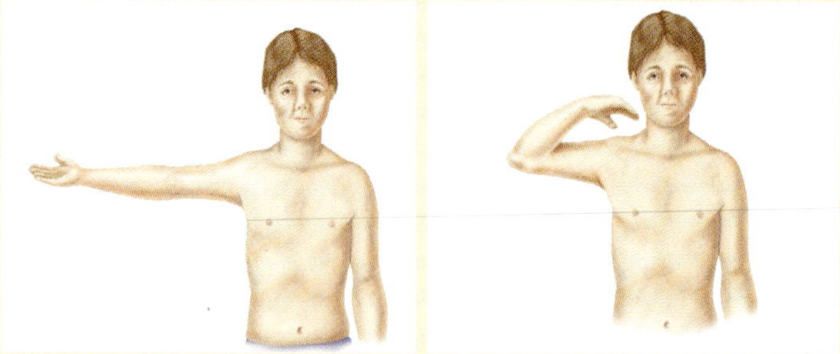	6. Hold arms out, completely bend and straighten elbows.	Reduced range of motion of elbow
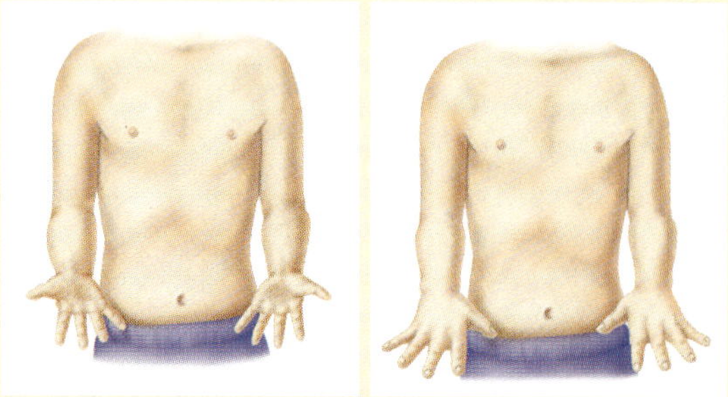	7. Hold arms down, bend elbows 90° and pronate and supinate forearm.	Reduced range of motion from injury to forearm, elbow, or wrist
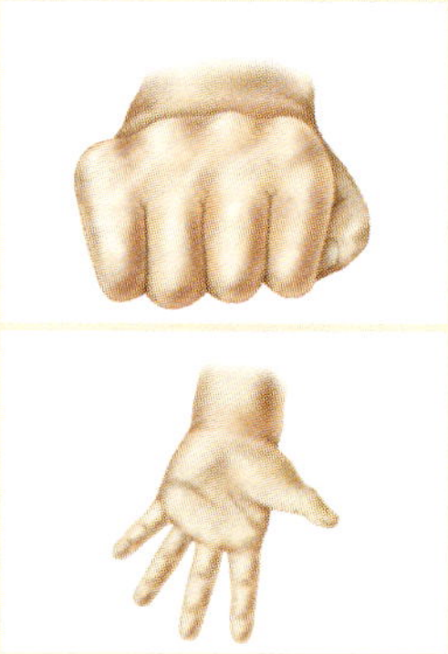	8. Make a fist, clench and then spread fingers.	Protruding knuckle, reduced range of motion of fingers from prior sprain or fracture

(continued)

Specific Components of the Musculoskeletal Examination: *Positioning*	*Instructions to Patients*	Common Abnormalities Due to Prior Injury
	9. Squat and duck-walk for four steps toward you.	Inability to fully flex knees and difficulty standing up due to prior knee or ankle injury
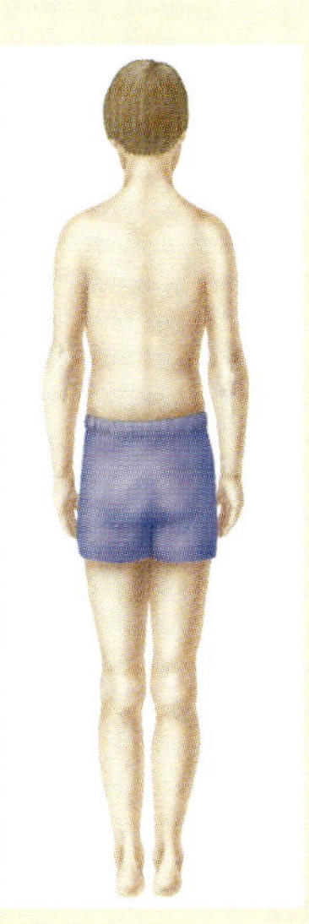	10. Stand straight with arms at sides, back to you.	Asymmetry from scoliosis, or leg-length discrepancy, or weakness from injury
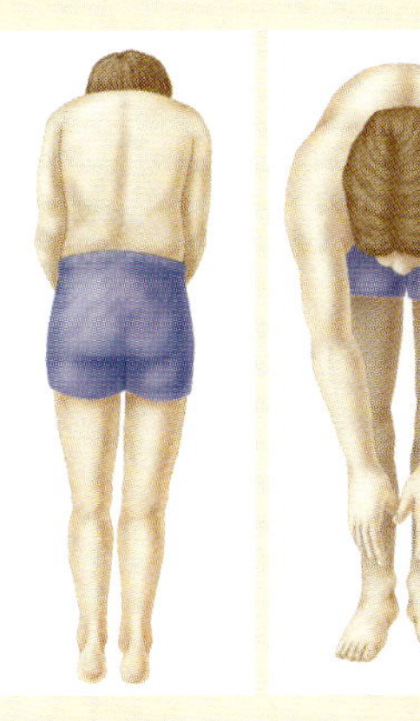	11. Bend forward with knees straight and touch toes.	Asymmetry from scoliosis, and twisting of back from low back pain
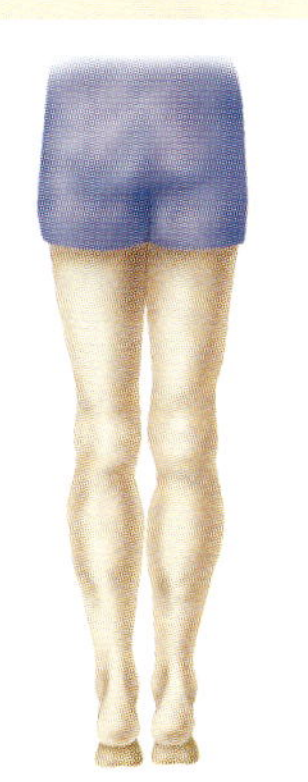 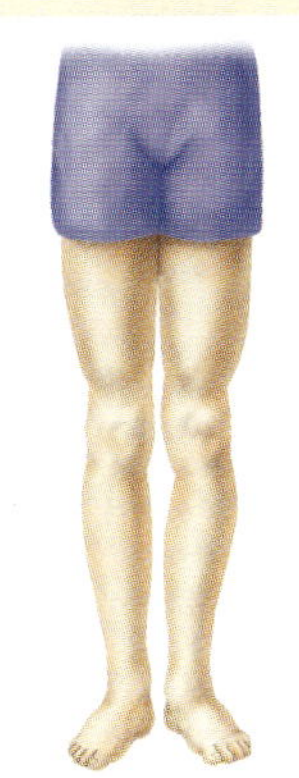	12. Stand on heels and rise to the toes.	Wasting of calf muscles from ankle or Achilles tendon injury

The Nervous System

The examination of the nervous system in infants and children has several special characteristics. The examination includes techniques that are highly specific to a particular age, especially for infants. Testing primitive reflexes is important in infants; they are only present at certain ages and then disappear. Absent reflexes or retention of these reflexes may signify abnormalities. In general, the examination of the nervous system of infants and young children is highly dependent on both internal and external factors listed here.

UNIQUE ASPECTS OF THE PEDIATRIC NEUROLOGIC EXAMINATION

- Age-specific
- Some reflexes are only present at certain ages.
- Findings are greatly affected by factors:
  - Internal: alertness, timing with respect to feeding and sleeping
  - External: presence of parents, fearful stimuli
- Neurologic changes often present as developmental abnormalities.
- Neurologic and developmental examinations often are combined.

It is important to note that while many neurologic abnormalities in adults produce asymmetric localized findings, neurologic abnormalities in infants and young children often present as developmental abnormalities, such as failure to do age-appropriate tasks. Therefore, the neurologic and developmental examinations need to proceed hand in hand. Finding a developmental abnormality should prompt you to pay particular attention to the neurologic examination.

NEWBORN PERIOD AND INFANCY

The neurologic screening examination of all newborns should include assessment of mental status, gross and fine motor function, tone, cry, deep tendon reflexes, and primitive reflexes. More detailed examination of cranial nerve function, sensory function, and less common primitive reflexes are indicated if you suspect any abnormalities from the history or screening. The neurologic examination can reveal extensive disease but will not pinpoint specific functional deficits or minute lesions.

Assess the *mental status* of newborns by observing many of the newborn activities discussed on pp. 644–645 ("What newborns can do"). Make sure you test the newborn during alert periods, and, if possible, return at a later time if the baby is transiently too drowsy.

Persistent irritability in the newborn may be a sign of *neurologic insult,* or may reflect a variety of *metabolic, infectious,* or other *constitutional abnormalities,* or environmental conditions such as *drug withdrawal.*

Assess the *motor tone* of newborns and infants, first by carefully watching their position at rest and testing their resistance to passive movement.

Then assess *tone* as you move each major joint through its range of motion, noting any spasticity or flaccidity. Hold the baby in your hands, as shown

Newborns with *hypotonia* often lie in a frog-leg position, with arms

below, to determine if the tone is normal, increased, or decreased. Either increased or decreased tone may indicate intracranial disease, although such disease is usually accompanied by a number of other signs.

flexed and hands near the ears. Hypotonia can be caused by a variety of *central nervous system abnormalities* and *disorders of the motor unit.*

SIGNS OF SEVERE NEUROLOGIC DISEASE

- Extreme irritability
- Persistent asymmetry of posture
- Persistent extension of extremities
- Constant turning of head to one side
- Marked extension of head, neck, and extremities (opisthotonus)
- Severe flaccidity
- Limited response to pain

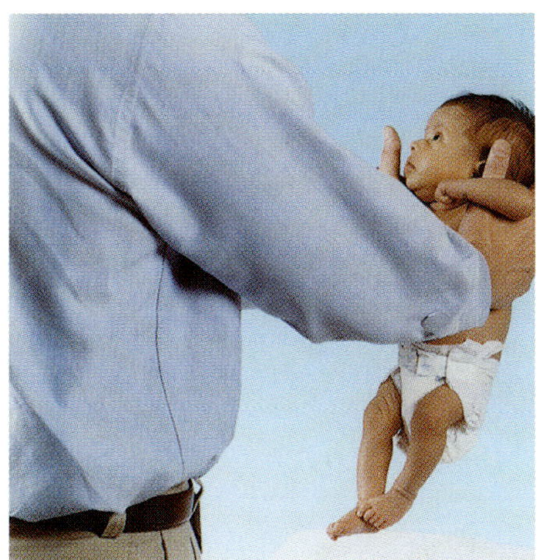

You can only test for *sensory function* of the newborn in a limited way. Test for pain sensation by flicking the infant's palm or sole with your finger. Observe for withdrawal, arousal, and change in facial expression. Do not use a pin to test for pain.

The *cranial nerves* of the newborn or infant can be tested, although you will have to open your bag of tricks for special methods that differ from those used for the older child or adult. The table on the next page provides some useful strategies.

Persistent effects of anesthesia may limit a newborn's response to pain. If changes in facial expression or cry follow a painful stimulus but no withdrawal occurs, *paralysis* may be present.

The *deep tendon reflexes* are variable in newborns and infants because the corticospinal pathways are not fully developed. Thus, their exaggerated presence or their absence has little diagnostic significance unless this response is different from results of previous testing, or extreme responses are observed.

A progressive increase in deep tendon reflexes during the first year of life may indicate central nervous system disease such as *cerebral palsy,* especially if it is coupled with increased tone.

Strategies to Assess Cranial Nerves in Newborns and Infants

Cranial Nerve		Strategy
I	Olfactory	Difficult to test
II	Visual acuity	Have baby regard your face and look for facial response and tracking.
II, III	Response to light	Darken room, raise baby to sitting position to open eyes. Use light and test for *optic blink reflex* (blinking in response to light). Use the otoscope (without a speculum) to assess papillary responses.
III, IV, VI	Extraocular movements	Observe tracking as the baby regards your smiling face move side-to-side. Use light if needed.
V	Motor	Test rooting reflex. Test sucking reflex (watch baby suck breast, bottle, or possibly pacifier).
VII	Facial	Observe baby crying and smiling, note symmetry of face and forehead.
VIII	Acoustic	Test acoustic blink reflex (blinking of both eyes in response to loud noise). Observe tracking in response to sound.
IX, X	Swallow Gag	Observe coordination during swallowing. Test for gag reflex.
XI	Spinal accessory	Observe symmetry of shoulders.
XII	Hypoglossal	Observe coordination of swallowing, sucking, and tongue thrusting. Pinch nostrils, observe reflex opening of mouth with tip of tongue to midline.

Use the same techniques to elicit deep tendon reflexes as you would for an adult. You can substitute your index or middle finger for the neurologic hammer, as shown below.

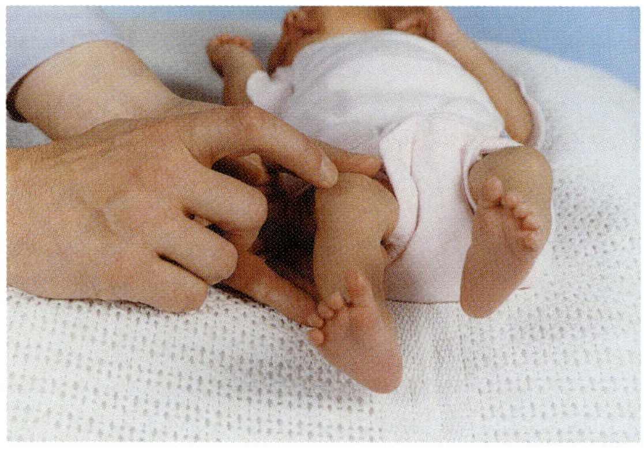

The triceps, brachioradialis, and abdominal reflexes are difficult to elicit before 6 months of age. The *anal reflex* is present at birth and important to elicit if a spinal cord lesion is suspected.

An absent anal reflex suggests loss of innervation of the external sphincter muscle caused by a

Although a normal flexion plantar response is obtained in 90% of infants, a *positive Babinski response* to plantar stimulation (dorsiflexion of big toe and fanning of other toes) can be elicited in some normal infants until 2 years of age.

spinal cord abnormality such as a congenital anomaly (e.g., *spina bifida*), *tumor*, or *injury*.

You can try to elicit the ankle reflex as for adults by tapping on the Achilles tendon but often will not get a response. Another method shown below is to grasp the infant's malleolus with one hand and abruptly dorsiflex the ankle. Don't be surprised if you note rapid, rhythmic plantar flexion of the newborn's foot (*ankle clonus*) in response to this maneuver. Up to 10 beats are normal in newborns and young infants; this is *unsustained ankle clonus*.

When the contractions are continuous (*sustained ankle clonus*), *central nervous system disease* should be suspected.

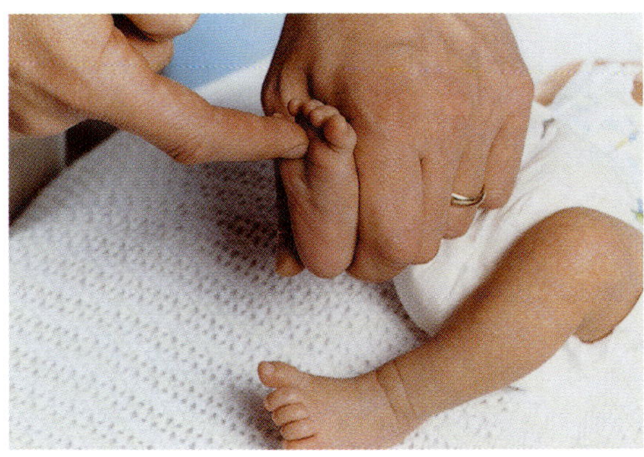

The newborn and infant's developing central nervous system can be evaluated by assessing *infantile automatisms*, called *primitive reflexes*. These develop during gestation, are generally demonstrable at birth, and disappear at defined ages. Abnormalities in these primitive reflexes suggest neurologic disease and merit more intensive investigation. The most important primitive reflexes are illustrated on the next page.

A *neurologic or developmental abnormality* is suspected if primitive reflexes are

- Absent at appropriate age
- Present longer than normal
- Asymmetric
- Associated with posturing or twitching

There are additional primitive reflexes shown on p. 731 not usually used in the general examination but helpful in a more extensive evaluation of an infant with abnormal neurologic findings. A summary of some general indicators of central nervous system disease in newborns and infants, including mild disease, is provided here.

GENERAL INDICATORS OF CENTRAL NERVOUS SYSTEM DISEASE DURING INFANCY

1. Abnormal localized neurologic findings
2. Asymmetry of movement of extremities
3. Failure to elicit expected primitive reflexes
4. Late persistence of primitive reflexes
5. Reemergence of vanished primitive reflexes
6. Delays in reaching developmental milestones
    - Gross motor
    - Fine motor
    - Cognitive and language
    - Social and emotional

Primitive Reflexes That Should Be Part of the Routine Neurologic Examination of Infants

Primitive Reflex	Maneuver	Ages	Examples of Abnormalities
Palmar Grasp Reflex	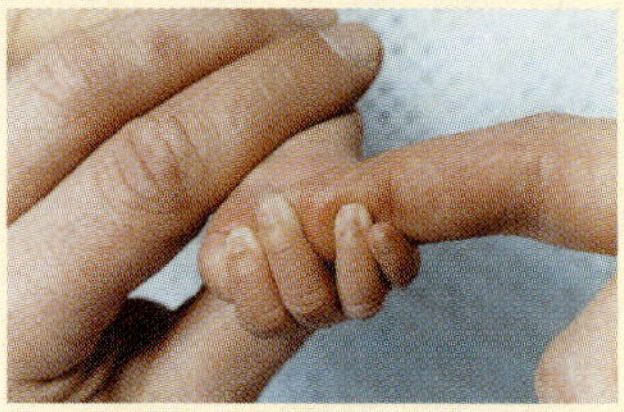 Place your fingers into the baby's hands and press against the palmar surfaces. The baby will flex all fingers to grasp your fingers.	Birth to 3–4 mos	Persistence beyond 4 mos suggests cerebral dysfunction. Persistence of clenched hand beyond 2 mos suggests central nervous system damage, especially if fingers overlap thumb.
Plantar Grasp Reflex	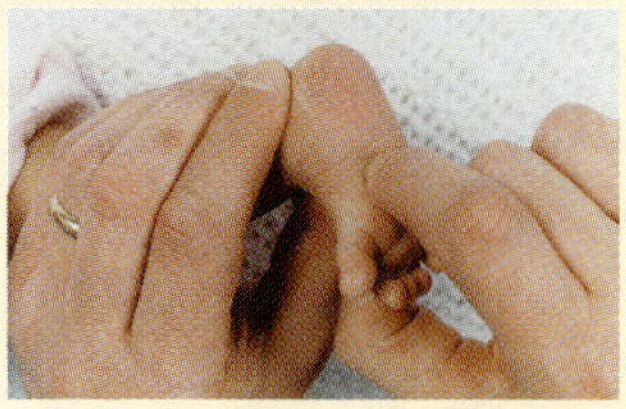 Touch the sole at the base of the toes. The toes curl.	Birth to 6–8 mos	Persistence beyond 8 mos suggests cerebral dysfunction.
Moro Reflex (Startle Reflex)	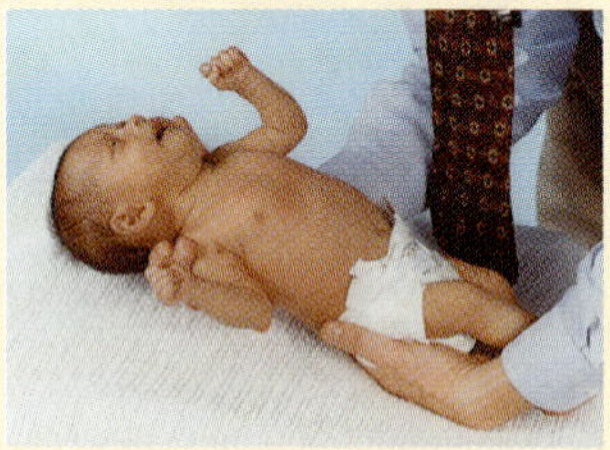 Hold the baby supine, supporting the head, back, and legs. Abruptly lower the entire body about 2 feet. The arms abduct and extend, hands open, and legs flex. Baby may cry.	Birth to 4–6 mos	Persistence beyond 4 mos suggests neurologic disease; beyond 6 mos strongly suggests it. Asymmetric response suggests fracture of clavicle or humerus or brachial plexus injury.
Asymmetric Tonic Neck Reflex	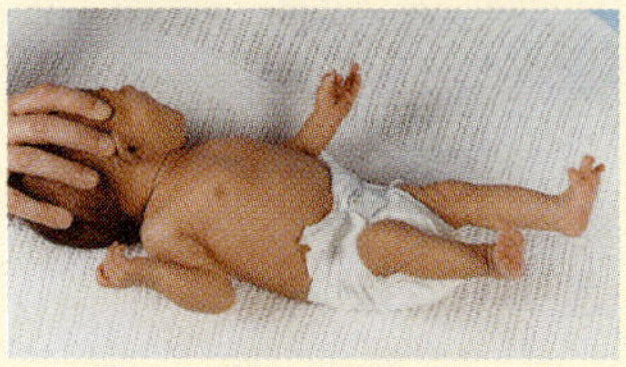 With baby supine, turn head to one side, holding jaw over shoulder. The arms/legs on side to which head is turned extend while the opposite arm/leg flex. Repeat on other side.	Birth to 2 mos	Persistence beyond 2 mos suggests neurologic disease.
Positive Support Reflex	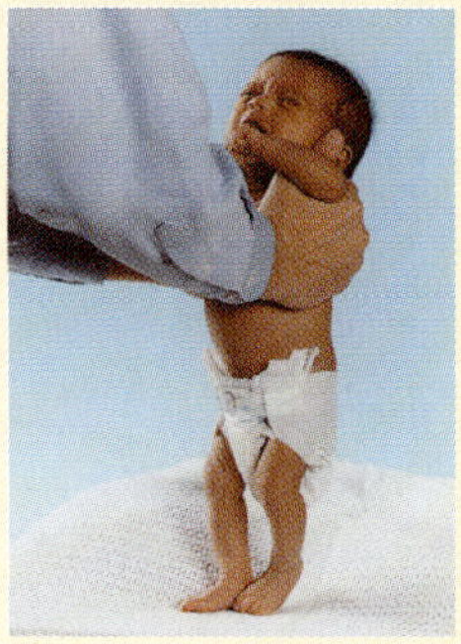 Hold the baby around the trunk and lower until the feet touch a flat surface. The hips, knees, and ankles extend, the baby stands up, partially bearing weight, sags after 20–30 seconds.	Birth or 2 mos until 6 mos	Lack of reflex suggests hypotonia or flaccidity. Fixed extension and adduction of legs (scissoring) suggests spasticity due to neurologic disease.

Additional Primitive Reflexes That Should Be Tested If Neurologic Abnormality Is Suspected

Primitive Reflex	Maneuver	Ages	
Rooting Reflex	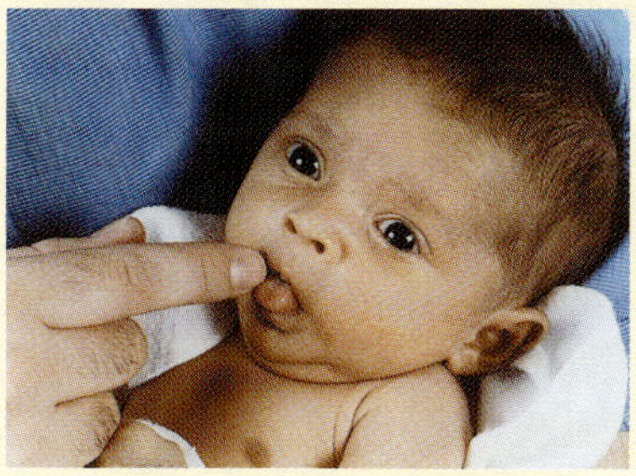 Stroke the perioral skin at the corners of the mouth. The mouth will open and baby will turn the head toward the stimulated side and suck.	Birth to 3–4 mos	Absence of rooting indicates severe generalized or central nervous system disease.
Trunk Incurvation (Galant's) Reflex	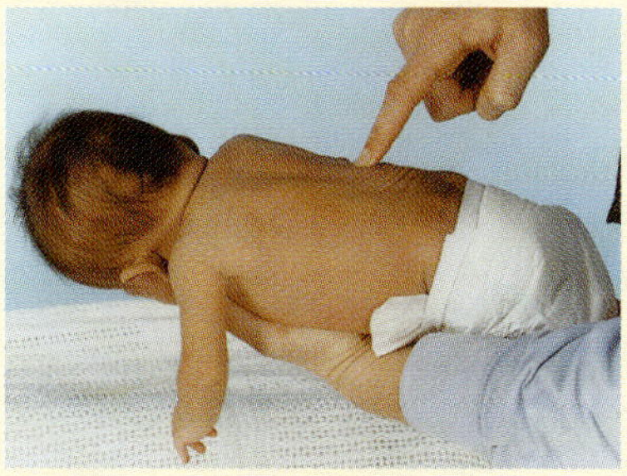 Support the baby prone with one hand, and stroke one side of the back 1 cm from midline, from shoulder to buttocks. The spine will curve toward the stimulated side.	Birth to 2 mos	Absence suggests a transverse spinal cord lesion or injury. Persistence may indicate delayed development.
Placing and Stepping Reflexes	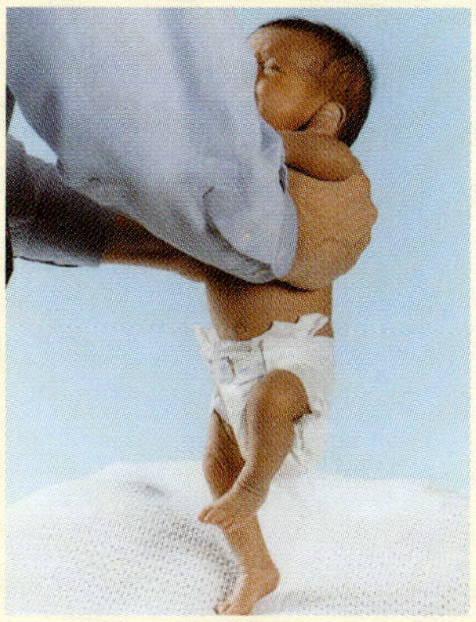 Hold baby upright from behind as in positive support reflex. Have one sole touch the tabletop. The hip and knee of that foot will flex and the other foot will step forward. Alternate stepping will occur.	Birth (best after 4 days). Variable age to disappear	Absence of placing may indicate paralysis. Babies born by breech delivery may not have placing reflex.
Landau Reflex	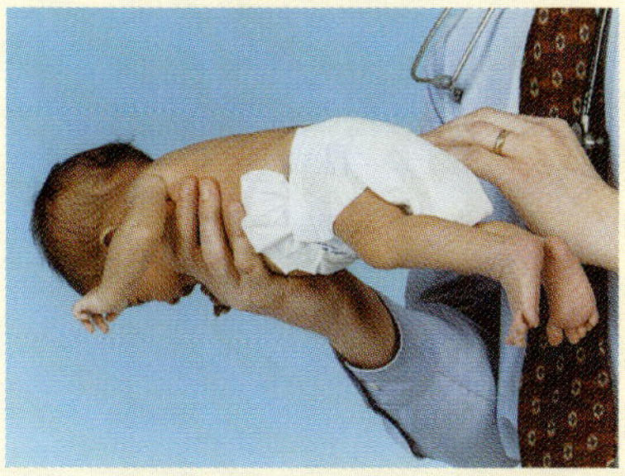 Suspend the baby prone with one hand. The head will lift up and the spine will straighten.	Birth to 6 mos	Persistence may indicate delayed development.
Parachute Reflex	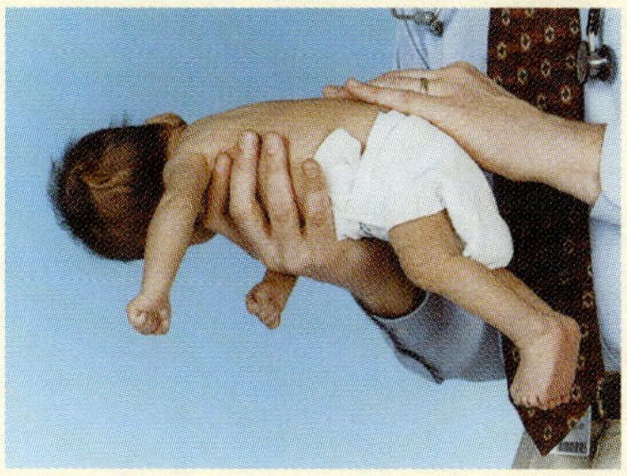 Suspend the baby prone and slowly lower the head toward a surface. The arms and legs will extend in a protective fashion.	4–6 mos and does not disappear	Delay in appearance may predict future delays in voluntary motor development

Refer to the developmental milestones on pp. 626–628 and to the DDST on pp. 738–739 to learn which age-specific developmental tasks to evaluate. The figure on this page pictorially displays the development of *gross motor skills* in the first year of life. By observation and play with the infant, you can do both a developmental screening examination and an assessment for gross and fine motor achievement. Specifically, look for *weakness* by observing sitting, standing, and transitions. Note *station,* or the posture of sitting or standing. Carefully observe the *gait* of the toddler, including balance and fluidity of movements. Fine motor development can be assessed in a similar way, combining the neurologic and developmental exam. Again, refer to the milestones on pp. 626–628 and 738–739. Key milestones include the development of the pincer grasp, ability to manipulate objects with the hands, and more precise tasks, such as building a tower of cubes or scribbling, as fine motor development progresses in a proximal to distal direction.

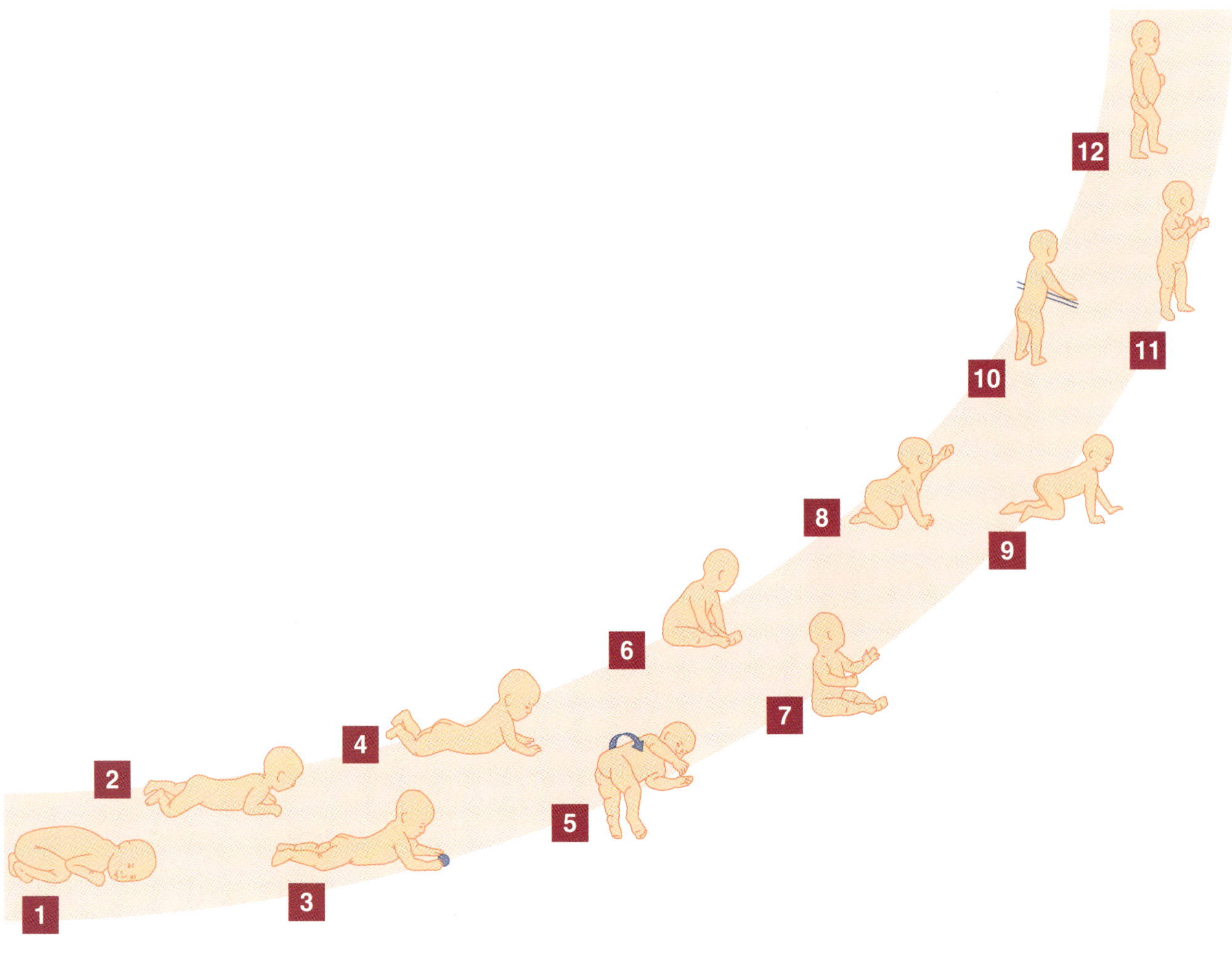

Cognitive and social/emotional development should also be assessed as you proceed with the comprehensive neurologic and developmental examination. Some neurologic abnormalities produce deficits or slowing in cognitive and social development. As stated, infants who have developmental delay may have abnormal findings on the neurologic examination because much of the examination is based on age-specific norms.

A normative measure of development is the developmental quotient, which is shown here:

$$\text{Developmental quotient} = \frac{\text{Developmental age}}{\text{Chronologic age}} \times 100$$

The development of an infant or child can be assessed using standard scales such as the DDST for each of the types of development. For example, you can assign to a child a gross motor developmental quotient, a fine motor developmental quotient, a cognitive developmental quotient, and so forth.

DEVELOPMENTAL QUOTIENTS

>85	Normal
70–85	Possibly delayed; follow-up needed
<70	Delayed

CASE EXAMPLES OF GROSS AND FINE MOTOR DEVELOPMENT

Gross Motor Development

A 12-month-old child who is just pulling to stand (gross motor developmental age of 9 mos), cruising (10 mos), and walking when both hands are held (10 mos) has a gross motor developmental age of 10 months. This child's gross motor developmental quotient is:

$(\frac{10}{12} \times 100) = 83$

This child is in the gray zone, is likely to do well without intervention, but requires close follow-up.

Fine Motor Development

A 12-month-old child can transfer objects from hand to hand (a fine motor developmental age of 6 mos), rake objects into his palm (7 mos), and pull things (7 mos). He cannot hold blocks in each hand and does not have thumb and finger grasp (8–9 mos).

He has normal primitive reflexes (most absent), increased tone, scissoring of legs when held, spasticity, and delays on the gross motor part of the DDST.

This child's fine motor developmental quotient is:

$(\frac{7}{12} \times 100) = 58$

This child is delayed in fine motor development and has signs of *cerebral palsy.*

EARLY AND LATE CHILDHOOD

Beyond infancy, when the primitive reflexes have disappeared, the neurologic examination includes the components evaluated in adults. Again, you should combine the neurologic and developmental assessment and will need to turn this into a game with the child. The goal is to assess optimal development and neurologic performance, and this requires the child to be cooperative.

Children with *spastic diplegias* will often have hypotonia as infants and then excessive tone with spasticity, scissoring, and perhaps clenched fists as toddlers and young children.

Perform the DDST as described and shown on pp. 738–739. Children usually enjoy this component, and you can too. Remember that the DDST is better at detecting delays in motor skills than in language or cognitive milestones.

The cranial nerves can be assessed quite well using developmentally appropriate strategies as shown in the following table:

Strategies to Assess Cranial Nerves in Young Children

Cranial Nerve		Strategy
I	Olfactory	Testable in older children.
II	Visual acuity	Use Snellen chart after age 3 years. Test visual fields as for an adult. A parent may need to hold the child's head.
III, IV, VI	Extraocular movements	Have the child track a light or an object (a toy is preferable). A parent may need to hold the child's head.
V	Motor	Play a game with a soft cotton ball to test sensation. Have the child clench the teeth and chew or swallow some food.
VII	Facial	Have the child "make faces" or imitate you as you make faces (including moving your eyebrows), and observe symmetry and facial movements.
VIII	Acoustic	Perform auditory testing after age 4 years. Whisper a word or command behind the child's back and have the child repeat it.
IX, X	Swallow and gag	Have the child stick the "whole tongue out" or "say 'ah'." Observe movement of the uvula and soft palate. Test the gag reflex.
XI	Spinal accessory	Have the child push your hand away with his head. Have the child shrug his shoulders while you push down with your hands to "see how strong you are."
XII	Hypoglossal	Ask the child to "stick out your tongue all the way."

An important part of the motor examination is to observe the child's gait while the child is walking and, optimally, running. Note any asymmetries, weakness, undue tripping or clumsiness. Follow the DDST examination

In children with uncoordinated gait, be sure to distinguish *orthopedic causes* such as positional

milestones to test for appropriate maneuvers such as heel-to-toe walking (photo below), hopping, and jumping. Use a toy to test for coordination and strength of the upper extremities.

deformities of the hip, knee, or foot from *neurologic* abnormalities such as *cerebral palsy, ataxia, neuromuscular conditions* producing weakness, or *degenerative diseases.*

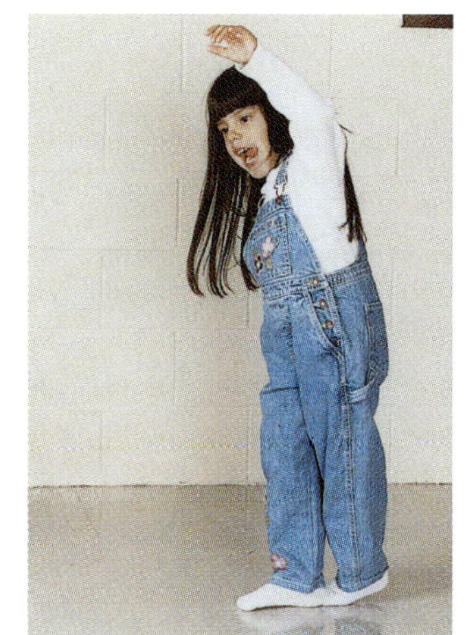

If you are concerned about the child's strength, have the child lie on the floor and then stand up, and closely observe the stages. Most normal children will first sit up, then flex the knees and extend the arms to the side to push off from the floor and stand up.

In certain forms of *muscular dystrophy* with weakness of the pelvic girdle muscles, children will rise to standing by rolling over prone and pushing off the floor with the arms while the legs remain extended (*Gower's sign*).

Hand preference is demonstrated in most children by age 2 and rarely before 18 months of age.

The sensory examination can be performed using a cotton ball or tickling the child. This is best performed with the child's eyes closed. Do not use pin pricks to evaluate sensation or else you will have a very uncooperative and unhappy patient!

Deep tendon reflexes can be tested as in adults. First demonstrate the use of the reflex hammer on the child's hand, assuring the child that it will not hurt. Children love to feel their legs bounce when you test their patellar reflexes. You will need to have the child cooperate and keep the eyes closed during some of this examination because tensing will disrupt the results.

You can ask children older than 3 years to draw a picture, copy objects as is done in the DDST, and then discuss their pictures to test simultaneously for fine motor coordination, cognition, and language.

It is important to distinguish between isolated delays in one aspect of development (e.g., coordination or language) and more generalized delays that occur in several components. The latter is more likely to reflect global neurologic disorders such as *mental retardation* that can be caused by a large number of etiologies.

The cerebellar examination can be tested using finger to nose and rapid alternating movements of the hands or fingers. Children enjoy this game. Children older than 5 years should be able to tell right from left, so you can assign them right–left discrimination tasks as is done in the adult patient.

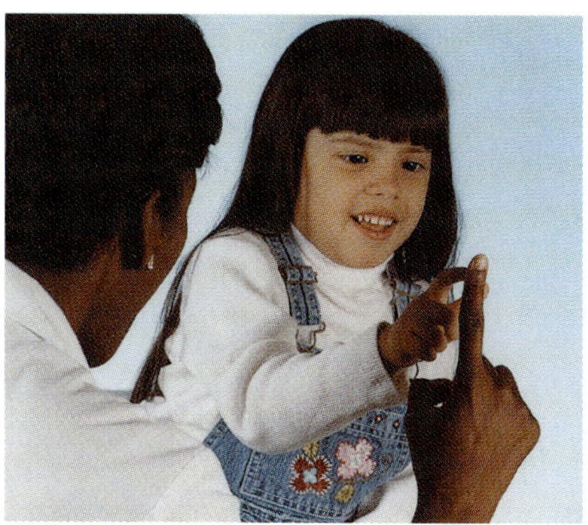

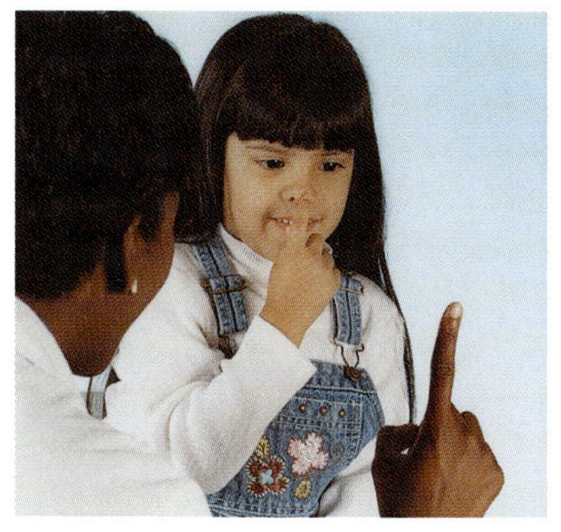

Use the expected milestones on the DDST and on pp. 628–631 to test for language, cognitive, and social and emotional development. Remember that the neurologic and developmental examinations require a cooperative child, so be patient, have fun, and don't be embarrassed to play and innovate as you refine your examination skills to the developmental level of your pediatric patient.

Some children who have *attention deficit disorder with hyperactivity (ADHD)* will have a great deal of difficulty cooperating with your neurologic and developmental examination due to problems focusing. These children often have high energy levels, cannot stay still for extended periods, and have a history of difficulty in school or structured situations.

THE ADOLESCENT

The neurologic examination of the adolescent and the adult is the same. Still, it is important to assess the adolescent's developmental achievement according to age-specific milestones as described on pp. 631–633.

TABLE 17-1 ■ Ballard Scoring System for Determining Gestational Age in Weeks

Neuromuscular Maturity

	-1	0	1	2	3	4	5
Posture							
Square Window (wrist)	>90°	90°	60°	45°	30°	0°	
Arm Recoil		180°	140°-180°	110°-140°	90-110°	<90°	
Popliteal Angle	180°	160°	140°	120°	100°	90°	<90°
Scarf Sign							
Heel to Ear							

Physical Maturity

Skin	sticky friable transparent	gelatinous red, translucent	smooth pink, visible veins	superficial peeling &/or rash. few veins	cracking pale areas rare veins	parchment deep cracking no vessels	leathery cracked wrinkled
Lanugo	none	sparse	abundant	thinning	bald areas	mostly bald	
Plantar Surface	heel-toe 40-50 mm: -1 <40 mm: -2	>50mm no crease	faint red marks	anterior transverse crease only	creases ant. 2/3	creases over entire sole	
Breast	imperceptible	barely perceptible	flat areola no bud	stippled areola 1-2mm bud	raised areola 3-4mm bud	full areola 5-10mm bud	
Eye/Ear	lids fused loosely: -1 tightly: -2	lids open pinna flat stays folded	sl. curved pinna; soft; slow recoil	well-curved pinna; soft but ready recoil	formed & firm instant recoil	thick cartilage ear stiff	
Genitals male	scrotum flat, smooth	scrotum empty faint rugae	testes in upper canal rare rugae	testes descending few rugae	testes down good rugae	testes pendulous deep rugae	
Genitals female	clitoris prominent labia flat	prominent clitoris small labia minora	prominent clitoris enlarging minora	majora & minora equally prominent	majora large minora small	majora cover clitoris & minora	

Maturity Rating

score	weeks
-10	20
-5	22
0	24
5	26
10	28
15	30
20	32
25	34
30	36
35	38
40	40
45	42
50	44

The Neuromuscular Maturity Criteria are depicted in the top half of the figure. Asphyxiated neonates or neonates obtunded by anesthetic agents or drugs will score lower on neuromuscular maturity criteria. In such instances, scoring should be repeated at 24 to 48 hours of age. The Physical Maturity Criteria are shown in the bottom half of the figure and are self-explanatory. The scores for each criterion are again the numbers at the top of the columns. The sum of the scores for all of the neuromuscular and physical maturity items provides an estimate of gestational age in weeks, using the maturity rating scale at the lower right portion of the figure. (Figure from Ballard JL, et. al. J. Pediatr 119:417, 1991.)

TABLE 17-2 ■ Denver Developmental Screening Test

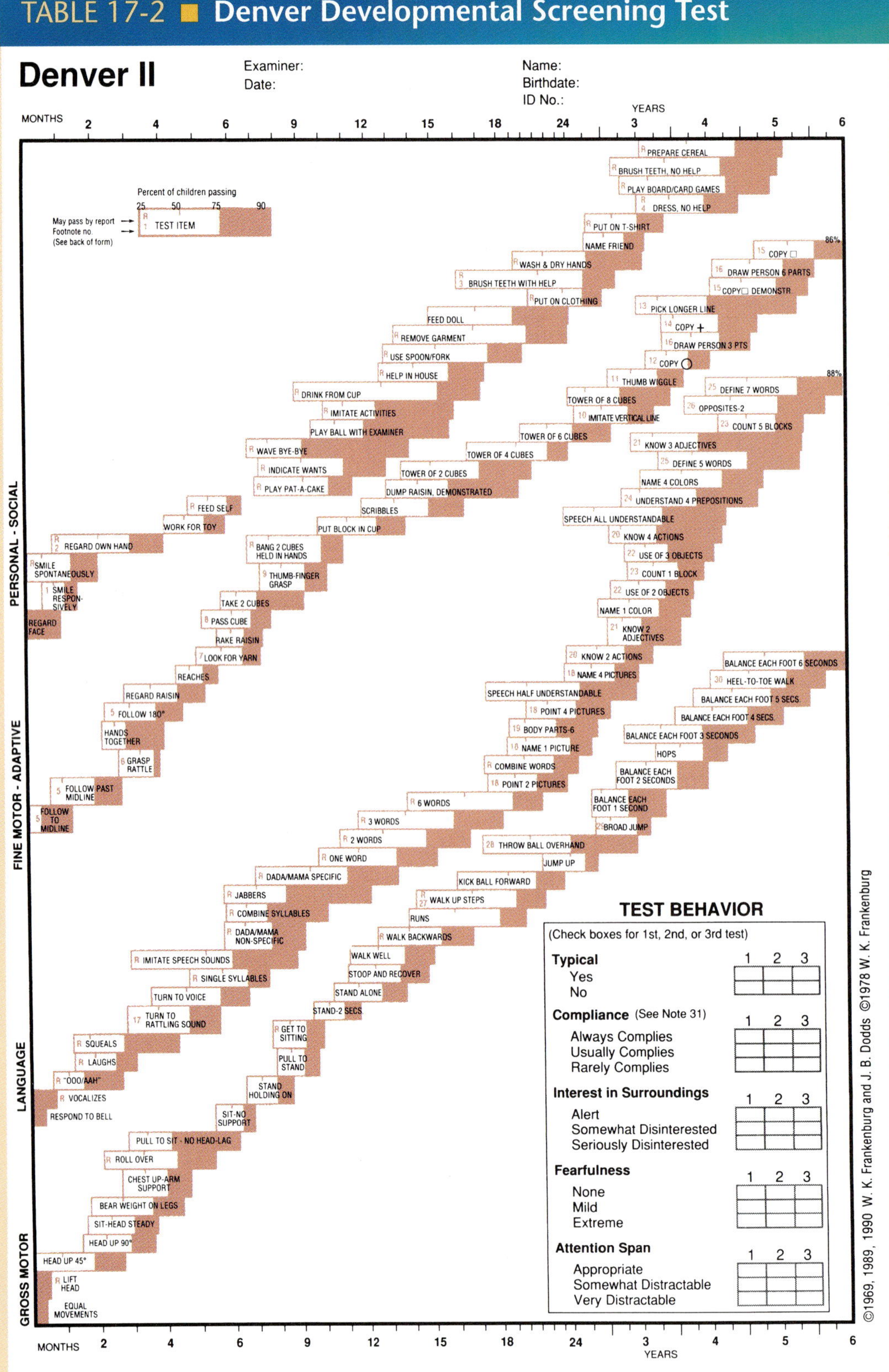

Testing kits, test forms, and reference manuals (which must be used to ensure accuracy in administration of the test) for the DDST may be ordered from Denver Developmental Materials Incorporated, P.O. Box 6919, Denver, CO 80206-0919. (Reprinted with permission from William K. Frankenburg, M.D.)

TABLE 17-2 ■ Denver Developmental Screening Test *(Continued)*

DIRECTIONS FOR ADMINISTRATION

1. Try to get child to smile by smiling, talking or waving. Do not touch him/her.
2. Child must stare at hand several seconds.
3. Parent may help guide toothbrush and put toothpaste on brush.
4. Child does not have to be able to tie shoes or button/zip in the back.
5. Move yarn slowly in an arc from one side to the other, about 8″ above child's face.
6. Pass if child grasps rattle when it is touched to the backs or tips of fingers.
7. Pass if child tries to see where yarn went. Yarn should be dropped quickly from sight from tester's hand without arm movement.
8. Child must transfer cube from hand to hand without help of body, mouth, or table.
9. Pass if child picks up raisin with any part of thumb and finger.
10. Line can vary only 30 degrees or less from tester's line.
11. Make a fist with thumb pointing upward and wiggle only the thumb. Pass if child imitates and does not move any fingers other than the thumb.

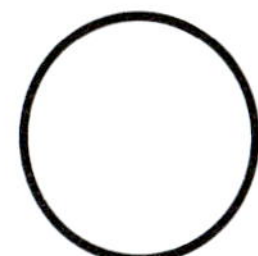

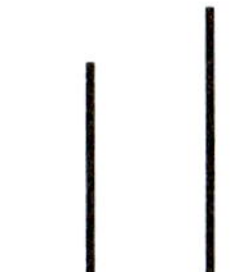

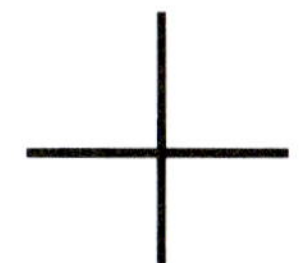

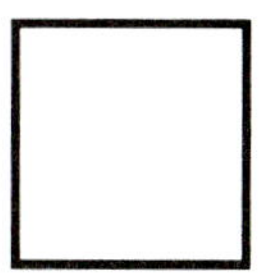

12. Pass any enclosed form. Fail continuous round motions.
13. Which line is longer? (Not bigger.) Turn paper upside down and repeat. (pass 3 of 3 or 5 of 6)
14. Pass any lines crossing near midpoint.
15. Have child copy first. If failed, demonstrate.

When giving items 12, 14, and 15, do not name the forms. Do not demonstrate 12 and 14.

16. When scoring, each pair (2 arms, 2 legs, etc.) counts as one part.
17. Place one cube in cup and shake gently near child's ear, but out of sight. Repeat for other ear.
18. Point to picture and have child name it. (No credit is given for sounds only.) If less than 4 pictures are named correctly, have child point to picture as each is named by tester.

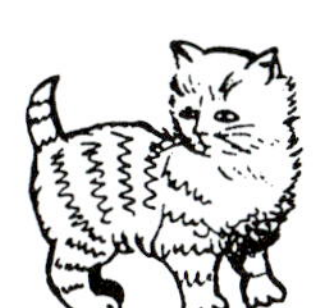

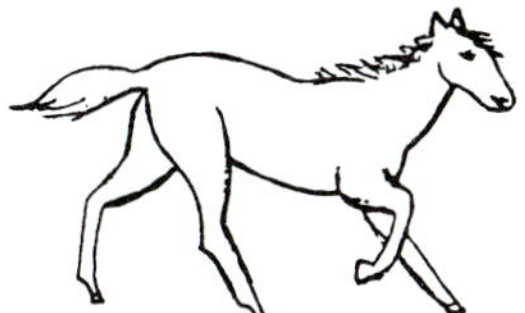

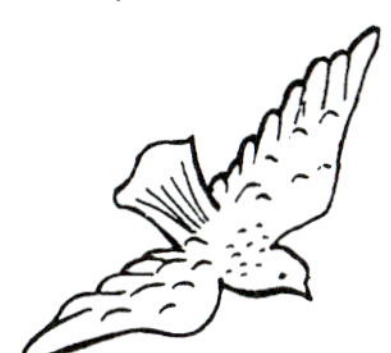

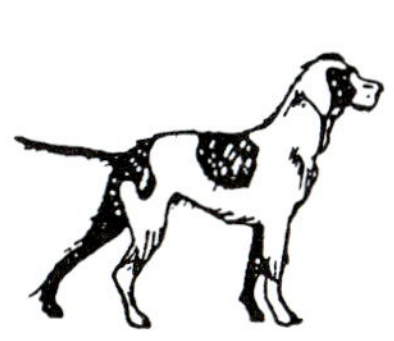

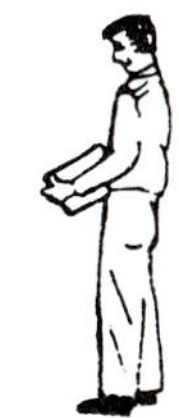

19. Using doll, tell child: Show me the nose, eyes, ears, mouth, hands, feet, tummy, hair. Pass 6 of 8.
20. Using pictures, ask child: Which one flies?... says meow?... talks?... barks?... gallops? Pass 2 of 5, 4 of 5.
21. Ask child: What do you do when you are cold?... tired?... hungry? Pass 2 of 3, 3 of 3.
22. Ask child: What do you do with a cup? What is a chair used for? What is a pencil used for? Action words must be included in answers.
23. Pass if child correctly places and says how many blocks are on paper. (1, 5)
24. Tell child: Put block **on** table; **under** table; **in front of** me, **behind** me. Pass 4 of 4. (Do not help child by pointing, moving head or eyes.)
25. Ask child: What is a ball?... lake?... desk?... house?... banana?... curtain?... fence?... ceiling? Pass if defined in terms of use, shape, what it is made of, or general category (such as banana is fruit, not just yellow). Pass 5 of 8, 7 of 8.
26. Ask child: If a horse is big, a mouse is __? If fire is hot, ice is __? If the sun shines during the day, the moon shines during the __? Pass 2 of 3.
27. Child may use wall or rail only, not person. May not crawl.
28. Child must throw ball overhand 3 feet to within arm's reach of tester.
29. Child must perform standing broad jump over width of test sheet (8½ inches).
30. Tell child to walk forward, heel within 1 inch of toe. Tester may demonstrate. Child must walk 4 consecutive steps.
31. In the second year, half of normal children are noncompliant.

OBSERVATIONS:

Instructions printed on the back of the DDST form for administering some of the items contained in the Denver Developmental Screening Test. (Reprinted with permission from William K. Frankenburg, M.D.)

TABLE 17-3 ■ Blood Pressure Levels for the 90th and 95th Percentiles of Blood Pressure for Boys Aged 1 to 17 Years by Percentiles of Height

Age, y	Blood Pressure Percentile*	Systolic Blood Pressure by Percentile of Height, mm Hg†							Diastolic Blood Pressure by Percentile of Height, mm Hg†						
		5%	10%	25%	50%	75%	90%	95%	5%	10%	25%	50%	75%	90%	95%
1	90th	94	95	97	98	100	102	102	50	51	52	53	54	54	55
	95th	98	99	101	102	104	106	106	55	55	56	57	58	59	59
2	90th	98	99	100	102	104	105	106	55	55	56	57	58	59	59
	95th	101	102	104	106	108	109	110	59	59	60	61	62	63	63
3	90th	100	101	103	105	107	108	109	59	59	60	61	62	63	63
	95th	104	105	107	109	111	112	113	63	63	64	65	66	67	67
4	90th	102	103	105	107	109	110	111	62	62	63	64	65	66	66
	95th	106	107	109	111	113	114	115	66	67	67	68	69	70	71
5	90th	104	105	106	108	110	112	112	65	65	66	67	68	69	69
	95th	108	109	110	112	114	115	116	69	70	70	71	72	73	74
6	90th	105	106	108	110	111	113	114	67	68	69	70	70	71	72
	95th	109	110	112	114	115	117	117	72	72	73	74	75	76	76
7	90th	106	107	109	111	113	114	115	69	70	71	72	72	73	74
	95th	110	111	113	115	116	118	119	74	74	75	76	77	78	78
8	90th	107	108	110	112	114	115	116	71	71	72	73	74	75	75
	95th	111	112	114	116	118	119	120	75	76	76	77	78	79	80
9	90th	109	110	112	113	115	117	117	72	73	73	74	75	76	77
	95th	113	114	116	117	119	121	121	76	77	78	79	80	80	81
10	90th	110	112	113	115	117	118	119	73	74	74	75	76	77	78
	95th	114	115	117	119	121	122	123	77	78	79	80	80	81	82
11	90th	112	113	115	117	119	120	121	74	74	75	76	77	78	78
	95th	116	117	119	121	123	124	125	78	79	79	80	81	82	83
12	90th	115	116	117	119	121	123	123	75	75	76	77	78	78	79
	95th	119	120	121	123	125	126	127	79	79	80	81	82	83	83
13	90th	117	118	120	122	124	125	126	75	76	76	77	78	79	80
	95th	121	122	124	126	128	129	130	79	80	81	82	83	83	84
14	90th	120	121	123	125	126	128	128	76	76	77	78	79	80	80
	95th	124	125	127	128	130	132	132	80	81	81	82	83	84	85
15	90th	123	124	125	127	129	131	131	77	77	78	79	80	81	81
	95th	127	128	129	131	133	134	135	81	82	83	83	84	85	86
16	90th	125	126	128	130	132	133	134	79	79	80	81	82	82	83
	95th	129	130	132	134	136	137	138	83	83	84	85	86	87	87
17	90th	128	129	131	133	134	136	136	81	81	82	83	84	85	85
	95th	132	133	135	136	138	140	140	85	85	86	87	88	89	89

*Blood pressure percentile was determined by a single measurement.

†Height percentile was determined by standard growth curves.

Reproduced with permission from Update on the 1987 Task Force Report on High Blood Pressure in Children and Adolescents: A Working Group Report from the National High Blood Pressure Education Program. Pediatrics 98:649, 1996.

TABLE 17-3 ■ Blood Pressure Levels for the 90th and 95th Percentiles of Blood Pressure for Girls Aged 1 to 17 Years by Percentiles of Height

Age, y	Blood Pressure Percentile*	Systolic Blood Pressure by Percentile of Height, mm Hg†							Diastolic Blood Pressure by Percentile of Height, mm Hg†						
		5%	10%	25%	50%	75%	90%	95%	5%	10%	25%	50%	75%	90%	95%
1	90th	97	98	99	100	102	103	104	53	53	53	54	55	56	56
	95th	101	102	103	104	105	107	107	57	57	57	58	59	60	60
2	90th	99	99	100	102	103	104	105	57	57	58	58	59	60	61
	95th	102	103	104	105	107	108	109	61	61	62	62	63	64	65
3	90th	100	100	102	103	104	105	106	61	61	61	62	63	63	64
	95th	104	104	105	107	108	109	110	65	65	65	66	67	67	68
4	90th	101	102	103	104	106	107	108	63	63	64	65	65	66	67
	95th	105	106	107	108	109	111	111	67	67	68	69	69	70	71
5	90th	103	103	104	106	107	108	109	65	66	66	67	68	68	69
	95th	107	107	108	110	111	112	113	69	70	70	71	72	72	73
6	90th	104	105	106	107	109	110	111	67	67	68	69	69	70	71
	95th	108	109	110	111	112	114	114	71	71	72	73	73	74	75
7	90th	106	107	108	109	110	112	112	69	69	69	70	71	72	72
	95th	110	110	112	113	114	115	116	73	73	73	74	75	76	76
8	90th	108	109	110	111	112	113	114	70	70	71	71	72	73	74
	95th	112	112	113	115	116	117	118	74	74	75	75	76	77	78
9	90th	110	110	112	113	114	115	116	71	72	72	73	74	74	75
	95th	114	114	115	117	118	119	120	75	76	76	77	78	78	79
10	90th	112	112	114	115	116	117	118	73	73	73	74	75	76	76
	95th	116	116	117	119	120	121	122	77	77	77	78	79	80	80
11	90th	114	114	116	117	118	119	120	74	74	75	75	76	77	77
	95th	118	118	119	121	122	123	124	78	78	79	79	80	81	81
12	90th	116	116	118	119	120	121	122	75	75	76	76	77	78	78
	95th	120	120	121	123	124	125	126	79	79	80	80	81	82	82
13	90th	118	118	119	121	122	123	124	76	76	77	78	78	79	80
	95th	121	122	123	125	126	127	128	80	80	81	82	82	83	84
14	90th	119	120	121	122	124	125	126	77	77	78	79	79	80	81
	95th	123	124	125	126	128	129	130	81	81	82	83	83	84	85
15	90th	121	121	122	124	125	126	127	78	78	79	79	80	81	82
	95th	124	125	126	128	129	130	131	82	82	83	83	84	85	86
16	90th	122	122	123	125	126	127	128	79	79	79	80	81	82	82
	95th	125	126	127	128	130	131	132	83	83	83	84	85	86	86
17	90th	122	123	124	125	126	128	128	79	79	79	80	81	82	82
	95th	126	126	127	129	130	131	132	83	83	83	84	85	86	86

*Blood pressure percentile was determined by a single reading.

†Height percentile was determined by standard growth curves.

Reproduced with permission from Update on the 1987 Task Force Report on High Blood Pressure in Children and Adolescents: A Working Group Report from the National High Blood Pressure Education Program. Pediatrics 98:649, 1996.

TABLE 17-4 ■ Growth Charts

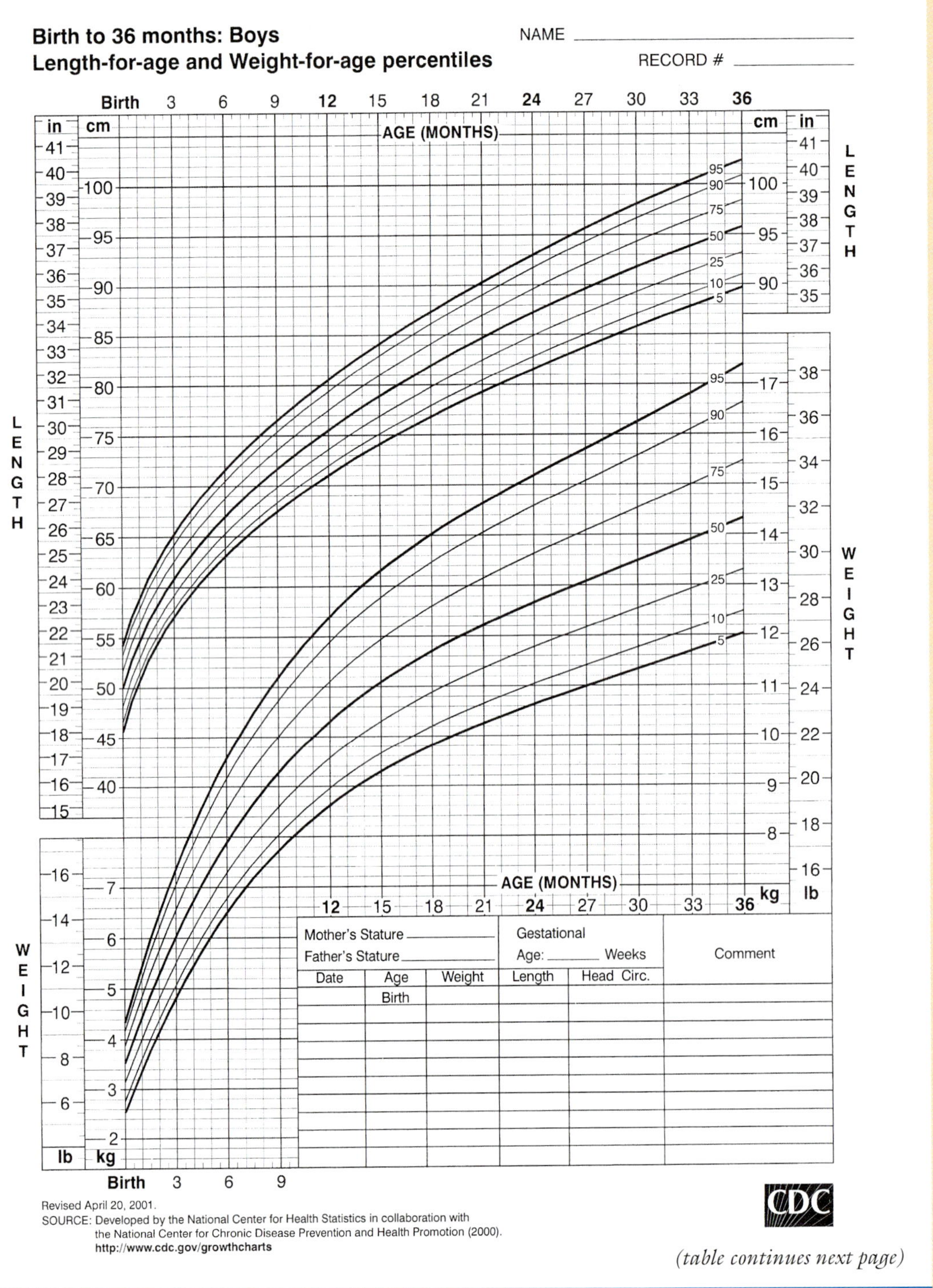
Birth to 36 months: Boys
Length-for-age and Weight-for-age percentiles
NAME
RECORD #
Birth 3 6 9 12 15 18 21 24 27 30 33 36
AGE (MONTHS)
in
cm
LENGTH
WEIGHT
95
90
75
50
25
10
5
lb
kg
Mother's Stature
Father's Stature
Gestational Age: Weeks
Comment
Date
Age
Weight
Length
Head Circ.
Birth
Revised April 20, 2001.
SOURCE: Developed by the National Center for Health Statistics in collaboration with the National Center for Chronic Disease Prevention and Health Promotion (2000).
http://www.cdc.gov/growthcharts
CDC

(table continues next page)

TABLE 17-4 ■ **Growth Charts** *(Continued)*

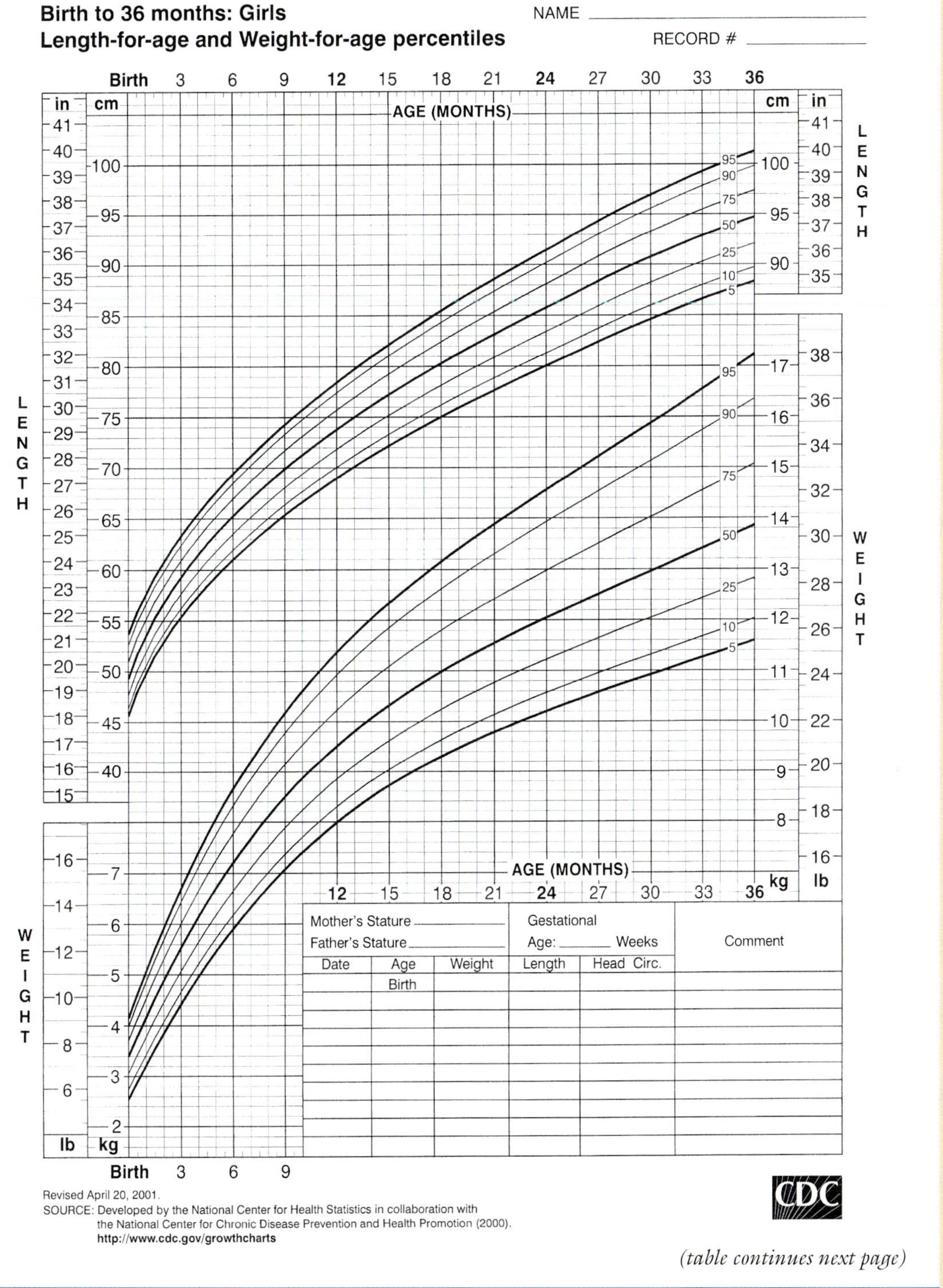

(table continues next page)

TABLE 17-4 ■ Growth Charts *(Continued)*

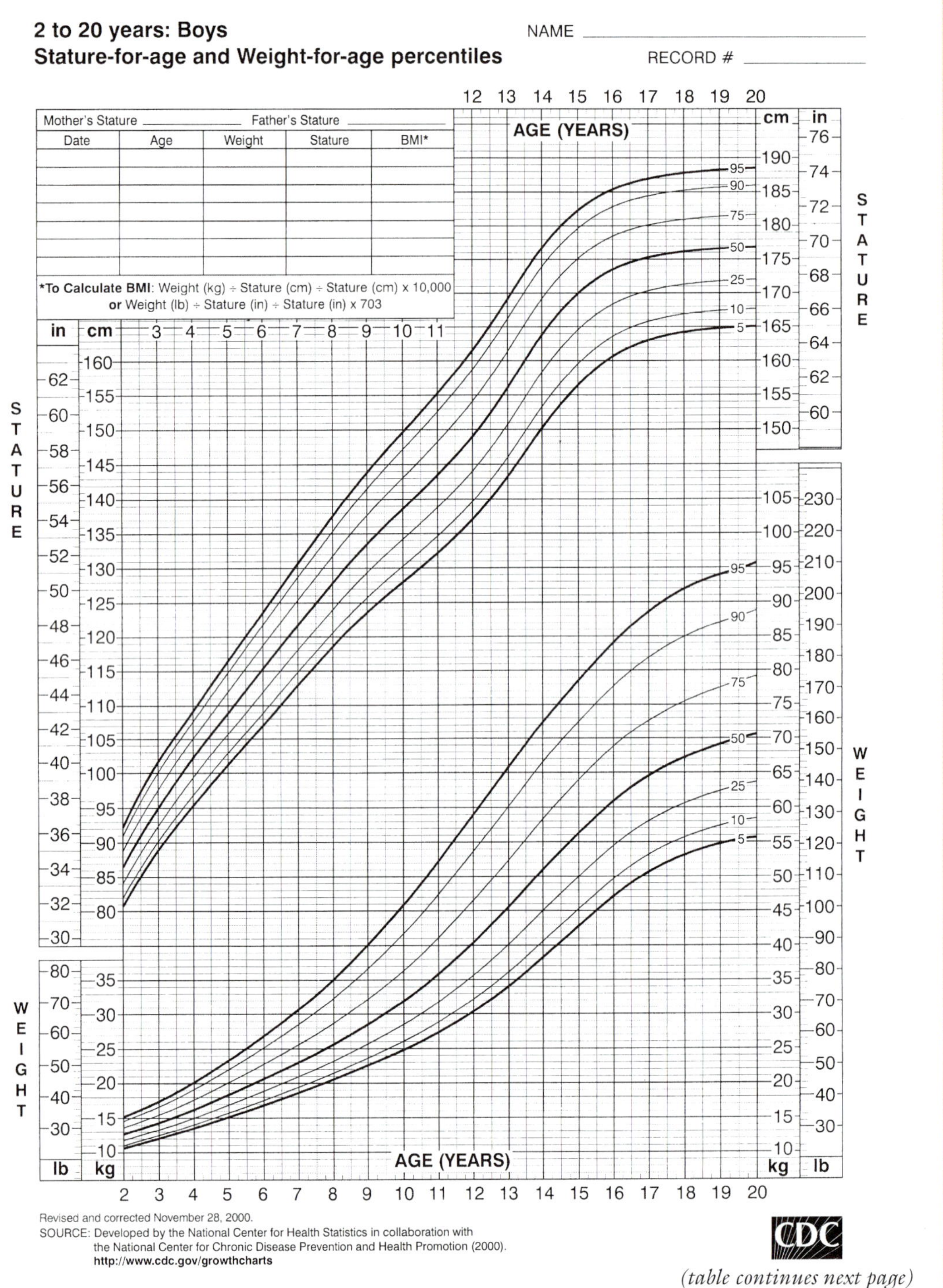

(table continues next page)

TABLE 17-4 ■ Growth Charts *(Continued)*

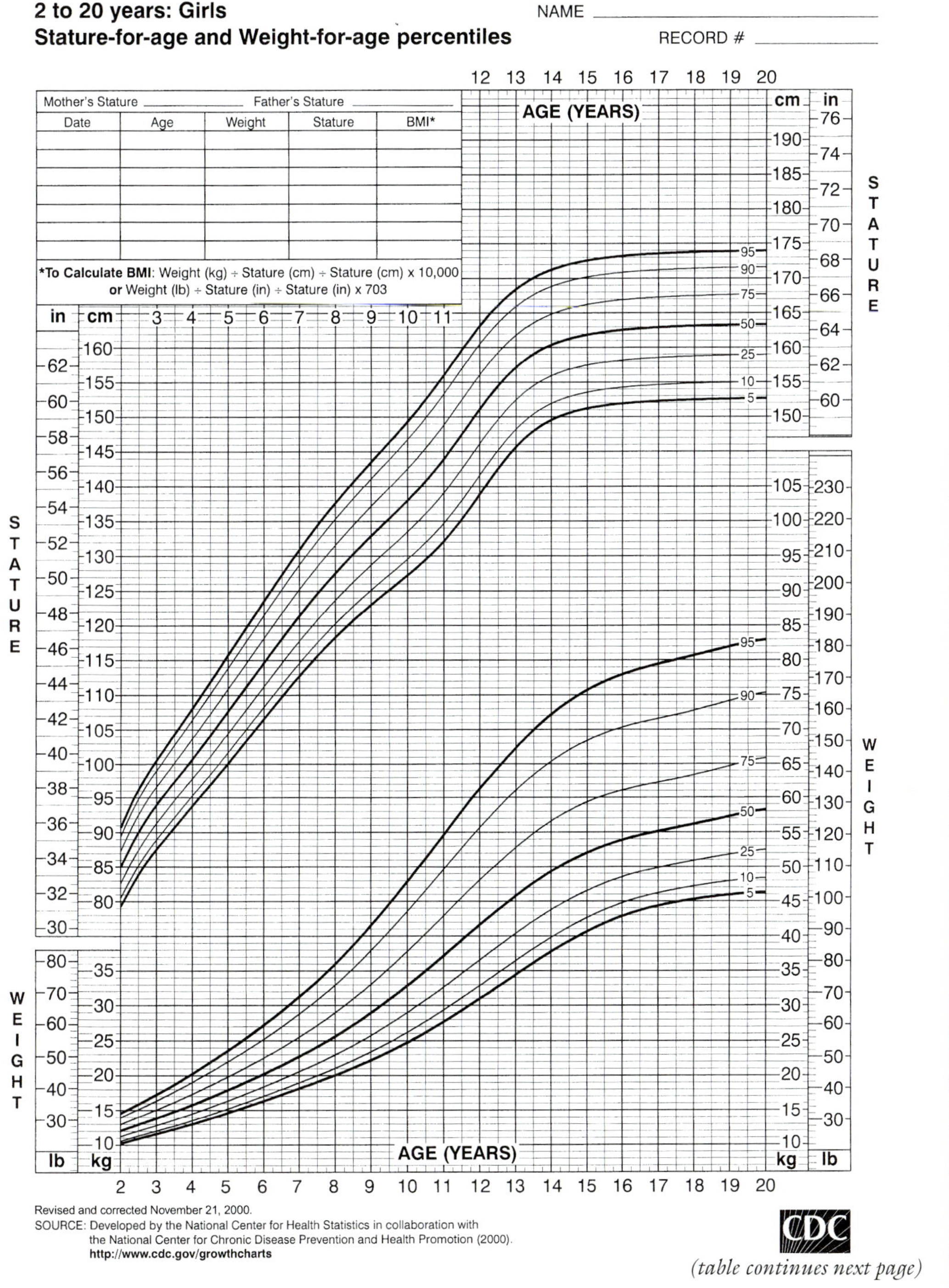

(table continues next page)

TABLE 17-4 ■ Growth Charts *(Continued)*

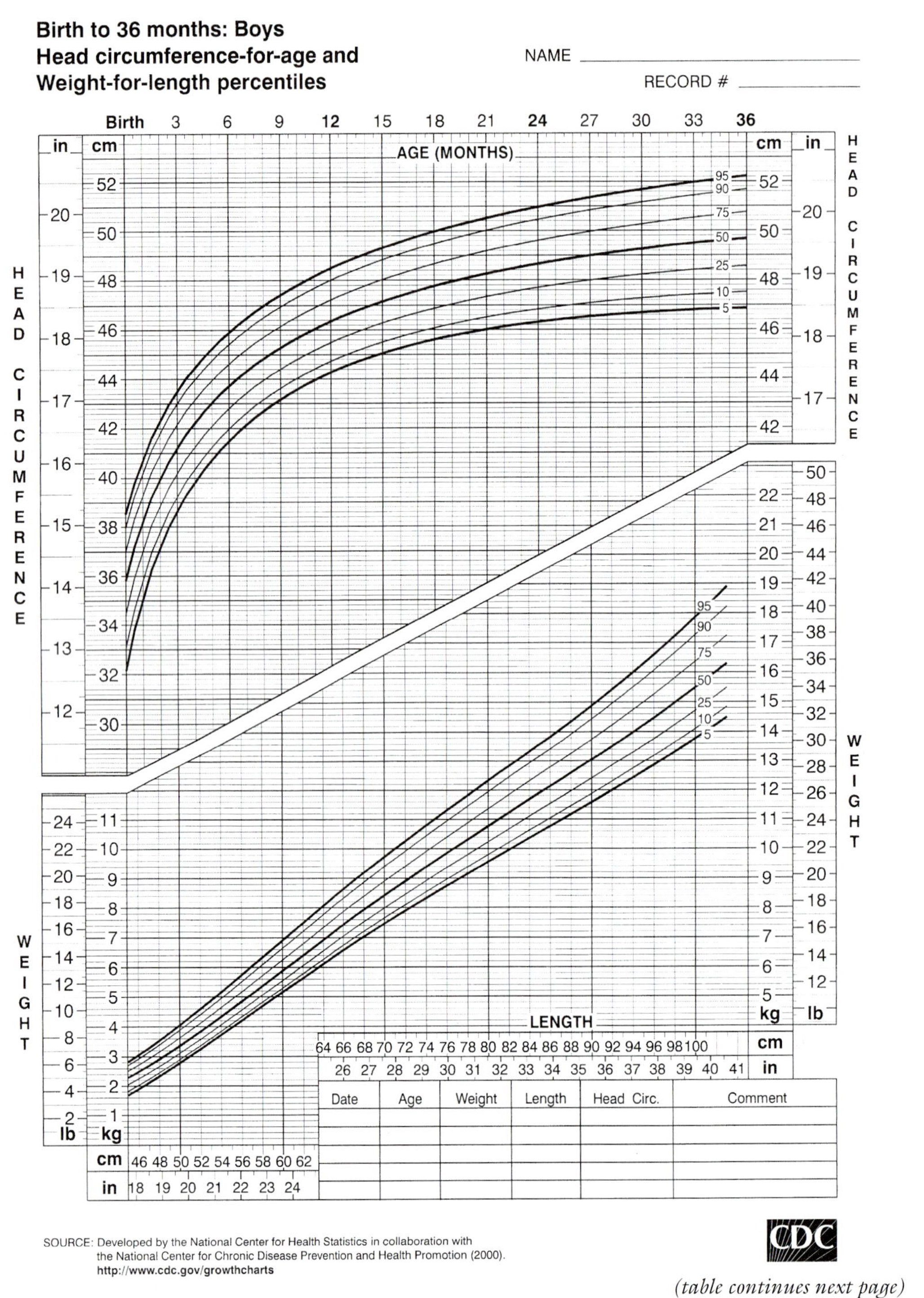

(table continues next page)

TABLE 17-4 ■ Growth Charts *(Continued)*

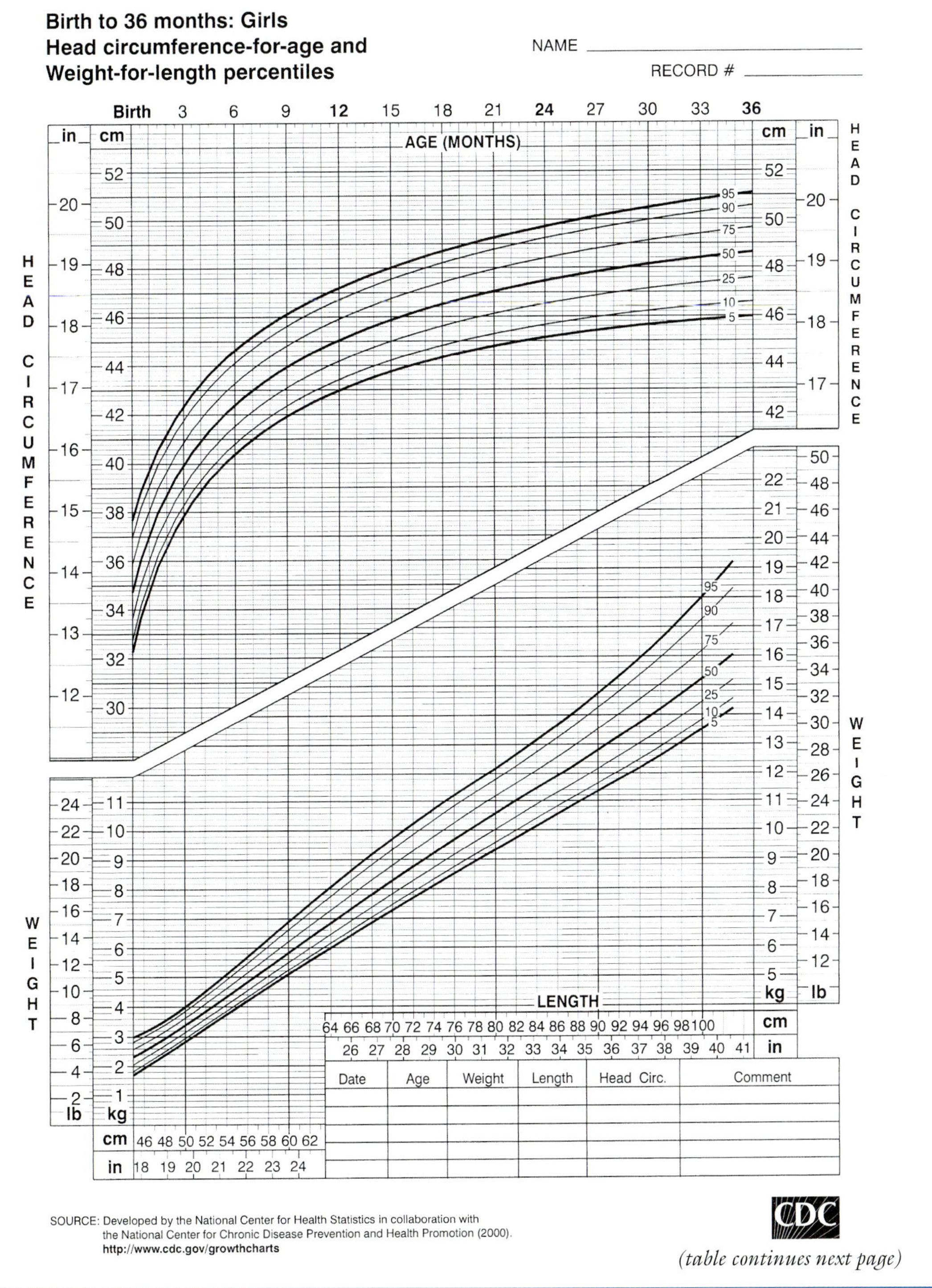
Birth to 36 months: Girls
Head circumference-for-age and
Weight-for-length percentiles
NAME
RECORD #
Birth 3 6 9 12 15 18 21 24 27 30 33 36
AGE (MONTHS)
HEAD CIRCUMFERENCE
in cm
95 90 75 50 25 10 5
WEIGHT
LENGTH
lb kg
cm 46 48 50 52 54 56 58 60 62
in 18 19 20 21 22 23 24
64 66 68 70 72 74 76 78 80 82 84 86 88 90 92 94 96 98 100 cm
26 27 28 29 30 31 32 33 34 35 36 37 38 39 40 41 in
Date
Age
Weight
Length
Head Circ.
Comment
SOURCE: Developed by the National Center for Health Statistics in collaboration with the National Center for Chronic Disease Prevention and Health Promotion (2000).
http://www.cdc.gov/growthcharts
CDC

(table continues next page)

TABLE 17-4 ■ Growth Charts *(Continued)*

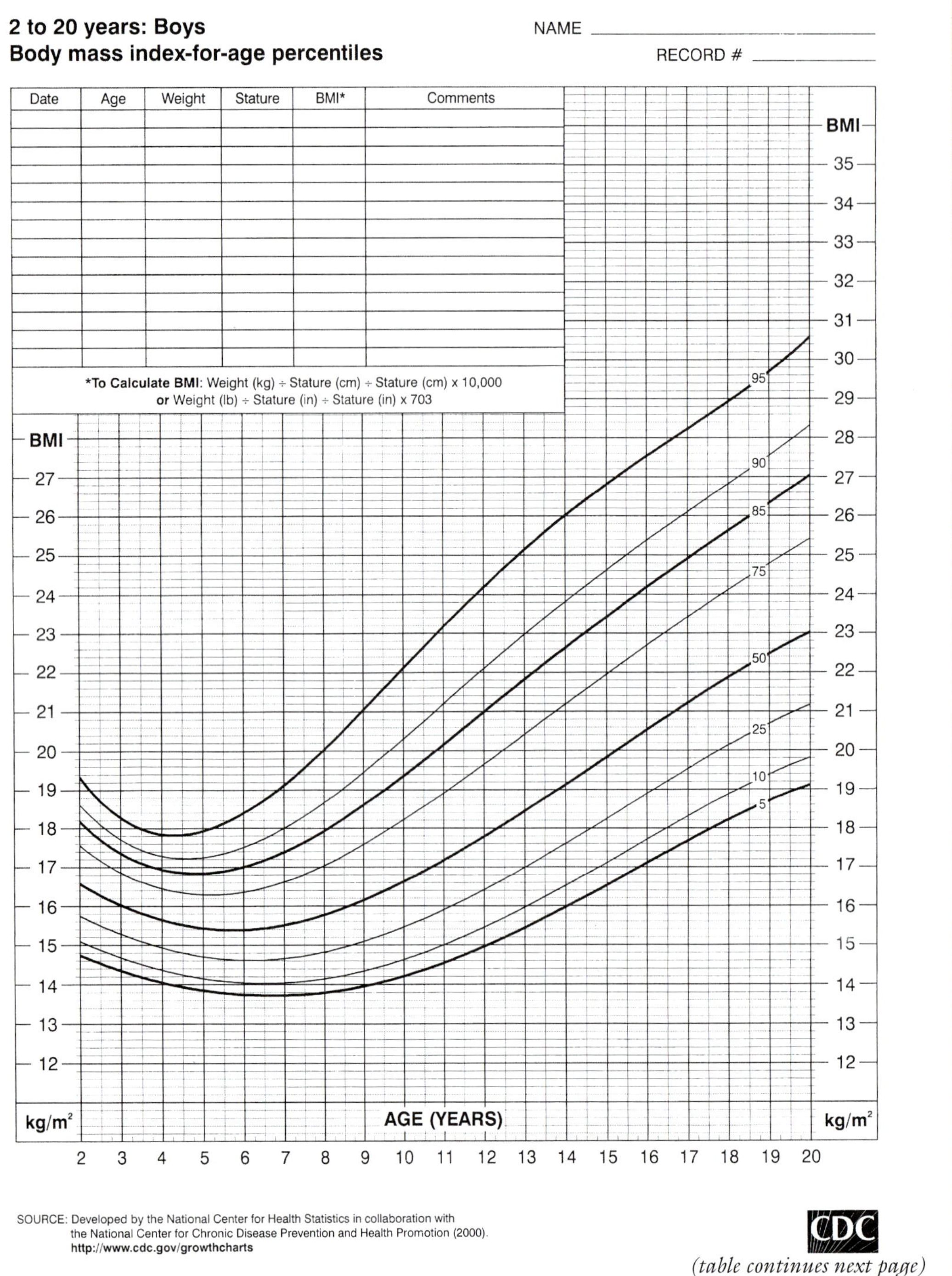

SOURCE: Developed by the National Center for Health Statistics in collaboration with the National Center for Chronic Disease Prevention and Health Promotion (2000). http://www.cdc.gov/growthcharts

CDC

(table continues next page)

TABLE 17-4 ■ Growth Charts *(Continued)*

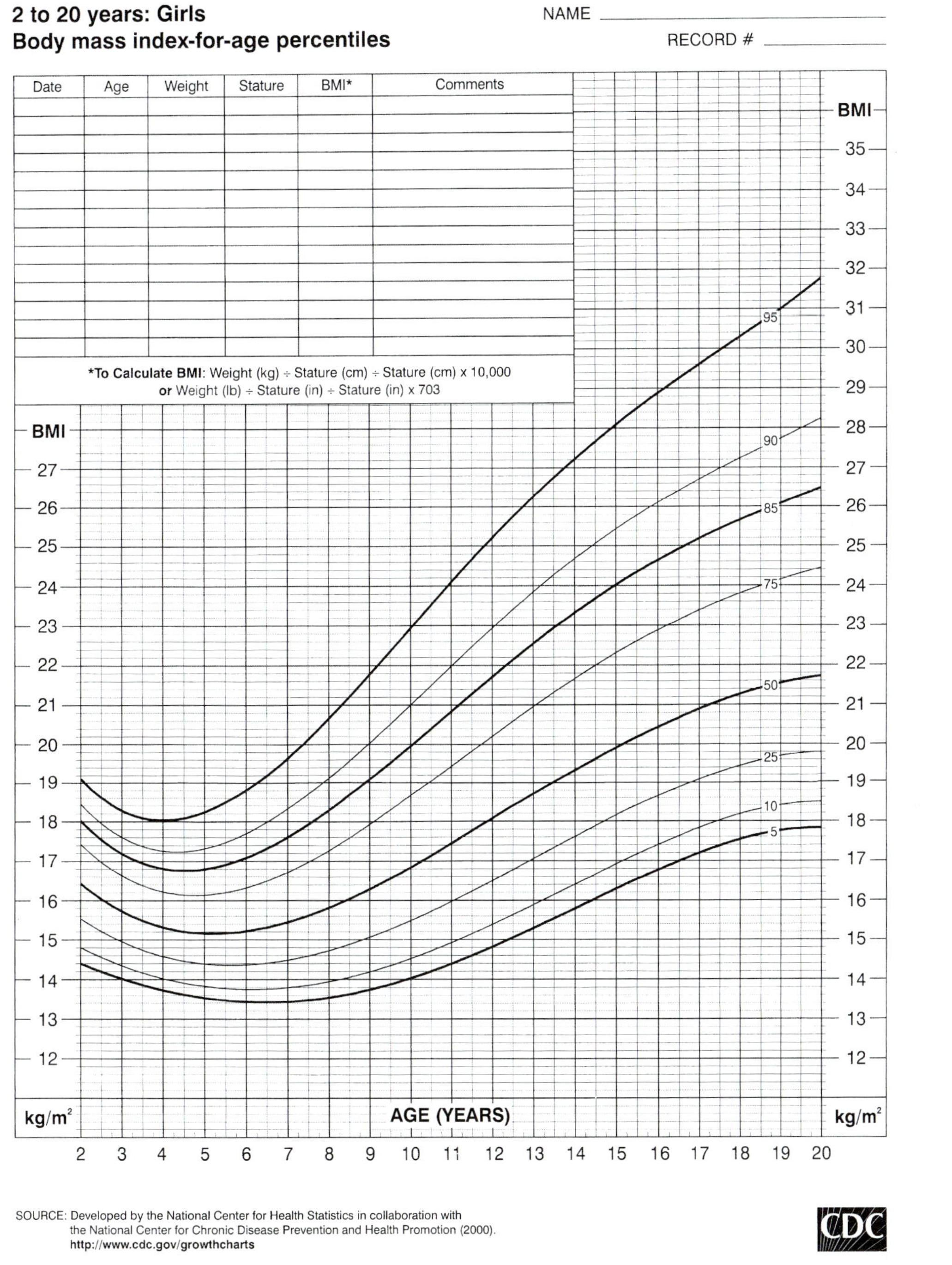

SOURCE: Developed by the National Center for Health Statistics in collaboration with the National Center for Chronic Disease Prevention and Health Promotion (2000). http://www.cdc.gov/growthcharts

CDC

TABLE 17-5 ■ Abnormal Growth Patterns in Infancy and Childhood

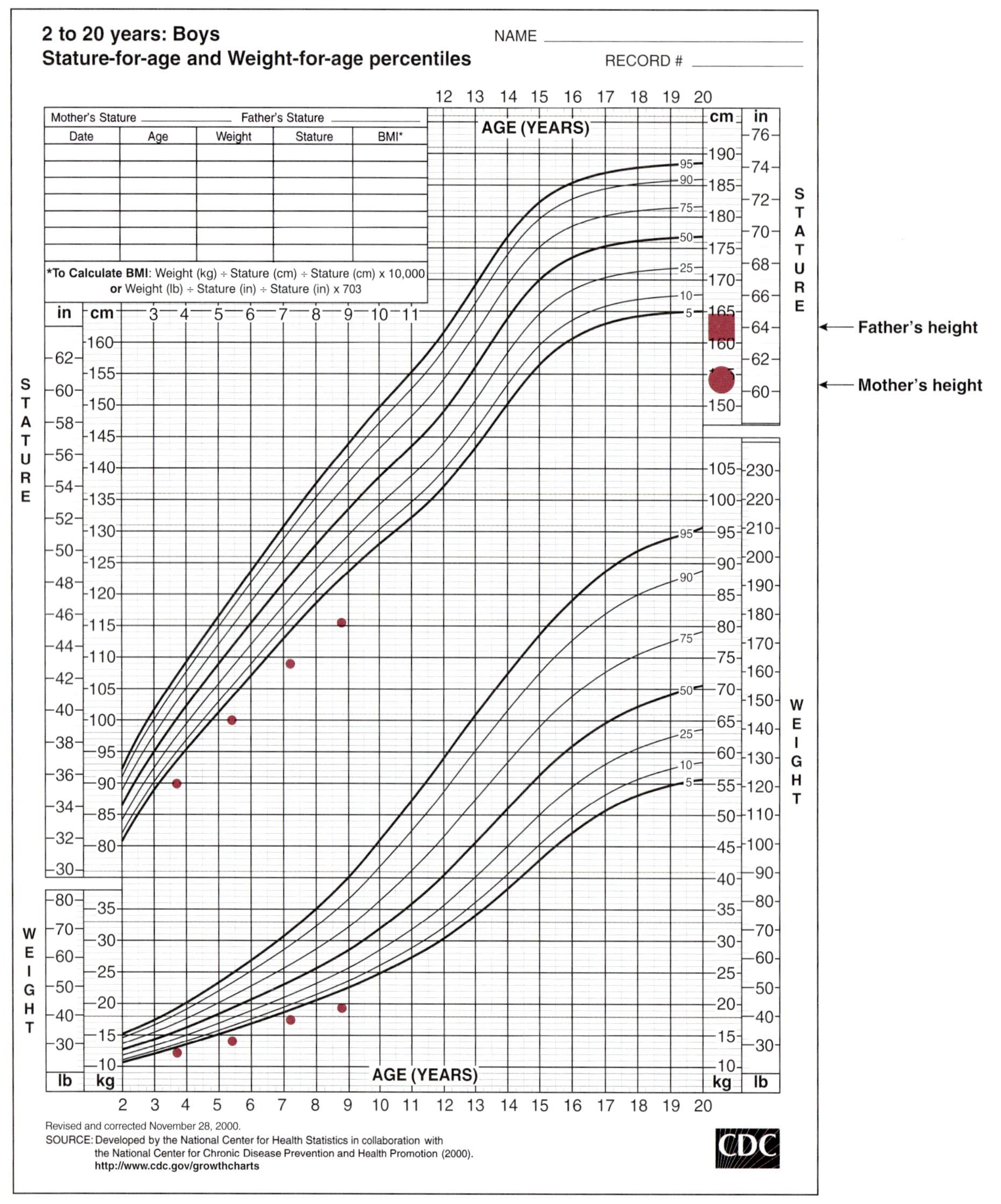

Genetic (familial) Short Stature

Normal birth size, deceleration by 2 yrs, then steady growth. Short adult height, like parents.

TABLE 17-5 ■ Abnormal Growth Patterns in Infancy and Childhood *(Continued)*

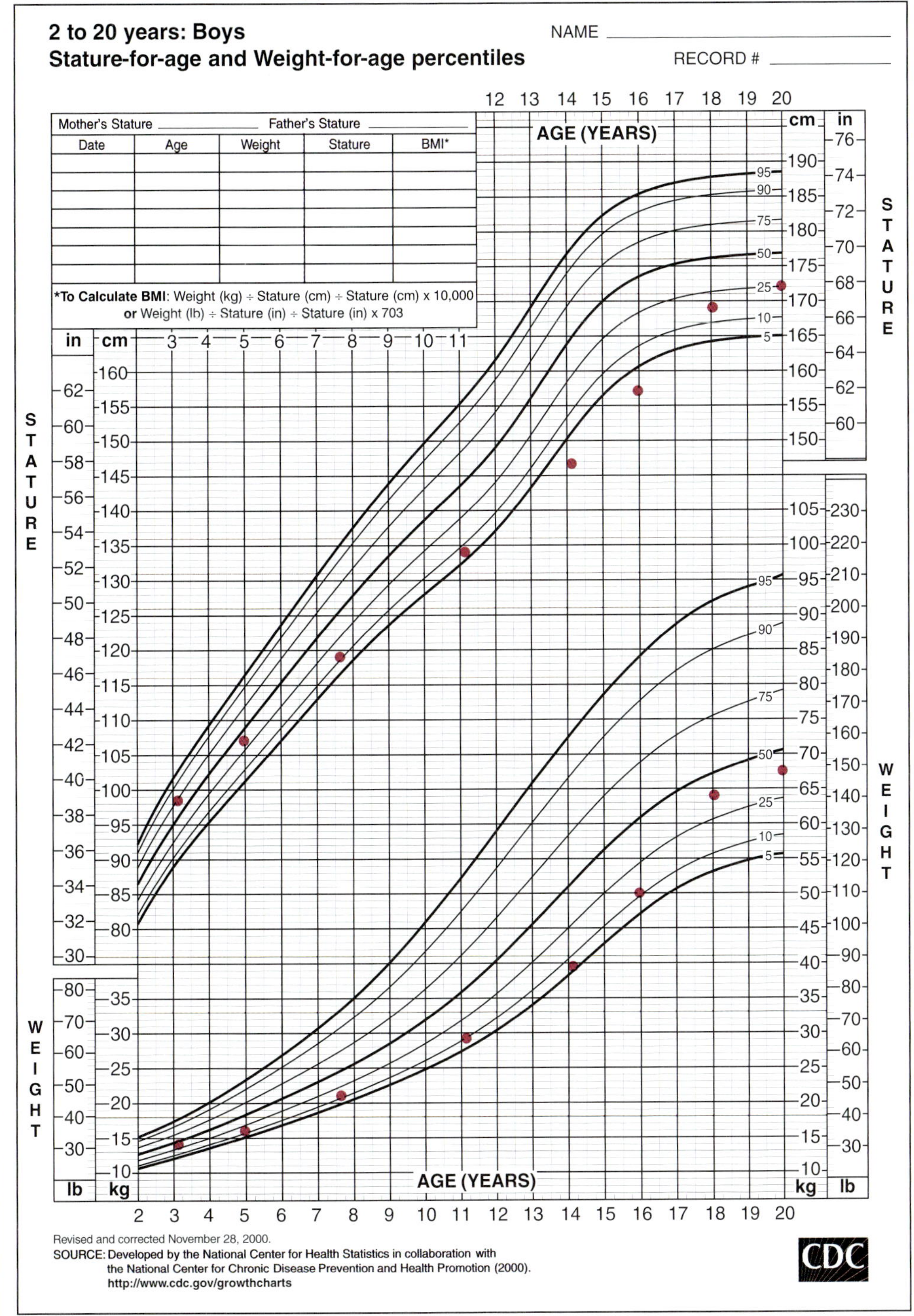

Constitutional Delay of Puberty

Slowing growth from 3–10 yrs, delayed puberty, and normal final adult height.

(table continues next page)

TABLE 17-5 ■ Abnormal Growth Patterns in Infancy and Childhood *(Continued)*

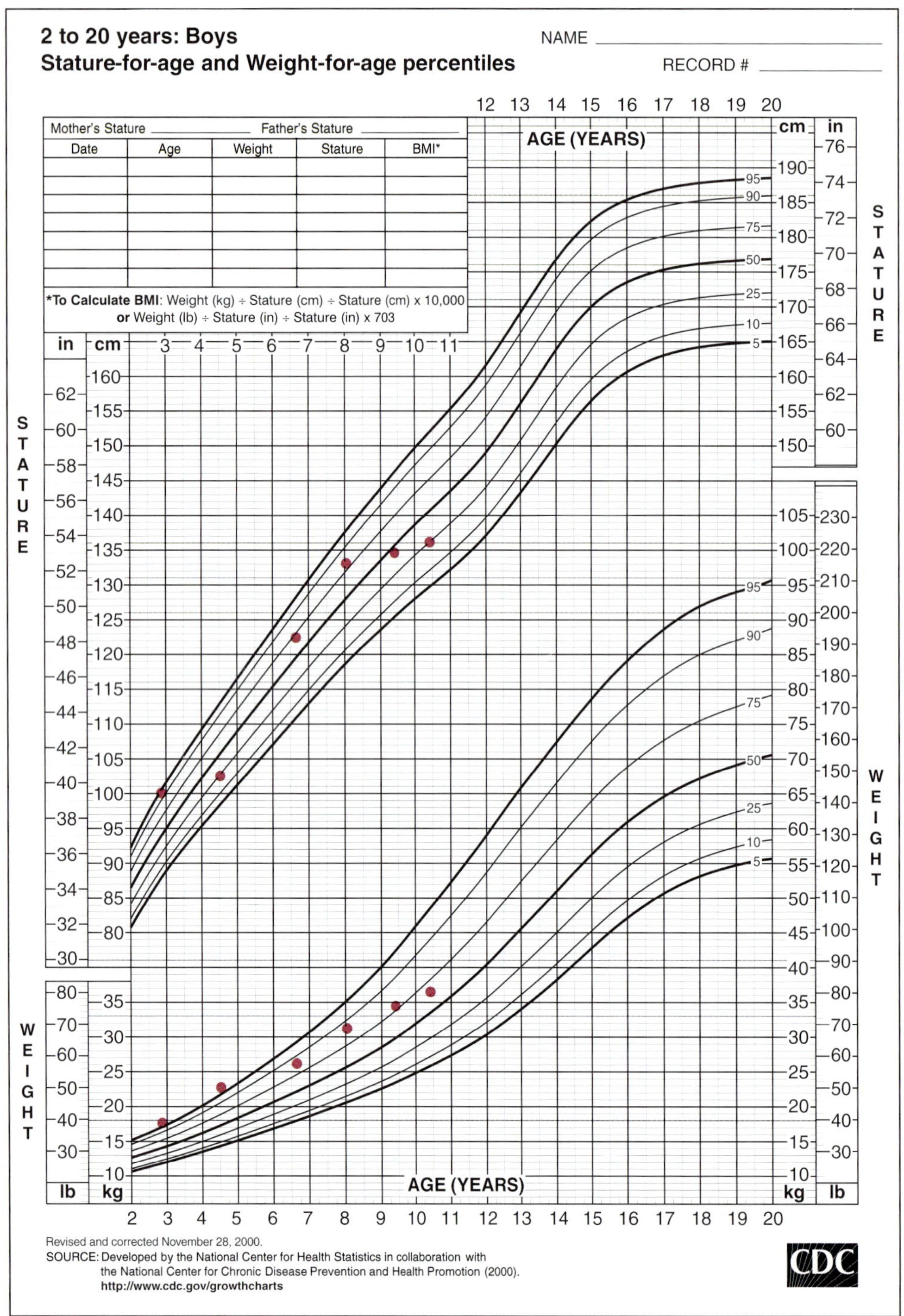

Acquired Growth Hormone Deficiency

Profound deceleration in linear growth is noted, here starting at age 8 yrs.

TABLE 17-5 ■ Abnormal Growth Patterns in Infancy and Childhood *(Continued)*

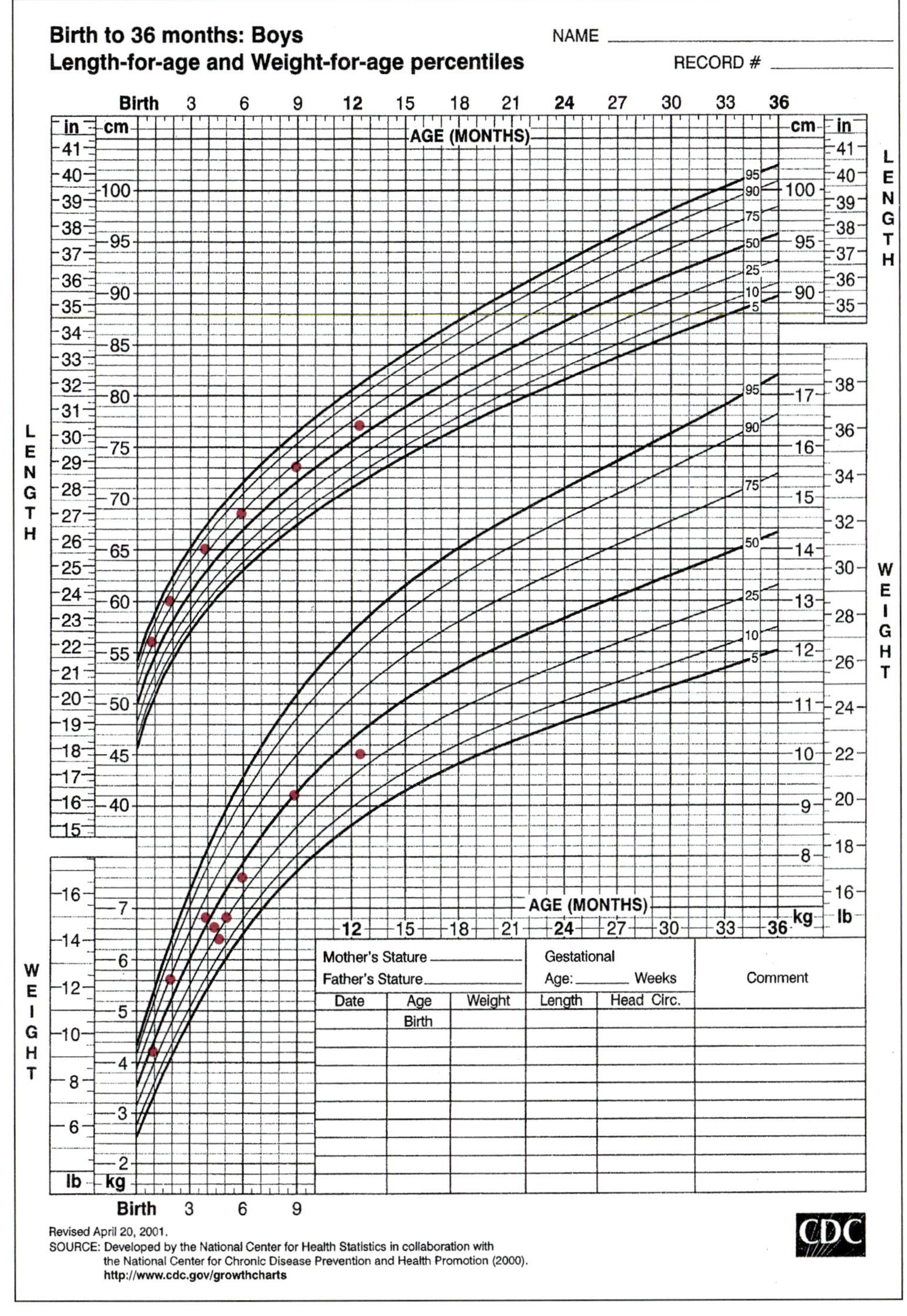

Acute Weight Loss Due to Illness at 2 Months

The weight was regained rapidly, and there was no loss of height.

(table continues next page)

TABLE 17-5 ■ Abnormal Growth Patterns in Infancy and Childhood *(Continued)*

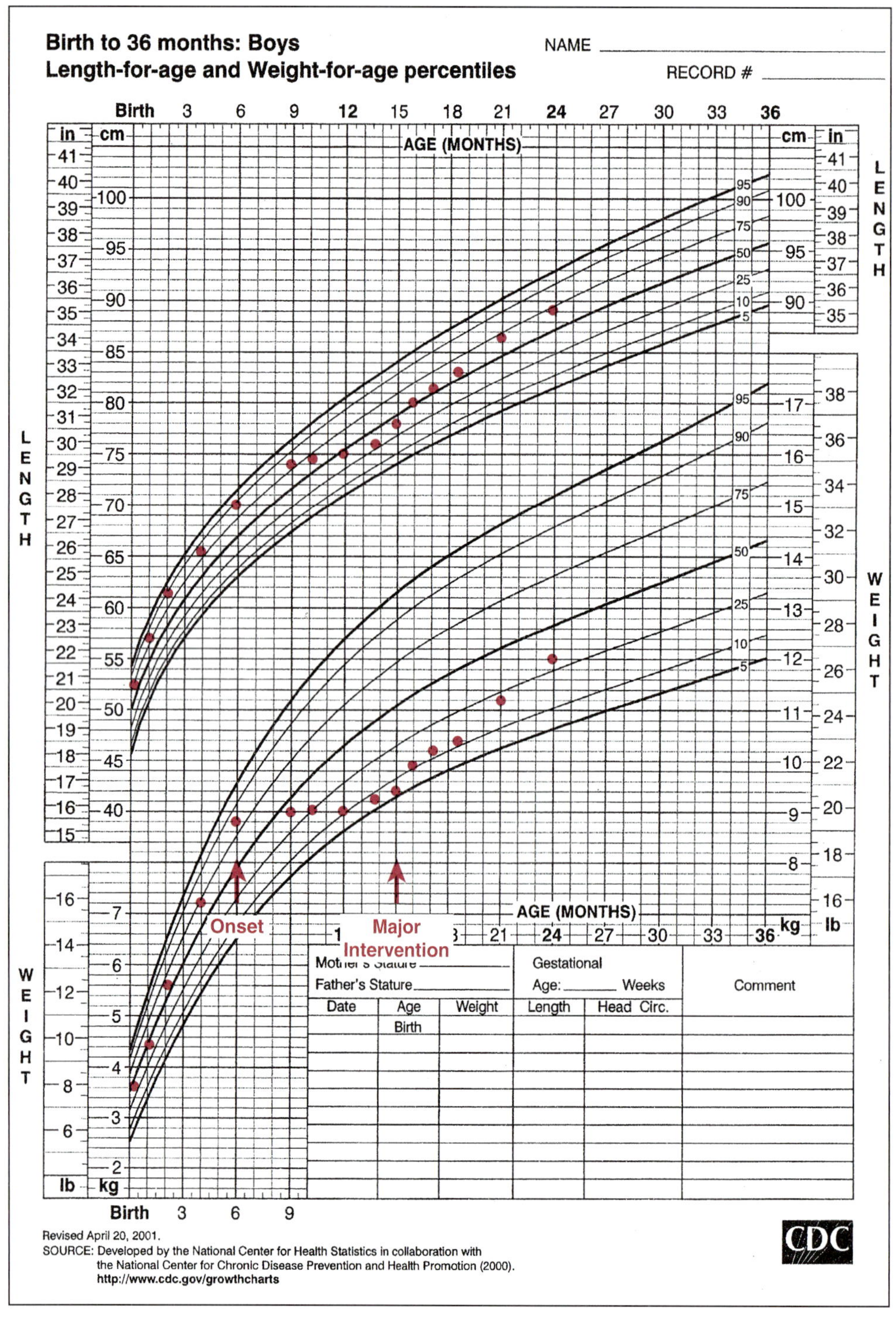

Failure to Thrive

Beginning at 6 mos, the weight dropped off before the height. Intervention occurred at 12 mos.

TABLE 17-5 ■ Abnormal Growth Patterns in Infancy and Childhood *(Continued)*

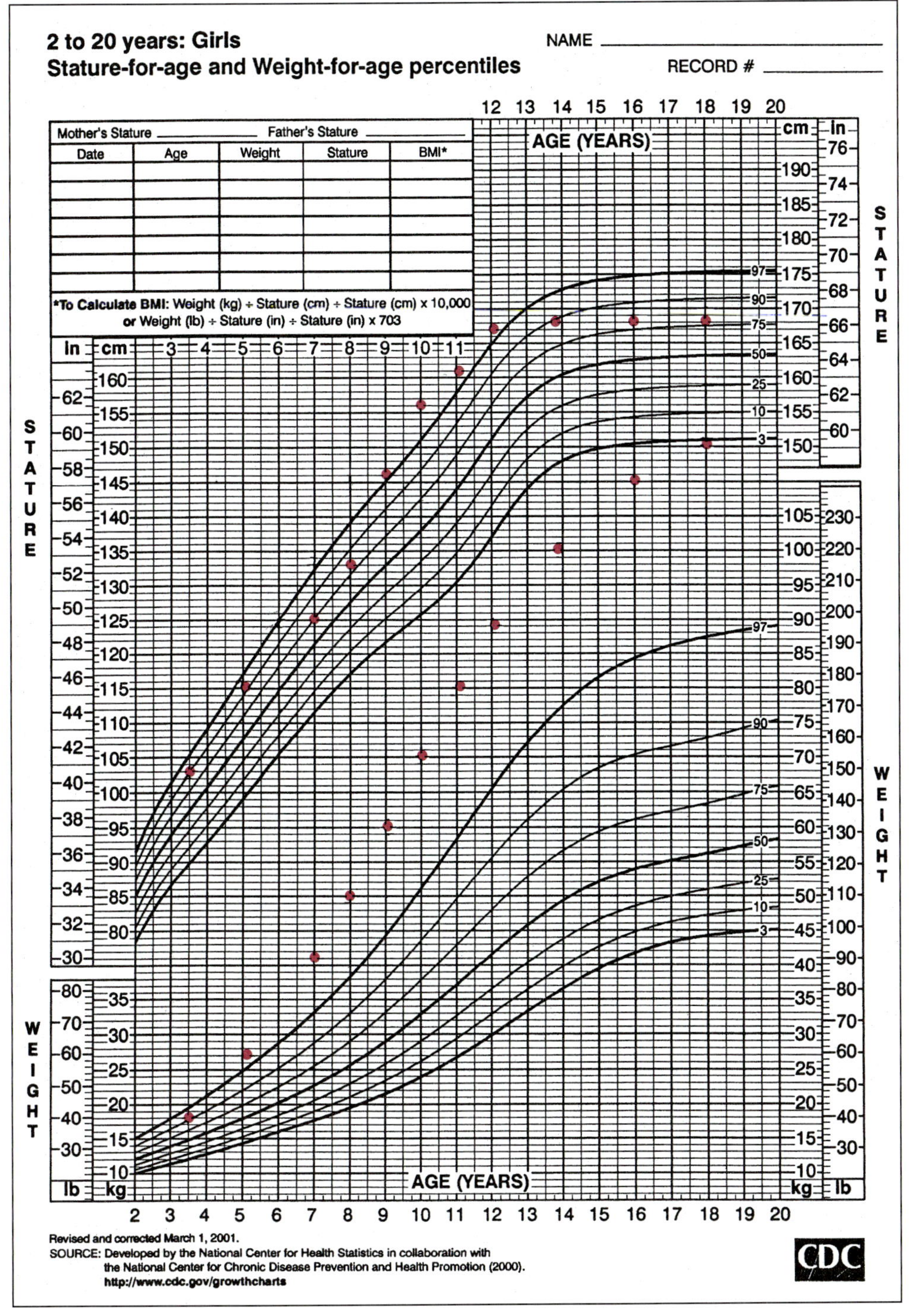

Exogenous Obesity

Note that in this child, obesity started by 5 yrs. The child is also tall and enters puberty at an early age.

(table continues next page)

TABLE 17-5 ■ Abnormal Growth Patterns in Infancy and Childhood *(Continued)*

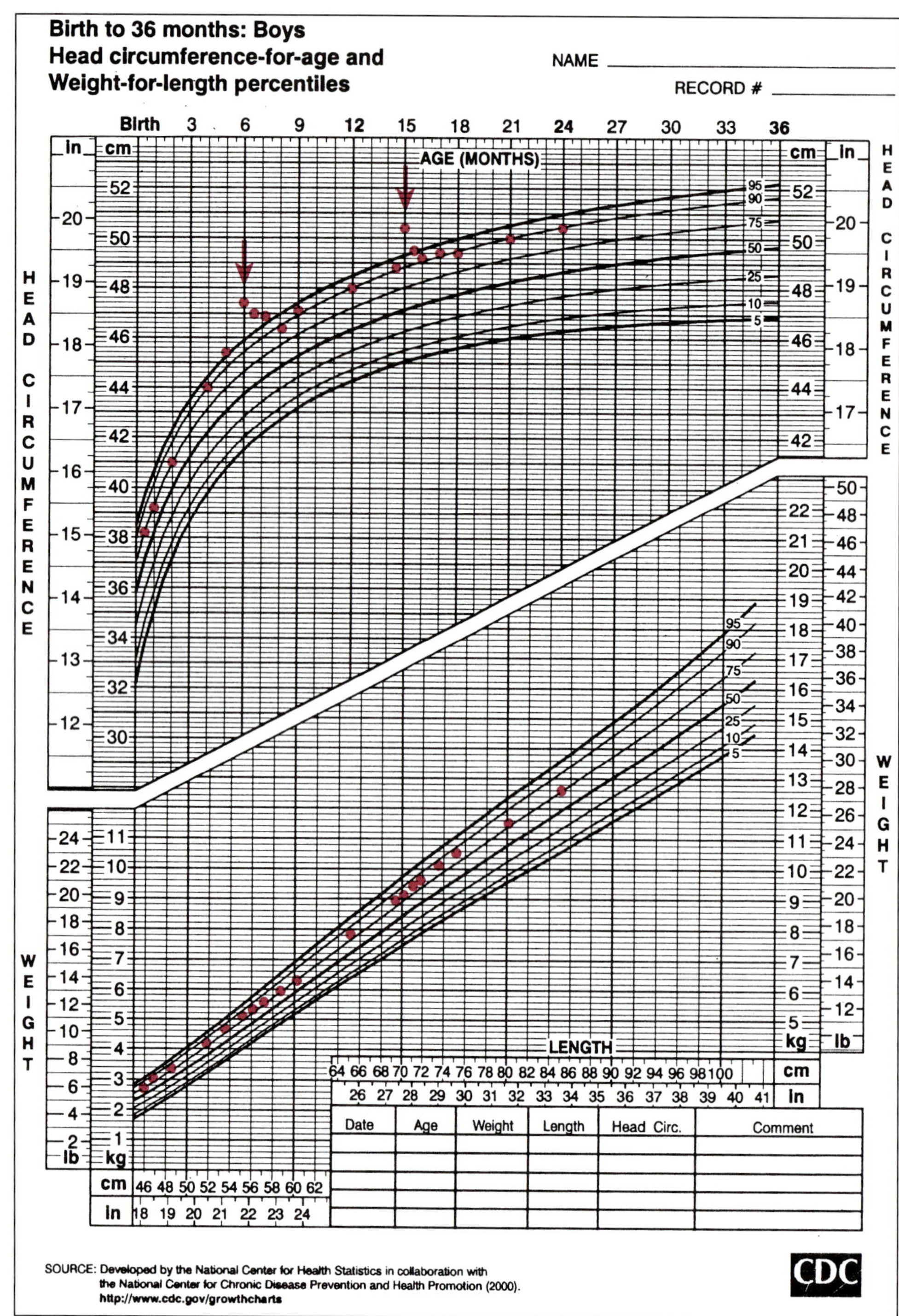

Hydrocephalus

Head circumference of a child with communicating hydrocephalus. A ventriculo-peritoneal shunt was placed at 6 mos of age; it became nonfunctional at 15 mos and was revised.

TABLE 17-5 ■ Abnormal Growth Patterns in Infancy and Childhood *(Continued)*

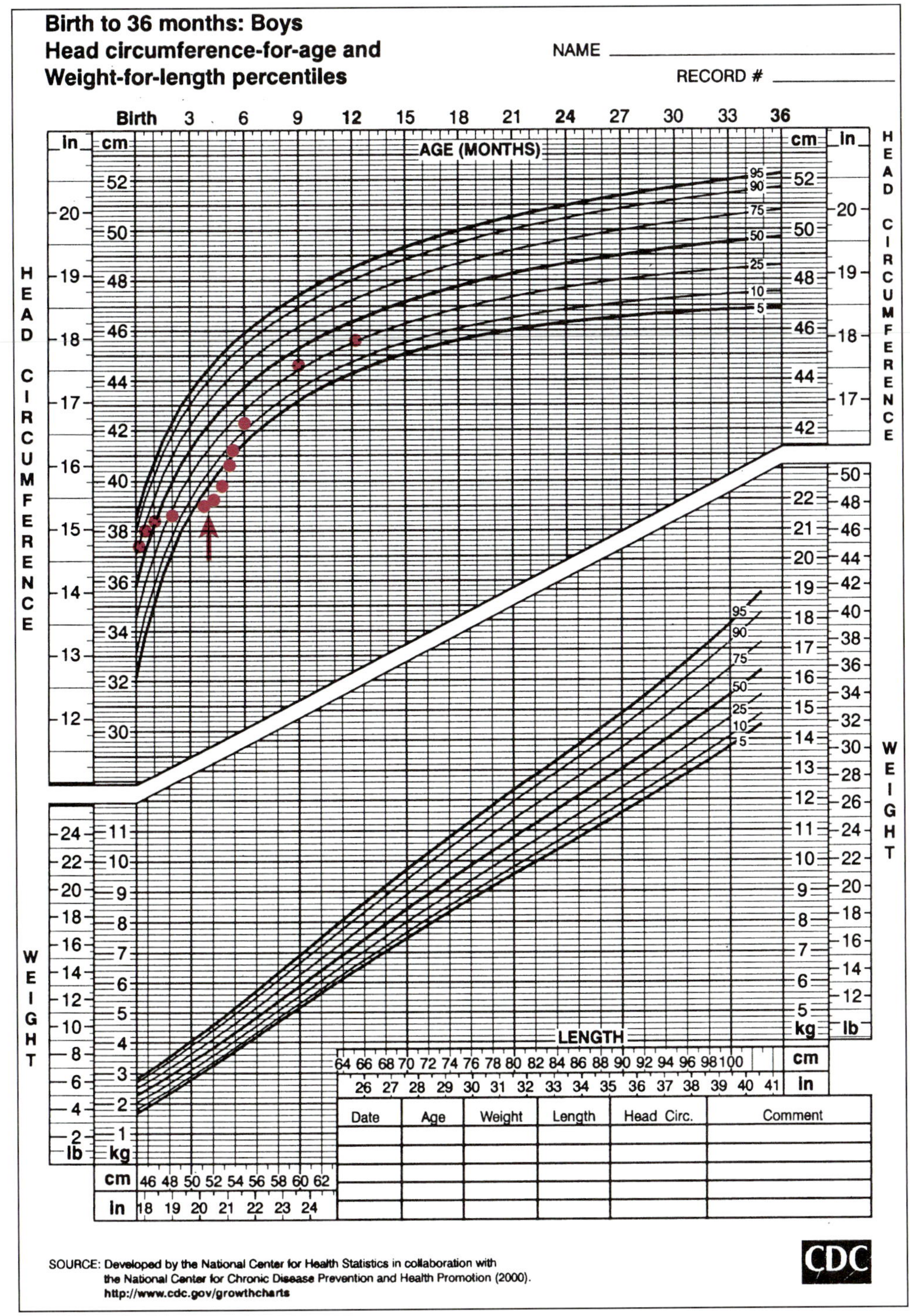

Craniosynostosis

Premature closure of one or more sutures causes microcephaly, deceleration of head growth, and abnormal head shape. Surgical repair occurred at 4 mos in this child.

(table continues next page)

TABLE 17-5 ■ Abnormal Growth Patterns in Infancy and Childhood *(Continued)*

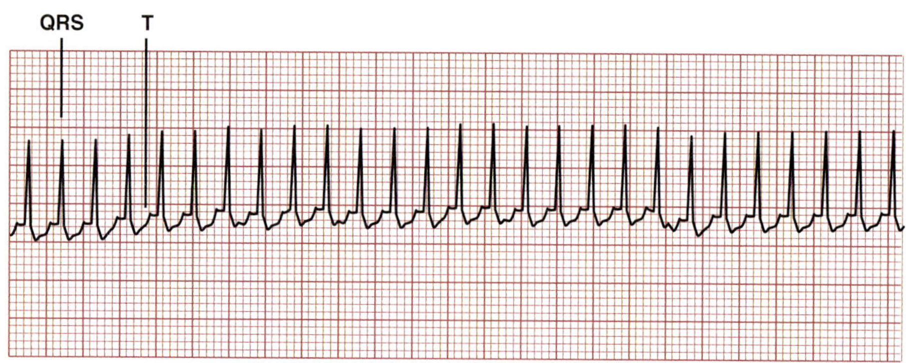

Supraventricular Tachycardia

Paroxysmal supraventricular tachycardia (SVT) is the most common dysrhythmia in children. Some infants with SVT look quite well or may be somewhat pale with tachypnea, but have a heart rate of 240 beats per min or greater. Others are quite ill and in cardiovascular collapse.

SVT in infants is usually sustained, requiring medical therapy for conversion to a normal rate and rhythm. In older children, it is more likely to be truly paroxysmal, with episodes of varying duration and frequency.

TABLE 17-5 ■ Abnormal Growth Patterns in Infancy and Childhood *(Continued)*

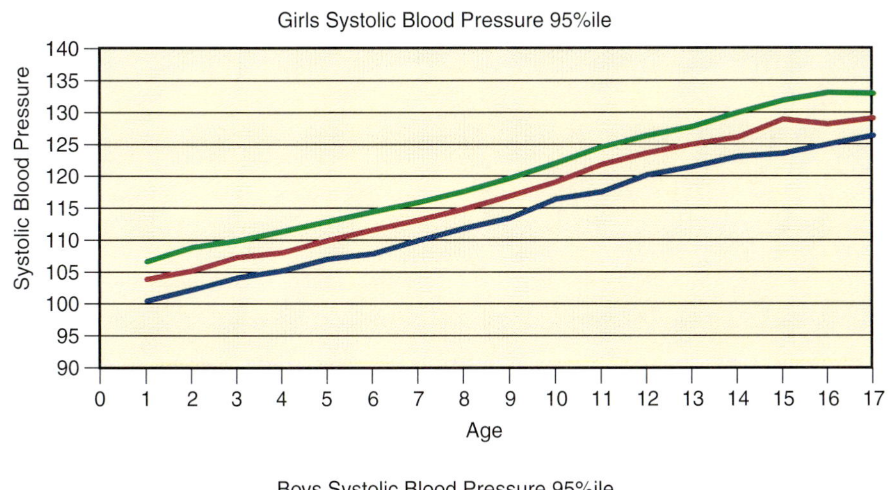

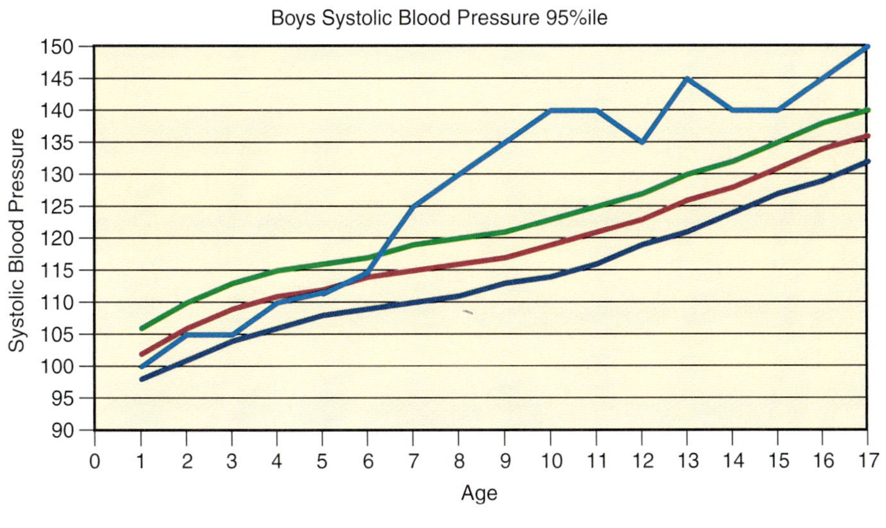

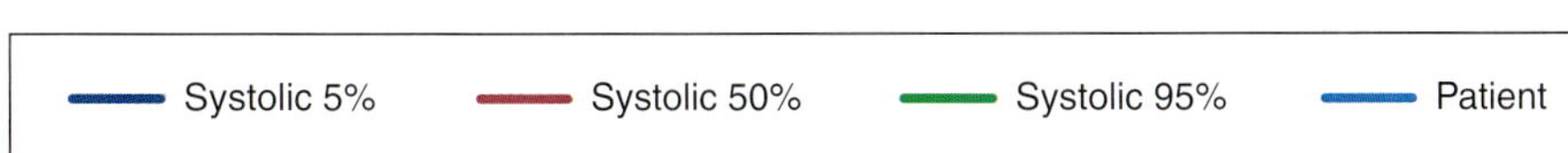

Hypertension in Childhood

Hypertension can start in childhood. While young children with elevated blood pressure are more likely to have a renal, cardiac, or endocrine cause, adolescents with hypertension are most likely to have primary or essential hypertension.

This child developed hypertension during adolescence, and it "tracked" into adulthood. Children tend to remain in the same percentile for blood pressure as they grow. This tracking of blood pressure continues into adulthood, supporting the concept that adult essential hypertension begins during childhood.

The consequences of untreated hypertension can be severe.

TABLE 17-6 ■ Benign Birthmarks Versus Pathologic Neurocutaneous Syndromes

When you detect a birthmark on a newborn or infant, you will need to differentiate common, benign birthmarks from uncommon but neurologically significant neurocutaneous syndromes. Use these photographs to help you make this distinction.

Benign Birthmarks

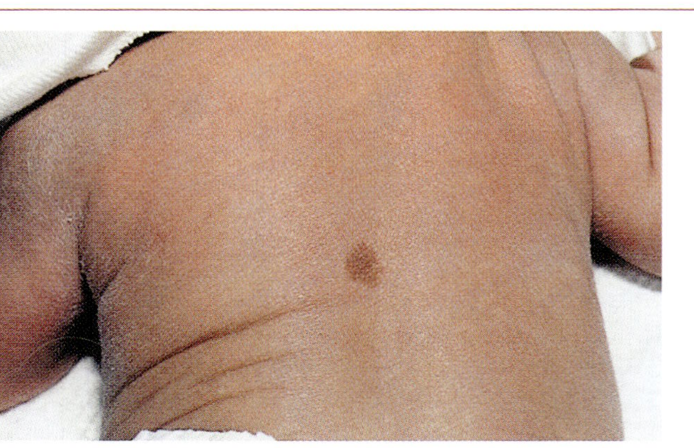

Café-au-lait spots
These light-brown pigmented lesions usually have ragged borders and are uniform. They are noted in more than 10% of black infants.

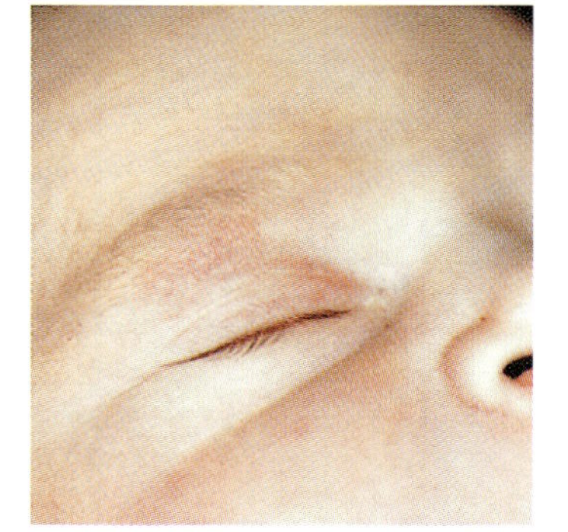

Eyelid Patch
This birthmark fades, usually in the first year.

Salmon Patch
Also called "stork bite," this splotchy pink mark fades with age.

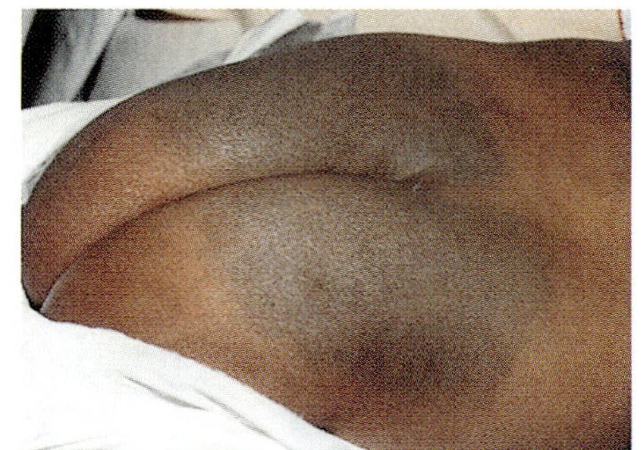

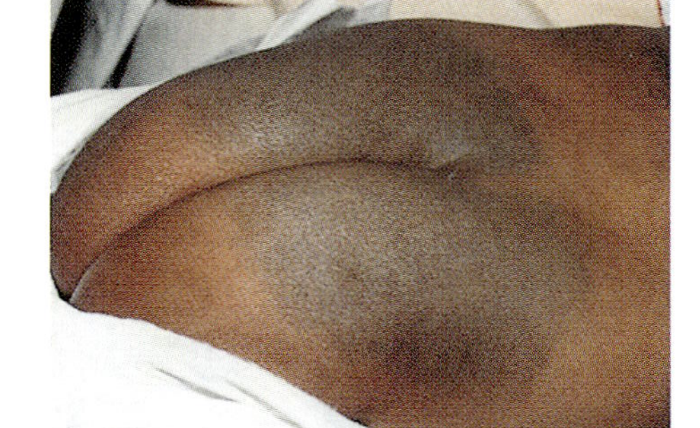

Mongolian Spots
These are more common among dark-skinned babies. It is important to note them so that they are not mistaken for bruises.

Neurocutaneous Syndromes

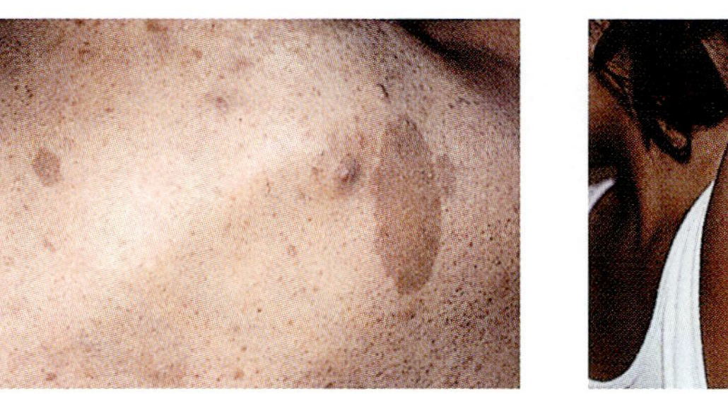

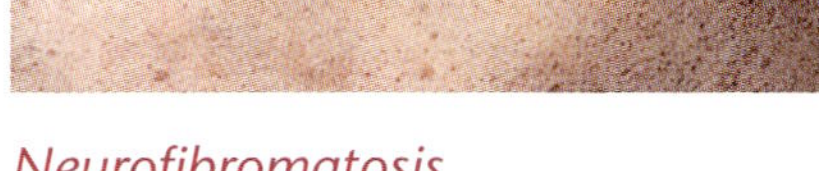

Neurofibromatosis

Characteristic features include more than 5 café-au-lait spots and axillary freckling, both shown above. Later findings include neurofibromas and Lish nodules (not shown).

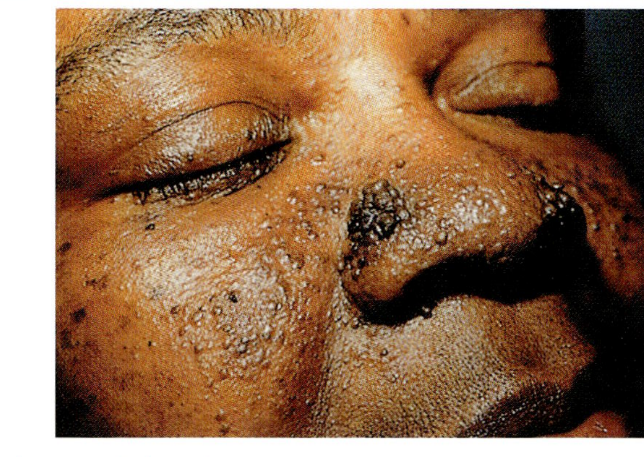

Tuberous Sclerosis

Findings in young children include adenoma sebaceum as shown here (angiofibromas surrounding sweat glands). Older children may have oval, depigmented ash-leaf spots (not shown).

(Sources of photos: *Café-au-lait Spots, Salmon Patch, Eyelid Patch, Mongolian Spots*—Fletcher M: Physical Diagnosis in Neonatology, Philadelphia, Lippincott-Raven Publishers, 1998; *Neurofibromatosis*—Goodheart H: A Photoguide of Common Skin Disorders, Baltimore, Williams & Wilkins, 1999; *Tuberous Sclerosis*—Hall J: Sauer's Manual of Skin Diseases, 8th ed., Philadelphia, Lippincott Williams & Wilkins, 2000.)

TABLE 17-7 ■ Common Skin Rashes and Skin Findings in Newborns and Infants

Newborns

Jaundice
More than half of newborns have jaundice. This is best noted by pressing your finger or a glass slide against the skin.

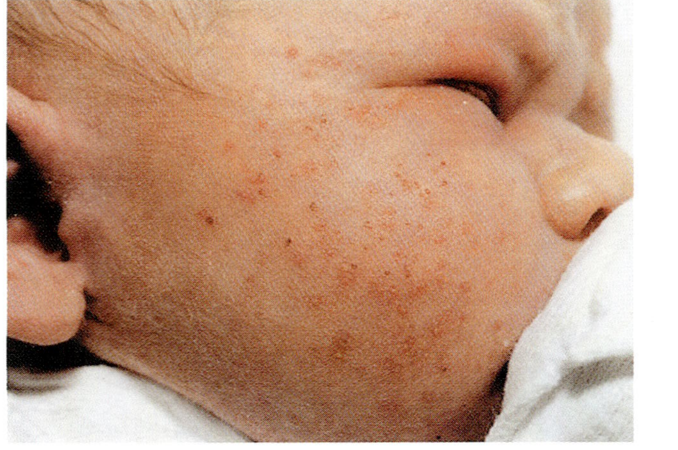
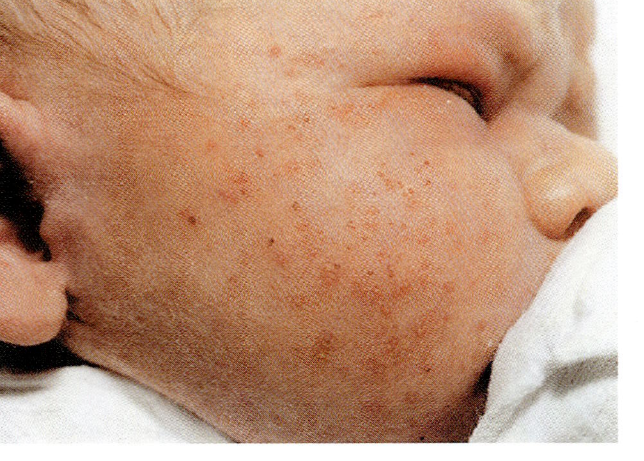

Erythema Toxicum
These yellow or white pustules are surrounded by a red base and are commonly noted in normal newborns.

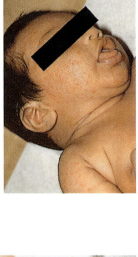

Neonatal Acne
Red pustules and papules are most prominent over the cheeks and nose of some normal newborns.

Infants

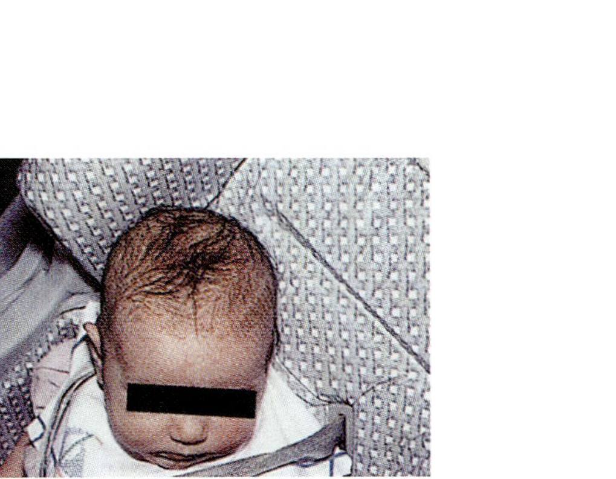

Seborrhea
The salmon red, scaly eruption often involves the face, neck, axilla, diaper area, and behind the ears.

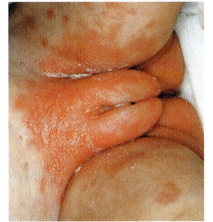

Candidal Diaper Dermatitis
This bright red rash involves the intertriginous folds, with small "satellite lesions" along the edges.

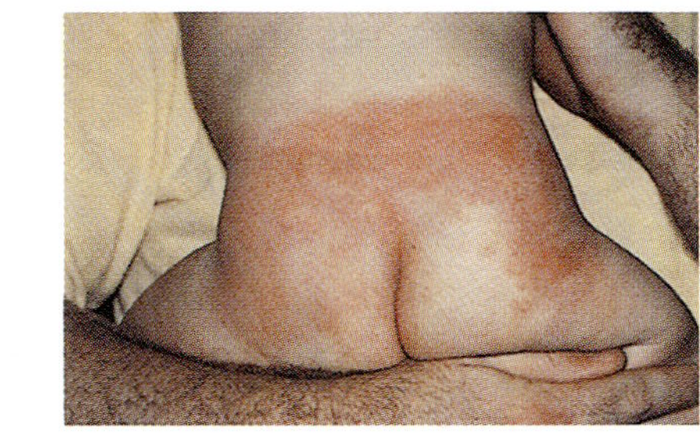

Contact Diaper Dermatitis
This irritant rash is secondary to diarrhea or irritation and is noted along contact areas (here, the area touching the diaper).

(Sources of photos: *Erythema Toxicum, Candidal Diaper Dermatitis*—Fletcher M: Physical Diagnosis in Neonatology, Philadelphia, Lippincott-Raven Publishers, 1998; *Neonatal Acne, Seborrhea, Contact Diaper Dermatitis*—Goodheart H: A Photoguide of Common Skin Disorders, Baltimore, Williams & Wilkins, 1999.)

TABLE 17-8 ■ Warts, Lesions that Resemble Warts, and Other Raised Lesions

Warts are commonly found in children. Since they often appear on the fingers or the hands and on the soles of the feet, you will need to examine the skin of children carefully.

Warts and Lesions that May Resemble Warts

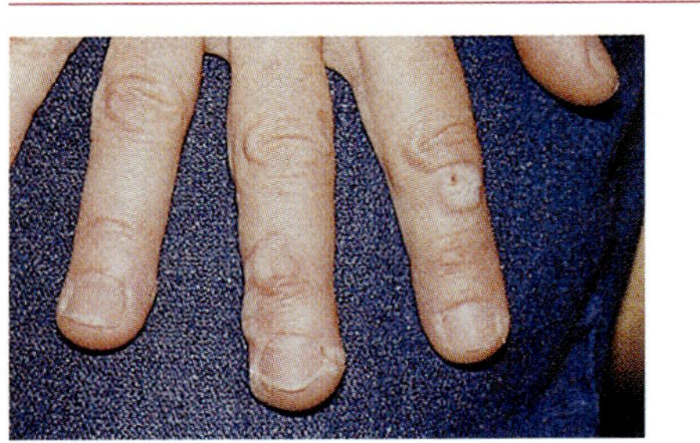

Verruca Vulgaris
Dry, rough warts on hands

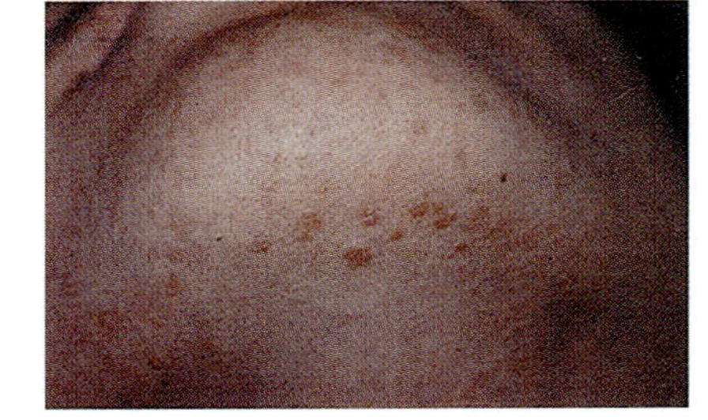

Verruca Plana
Small, flat warts

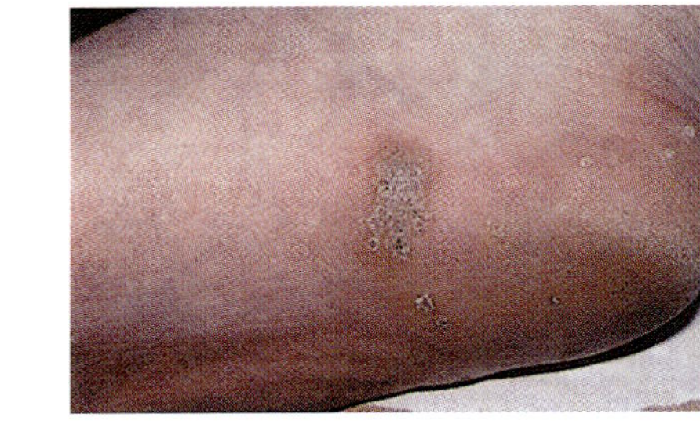

Plantar Warts
Tender warts on feet

Other Raised Lesions in Children

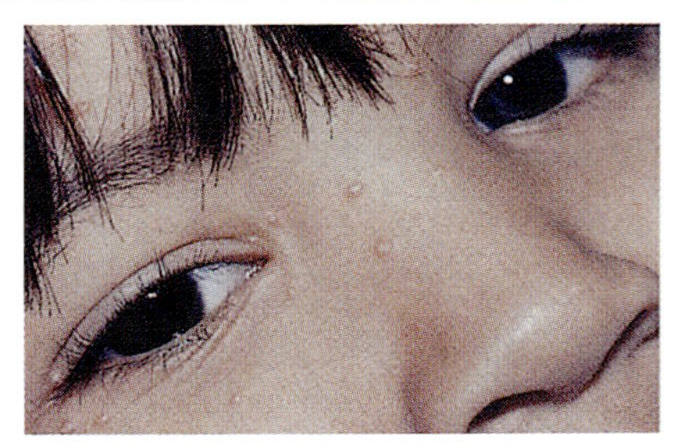

Molluscum Contagiosum
Dome-shaped, fleshy lesions

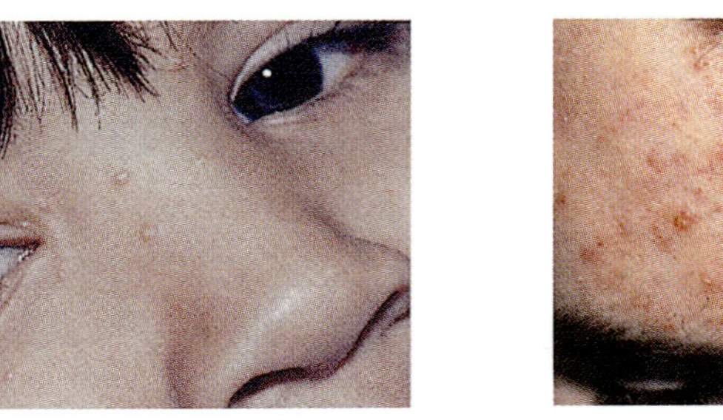

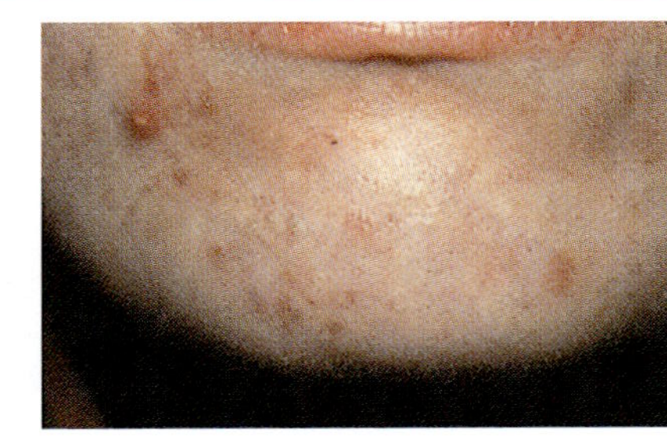

Adolescent Acne
You will frequently note acne in adolescents. Differentiate between open comedones (blackheads) and closed comedones (whiteheads) shown at the left, and inflamed pustules (right).

(Source of photos: Goodheart H: A Photoguide of Common Skin Disorders, Baltimore, Williams & Wilkins, 1999.)

TABLE 17-9 ■ Common Skin Lesions During Childhood

This table shows examples of common lesions of the skin, scalp, and hair of children. While these lesions are relatively mild, all will respond to appropriate treatment.

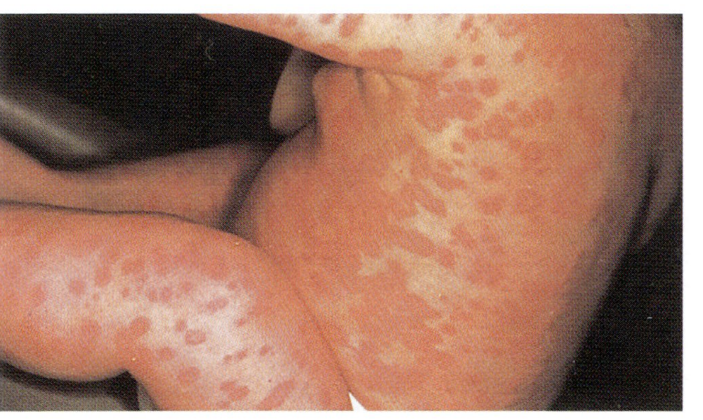

Urticaria (hives)
This pruritic, allergic sensitivity reaction changes shape quickly.

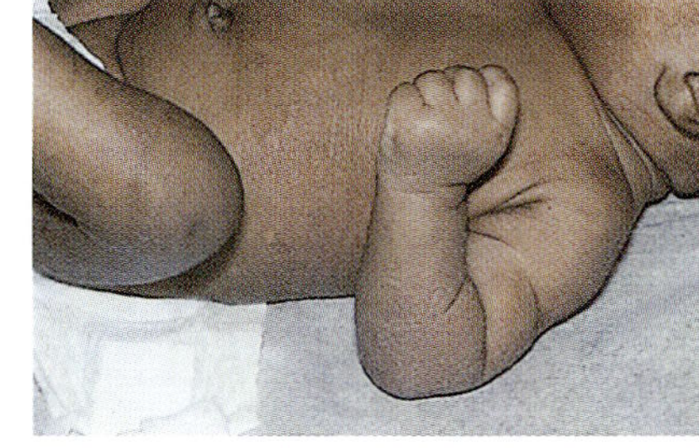
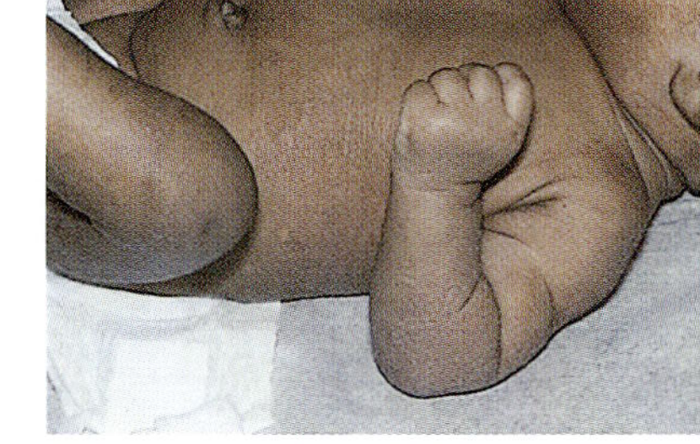

Atopic Dermatitis (eczema)
Erythema, scaling, dry skin, and intense itching characterize this condition in children.

Tinea Capitis
Scaling, crusting, and hair loss are seen in the scalp, along with a painful plaque (kerion) and occipital lymph node (arrow).

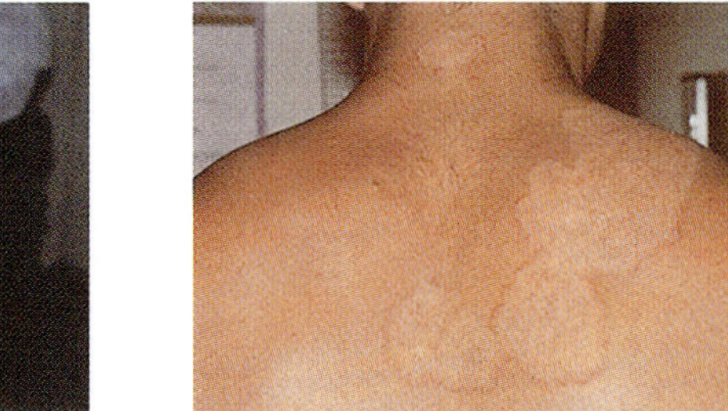

Tinea Corporis
This annular lesion has central clearing and papules along the border.

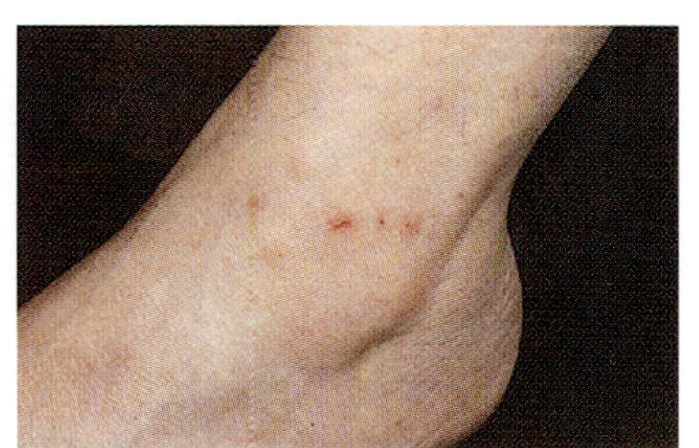
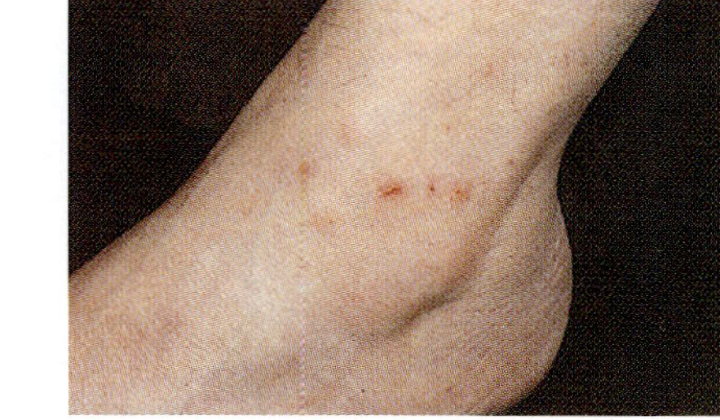

Insect Bites
Intensely pruritic, red, distinct papules characterize these lesions.

(Source of all photos except *Urticaria:* Goodheart H: A Photoguide of Common Skin Disorders, Baltimore, Williams & Wilkins, 1999.)

TABLE 17-10 ■ Cyanosis in Children

It is important for you to be able to recognize cyanosis. The best location to examine is the mucous membranes. Cyanosis is a "raspberry" color, while normal mucous membranes should have a "strawberry color." Try to identify the cyanosis in these photographs before reading the captions.

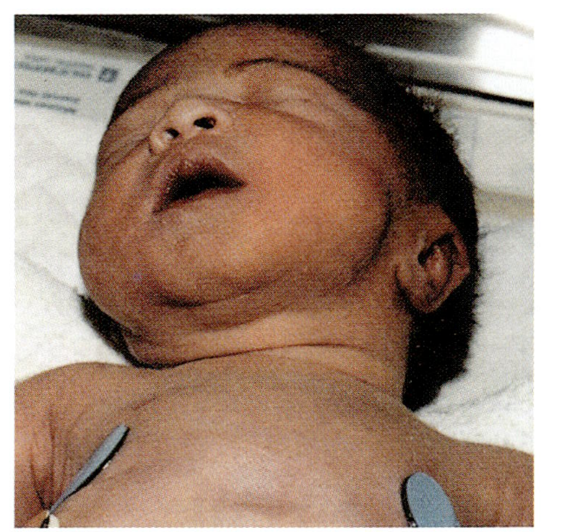

Generalized Cyanosis
This baby had total anomalous pulmonary venous return and an oxygen saturation level of 80%.

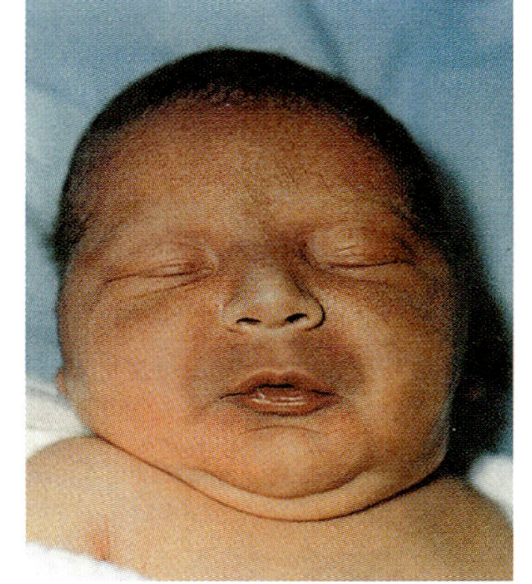

Perioral Cyanosis
This baby has mild cyanosis above the lips, but the mucous membranes remain pink.

Bluish Lips, Giving Appearance of Cyanosis
Normal pigment deposition in the vermilion border of the lips gives them a bluish hue, but the mucous membranes are pink.

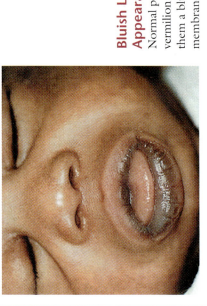

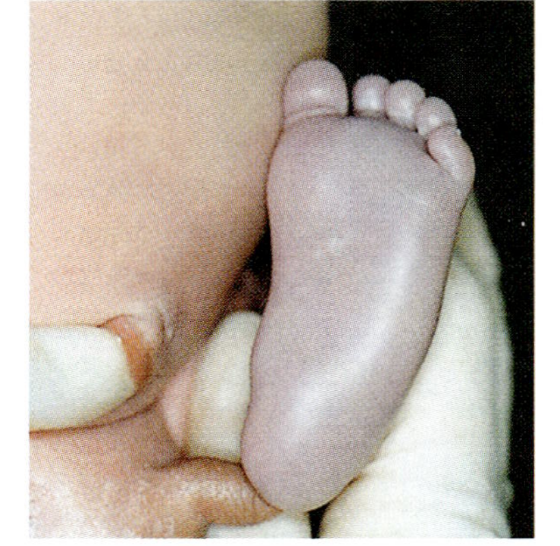

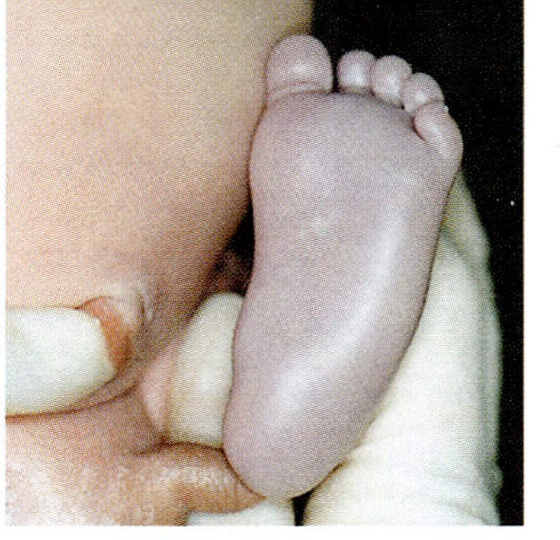

Acrocyanosis
This commonly appears on the feet and hands of babies shortly after birth. This infant is a 32-week newborn.

(Source of photos: Fletcher M: Physical Diagnosis in Neonatology, Philadelphia, Lippincott-Raven Publishers, 1998.)

TABLE 17-11 ■ Abnormalities of the Head

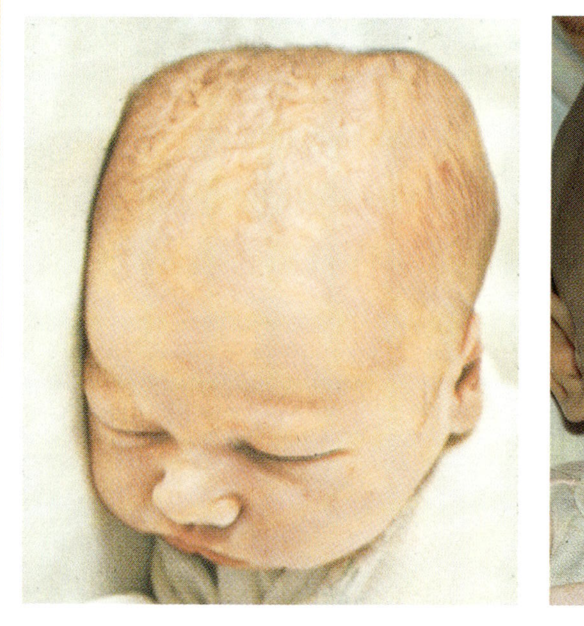

Cephalohematoma

Although not present at birth, cephalohematomas appear within the first 24 hours and are due to subperiosteal hemorrhage involving the outer table of one of the cranial bones. The swelling, as above, does not extend across a suture, though it is occasionally bilateral following a difficult delivery. The swelling is initially soft, then develops a raised bony margin within a few days due to calcium deposits at the edge of the periosteum, and tends to resolve within several weeks.

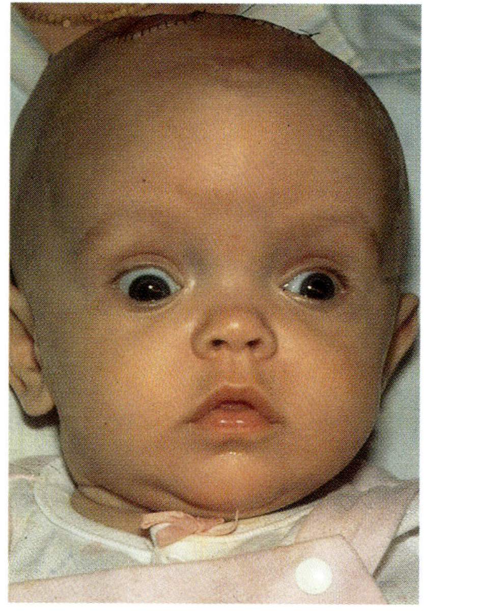

Hydrocephalus

In hydrocephaly, the anterior fontanelle is bulging and the eyes may be deviated downward, revealing the upper scleras and creating the *"setting sun"* sign, as shown in the figure above. The setting sun sign is also seen briefly in some normal newborns. (From Zitelli, BJ & Davis, HW. [1997]. Atlas of Pediatric Physical Diagnosis, 3rd ed., St. Louis: Mosby–Year Book. Courtesy of Dr. Albert Briglan, Children's Hospital of Pittsburgh.)

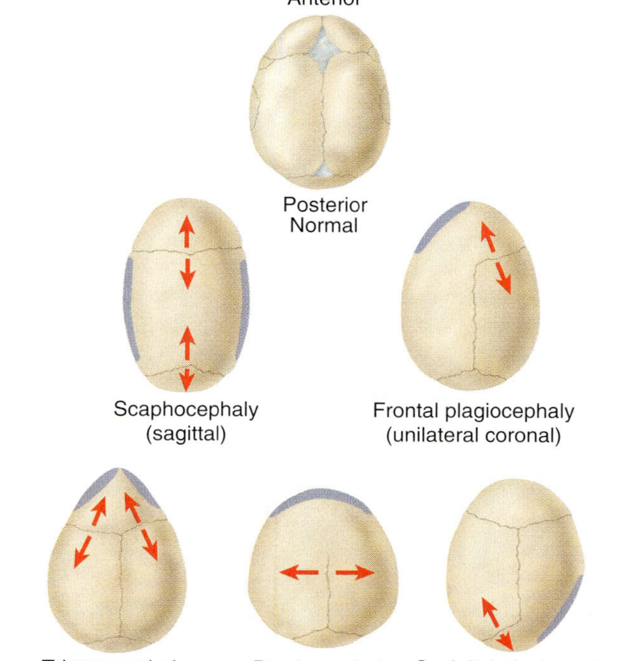

Craniosynostosis is a condition of premature closure of one or more sutures of the skull. This results in an abnormal growth and shape of the skull since growth will occur across sutures that are not affected but not across sutures that are affected. The figures above demonstrate different skull shapes associated with the various types of craniosynostosis. Scaphocephaly and frontal plagiocephaly are the more common types. The blue shading shows areas of maximal flattening. The red arrows show the direction of continued growth across the sutures, which is normal.

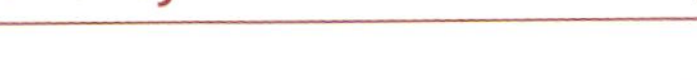

TABLE 17-12 ■ Diagnostic Facies in Infancy and Childhood

Fetal Alcohol Syndrome

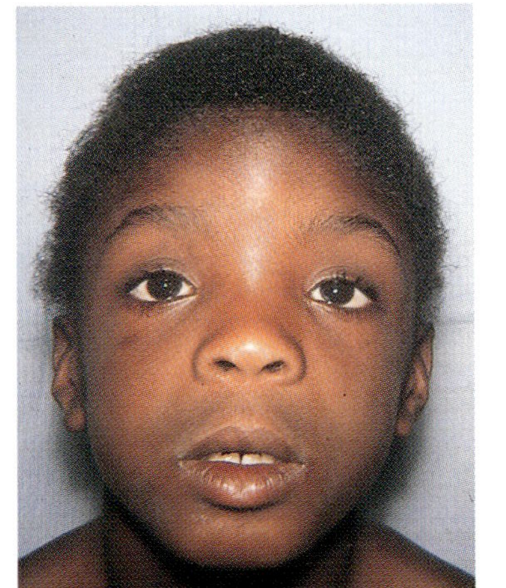

Babies born to women who are chronic alcoholics are at increased risk for growth deficiency, microcephaly, and mental retardation. Facial characteristics shown here include short palpebral fissures, a wide and flattened philtrum (the vertical groove in the midline of the upper lip), and thin lips.

Congenital Syphilis

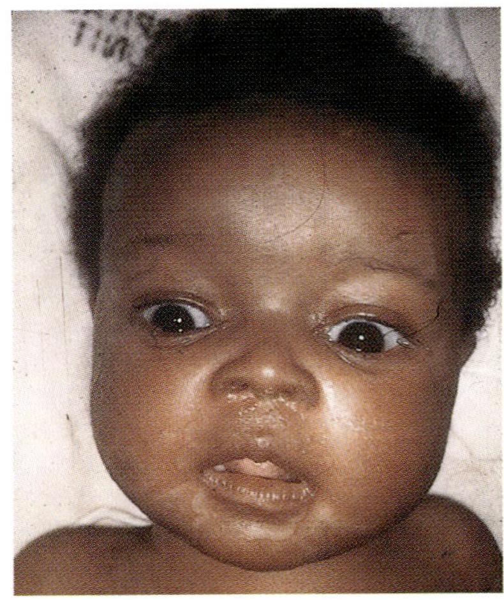

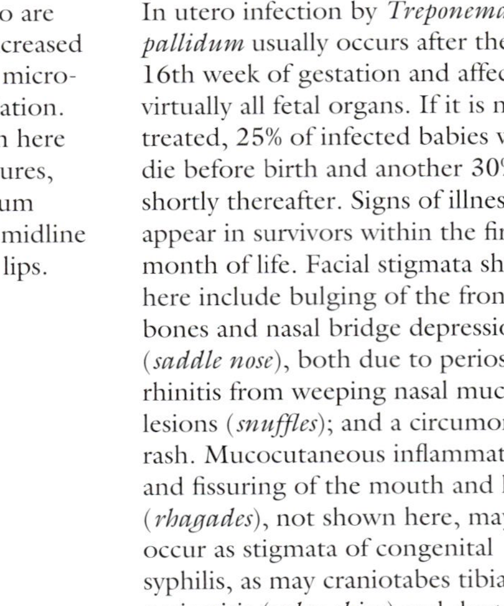

In utero infection by *Treponema pallidum* usually occurs after the 16th week of gestation and affects virtually all fetal organs. If it is not treated, 25% of infected babies will die before birth and another 30% shortly thereafter. Signs of illness appear in survivors within the first month of life. Facial stigmata shown here include bulging of the frontal bones and nasal bridge depression (*saddle nose*), both due to periostitis; rhinitis from weeping nasal mucosal lesions (*snuffles*); and a circumoral rash. Mucocutaneous inflammation and fissuring of the mouth and lips (*rhagades*), not shown here, may also occur as stigmata of congenital syphilis, as may craniotabes tibial periostitis (*saber shins*) and dental dysplasia (*Hutchinson's teeth*—see p. 205).

Congenital Hypothyroidism

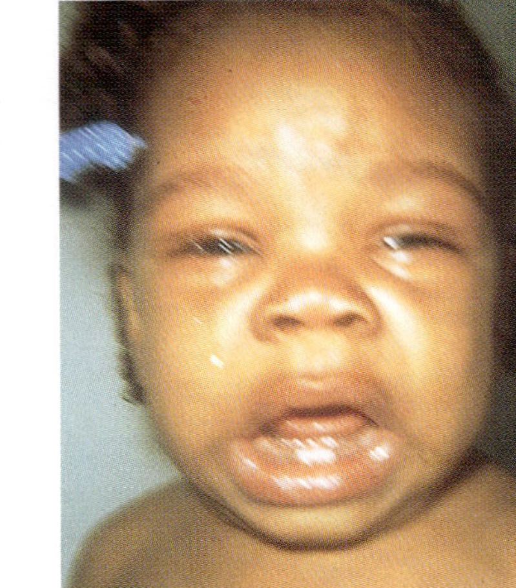

The child with congenital hypothyroidism (cretinism) has coarse facial features, a low-set hair line, sparse eyebrows, and an enlarged tongue. Associated features include a hoarse cry, umbilical hernia, dry and cold extremities, myxedema, mottled skin, and mental retardation. It is important to note that the majority of infants with congenital hypothyroidism have no physical stigmata; this has led to screening of all newborns in the United States and in most other developed countries, for depressed thyroxin or elevated thyroid-stimulating hormone levels.

Facial Nerve Palsy

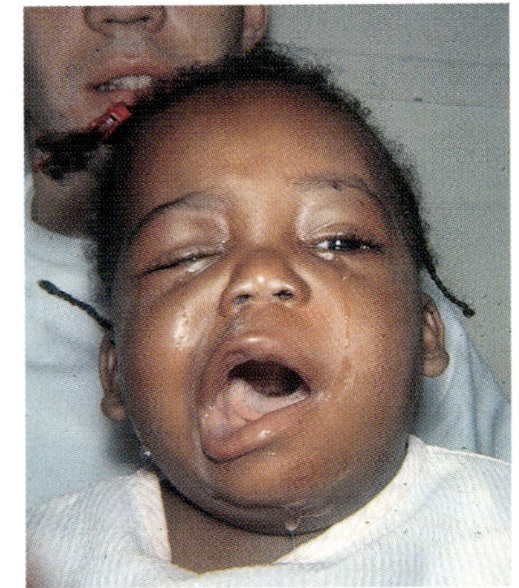

Peripheral (lower motor neuron) paralysis of the facial nerve may be due to (1) an injury to the nerve from pressure during labor and delivery, (2) inflammation of the middle ear branch of the nerve during episodes of acute or chronic otitis media, or (3) unknown causes (Bell's palsy). See p. 612 and p. 613. The nasolabial fold on the affected left side is flattened and the eye does not close. This is accentuated during crying, as shown here. Full recovery occurs in ≥90% of those affected, usually within a few weeks.

Down Syndrome

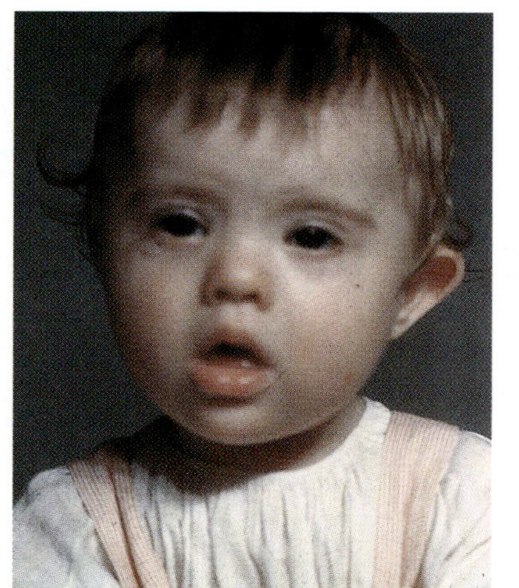

The child with Down syndrome (trisomy 21) usually has a small, rounded head, a flattened nasal bridge, oblique palpebral fissures, prominent epicanthal folds, small, low-set, shell-like ears, and a relatively large tongue. Associated features include generalized hypotonia, transverse palmar creases (*simian lines*), shortening and incurving of the 5th fingers (*clinodactyly*), Brushfield's spots (see p. 771), and mental retardation.

Battered-Child Syndrome

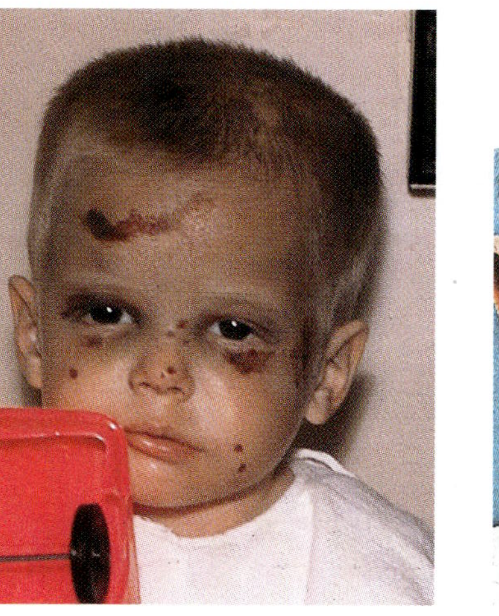

The child who has been physically abused (battered) may have old *and* fresh bruises about the head and face and may either look sad and forlorn or be actively seeking to please, sometimes even particularly involved with and attentive to the abusing parent. Other stigmata include: bruises in areas (axilla and groin) not usually subject to injury rather than the bony prominences, x-ray evidence of fractures of the skull, ribs, and long bones in various stages of healing, and skin lesions that are morphologically similar to implements used to inflict trauma (hand, belt buckle, strap, rope, coat hanger, or lighted cigarette).

Perennial Allergic Rhinitis

The child suffering from perennial allergic rhinitis has an open mouth (cannot breathe through the nose) and edema and discoloration of the lower orbitopalpebral grooves ("allergic shiners"). Such a child is often seen to push the nose upward and backward with a hand ("allergic salute") and to grimace (wrinkle the nose and mouth) to relieve nasal itching and obstruction. (Photograph reproduced with permission from Marks MB: Allergic shiners: Dark circles under the eyes in children. Clin Pediatr 5:656, 1966)

Hyperthyroidism

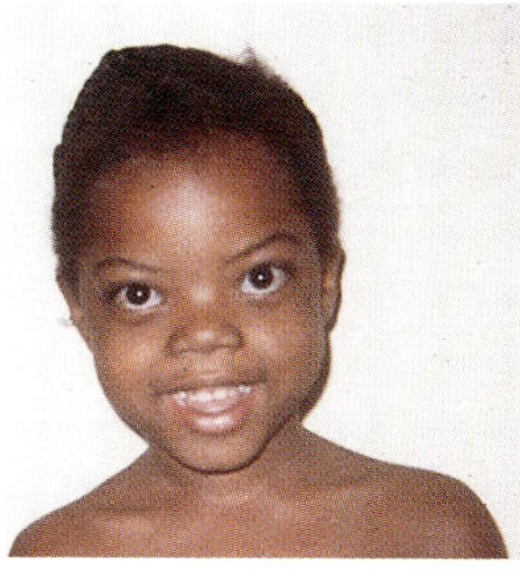

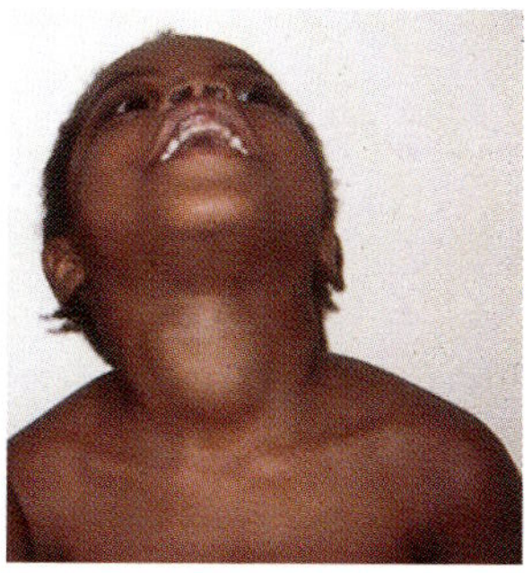

Thyrotoxicosis (*Graves' disease*) occurs in approximately 2 per 1,000 children under the age of 10 years. Affected children exhibit hypermetabolism and accelerated linear growth. Facial characteristics shown in this 6-year-old girl are "staring" eyes (not true exophthalmos, which is rare in children) and an enlarged thyroid gland (*goiter*). See p. 208.

TABLE 17-13 ■ Abnormalities of the Neck

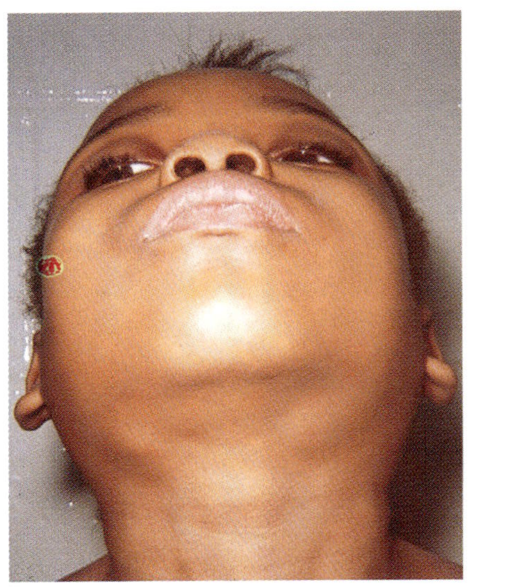

Lymphadenopathy

Enlarged and tender cervical lymph nodes are common in children. The most likely causes are viral and bacterial infections. Lymph node enlargement can be bilateral, as shown above.

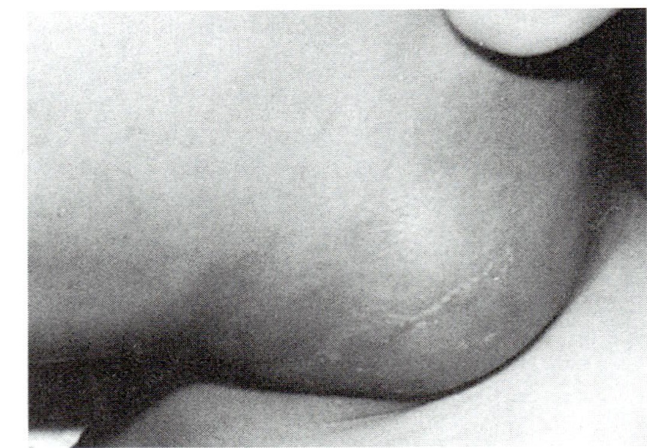

Lymphadenitis and Abscess

An infected cervical lymph node may turn into an abscess, with fluctuance.

(Source of photo for: *Lymphadenitis and Abscess*—Fleisher G, Ludwig S: Textbook of Pediatric Emergency Medicine, 4th ed. Philadelphia, Lippincott Williams & Wilkins, 2000.)

TABLE 17-14 ■ Abnormalities of the Eyes and Ears

Eye Abnormalities

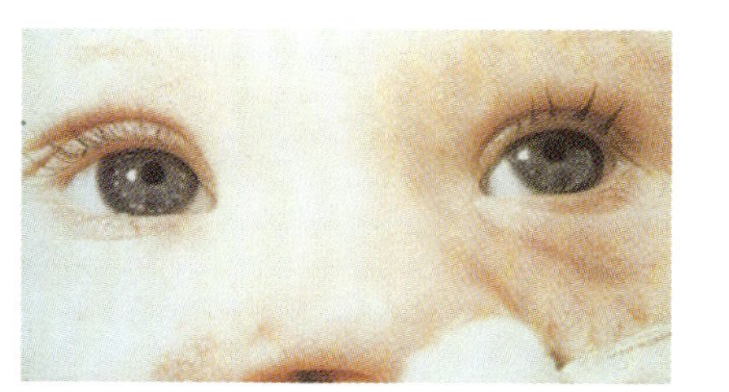

Brushfield's Spots
These abnormal speckling spots on the iris suggest Down syndrome.

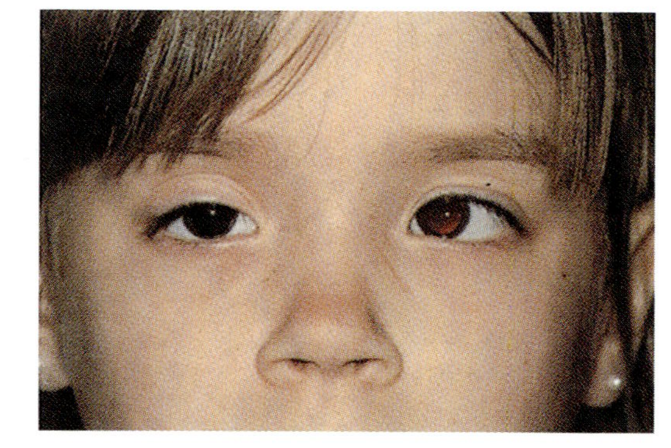

Strabismus
Strabismus, or misalignment of the eyes, can lead to visual impairment. Esotropia, shown here, is an inward deviation.

Ear Abnormalities

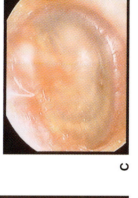

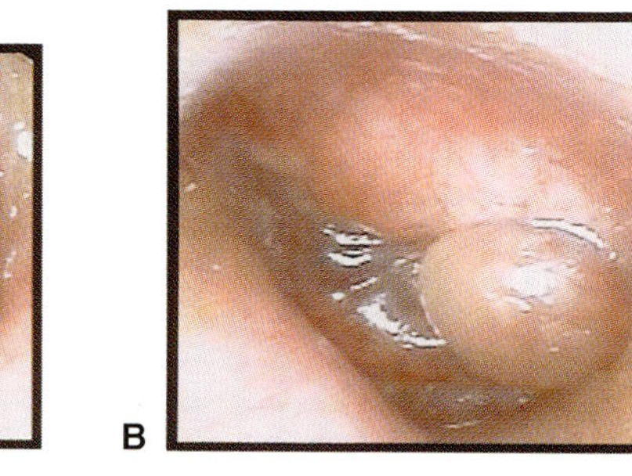

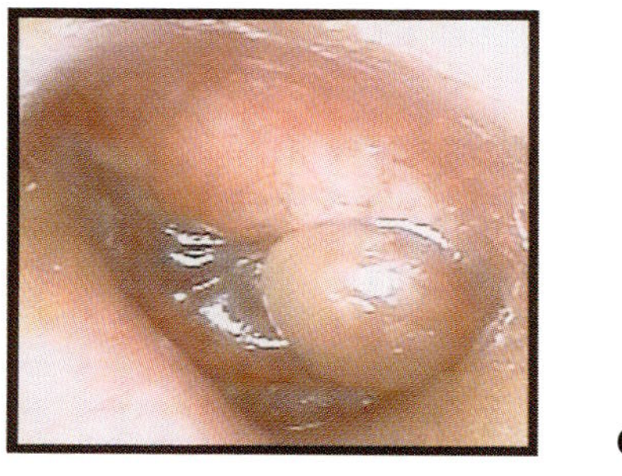

A B C

Otitis Media
Otitis media is one of the most common conditions in young children. The spectrum of otitis media is shown here. **(A)** Typical acute otitis media with a red, distorted, bulging tympanic membrane in a highly symptomatic child. **(B)** Acute otitis media with bullae formation and fluid visible behind the tympanic membrane. **(C)** Otitis media with effusion, showing a yellowish fluid behind a retracted and thickened tympanic membrane.

Source of photos: *Estropia*—Fleisher G, Ludwig S: Textbook of Pediatric Emergency Medicine, 4th ed., Philadelphia, Lippincott Williams & Wilkins, 2000; *Otitis Media*—Courtesy of Alejandro Hoberman, Children's Hospital of Pittsburgh, University of Pittsburgh.

TABLE 17-15 ■ Abnormalities of the Mouth and Teeth

Mouth Abnormalities

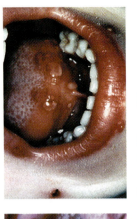

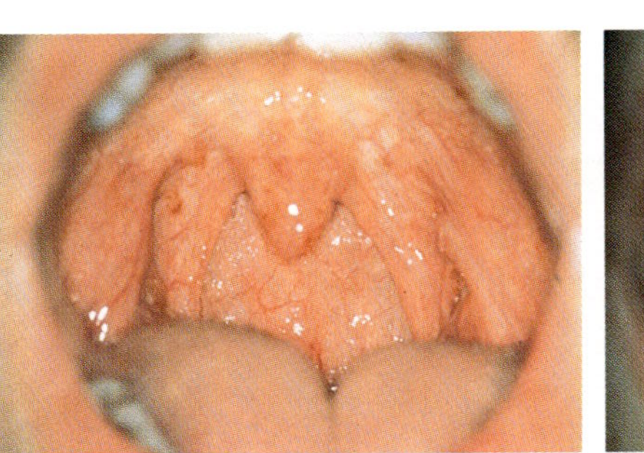

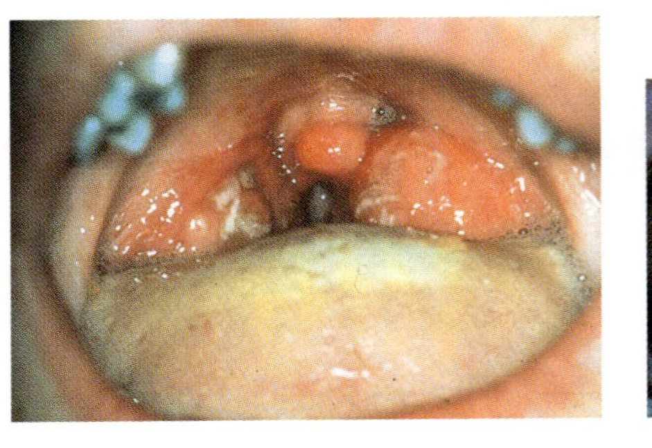

Streptococcal Pharyngitis ("strep throat")
This common childhood infection has a classic presentation of erythema of the posterior pharynx and palatal petechiae (left). A foul-smelling exudate (right) is also commonly noted.

Oral Candidiasis ("thrush")
This infection is common in infants. The white plaques do not rub off.

Herpetic Stomatitis
Tender ulcerations on the oral mucosa are surrounded by erythema.

Dental Abnormalities

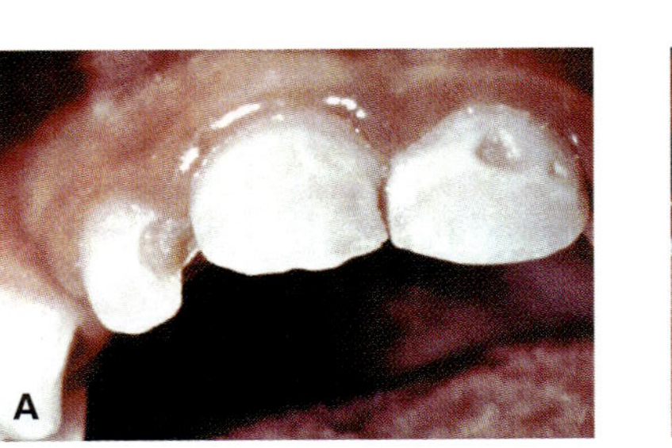

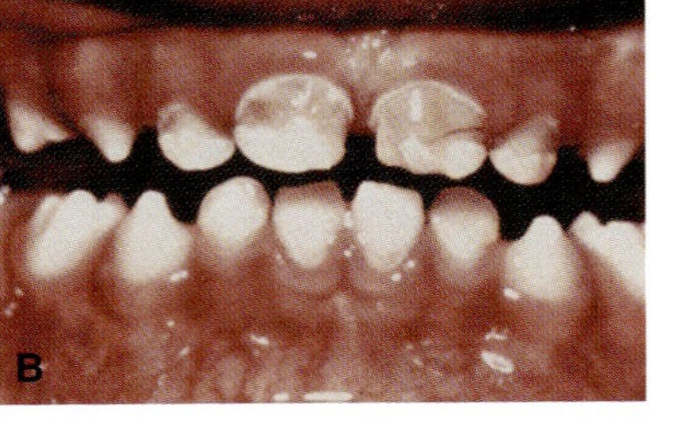

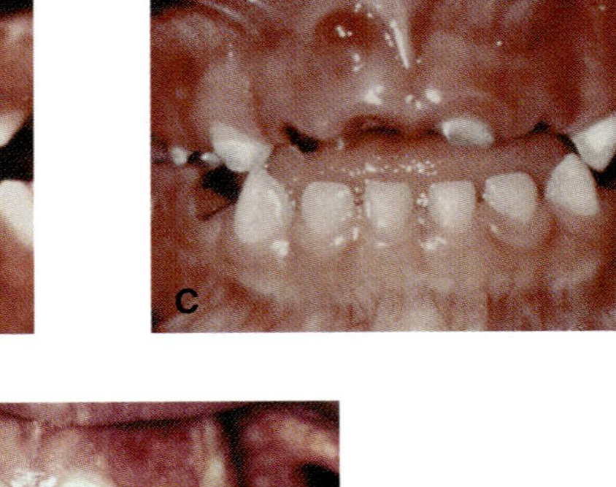

Dental Caries
Dental caries is a major public health and pediatric problem throughout the world. The photographs on the left show different characteristics of caries. **(A)** Early nursing-bottle caries with discoloration on the inside of the upper incisors. **(B)** Erosion of several teeth. **(C)** Severe erosion and abscess formation.

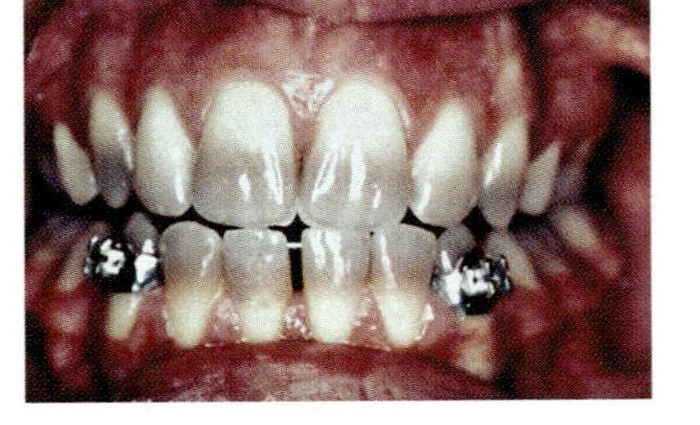

Staining of the Teeth
The teeth of children can become stained from a variety of causes, including intrinsic stains such as tetracycline (right) or extrinsic stains such as poor oral hygiene (not shown). Extrinsic stains can be removed.

Photos courtesy of American Academy of Pediatrics.

TABLE 17-16 ■ Pathologic Findings of Some Common Congenital Cardiac Defects: Heart Murmurs

Some heart murmurs reflect underlying heart disease. If you understand the physiologic causes for these heart murmurs, you will more readily be able to identify them and distinguish them from innocent heart murmurs. Obstructive lesions are caused by normal blood flow through valves that are too small for normal flow. Since this problem is not dependent on the drop in pulmonary vascular resistance that occurs following birth, these murmurs are audible at birth. Defects with left-to-right shunts, on the other hand, are dependent on the drop in pulmonary vascular resistance and are, therefore, not heard until a week or more after birth in the case of high-pressured shunts such as ventricular septal defect, patent ductus arteriosus, and persistent truncus arteriosus. Low-pressured left-to-right shunts, such as in atrial septal defects, may not be heard for a considerably longer time, usually first being noted at a year or more of age. It is important to note that many children with congenital cardiac defects have combinations of defects or variations of abnormalities, so that findings on cardiac examination will not follow these classic patterns. This table shows a limited selection of the more common defects.

Congenital Defect	Mechanism	Characteristics of the Murmur	Associated Findings
Pulmonary Valve Stenosis			
Mild S_1 A_2 P_2	Usually a normal valve anulus with fusion of some or most of the valve leaflets, restricting flow across the valve	*Location.* Upper left sternal border *Radiation.* In mild degrees of stenosis, the murmur may be heard over the course of the pulmonary arteries in the lung fields. *Intensity.* Increases in intensity and duration as the degree of obstruction increases *Quality.* Ejection, peaking later in systole as the obstruction increases	Usually a prominent ejection click in early systole The pulmonary component of the second sounds at the base (P_2) becomes delayed and softer, disappearing as obstruction increases. Inspiration may increase the murmur and expiration may increase the click. Growth is usually normal. Newborns with severe stenosis may be cyanotic from right-to-left shunting at atrial level and rapidly develop congestive heart failure.
Moderate S_1 A_2 P_2			
Severe S_1 A_2 P_2			
Aortic Valve Stenosis S_1 A_2 P_2	Usually a bicuspid valve with progressive obstruction, but there may be a dysplastic valve or damage from rheumatic fever or degenerative disease.	*Location.* Midsternum, upper right sternal border *Radiation.* To the carotid arteries and suprasternal notch; may also be a thrill *Intensity.* Varies, louder with increasingly severe obstruction *Quality.* An ejection, often harsh, systolic murmur	May be an associated ejection click The aortic closure sound may be increased in intensity. There may be a diastolic murmur of aortic valve regurgitation. Children and adolescents are seldom symptomatic, but newborns with severe stenosis may have weak or absent pulses and severe congestive heart failure. Unless heart failure, growth is normal. May not be audible until adulthood even though the valve is congenitally abnormal

(table continues next page)

TABLE 17-16 ■ Pathologic Findings of Some Common Congenital Cardiac Defects: Heart Murmurs *(Continued)*

Congenital Defect	Mechanism	Characteristics of the Murmur	Associated Findings
Tetralogy of Fallot *With pulmonic stenosis* *With pulmonic atresia*	Complex defect with ventricular septal defect, infundibular and usually valvular right ventricular outflow obstruction, malrotation of the aorta, and right-to-left shunting at ventricular septal level.	*General.* Variable cyanosis, increasing with activity *Location.* Mid-to-upper left sternal border. If pulmonary atresia, there is no systolic murmur but the continuous murmur of ductus arteriosus flow at upper left sternal border or in the back. *Radiation.* Little, to upper left sternal border, occasionally to lung fields *Intensity.* Usually Grade III-IV *Quality.* Midpeaking, systolic ejection murmur	Normal pulses The pulmonary closure sound is usually not heard. May have abrupt hypercyanotic spells with sudden increase in cyanosis, air hunger, altered level of awareness Failure to gain weight with persistent and increasingly severe cyanosis Long-term persistence of cyanosis accompanied by clubbing of fingers and toes Persistent hypoxemia leads to polycythemia, which will accentuate the cyanosis.
Transposition of the Great Arteries	A severe defect with failure of rotation of the great vessels, leaving the aorta to arise from the right ventricle and the pulmonary artery from the left ventricle	*General.* Intense generalized cyanosis *Location.* No characteristic murmur. If a murmur is present, it may reflect an associated defect such as VSD or patent ductus arteriosus. *Radiation.* Depends on associated abnormalities *Quality.* Depends on associated abnormalities	Single loud second sound of the anterior aortic valve Frequent rapid development of congestive heart failure Frequent associated defects as described at the left
Ventricular Septal Defect *Small to moderate* 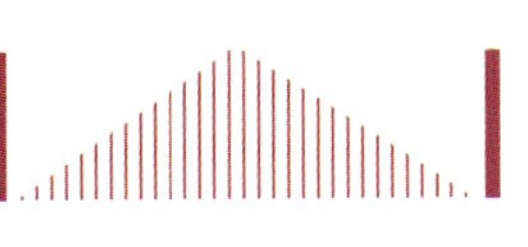	Blood going from a high-pressured left ventricle through a defect in the septum to the lower-pressured right ventricle creates turbulence, usually throughout systole.	*Location.* Lower left sternal border *Radiation.* Little *Intensity.* Variable, only partially determined by the size of the shunt. Small shunts with a high pressure gradient may have very loud murmurs. Large defects with elevated pulmonary vascular resistance may have no murmur. Grade II-IV/VI with a thrill if Grade IV/VI or higher.	With large shunts, there may be a low-pitched middiastolic murmur of relative mitral stenosis at the apex. As pulmonary artery pressure increases, the pulmonic component of the second sounds at the base increases in intensity. When pulmonary artery pressure equals aortic pressure, there may be no murmur, and P_2 will be very loud. In low-volume shunts, growth is normal.

		Quality. Pansystolic, usually harsh, may obscure S_1 and S_2 if loud enough	In larger shunts, congestive heart failure may occur by 6–8 weeks; poor weight gain. Associated defects are frequent.
Patent Ductus Arteriosus *Small to moderate* 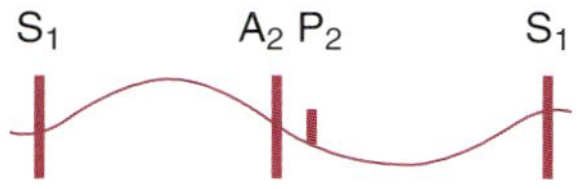 S_1 A_2 P_2 S_1	Continuous flow from aorta to pulmonary artery throughout the cardiac cycle when ductus arteriosus does not close after birth	*Location.* Upper left sternal border and to left *Radiation.* Sometimes to the back *Intensity.* Varies depending on size of the shunt, usually Grade II-III/VI. *Quality.* A rather hollow, sometimes machinerylike murmur that is continuous throughout the cardiac cycle, although occasionally almost inaudible in late diastole, uninterrupted by the heart sounds, louder in systole	Full to bounding pulses Noticed at birth in the premature infant who may have bounding pulses, a hyperdynamic precordium, and an atypical murmur Noticed later in the full-term infant as pulmonary vascular resistance falls May develop congestive heart failure at 4 to 6 weeks if large shunt Poor weight gain related to size of shunt Pulmonary hypertension affects murmur as above.
Atrial Septal Defect 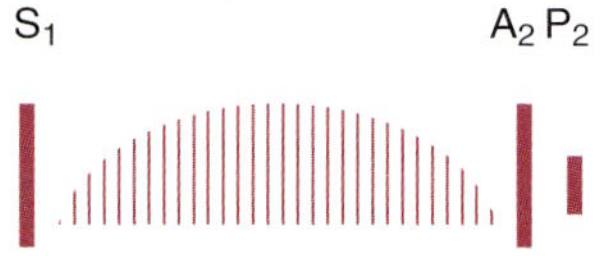 S_1 A_2 P_2	Left-to-right shunt through an opening in the atrial septum, possible at various levels	*Location.* Upper left sternal border *Radiation.* To the back *Intensity.* Variable, usually Grade II-III/VI *Quality.* Ejection but without the harsh quality	Widely split second sounds throughout all phases of respiration, normal intensity Usually not heard until after age of 1 year Gradual decrease in weight gain as shunt increases Decreased exercise tolerance, subtle, not dramatic Congestive heart failure is rare.

TABLE 17-17 ■ The Male Genitourinary System

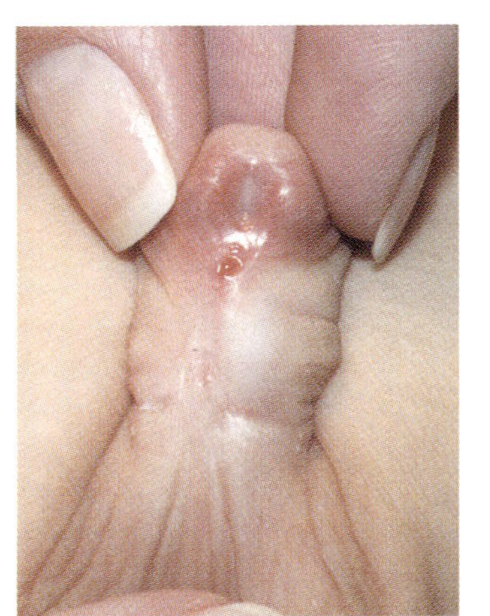

Hypospadius

Hypospadius is the most common congenital penile abnormality. The urethral meatus opens abnormally on the ventral surface of the penis. One form is shown above; more severe forms involve openings on the lower shaft or scrotum.

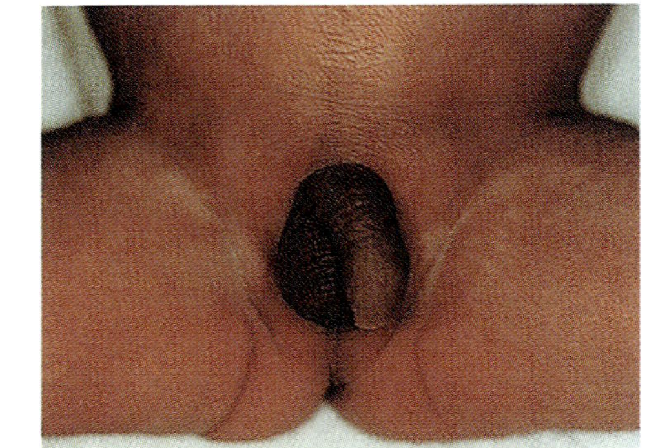

Undescended Testicle

You should distinguish between undescended testes, shown above (with testes in the inguinal canals), from highly retractile testes due to an active cremasteric reflex.

Torsion

In school-age and adolescent boys, two types of torsion can occur: torsion of the testis and torsion of the appendix testis. In torsion of the testis, boys have acute severe testicular pain. Examination shows a swollen, tender testis and an absent cremasteric reflex. In torsion of the appendix testis (not shown), there is also acute pain, although generally not as sever as with torsion of the testis. You may note a bluish discoloration (blue dot sign) at the infarcted appendage. In these cases, the cremasteric reflex is usually present

Source of photos: *Hypospadius*—Courtesy of Warren Snodgrass, MD, UT–Southwestern Medical Center at Dallas; *Undescended Testicle*—Fletcher M: Physical Diagnosis in Neonatology, Philadelphia, Lippincott-Raven Publishers, 1998.

TABLE 17-18 ■ Abnormalities of the Female Genitourinary System

Ambiguous Genitalia

Some rare conditions result in ambiguous genitalia. This is a case of congenital adrenal hyperplasia.

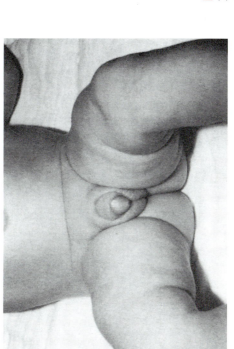

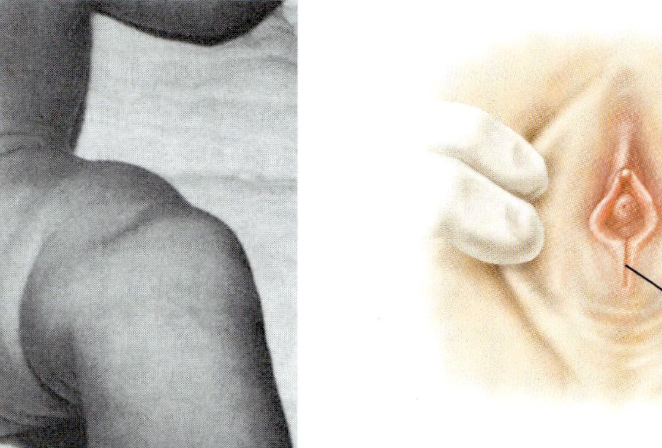

Labial Adhesions

Fusion of the labia minora can obscure part or all of the vaginal orifice.

(table continues next page)

TABLE 17-18 ■ Abnormalities of the Female Genitourinary System *(Continued)*

Physical Signs of Sexual Abuse in Girls

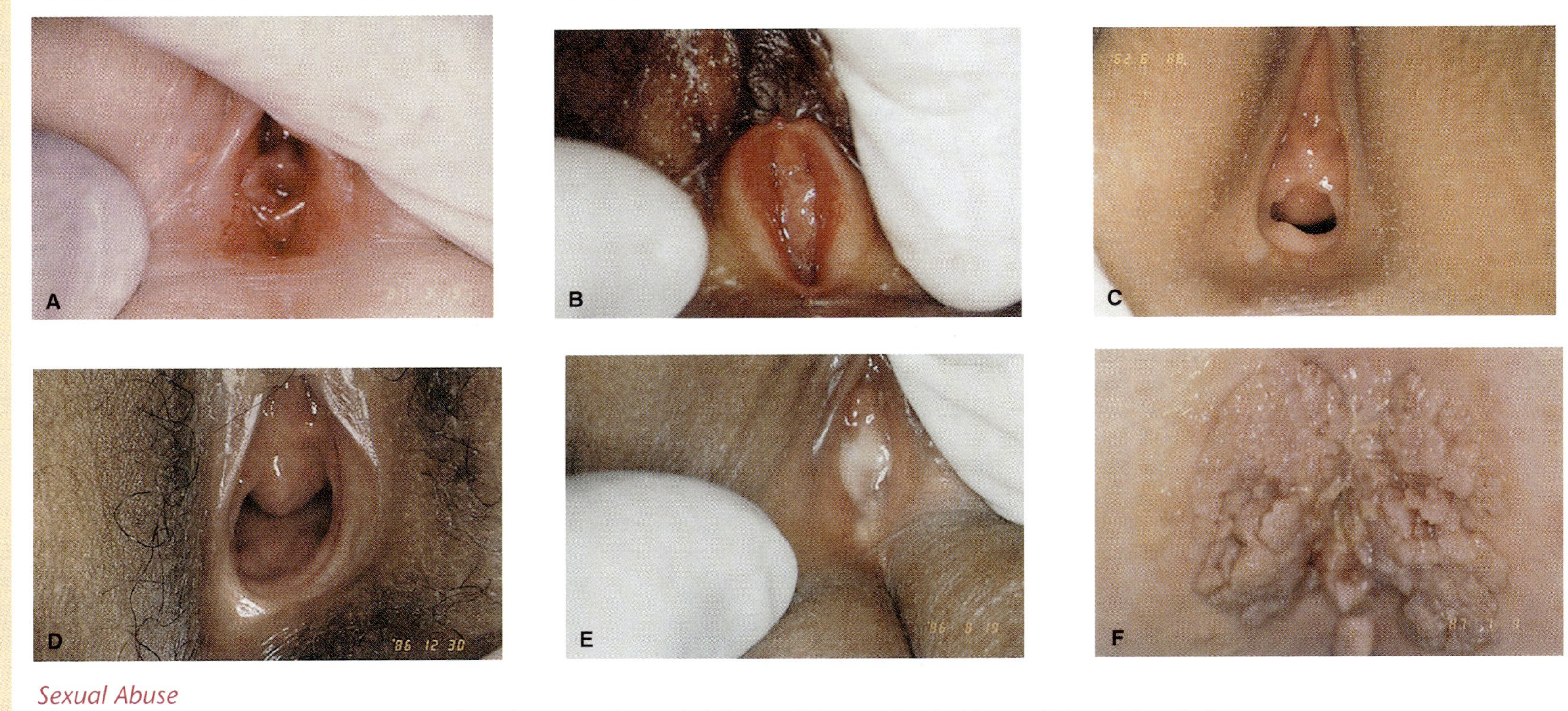

Sexual Abuse

Since sexual abuse is all too common, you will need to recognize genital abnormalities associated with sexual abuse. These include:

(A) Acute hemorrhage and ecchymoses of tissues (10-mo old)
(B) Erythema and superficial abrasions to the labia minora (5-yr old)
(C) Healed interruption of hymenal membrane at 9 o'clock (4-yr old)
(D) Narrowed posterior ring continuous with floor of vagina (12-yr old)
(E) Copious vaginal discharge and erythema (9-yr old)
(F) Extensive condylomata around the anus (2-yr old)

(Sources of photos: *Ambiguous Genitalia*—McMillan J, DeAngelis C, Feigin R, Warshaw J: Oski's Pediatrics, 3rd ed., Philadelphia, Lippincott Williams & Wilkins, 1999; *Sexual Abuse, (A), (B), (C), (D), (E), (F)*—Reece R, Ludwig S (eds.): Child Abuse Medical Diagnosis and Management, 2nd ed., Philadelphia, Lippincott Williams & Wilkins, 2001.)

TABLE 17-19 ■ Abnormalities of the Musculoskeletal and Nervous Systems

Orthopedic Abnormalities in Children

Scoliosis
Idiopathic scoliosis occurs most often in adolescent girls. The rotation of the spine usually results in a right-sided prominence.

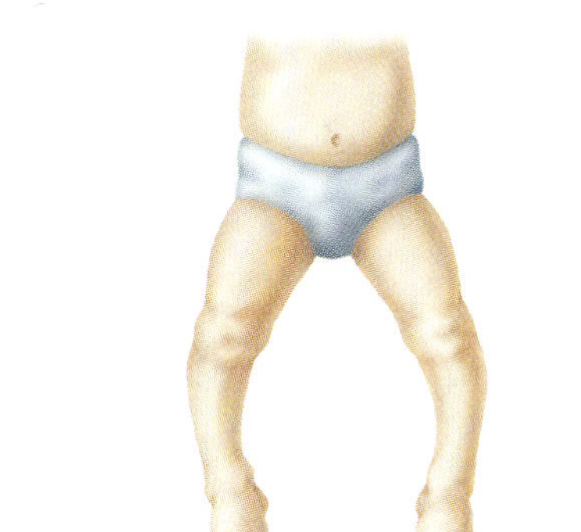

Bowing of Knees from Rickets
Severe bowing of the knees may be due to rickets. Other clinical signs are usually present in this condition.

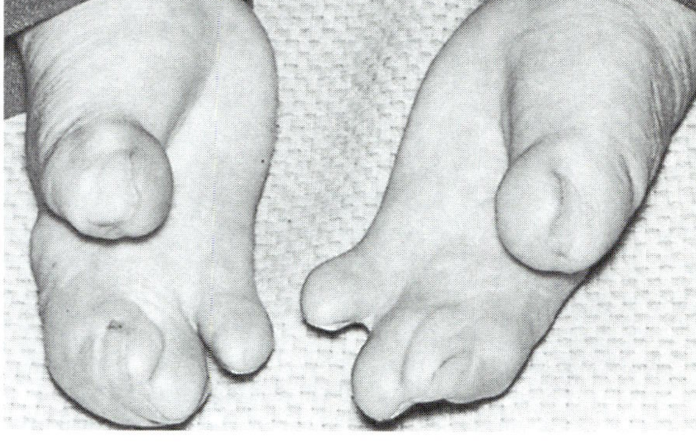

Syndactyly
A number of conditions occur involving congenital failure of differentiation, such as synostosis of the middle and ring fingers shown here. (From: McMillan J, DeAngelis C, Feigin R, Warshaw J: Oski's Pediatrics, 3rd ed., Philadelphia, Lippincott Williams & Wilkins, 1999.)

(table continues next page)

TABLE 17-19 ■ Abnormalities of the Musculoskeletal and Nervous Systems *(Continued)*

Neurologic Abnormalities in Children

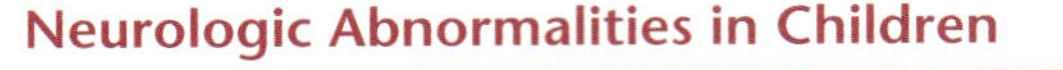

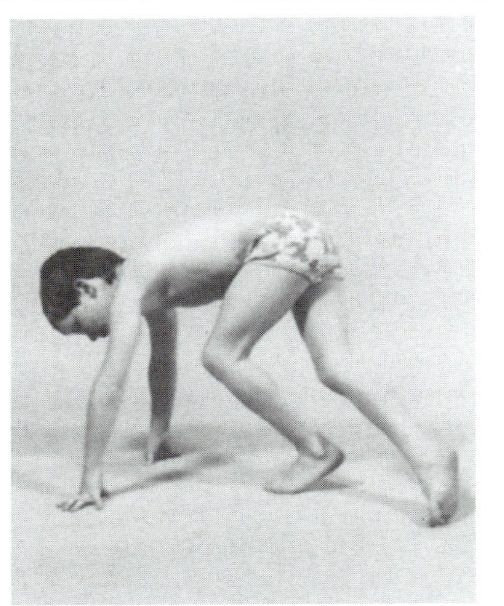

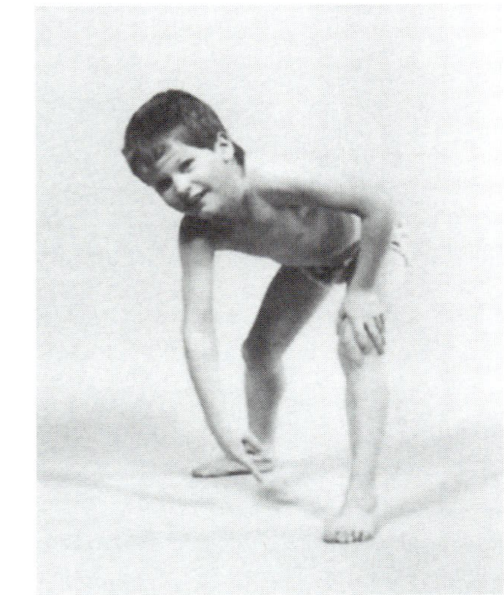

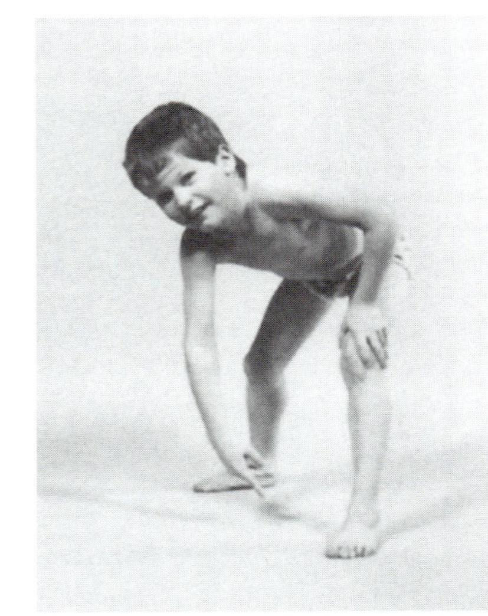

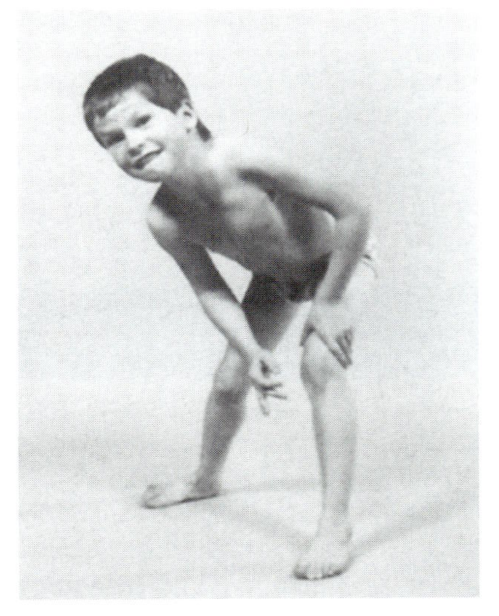

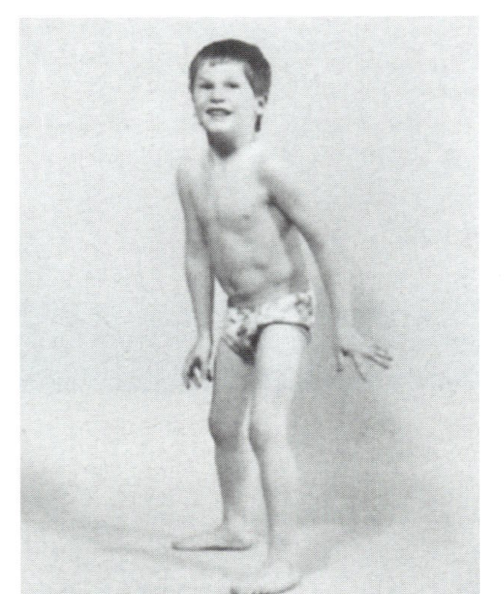

The Gower Maneuver

Certain forms of muscular dystrophy involve weakness of the pelvic girdle muscles. Children with this disease rise from a supine to a standing position in a characteristic manner, by rolling over to a prone position, pushing off the floor with the arms, bringing the legs to a flexed position under the trunk, and extending the legs with help of the hands.

TABLE 17-20 ■ The Power of Prevention: Vaccine-Preventable Diseases

This table shows photographs of children with vaccine-preventable diseases. Childhood vaccines have been named the single most important medical intervention in the world from the standpoint of impact on public health. Because of vaccinations, we hope you will never see many of these conditions, but you should be able to identify them. Try to identify the diseases before reading the captions.

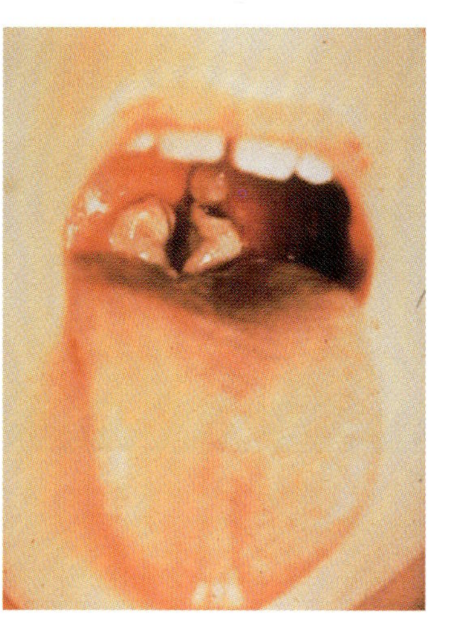

Diphtheria
This child has the characteristic gray coating on the posterior pharynx.

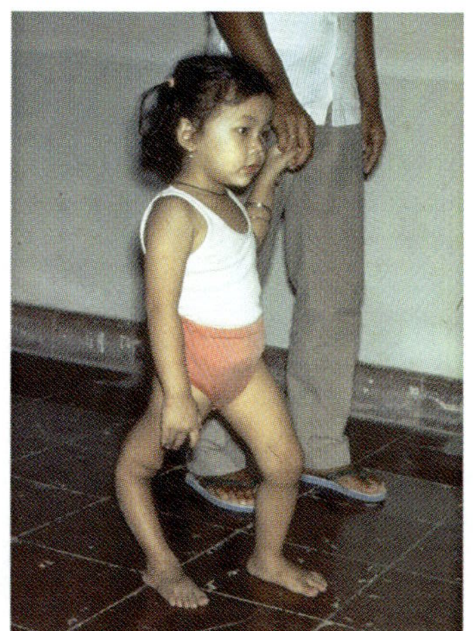

Polio
The deformed leg of this child is due to polio.

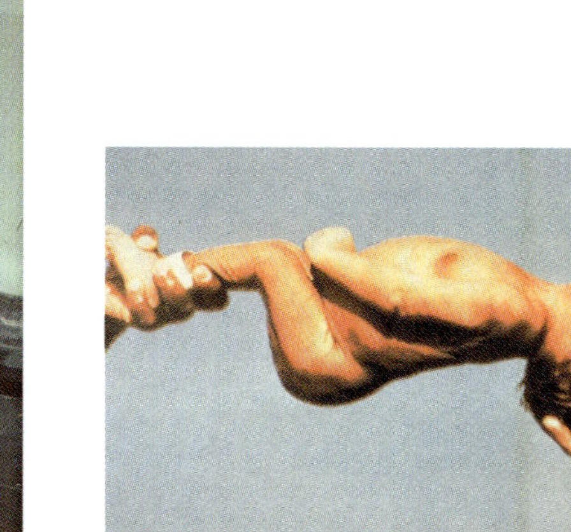

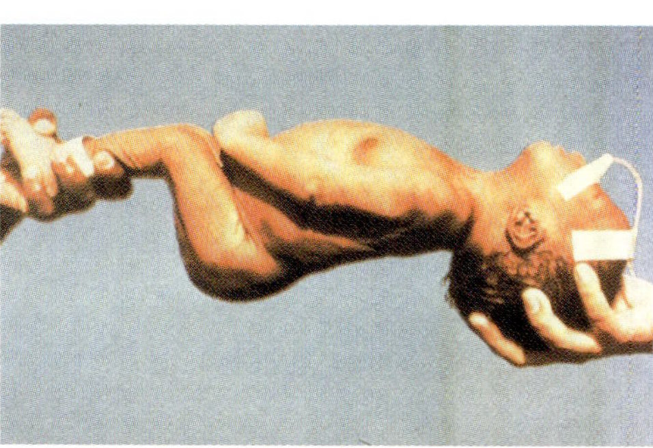

Tetanus
Rigid newborn with neonatal tetanus

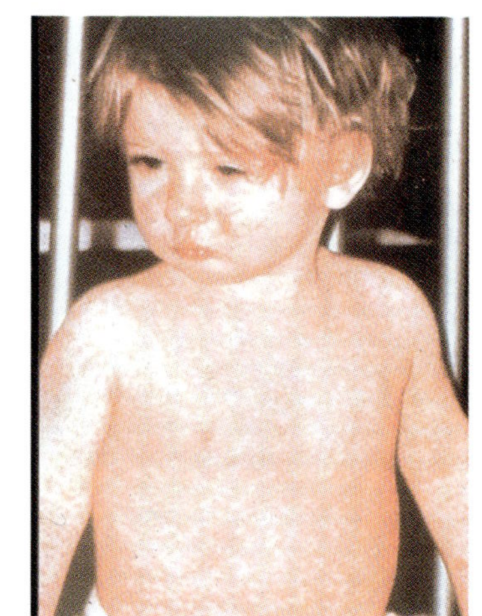

Measles
Characteristic rash of measles

(table continues next page)

TABLE 17-20 ■ The Power of Prevention: Vaccine-Preventable Diseases *(Continued)*

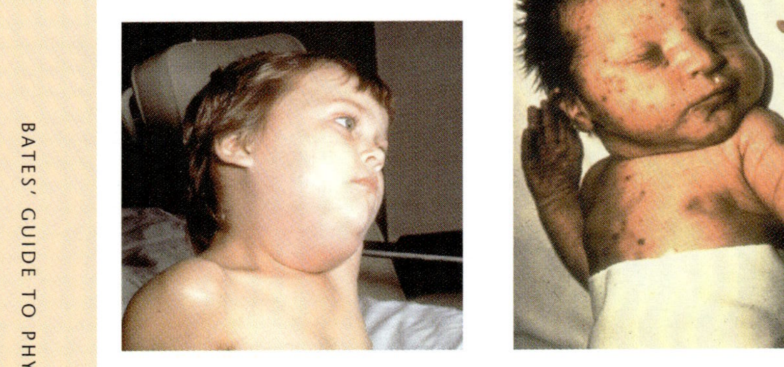

Mumps
Submandibular lymphadenopathy, extensive edema and erythema from mumps.

Rubella
Infant born with congenital rubella syndrome

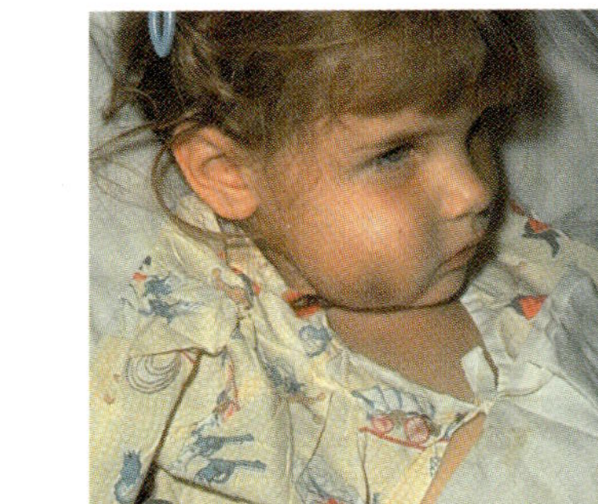

***Haemophilus influenzae* type b**
Periorbital cellulitis due to this invasive bacterial disease

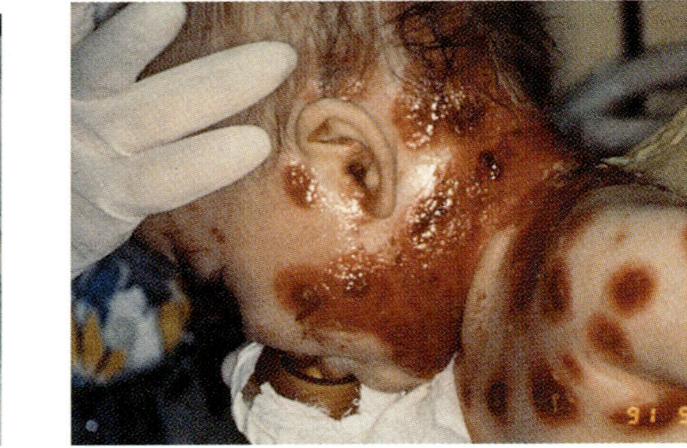

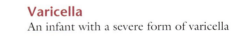

Varicella
An infant with a severe form of varicella

(Sources of photos: *Polio* courtesy of World Health Organization; *Haemophilus influenzae*, courtesy of American Academy of Pediatrics; *Varicella*, courtesy of Barbara Watson, MD, Albert Einstein Medical Center and Division of Disease Control, Philadelphia Department of Health; all others courtesy of Centers for Disease Control and Prevention.)

CHAPTER

18

Clinical Reasoning, Assessment, and Plan

Now that you have gained your patient's trust, gathered a detailed history, and completed the requisite portions of the physical examination, you have reached the critical step of formulating your *Assessment(s)* and *Plan*. It is your task to analyze your findings and identify the patient's problems. Furthermore, you must share your impressions with the patient, eliciting any concerns and making sure that he or she understands and agrees to the steps ahead. Finally, you must document your findings in the patient's record in a succinct and legible format. A clear and well-organized record is essential for communicating the patient's story and your clinical reasoning and plan to other members of the health care team.

The comprehensive data you have collected, both *subjective* (the history, or what the patient or family have told you) and *objective* (the physical examination and laboratory tests), make up the core elements of your patient's database. This information is primarily factual and descriptive. As you move to *Assessment*, you go beyond description and observation to analysis and interpretation. You select and cluster relevant pieces of information, analyze their possible meanings, and try to explain them logically using principles of biopsychosocial and biomedical science. The *Assessment* and *Plan* include the patient's responses to the problems identified and to your diagnostic and therapeutic plans. A successful *Plan* requires good interpersonal skills and sensitivity to the patient's goals, economic means, competing responsibilities, and family structure and dynamics.

In this chapter, we describe the process of clinical reasoning and illustrate the written *Assessment* and *Plan* using the case of Mrs. N from Chapter 1, pp. 14–18. A series of guidelines outline principles for developing an accurate, clear, and logical patient record. A well-organized record facilitates clinical thinking, promotes communication and coordination among the many professionals caring for your patient, and documents that patient's problems and management for medicolegal purposes. There is also a section describing quantitative tools such as sensitivity and specificity to help strengthen your skills of clinical reasoning.

Assessment and Plan: The Process of Clinical Reasoning

Generating Your Assessment. Because assessment takes place in the clinician's mind, the process of clinical reasoning often seems inaccessible and even mysterious to the beginning student. Experienced clinicians often think quickly, with little overt or conscious effort. They differ widely in personal style, communication skills, clinical training, experience, and interests. Some clinicians may find it difficult to explain the logic behind their clinical thinking. As an active learner, it is expected that you will ask teachers and clinicians to elaborate on the fine points of their clinical reasoning and decision making.

As you gain experience, your thinking process will begin at the outset of the patient encounter, not at the end. Listed below are a set of principles that underlie the process of clinical reasoning and certain explicit steps to help guide your thinking as you analyze the information you have compiled. After reading through this section, review the case of Mrs. N, introduced in Chapter 1, and use this as a sample database to practice the process of clinical reasoning and assessment. As with all patients, focus on finding answers to the questions "What is wrong with this patient?" "What are the problems and diagnoses?" To reach these answers, try following the steps discussed below. Then turn to the *Assessment and Plan* for Mrs. N on pp. 14–18 and compare them to your own insights and clinical thinking.

IDENTIFYING PROBLEMS AND MAKING DIAGNOSES: STEPS IN CLINICAL REASONING

- Identify abnormal findings
- Localize findings anatomically
- Interpret findings in terms of probable process
- Make hypotheses about the nature of the patient's problem
- Test the hypotheses and establish a working diagnosis
- Develop a plan agreeable to the patient

- **Identify abnormal findings.** Make a list of the patient's *symptoms,* the *signs* you observed during the physical examination, and any laboratory reports that are available to you.

- **Localize these findings anatomically.** This step may be easy. The symptom of scratchy throat and the sign of an erythematous inflamed pharynx, for example, clearly localize the problem to the pharynx. For Mrs. N, the complaint of headache leads you quickly to the structures of the skull and brain. Other symptoms, however, may present greater difficulty. Chest pain, for example, can originate in the coronary arteries, the stomach and esophagus, or the muscles and bones of the chest. If the pain is exertional and relieved by rest, either the heart or the musculoskeletal components of the chest wall may be involved. If the patient notes pain only when carrying groceries with the left arm, the musculoskeletal system becomes the likely culprit. When localizing findings, be as specific as your data allow, but bear in mind that you may have to settle for a body region, such as the chest, or a body system, such as the musculoskeletal system. On the other hand, you may be able to define the exact structure involved, such as the left pectoral muscle. Some symptoms and signs cannot be localized, such as fatigue or fever, but are useful in the next set of steps.

- **Interpret the findings in terms of the probable process.** Patient problems often stem from a *pathologic process* involving diseases of a body structure. There are a number of such processes, variably classified, including congenital, inflammatory or infectious, immunologic, neoplastic, metabolic, nutritional, degenerative, vascular, traumatic, and toxic. Possible pathologic causes of headache, for example, include concussion from trauma, subarachnoid hemorrhage, or even compression from a brain tumor. Fever and stiff neck, or nuchal rigidity, are two of the classic signs of headache from meningitis. Even without other signs such as rash or papilledema, they strongly suggest an infectious process.

  Other problems are *pathophysiologic,* reflecting derangements of biologic functions, such as congestive heart failure or migraine headache. Still other problems are *psychopathologic,* such as disorders of mood like depression or headache as an expression of a somatization disorder.

- **Make hypotheses about the nature of the patient's problem.** Here you will draw on all the knowledge and experience you can muster, and it is here that reading will be most helpful in learning about patterns of abnormalities and diseases, and clustering your patient's findings accordingly. Until you gain broader knowledge and experience, you may not be able to develop highly specific hypotheses, but proceed as far as you can with the data and knowledge you have. The following steps should help:

  1. *Select the most specific and critical findings to support your hypothesis.* If the patient reports "the worst headache of her life," nausea, and vomiting, for example, and you find mental status change, papilledema, and meningismus, build your hypothesis around elevated intracranial pressure rather than gastrointestinal disorders. Although other symptoms are useful diagnostically, they are much less specific.

  2. Using your inferences about the structures and processes involved, *match your findings against all the conditions you know that can produce them.* For example, you can match your patient's papilledema with a list of conditions affecting intracranial pressure. Or you can compare the symptoms and signs associated with the patient's headache with the various infectious, vascular, metabolic, or neoplastic conditions that might produce this kind of clinical picture.

  3. *Eliminate the diagnostic possibilities that fail to explain the findings.* You might consider cluster headache as a cause of Mrs. N's headaches, but eliminate this hypothesis because it fails to explain the patient's throbbing bifrontal localization with intermittent nausea and vomiting. Also, the pain pattern is atypical for cluster headache—it is not unilateral, boring, occurring repetitively at the same time over a period of days, nor is it associated with lacrimation or rhinorrhea.

4. *Weigh the competing possibilities and select the most likely diagnosis* from among the conditions that might be responsible for the patient's findings. You are looking for a *close match* between the patient's clinical presentation and a typical case of a given condition. Other clues help in this selection, too. The *statistical probability* of a given disease in a patient of this age, sex, ethnic group, habits, lifestyle, and locality should greatly influence your selection. You should consider the possibilities of osteoarthritis and metastatic prostate cancer in a 70-year-old man with back pain, for example, but not in a 25-year-old woman with the same complaint. The *timing of the patient's illness* also makes a difference. Headache in the setting of fever, rash, and stiff neck that develops suddenly over 24 hours suggests quite a different problem than recurrent headache over a period of years associated with stress, visual scotoma, and nausea and vomiting relieved by rest.

5. Finally, as you develop possible explanations for the patient's problem, *give special attention to potentially life-threatening and treatable conditions* such as meningococcal meningitis, bacterial endocarditis, pulmonary embolus, or subdural hematoma. Here you make every effort to minimize the risk of missing conditions that may occur less frequently or be less probable but that, if present, would be particularly ominous. *One rule of thumb is always to include "the worst case scenario" in your list of differential diagnoses* and make sure you have ruled out that possibility based on your findings and patient assessment.

- **Test your hypotheses.** Now that you have made a hypothesis about the patient's problem, you will usually want to *test your hypothesis.* You are likely to need further history, additional maneuvers on physical examination, or laboratory studies or x-rays to confirm or rule out your tentative diagnosis or to clarify which of two or three possible diagnoses are most likely. When the diagnosis seems clear-cut—a simple upper respiratory infection or a case of hives, for example—these steps may not be necessary.

- **Establish a working diagnosis.** You are now ready to establish a working definition of the problem. Make this at the highest level of explicitness and certainty that the data allow. You may be limited to a symptom, such as "tension headache, cause unknown." At other times, you can define a problem explicitly in terms of its structure, process, and cause. Examples include "bacterial meningitis, pneumococcal," "subarachnoid hemorrhage, left temporoparietal lobe," or "hypertensive cardiovascular disease with left ventricular enlargement and congestive heart failure."

Although medical diagnosis is based primarily on identifying abnormal structures, altered processes, and specific causes, you will frequently see patients whose complaints do not fall neatly into these categories. Some symptoms defy analysis, and you may never be able to move beyond simple descriptive categories such as "fatigue" or "anorexia." Other problems relate to the patient's life, rather than to the body. Events such as losing a job or loved one may increase the risk of subsequent illness. Identifying these events and helping the patient develop coping strategies are just as important as managing a headache or a duodenal ulcer.

Another increasingly prominent item on problem lists is *Health Maintenance*. Routinely listing this category helps you track several important health concerns more effectively: immunizations, screening measures (e.g., mammograms, prostate examinations), instructions regarding nutrition and breast or testicular self-examinations, recommendations about exercise or use of seat belts, and responses to important life events.

- **Develop a plan agreeable to the patient.** You should identify and record a *Plan* for each patient problem. Your *Plan* will flow logically from the problems or diagnoses you have identified and specify which steps are needed next. These steps range from tests to confirm or further evaluate a diagnosis, to consultations for subspecialty evaluation, to additions, deletions, or changes in medication, to arranging a family meeting. You will find that you will follow many of the same diagnoses over time; however, your *Plan* is often more fluid, encompassing changes and modifications that emerge from each patient visit. The *Plan* should make reference to diagnosis, therapy, and patient education.

  Before finalizing your *Plan*, it is important to share your assessment and clinical thinking with the patient and seek out his or her opinions, concerns, and willingness to proceed with any further testing or evaluation. Remember that patients may need to hear the same information multiple times and ways before they comprehend it. Your relationship with the patient will be enhanced if the patient is an active participant in the plan of care.

The Case of Mrs. N: Assessment and Plan

As you study the *Assessment* and *Plan* for Mrs. N, think carefully about the clarity and organization of the clinical record. When creating a record, you do more than simply list the patient's story and your physical findings. You must review and organize your data, evaluate the importance and relevance of each item, and construct a clear, concise, yet comprehensive report. At first, it will be challenging to clearly and logically organize your patient assessment. Let the patient's story and symptoms serve as guides, examine the appropriate areas of the body, and apply the steps of clinical reasoning to deepen your knowledge, judgment, and clinical acumen.

Using Mrs. N's record, begin to make a checklist of the features of a good medical record. Later, compare your list with the checklist on pp. 796–798. The following questions may help: Are the data easy to follow, orderly, and presented in a readable format? Is there sufficient detail, both positive and negative, to formulate an Assessment and Plan? Is there excess repetition of information or redundancy? Is the tone professional, avoiding disapproving or moralizing comments?

ASSESSMENT AND PLAN FOR MRS. N

1. **Migraine headaches.** 54-year-old woman with migraine headaches since childhood, with a throbbing vascular pattern and frequent nausea and vomiting. Headaches are associated with stress and relieved by sleep and cold compresses. There is no papilledema, and there are no motor or sensory deficits on the neurologic examination. The differential diagnosis includes tension headache, also associated with stress, but there is no relief with massage, and the pain is more throbbing than aching. There are no fever, stiff neck, or focal findings to suggest meningitis, and lifelong recurrent pattern makes subarachnoid hemorrhage unlikely (usually described as "the worst headache of my life").

   Plan:

   - Discuss features of migraine vs. tension headaches.
   - Discuss biofeedback and stress management.
   - Advise patient to avoid caffeine, including coffee, colas, and other carbonated beverages.
   - Start NSAIDs for headache, as needed.
   - If needed next visit, begin prophylactic medication, because patient is having more than three migraines per month.

2. **Elevated blood pressure.** Systolic hypertension with wide cuff is present. May be related to obesity, also to anxiety from first visit. No evidence of end-organ damage to retina or heart.

   Plan:

   - Discuss standards for assessing blood pressure.
   - Recheck blood pressure in 1 month, using wide cuff.
   - Review urinalysis.
   - Introduce weight reduction and/or exercise programs (see #4).
   - Reduce salt intake.

3. **Cystocele with occasional stress incontinence.** Cystocele on pelvic examination, probably related to bladder relaxation. Patient is perimenopausal. Incontinence reported with coughing, suggesting alteration in bladder neck anatomy. No dysuria, fever, flank pain. Not on any contributing medications. Usually involves small amounts of urine, no dribbling, so doubt urge or overflow incontinence.

   Plan:

   - Explain cause of stress incontinence.
   - Review urinalysis.
   - Recommend Kegel's exercises.
   - Consider topical estrogen cream to vagina next visit if no improvement.

4. **Overweight.** Patient 5′2″, weighs 143 lbs. BMI is ~26.

   Plan:

   - Explore diet history, ask patient to keep food intake diary.
   - Explore motivation to lose weight, set target for weight loss by next visit.
   - Schedule visit with dietician.
   - Discuss exercise program, specifically, walking 30 minutes at least three times a week.

5. **Family stress.** Son-in-law with alcohol problem; daughter and grandchildren seeking refuge in patient's apartment, leading to tensions in these relationships. Patient also has financial constraints. Stress currently situational. No evidence of major depression at present.

Plan:

- Explore patient's views on strategies to cope with sources of stress.
- Explore sources of support, including Al-Anon for daughter and financial counseling for patient.
- Continue to monitor for depression.

6. **Occasional musculoskeletal low back pain.** Usually with prolonged standing. No history of trauma or motor vehicle accident. Pain does not radiate; no tenderness or motor-sensory deficits on examination. Doubt disc or nerve root compression, trochanteric bursitis, sacroiliitis.

   Plan:

   - Review benefits of weight loss and exercises to strengthen low back muscles.

7. **Tobacco abuse.** 1 pack per day for 36 years.

   Plan:

   - Check peak flow or FEV_1/FVC on office spirometry.
   - Give strong warning to stop smoking.
   - Offer referral to tobacco cessation program.
   - Offer patch, current treatment to enhance abstinence.

8. **Varicose veins, lower extremities.** No complaints currently.
9. **History of right pyelonephritis, 1982.**
10. **Ampicillin allergy.** Developed rash but no other allergic reaction.
11. **Health maintenance.** Last Pap smear 1998; has never had a mammogram.

    Plan:

    - Teach patient breast self-examination; schedule mammogram.
    - Schedule Pap smear next visit.
    - Provide three stool guaiac cards; next visit discuss screening flexible sigmoidoscopy.
    - Suggest dental care for mild gingivitis.
    - Advise patient to move medications and caustic cleaning agents to locked cabinet, if possible, above shoulder height.

Approaching the Challenges of Clinical Data

As you can see from the case of Mrs. N, organizing the patient's clinical data poses several challenges. The beginning student must decide whether to cluster the patient's symptoms and signs into one problem or into several problems. The amount of data may appear unmanageable. The quality of the data may be prone to error. Guidelines to help you address these challenges are provided in the following paragraphs.

Clustering Data Into Single Versus Multiple Problems. One of the greatest difficulties facing students is how to cluster the clinical data. Do selected data fit into one problem or several problems? The patient's *age* may help—young people are more likely to have a single disease, while older people tend to have multiple diseases. The *timing* of symptoms is often useful. For example, an episode of pharyngitis 6 weeks ago is probably unrelated to fever, chills, pleuritic chest pain, and cough that prompt an office visit today. To use timing effectively, you need to know the natural history of various diseases and conditions. A yellow penile discharge followed 3 weeks later by a painless penile ulcer suggests two problems: gonorrhea and primary syphilis. In contrast, a penile ulcer followed in 6 weeks by a maculopapular skin rash and generalized lymphadenopathy suggest two stages of the same problem: primary and secondary syphilis.

Involvement of *different body systems* may help you to cluster the clinical data. If symptoms and signs occur in a single system, one disease may explain them. Problems in different, apparently unrelated systems often require more than one explanation. Again, knowledge of disease patterns is necessary. You might decide, for example, to group a patient's high blood pressure and sustained apical impulse together with flame-shaped retinal hemorrhages, place them in the cardiovascular system, and label the constellation "hypertensive cardiovascular disease with hypertensive retinopathy." You would develop another explanation for the patient's mild fever, left lower quadrant tenderness, and diarrhea.

Some diseases involve more than one body system. As you gain knowledge and experience, you will become increasingly adept at recognizing *multisystem conditions* and building plausible explanations that link together their seemingly unrelated manifestations. To explain cough, hemoptysis, and weight loss in a 60-year-old plumber who has smoked cigarettes for 40 years, you probably even now would rank lung cancer high in your differential diagnosis. You might support your diagnosis with your observation of the patient's clubbed fingernails. With experience and continued reading, you will recognize that his other symptoms and signs can be linked to the same diagnosis. Dysphagia would reflect extension of the cancer to the esophagus, pupillary asymmetry would suggest pressure on the cervical sympathetic chain, and jaundice could result from metastases to the liver.

In another case of multisystem disease, a young man who presents with odynophagia, fever, weight loss, purplish skin lesions, leukoplakia, generalized lymphadenopathy, and chronic diarrhea is likely to have AIDS. Related risk factors should be explored promptly.

Sifting Through an Extensive Array of Data. It is common to confront a relatively long list of symptoms and signs, and an equally long list of potential explanations. One approach is to *tease out separate clusters of observations and analyze one cluster at a time,* as just described. You can also *ask a series of key questions* that may steer your thinking in one direction and allow you to temporarily ignore the others. For example, you may ask what produces and relieves the patient's chest pain. If the answer is exercise and rest, you can focus on the cardiovascular and musculoskeletal systems and set the gastrointestinal system aside. If the pain is substernal, burning, and occurs only after meals, you can logically focus on the gastrointestinal tract. A series of discriminating questions helps you form a decision tree or algorithm that is helpful in collecting and analyzing clinical data and reaching logical conclusions and explanations.

Assessing the Quality of the Data. Almost all clinical information is subject to error. Patients forget to mention symptoms, confuse the events of their illness, avoid recounting facts that are embarrassing, and often slant their stories to what the clinician wants to hear. Clinicians misinterpret patient statements, overlook information, fail to ask "the one key question," jump prematurely to conclusions and diagnoses, or forget an important part of the examination, such as the testicular examination in a young man with asymptomatic testicular carcinoma. You can avoid some of these errors by acquiring the habits of skilled clinicians, summarized below.

TIPS FOR ENSURING THE QUALITY OF PATIENT DATA

- Ask open-ended questions and listen carefully and patiently to the patient's story.
- Craft a thorough and systematic sequence to history-taking and physical examination.
- Keep an open mind toward both the patient and the data.
- Always include "the worst-case scenario" in your list of possible explanations of the patient's problem, and make sure it can be safely eliminated.
- Analyze any mistakes in data collection or interpretation.
- Confer with colleagues and review the pertinent medical literature to clarify uncertainties.
- Apply principles of data analysis to patient information and testing.

Symptoms, physical findings, tests, and x-rays should help you reduce uncertainty about whether a patient does or does not have a given condition. Clinical data, including laboratory work, however, are inherently imperfect. You can improve your assessment of clinical data and laboratory tests by applying several key principles for selecting and using clinical data and tests. Learn to apply the principles of *reliability, validity, sensitivity, specificity,* and *predictive value* to your clinical findings and the tests you order. These test characteristics will help you decide how confident you can be of your findings and test results as you assess the presence or absence of a disease or problem.

PRINCIPLES OF TEST SELECTION AND USE

Reliability

Indicates how well repeated measurements of the same relatively stable phenomenon will give the same result, also known as precision. Reliability may be measured for one observer or for more than one observer.

Example: If on several occasions one clinician consistently percusses the same span of a patient's liver dullness, *intraobserver reliability* is good. If, on the other hand, several observers find quite different spans of liver dullness on the same patient, *interobserver reliability* is poor.

Validity

Indicates how closely a given observation agrees with "the true state of affairs," or the best possible measure of reality.

Example: Blood pressure measurements by mercury-based sphygmomanometers are less valid than intra-arterial pressure tracings.

Sensitivity

Identifies the proportion of people who test positive in a group of people known to have the disease or condition, or the proportion of people who are *true positives* compared to the total number of people who actually have the disease. When the observation or test is negative in persons who have the disease, the result is termed *false negative. Good observations or tests have a sensitivity of over 90%, and help rule out disease because there are few false negatives. Such observations or tests are especially useful for screening.*

Example: The sensitivity of Homan's sign in the diagnosis of deep venous thrombosis of the calf is 50%. In other words, compared to a group of patients with deep venous thrombosis confirmed by phlebogram, a much better test, only 50% will have a positive Homan's sign, so this sign, if absent, is not helpful, since 50% of patients may have a DVT.

Specificity

Identifies the proportion of people who test negative in a group of people known to be *without* a given disease or condition, or the proportion of people who are "true negatives" compared to the total number of people without the disease. When the observation or test is positive in persons without the disease, the result is termed "false positive." Good observations or tests have a specificity of over 90% and help "rule in" disease, because the test is rarely positive when disease is absent, and there are few false positives.

Example: The specificity of serum amylase in patients with possible acute pancreatitis is 70%. In other words, of 100 patients without pancreatitis, 70% will have a normal serum amylase; in 30%, the serum amylase will be falsely elevated.

Predictive Value

Indicates how well a given symptom, sign, or test result—either positive or negative—predicts the presence or absence of disease.

Positive predictive value is the probability of disease in a patient with a positive (abnormal) test, or the proportion of "true positives" out of the total population tested.

Example: In a group of women with palpable breast nodules in a cancer screening program, the proportion with confirmed breast cancer would constitute the *positive predictive value* of palpable breast nodules for diagnosing breast cancer.

Negative predictive value is the probability of not having the condition or disease when the test is negative, or normal, or the proportion of "true negatives" out of the total population tested.

Example: In a group of women without palpable breast nodules in a cancer screening program, the proportion without confirmed breast cancer constitutes the *negative predictive value* of absence of breast nodules.

Displaying Clinical Data. To use these principles, it is important to display the data in the 2 × 2 format diagrammed on the following page. Always using this format will ensure the accuracy of your calculations of sensitivity, specificity, and predictive value. Note that the presence or absence of disease implies use of a "*gold standard*" to establish whether the disease is truly present or absent. This is usually the best test available, such as a coronary angiogram for assessing coronary artery disease or a tissue biopsy for malignancy.

Note that the numbers related to presence or absence of disease, as determined by the "gold standard," are always displayed **down the table** in the left and right columns (*present* = *a* + *c*; *absent* = *b* + *d*). Numbers related to the observation or test are always displayed **across the table** in the upper and lower rows (*test positive* = *a* + *b*; *test negative* = *c* + *d*).

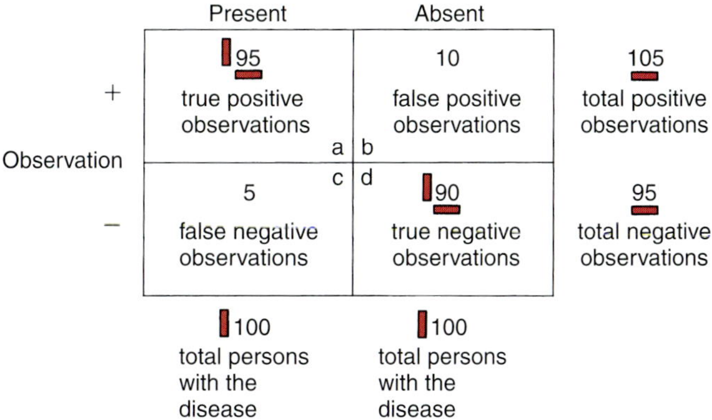

Now you are ready to make your calculations:

$$\textbf{Sensitivity} = \frac{a}{a+c} = \frac{\text{true positive observations (95)}}{\text{total persons with disease (95 + 5)}} \times 100 = 95\%$$

$$\textbf{Specificity} = \frac{d}{b+d} = \frac{\text{true negative observations (90)}}{\text{total persons with disease (90 + 10)}} \times 100 = 90\%$$

$$\textbf{Positive predictive value} = \frac{a}{a+b} = \frac{\text{true positive observations (95)}}{\text{total positive observations (95 + 10)}} \times 100 = 90.5\%$$

$$\textbf{Negative predictive value} = \frac{d}{c+d} = \frac{\text{true negative observations (90)}}{\text{total negative observations (90 + 5)}} \times 100 = 94.7\%$$

Now return to the table. *The **vertical red bars** designate sensitivity (a/a + c) and specificity (d/b + d), and the **horizontal red bars** designate positive predictive value (a/a + b) and negative predictive value (d/c + d).* The data displayed indicate that the hypothetical test has excellent test characteristics. The sensitivity and specificity of the test are both over 90%, as are the positive and negative predictive values. Such a test would be clinically useful for assessing a disease or condition in your patient.

Note that the predictive value of a test or observation depends heavily on the *prevalence* of the condition within the population studied. Prevalence is the proportion of people in a defined population at any given point in time who have the condition in question. When the prevalence of a condition is *low*, the positive predictive value of the test will fall. When the prevalence is *high*, the sensitivity, specificity, and positive predictive value are high, and the negative predictive value approaches zero. To work further on these relationships, turn to the Appendix, Prevalence and Predictive Value, on pp. 801–802 to practice making the calculations described.

Building Your Case: The Interplay of Clinical Reasoning and Assessment of Clinical Data

The concepts of sensitivity and specificity help in both the collection and analysis of data. They even underlie some of the basic strategies of interviewing. Questions with high sensitivity, if answered in the affirmative, may be particularly useful for screening and for gathering evidence to support a hypothesis. For example, "Have you had any discomfort or pain in your chest?" is a highly sensitive question for diagnosing angina pectoris. For patients with this condition, there would be few false-negative responses. Thus, it is a good first screening question. However, because there are many other causes of chest discomfort, it is not all that specific. Pain that is retrosternal, pressing, and less than 10 minutes in duration—each a reasonably sensitive attribute of angina—would add importantly to your growing evidence for the diagnosis. To confirm your hypothesis, a more specific question, if answered in the affirmative, is needed, such as "Is the pain precipitated by exertion?" or "Is the pain relieved by rest?"

Data for testing hypotheses also come from the physical examination. Heart murmurs are good examples of findings with varying sensitivity and specificity. The vast majority of patients with significant valvular *aortic stenosis* have systolic ejection murmurs audible in the aortic area. Presence of a systolic murmur has a high sensitivity for aortic stenosis. This finding is present in most cases. The false-negative rate is low. On the other hand, many other conditions produce systolic murmurs, such as increased blood flow across a normal valve, or the sclerotic changes associated with aging, termed aortic sclerosis, so the finding of a systolic murmur is not very specific . . . there are many false positives. Using such a murmur as your only criterion for diagnosing aortic stenosis would lead to many false positives.

In contrast, a high-pitched, soft blowing decrescendo diastolic murmur best heard along the left sternal border is quite specific for *aortic regurgitation*. Such a murmur is almost never heard in normal people, and it is present in very few other conditions, so there are few false positives.

Combining data from the history and physical examination allows you to test your hypotheses, screen for selected conditions, build your case, and clinch a diagnosis even before obtaining further diagnostic tests. Consider the following list of evidence: cough, fever, a shaking chill, left-sided pleuritic chest pain, dullness throughout the left lower posterior lung field with crackles, bronchial breathing, and egophony. Cough and fever are good screening items for pneumonia, the next items support the hypothesis, and bronchial breathing with egophony in this distribution is very specific for lobar pneumonia. A chest x-ray would confirm the diagnosis.

Absence of selected symptoms and signs is also diagnostically useful, especially when they are usually present in a given condition (i.e., their sensitivity is high). For example, if a patient with cough and left-sided pleuritic chest pain does not have fever, bacterial pneumonia becomes much less likely (except possibly in infancy and old age). Likewise, in a patient with severe dyspnea, the absence of orthopnea makes left ventricular failure less probable as an explanation for shortness of breath.

Skilled clinicians use this kind of logic even if they are unaware of its statistical underpinnings. They start to generate tentative hypotheses as soon as the patient describes the *Chief Complaint,* then build evidence for one or more of these hypotheses and discard others as they continue with the history and examination. In developing a *Present Illness,* they borrow items from other parts of the history, such as the *Past Medical History,* the *Family History,* and the *Review of Systems.* In a 55-year-old man with chest pain, the skilled clinician does not stop with the attributes of pain, but moves on to probe risk factors from coronary artery disease such as family history, hypertension, diabetes, lipid abnormalities, and smoking. In both the history and physical examination, the clinician searches explicitly for other possible manifestations of cardiovascular disease such as congestive heart failure or the claudication or diminished lower extremity pulses of atherosclerotic peripheral vascular disease. By generating hypotheses early and testing them sequentially, experienced clinicians improve their efficiency and enhance the relevance and value of the data they collect. They dig and collect less ore but find more gold.

This sequence of collecting data and testing hypotheses is diagrammed below.

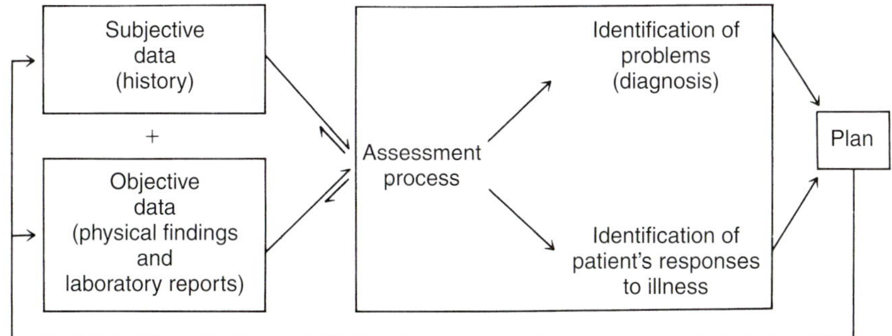

After the plan has been implemented, the process recycles. The clinician gathers more data, assesses the patient's progress, modifies the problem list if indicated, and adjusts the plan accordingly. As you gain experience, the interplay of assessment and data collection will become increasingly familiar. You will come to value the challenges and rewards of clinical reasoning and assessment that make patient care so meaningful.

Organizing the Patient Record

A clear, well-organized clinical record is one of the most important adjuncts to your patient care. Your skill in recording your patient's history and physical examination should evolve in parallel with your growing skills in clinical reasoning and your ability to formulate the patient's *Assessment* and *Plan.* Your goal should be a clear, concise, but comprehensive report that documents the key findings of your patient assessment and communicates the patient's problems in a succinct and *legible* format to other providers and members of the health care team. Note that a good record provides the supporting data for the problems or diagnoses identified.

Regardless of your experience, certain principles will help you to organize a good record. Think especially about the *order and readability* of the record and the *amount of detail* needed. How much detail to include often poses a vexing problem. As a student, you may wish (or you may be required) to be quite detailed. This helps to build your descriptive skills, vocabulary, and speed—admittedly a painful and tedious process. Pressures of time, however, will ultimately force some compromises.

Run through the following checklist to make sure your record is clear, informative, and easy to follow.

CHECKLIST FOR YOUR PATIENT RECORD

Is the order clear?	Order is imperative. Make sure that future readers, including yourself, can easily find specific points of information. Keep the *subjective* items of the history, for example, in the history; do not let them stray into the physical examination. Did you . . . ■ Make the headings clear? ■ Accent your organization with indentations and spacing? ■ Arrange the *Present Illness* in chronologic order, starting with the current episode, then filling in relevant background information?
Do the data included contribute directly to the assessment?	You should spell out the supporting data—both positive and negative—for every problem or diagnosis that you identify.
Are pertinent negatives specifically described?	Often portions of the history or examination suggest that an abnormality might exist or develop in that area. *Examples:* For the patient with notable bruises, record the "pertinent negatives," such as the absence of injury or violence, familial bleeding disorders, or medications or nutritional deficits that might lead to bruising. For the patient who is depressed but not suicidal, record both facts. In the patient with a transient mood swing, on the other hand, a comment on suicide is unnecessary.
Are there overgeneralizations or omissions of important data?	*Remember that data not recorded are data lost.* No matter how vividly you can recall selected details today, you will probably not remember them in a few months. The phrase "neurologic exam negative," even in your own handwriting, may leave you wondering in a few months' time, "Did I really do the sensory exam?"

Is there too much detail?	Avoid burying important information in a mass of excessive detail, to be discovered by only the most persistent reader. *Omit most of your negative findings* unless they relate directly to the patient's complaints or to specific exclusions in your diagnostic assessment. *Do not list abnormalities that you did not observe. Instead, concentrate on a few major ones, such as* "no heart murmurs," and try to describe structures in a concise, positive way. *Examples:* "Cervix pink and smooth" indicates you saw no redness, ulcers, nodules, masses, cysts or other suspicious lesions, but the description is shorter and much more readable. You can omit certain body structures even though you examined them, such as normal eyebrows and eyelashes.
Are phrases and short words used appropriately? Is there unnecessary repetition of data?	Omit unnecessary words, such as those in parentheses in the examples below. This saves valuable time and space. *Examples:* "Cervix is pink (in color)." "Lungs are resonant (to percussion)." "Liver is tender (to palpation)." "Both (right and left) ears with cerumen." "II/VI systolic ejection murmur (audible)." "Thorax symmetric (bilaterally)." Omit repetitive introductory phrases such as "The patient reports no . . . ," since readers assume the patient is the source of the history unless otherwise specified. Use short words instead of longer, fancier ones when they mean the same thing, such as "felt" for "palpated" or "heard" for "auscultated." *Describe what you observed, not what you did.* "Optic discs seen" is less informative than "disc margins sharp," even if it marks your first glimpse as an examiner!
Is the written style succinct? Is there excessive use of abbreviations?	Records are scientific and legal documents, so they should be clear and understandable. Using words and brief phrases instead of whole sentences is common, but abbreviations and symbols should be used only if they are readily understood. Likewise, an overly elegant style is less appealing than a concise summary. Be sure your record is legible, otherwise all that you have recorded is worthless to your readers.

Are diagrams and precise measurements included where appropriate?

Diagrams add greatly to the clarity of the record. *Examples:* Study the examples below:

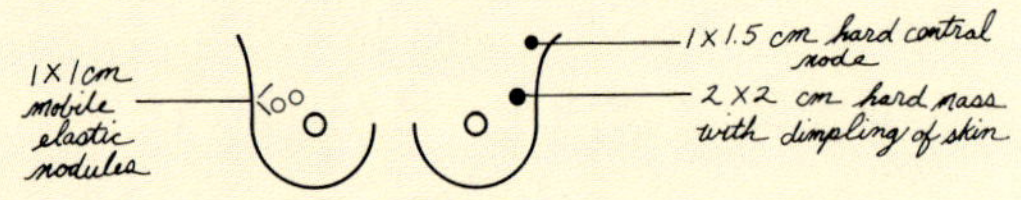

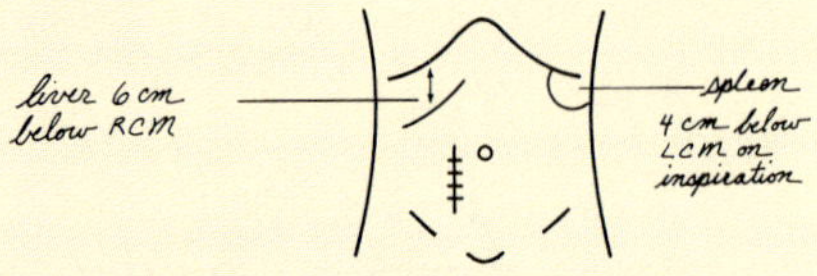

To ensure accurate evaluations and future comparisons, make measurements in centimeters, not in fruits, nuts, or vegetables.
Examples: "1 × 1 cm lymph node" versus a "pea-sized lymph node . . ." Or "2 × 2 cm mass on the left lobe of the prostate" versus a "walnut-sized prostate mass."

Is the tone of the write-up neutral and professional?

It is important to be objective. Hostile, moralizing, or disapproving comments have no place in the patient's record. Never use words, penmanship, or punctuation that are inflammatory or demeaning.
Example: Comments such as "Patient DRUNK and LATE TO CLINIC AGAIN!!" are unprofessional and set a bad example for other providers reading the chart. They also might prove difficult to defend in a legal setting.

Your institution or agency may have printed forms for recording patient information, but you should always be able to create your own record. The record of Mrs. N may be longer than what you might see in patient charts, yet it still does not reflect every question and technique that you have learned to use. The amount of detail varies, depending on the patient's symptoms and signs and the complexity of the clinician's diagnoses and plans for management.

Generating the Problem List. Once you have completed your assessment and written record, you will find it helpful to generate a *Problem List* that summarizes the patient's problems for the front of the office or hospital chart. List the most active and serious problems first, and record their date of onset. Some clinicians make separate lists for active or inactive problems; others make one list in order of priority. You will find that on follow-up visits the *Problem List* helps you remember to check the status of problems the patient may not mention. The *Problem List* also allows other members of the health care team to review the patient's health status at a glance.

A sample *Problem List* for Mrs. N is provided on the following page. You may wish to give each problem a number and use the number when referring to specific problems in subsequent notes.

Sample Problem List

Date Entered	Problem No.	Problem
8/30/02	1	Migraine headaches
	2	Elevated blood pressure
	3	Cystocele with occasional stress incontinence
	4	Overweight
	5	Family stress
	6	Low back pain
	7	Tobacco abuse
	8	Varicose veins
	9	History of right pyelonephritis
	10	Allergy to ampicillin
	11	Health maintenance

Clinicians organize problem lists differently, even for the same patient. Your problem list for Mrs. N may look somewhat different from the one above. Note that problems can be symptoms, signs, or conditions. Good lists vary in emphasis, length, and detail, depending on the clinician's philosophy, specialty, and role as a provider. The list illustrated here includes problems that need attention now, such as the headaches, as well as problems that need future observation or attention, such as the blood pressure and cystocele. Listing the allergy to ampicillin warns you not to prescribe medications in the penicillin family.

Some of the items noted in the history and physical examination, such as the canker sores and hard stools, do not appear in this problem list because they are relatively common phenomena that do not currently demand attention. Such judgments may prove to be wrong; however, problem lists that are cluttered with relatively insignificant items diminish in value. Some clinicians would find this list too long; others would be more explicit about such problems as "family stress" or "varicose veins."

Writing the Progress Note. A month later, Mrs. N returns for a follow-up visit. The style of the progress note is also quite variable, but it should follow the same standards as the initial assessment. It should be clear, sufficiently detailed, and easy to follow. It should reflect your clinical thinking and delineate your assessment and plan. The following note follows the SOAP note format (**S**ubjective, **O**bjective, **A**ssessment, and **P**lan), but you will see many other styles. Often clinicians record the history and physical examination, then break out the patient's problems into separate *Assessments* and *Plans.*

SAMPLE SOAP NOTE

1. Migraine headaches.
   S: Has had only two headaches, both mild and without associated symptoms. These are less troubling. Cannot detect any precipitating factors.
   O: No tenderness over the temporal muscles. No papilledema.
   A: Headaches improved, now without migraine features.
   P: Call if symptoms recur.

Clinical Assessment: The Journey to Excellence

The process of learning about a patient continues far beyond the first few encounters. Your understanding of patient care will grow in depth and complexity throughout your clinical career. Your prowess in history taking, physical examination, clinical reasoning, and documenting the patient record is launched. Now you must embark on repetitive practice, with supervision, and on the lifelong pursuit of polishing your newly acquired skills.

APPENDIX

PREVALENCE AND PREDICTIVE VALUE

Two examples further illustrate these principles and show *how predictive values vary with prevalence.* Consider first (*Example 1*) an imaginary population *A* with 1000 people. The prevalence of disease *X* in this population is high—40%. You can quickly calculate that 400 of these people have *X*. You then set out to detect these cases with an observation that is 90% sensitive and 80% specific. Of the 400 people with *X*, the observation reveals .90 × 400, or 360 (the true positives). It misses the other 40 (400 – 360, the false negatives). Out of the 600 people without *X*, the observation proves negative in .80 × 600, or 480. These people are truly free of *X*, as the observation suggests (the true negatives). But the observation misleads you in the remaining 120 (600 – 480). These people are falsely labeled as having *X* when they are really free of it (the false positives). These figures are summarized below:

Example 1. Prevalence of Disease X = 40%

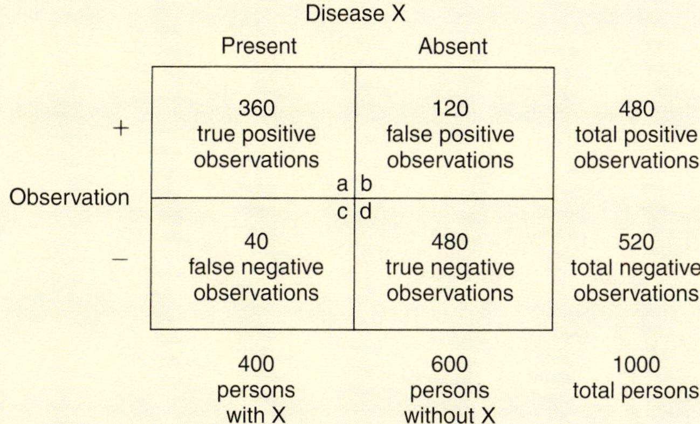

Observation	Disease X: Present	Disease X: Absent	
+	360 true positive observations (a)	120 false positive observations (b)	480 total positive observations
–	40 false negative observations (c)	480 true negative observations (d)	520 total negative observations
	400 persons with X	600 persons without X	1000 total persons

As a clinician who does not have perfect knowledge of who really does or does not have disease *X*, you are faced with a total of 480 people with positive observations. You must try to distinguish between the true and the false positives and will undoubtedly use additional kinds of data to help you in this task. Given only the sensitivity and specificity of your observation, however, you can determine the probability that a positive observation is a true positive, and you may wish to explain it to the concerned patient. This probability is calculated as follows:

$$\textit{Positive predictive value} = \frac{a}{a + b} = \frac{\text{true positives (360)}}{\text{total positives (360 + 120)}} \times 100 = 75\%$$

Thus, 3 out of 4 of the persons with positive observations really have the disease, and 1 out of 4 does not.

By a similar calculation, you can determine the probability that a negative observation is a true negative. The results here are reasonably reassuring to the involved patient:

$$\textit{Negative predictive value} = \frac{d}{c + d} = \frac{\text{true negatives (480)}}{\text{total negatives (40 + 480)}} \times 100 = 92\%$$

As *prevalence* of the disease in a population diminishes, however, the predictive value of a positive observation diminishes remarkably, while the predictive value of a negative observation rises further. In *Example 2,* in a second population, *B,* of 1000 people, only 1% have disease *X*. Now there are only 10 cases of *X* and 990 people without *X*. If this population is screened with the same observation, which has a 90% sensitivity and an 80% specificity, here are the results:

Example 2. Prevalence of Disease X = 1%

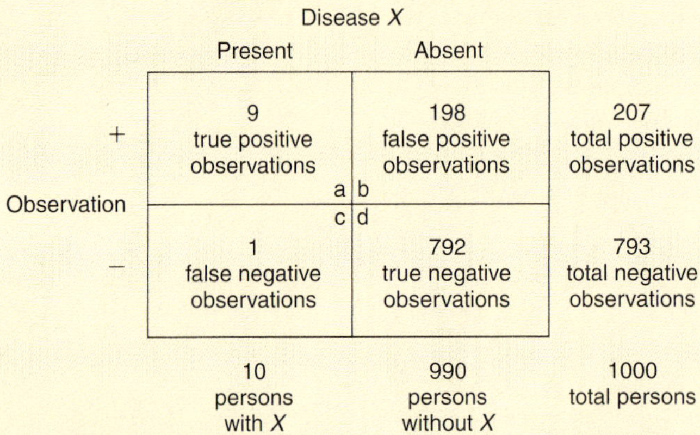

		Disease *X* Present	Disease *X* Absent	
Observation	+	9 true positive observations (a)	198 false positive observations (b)	207 total positive observations
	−	1 false negative observations (c)	792 true negative observations (d)	793 total negative observations
		10 persons with *X*	990 persons without *X*	1000 total persons

You are now confronted with possibly upsetting 207 people (all those with positive observations) to detect 9 out of the 10 real cases. The predictive value of a positive observation is only 4%. Improving the specificity of your observation without diminishing its sensitivity would be very helpful, if it were possible. For example, if you could increase the specificity of the observation from 80% to 98% (given the same prevalence of 1% and sensitivity of 90%), the positive predictive value of the observation would improve from 4% to 31%—scarcely ideal but certainly better. Good observations or tests have a sensitivity and specificity of 90%.

Because prevalence strongly affects the predictive value of an observation, prevalence too influences the assessment process. Because coronary artery disease is much more common in middle-aged men than in young women, you should pursue angina as a cause of chest pain more actively in the former group. The effect of prevalence on predictive value explains why your odds of making a correct assessment are better when you hypothesize a common condition rather than a rare one. The combination of fever, headache, myalgias, and cough probably has the same sensitivity and specificity for influenza throughout the year, but your chance of making this diagnosis correctly by using this cluster of symptoms is much greater during a winter flu epidemic than it is during a quiet August.

Prevalence varies importantly with clinical setting as well as with season. Chronic bronchitis is probably the most common cause of hemoptysis among patients seen in a general medical clinic. In the oncology clinic of a tertiary medical center, however, lung cancer might head the list, while in a group of postoperative patients on a general surgical service, irritation from an endotracheal tube or pulmonary infarction might be most likely. In certain parts of Asia, in contrast, one should think first of a worm called a lung fluke. When you hear hoofbeats in the distance, according to the familiar saying, bet on horses, not on zebras, unless, of course, you're visiting the zoo.

Bibliography

General References

Anatomy and Physiology

Agur AMR: Grant's Atlas of Anatomy, 10th ed. Philadelphia, Lippincott Williams & Wilkins, 1999.

Berne RM, Levy MN (eds): Physiology, 4th ed. St. Louis, Mosby–Year Book, 1998.

Gray H, Williams PL, Bannister LH: Gray's Anatomy, 38th ed. New York, Churchill Livingstone, 1995.

Guyton AC: Textbook of Medical Physiology, 10th ed. Philadelphia, WB Saunders, 1998.

Moore KL: Clinically Oriented Anatomy, 4th ed. Philadelphia, Lippincott Williams & Wilkins, 1999.

Netter FH, Dalley AF: Atlas of Human Anatomy. East Hanover New Jersey, Novartis, 1997.

Medicine, Surgery, and Physical Examination

Barker LR, Burton JR, Zieve PD: Principles of Ambulatory Medicine, 5th ed. Baltimore, Williams & Wilkins, 1999.

Clain A (ed): Hamilton Bailey's Demonstration of Physical Signs in Clinical Surgery, 17th ed. Bristol, England, John Wright, 1986.

Fauci AS, Braunwald E, Isselbacher KJ, et al (eds): Harrison's Principles of Internal Medicine, 15th ed. New York, McGraw-Hill, 2002.

Goldman L, Bennett JC (eds): Cecil Textbook of Medicine, 21st ed. Philadelphia, WB Saunders, 2000.

Hazzard WR, Bierman EL, Blass JP, et al: Principles of Geriatric Medicine and Gerontology, 4th ed. New York, McGraw-Hill, 1999.

Judge RD, Zuidema GD, Fitzgerald FT (eds): Clinical Diagnosis: A Physiologic Approach, 5th ed. Boston, Little, Brown and Co, 1989.

Kane RL, Ouslander JG, Abrass IB: Essentials of Clinical Geriatrics, 4th ed. New York, McGraw-Hill, 1999.

Mandell GL, Mildran D (eds): Atlas of AIDS. Philadelphia, Current Medicine, 2001.

Nathan DM: Long-term complications of diabetes mellitus. N Engl J Med 328:1676, 1993.

Noble J, Greene HL, Levinson W, et al (eds): Primary Care Medicine, 3rd ed. St. Louis, Mosby, 2001.

Orient JA, Sapira JD: The Art and Science of Bedside Diagnosis. Philadelphia, Lippincott Williams & Wilkins, 2000.

Sabiston DC, Lyerly HR (eds): Textbook of Surgery: The Biological Basis of Modern Surgical Practice, 15th ed. Philadelphia, WB Saunders, 1997.

Sande MA, Volberding PA: The Medical Management of AIDS, 6th ed. Philadelphia, WB Saunders, 1999.
Schwartz SI (ed): Principles of Surgery, 7th ed. New York, McGraw-Hill, 1999.
Youngkin EQ, Davis MS: Women's Health: A Primary Care Clinical Guide. Stamford, CT, Appleton and Lange, 1998.

Health Promotion and Counseling

American Nurses Association: Clinician's Handbook on Preventive Services: Put Prevention into Practice. Waldorf, MD, American Nurses Publishing, 1994.
Dowd R: Role of calcium, vitamin D, and other essential nutrients in the prevention and treatment of osteoporosis. Nurs Clin North Am 36:417, 2001.
Ernst E: The risk–benefit profile of commonly used herbal therapies: ginko, St. John's wort, ginseng, echinacea, saw palmetto, and kava. Ann Intern Med 136:42, 2002.
Palmer RM: Geriatric assessment. Med Clin N Am 83:1503, 1999.
Reid KC, Grizzard TA, Poland GA: Adult immunizations: recommendations for practice. Mayo Clinc Proc 74:377, 1999.
Sox HC: Editorial. Disease prevention guidelines from the US Preventive Services Task Force. Ann Intern Med 136:155, 2002.
U.S. Department of Health and Human Services, Public Health Service: Treating tobacco use and dependence. A clinical practice guideline. June 2000. Available at: www.clearinghouse.gov. Accessed January 31, 2002.
U.S. Preventive Services Task Force: Guide to Clinical Preventive Services, 2nd ed. Baltimore, Williams & Wilkins, 1996.
Woolf SH, Jonas S, Lawrence RS: Health Promotion and Disease Prevention in Clinical Practice. Baltimore, Williams & Wilkins, 1996.

Chapter 1. An Overview of Physical Examination and History Taking

Beckman HB, Frankel RM: The effect of physician behavior on the collection of data. Ann Intern Med 101:693, 1984.
Hensrud DD: Clinical preventive medicine in primary care: background and practice: rationale and current preventive practices. Mayo Clin Proc 75:165–172, 2000.
Moore AA, Siu AI: Screening for common problems in ambulatory elderly: clinical confirmation of a screening instrument. Am J Med 100:438, 1996.
Oboler SK, LaForce FM: The periodic physical examination in asymptomatic adults. Ann Intern Med 110:214, 1989.
Platt FW, Gaspar DL, Coulehan JL, et al: "Tell me about yourself": The patient-centered interview. Ann Intern Med 134:1079, 2001.
Sackett DL: A primer on the precision and accuracy of the clinical examination. JAMA 267:2638, 1992.
Sager MA, Franke T, Inouye S, et al: Functional outcomes of acute medical illness and hospitalization in older persons. Arch Intern Med 156:645, 1996.
Schneiderman H, Peixoto AJ: Bedside Diagnosis, 3rd ed. Philadelphia, American College of Physicians, 1997.
Sox HC Jr: Preventive Services Task Force: Guide to Clinical Preventive Services: An Assessment of the Effectiveness of 169 Interventions. Baltimore, Williams & Wilkins, 1989.

Chapter 2. Interviewing and the Health History

Billings JA, Stoeckle JD: The Clinical Encounter: A Guide to the Medical Interview and Case Presentation. Chicago, Year Book Medical Publishers, 1989.

Bird J, Cohen-Cole SA: The three-function model of the medical interview. Adv Psychosom Med 65:20, 1990.

Conant EB: Addressing patients by their first names. N Engl J Med 308:226, 1983. [*A patient's view*]

Delbanco TL: Enriching the doctor–patient relationship by inviting the patient's perspective. Ann Intern Med 116:414, 1992.

Engel GL, Morgan WL Jr: Interviewing the Patient. Philadelphia, WB Saunders, 1973.

Fadiman A: The Spirit Catches You and You Fall Down. New York, Farrar, Straus and Giroux, 1997.

Heller ME: Addressing patients by their first names. N Engl J Med 308:1107, 1987. *[Short report of a survey of obstetrical outpatients]*

McDaniel SH, Hepworth J, Doherty WJ: Medical family therapy: a biopsychosocial approach to families with health problems. New York, Basic Books, 1992.

Facilitating the Patient's Story: The Techniques of Skilled Interviewing

Branch WT, Malik TK: Using 'windows of opportunities' in brief interviews to understand patients' concerns. JAMA 269:1667, 1993.

Brown JB, Weston WW, Stewart AM: Patient-centered interviewing, Part I: Understanding patients' experiences. Can Fam Physician 147:35, 1989.

Brown JB, Weston WW, Stewart AM: Patient-centered interviewing, Part II: Finding common ground. Can Fam Physician 153:35, 1989.

Silverman J, Kurtz S, Draper J: Skills for Communicating with Patients. Abingdon, UK: Radcliffe Medical Press, Ltd., 1998.

Smith RC: The Patient's Story, Integrated Patient–Doctor Interviewing. Boston, Little, Brown and Company, 1996.

Waitzkin H: Doctor–patient communication: clinical implications of social scientific research. JAMA 252:2441, 1984.

Adapting Interviewing Techniques to Specific Situations

Committee on Disabilities of the Group for the Advancement of Psychiatry: Issues to consider in deaf and hard-of-hearing patients. Am Fam Physician 56(8):2057–2066, 1997.

Davis TC, Long SW, Jackson RH, et al: Rapid estimate of adult literacy in medicine: a shortened screening instrument. Family Medicine 25(6):391, 1993.

Goldoft M: A piece of mind: another language. JAMA 268(24):23, 1992.

Mayeaux EJ Jr., Murphy PW, Arnold C, et al: Improving patient education for patients with low literacy skills. Am Fam Physician 53(1):205, 1996.

National Work Group on Literacy and Health: Communicating with patients who have limited literacy skills. Report of the National Work Group on Literacy and Health. J Fam Prac 46:168, 1998.

Putsch RW:Cross-cultural communication: the special case of interpreters in health Care. JAMA 254(23):3344, 1985.

Rivadeneyra R, Elderkin-Thompson V, Silver RC, et al: Patient centeredness in medical encounters requiring an interpreter. Am J Med 108:470, 2000.

Special Task Interpreters for the Deaf (STID), Inc. Available at: www.stid.org. Accessed April 30, 2002.

Special Aspects of Interviewing

Carrillo JE, Green AR, Betancourt JR: Cross-cultural primary care: a patient-based approach. Ann Intern Med 130:829, 1999.

Council on Scientific Affairs, American Medical Association: Health care needs of gay men and lesbians in the U.S. JAMA 275:1354, 1996.

Cyr MG, Wartman SA: The effectiveness of routine screening questions in the detection of alcoholism. JAMA 259:51, 1998.

Ewing JA: Detecting alcoholism: the CAGE questionnaire. JAMA 252:1905,1984.

Harrison AE: Primary care of lesbian and gay patients: educating ourselves and our students. Fam Med 28(1):10, 1996.

Helman CG: Culture Health and Illness. 4th ed. Boston, Butterworth-Heinemann, 2000.

Kleinman A, Eisenberg L, Good B: Culture, illness, and care: clinical lessons from anthropologic and cross-cultural research. Ann Intern Med 88:251, 1978.

Neisson O and Cone H: Screening patients for alcohol problems in primary health care settings. Am J Addictions 5 (suppl 4):53, 1996.

The Sexual History and Domestic and Physical Violence

Flitcraft AH, Hadley SM, Hendricks-Matthews MK, et al: American Medical Association diagnostic and treatment guidelines on domestic violence. Arch Fam Med 1:39–47, 1992.

Institute for Clinical Systems Improvement (ICSI): ICSI health care guidelines; No. GHM02. May 2000 (revision); original release date June 1996.

Maurice WL: Sexual Medicine in Primary Care. St. Louis, Mosby, 1998.

Ethical Considerations

Christakis DA, Feudtner C: Ethics in a short white coat: the ethical dilemmas that medical students confront. Acad Medic 68:249–254, 1993.

Council on Ethical and Judicial Affairs, AMA: Sexual misconduct in the practice of medicine. JAMA 266:2741, 1991.

Davidoff, F: Editorial. Changing the subject: ethical principles for everyone in health care. Ann Intern Med 133(5):386–398, 2000.

Doyal L: Closing the gap between professional teaching and practice. BMJ 322:685–686, 2001.

Gabbard GO, Nadelson C: Professional boundaries in the physician–patient relationship. JAMA 273(18):1445, 1995.

Lo B: Resolving Ethical Dilemmas: A Guide for Clinicians. Philadelphia, Lippincott Williams & Wilkins, 2000.

Interviewing Patients of Different Ages

Talking With Children and Adolescents

See references for Chapter 17.

Talking With Aging Patients

Buckman R, Kason Y: How to Break Bad News: A Guide for Health Care Professionals. Baltimore, The Johns Hopkins University Press, 1992.

Casarett D, Kutner JS, Abrahm J: Life after death: a practical approach to grief and bereavement. Ann Intern Med 134:208, 2001.

Kubler-Ross E: On Death and Dying. New York, Macmillan, 1997.

Magilvy JK, Congdon JG: The crisis nature of health care transitions for rural older adults. Pub Health Nurs 17:336, 2000.

Miller KE, Zylstra RG, Standridge JB: The geriatric patient: a systematic approach to maintaining health. Am Fam Physician 61:1089, 2000.

Von Gunten CF, Ferris FD, Emanuel LL: Ensuring competency in end-of-life care. JAMA 284:3051–3057, 2000.

Chapter 3. Beginning the Physical Examination: General Survey and Vital Signs

Weight and Nutrition

Andres R, Muller DC, Sorkin JD: Long-term effects of change in body weight on all-cause mortality: a review. Ann Intern Med 119:737, 1993.

Becker AE, Grinspoon SK, Klibanski A, et al: Eating disorders. N Engl J Med 340:1092, 1999.

Blair SN, Shaten J, Brownell K, et al: Body weight change, all-cause mortality, and cause-specific mortality in the Multiple Risk Factor Intervention Trial. Ann Intern Med 119:749, 1993.

Dietary Guidelines Committee 2000 Report: Nutrition and your health: dietary guidelines for Americans. Agricultural Research Service, U.S. Department of Agriculture.

Executive Summary, Clinical Guidelines on the Identification, Evaluation, and Treatment of Overweight and Obesity in Adults. National Heart, Lung, and Blood Institute. Available at: www.nhlbi.gov/guidelines/obesity. Accessed January 26, 2002.

Mehler PS: Diagnosis and care of patients with anorexia nervosa in primary care settings. Ann Intern Med 134:1046, 2001.

Rosenbaum M, Leibel RL, Hirsch J: Obesity. N Engl J Med 337:396, 1997.

Sacks FM, Svetkey LP, Vollmer WM, et al: Effects on blood pressure of reduced dietary sodium and the dietary approaches to stop hypertension (DASH) diet. N Engl J Med 344:3, 2001.

Stevens VJ, Obarzanek E, Cook NR, et al: Long-term weight loss and changes in blood pressure: results of the trials of hypertension prevention, Phase II. Ann Intern Med 134:1, 2001.

Blood Pressure

Appel LJ, Moore TJ, et al: A clinical trial of the effects of dietary patterns on blood pressure. N Engl J Med 336:1117, 1997.

Cavallini MC, Roman MJ, Blank SG, et al: Association of the auscultatory gap with vascular disease in hypertensive patients. Ann Intern Med 124:877, 1996.

Franklin SS, Shehzad A, Khan A, et al: Is pulse pressure useful in predicting risk for coronary heart disease? The Framingham Heart Study. Circulation 100:354–360, 1999.

Joint National Commission on Prevention, Detection, Evaluation, and Treatment of High Blood Pressure and the National High Blood Pressure Education Program Coordinating Committee: The Sixth Report on Prevention, Detection, Evaluation, and Treatment of High Blood Pressure. Arch Intern Med 157:2413, 1997.

Reeves RA: Does this patient have hypertension? JAMA 273:1211, 1995.

Sague A, Larson MG, Levy D: The natural history of borderline isolated systolic hypertension. N Engl J Med 329:1912, 1993.

Schmieder RE, Martus P, Klingbeil A: Reversal of left ventricular hypertrophy in essential hypertension. JAMA 275:1507, 1996.

SHEP Cooperative Research Group: Prevention of stroke by anti-hypertensive drug treatment in older persons with isolated systolic hypertension. JAMA 265:3255, 1991.

Smulyan H, Safar ME: The diastolic blood pressure in systolic hypertension. Ann Intern Med 132:233, 2000.

Fever

Mackowiak PA, Bartlett JG, Borden EC, et al: Concepts of fever: recent advances and lingering dogma. Clin Infect Dis 25:120–138, 1997.

Pizzo PA: Fever in immunocompromised patients. N Engl J Med 341:893, 1999.

Chapter 4. The Skin

Agency for Health Care Policy and Research, U.S. Department of Health and Human Services: Treatment of Pressure Ulcers. Clinical Practice Guideline Number 15. Rockville, MD, AHCPR Publication Number 95-0652, 1994.

Bisno AL, Stevens DL: Streptococcal infections of the skin and soft tissues. N Engl J Med 334:240, 1996.

Drake LA, Dinehart SM, Farmer ER, et al: Guidelines of care for superficial mycotic skin infections of the skin: onychomycosis. J Am Acad Dermatol 34:116, 1996.

Fife C, Otto G, Capsuto EG, et al: Incidence of pressure ulcers in a neurologic intensive care unit. Crit Care Med 29:283–290, 2001.

Fine JD: Management of acquired bullous skin diseases. N Engl J Med 333:1475, 1995.

Fitzpatrick TB: Color Atlas and Synopsis of Clinical Dermatology: Common and Serious Diseases, 4th ed. New York, McGraw-Hill, 2001.

Freedberg IM, Fitzpatrick TB: Dermatology in General Medicine, 5th ed. New York, McGraw-Hill, 1999.

Goldsmith LA, Lazarus GS, Thorp MD: Adult and Pediatric Dermatology: A Color Guide to Diagnosis and Treatment. Philadelphia, FA Davis, 1997.

Hacker SM: Common disorders of pigmentation. Postgrad Med 99:177, 1996.

Habif TP: Clinical Dermatology: A Color Guide to Diagnosis and Therapy, 3rd ed. St. Louis, CV Mosby, 1996.

Jeghers H, Edelstein LM: Skin color in health and disease. In Blacklow RS: MacBryde's Signs and Symptoms: Applied Pathologic Physiology and Clinical Interpretation, 6th ed. Philadelphia, JB Lippincott, 1983.

Kalve E, Klein JE: Evaluation of women with hirsutism. Am Fam Physician 54:117, 1996.

Myers KA, Farquhar DRE: The rational clinical examination: does this patient have clubbing? JAMA 286:341–347, 2001.

Noronha PA, Zubkov B: Nails and nail disorders in children and adults. Am Fam Med 55:2129, 1997.

Sauer GC: Manual of Skin Diseases, 7th ed. Philadelphia, Lippincott-Raven, 1996.

Sawaya ME: Clinical updates in hair. Dermatol Clin 15:37, 1997.

Sumpio BE: Foot ulcers. N Engl J Med 343:787–793, 2000.

Talbot, Land-Curtis L: The challenges of assessing skin indicators in people of color. Home Healthcare Nurse 14:167, 1996.

Tucker MA, Halpern A, Holly EA, et al: Clinically recognized dysplastic nevi: a central risk factor for cutaneous melanoma. JAMA 277:1439, 1997.

Whited JD, Grichnik JM. Does this patient have a mole or a melanoma? JAMA 279:696, 1998.

Witman PM: Topical therapies for localized psoriasis. Mayo Clin Proc 76:943, 2001.

Young EM Jr, Newcomer VD, Kligman AM: Geriatric Dermatology: Color Atlas and Practitioner's Guide. Philadelphia, Lea & Febiger, 1993.

Chapter 5. The Head and Neck

The Head

Goadsby PJ, Lifton RB, Ferrari MD: Migraine—current understanding and treatment. N Engl J Med 346:257, 2002.

Smetana GW, Slumerling RH: Does this patient have temporal arteritis? JAMA 287:92, 2002.

Spector SL, Bernstein IL, Li JT, et al: Parameters for the diagnosis and management of sinusitis. J Allergy Clin Immunol 102 (6 Pt 2):S107, 1998.

Williams JW, Simel DL, Roberts L, et al: Clinical evaluation for sinusitis: making the diagnosis by history and physical examination. Ann Intern Med 117:705, 1992.

The Eye

Adams GGW, Hubbard AD, Bankes JLK: Kennerly Bankes's Clinical Ophthalmology: A Text and Colour Atlas. Boston, Butterworth-Heinemann, 1999.

Albert DM: Principles and Practice of Ophthalmology, 2nd ed. Philadelphia, WB Saunders, 2000.

American Diabetes Association: Diabetic retinopathy. Diabetes Care 25 (suppl 1):S90, 2002.

Coleman AC: Glaucoma. Lancet 20:1803, 1999.

Fine SL, Berger JW, Maguire MG, et al: Age-related macular degeneration. N Engl J Med 342:483–492, 2000.

Gaston H: Ophthalmology for Nurses. London, Croom Helar, 1986.

Gold DH, Weingeist TA: Color Atlas of the Eye in Systemic Disease. Philadelphia, Lippincott Williams & Wilkins, 2001.

Kritzinger EE, Beaumont HM: A Colour Atlas of Optic Disc Abnormalities. London, Wolfe Medical Publications, 1987.

Leibowitz HM: The red eye. N Engl J Med 343:345–351, 2000.

McCluskey PJ, Towler HM, Lightman S: Management of chronic uveitis. BMJ 320:555, 2000.

Newell FW: Ophthalmology: Principles and Concepts, 8th ed. St. Louis, Mosby–Year Book, 1996.

O'Neill D: Perkin's & Hansell's Atlas of Diseases of the Eye, 4th ed. Edinburgh, Churchill Livingstone, 1994.

Rosenthal BP: Ophthalmologic screening and treatment of age-related and pathological visions changes. Geriatrics 56:27, 2001.

Shields SR: Managing eye disease in primary care. Part 1. How to screen for occult disease. Postgrad Med 108:69, 2000.

Shingleton BJ, O'Donoghue MW: Blurred vision. N Engl J Med 343:556–562, 2000.

Sommers A, Tielsch JM, Katz J, et al: Racial differences in the cause-specific prevalence of blindness in East Baltimore. N Engl J Med 325:1412, 1991.

Tasman W, Jaeger EA: The Wills Eye Hospital Atlas of Clinical Ophthalmology. Philadelphia, Lippincott-Raven, 1996.

Walsh TJ (ed): Neuro-ophthalmology: Clinical Signs and Symptoms, 4th ed. Baltimore, Williams & Wilkins, 1997.

Yanoff M: Ocular Pathology: A Text and Atlas, 2nd ed. Philadelphia, Harper and Row, 1992.

The Ears, Nose, and Throat

Bain J, Carter P, Morton R: Colour Atlas of Mouth, Throat and Ear Disorders in Children. San Diego, CA, College-Hill Press, 1985.

Bisno AL: Acute pharyngitis. N Engl J Med 344:205–211, 2001.

Bull TR: A Colour Atlas of E.N.T. Diagnosis, 3rd ed. Baltimore, Mosby–Wolfe, 1995.

Corren J: Allergic rhinitis: treating the adult. J Allergy Clin Immunol 105 (6 Pt 2):S610, 2000.

Cummings C, Harker LA, Krause CJ, et al: Head and Neck Surgery, 3rd ed. St. Louis, Mosby, 1998.

Hawke M, Bruce B: A Color Atlas of Otorhinolaryngology. Philadelphia, JB Lippincott, 1995.

Lalwani AK, Snow JB: Disorders of smell, taste, and hearing (Ch 29). In Braunwald E, Fauci AS, Kasper DL, et al (eds): Harrison's Principles of Internal Medicine, 15th ed. New York, McGraw-Hill, 2001.

O'Donoghue GM, Narula AA, Bates GJ: Clinical ENT: An Illustrated Textbook. San Diego, Singular Publishing Group, 2000.

Russell J: Ear screening. Comm Nurse 1:14, 1995.

The Mouth

Beaven DW, Brooks SE: Color Atlas of the Tongue in Clinical Diagnosis. Chicago, Year Book Medical Publishers, 1988.

Cawson RA, Binnie WH, Eveson JW: Oral Pathology and Diagnosis: Colour Atlas with Integrated Text, 2nd ed. London, Wolfe, 1994.

Langlais RP, Miller CS: Color Atlas of Common Oral Diseases, 2nd ed. Baltimore, Williams & Wilkins, 1998.

Neville BW, Damm DD, White DK, et al: Color Atlas of Clinical Oral Pathology. Philadelphia, Lea & Febiger, 1991.

Newman MG, Carranza FA, Takei H: Carranza's Clinical Periodontology, 9th ed. Philadelphia, WB Saunders, 2002.

Regezi JA, Sciubba JJ: Oral Pathology: Clinical–Pathologic Correlations, 3rd ed. Philadelphia, WB Saunders, 1999.

Robinson HBG, Miller AS: Colby, Kerr, and Robinson's Atlas of Oral Pathology, 5th ed. Philadelphia, JB Lippincott, 1990.

Rogers RS: Common lesions of the oral mucosa. Postgrad Med 91:141, 1992.

Tyldesley WR: Color Atlas of Orofacial Diseases, 2nd ed. St. Louis, Mosby–Year Book, 1991.

The Neck

Henry PH, Longo DL: Enlargement of the lymph nodes and spleen (Chapter 63). In Harrison's Principles of Internal Medicine, 15th ed. New York, McGraw-Hill, 2001.

McGuirt WF: The neck mass. Med Clin N Am 83:219, 1999.
Siminoski K: Does this patient have a goiter? JAMA 273: 813, 1995.
Trivalle C, Doucet J, Chassagne P, et al: Differences in the signs and symptoms of hyperthyroidism in older and younger patients. J Am Geriatr Soc 44:50, 1996.
Walsh RM: The management of a solitary thyroid nodule: a review. Clin Otolaryngol 24:388, 1999.
Woeber KA: Update on the management of hyperthyroidism and hypothyroidism. Arch Intern Med 160:1067, 2000.

Chapter 6. The Thorax and Lungs

Examination of the Lungs

Badgett RG, et al: Can moderate obstructive pulmonary disease be diagnosed by historical and physical findings alone? Am J Med 94:188, 1993.
Bettancourt PE, DelBono EA, Speigelman D, et al: Clinical utility of chest auscultation in common pulmonary disease. Am J Resp Crit Care Med 150:1921, 1994.
Cugell DW: Lung sound nomenclature. Am Rev Respir Dis 136:1016, 1987.
Epler GR, Carrington CB, Gaensler EA: Crackles (rales) in the interstitial pulmonary diseases. Chest 73:333, 1978.
Holleman DR, Simel DL: Does the clinical examination predict airflow limitation? JAMA 273:313, 1995.
Koster MEY, Baughmann RP, Loudon RG: Continuous adventitious lung sounds. J Asthma 27:237, 1990.
Kraman SS: Lung sounds for the clinician. Arch Intern Med 146:1411, 1986.
Lehrer S: Understanding Lung Sounds, 2nd ed. Philadelphia, WB Saunders, 1993. (With audiocassette)
Loudon RG: The lung exam. Clin Chest Med 8:265, 1987.
Metlay JP, Kapoor WN, Fine MJ: Does this patient have community-acquired pneumonia? Diagnosing pneumonia by history and physical examination. JAMA 278:1440, 1997.
Nath AR, Carpel LH: Inspiratory crackles—early and late. Thorax 29:223, 1974.
Nath AR, Carpel LH: Lung crackles in bronchiectasis. Thorax 35:694, 1980.
Schapira RM, et al: The value of the forced expiratory time in the physical diagnosis of obstructive airways disease. JAMA 270:731, 1993.

Pulmonary Conditions

Abenhaim L, Moride Y, Brenot F, et al: Appetite-suppressant drugs and the risk for primary pulmonary hypertension. N Engl J Med 335:609, 1996.
American Thoracic Society and Centers for Disease Control and Prevention: Diagnostic standards and classification of tuberculosis in adults and children. Am J Respir Crit Care Med 161 (4 Pt 1):1376, 2000.
Baum GL, Wolinsky E (eds): Textbook of Pulmonary Diseases, 6th ed. Philadelphia, Lippincott Williams & Wilkins, 1998.
Bochud PY, Moser F, Erard P, et al: Community-acquired pneumonia. A prospective outpatient study. Medicine 80:75, 2001.
Busse WW, Lemanske RF: Asthma. N Engl J Med 5:350, 2001.
Irwin RS, Madison JM: The diagnosis and treatment of cough. N Engl J Med 343:1715, 2000.
National Heart, Lung, and Blood Institute/World Health Organization: Global initiative for chronic obstructive lung disease (GOLD). Available at: www.nhlbi.nih.gov/guidelines/index.htm. Accessed January 29, 2002.

Weinberger SE: Principles of Pulmonary Medicine, 3rd ed. Philadelphia, WB Saunders, 1998.

Chapter 7. The Cardiovascular System

Chest Pain and Syncope

Alpert JS: The patient with angina: the importance of careful listening. J Am Coll Cardiol 11:27, 1988.

Calkins H, Shyr Y, Frumin H, et al: The value of the clinical history in the differentiation of syncope due to ventricular tachycardia, atrioventricular block and neurocardiogenic syncope. Am J Med 98:365, 1995.

Douglas PS, Ginsburg GS: The evaluation of chest pain in women. N Engl J Med 334:1311, 1996.

Lee TH, Goldman L: Evaluation of the patient with acute chest pain. N Engl J Med 342:1187–1195, 2000.

Yeghiazarians Y, Braunstein JB, Askari A, et al: Unstable angina pectoris. N Engl J Med 342:101–114, 2000.

Examination of the Cardiovascular System

Badgett RG, Lucey CR, Mulrow CD: Can the clinical examination diagnose left-sided heart failure in adults? JAMA 277:1712, 1997.

Butman SM, Ewy GA, et al: Bedside cardiovascular examination in patients with severe chronic heart failure: importance of rest or inducible jugular venous distension. J Am Coll Card 22:968, 1993.

Cook DJ, Simel DL: Does this patient have abnormal central venous pressure? JAMA 275:630, 1996.

Don Michael TA: Auscultation of the Heart: A Cardiophonetic Approach. New York, McGraw-Hill, 1998.

Etchells E, Bell C, Robb K: Does this patient have an abnormal systolic murmur? JAMA 277:564,1997.

Folland ED, Kriegel BJ, Henderson WG, et al: Implications of third heart sounds in patients with valvular heart disease. N Engl J Med 327:458, 1992.

Harvey WP, Canfield DC: Clinical auscultation of the cardiovascular system. Newton, New Jersey. Laennec Publishing, 1996.

Hulley S, Grady D, Bush T, et al: Randomized trial of estrogen plus progestin for secondary prevention of coronary heart disease in postmenopausal women. JAMA 280:605, 1998.

Kupari M, Koskinen P, Virolainen J, et al: Prevalence and predictors of audible physiological third heart sound in a population sample aged 36 to 37 years. Circulation 89:1189, 1994.

Lembo NJ, Dell'Italia LJ, Crawford MH, et al: Bedside diagnosis of systolic murmurs. N Engl J Med 318:1572, 1988.

Novey DW, Pencak M, Stang JM: The Guide to Heart Sounds: Normal and Abnormal. Boca Raton, FL, CRC Press, 1988. (Audiocassette with pamphlet)

Perloff JK: Physical Examination of the Heart and Circulation, 3rd ed. Philadelphia, WB Saunders, 2000.

Sauve JS, Laupacis A, Ostbye T, et al: Does this patient have a clinically important carotid bruit? JAMA:2843, 1993.

Weibers PO, Whisnant JP, Sandok BA, et al: Prospective comparison of a cohort of asymptomatic carotid bruit and a population-based cohort without carotid bruit. Stroke 21:984, 1990.

Cardiovascular Conditions

Alexander RW, Schlant RC, Fuster V, et al (eds): Hurst's The Heart, Arteries, and Veins, 9th ed. New York, McGraw-Hill, 1998.

American Diabetes Association: Treatment of hypertension in adults with diabetes. Diabetes Care 25 (suppl 1):S71, 2002.

Braunwald E, Zipes DP, Libby P (eds): Heart Disease. A Textbook of Cardiovascular Medicine, 6th ed. Philadelphia, WB Saunders, 2001.

Carabello BA, Crawford FA: Valvular heart disease. N Engl J Med 337:32, 1997.

Dajani AS, Taubert KA, Wilson W, et al: Prevention of bacterial endocarditis. Recommendations by the American Heart Association. JAMA 277:1794, 1997.

Expert Panel on Detection, Evaluation, and Treatment of High Blood Cholesterol in Adults (Adult Treatment Panel III): Executive summary of the third report of the National Cholesterol Education Program (NCEP). JAMA 285:2486, 2001.

Hall WD: Risk reduction associated with lowering systolic blood pressure: a review of clinical trial date. Am Heart J 138 (3 Pt 2):225, 1999.

Mosca L, Grundy SM, Judelson D, et al: Guide to preventive cardiology for women. Circulation 99:2480, 1999.

Pignone M, Mulrow C: Using cardiovascular risk profiles to individualise hypertensive treatment. BMJ 322:1164, 2001.

Taylor HA: Sexual activity and the cardiovascular patient: guidelines. Am J Cardiol 84(5B):6N, 1999.

Chapter 8. The Breasts and Axillae

Examination of the Breasts

Barton MB, Harris R, Fletcher SW: The rational clinical examination: does this patient have breast cancer? JAMA 282:1270, 1999.

Ely KA, Tse G, Simpson JF, et al: Diabetic mastopathy. Am J Clin Pathol 113:541–545, 2000.

Harris JR, Morrow M, Bonadonna G: Cancer of the Breast. In DeVita VT, Hellman S, Rosenberg SA (eds): Cancer Principles & Practice of Oncology, 6th ed. Philadelphia, Lippincott Williams & Wilkins, 2001.

Love SM: Dr. Susan Love's Breast Book, 2nd ed. Reading, MA, Addison-Wesley Publishing, 1995. *(Although this book is written for general readers, professionals can learn much from it.)*

Pennypacker HS, Naylor L, Sander AA, et al: Why can't we do better breast examinations? Nurse Pract 10:122, 1999.

Pruthi S: Detection and evaluation of a palpable breast mass. Mayo Clin Proc 76:641, 2001.

Rutter CM, Mandelson MT, Laya MB, et al: Changes in breast density associated with initiation, discontinuation, and continuing use of hormone replacement therapy. JAMA 285:171, 2001.

Schultz MZ, Ward BA, Reiss M: Breast Diseases (Chapter 149). In Noble J, Greene HL, Levinson W, et al (eds): Primary Care Medicine, 3rd ed. St. Louis, Mosby, 2001.

Sirovich BE, Sox HC: Breast cancer screening. Surg Clin North Am 79:961, 1999.

Breast Conditions and Diseases

Breast Mass

Bland KI, Vezerdis MP, Copeland EM: Breast (Chapter 14). In Schwarts SI, Shires GT, Spencer F, et al (eds): Principles of Surgery, 7th ed. New York, McGraw-Hill, 1998.

Cancer Committee of the College of American Pathologists: Is fibrocystic disease of the breast precancerous? Arch Pathol Lab Med 110:171, 1986.

Donegan WL: Evaluation of the palpable breast mass. N Engl J Med 327:937, 1992.

Dupont WD, Page DL: Risk factors for breast cancer in women with proliferative breast disease. N Engl J Med 312:146, 1985.

Dupont WD, Page DL, Parl FF: Long-term risk of breast cancer in women with fibroadenoma. N Engl J Med 331:10, 1994.

Breast Cancer

Baquest CR, Commiskey P: Socioeconomic factors and breast carcinoma in multicultural women. Cancer 88 (5 suppl):1256, 2000.

Bilmoria MM, Morrow M: The woman at increased risk for breast cancer. Evaluation and management strategies. Cancer 45:263, 1995.

Clemons M, Goss P: Estrogen and the risk of breast cancer. N Engl J Med 344:276, 2001.

Jaiyesimi IA, Buzday, Sahin AA, et al: Carcinoma of the male breast. Ann Intern Med 117:771, 1992.

Marchant DJ: Risk factors in contemporary management of breast disease, II: Breast cancer. Obstet Gynecol Clin North Am 21:561, 1994.

Marcus JN, Watson P, Page DL, et al: Pathology and heredity of breast cancer in younger women. Monogr Natl Cancer Inst 16:23, 1994.

McPherson K, Steel CM, Dixon JM: Breast cancer–epidemiology, risk factors, and genetics. BMJ 321:624–628, 2000.

Miller AB, Baines CJ, To T, et al: Canadian National Breast Screening Study: 1. Breast cancer detection and death rates among women aged 40 to 49 years; 2. Breast cancer detection and death rates among women aged 50 to 59 years. Can Med Assoc J 147:1459, 1477, 1992.

Velentgas P, Daline JR: Risk factors for breast cancer in younger women. Monogr Natl Cancer Inst 16:15, 1994.

Chapter 9. The Abdomen

Arnell TD, DeVirgilio C, Doneyre C, et al: Abdominal aortic aneurysm in elderly males with atherosclerosis: the value of physical exam. Am Surgeon 62:661, 1996.

Feldman M, Scharschmidt BF, Sleisinger MH (eds): Sleisenger's and Fortran's Gastrointestinal and Liver Disease: Pathophysiology/Diagnosis/Management, 6th ed. Philadelphia, WB Saunders, 1998.

Heitkemper M, Jarrett M, Taylor P, et al: Effect of sexual and physical abuse on symptom experiences in women with irritable bowel syndrome. Nurs Res 50:15, 2001.

Lederle FA, Simel DL: Does this patient have abdominal aortic aneurysm? JAMA 281:77–82, 1999.

Sherlock SD, Summerfield JA: Color Atlas of Liver Disease, 2nd ed. St. Louis Mosby–Year Book, 1991.

Silen, W: Cope's Early Diagnosis of the Acute Abdomen, 20th ed. New York, Oxford University Press, 2000.

Turnbull JM: Is listening for abdominal bruits useful in the evaluation of hypertension? JAMA 274:1299, 1995.

Williams JW Jr, Simel DL: Does this patient have ascites? How to divine fluid in the abdomen. JAMA 267:2645, 1992.

Examination of the Liver

Meidl EJ, Ende J: Evaluation of liver size by physical examination. J Gen Intern Med 8:835, 1993.

Naylor CD: Physical examination of the liver. JAMA 271:1859, 1994.

Zoli M, Magliotti D, Grimaldi M, et al: Physical examination of the liver: is it still worth it? Am J Gastroenterol 90:1428, 1995.

Examination of the Spleen

Barkun AN, Camus M, Green L, et al: The bedside assessment of splenic enlargement. Am J Med 91:512, 1991.

Grover SA, Barkun AN, Sackett DL: Does this patient have splenomegaly? JAMA 270:2218, 1993.

Sullivan S, Williams R: Reliability of clinical techniques for detecting splenic enlargement. BMJ 2:1043, 1976.

Tamayo SG, Rickman LS, Matthews WC, et al: Examiner dependence on physical diagnostic tests of splenomegaly: a prospective study with multiple observers. J Gen Intern Med 8:69, 1993.

Chapter 10. Male Genitalia and Hernias

Pubertal Changes

See references for Chapter 17.

Urology

Gillenwater TY, Grayhack JT, Howards SS, et al: Adult and Pediatric Urology, 3rd ed. St Louis, Mosby, 1996.

Smoger SH, Felice TL, Kloecker GH: Urinary incontinence among male veterans receiving care in primary care clinics. Ann Intern Med 1342:547, 2000.

Tanagho EA, McAninch JW: Smith's General Urology, 15th ed. New York, Lange Medical Books, McGraw-Hill, 2000.

Walsh PC, Retik AB, Staney TA, et al (eds): Campbell's Urology, 7th ed. Philadelphia, WB Saunders, 1998.

Hernias

Eubanks S: Hernias (Chapter 40). In Townsend CM, Beauchamp RB, Evers BM, et al (eds): Sabiston Textbook of Surgery: The Biological Basis of Modern Surgical Practice, 16th ed. Philadelphia, WB Saunders, 2001.

Wantz GE: Abdominal wall hernias (Chapter 34). In Schwartz SI, Shires GT, Spencer F, et al (eds): Principles of Surgery, 7th ed. New York, McGraw-Hill, 1998.

Genito-Urinary Conditions

Barry MJ: Prostate specific-antigen testing for early diagnosis of prostate cancer. N Engl J Med 344:1373, 2001.

Davis-Joseph B, Tiefer L, Melman A: Accuracy of the initial history and physical examination to establish the etiology of erectile dysfunction. Urology 40:498, 1995.

Handsfield HH: Color Atlas and Synopsis of Sexually Transmitted Diseases, 2nd ed. New York, McGraw-Hill, 2001.
Hargreave TB: Investigating and managing infertility in general practice. BMJ 316:1438, 1998.
Holmes KK, Mardh PA, Sparling PF (eds): Sexually Transmitted Diseases, 3rd ed. New York, McGraw-Hill, 1999.
Whitman G: Patients with urinary incontinence and falls. J Am Geriatr Soc 49:336, 2001.
Wisdom A, Hawkins DA: Colour Atlas of Sexually Transmitted Diseases, 2nd ed. London/Philadelphia, Mosby-Wolfe, 1997.

Chapter 11. Female Genitalia

Pubertal Changes

See references for Chapter 17.

The Pelvic Examination

Brink CA, Sampselle CM, Wells TJ, et al: A digital test for pelvic muscle strength in older women with urinary incontinence. Nurs Res 38:196, 1989.
Pearce KF, et al: Cytopathological findings on vaginal Papanicolaou smears after hysterectomy for benign gynecologic disease. N Engl J Med 335:1559, 1996.
Primrose RB: Taking the tension out of a pelvic exam. Am J Nurs 84:72, 1984.
Rimsza ME: An illustrated guide to adolescent gynecology. Pediatr Clin North Am 36:639, 1989.
Willard MA, Heaberg GL, Pack JB: The educational pelvic examination: women's responses to a new approach. J Obstet Gynecol Neonatal Nurs 15:135, 1986.

Gynecology

Berek JS (ed): Novak's Gynecology, 13th ed. Philadelphia, Lippincott Williams & Wilkins, 2002.
Herbst AL, Mishell DR Jr, Stenchever MA, et al (eds): Comprehensive Gynecology, 4th ed. St. Louis, Mosby, 2001.
Sawaya GF, Brown AD, Washington AE, et al: Current approaches to cervical cancer screening. N Engl J Med 344:1603, 2001.
Scott JR, DiSaia PJ, Hammond CB, et al (eds): Danforth's Obstetrics and Gynecology, 8th ed. Philadelphia, Lippincott Williams & Wilkins, 1999.

Vaginal and Pelvic Conditions

Bickley LS: Acute vaginitis. In Black ER, Panzer RJ, Bordley DR, et al (eds): Diagnostic Strategies for Common Medical Problems, 2nd ed. Philadelphia, American College of Physicians, 1999.
Ho GYF, Bierman R, Beardsley L, et al: Natural history of cervicovaginal papillomavirus infection in young women. N Engl J Med 338:423, 1998.
Piepert JF, Ness RB, Blume J, et al. Clinical predictors of endometritis in women with symptoms and signs of pelvic inflammatory disease. Am J Obstet Gynecol 184:856, 2001.
Scholes D, et al: Prevention of pelvic inflammatory disease by screening for cervical chlamydial infection. N Engl J Med 334:1362, 1996.

Genito-Urinary Conditions

See references listed on this topic in Chapter 10.
Brown JS, Steely DG, Fong J, et al: Urinary incontinence in older women: who is at risk? Obstet Gynecol 87:715, 1996.

Weiss BD: Diagnostic evaluation of urinary incontinence in geriatric patients. Am Fam Physician 57:2675–2682, 1998.

Chapter 12. The Pregnant Woman

General

American Diabetes Association: Preconception care of women with diabetes. Diabetes Care 25 (suppl 1):S82, 2002.

Baron TH, Ramirez B, Richter JE: Gastrointestinal motility disorders during pregnancy. Ann Intern Med 118:366, 1993.

Beebe JE, Duperret M (consultants): Programmed instruction: examination of the female pelvis, Part I. Am J Nurs 78:10, 1978.

Bennet R, Brown LK: Myles Textbook for Midwives, 13th ed. Edinburgh/New York, Churchill Livingstone, 1999.

Cunningham FG, Whitridge J, et al: Williams Obstetrics, 21st ed. New York, McGraw-Hill, 2001.

Thompson JE: Primary health care nursing for women. In Mezey MD, McGivern DO: Nurses, Nurse Practitioners, 3rd ed. New York, Springer Publishing Co., 1999.

Vaney HJ: Nurse Midwifery, 3rd ed. Boston, Jones & Bartlett, 1997.

Nutrition

Enkin M, Keirse MJNC, Renfrew M, et al: A Guide to Effective Care in Pregnancy and Childbirth, 3rd ed. New York, Oxford University Press, 2000.

Food and Nutrition Board: Recommended Dietary Allowances, 10th ed. National Research Council, National Academy of Sciences, Washington, DC, 1989.

Institute of Medicine: Nutrition During Pregnancy. Part I, Weight Gain; Part II, Nutrient Supplements. Committee on Nutritional Status During Pregnancy and Lactation, Food and Nutrition Board, National Academy Press, Washington, DC, 1990.

Institute of Medicine: Nutrition During Pregnancy and Lactation: An Implementation Guide. Subcommittee for a Clinical Application Guide, Committee on Nutritional Status During Pregnancy and Lactation, Food and Nutrition Board, National Academy Press, Washington, DC, 1992.

Worthington-Roberts B: Nutrition. In Fogel CI, Woods NF (eds): Women's Health Care: A Comprehensive Handbook. Thousand Oaks, California, Sage Publications, 1995.

Exercise

ACOG: Technical Bulletin No. 189, February 1994.

Bell R, O'Neill M: Exercise and pregnancy: a review. Birth 2:85, 1994.

Yeo S: Exercise guidelines for pregnant women. Image 26:265, 1994.

Domestic Violence and Pregnancy

Adler C: Unheard and unseen: rural women and domestic violence. J Nurse Midwifery 41:463, 1996.

Campbell J, Soeken K: Forced sex and intimate partner violence: effects on women's health. Violence Against Women 5:1017, 1999.

McFarlane J, Campbell JC, Wilt S, et al: Stalking and intimate partner femicide. Homicide Studies 3:300, 1999.

McFarlane J, Parker B, Soeken K: Abuse during pregnancy: associations with maternal health and infant birth weight. Nurs Res 45:37, 1996.

Paluzzi PA, Houde-Quimby C: Domestic violence: implications for the American College of Nurse-Midwives and its members. J Nurse Midwifery 41:430, 1996.

United Nations Population Fund (UNFPA) (2001 Pilot Edition): A practical approach to gender-based violence: a programme guide for health care providers and managers. New York, UNFPA, 2001.

Chapter 13. The Anus, Rectum, and Prostate

American College of Physicians: Suggested technique for fecal occult blood testing and interpretation of colorectal cancer screenings. Ann Intern Med 126:808, 1997.

Donowitz M, Kokke FT, Saidi R: Evaluation of patients with chronic diarrhea. N Engl J Med 332:725, 1995.

Hanauer SB: Inflammatory bowel disease. N Engl J Med 334:841, 1996.

Madoff RD, William JG, Caushaj PF: Fecal incontinence. N Engl J Med 326:1002, 1992.

Schrock TR: Examination and diseases of the anorectum. In Feldmen M, Scharschmidt BF, Sleisinger MH (eds): Sleisinger's and Fortran's Gastrointestinal and Liver Disease: Pathophysiology/Diagnosis/Management, 6th ed. Philadelphia, WB Saunders, 1998.

Chapter 14. The Peripheral Vascular System

Anand SS, Wells PS, Hunt D, et al: Does this patient have a deep vein thrombosis? JAMA 279:1094, 1998.

Baraff LJ: Capillary refill: is it a useful sign? Pediatrics 92:723, 1993.

Coleman RW, Hirsh J, Marder VJ, et al: Hemostasis and Thrombosis: Basic Principles and Clinical Practice, 4th ed. Philadelphia, Lippincott Williams & Wilkins, 2000.

Geerts WH, Heit JA, Clagett GP, et al: Prevention of venous thromboembolism. Chest 119 (1 suppl):325, 2001.

Harris AH, Brown-Etris M, Troyer-Caudle J: Managing vascular leg ulcers. Part I. Am J Nurs 96:38, 1996.

Hiatt WR: Medical treatment of peripheral arterial disease and claudication. N Engl J Med 344:1608, 2001.

Hirsch AT, Criqui MH, Treat-Jacobson D, et al: Peripheral arterial disease detection, awareness, and treatment in primary care. JAMA 286:1317, 2001.

Loscalzo J, Creager MA, Dzau VJ (eds): Vascular Medicine: A Textbook of Vascular Biology and Diseases, 2nd ed. Boston, Little, Brown and Co. 1996.

Tibbs DJ: Varicose Veins and Related Disorders. Boston, Butterworth-Heinemann, 1992.

Chapter 15. The Musculoskeletal System

Alexander NB: Gait disorders in older adults. J Am Geriatr Soc 44:434, 1996.

Baker DG, Schumacher HR Jr: Acute monoarthritis. N Engl J Med 329:1013, 1993.

Bland JH: Disorders of the shoulder (Chapter 71). In Noble J (ed): Primary Care Medicine, 2nd ed. St. Louis, Mosby, 1996.

D'Arcy CA, McGee S: Does this patient have carpal tunnel syndrome? JAMA 283:3110, 2000.

Deyo RA, Rainville J, Kent DL: What can the history and physical examination tell us about low back pain? JAMA 268:760, 1992.
Deyo RA, Weinstein JN: Low back pain. N Engl J Med 344:363, 2001.
Doherty M, Doherty J: Clinical Examination in Rheumatology. London, Wolfe Publishing, 1992.
Emerson BT: The management of gout. N Engl J Med 334:445, 1996.
Heinemann DF: Osteoporosis. An overview of the National Osteoporosis Foundation clinical practice guide. Geriatrics 55:31, 2000.
Hoppenfeld S: Physical Examination of the Spine and Extremities. Norwalk, CT, Appleton-Century-Crofts, 1976.
Johnson M, Cusick A, Chang S, et al: Home-screen: a short scale to measure fall risk in the home. Pub Health Nurs 18:169, 2001.
Klippel JH, Weyand CM, Wortmann RL (eds): Primer on the Rheumatic Diseases, 11th ed. Atlanta, Arthritis Foundation, 1997.
Koopman WJ: Arthritis and Allied Conditions: A Textbook of Rheumatology, 14th ed. Philadelphia, Lippincott Williams & Wilkins, 2000.
Polley HF, Hunder GG: Rheumatologic Interviewing and Physical Examination of the Joints, 2nd ed. Philadelphia, WB Saunders, 1978.
Ruddy S, Harris ED, Sledge CB, et al: Kelley's Textbook of Rheumatology, 6th ed. Philadelphia, WB Saunders, 2001.
Snider RK (ed): Essentials of Musculoskeletal Care. Rosemont, IL, American Academy of Orthopedic Surgeons, 1997.

Chapter 16. The Nervous System

Mental Status

American Psychiatric Association: Diagnostic and Statistical Manual of Mental Disorders, 4th ed. Text Revision. Washington DC, American Psychiatric Association, 2000.
Beck AT, Ward CH, Mendelson M, et al: An inventory for measuring depression. Arch Gen Psychiatry 4:561, 1961.
Coffey E, Cummings JL: Textbook of Geriatric Neuropsychiatry. Washington DC, The American Psychiatric Press, 2000.
Folstein M, Folstein SE, McHugh PR: Mini-mental state. J Psych Res 12:189, 1975.
Hales RE, Hilty DA, Hise MG: A treatment algorithm for the management of anxiety. J Clin Psychiatry 58 (suppl 3):76, 1997.
Hales RE, Yudofsky SC, Talbott JA: The American Psychiatric Press Textbook of Psychiatry, 3rd ed. Washington, DC, The American Psychiatric Press, 1997.
Hamilton NG: Suicide prevention in primary care. Careful questioning, prompt treatment can save lives. Postgrad Med 108:81, 2000.
Kaplan HI, Sadock BJ, Grebb JA: Kaplan and Sadock's Synopsis of Psychiatry, 8th ed. Baltimore, Williams & Wilkins, 1998.
Kroenke K, Spitzer RL, Willans JBW, et al: Physical symptoms in primary care: predictors of psychiatric disorders and functional impairment. Arch Fam Med 3:774, 1993.
Kupfer DJ, Reynolds CF: Management of insomnia. N Engl J Med 336:341, 1997.
Lawlor P, Fainsinger RL, Bruera ED: Delerium at the end of life: critical issues in clinical practice and research. JAMA 284:2427, 2000.

Lipowski ZJ: Delirium in the elderly patient. N Engl J Med 320:578, 1989.
Schiffer RB, Rao S (eds): Neuropsychiatry. Philadelphia, Lippincott Williams & Wilkins, 2002.
Some drugs that cause psychiatric symptoms. Med Lett Drugs Ther 40:21, 1998.
Waldinger RJ: Psychiatry for Medical Students, 3rd ed. Washington DC, American Psychiatric Press, 1997.
Whooley MA, Simon GE: Managing depression in medical outpatients. N Engl J Med 343:1942, 2000.
Zimmerman M: Diagnosing DSM IV Psychiatric Disorders in Primary Care Settings: An Interview Guide for the Nonpsychiatrist Physician. Providence, Rhode Island, Psych Products Press, 1994.

Neurology

Bennett DA, et al: Prevalence of parkinsonian signs and associated mortality in a community population of older people. N Engl J Med 334:71, 1996.
Damasio AR: Aphasia. N Engl J Med 326:531, 1992.
DeGroot J, Waxman SG: Correlative Neuroanatomy, 22nd ed. Norwalk, CT: Appleton & Lange, 1995.
Gilman SG, Newman SW: Manter and Gatz's Essential of Clinical Neuroanatomy and Neurophysiology, 10th ed. Philadelphia, FA Davis, 2001.
Hughes RA, Rees JH: Clinical and epidemiologic features of Guillain-Barre syndrome. J Infec Dis 176 (suppl 2):S92, 1997.
Joynt RJ, Griggs RC: Baker's Clinical Neurology on CD-ROM. Philadelphia, Lippincott Williams & Wilkins, 2000.
Kapoor WN: Syncope. N Engl J Med 343:1856, 2000.
Kroenke K, Lucas CA, Rosenberg ML, et al: Causes of persistent dizziness: a prospective study of 100 patients in ambulatory care. Ann Intern Med 117:898, 1992.
Lipowski ZJ: Delirium (acute confusional states). JAMA 258:1789, 1987.
Louis ED: Essential tremor. N Engl J Med 345:887, 2001.
Rowland LP (ed): Merritt's Textbook of Neurology, 10th ed. Philadelphia, Lippincott Williams & Wilkins, 2001.
Sacco RL: Extracranial carotid stenosis. N Engl J Med 345:1113, 2001.
Santacruz KS, Swagerty D: Early diagnosis of dementia. Am Fam Physician 63:620, 2001.
Solomon S: Diagnosis of primary headache disorders. Neuro Clinics 15:15, 1997.
Tinetti ME, Williams CS, Gill TM: Dizziness among older adults: a possible geriatric syndrome. Ann Intern Med 132:337, 2000.
Victor M, Ropper AH: Adam's and Victor's Principles of Neurology, 7th ed. New York, McGraw-Hill, 2001.
Willoughby D, Sanders L, Privette A: The impact of a stroke screening program. Pub Health Nurs 18:418, 2001.

Examination of the Nervous System

Aids to the Examination of the Peripheral Nervous System: Medical Research Council Memorandum No. 45. London, Her Majesty's Stationery Office, 1976.
Dawson DM: Entrapment neuropathies of the upper extremities. N Engl J Med 329:2013, 1993.
DeMyer WE: Technique of the Neurologic Examination, A Programmed Text, 4th ed. New York, McGraw-Hill, 1994.

Edwards RH, Simon RP: Coma. Vol 2 (19). In Joynt RJ, Griggs RC (eds): Clinical Neurology. Philadelphia, Lippincott-Raven, 1996.

Haerer AF: DeJong's The Neurologic Examination, 5th ed. Philadelphia, JB Lippincott, 1992.

Plum F, Posner JB: The Diagnosis of Stupor and Coma, 3rd ed. Philadelphia, FA Davis, 1980.

Chapter 17. Assessing Children: Infancy Through Adolescence

Allen HD, Moss AJ, Adams FH: Moss and Adams' Heart Disease in Infants, Children, and Adolescents, 6th ed. Philadelphia, Lippincott Williams & Wilkins, 2001.

American Academy of Family Physicians: Preparticipation Examination. Appendix. Available at: http://www.aafp.org/afp/20000501/2696.html. Accessed January 29, 2002.

American Academy of Pediatrics: Recommendations for Preventive Pediatric Health Care. Available at: http://www.aap.org/policy/re9939.html. Accessed January 29, 2002.

Andrews JS: Making the most of the sports physical. Contemp Pediatr 14(3):183–205, 1997.

Blake J: Gynecologic examination of the teenager and young child. Obstet Gynecol Clin North Am 19:27, 1992.

Bright Futures: Guidelines for Health Supervision of Infants, Children, and Adolescents. 2nd ed. Available at: http://www.brightfutures.org/. Accessed January 29, 2002.

Colson ER, Dworkin PH: Toddler development. Pediatr in Rev 18(8):255–259, 1997.

Copelan J: Normal speech and development. Pediatr in Rev 18:91–100, 1995.

Coupey SM: Interviewing adolescents. Pediatr Clin of North Am 44(6): 1349–1364, 1997

Emmanouilides GC, et al (eds): Heart Disease of Infants, Children and Adolescents, including the Fetus and Young Adult, 5th ed. Baltimore, Williams & Wilkins, 1994.

Fanaroff AA, Martin RJ: Neonatal–Perinatal Medicine: Diseases of the Fetus and Infants, 7th ed. St. Louis, Mosby, 2002.

Fletcher MA: Physical Diagnosis in Neonatology. Philadelphia, Lippincott-Raven, 1997.

Goodheart HP: A Photoguide of Common Skin Disorders: Diagnosis and Management. Philadelphia, Lippincott Williams & Wilkins, 1999.

Green M: Bright Futures: Guidelines for Health Supervision of Infants, Children, and Adolescents. Arlington, VA, National Center for Education in Maternal and Child Health. 2000.

Harlan WR, Grillo GP, Comoni-Huntley J, et al: Secondary sex characteristics of boys 12 to 17 years of age. The U.S. Health Examination Survey. J Pediatr 95:293, 1979.

Harlan WR, Harlan EA, Grillo GP: Secondary sex characteristics of girls 12 to 17 years of age. The U.S. Health Examination Survey. J Pediatr 96:1074, 1980.

Harris JP: Consultation with the specialist. Evaluation of heart murmurs. Pediatr in Rev 15(12):490–494, 1994.

Herman-Giddens ME, Wang L, Koch G: Secondary sexual characteristics in boys: estimates from the national health and nutrition examination survey III, 1988–1994. Arch Pediatr & Adolesc Med. 155(9):1022–1028, 2001.

Herring JA, Tachdjian MO: Tachdjian's Pediatric Orthopedics, 3rd ed. (3 vols). Philadelphia, WB Saunders, 2002.

Hoekelman RA, et al (eds): Primary Pediatric Care, 4th ed. St. Louis, Mosby–Year Book, 2001.

Johnson CP, Blasco PA: Infant growth and development. Pediatr in Rev 18(7):224–242, 1997.

Kreipe RE, McAnarney ER: Adolescent growth and development. In Behrman RE and Kliegman R: Nelson Essentials of Pediatrics, 4th ed. Philadelphia, WB Saunders. 2002.

Levine MD, Carey WB, Crocker AC: Developmental–Behavioral Pediatrics, 3rd ed. Philadelphia, WB Saunders, 2002.

McAnarney ER, Kreipe RE, Orr DP, et al: Textbook of Adolescent Medicine. Philadelphia, WB Saunders, 1992.

Margolis P, Gadomski A: Does this infant have pneumonia? JAMA 279(4):308–313. 1998.

Myers GJ, McBride MC: Clinical neurologic examination of the preterm and term neonate. Semin Neurol 13(1): 1993.

Nelson LB, Calhoun JH, Harley RD: Pediatric Ophthalmology, 3rd ed. Philadelphia, WB Saunders, 1991.

Park MK: Pediatric Cardiology for Practitioners. 4th ed. St Louis, Mosby, 2002.

Piper MC, Darrah J: Motor Assessment of the Developing Infant. Philadelphia, WB Saunders, 1994.

Pizzutillo PD: Practical Orthopaedics in Primary Practice. New York, McGraw-Hill, 1997.

Reece RM, Ludwig S: Child Abuse: Medical Diagnosis and Management. 2nd ed. Philadelphia, Lippincott Williams & Wilkins, 2001.

Smith DM, Kovan JR, Rich BSE, et al: Preparticipation Physical Evaluation, 2nd ed. Minneapolis, McGraw-Hill Co., 1997.

Swaiman KF, Ashwal S: Pediatric Neurology: Principles and Practice, 3rd ed, (2 vols). St. Louis, Mosby–Year Book, 1999.

Tanner JM: Growth at Adolescence, 2nd ed. Oxford, Blackwell Scientific Publications, 1962.

Chapter 18. Clinical Reasoning, Assessment and Plan

Alfaro-Lefevre R: Critical Thinking in Nursing: A Practical Approach. 2nd ed. Philadelphia, WB Saunders, 1999.

Black ER, Panzer RJ, Bordley DR, et al (eds): Diagnostic Strategies for Common Medical Problems, 2nd ed. Philadelphia, American College of Physicians, 1999.

Carpenito LJ: Nursing Diagnosis: Application to Clinical Practice, 9th ed. Philadelphia, Lippincott Williams & Wilkins, 2001.

Cutler P: Problem Solving in Clinical Medicine; From Data to Diagnosis, 3rd ed. Philadelphia, Lippincott Williams & Wilkins, 1998.

Fletcher RH: Clinical Epidemiology: The Essentials. 3rd ed. Baltimore, Williams & Wilkins, 1996.

Hurst JW, Walker HK (eds): The Problem-Oriented System. New York, Medcom, 1972.

Nettina SM: The Lippincott Manual of Nursing Practice, 7th ed. Philadelphia, Lippincott Williams & Wilkins, 2001.

Orem DE, Taylor SG, Renpenning KM: Nursing Concepts of Practice, 6th ed. St. Louis, Mosby, 2001.

Rubenfield MG, Scheffer BK: Critical Thinking in Nursing: An Interactive Approach. Philadelphia, JB Lippincott, 1995.

Sackett DL: A primer on the precision and accuracy of the clinical examination. JAMA 267:2638, 1992.

Sackett DL, Haynes RB, Tugwell P: Clinical Epidemiology: A Basic Science for Clinical Medicine, 2nd ed. Boston, Little, Brown and Co, 1991.

Subject Index

NOTE: A *b* following a page number indicates in-chapter boxed material and a *t* following a page number indicates an end-of-chapter table.

B

E

F

G

H

I

N

O

S

T

U

V

W

X

Y

Z

CD-ROM TO ACCOMPANY BATES' GUIDE TO PHYSICAL EXAMINATION AND HISTORY TAKING, 8th EDITION

PROGRAM LICENSE AGREEMENT

Read carefully the following terms and conditions before using the Software. Use of the Software indicates you and, if applicable, your Institution's acceptance of the terms and conditions of this License Agreement. If you do not agree with the terms and conditions, you should promptly return this package to the place you purchased it and your payment will be refunded.

Definitions

As used herein, the following terms shall have the following meanings:

"Software" means the software program contained on the diskette(s) or CD-ROM or preloaded on a workstation and the user documentation, which includes all accompanying printed material.

"Institution" means a nursing or professional school, a single academic organization that does not provide patient care and is located in a single city and has one geographic location/address.

"Geographic location" means a facility at a specific location; geographic locations do not provide for satellite or remote locations that are considered a separate facility.

"Facility" means a health care facility at a specific location that provides patient care and is located in a single city and has one geographic location/address.

"Publisher" means Lippincott Williams & Wilkins, Inc., with its principal office in Philadelphia, Pennsylvania.

"Developer" means the company responsible for developing the software as noted on the product.

License

You are hereby granted a nonexclusive license to use the Software in the United States. This license is not transferable and does not authorize resale or sublicensing without the written approval or an authorized officer of Publisher.

The Publisher retains all rights and title to all copyrights, patents, trademarks, trade secrets, and other proprietary rights in the Software. You may not remove or obscure the copyright notices in or on the Software. You agree to use reasonable efforts to protect the Software from unauthorized use, reproduction, distribution or publication.

Single-User license

If you purchased this Software program at the Single-User License price or a discount of that price, you may use this program on one single-user computer. You may not use the Software in a time-sharing environment or otherwise to provide multiple, simultaneous access. You may not provide or permit access to this program to anyone other than yourself.

Institutional/Facility license

If you purchased the Software at the Institutional or Facility License Price or at a discount of that price, you have purchased the Software for use within your Institution/Facility on a single workstation/computer. You may not provide copies of or remote access to the Software. You may not modify or translate the program or related documentation. You agree to instruct the individuals in your Institution/Facility who will have access to the Software to abide by the terms of this License Agreement. If you or any member of your Institution fail to comply with any of the terms of this License Agreement, this license shall terminate automatically.

Network license

If you purchased the Software at the Network License Price, you may copy the Software for use within your Institution/Facility on an unlimited number of computers within one geographic location/address. You may not provide remote access to the Software over a value-added network or otherwise. You may not provide copies of or remote access to the Software to individuals or entities who are not members of your Institution/Facility. You may not modify or translate the program or related documentation. You agree to instruct the individuals in your Institution/Facility who will have access to the

Software to abide by the terms of this License Agreement. If you or any member of your Institution/Facility fail to comply with any of the terms of this License Agreement, this license shall terminate automatically.

Limited warranty

The Publisher warrants that the media on which the Software is furnished shall be free from defects in materials and workmanship under normal use for a period of 90 days from the date of delivery to you, as evidenced by your receipt of purchase.

The Software is sold on a 30-day trial basis. If, for whatever reason, you decide not to keep the software, you may return it for a full refund within 30 days of the invoice date or purchase, as evidenced by your receipt of purchase by returning all parts of the Software and packaging in saleable condition with the original invoice, to the place you purchased it. If the Software is not returned in such condition, you will not be entitled to a refund. When returning the Software, we suggest that you insure all packages for their retail value and mail them by a traceable method.

The Software is a computer assisted instruction (CAI) program that is not intended to provide medical consultation regarding the diagnosis or treatment of any specific patient.

The Software is provided without warranty of any kind, either expressed or implied, including but not limited to any implied warranty of fitness for a particular purpose of merchantability. Neither Publisher nor Developer warrants that the Software will satisfy your requirements or that the Software is free of program or content errors. Neither Publisher nor Developer warrants, guarantees, or makes any representation regarding the use of the Software in terms of accuracy, reliability or completeness, and you rely on the content of the programs solely at your own risk.

The Publisher is not responsible (as a matter of products liability, negligence or otherwise) for any injury resulting from any material contained herein. This Software contains information relating to general principles of patient care that should not be construed as specific instructions for individual patients.

Manufacturers' product information and package inserts should be reviewed for current information, including contraindications, dosages and precautions.

Some states do not allow the exclusion of implied warranties, so the above exclusion may not apply to you. This warranty gives you specific legal rights and you may also have other rights that vary from state to state.

Limitation of remedies

The entire liability of Publisher and Developer and your exclusive remedy shall be: (1) the replacement of any CD which does not meet the limited warranty stated above which is returned to the place you purchased it with your purchase receipt; or (2) if the Publisher or the wholesaler or retailer from whom you purchased the Software is unable to deliver a replacement CD free from defects in material and workmanship, you may terminate this License Agreement by returning the CD, and your money will be refunded.

In no event will Publisher or Developer be liable for any damages, including any damages for personal injury, lost profits, lost savings or other incidental or consequential damages arising out of the use or inability to use the Software or any error or defect in the Software, whether in the database or in the programming, even if the Publisher, Developer, or an authorized wholesaler or retailer has been advised of the possibility of such damage.

Some states do not allow the limitation or exclusion of liability for incidental or consequential damages. The above limitations and exclusions may not apply to you.

General

This License Agreement shall be governed by the laws of the State of Pennsylvania without reference to the conflict of laws provisions thereof, and may only be modified in a written statement signed by an authorized officer of the Publisher. By opening and using the Software, you acknowledge that you have read this License Agreement, understand it, and agree to be bound by its terms and conditions. You further agree that it is a complete and exclusive statement of the agreement between the Institution/Facility and the Publisher, which supersedes any proposal or prior agreement, oral or written, and any other communication between you and Publisher or Developer relative to the subject matter of the License Agreement.

Note

Attach a paid invoice to the License Agreement as proof of purchase.

About HeartSounds

Welcome to HeartSounds—An Interactive Auscultation Tutorial. The contents of this CD-ROM are meant to serve as an introduction to the basic heart sounds that might be encountered in clinical practice. Care has been taken to accurately present these basic cardiac sounds. To emphasize certain aspects, some of the sounds were artificially generated. Other sounds are from real patients.

SYSTEM REQUIREMENTS

Windows 98, Windows NT, or Windows 2000 with 16 Mb RAM, 8X CD-ROM drive, video card capable of 256 colors, and compliant sound card.

Apple Macintosh with PowerPC 132 Mhz or higher, 32 Mb of RAM, 8X CD-ROM drive, video card capable of 256 colors, and sound capability. OS 7.6 to 9.2 is supported. **OSX is not supported in this release.** If running OSX, restart in OS 9.2. Problems have arisen while running HeartSounds in classic mode within OSX. A demo that runs in a shockwave compliant Web browser within OSX is provided without guarantee.

General: External speakers with a wide frequency range are highly recommended to fully appreciate the dynamic range of cardiac sounds.

OPERATING INSTRUCTIONS

Windows and Macintosh: The CD-ROM is configured to autorun when inserted. Alternatively, you may copy the contents of the CD-ROM to your hard drive.

Questions or comments about how we can improve the program are welcome. Please email Brian Pitts, M.D., at pittbria@earthlink.net. Technical support with operation or installation is NOT provided at this email address.

TECHNICAL SUPPORT

LWW Technical Support @ 1-800-638-3030 or at techsupp@lww.com

Thanks for using HeartSounds, and best wishes.